D1596471

EXPERTddx™

CHEST

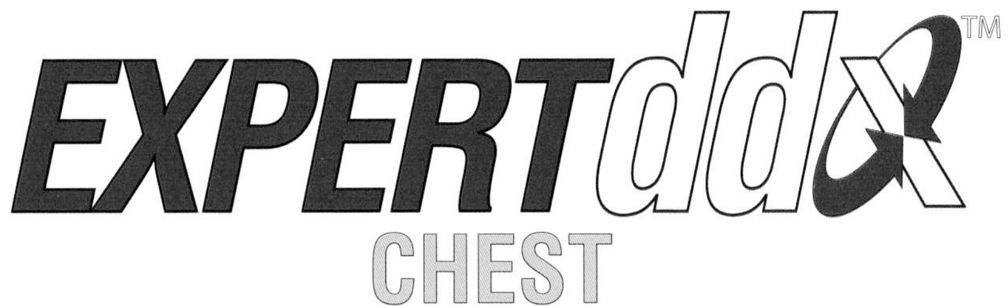

Eric J. Stern, MD

Vice Chair, Academic Affairs
Professor of Radiology
Adjunct Professor of Medicine
Adjunct Professor of Medical Education and Bioinformatics
Adjunct Professor of Global Health
University of Washington
Seattle, Washington

Jud W. Gurney, MD

Charles A. Dobry Professor of Radiology
University of Nebraska Medical Center
Omaha, Nebraska

Christopher M. Walker, MD

Radiology Resident
Radiology Department, Thoracic Imaging Division
University of Washington
Seattle, Washington

Jeffrey P. Kanne, MD

Associate Professor of Radiology
University of Wisconsin School of Medicine and Public Health
Madison, Wisconsin

Tomás Franquet, MD, PhD

Associate Professor of Radiology
Universitat Autónoma de Barcelona
Chief of Thoracic Imaging
Department of Radiology
Hospital de Sant Pau
Barcelona, Spain

Sudhakar Pipavath, MD

Assistant Professor
Department of Radiology
University of Washington
Seattle, Washington

Jonathan H. Chung, MD

Assistant Professor
Institute for Advanced Biomedical Imaging
National Jewish Health
Denver, Colorado
Fellow in Cardiothoracic Imaging
Department of Radiology
Massachusetts General Hospital
Boston, Massachusetts

Gregory Kicska, MD, PhD

Assistant Professor
Thoracic Imaging
University of Washington
Seattle, Washington

Robert B. Carr, MD

Radiology Resident
University of Washington
Seattle, Washington

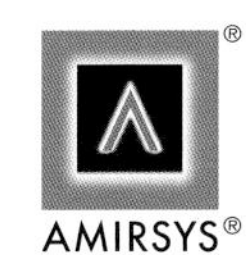

AMIRSYS®
Names you know. Content you trust.®

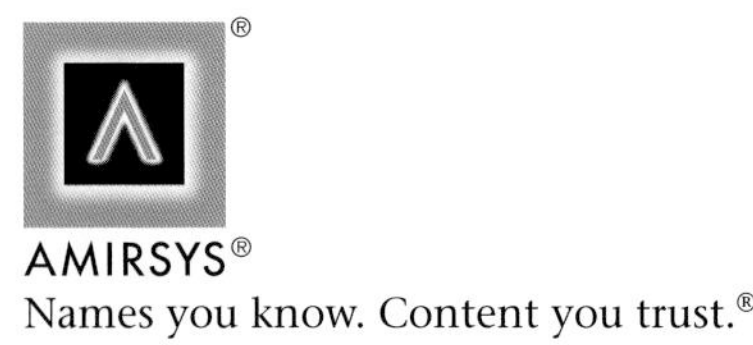

AMIRSYS®
Names you know. Content you trust.®

First Edition

Printed in Canada by Friesens, Altona, Manitoba, Canada

ISBN: 978-1-931884-12-9

Notice and Disclaimer

Library of Congress Cataloging-in-Publication Data

Expertddx. Chest / [edited by] Eric J. Stern. -- 1st ed.
p. ; cm.
Chest
Includes index.
ISBN 978-1-931884-12-9
1. Chest--Diseases--Diagnosis--Atlases. 2. Differential diagnosis--Atlases.
I. Stern, Eric J. II. Title: Chest.
[DNLM: 1. Lung Diseases--diagnosis--Handbooks. 2. Lung Diseases--radiography--Handbooks. 3. Diagnosis, Differential--Handbooks. 4. Thoracic Diseases--diagnosis--Handbooks. 5. Thoracic Diseases--radiography--Handbooks. WF 39]

RC941.E97 2011
617.5'4--dc22

2010038964

This book is dedicated to the memory and legacy of Jud Gurney, my friend and colleague.

Jud was a renowned educator and extraordinary teacher, both at the University of Nebraska Radiology and in worldwide thoracic imaging communities. His elegant, yet simple and easy to understand approach to teaching radiology, as manifest in this book, is part of his lasting legacy. Jud did his best and made a difference. We have lost a radiology superstar. He will be dearly missed.
EJS

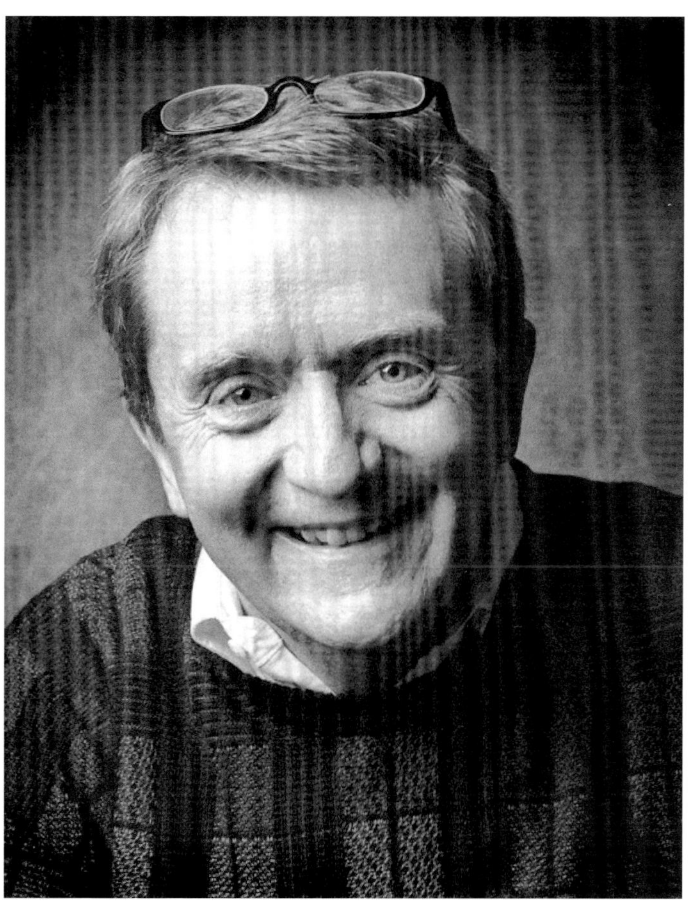

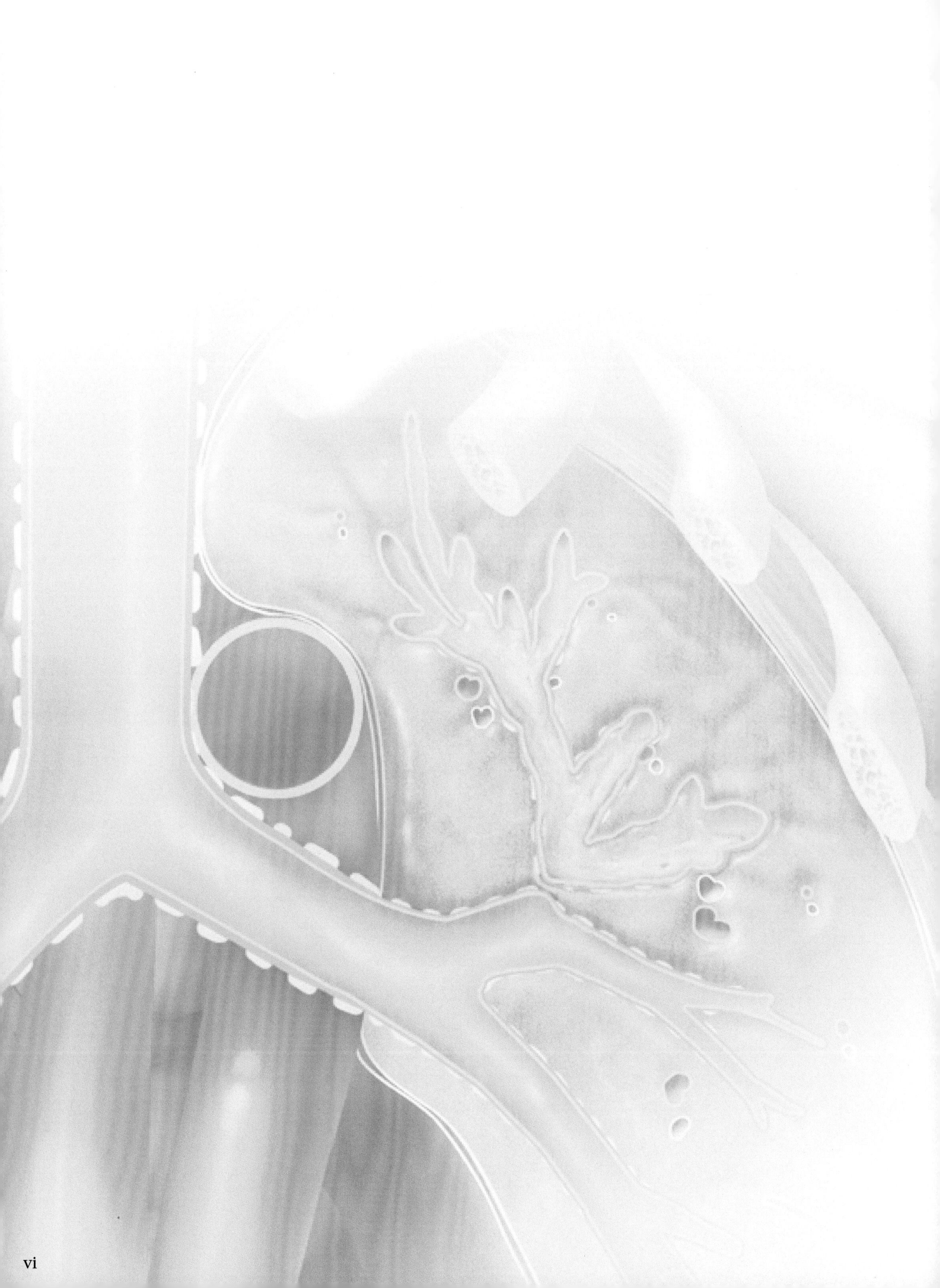

To my beautiful wife, Eunhee. Thank you for your continuned support and guidance. You make the journey fun and exciting.
CW

To my parents, Kyu Youl and Bok Hee, and my wife, Aimee-Sue.
JHC

To Elizabeth, who makes everything possible.
JPK

I am grateful to Eric Stern for the opportunity to participate in this project. I would like to thank Gautham Reddy for his professional support. I would like to dedicate this endeavor to my daughter, Tess, who fills me with smiles, and to my wife, Kat, with whom I share them.
GK

To my children, Tomás, Pablo, and Elisa, and my loving wife, Salomé.
TF

To Sarah.
RC

To Bhavana and Sai, who supported and inspired me in every way, and J.D. Godwin, a phenomenal mentor.
SP

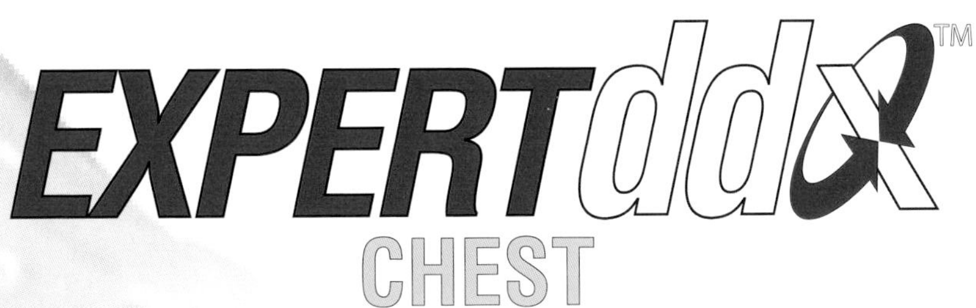

Once the appropriate technical protocols have been delineated, the best quality images obtained, and the cases queued up on PACS, the diagnostic responsibility reaches the radiology reading room. The radiologist must do more than simply "lay words on" but reach a real conclusion. If we cannot reach a definitive diagnosis, we must offer a reasonable differential diagnosis. A list that's too long is useless; a list that's too short may be misleading. To be useful, a differential must be more than a rote recitation from some dusty book or a mnemonic from a lecture way back when. Instead, we must take into account key imaging findings and relevant clinical information.

With these considerations in mind, we at Amirsys designed our Expert Differential Diagnoses series—EXPERTddx for short. Leading experts in every subspecialty of radiology identified the top differential diagnoses in their respective fields, encompassing specific anatomic locations, generic imaging findings, modality-specific findings, and clinically based indications. Our experts gathered multiple images, both typical and variant, for each EXPERTddx. Each features at least eight beautiful images that illustrate the possible diagnoses, accompanied by captions that highlight the pertinent imaging findings. Hundreds more are available in the eBook feature that accompanies every book. In classic Amirsys fashion, each EXPERTddx includes bulleted text that distills the available information to the essentials. You'll find helpful clues for diagnoses, ranked by prevalence as Common, Less Common, and Rare but Important.

Our EXPERTddx series is designed to help radiologists reach reliable—indeed, expert—conclusions. Whether you are a practicing radiologist or a resident/fellow in training, we think the EXPERTddx series will quickly become your practical "go-to" reference.

Anne G. Osborn, MD
CEO, Amirsys Publishing, Inc.

Paula J. Woodward, MD
President, Amirsys Publishing, Inc.

H. Ric Harnsberger, MD
CEO, Amirsys, Inc.

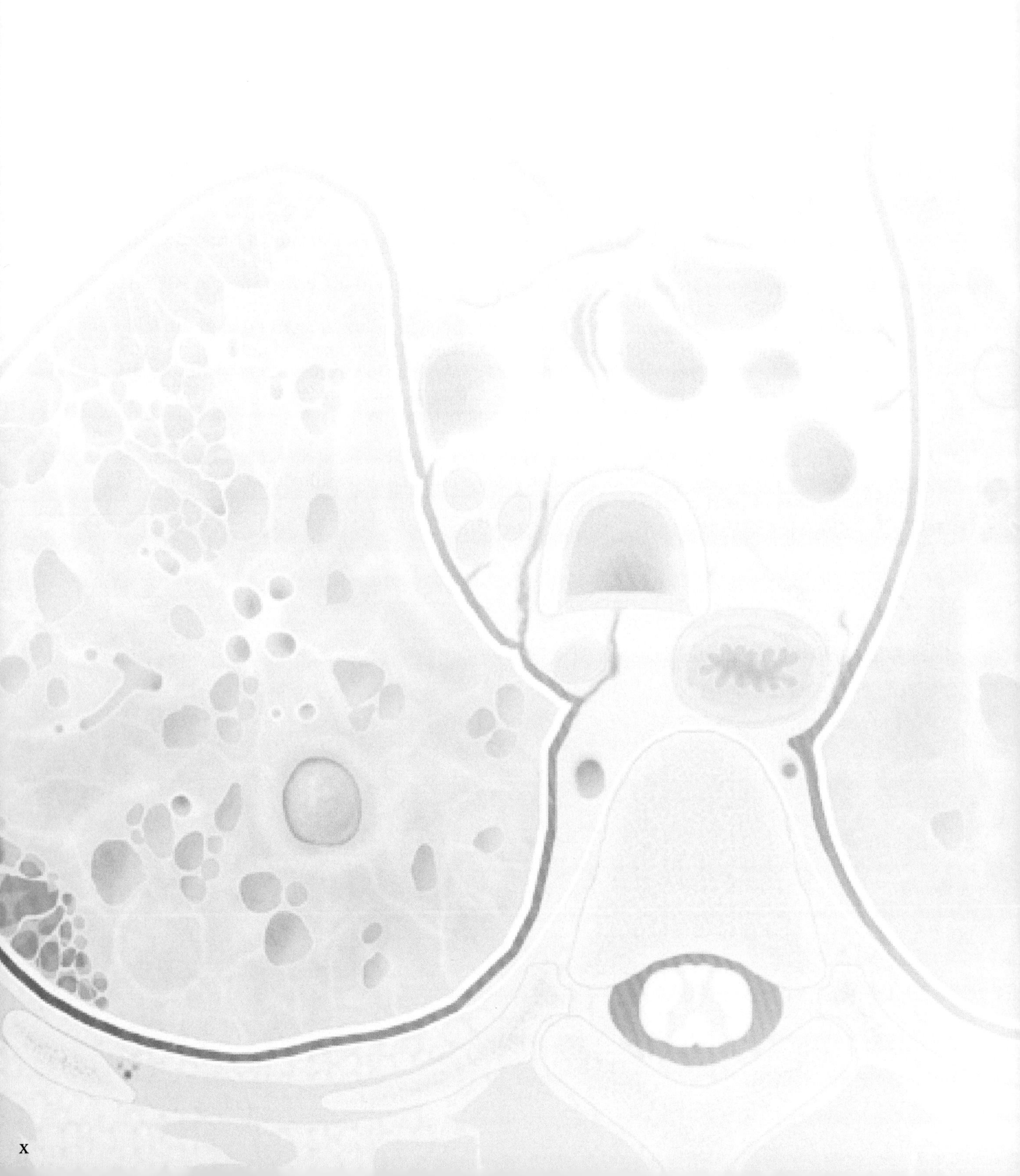

PREFACE

EXPERTddx: Chest focuses on observed radiographic findings and specific patient complaints, much like real-life clinical practice. Rather than focusing on a particular disease topic, this book focuses more on observed radiographic findings and specific patient complaints. We developed the contents to help you generate focused, specific, and accurate differential diagnoses. Based upon the collective wisdom and experiences of the authors at several major academic medical institutions across the United States and Europe, the possible diagnoses for each of the titled radiographic findings are ranked from most common or likely, to rare, but still important. The very nature of this book precludes an exhaustive differential diagnosis for each entity; our focus was on providing important and practical differential diagnostic considerations rather than minutia and esoterica. Keenly aware of the subtleties and art of radiology, we offer helpful clues in distinguishing diagnostic possibilities and provide key points on how best to provide the most accurate diagnosis possible. The key distinguishing features we provide are the same that we might offer to our trainees and clinical colleagues in our daily practice, teaching rounds, and consultations.

The table of contents is organized into logical anatomic groupings including large airways, small airways, alveolar spaces, the pulmonary interstitium, the pulmonary vasculature, the mediastinum/hilum, the pleura, chest wall, diaphragm, and heart. In addition, there is a separate section devoted to patient symptoms or presentation. Within these sections, you will find 116 chapters covering all gamuts of chest disorders, based upon observed findings rather than a specific disease. In each chapter you will find a focused and succinct list of differential diagnostic possibilities and the key features that distinguish among them. For example, in the large airways section, you'll find a chapter titled, "Tracheal Dilatation," rather than a chapter on tracheobronchomegaly. In the section on the hilum, you will find a specific chapter devoted to the differential diagnosis of the radiographic finding of the pattern of eggshell calcification of hilar lymph nodes rather than a chapter on sarcoidosis. Differential diagnostic possibilities are beautifully illustrated with multiple examples of typical and variant cases. All of the images are annotated and labeled to provide as much clarity as possible.

The easy-to-read bulleted content is distilled to the essential information necessary to be easy to use on a day-to-day basis. Case material used to illustrate the diagnostic possibilities has been derived from state-of-the-art imaging techniques, equipment, and modalities, and include appropriate imaging examples from digital radiography, to multi-detector CT scanning, to high field strength MRI.

This book is intended primarily for radiologists at all levels of training and experience who have an interest in chest imaging. We hope that it will serve you well in your practices to improve human health.

Eric J. Stern, MD
Vice Chair, Academic Affairs
Professor of Radiology
Adjunct Professor of Medicine
Adjunct Professor of Medical Education and Bioinformatics
Adjunct Professor of Global Health
University of Washington
Seattle, Washington

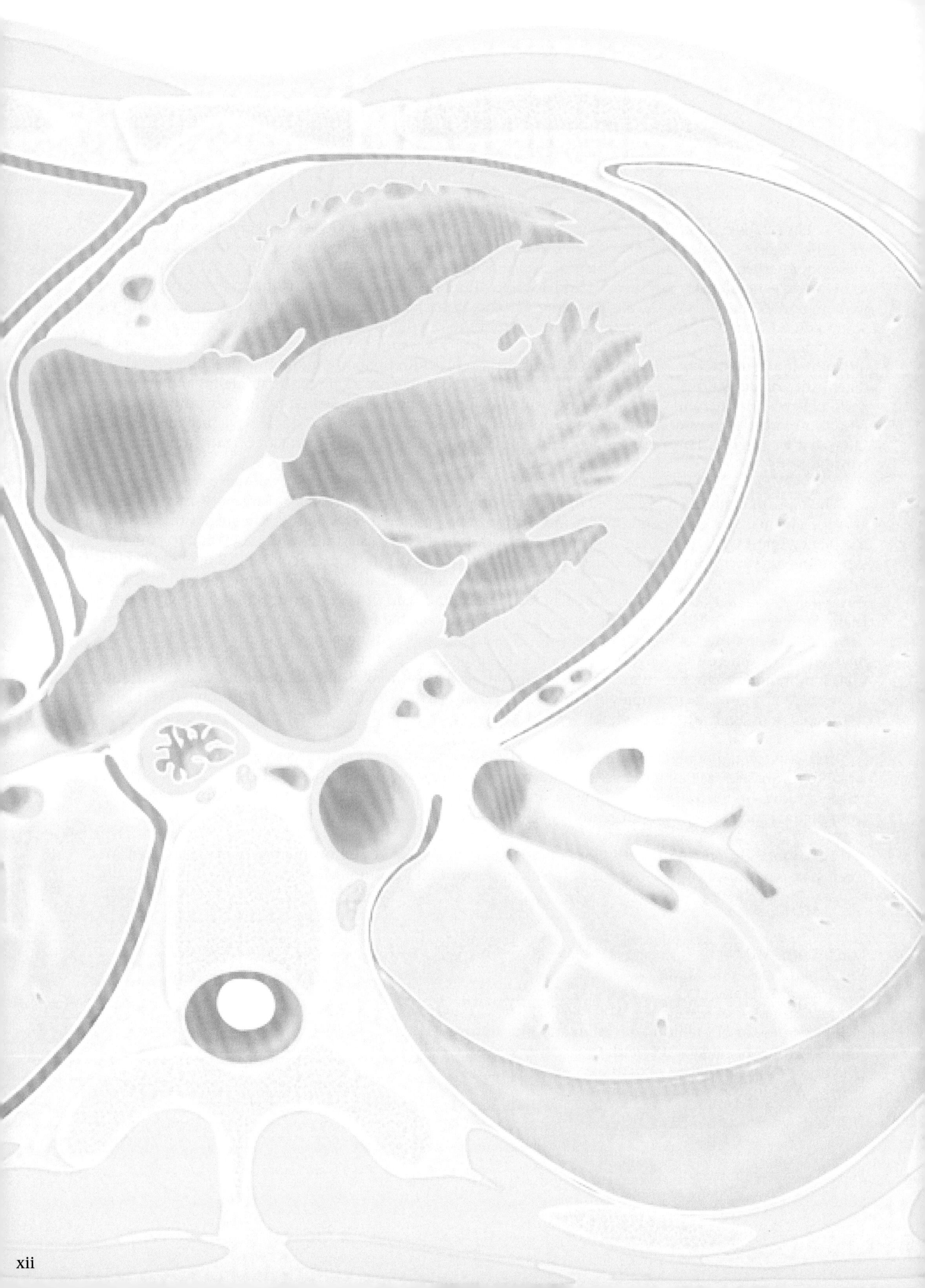

ACKNOWLEDGMENTS

Contributing Author

Dharshan Vummidi, MD
Acting Instructor/Senior Fellow
University of Washington
Seattle, Washington

Text Editing

Arthur G. Gelsinger, MA
Katherine Riser, MA
Dave L. Chance, MA
Matthew C. Connelly, MA

Image Editing

Jeffrey J. Marmorstone

Medical Text Editing

Laura K. Nason, MD

Art Direction and Design

Laura C. Sesto, MA

Associate Editor

Ashley R. Renlund, MA

Production Lead

Kellie J. Heap

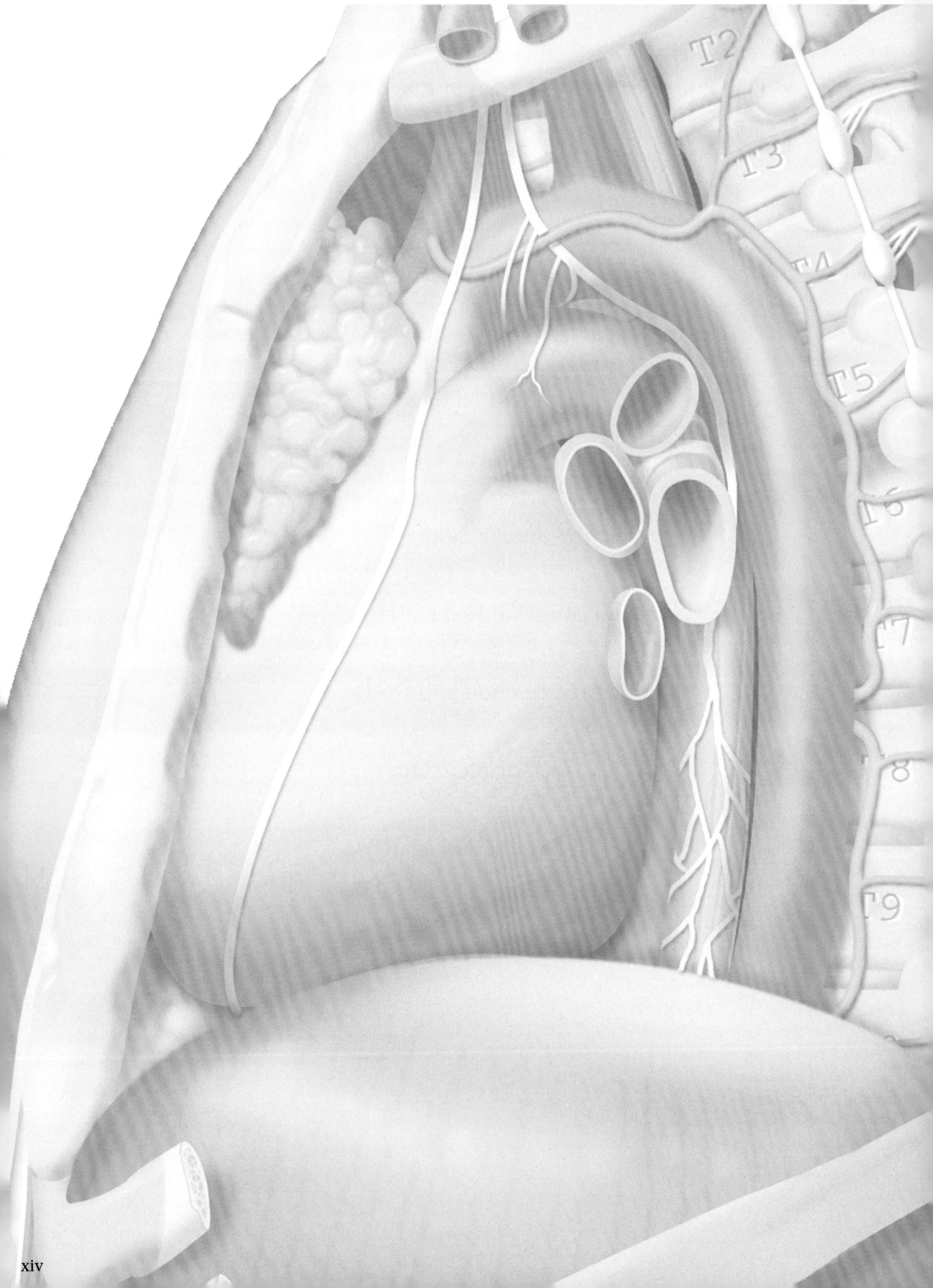
T2
T3
T4
T5
T6
T7
T8
T9

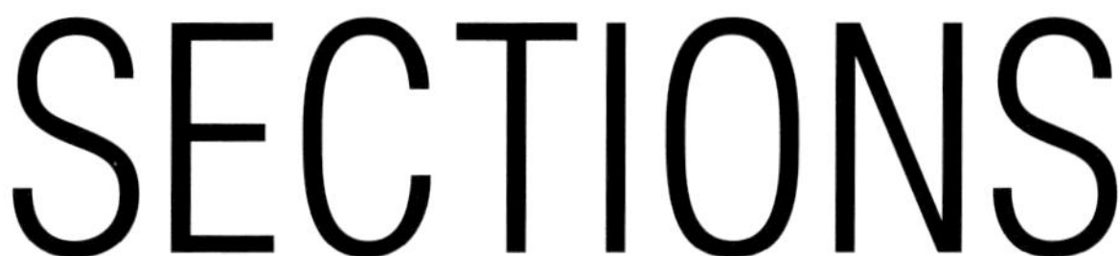
SECTIONS

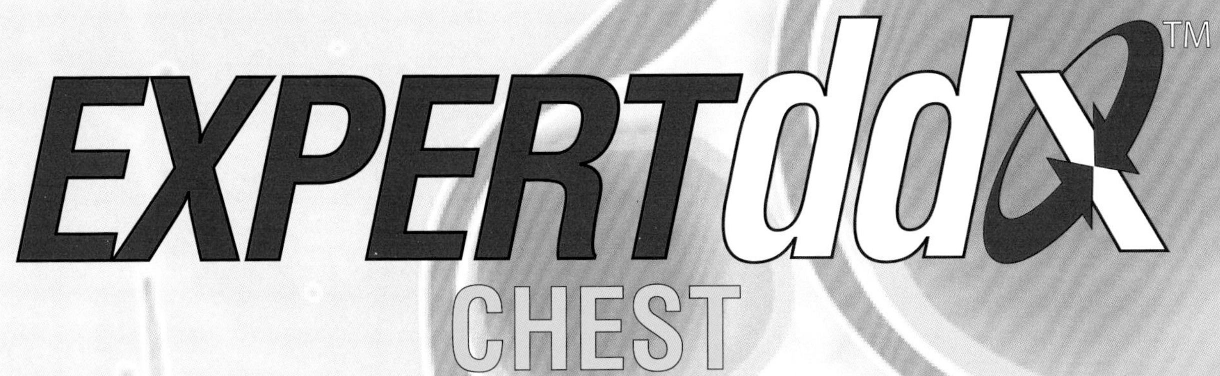
EXPERTddx™
CHEST

TABLE OF CONTENTS

SECTION 1
Thorax

SECTION 2
Large Airways

SECTION 3
Small Airways

SECTION 4
Symptoms

SECTION 5
Airspace

SECTION 6
Interstitium

SECTION 7
Pulmonary Vasculature

SECTION 8
Mediastinum and Hilum

SECTION 9
Pleura, Chest Wall, Diaphragm

SECTION 10
Heart

SECTION 1
Thorax

UNILATERAL HYPERLUCENT HEMITHORAX

DIFFERENTIAL DIAGNOSIS

Common

- Pneumothorax
- Mastectomy
- Prior Surgery
- Bronchial Obstruction

Less Common

- Swyer-James Syndrome
- Bronchial Atresia
- Congenital Lobar Emphysema

ESSENTIAL INFORMATION

Key Differential Diagnosis Issues

- Check for central airway obstruction
    - Endobronchial tumors, extrinsic compression, foreign bodies
- Check lung parenchyma for focal air-trapping
    - Exhalation CT helpful to increase confidence
- Check chest wall for evidence of prior surgery or deformities

Helpful Clues for Common Diagnoses

- **Pneumothorax**
    - Look for "deep sulcus" sign on supine radiographs
- **Mastectomy**
    - Breast asymmetry; surgical clips in axilla
- **Prior Surgery**
    - Single lung transplant
    - Ipsilateral lobectomy
- **Bronchial Obstruction**
    - Hyperlucency from air-trapping, ball-valve effect
    - Lobar collapse and hyperinflation of other lobes
    - Foreign body in children
    - Endobronchial tumors in adults
        - Primary malignancy > endobronchial metastases
        - Carcinoids commonly have central, chunky calcifications

Helpful Clues for Less Common Diagnoses

- **Swyer-James Syndrome**
    - Unilateral postinfectious constrictive bronchiolitis
    - Decreased vascular markings; air-trapping on exhalation
    - CT: Bronchiectasis often present; more extensive air-trapping than on radiograph
- **Bronchial Atresia**
    - Collateral ventilation; air-trapping on expiratory imaging
    - Mucocele common in airway distal to obliteration
    - Left upper lobe > right middle lobe > lower lobes
- **Congenital Lobar Emphysema**
    - Focal overinflation and air-trapping in disorganized parenchyma
    - Left upper lobe > right middle lobe > right lower lobe

Pneumothorax

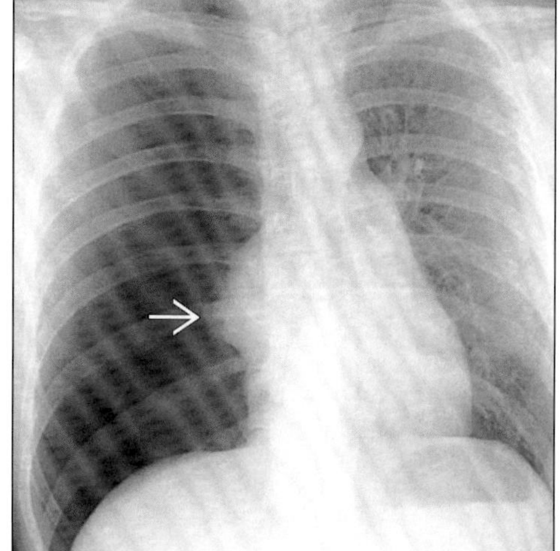

Frontal radiograph shows typical radiographic features of tension pneumothorax. Note the hyperlucent right hemithorax and collapsed right lung →, as well as mediastinum shifted to the left.

Pneumothorax

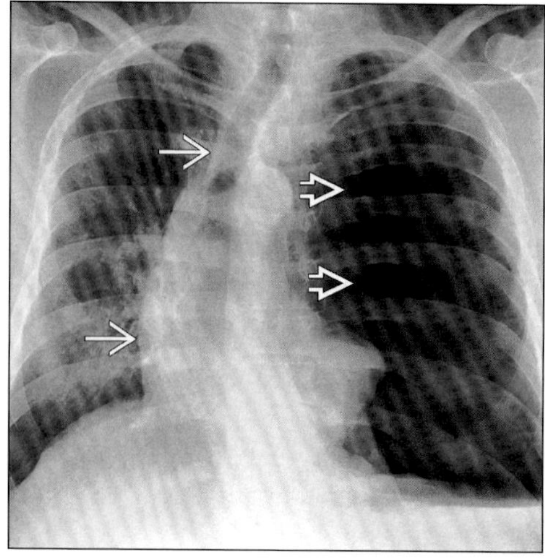

Anteroposterior radiograph shows typical radiograph features of lucent hemithorax → due to tension pneumothorax with contralateral mediastinal shift →.

UNILATERAL HYPERLUCENT HEMITHORAX

Mastectomy

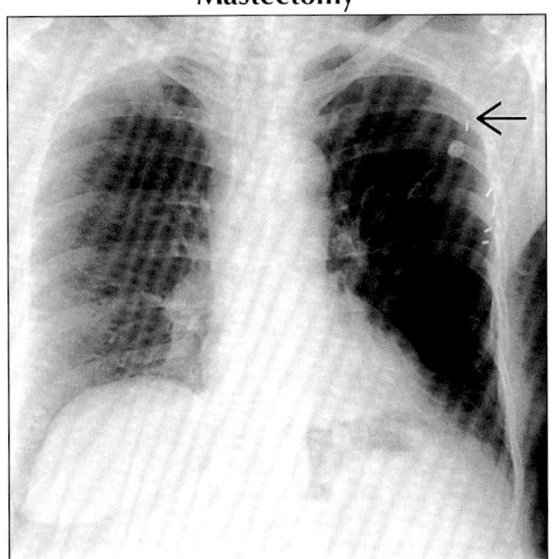

Bronchial Obstruction

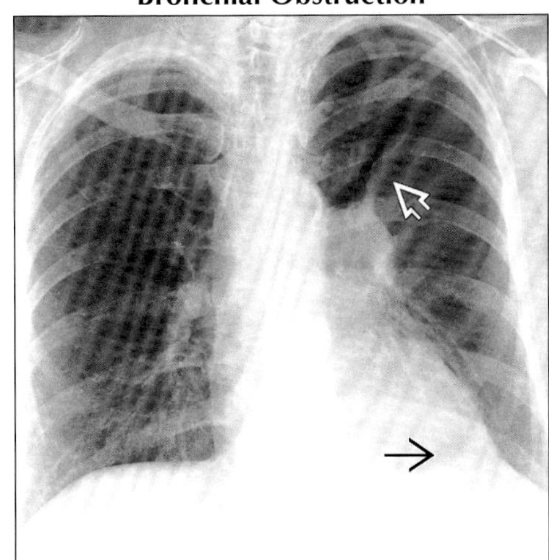

(Left) *Frontal radiograph shows a unilateral hyperlucent-appearing left hemithorax, in this case due to a prior left mastectomy. Note the surgical clips in the left axilla* →. ***(Right)*** *Frontal radiograph shows typical radiographic features of left upper lobe collapse from carcinoid tumor. Note the elevated left hilum, juxtaphrenic peak* →*, and Luftsichel (air-crescent) sign* ➡.

Swyer-James Syndrome

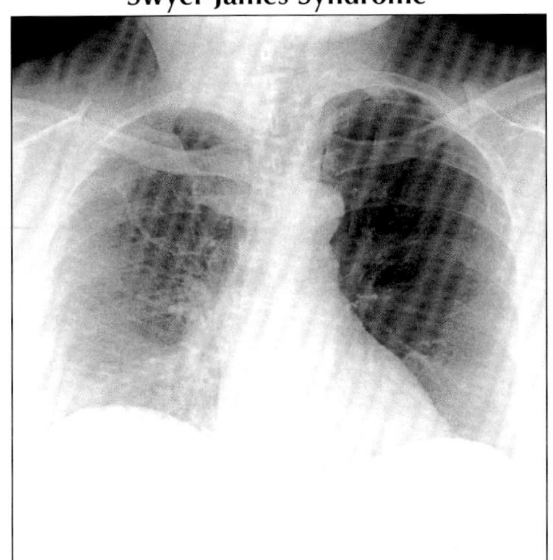

Swyer-James Syndrome

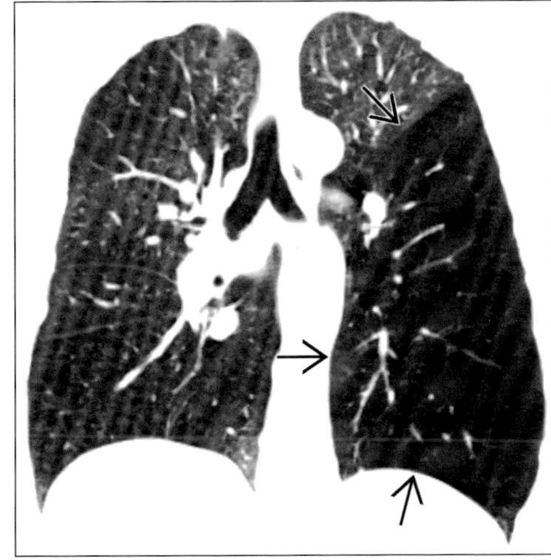

(Left) *Frontal radiograph shows a unilateral lucent left hemithorax secondary to postinfectious constrictive bronchiolitis, Swyer-James syndrome. Note small left pulmonary artery and the relative paucity of left-sided pulmonary vascular markings.* ***(Right)*** *Coronal NECT shows focal hyperinflation and vascular attenuation in left lower lobe* → *from postinfectious constrictive bronchiolitis, Swyer-James syndrome, as sequelae of a childhood adenovirus infection.*

Bronchial Atresia

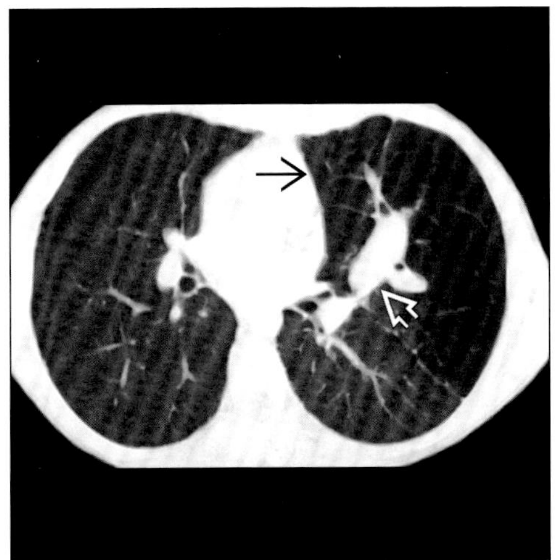

Bronchial Atresia

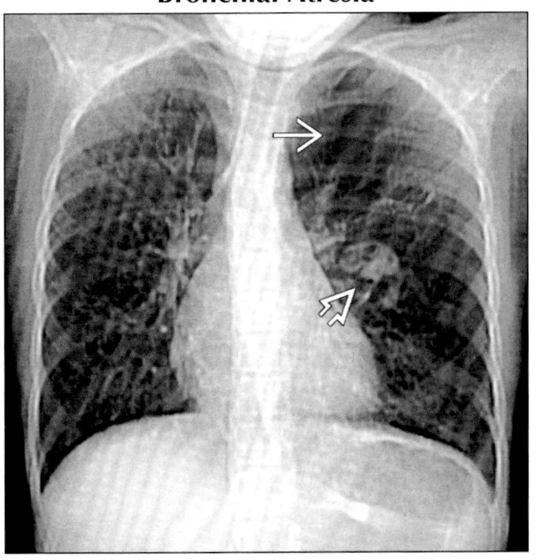

(Left) *Axial NECT shows paucity of vessels in the left upper lobe* → *and central tubular opacity* ➡*, representing the obstructed, dilated, and mucus-impacted distal airway.* ***(Right)*** *Frontal NECT shows typical CT scanogram features of hyperlucent lung due to bronchial atresia. Note the focal hyperlucent lung* ➡ *in the left upper lobe and elliptical opacity in the left hilum* ➡.

BILATERAL HYPERLUCENT HEMITHORAX

DIFFERENTIAL DIAGNOSIS

Common
- Centrilobular Emphysema
- Panlobular Emphysema
- Bronchiectasis
- Bronchiolitis

Less Common
- Constrictive Bronchiolitis
- Asthma
- Pulmonary Langerhans Cell Histiocytosis
- Lymphangiomyomatosis

Rare but Important
- Pulmonary Atresia

ESSENTIAL INFORMATION

Key Differential Diagnosis Issues
- Pulmonary causes
  - Usually related to airways disease
  - Pulmonary vascular causes much less common
- Extrapulmonary causes
  - Congenital or developmental lack of chest wall soft tissue
  - Bilateral mastectomy
- Technical
  - Overexposure
    - Uncommon with digital radiography
  - Incorrect window and level settings on CT

Helpful Clues for Common Diagnoses
- **Centrilobular Emphysema**
  - Most common type of emphysema
  - Almost always smoking related
  - Predominates in upper lobes and superior segments of lower lobes
  - Radiography: Hyperinflation, attenuation of vessels in affected areas
  - CT: Centrilobular foci of low attenuation without perceptible walls
  - Bulla: Emphysematous space > 1 cm
- **Panlobular Emphysema**
  - Most commonly associated with α-1-antitrypsin deficiency
  - Rarely associated with intravenous drug abuse (e.g., methylphenidate [Ritalin])
  - Predominates in basal portions of lungs
  - Radiography
    - Hyperinflation
    - Attenuation of vessels in affected areas, particularly lower lung zones
  - CT
    - Hyperinflation, particularly of lower lobes
    - Diffusely decreased attenuation of affected lung parenchyma with small vessels
- **Bronchiectasis**
  - Hyperinflation and air-trapping from associated small airways disease
  - Related to chronic or recurrent infection
    - Rarely result of congenital cartilage abnormality (Williams-Campbell syndrome)
  - Radiography
    - Pulmonary hyperinflation
    - Dilated bronchi
    - "Tram-tracking": Parallel lines representing nontapering walls of ectatic bronchi seen in profile
    - Mucoid impaction may be present
  - CT
    - Bronchial abnormalities clearly shown
    - Diffuse low attenuation and small vessels often present in parenchyma supplied by dilated and inflamed bronchi
    - Extensive air-trapping may be apparent on expiratory CT
- **Bronchiolitis**
  - Usually infectious
    - Viral
    - *Mycoplasma*
  - Radiography: Hyperinflation, small lung nodules
  - CT: Centrilobular nodules, tree in bud opacities

Helpful Clues for Less Common Diagnoses
- **Constrictive Bronchiolitis**
  - Submucosal and peribronchial fibrosis resulting in luminal narrowing or occlusion
  - Numerous causes
    - Infection: Viral (adenovirus and respiratory syncytial virus), *Mycoplasma*, *Pneumocystis*
    - Connective tissue diseases, especially rheumatoid arthritis and Sjögren syndrome
    - Drug reaction
    - Inhalational injury (toxic fumes, smoke)

- Transplant: Lung and blood stem cell
  - Radiography: Normal lung volume to hyperinflation
  - CT: Heterogeneity of lung with smaller vessels in areas of low attenuation
    - Expiratory imaging confirms presence of air-trapping
- **Asthma**
  - Chronic airway inflammation with remodeling
  - Radiography
    - Most patients have normal or near normal radiographs
    - Bronchial wall thickening may be evident
    - Pulmonary hyperinflation in severe cases
  - CT
    - Bronchial wall thickening
    - Bronchial luminal narrowing
    - Air-trapping (expiratory CT)
    - Allergic bronchopulmonary aspergillosis should be considered with central bronchiectasis and mucoid impaction
- **Pulmonary Langerhans Cell Histiocytosis**
  - Nearly all patients are smokers
  - Radiography
    - Hyperinflation
    - Reticular or reticulonodular abnormality sparing costophrenic sulci
  - CT
    - Upper lobe predominant cysts: Vary in size and shape
    - Small nodules ± central lucency progressing to cysts over time
    - Ground-glass opacity
  - Spontaneous pneumothorax in < 10%
- **Lymphangiomyomatosis**
  - Occurs exclusively in women of child-bearing age or patients with tuberous sclerosis
  - Radiography
    - Hyperinflation
    - Diffuse reticular abnormality (from superimposition of cysts)
    - Pleural effusion (chylous)
  - CT
    - Diffuse lung cysts ranging 2-20 mm with thin, smooth walls
    - Associated findings: Renal angiomyolipomas, retroperitoneal and mediastinal lymphangiomas, chylous pleural effusion
  - Patients may present with recurrent or chronic pneumothoraces

Helpful Clues for Rare Diagnoses

- **Pulmonary Atresia**
  - Presents in neonatal period: Cyanosis
  - Associated with other congenital cardiac malformations (e.g., tetralogy of Fallot)
  - Radiography
    - Cardiomegaly
    - Concave pulmonary artery segment
    - Pulmonary oligemia
  - Diagnosis usually confirmed by echocardiography or cardiac MR

Centrilobular Emphysema

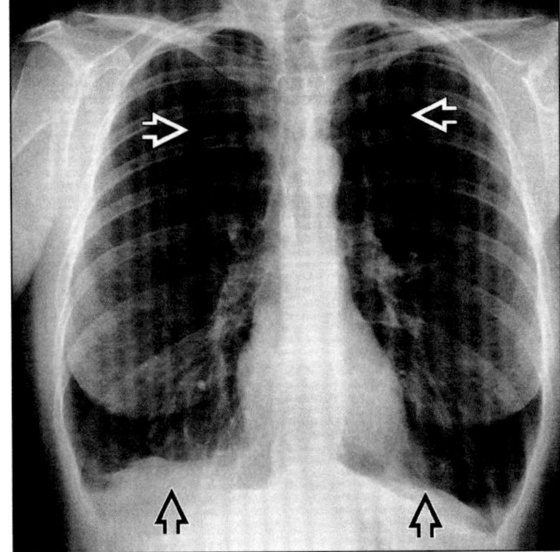

Frontal radiograph shows bilateral pulmonary hyperinflation with marked attenuation of the pulmonary vessels ➡ in the mid and upper lung zones. Note the depressed hemidiaphragms ⇨.

Centrilobular Emphysema

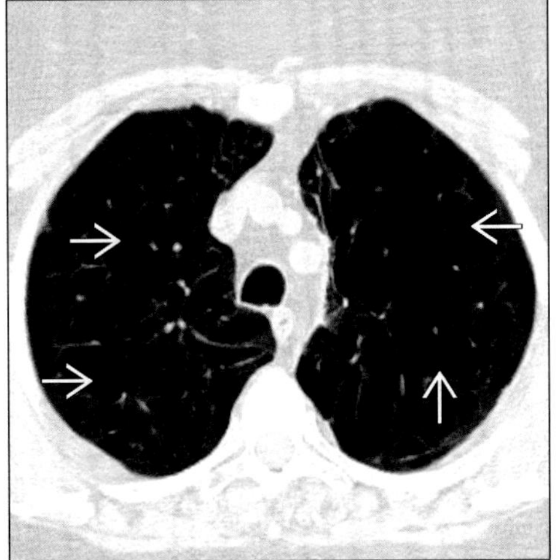

Axial HRCT shows severe, predominantly centrilobular emphysema ➡ in this heavy cigarette smoker. Note relative sparing of the lung periphery.

BILATERAL HYPERLUCENT HEMITHORAX

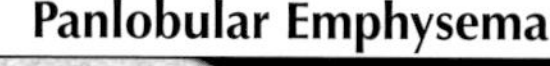

*(**Left**) Axial HRCT shows severe panlobular emphysema → predominantly in the lower lobes characterized by decreased lung attenuation and small vessels →. The right middle lobe → is compressed but is otherwise relatively spared. (**Right**) Coronal CT reconstruction shows markedly decreased parenchymal attenuation → in the lower lobes as compared to the upper lobes, which contain a small amount of centrilobular emphysema →.*

Panlobular Emphysema

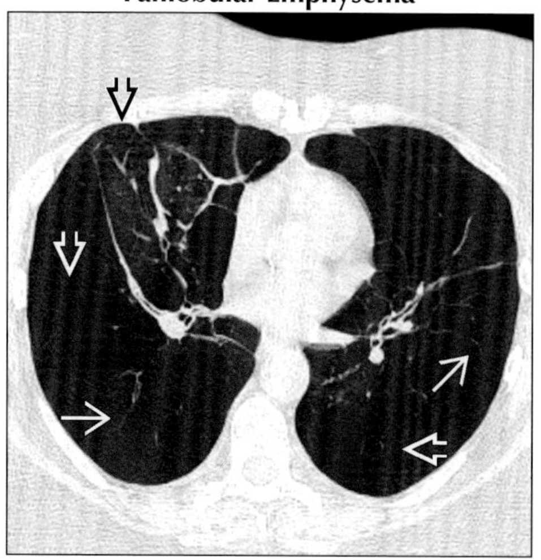

Panlobular Emphysema

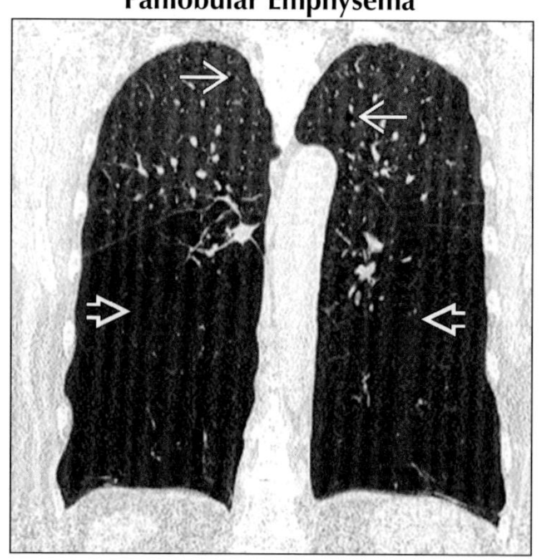

*(**Left**) Coronal HRCT shows multiple foci of cylindrical bronchiectasis → associated with low-attenuation oligemic regions of lung → in this patient who also had small airways disease. Patchy ground-glass opacity → reflects the normal lung. (**Right**) Axial HRCT shows extensive cylindrical bronchiectasis → with bronchial wall thickening and foci of mucoid impaction →. Note the relatively low-attenuation, oligemic areas of lung →.*

Bronchiectasis

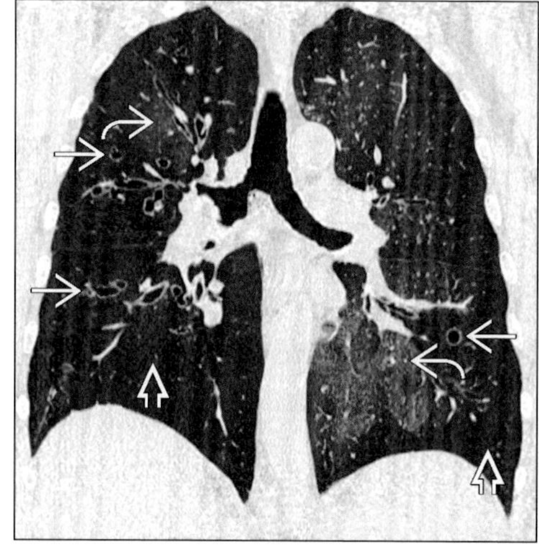

Bronchiectasis

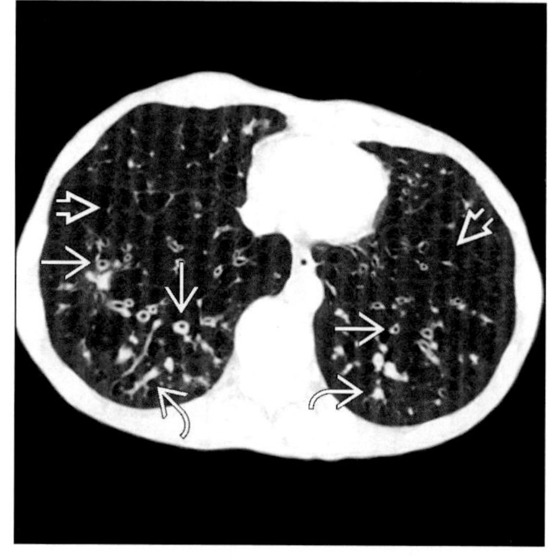

*(**Left**) Axial CT reconstruction shows numerous centrilobular nodules and tree in bud opacities → in this transplant recipient with infectious bronchiolitis. Note the relative low attenuation of lung →, reflecting air-trapping, in areas with highest profusion of nodules. (**Right**) Coronal CT reconstruction shows a mosaic pattern of attenuation with multiple areas of low attenuation and oligemic lung →, reflecting small airways disease.*

Bronchiolitis

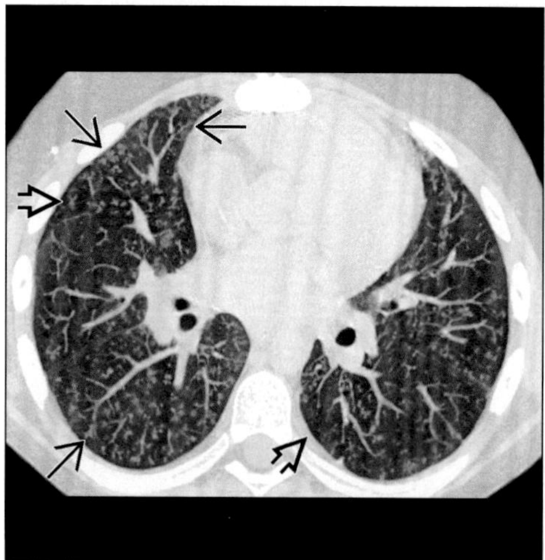

Constrictive Bronchiolitis

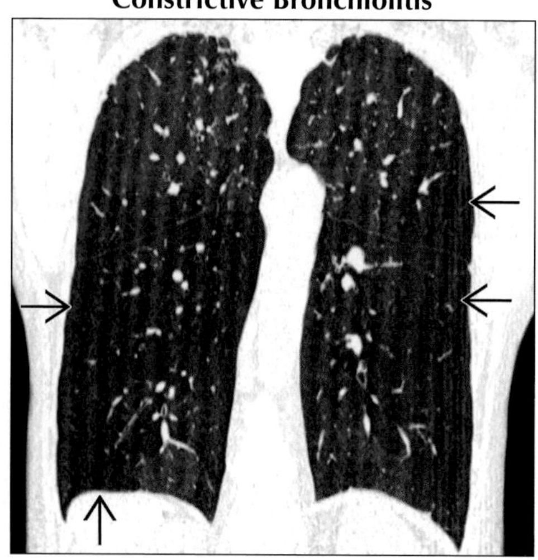

BILATERAL HYPERLUCENT HEMITHORAX

Asthma

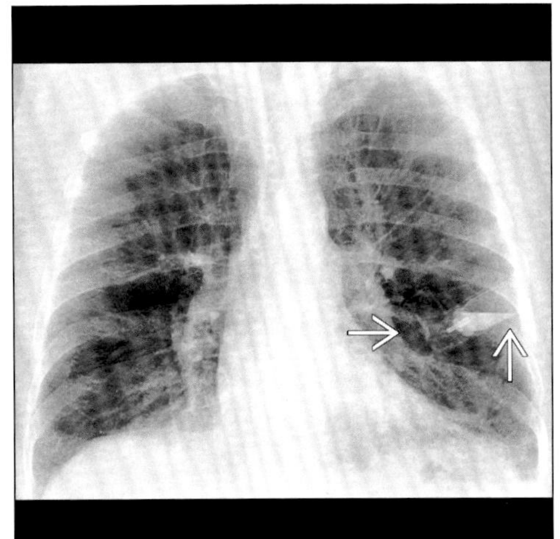

Pulmonary Langerhans Cell Histiocytosis

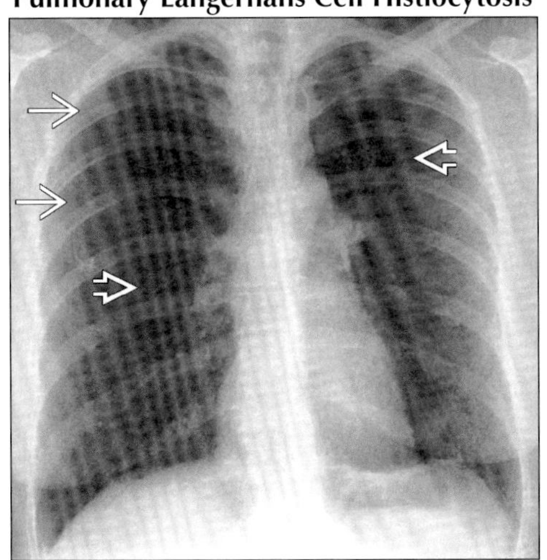

*(**Left**) Frontal radiograph shows diffuse pulmonary hyperinflation. Note the inhaler ➡ is in the patient's pocket. Many patients with asthma have normal or near normal chest radiographs. Occasionally, bronchial wall thickening may be present. (**Right**) Frontal radiograph shows a faint reticulonodular pattern ➡ in both lungs and pneumothorax on the right ➡. The lungs are mildly hyperinflated. Overlap of cyst walls contributes to the reticular abnormality.*

Pulmonary Langerhans Cell Histiocytosis

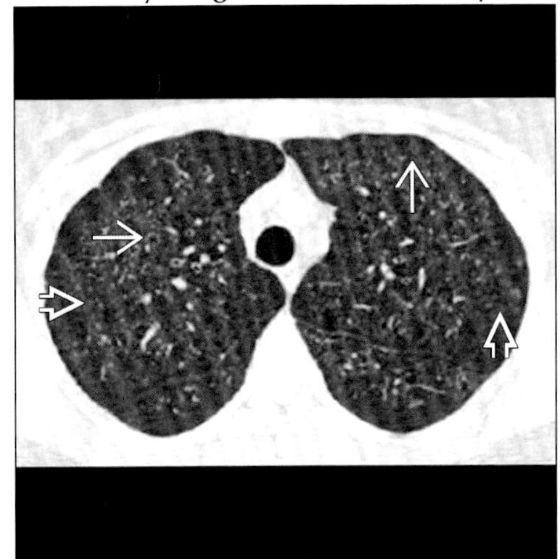

Lymphangiomyomatosis

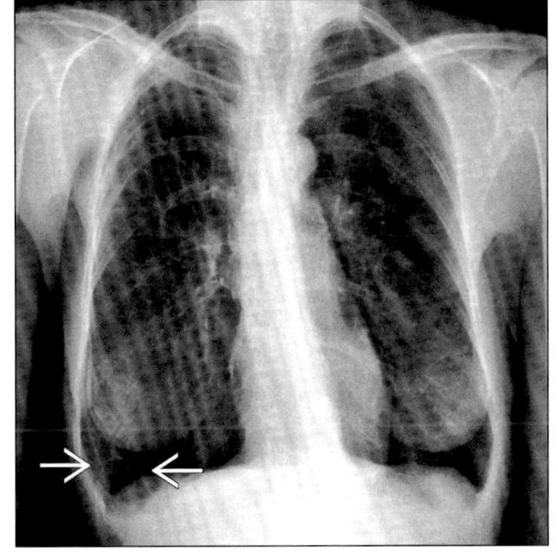

*(**Left**) Axial NECT shows faint, predominantly centrilobular nodules ➡ and a few small cysts ➡ in this smoker. With progression, nodules cavitate and form cysts. (**Right**) Frontal radiograph shows marked pulmonary hyperinflation and decreased attenuation of the lungs. Curvilinear opacities ➡ reflect overlapping walls of cysts. The walls of smaller cysts superimpose to create a fine reticular pattern.*

Lymphangiomyomatosis

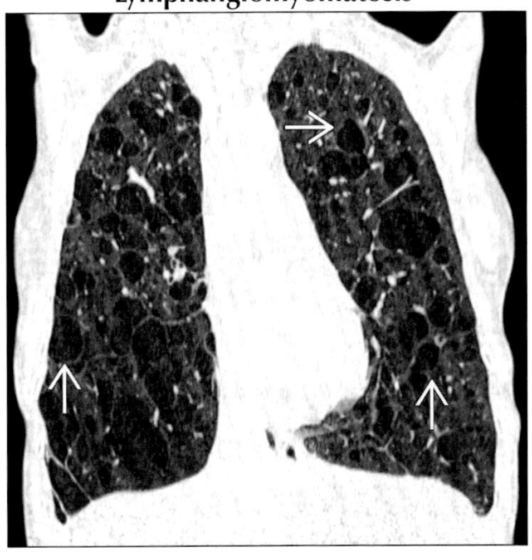

Pulmonary Atresia

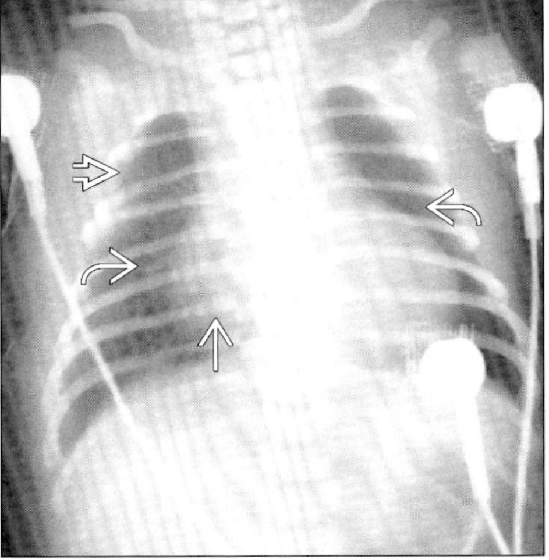

*(**Left**) Coronal CT reconstruction shows diffuse lung cysts ➡ without a zonal predominance. Note the relative uniformity of size and thin walls, typical of lymphangioleiomyomatosis. The lungs are hyperinflated. Patients may develop recurrent and chronic pneumothoraces. (**Right**) Anteroposterior radiograph shows right cardiomegaly ➡ and pulmonary oligemia ➡ following creation of a Blalock-Taussig shunt (note splaying of ribs on right ➡).*

UNILATERAL OPAQUE HEMITHORAX

DIFFERENTIAL DIAGNOSIS

Common
- Pleural Effusion
- Empyema
- Hemothorax
- Pneumonectomy
- Community Acquired Pneumonia

Less Common
- Endobronchial Tumor
- Non-Small Cell Lung Cancer
- Small Cell Lung Cancer
- Pleural Metastasis

Rare but Important
- Pulmonary Agenesis
- Fibrous Tumor of Pleura
- Malignant Mesothelioma

ESSENTIAL INFORMATION

Key Differential Diagnosis Issues
- Chest wall
  - CT and MR usually definitive
  - Absent mediastinal shift
  - Associated osseous lesions (e.g., fracture with chest wall hematoma)
- Pleural
  - Obtuse margins with pleural interfaces
  - Contralateral mediastinal shift
  - CT and MR usually definitive
- Pulmonary
  - Acute margins with pleural surface
  - Mediastinal shift varies depending on etiology
  - CT usually definitive

Helpful Clues for Common Diagnoses
- **Pleural Effusion**
  - Contralateral mediastinal shift
  - Atelectasis of underlying lung
  - Meniscus sign: Lateral concave border where effusion meets costal pleura
  - Downward displacement of hemidiaphragm on left
- **Empyema**
  - Lenticular shape
  - Nondependent location with clear demarcation from adjacent lung
  - Split pleura sign
    - Pleural fluid separates enhancing visceral and parietal pleura
    - Not specific for empyema: Occurs with any form of pleural inflammation
  - Haziness in adjacent extrapleural fat
  - Compresses adjacent lung and vessels
  - Presence of gas in absence of thoracentesis
  - Contralateral mediastinal shift
- **Hemothorax**
  - High-attenuation pleural fluid (> 50 HU)
  - Usually unilateral
  - Blunt or penetrating trauma
  - Iatrogenic
  - Spontaneous causes include rupture of aneurysms, coagulopathy, pleural metastases, and pleural endometriosis
- **Pneumonectomy**
  - Pneumonectomy space fills with fluid within 30 days
  - Ipsilateral mediastinal shift
  - New or increased gas in existing pneumonectomy space indicates bronchopleural fistula
- **Community Acquired Pneumonia**
  - Lobar consolidation
    - *S. pneumoniae* most common
    - TB, *H. influenzae*, *Legionella* less common
  - Parapneumonic effusion
    - Can develop into empyema

Helpful Clues for Less Common Diagnoses
- **Endobronchial Tumor**
  - Whole lung collapse less common than lobar collapse
  - Primary lung carcinoma: Squamous cell carcinoma most common
  - Metastasis: Breast, colon, and renal cell carcinoma; melanoma
  - Ipsilateral mediastinal shift
- **Non-Small Cell Lung Cancer**
  - Extrinsic compression of main bronchus
    - Primary tumor, lymph node metastases, or both
- **Small Cell Lung Cancer**
  - Extrinsic compression of main bronchus
    - Bulky lymph node metastases common
  - May also invade mediastinum
- **Pleural Metastasis**
  - ~ 90% of all pleural neoplasms
    - Lung carcinoma leading cause
    - Breast, ovary, and gastric carcinomas and lymphoma also common causes
  - Usually multiple
  - Can simulate benign pleural disease

- Nodular, circumferential, and mediastinal pleural involvement suggestive of malignancy
- Associated pleural effusion common
- Can have lung or thoracic lymph node metastases

Helpful Clues for Rare Diagnoses

- **Pulmonary Agenesis**
  - Complete absence of lung with no bronchial or vascular tissue
  - Often associated with other congential anomalies, resulting in neonatal death
  - Adults with isolated pulmonary hypoplasia often asymptomatic
  - Identical imaging appearance to patients with childhood pneumonectomy
- **Fibrous Tumor of Pleura**
  - 5-10% of primary pleural neoplasms, 12% malignant
    - Imaging alone cannot determine whether malignant or not
  - Peak incidence: 6th and 7th decades
  - Approximately 50% patients symptomatic
    - Clubbing (4%)
    - Symptomatic hypoglycemia (4-5%)
  - Radiography
    - Solitary peripheral pleural mass with smooth margins
    - May develop within pulmonary fissure
    - Can change orientation with changes in patient position
  - CT
    - Smaller tumors homogeneous
    - Larger tumors heterogeneous with necrosis, cystic degeneration, and hemorrhage
    - Calcification (7-25%) (more common in larger tumors)
    - Has smooth margins, abuts pleural surface, and may form obtuse angles with adjacent pleura
    - Intense, uniform enhancement except in areas of necrosis
  - MR
    - Fibrous tissue: Low to intermediate signal intensity on T1- and T2-weighted imaging
    - Cystic degeneration, necrosis, myxoid: Foci of high T2 signal intensity
    - Low signal septa on T2-weighted imaging
    - Blood products: T1 and T2 signal intensity vary depending on age of hemorrhage
- **Malignant Mesothelioma**
  - Most result from asbestos exposure
    - Latency of up to 40 years
  - Can simulate benign pleural disease
  - Nodular, circumferential, and mediastinal pleural involvement suggestive of malignancy
  - Mediastinum relatively "fixed" with little or no shift
  - Associated pleural effusion may be present
  - Extrapleural spread
    - Chest wall, mediastinum, diaphragm

Pleural Effusion

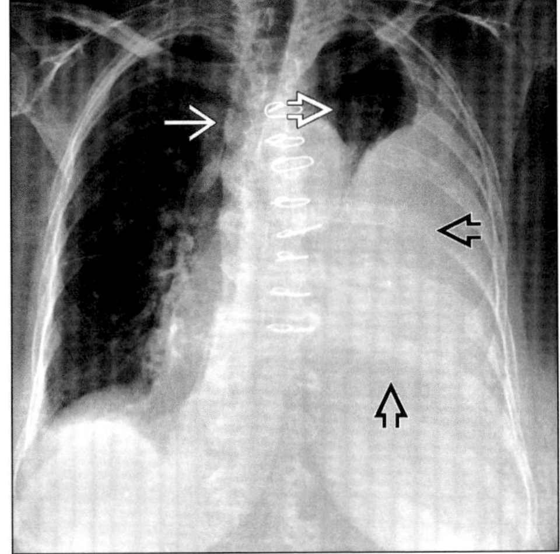

Frontal radiograph shows a large left pleural effusion ➩ causing marked left lung atelectasis with aeration of a small portion of the left upper lobe ➡. Note rightward mediastinal shift ➡.

Pleural Effusion

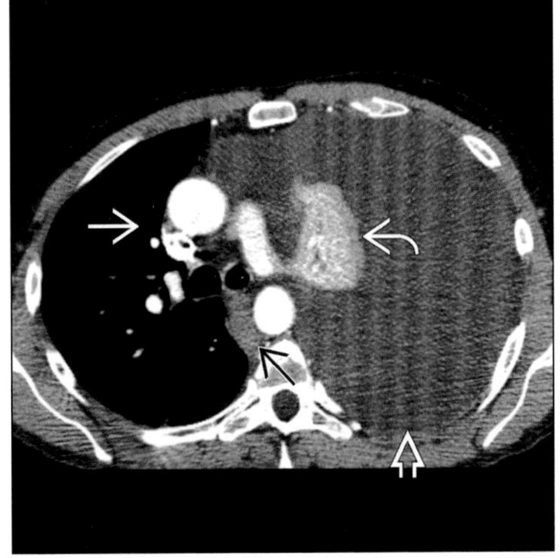

Axial CECT shows tension hydrothorax ➡ displacing the mediastinum ➡ to the right and collapsing the left lung ➡. Note right paraspinal lymphadenopathy →.

UNILATERAL OPAQUE HEMITHORAX

(Left) Axial CECT shows lobulated right pleural empyema ➔, lung abscess ➔, & pleural enhancement ➔. Fluid attenuation and pleural enhancement cannot determine whether or not pleural fluid is infected. ***(Right)*** *Transverse CECT shows enhancement of the thickened pleura ➔ & liquid ➔ & air ➔ collections. The presence of pleural gas in the absence of recent instrumentation is highly suggestive of empyema from gas-forming organisms.*

Empyema

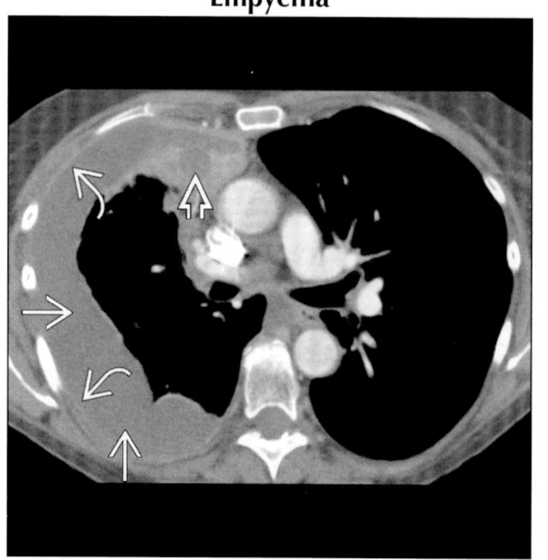

Empyema

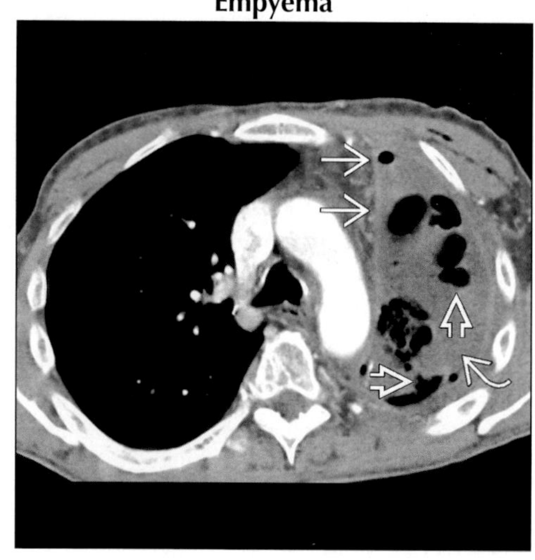

(Left) Axial NECT shows a large, heterogeneous and high-attenuation pleural collection ➔. Attenuation of the blood products will decrease as the hematoma breaks down. Pleural thickening and fibrothorax can develop when hemothorax is not properly drained. ***(Right)*** *Axial CECT shows right pneumonectomy space with calcification ➔ within markedly thickened parietal pleura ➔. There is compensatory hyperexpansion of the left lung.*

Hemothorax

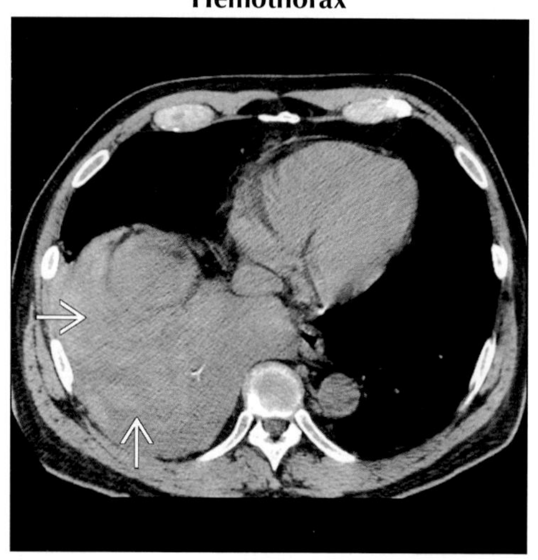

Pneumonectomy

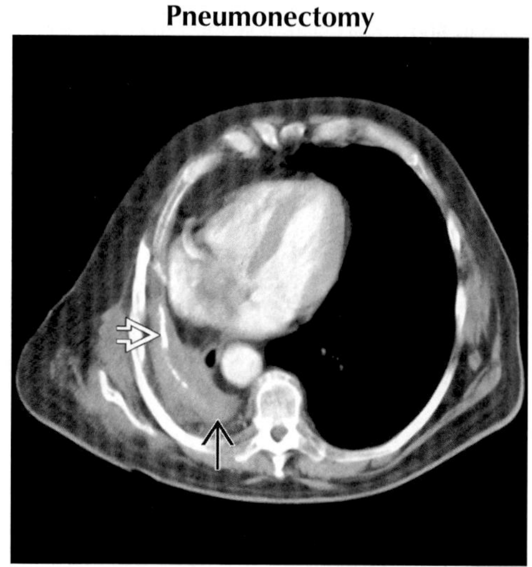

(Left) Frontal radiograph shows diffuse consolidation ➔ in the right lung. Mild focal consolidation ➔ is present in the left lung. ***(Right)*** *Frontal radiograph shows complete right lung collapse ➔ with rightward shift of the mediastinum ➔. Note the abrupt cutoff of the right main bronchus from an endobronchial lesion ➔. Ipsilateral mediastinal shift helps distinguish obstructive collapse from a large pleural effusion or mass.*

Community Acquired Pneumonia

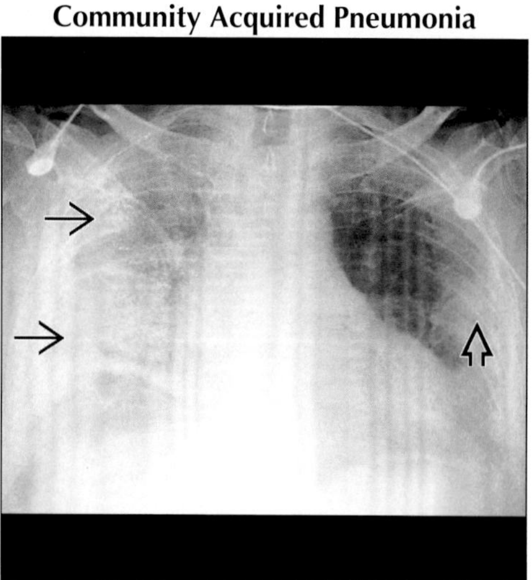

Endobronchial Tumor

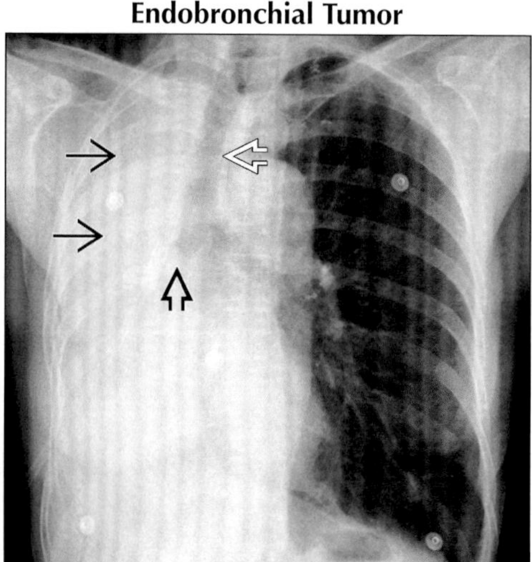

Non-Small Cell Lung Cancer

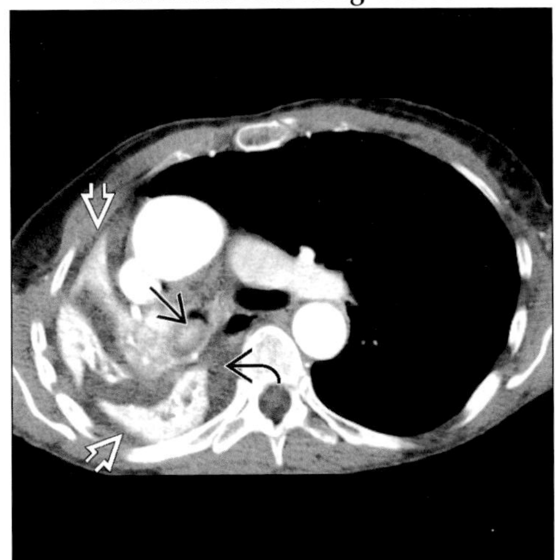

Small Cell Lung Cancer

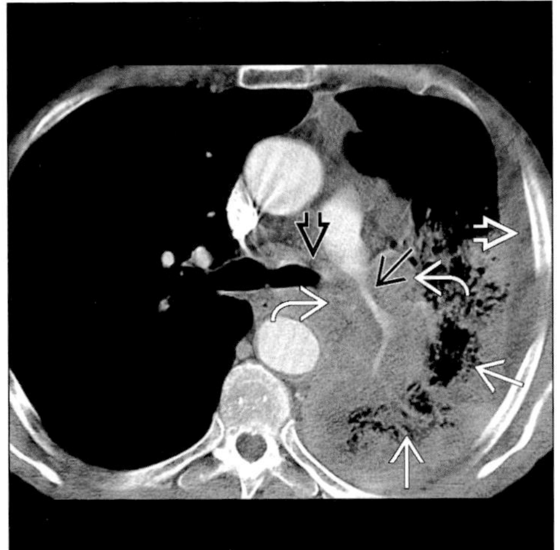

*(**Left**) Axial CECT shows an enhancing collapsed right lung ➡ resulting from an endobronchial primary lung carcinoma ➡. A small right pleural effusion ➡ is present. (**Right**) Axial CECT shows a large left hilar mass ➡ compressing the left pulmonary artery ➡ and left main bronchus ➡. Note obstructive pneumonia ➡ and a small pleural effusion ➡. Patients with small cell carcinoma often present with advanced disease.*

Pleural Metastasis

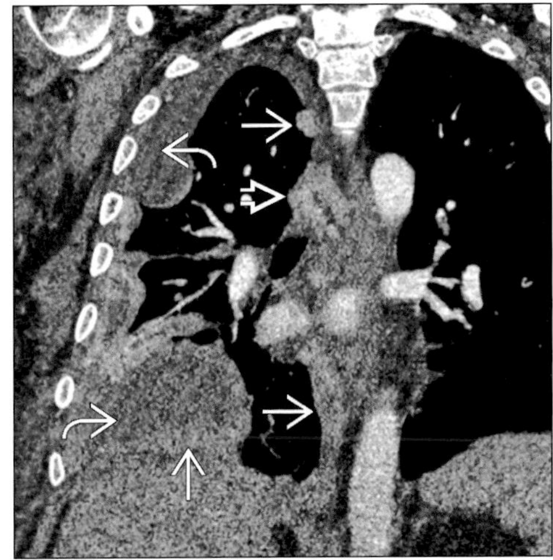

Pulmonary Agenesis

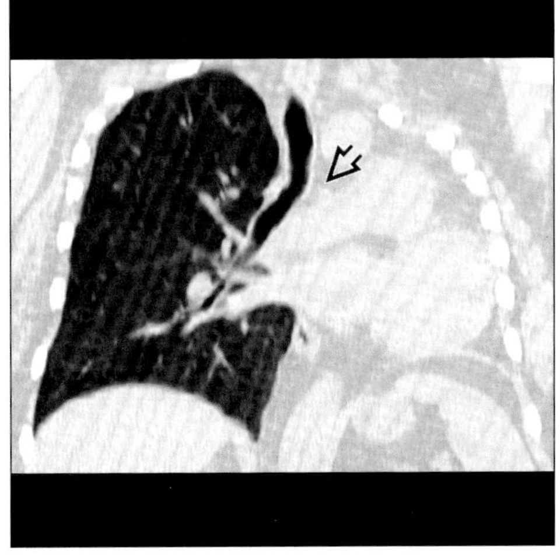

*(**Left**) Coronal CT reconstruction shows extensive right pleural metastases ➡ and associated effusion ➡ in this patient with metastatic renal cell carcinoma. Mediastinal lymphadenopathy ➡ is also present. (**Right**) Coronal NECT shows a small right hemithorax with no pulmonary, arterial, or airway structures. In contrast to pulmonary aplasia, which is slightly more common, no bronchial stump ➡ is present.*

Fibrous Tumor of Pleura

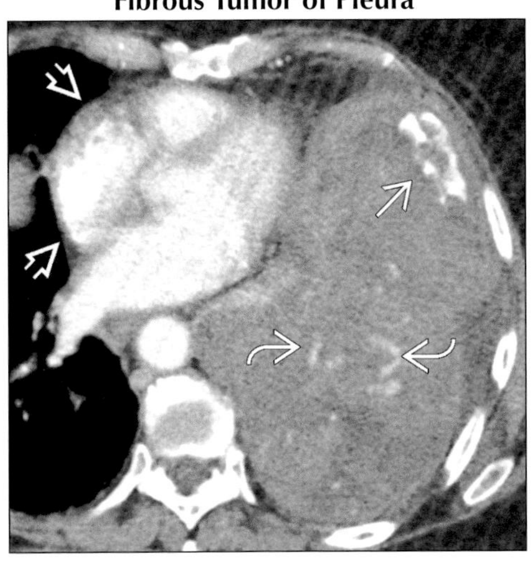

Malignant Mesothelioma

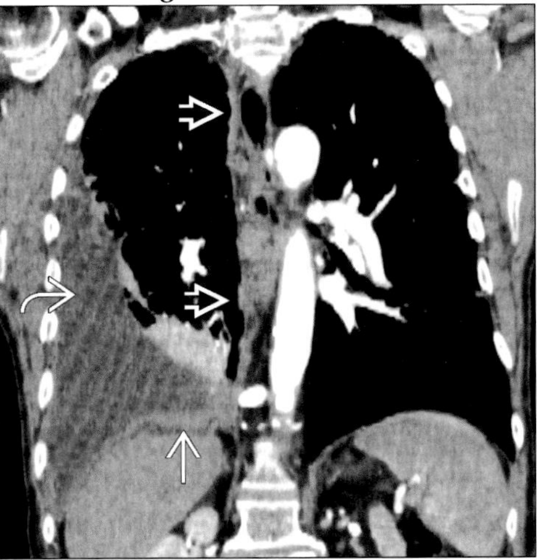

*(**Left**) Axial CECT shows a heterogeneous, lobulated pleural mass with focal enhancement ➡ and dense calcification ➡. The mass displaces the mediastinum ➡ to the right. (**Right**) Coronal CT reconstruction shows a large right pleural effusion ➡ and irregular pleural thickening ➡. Note involvement of the mediastinal pleura ➡, a finding suggestive of malignancy in the absence of previous instrumentation.*

BILATERAL OPAQUE HEMITHORAX

DIFFERENTIAL DIAGNOSIS

Common
- Pulmonary Edema
- Community Acquired Pneumonia
- Pleural Effusion

Less Common
- Diffuse Alveolar Hemorrhage
- Drug Reaction
- Acute Interstitial Pneumonia
- Pneumocystis Pneumonia
- Lung Contusion
- Bronchioloalveolar Carcinoma

Rare but Important
- Pulmonary Alveolar Proteinosis

ESSENTIAL INFORMATION

Key Differential Diagnosis Issues
- Acute
  - Pulmonary edema
  - Acute interstitial pneumonia
  - Diffuse alveolar hemorrhage
  - Pleural effusion
  - Drug reaction
  - Pneumocystis pneumonia
  - Lung trauma
- Chronic
  - Pleural metastasis
  - Bronchioloalveolar carcinoma
  - Pulmonary alveolar proteinosis

Helpful Clues for Common Diagnoses
- **Pulmonary Edema**
  - Bilateral diffuse patchy or confluent air space consolidation
    - More central
    - "Bat-wing" or "butterfly" perihilar distribution
  - Septal (Kerley B) lines
  - Cardiomegaly common, especially with congestive heart failure
  - CT: Smooth interlobular septal thickening with basal predominance
  - Associated pleural effusions
  - Radiological response to treatment
- **Community Acquired Pneumonia**
  - Diffuse bilateral disease usually from rapid spread of lobar pneumonia
    - *Legionella*
    - *Staphylococcus*
    - *Pneumococcus*
    - Viral
  - Immunocompromised patients at risk for disseminated infection
  - May develop acute respiratory distress syndrome (ARDS) or ARDS-like clinical picture
- **Pleural Effusion**
  - Bilateral effusions often related to congestive heart failure
  - Meniscus
  - Minimal or no mediastinal shift
  - Associated collapse of underlying lung (compressive atelectasis)
    - Air bronchograms common
    - Uniform enhancement of lung parenchyma on contrast-enhanced CT or MR

Helpful Clues for Less Common Diagnoses
- **Diffuse Alveolar Hemorrhage**
  - Usually related to capillaritis
    - Wegener granulomatosis
    - Microscopic polyangiitis
    - Systemic lupus erythematosus
    - Goodpasture syndrome
    - Drug reaction
  - Bilateral: Symmetric or asymmetric
  - Lung consolidation and ground-glass opacity
    - Peripheral sparing common
  - Elevated diffusing capacity (DLCO)
  - Bronchoalveolar lavage diagnostic
  - Usually clears within 7-10 days
- **Drug Reaction**
  - Wide range of reactions
    - Diffuse alveolar damage
    - Diffuse alveolar hemorrhage
    - Organizing pneumonia
    - Eosinophilic pneumonia
    - Hypersensitivity reaction
  - Numerous causative agents
    - Chemotherapeutic agents most commonly implicated
    - Amiodarone: Deposition and reaction
- **Acute Interstitial Pneumonia**
  - Diffuse alveolar damage
    - ARDS: Underlying cause known, common
    - Acute interstitial pneumonia (AIP): Idiopathic ARDS, rare
  - High mortality rate

- Perihilar and basal predominant lung consolidation and ground-glass opacity
  - Air bronchograms common
  - Septal lines and pleural effusions uncommon
- Slow evolution and response to treatment
  - Fibrosis may develop in spared areas

- **Pneumocystis Pneumonia**
  - Underlying immunosuppression
  - AIDS
    - More insidious onset than with other forms of immunosuppression
    - CD4(+) T-cell count < 200 cells/μL
  - Perihilar or diffuse ground-glass opacity
  - May progress to consolidation
  - May develop upper lobe predominant thin-walled pneumatoceles
  - Pleural effusions are uncommon
- **Lung Contusion**
  - Most common lung injury from blunt trauma
  - Hemorrhage into parenchyma
  - Marker of high-energy trauma
  - Radiography and CT
    - Nonanatomic distribution of consolidation and ground-glass opacity
    - Usually present on initial imaging
    - Should clear within 7 days
  - Extensive contusion associated with high mortality rate (> 25%)
- **Bronchioloalveolar Carcinoma**
  - Slowly progressive lung consolidation
  - Bilateral involvement typical of multicentric or disseminated disease
    - Least common manifestation (solitary lung nodule and focal consolidation more common)
  - CT often shows mixed consolidation and ground-glass opacity
    - Crazy-paving and septal thickening less common
    - Dilated airways within consolidation: "Pseudocavitation"

Helpful Clues for Rare Diagnoses

- **Pulmonary Alveolar Proteinosis**
  - Accumulation of periodic acid-Schiff (PAS) positive material in alveolar spaces
  - Primary (idiopathic)
    - Middle-aged men most commonly affected
  - Secondary
    - Blood stem cell recipients or patients with hematologic malignancies
  - Imaging abnormalities out of proportion to clinical signs and symptoms
    - Chest radiograph: Diffuse or patchy consolidation and ground-glass opacity
    - CT: Crazy-paving in geographic distribution with interspersed areas of normal lung
  - Bronchoalveolar lavage is both diagnostic and therapeutic
    - Clinical improvement promptly after therapeutic lavage
    - Radiograph improvement may lag behind clinical improvement

Pulmonary Edema

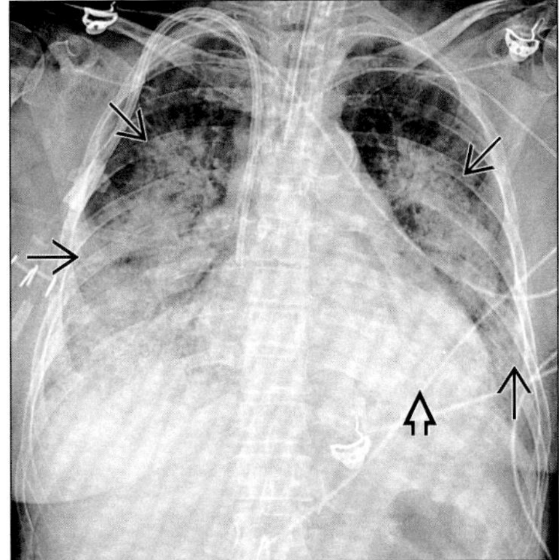

Frontal radiograph shows diffuse lung consolidation ➔ with relative peripheral sparing, typical of the "bat-wing" pattern. Note the enlarged heart ⇨.

Pulmonary Edema

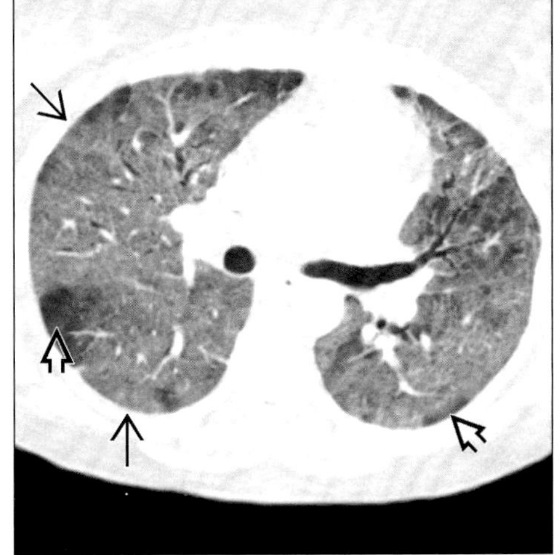

Axial HRCT shows diffuse ground-glass opacity ➔ from noncardiac pulmonary edema. Some peripheral lobules are spared ⇨. Note the lack of pleural effusion.

BILATERAL OPAQUE HEMITHORAX

Community Acquired Pneumonia

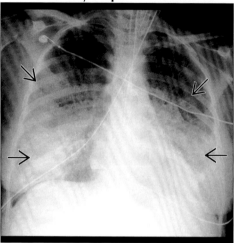

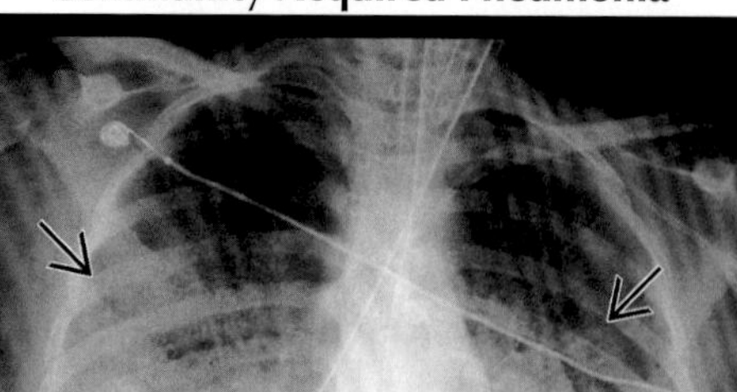

Pleural Effusion

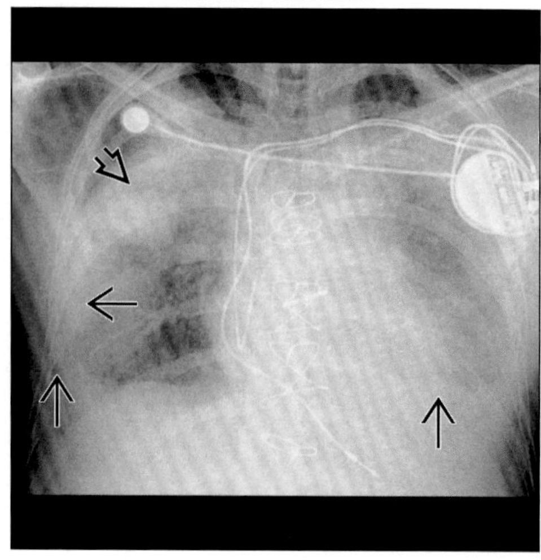

*(**Left**) Anteroposterior radiograph shows diffuse lung consolidation ➔ in this patient with viral pneumonia. Influenza virus and adenovirus are common causes of community acquired viral pneumonia. Patients may develop diffuse lung injury and progress to ARDS. (**Right**) Frontal radiograph shows bilateral hazy opacity secondary to layering pleural effusions ➔ in this supine patient. Some loculated fluid ⇨ is present in the upper right hemithorax.*

Diffuse Alveolar Hemorrhage

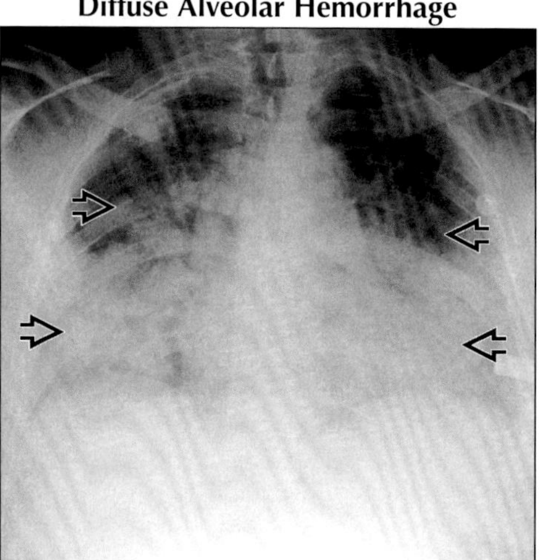

Diffuse Alveolar Hemorrhage

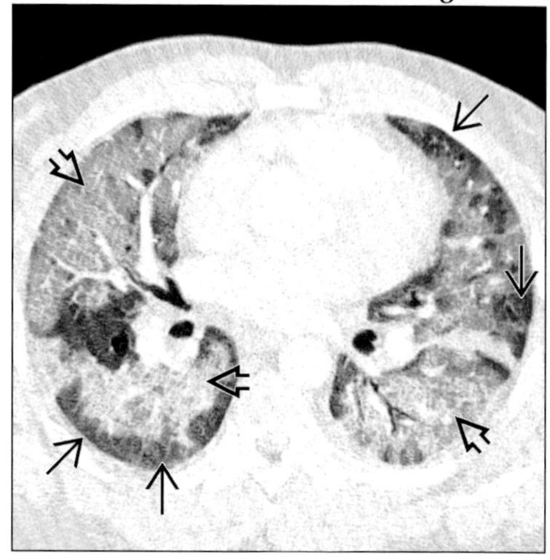

*(**Left**) Frontal radiograph shows extensive, fluffy lung consolidation ⇨ with some sparing of the apices in this patient with a history of cocaine abuse. (**Right**) Axial HRCT shows extensive ground-glass opacity ⇨ with some areas of peripheral sparing ➔ in this patient with a history of cocaine abuse. Peripheral sparing, while not specific, can be suggestive of diffuse alveolar hemorrhage in the correct setting.*

Drug Reaction

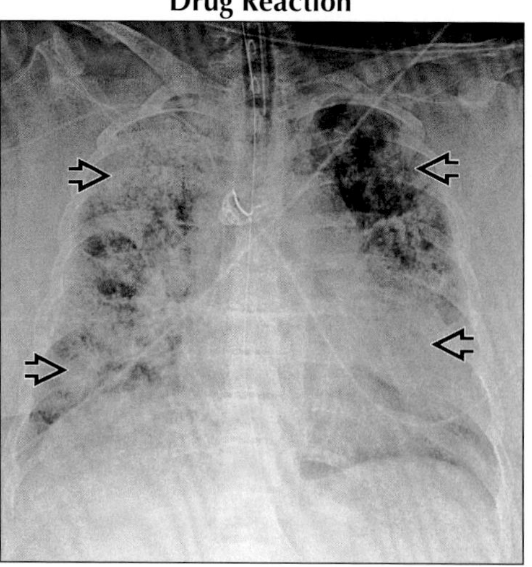

Acute Interstitial Pneumonia

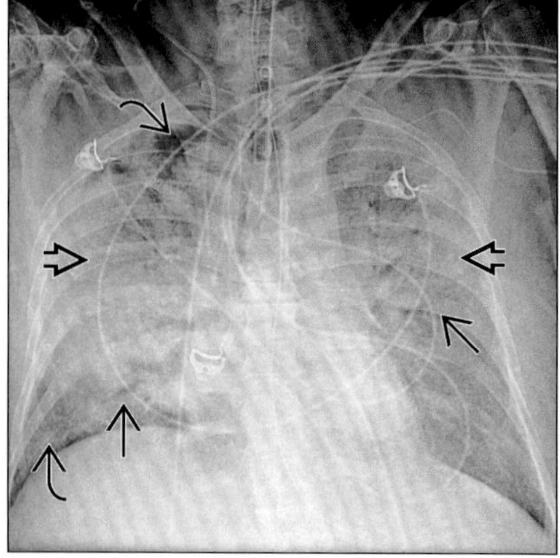

*(**Left**) Frontal radiograph shows extensive but patchy lung consolidation ⇨ in this patient who developed an acute lung injury from daptomycin therapy. Drug reactions can range from mild abnormalities to diffuse alveolar damage. (**Right**) Frontal radiograph shows diffuse lung opacity ⇨ with air bronchograms ➔ and a few foci of peripheral sparing ↷ in this patient with ARDS. Note the normal heart size and lack of pleural effusions.*

BILATERAL OPAQUE HEMITHORAX

Acute Interstitial Pneumonia

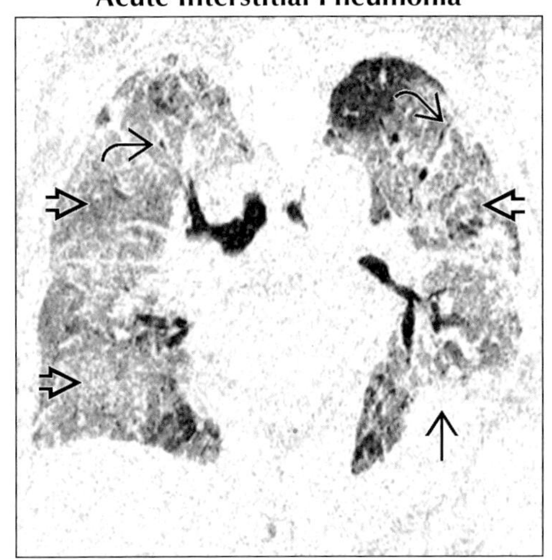

Pneumocystis Pneumonia

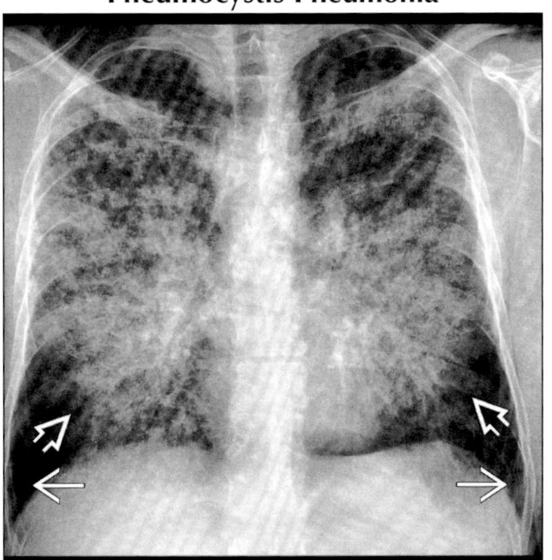

(Left) *Coronal CT reconstruction shows diffuse ground-glass opacity ⇨ in this patient with AIP. Focal consolidation → is in the left lower lobe. Note the presence of air bronchograms ↪.* ***(Right)*** *Frontal radiograph shows diffuse nodular perihilar consolidation ➡ in an AIDS patient with PCP. Note the relative sparing of the costophrenic sulci ➡ and lack of pleural effusion.*

Lung Contusion

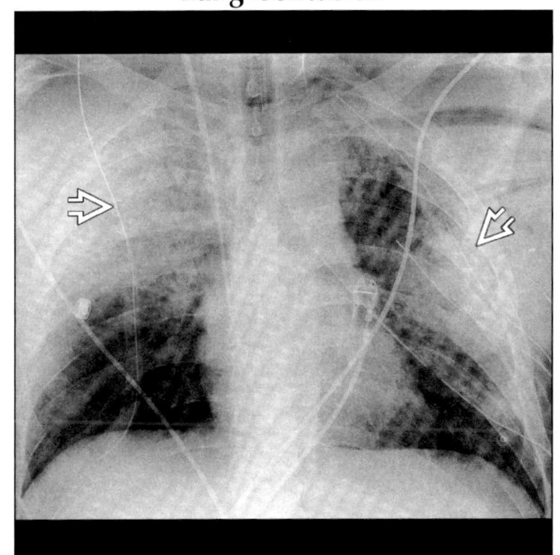

Bronchioloalveolar Carcinoma

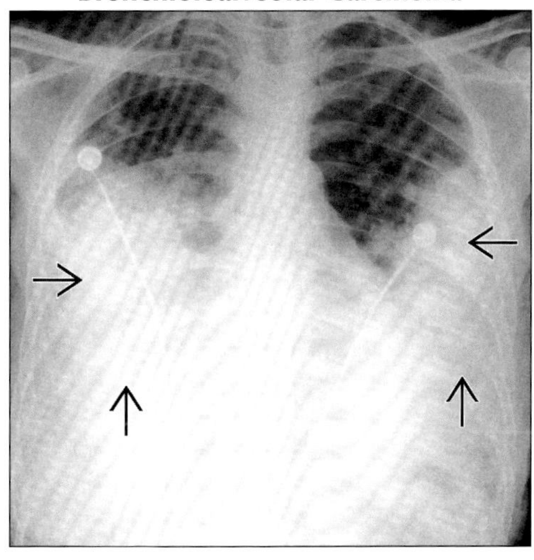

(Left) *Anteroposterior radiograph shows bilateral homogeneous consolidation ➡ from lung contusion following blunt trauma. Uncomplicated contusions rapidly resolve over 48 hours but may take up to 7 days.* ***(Right)*** *Frontal radiograph shows dense lung consolidation → from disseminated bronchioloalveolar carcinoma. Diffuse lung consolidation is the least common manifestation of bronchioloalveolar carcinoma.*

Bronchioloalveolar Carcinoma

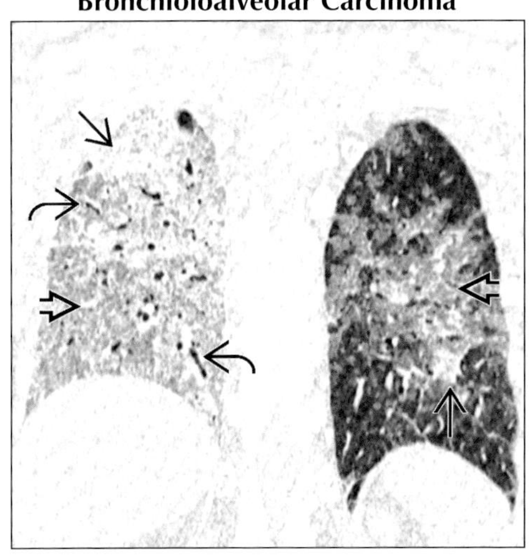

Pulmonary Alveolar Proteinosis

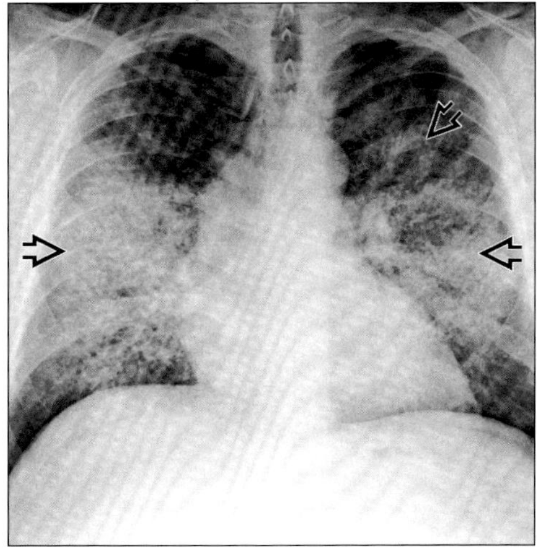

(Left) *Coronal CT reconstruction shows extensive bilateral ground-glass opacity ⇨ with more involvement of the right lung. Some foci of dense consolidation → are present. Note the presence of air bronchograms ↪.* ***(Right)*** *Frontal radiograph shows bilateral patchy lung consolidation ⇨ with relative sparing of the lung apices and bases. Patients with alveolar proteinosis often have radiographic findings out of proportion to signs and symptoms.*

SMALL LUNG VOLUMES

DIFFERENTIAL DIAGNOSIS

Common
- Lung Fibrosis
- Pleural Disease
- Lobectomy
- Skeletal Deformities
- Ascites

Less Common
- Neuromuscular Disorders

Rare but Important
- Pulmonary Hypoplasia

ESSENTIAL INFORMATION

Key Differential Diagnosis Issues
- Normal lungs vs. fibrotic
- Check for prior surgery
- Check for ascites
- Poor inspiratory effort vs. intrinsic disease

Helpful Clues for Common Diagnoses
- **Lung Fibrosis**
  - Reticulation or honeycombing in peripheral caudal lungs for interstitial pneumonias
  - Apical scarring from prior tuberculosis (or similar)
- **Pleural Disease**
  - Large pleural effusions frequently cause compressive atelectasis
  - Diffuse pleural thickening causes restrictive physiology
- **Lobectomy**
  - Surgical clips
  - Partial rib resection
- **Skeletal Deformities**
  - Congenital or acquired
    - Kyphosis
    - Scoliosis
    - Kyphoscoliosis
- **Ascites**
  - Abdominal fluid limits excursion of diaphragm
  - Abdominal distension on radiography and CT
  - Free fluid on CT

Helpful Clues for Less Common Diagnoses
- **Neuromuscular Disorders**
  - Respiratory muscle involvement
  - "Shrinking lungs" in systemic lupus erythematosus from muscle weakness
  - Muscular dystrophy
  - Polymyositis
  - Myasthenia gravis
    - Association with thymomas
  - Diaphragm weakness, paralysis, or hernia
    - Unilateral or bilateral

Helpful Clues for Rare Diagnoses
- **Pulmonary Hypoplasia**
  - Abnormal lung development
  - Reduced alveolar branching
  - Decrease in number of lobes
  - Associated with hypogenetic lung and pulmonary artery interruption

Lung Fibrosis

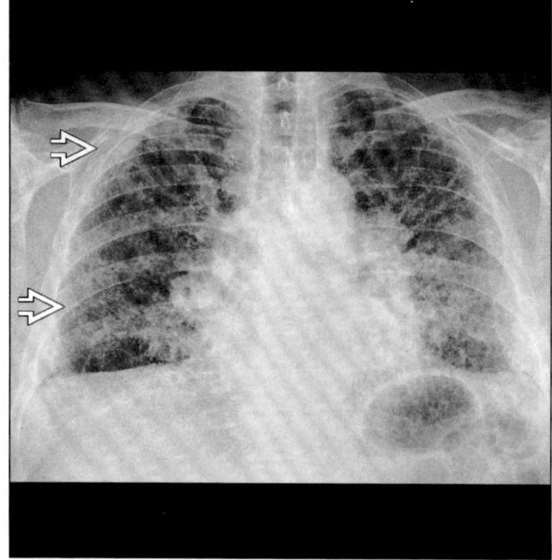

Frontal radiograph shows typical radiographic and CT features of honeycombing ➡ in idiopathic pulmonary fibrosis. Note the very low lung volumes due to the stiff lung fibrosis.

Lung Fibrosis

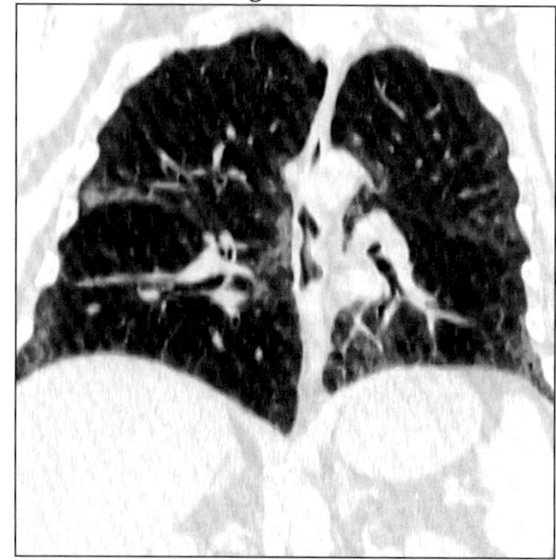

Coronal CT reconstruction from a different patient with usual interstitial pneumonia shows small lung volumes with a basilar, peripheral reticulation pattern.

SMALL LUNG VOLUMES

Pleural Disease

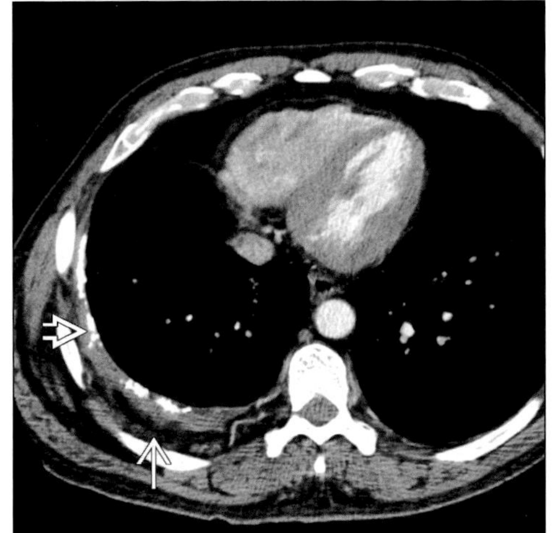

Pleural Disease

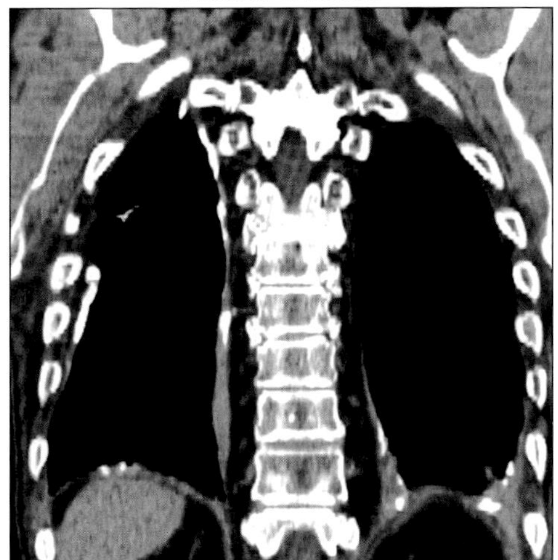

(Left) *Axial CECT shows diffuse, calcified, right-sided pleural thickening ➯ secondary to prior tuberculous empyema. Note the fatty hyperplasia of the extrapleural fat ➡.* ***(Right)*** *Coronal CT reconstruction from a patient with a long history of occupational asbestos exposure shows bilateral diffuse pleural thickening, with some calcification. This extensive pleural disease can be seen without lung fibrosis.*

Skeletal Deformities

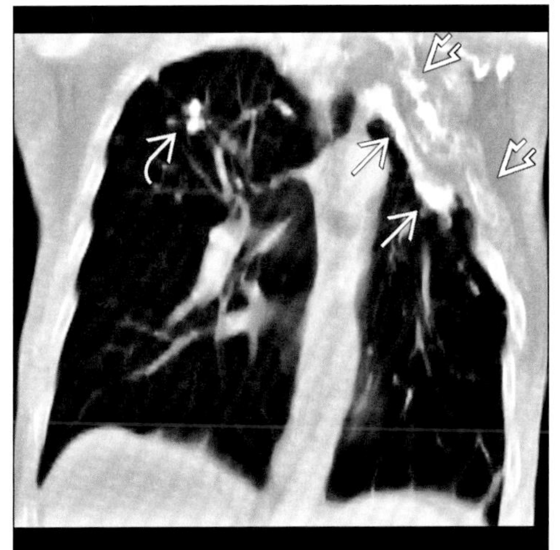

Ascites

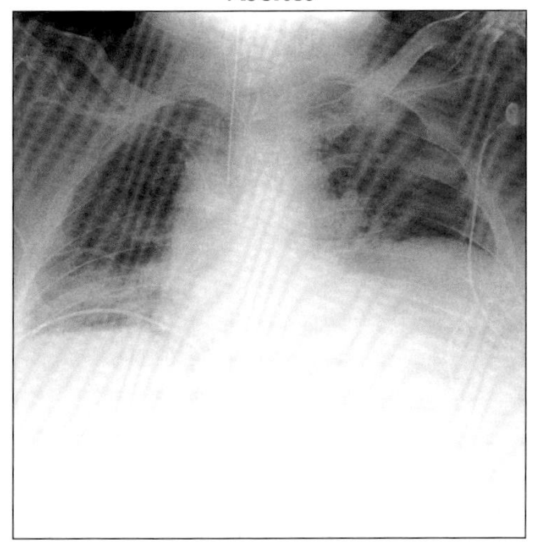

(Left) *Coronal CECT shows typical CT features of prior tuberculosis and tuberculous empyema, with old treatment of cavitary disease, known as thoracoplasty. Note the calcified granuloma ➦, thoracoplasty ➯, and calcified empyema ➡.* ***(Right)*** *Frontal radiograph shows very low lung volumes and dense opacity in the abdomen secondary to ascites. Note the paucity of bowel gas or visualization of any organs.*

Neuromuscular Disorders

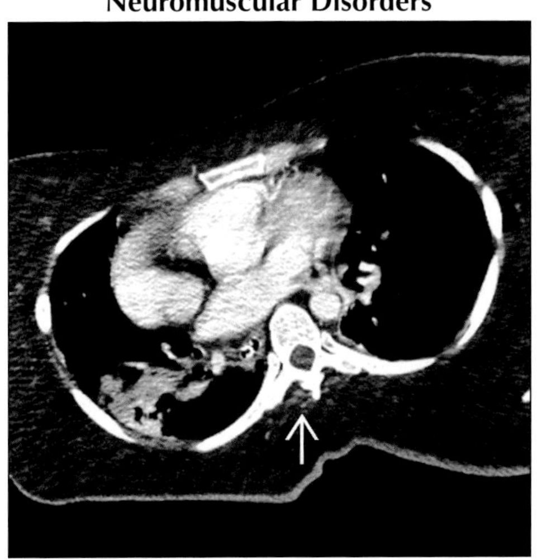

Pulmonary Hypoplasia

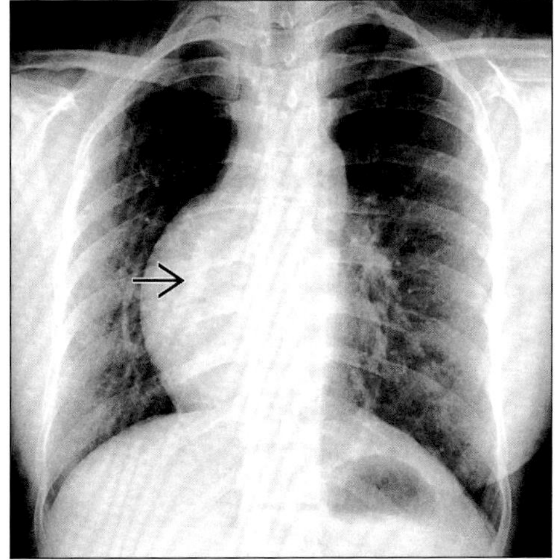

(Left) *Axial CECT from a patient with severe muscular dystrophy shows a near complete absence of any truncal musculature ➡. Note the minimal paraspinal muscles.* ***(Right)*** *Frontal radiograph shows a small right lung with shift of the mediastinum to the right in this patient with right-sided pulmonary hypoplasia and related anomalous pulmonary venous drainage ➡ (scimitar sign).*

LARGE LUNG VOLUMES

DIFFERENTIAL DIAGNOSIS

Common
- Pulmonary Emphysema
- Asthma
- Constrictive Bronchiolitis

Less Common
- Lymphangioleiomyomatosis (LAM)
- Langerhans Cell Histiocytosis

ESSENTIAL INFORMATION

Key Differential Diagnosis Issues
- Radiographs: Pruning of central vascular markings vs. increased reticulation

Helpful Clues for Common Diagnoses
- **Pulmonary Emphysema**
  - Centrilobular
    - Cigarette smokers
    - Upper lobe predominance
    - HRCT: Areas of abnormal low attenuation around centrilobular arteries, lack walls
  - Panlobular
    - α-1-antitrypsin deficiency, methylphenidate (Ritalin) crushed tablet IV injection
    - Diffuse emphysema with lower lung predominance
    - Decreased conspicuity of vessels
- **Asthma**
  - Increased lung lucency and bronchial wall thickening
  - Mild hilar prominence due to transient pulmonary hypertension
  - HRCT: Bronchial wall thickening, mosaic perfusion, and air-trapping on expiratory scanning
- **Constrictive Bronchiolitis**
  - Large or small lung volumes
  - Attenuation of pulmonary vasculature
  - HRCT: Mosaic perfusion and air-trapping on expiratory imaging
  - Bronchiectasis common

Helpful Clues for Less Common Diagnoses
- **Lymphangioleiomyomatosis (LAM)**
  - Almost exclusively in women of child-bearing age
  - CXR: Fine reticular pattern
    - Fine cysts with no zonal predominance
    - Lung bases are involved
    - Chylous effusions and pneumothoraces
  - HRCT
    - Thin-walled cysts
    - Diffuse lung involvement
    - Lung parenchyma between cysts is normal
- **Langerhans Cell Histiocytosis**
  - > 90% of affected adults are smokers
  - CXR
    - Reticulonodular pattern in upper lungs
  - HRCT
    - Bizarre-shaped cysts; thin and thick walls
    - Centrilobular nodules with irregular margins can coexist with cysts; may cavitate

Pulmonary Emphysema

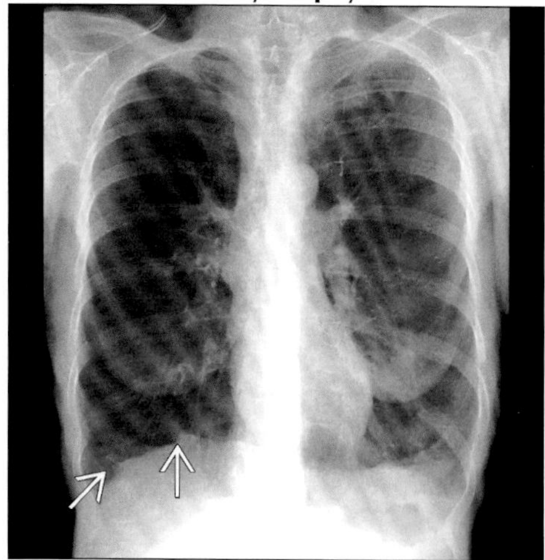

Frontal radiograph shows typical radiographic features of centrilobular emphysema with marked pulmonary hyperinflation. Note the flattened hemidiaphragms ➔ and peripheral pruning of the vasculature.

Pulmonary Emphysema

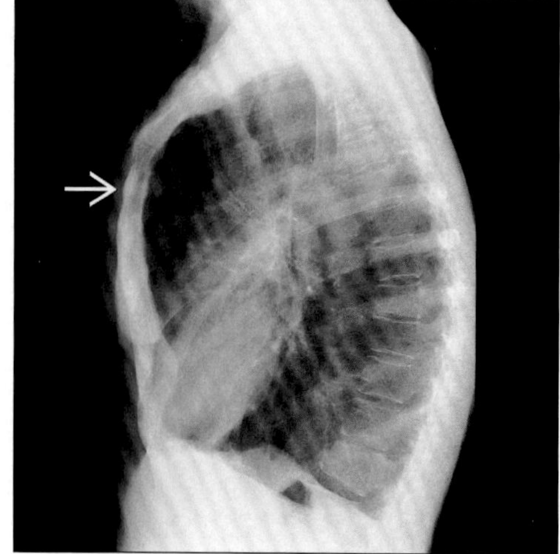

Lateral radiograph shows flattened hemidiaphragms with enlarged retrosternal clear space ➔.

LARGE LUNG VOLUMES

Asthma

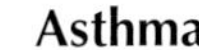

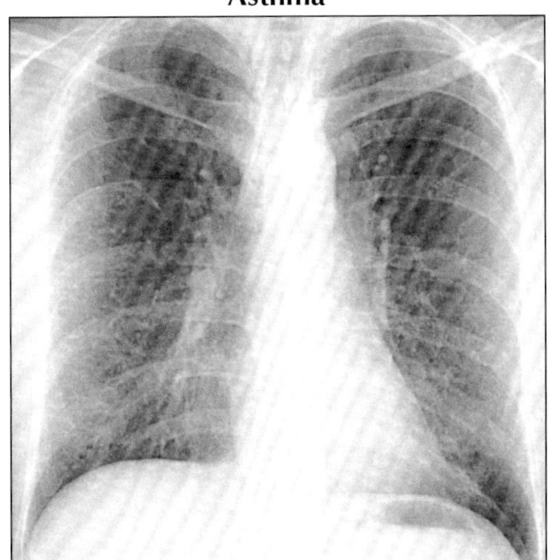

Constrictive Bronchiolitis

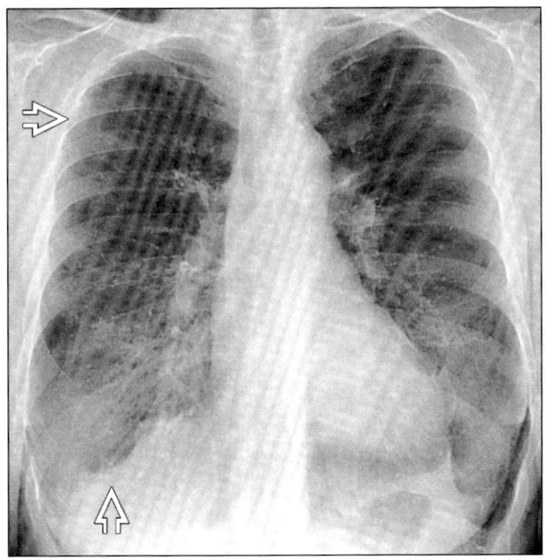

(Left) *Frontal radiograph from a patient with asthma shows bilateral large lung volumes with subtle diffuse increased reticular pattern and bronchial wall thickening. Asthmatics can have small, normal, or large lung volumes.* ***(Right)*** *Frontal radiograph shows typical radiographic features of hyperinflation from idiopathic constrictive bronchiolitis. Note marked pulmonary hyperinflation and paucity of blood vessels.*

Lymphangioleiomyomatosis (LAM)

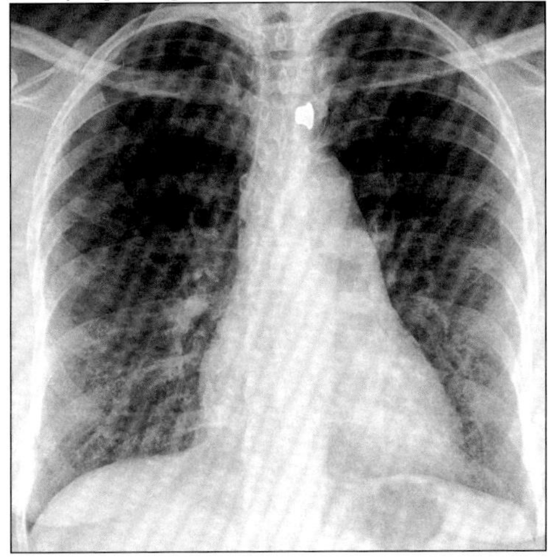

Lymphangioleiomyomatosis (LAM)

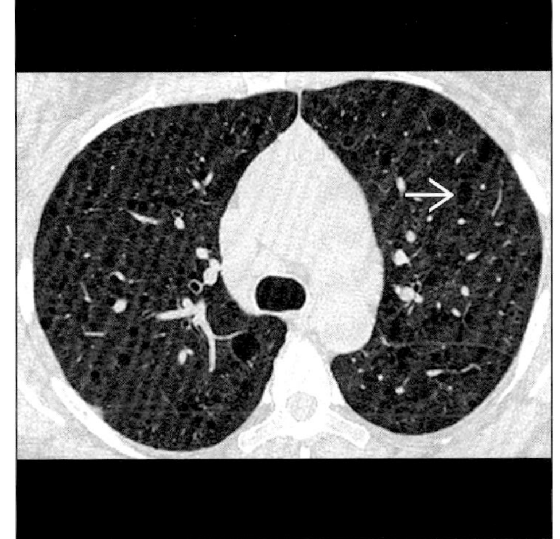

(Left) *Frontal radiograph from this patient with lymphangiomyomatosis demonstrates nearly normal radiographic features with large lung volumes and slight reticular prominence.* ***(Right)*** *Axial HRCT from the same patient shows innumerable thin-walled cysts that slightly vary in size and are uniformly distributed throughout the lungs.*

Langerhans Cell Histiocytosis

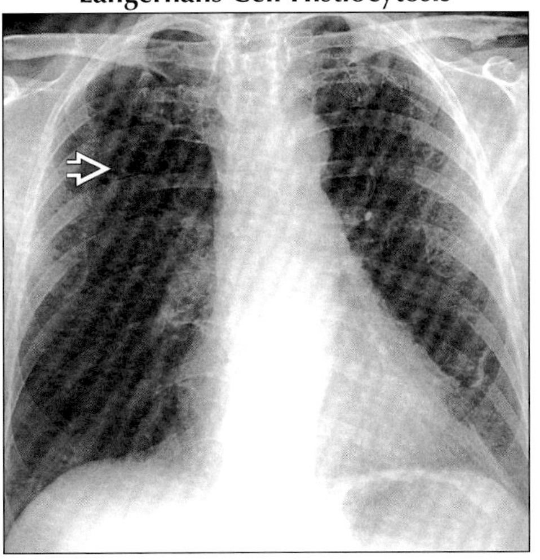

Langerhans Cell Histiocytosis

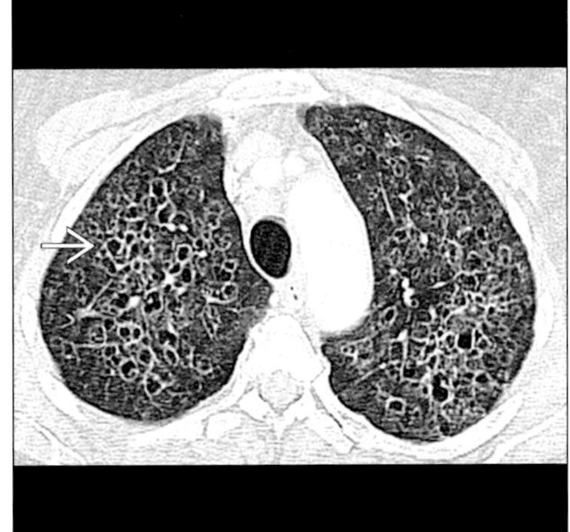

(Left) *Frontal radiograph shows typical radiographic features of cysts from Langerhans cell granulomatosis, manifested as subtle reticular lines in the upper lobes.* ***(Right)*** *Axial HRCT from the same patient shows typical CT features with innumerable thick-walled, irregularly shaped cysts, more profuse in upper lobes.*

SECTION 2
Large Airways

TRACHEAL DILATATION

DIFFERENTIAL DIAGNOSIS

Common

- Upper Lobe Fibrosis
  - Sarcoidosis
  - Hypersensitivity Pneumonitis, Chronic
  - Ankylosing Spondylitis
- Overdistension Endotracheal Balloon
- Saber-Sheath Trachea

Less Common

- Tracheobronchomegaly
  - Mounier-Kuhn Syndrome
  - Ehlers-Danlos Syndrome
- Tracheal Diverticuli

ESSENTIAL INFORMATION

Key Differential Diagnosis Issues

- Normal inspiratory shape
  - Round (= coronal and sagittal diameters)
  - Oval (elliptical shape)
  - Horseshoe (round anterior contour and flattened posterior membranous wall)
- Normal expiratory shape
  - Horseshoe shape ranging from slight to moderate anterior bowing of posterior tracheal membrane
    - Anterior convexity of the trachea may be narrow or broad
- Tracheal dilatation
  - Women: Tracheal transverse diameter > 21 mm, sagittal diameter > 23 mm
  - Men: Tracheal transverse diameter > 25 mm, sagittal diameter > 27 mm
- **Tracheal index** = (coronal diameter)/(sagittal diameter) measured 1 cm above aortic arch: **Normal index ~ 1**

Helpful Clues for Common Diagnoses

- **Upper Lobe Fibrosis**
  - Traction bronchiectasis seen with diseases causing upper lobe fibrosis
- **Overdistension Endotracheal Balloon**
  - More common with long-term intubation
  - Causes focal dilitation
- **Saber-Sheath Trachea**
  - 95% have chronic obstructive pulmonary disease (COPD)
  - Acquired disorder probably related to abnormal intrathoracic pressures
  - Affects intrathoracic trachea; extrathoracic trachea is normal

Helpful Clues for Less Common Diagnoses

- **Tracheobronchomegaly**
  - Tracheal wall corrugated due to mucosa herniating between tracheal rings
  - Central bronchi may be normal or mildly dilated (1st-4th order)
  - Distal lung may be normal, less common bronchiectasis or pulmonary fibrosis
- **Tracheal Diverticuli**
  - Mucosal herniation through tracheal wall from increased intraluminal pressure (COPD or professions like horn blowers)
  - Most common location: Right paratracheal region of thoracic inlet
  - Usually air-filled, < 2 cm in diameter, single or multiple

Ankylosing Spondylitis

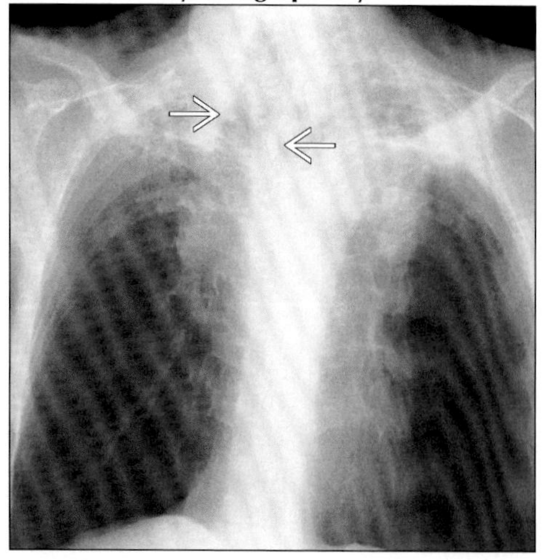

Frontal radiograph shows tracheal dilatation ➔ from upper lobe fibrosis in this patient with ankylosing spondylitis.

Overdistension Endotracheal Balloon

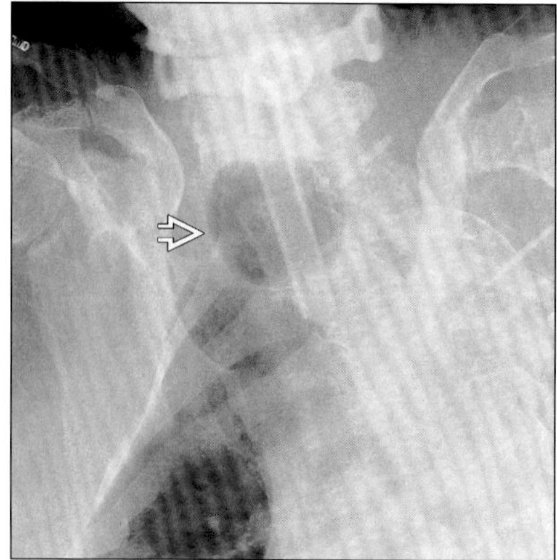

Anteroposterior radiograph shows an overdistension tracheostomy balloon ➔ causing focal tracheal dilatation.

TRACHEAL DILATATION

Mounier-Kuhn Syndrome

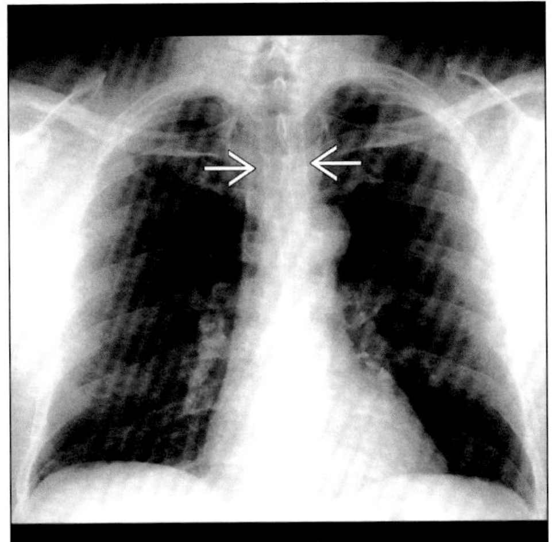

Mounier-Kuhn Syndrome

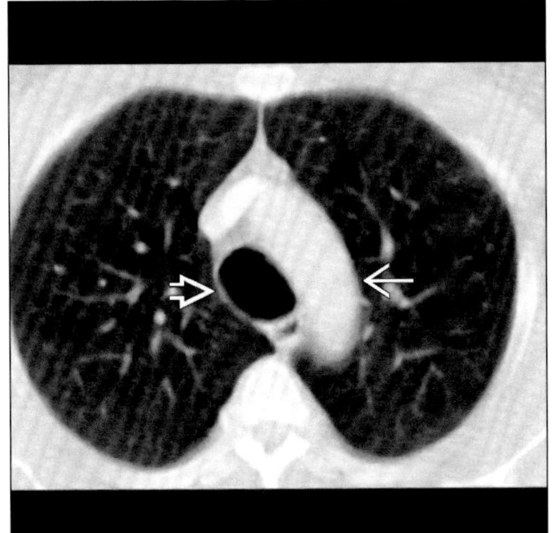

(Left) *Frontal radiograph shows widening of the trachea ➔. Dilatation is subtle and is easily missed.* ***(Right)*** *Axial CECT shows tracheal dilatation ➔ wider than the adjacent aorta ➔. Tracheal wall is of normal thickness. Note this rule of thumb: Tracheal diameter should be smaller than proximal aorta.*

Saber-Sheath Trachea

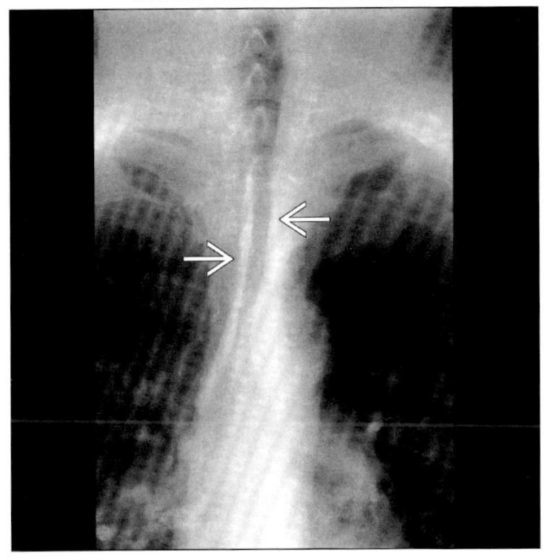

Saber-Sheath Trachea

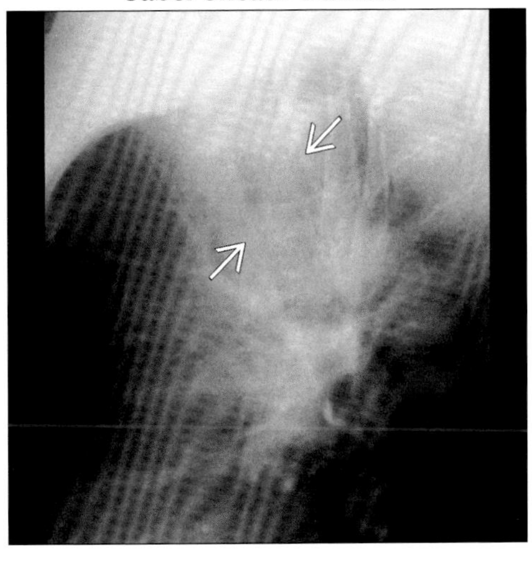

(Left) *Frontal radiograph shows typical saber-sheath deformity trachea with narrowing in the coronal dimension ➔.* ***(Right)*** *Lateral radiograph shows that the trachea is widened in the anteroposterior dimension ➔. Saber-sheath tracheal index is usually < 0.5.*

Saber-Sheath Trachea

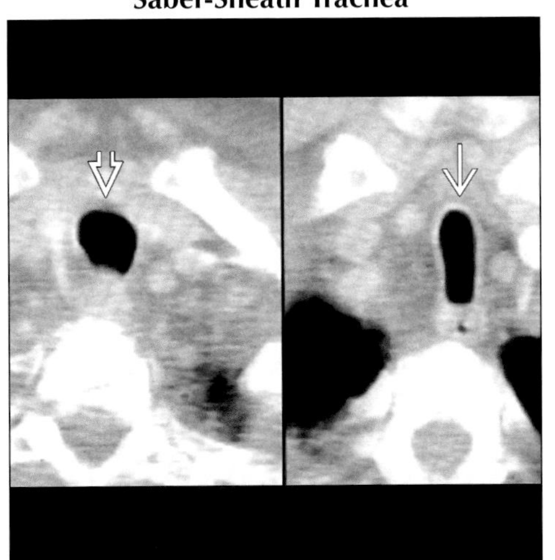

Tracheal Diverticuli

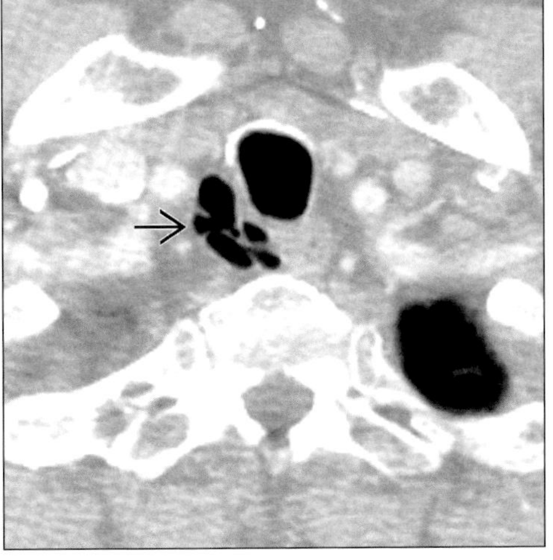

(Left) *Axial CECT shows the normal shape of the extrathoracic trachea ➔ and the saber-sheath deformity ➔ of the intrathoracic trachea.* ***(Right)*** *Axial CECT shows paratracheal diverticuli ➔ in the right thoracic inlet. Tracheal communication is rarely identified (10%) at CT and may not be found on bronchoscopy, either.*

TRACHEAL NARROWING

DIFFERENTIAL DIAGNOSIS

Common
- Extrinsic Compression
- Post-Traumatic Stenosis
- Tracheobronchomalacia
- Saber-Sheath Trachea

Less Common
- Tracheobronchopathia Osteochondroplastica
- Wegener Granulomatosis
- Relapsing Polychondritis
- Amyloidosis
- Laryngeal Papillomatosis

Rare but Important
- Tracheal Neoplasms
- Rhinoscleroma
- Complete Cartilaginous Rings

ESSENTIAL INFORMATION

Key Differential Diagnosis Issues
- Symptoms usually do not develop until tracheal lumen reduced > 50%
  - Even with fixed obstruction, symptoms often episodic, leading to misdiagnosis of asthma
- Normal tracheal size
  - Males: Coronal 13-25 mm; sagittal 13-27 mm; mean 20 mm
  - Females: Coronal 10-21 mm; sagittal 10-23 mm; mean 16 mm

Helpful Clues for Common Diagnoses
- **Extrinsic Compression**
  - Common etiology: Goiter, vascular rings, mediastinal fibrosis
  - Airway wall usually normal (except for mediastinal fibrosis)
  - Narrowing often concentric
  - May have secondary tracheomalacia
- **Post-Traumatic Stenosis**
  - Common causes: Prolonged intubation, penetrating or blunt chest trauma, post-surgery
  - Intubation: Location either at tracheal stoma or level of tube balloon
  - Airway wall usually thickened
  - CT coronal reconstructions more sensitive than axial imaging
- **Tracheobronchomalacia**
  - Defined as dynamic decrease in airway luminal diameter of > 70%
    - Crescent or lunate shape with ballooning of posterior tracheal membrane into airway lumen
  - May be primary or acquired
  - Confident diagnosis requires dynamic CT: Comparison of inspiratory and expiratory luminal diameters
    - Forced expiration or coughing more sensitive than tidal breathing
- **Saber-Sheath Trachea**
  - Associated with chronic obstructive pulmonary disease
  - Narrow side-to-side diameter, anteroposterior diameter increased
  - Extrathoracic trachea normal
  - Airway wall thickness normal

Helpful Clues for Less Common Diagnoses
- **Tracheobronchopathia Osteochondroplastica**
  - Nodular excrescences of cartilage spare posterior membrane and may be calcified
  - Size: 2-3 mm in diameter
  - Associated with elderly patients; usually incidental finding at autopsy
- **Wegener Granulomatosis**
  - Systemic necrotizing granulomatous vasculitis
  - Typical is subglottic narrowing with thickening of airway wall; may be diffuse or focal
  - May have thick-walled cavitary lung lesions
- **Relapsing Polychondritis**
  - Systemic autoimmune disorder with cartilage destruction
  - Airway involvement more common in women (M:F = 1:3); stenosis occurs late
  - Airway wall thickening either focal or diffuse and may have increased attenuation
  - Spares posterior tracheal membrane
- **Amyloidosis**
  - Airway involvement most common form of pulmonary amyloidosis
  - Airway involvement most common in localized amyloidosis
  - Focal or diffuse nodular soft tissue thickening of airway wall ± calcification/ossification

- **Laryngeal Papillomatosis**
  - Due to human papilloma virus
  - Younger patients
  - May seed lungs with solid to thin-walled cystic nodules
  - At risk to develop squamous cell carcinoma (2%)

Helpful Clues for Rare Diagnoses

- **Tracheal Neoplasms**
  - Rare tumors, 2/3 either squamous cell carcinoma or adenoid cystic carcinoma
  - More likely to have extraluminal extension and mediastinal adenopathy
  - Adenoid cystic carcinoma: Longitudinal extent > transaxial extent, and tumor usually more than 180° of airway circumference
  - Fat content suggests lipoma or hamartoma
- **Rhinoscleroma**
  - a.k.a. *Klebsiella rhinoscleromatis*
  - Chronic granulomatous infection of upper respiratory tract
    - Endemic in Central America and Africa
  - Diffuse airway wall thickening, nasal polyps, enlarged turbinates, and thickening nasopharynx common
- **Complete Cartilaginous Rings**
  - a.k.a. napkin rings
  - Associated with pulmonary artery sling
  - Complete rings may be diffuse or focal (most commonly distal trachea)

Alternative Differential Approaches

- **Focal narrowing**
  - Extrinsic compression
  - Post-traumatic stenosis
  - Tracheal neoplasms
  - **Subglottic narrowing**
    - Post-intubation stenosis
    - Wegener granulomatosis
    - Rhinoscleroma
    - Sarcoidosis
- **Diffuse narrowing**
  - Tracheomalacia
  - Saber-sheath trachea
  - Tracheobronchopathia osteochondroplastica
  - Relapsing polychondritis
- **Sparing posterior tracheal membrane**
  - Relapsing polychondritis
  - Tracheobronchopathia osteochondroplastica
- **Normal wall thickness**
  - Extrinsic compression
  - Tracheomalacia
  - Saber-sheath trachea
  - Complete cartilaginous rings
- **Tracheal wall calcification**
  - Normal process of aging
  - Tracheobronchopathia osteochondroplastica
  - Amyloidosis
  - Relapsing polychondritis
  - Long-term warfarin therapy

Extrinsic Compression

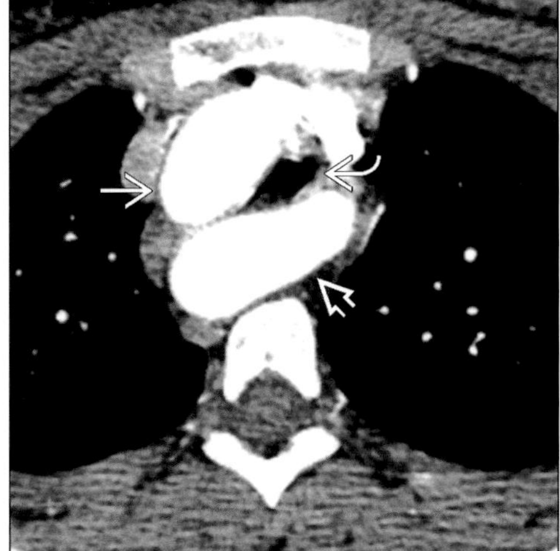

Axial CECT shows right cervical aortic arch ➔ and aberrant left subclavian artery ➔ extrinsically compressing the trachea ➔.

Extrinsic Compression

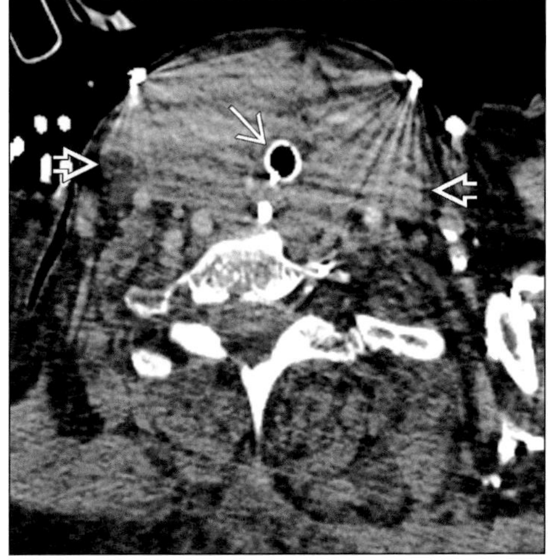

Axial CECT shows massive goiter ➔ extrinsically compressing the extrathoracic trachea around the ET tube ➔.

TRACHEAL NARROWING

*(**Left**) Axial NECT shows a trachea with irregular contour ➡. The trachea is narrowed, and the wall is thickened. (**Right**) Coronal NECT reconstruction better demonstrates short segment tracheal narrowing ➡ at the level of the thoracic inlet in this patient with stenosis due to endotracheal tube injury.*

Post-Traumatic Stenosis

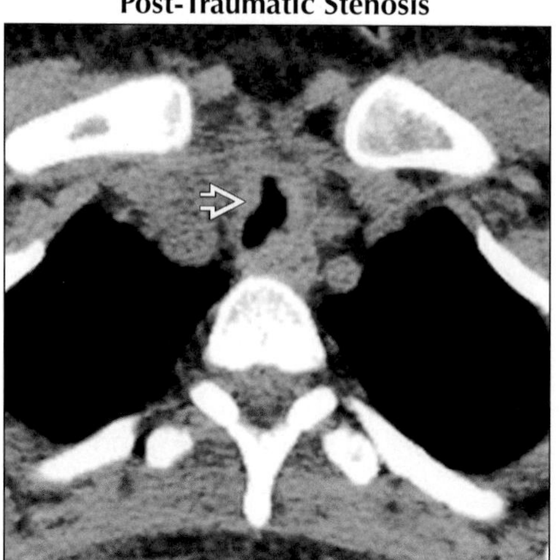

Post-Traumatic Stenosis

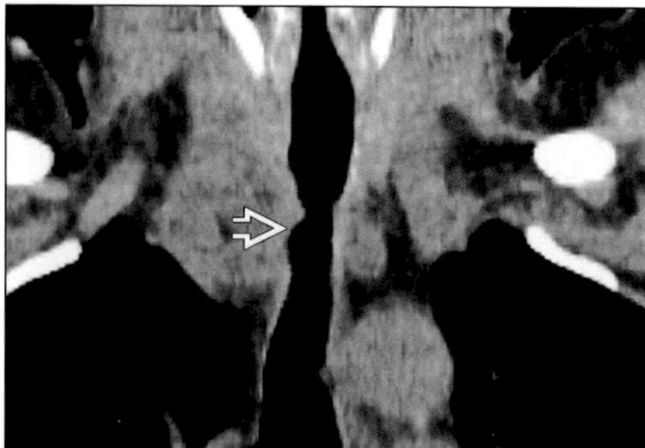

*(**Left**) Axial NECT at full inspiration shows the normal size and shape of the trachea ➡. (**Right**) Axial NECT at full expiration shows more than 50% narrowing of the distal trachea ➡. Marked invagination of posterior tracheal wall produces the "frown" sign.*

Tracheobronchomalacia

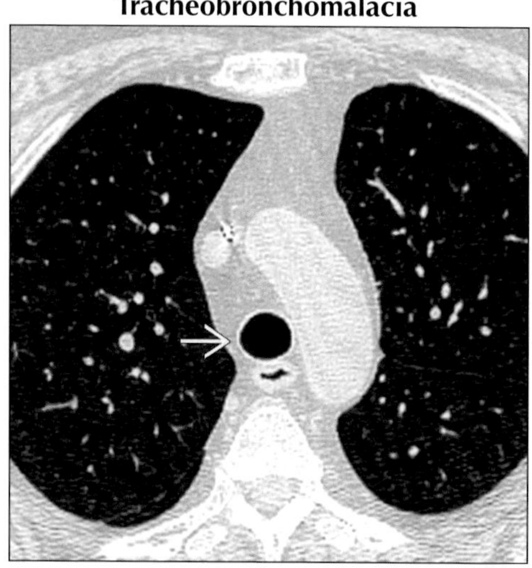

Tracheobronchomalacia

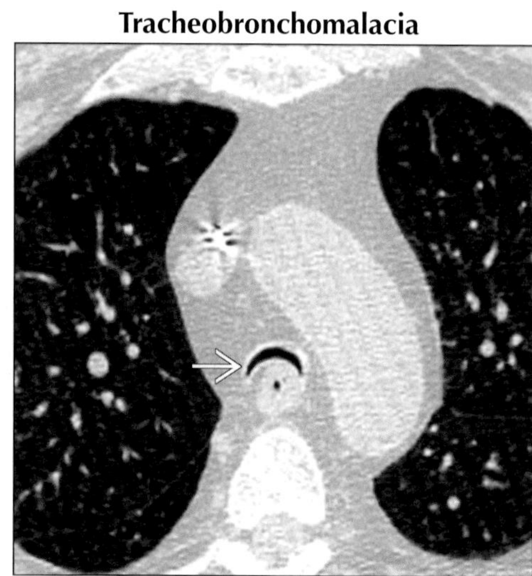

*(**Left**) Frontal radiograph shows diffuse narrowing ➡ of the intrathoracic trachea. The extrathoracic trachea is normal ➡. (**Right**) Axial CECT shows saber-sheath deformity ➡. The tracheal wall is of normal thickness in this patient who had severe obstruction on pulmonary function tests.*

Saber-Sheath Trachea

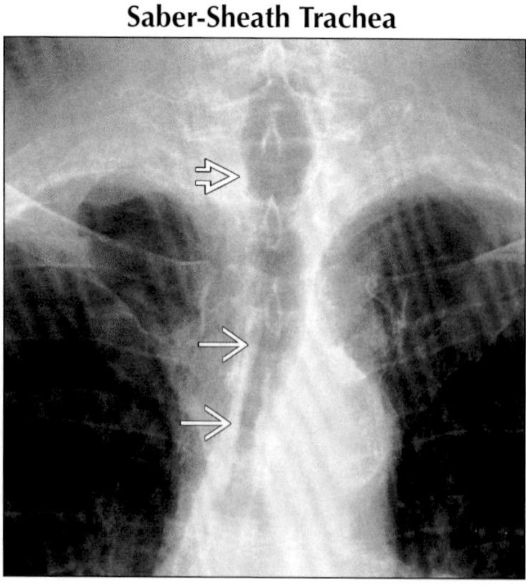

Saber-Sheath Trachea

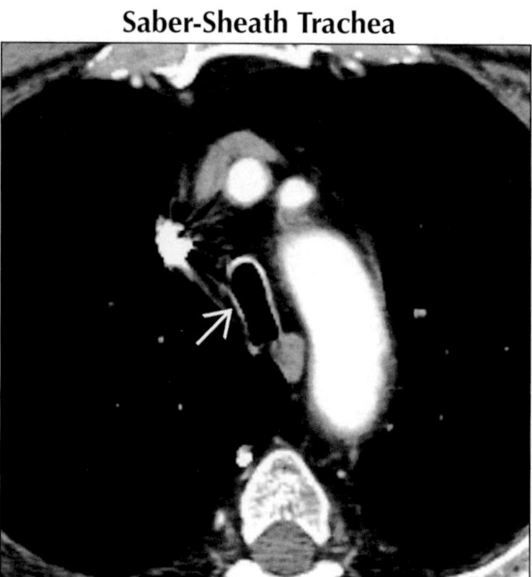

Tracheobronchopathia Osteochondroplastica

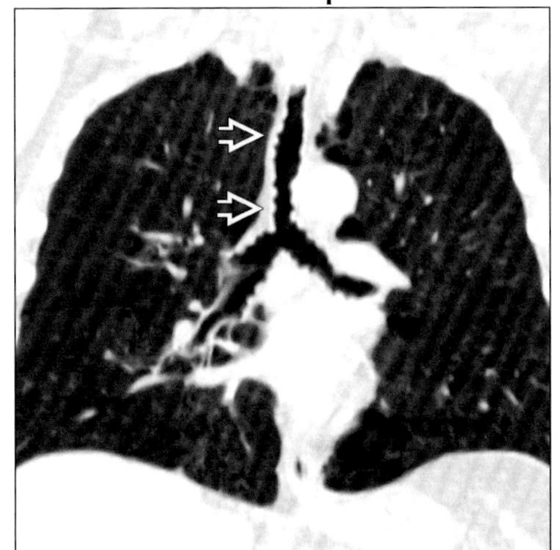

Tracheobronchopathia Osteochondroplastica

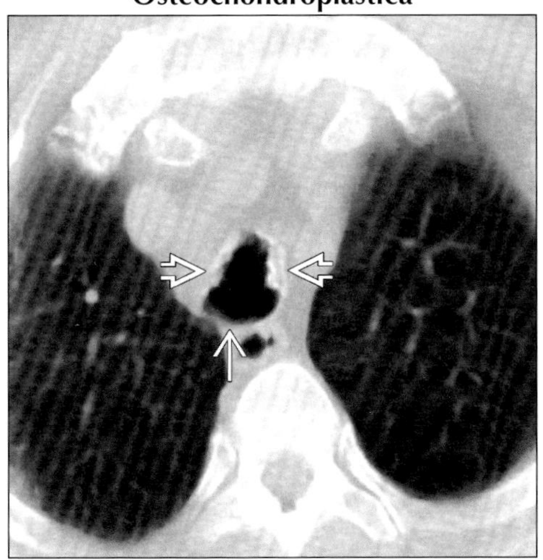

(Left) *Coronal NECT shows multiple nodular mucosal protrusions ➩ diffusely narrowing the trachea. Many of the nodules are calcified.* ***(Right)*** *Axial NECT in a different patient shows calcified nodules along the anterior and lateral walls of the trachea ➩. The posterior tracheal wall is spared ➡.*

Wegener Granulomatosis

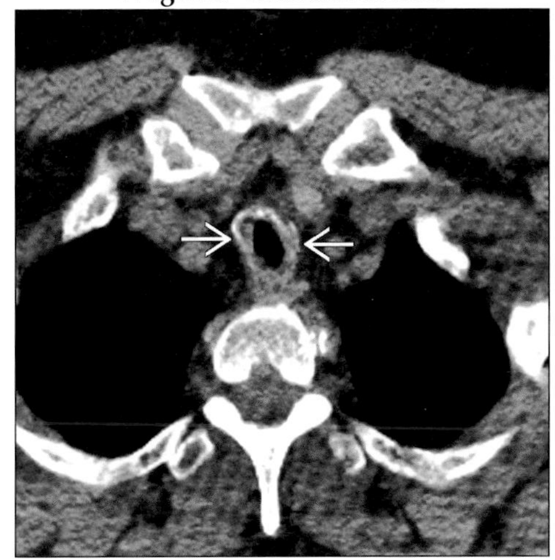

Wegener Granulomatosis

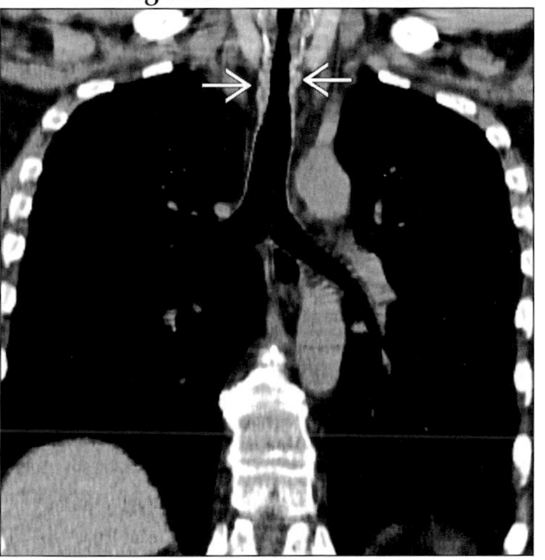

(Left) *Axial NECT shows smooth circumferential thickening ➡ of the subglottic trachea.* ***(Right)*** *Coronal NECT shows focal subglottic narrowing of the trachea ➡. The other airways and lungs were normal.*

Relapsing Polychondritis

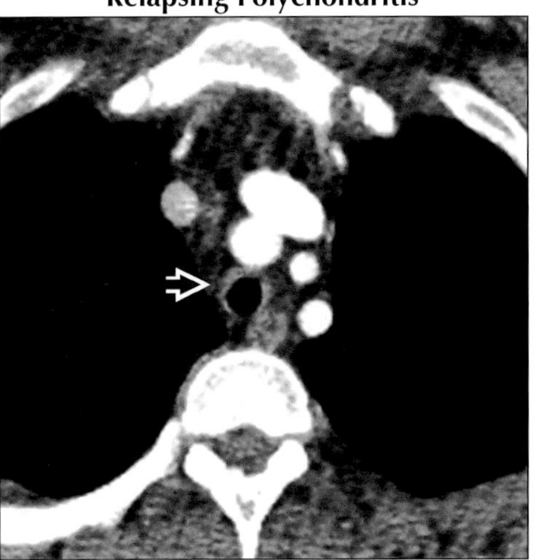

Relapsing Polychondritis

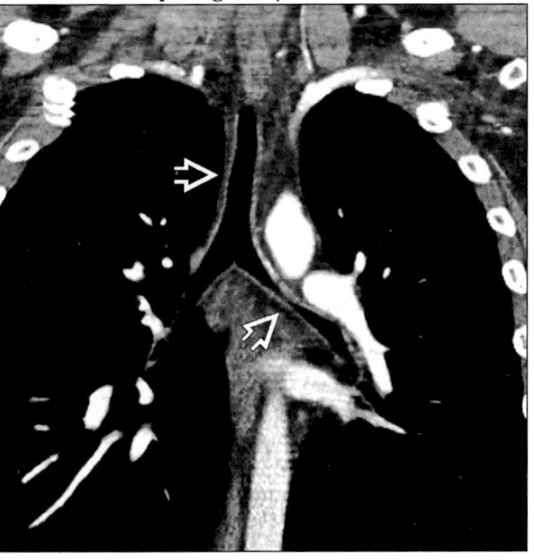

(Left) *Axial CECT shows diffuse narrowing of the trachea with thick anterior and lateral walls ➩; the posterior tracheal wall is spared. Consider this rule of thumb: Tracheal diameter should be larger than proximal great vessels.* ***(Right)*** *Coronal CECT shows diffuse tracheal narrowing extending into the left main bronchus ➩. Maximal tracheal diameter was 8 mm.*

TRACHEAL NARROWING

(Left) Axial CECT shows circumferential thickening of the tracheal wall ➡. Note the small focus of calcification. *(Right)* Coronal CECT shows diffuse tracheal wall thickening extending into the lobar bronchi ➡. The tracheal lumen is narrowed.

Amyloidosis

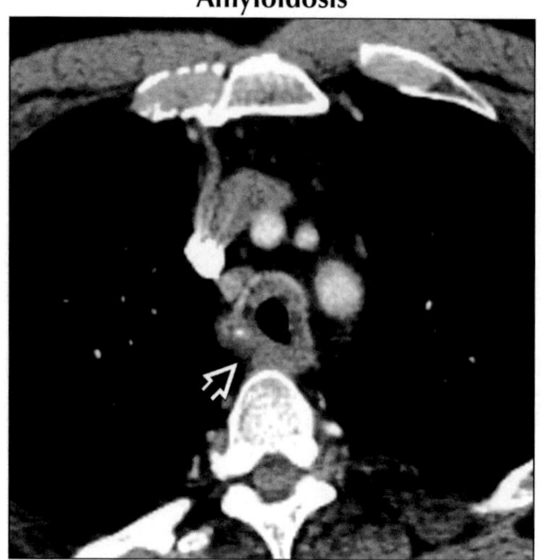

Amyloidosis

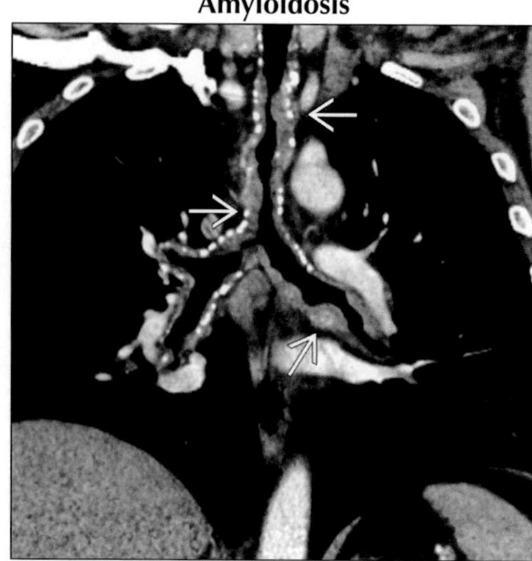

(Left) Axial NECT shows discrete tracheal nodules ➡ involving the posterior and lateral tracheal wall. *(Right)* Coronal NECT MIP reconstruction shows multiple discrete tracheal nodules ➡.

Laryngeal Papillomatosis

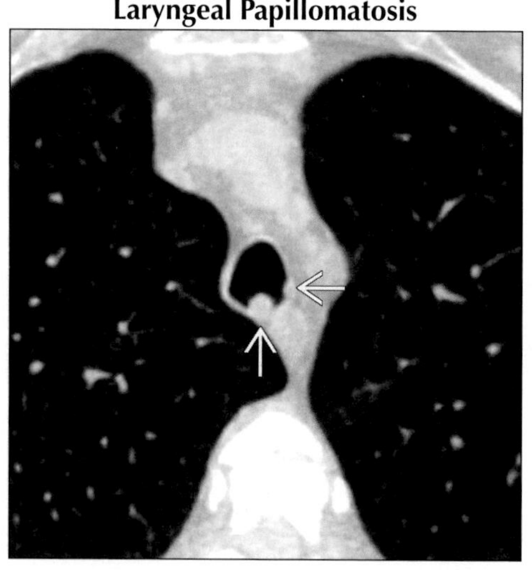

Laryngeal Papillomatosis

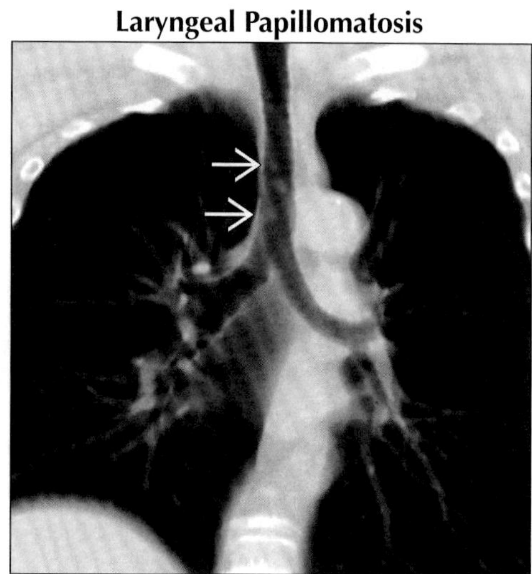

(Left) Axial CECT shows diffuse smooth circumferential tracheal wall thickening ➡. The tracheal lumen is narrowed. *(Right)* Coronal CECT shows the extent of the tumor along the trachea ➡. Histology was adenoid cystic carcinoma.

Tracheal Neoplasms

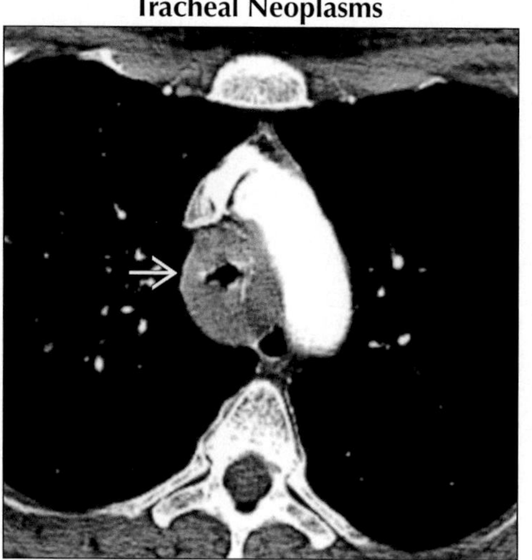

Tracheal Neoplasms

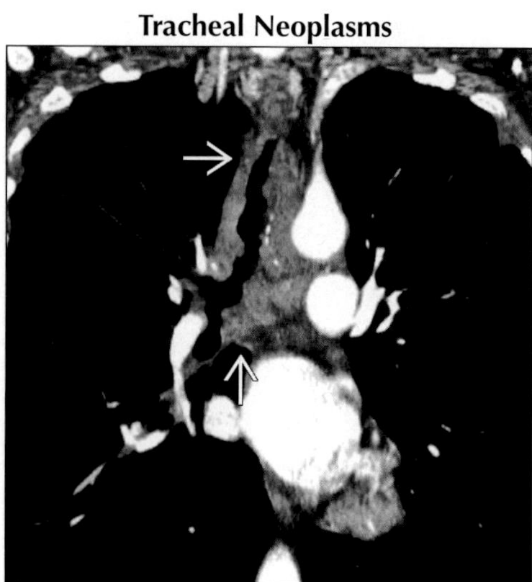

Tracheal Neoplasms

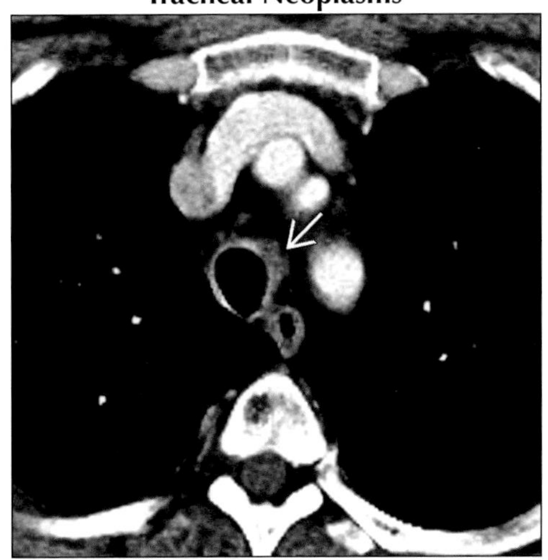

Tracheal Neoplasms

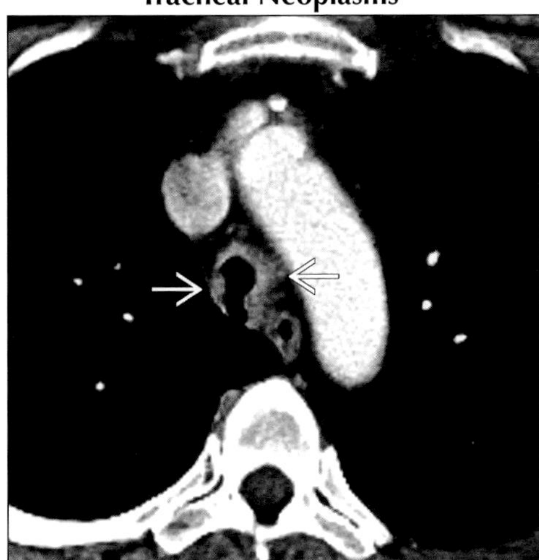

(Left) *Axial CECT shows focal nodular wall thickening of the trachea ➡.* ***(Right)*** *Axial CECT in the same patient shows nodular thickening of the tracheal wall ➡. The airway lumen is narrowed. Histology was adenoid cystic carcinoma.*

Rhinoscleroma

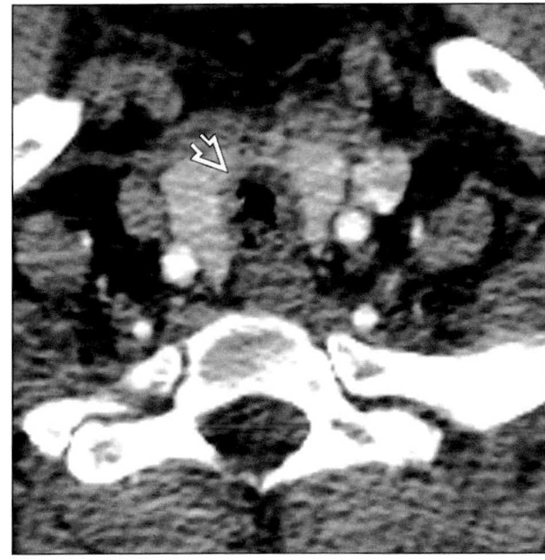

Rhinoscleroma

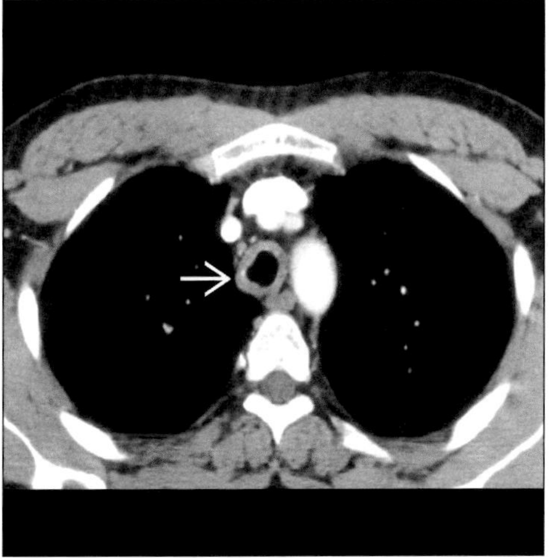

(Left) *Axial CECT shows circumferential subglottic narrowing containing crypt-like air spaces ➡. The remainder of the airways were normal.* ***(Right)*** *Axial CECT in a different patient shows diffuse circumferential tracheal wall thickening ➡, which involved the entire trachea and extended into the left main bronchus.*

Complete Cartilaginous Rings

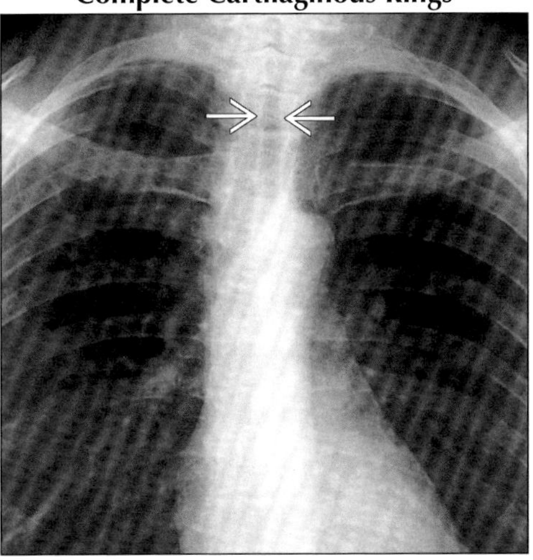

Complete Cartilaginous Rings

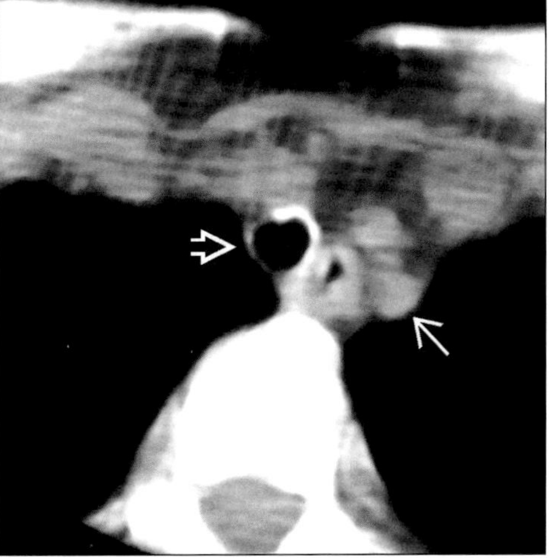

(Left) *Frontal radiograph shows a small-diameter trachea ➡ with a 10 mm diameter. This patient had a lifelong history of "asthma."* ***(Right)*** *Axial NECT shows the small size of the trachea ➡ just larger than the left subclavian artery ➡. The tracheal wall is normal in thickness. Bronchoscopy showed complete cartilaginous rings.*

TRACHEAL FISTULA

DIFFERENTIAL DIAGNOSIS

Common
- Congenital
- Neoplasm
  - Tracheal or Esophageal Cancer
  - Lymphoma

Less Common
- Trauma
  - Blunt or Penetrating Trauma
  - Iatrogenic
    - Endoscopy
    - Surgery
    - Chronic Endotracheal Intubation
- Infection
- Inflammation
  - Radiation
  - Corrosive Ingestion
  - Chronic Foreign Body

ESSENTIAL INFORMATION

Key Differential Diagnosis Issues
- In pediatric patients, tracheoesophageal fistulas (TEF) almost always congenital
- In adult patients, TEF most often due to malignancy and trauma
- Secondary findings in TEF: Esophageal dilation, aspiration in dependent portions of lungs

Helpful Clues for Common Diagnoses
- **Congenital**
  - Abnormal division of foregut into separate tracheal and esophageal lumens
  - High association with other congenital conditions including VACTERL
  - Most commonly associated with proximal esophageal atresia with distal TEF (over 80% of congenital cases)
- **Neoplasm**
  - History or imaging findings of tracheal or esophageal cancer
  - Focal chronic soft tissue thickening in association with TEF
  - Superimposed radiation potentiates local inflammation, predisposing to TEF

Helpful Clues for Less Common Diagnoses
- **Trauma**
  - History of imaging findings of blunt or penetrating trauma
  - History of recent procedure in region of TEF
  - Chronic intubation: Posterior wall erosion caused by excessive cuff pressures or abrasion by tube
- **Infection**
  - Tuberculosis or fungal infection
  - Superimposed pulmonary opacities (nodular opacities) with low-density lymphadenopathy
- **Inflammation**
  - Radiation: Adjacent radiation changes in lungs
  - Foreign body in airway; cross-sectional imaging highly sensitive

Congenital

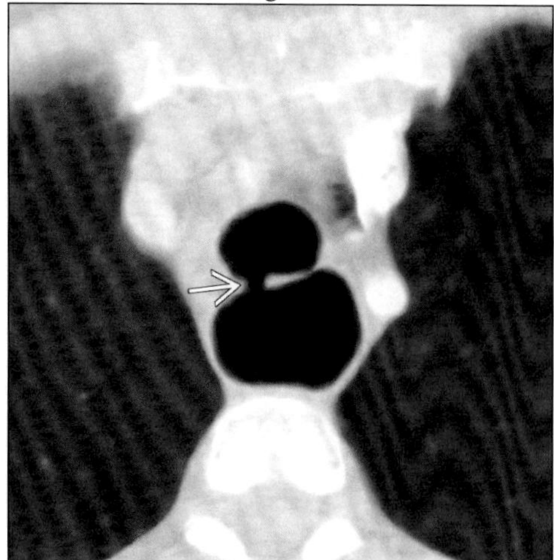

Axial CECT shows a small fistula ➔ between the trachea and esophagus. There is associated dilation of the esophagus.

Congenital

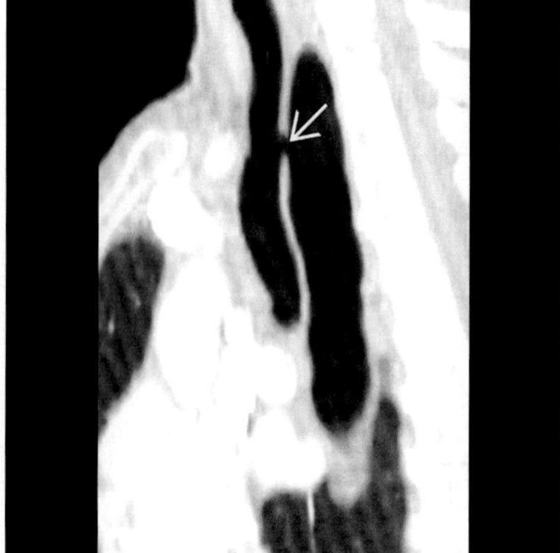

Sagittal CECT demonstrates the fistulous connection ➔ between the trachea and the esophagus in high detail. This is an H-type congenital tracheoesophageal fistula.

TRACHEAL FISTULA

Tracheal or Esophageal Cancer

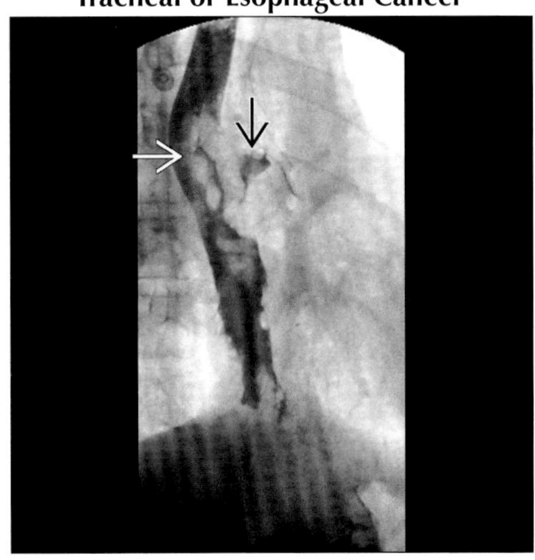

Tracheal or Esophageal Cancer

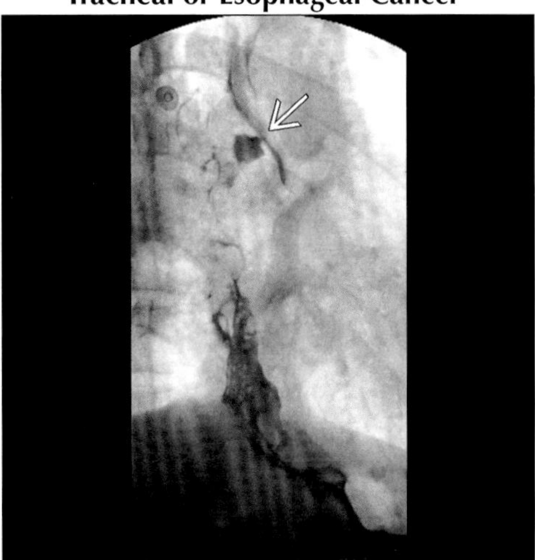

(Left) *Frontal esophagram shows an ulcerated mass ➡ in the esophagus consistent with esophageal carcinoma. There is extraluminal extension ➡ of contrast along the left aspect of the esophagus.* ***(Right)*** *Frontal esophagram shows fistulous extension of contrast from the esophagus into the left mainstem bronchus ➡; there is reflux of oral contrast into the more proximal aspect of the large airways.*

Radiation

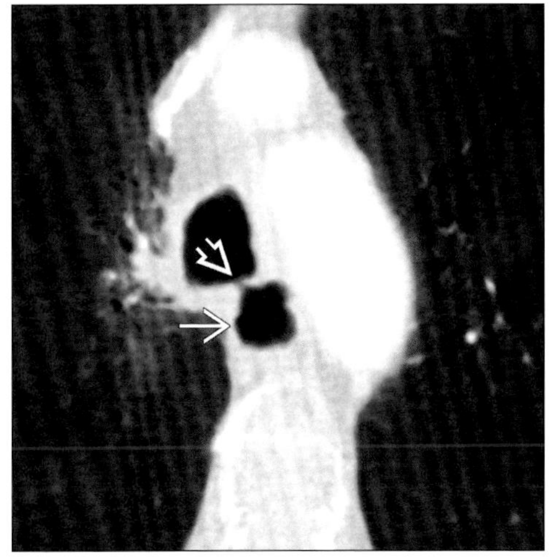

Radiation

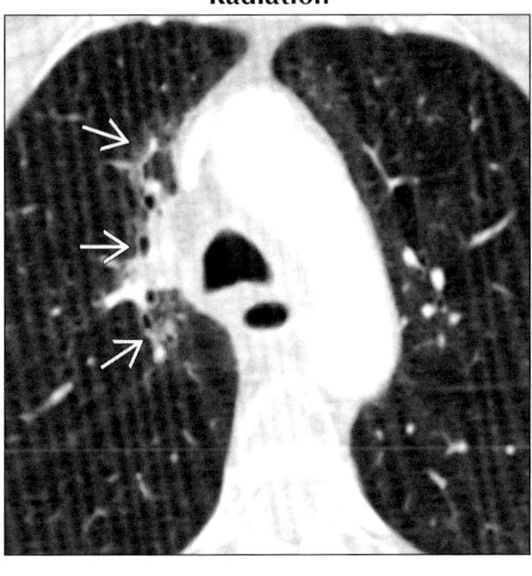

(Left) *Axial CECT minIP image shows a thin fistula ➡ between the trachea and esophagus. There is irregularity of the tracheal and esophageal contours from infiltrative esophageal cancer. There is mild dilation of the esophagus ➡, which is not uncommon in tracheoesophageal fistulas.* ***(Right)*** *Axial CECT in the same patient shows fibrosis ➡ in the medial aspect of the right upper lobe from radiation treatment.*

Radiation

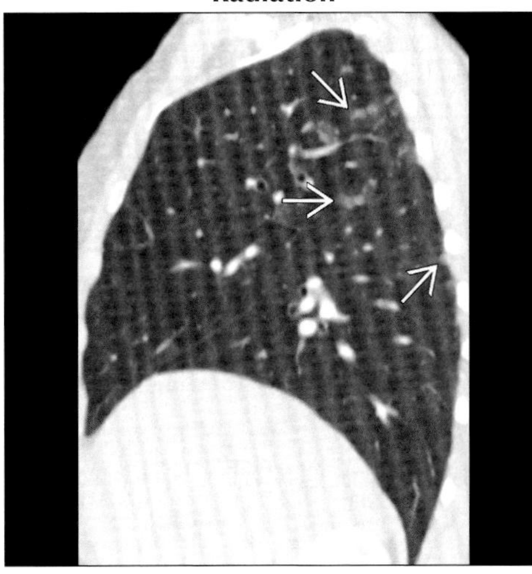

Radiation

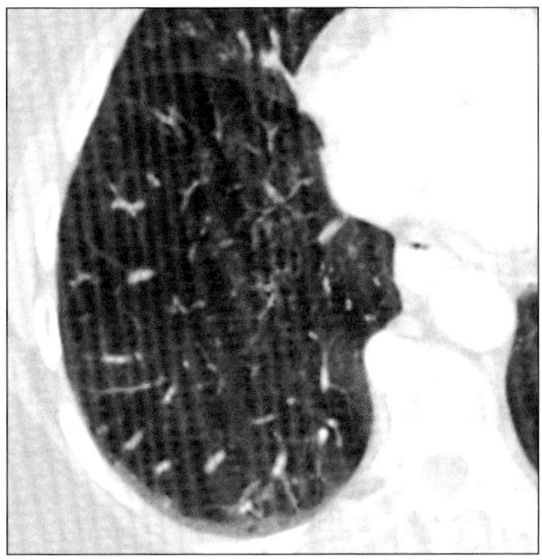

(Left) *Sagittal CECT in the same patient shows nodular opacities ➡ in the superior segment of the right lower lobe and posterior segment of the right upper lobe consistent with aspirated material from the tracheoesophageal fistula.* ***(Right)*** *Axial CECT in the same patient shows a cluster of tree in bud opacities in the right lower lobe consistent with aspiration through the tracheoesophageal fistula.*

FOCAL TRACHEOBRONCHIAL WALL THICKENING

DIFFERENTIAL DIAGNOSIS

Common
- Mucus
- Bronchial Neoplasm

Less Common
- Airway Stenosis
- Carcinoid

Rare but Important
- Metastasis
- Foreign Body
- Tracheal Neoplasm
- Infection
- Wegener Granulomatosis
- Fibrosing Mediastinitis
- Broncholith
- Tracheobronchial Amyloidosis

ESSENTIAL INFORMATION

Key Differential Diagnosis Issues
- Review focuses on diseases causing solitary/segmental wall thickening or nodularity
- Age of patient, smoking history, and history of malignancy are important considerations

Helpful Clues for Common Diagnoses
- **Mucus**
  - Common in emphysema, asthma, bronchitis, or cystic fibrosis
  - "Bubbly" or solid appearance on CT
  - Gravity-dependent location
  - Repeat CT after vigorous coughing helpful to differentiate from tumor
- **Bronchial Neoplasm**
  - Bronchogenic carcinoma
    - Polypoid nodule with endobronchial and extraluminal components
    - Postobstructive pneumonia/atelectasis
    - ± mediastinal and hilar lymphadenopathy
    - ± history of recurrent pneumonia
  - Hamartoma
    - Round and smooth nodule
    - ≤ 2 cm in diameter
    - ± internal fat
    - ± "popcorn" calcifications
  - Mucoepidermoid carcinoma
    - Intraluminal nodule
    - 50% of patients are ≤ 30 years old
    - Difficult to differentiate radiographically from carcinoid and bronchogenic carcinoma

Helpful Clues for Less Common Diagnoses
- **Airway Stenosis**
  - Progressive dyspnea following extubation or tracheostomy tube placement
    - Focal airway narrowing with circumferential wall thickening
    - Hourglass appearance
  - Prolonged endotracheal intubation
    - Subglottic narrowing at balloon cuff site
  - Tracheostomy tube
    - Stenosis at stoma site
  - Complete cartilaginous tracheal ring is an anomaly
  - Sarcoidosis; look for other typical features
- **Carcinoid**
  - Round or ovoid lobulated nodule
  - Occurs in lobar or segmental bronchi
  - ± intense contrast enhancement
  - 25% demonstrate chunky calcification
  - 80% are "typical"
    - Benign and slow growing
    - Metastases and carcinoid syndrome rare

Helpful Clues for Rare Diagnoses
- **Metastasis**
  - Invasion or compression from lymphoma, bronchogenic, thyroid, or esophageal carcinoma
    - Adjacent airway mass readily apparent
  - Hematogenous metastases from melanoma, breast, colon, or renal cell carcinoma
    - ± solitary or multiple endobronchial nodules
    - Lymph node metastases may cause airway compression
- **Foreign Body**
  - Most are radiolucent on radiographs
  - Easily mistaken for malignancy
  - History of aspiration and recurrent pneumonia
- **Tracheal Neoplasm**
  - Squamous cell carcinoma
    - Most common primary tracheal neoplasm
    - 33% have mediastinal or pulmonary metastases at diagnosis

- 40% with past, present, or future carcinoma of oropharynx, larynx, or lung
- Irregular-shaped polypoid or sessile lesion
- Predominates in lower trachea
  - Adenoid cystic carcinoma
    - Submucosal or circumferential wall thickening
    - ± long tracheal segment involvement
    - Disease recurs locally
    - Metastases are rare
- **Infection**
  - Tuberculosis
    - Distal trachea and proximal bronchi
    - Irregular circumferential wall thickening
    - Tracheal narrowing
    - Secondary to "endobronchial spread" or extension from involved lymph nodes
    - Infection rarely isolated to trachea
  - Histoplasmosis
    - Endobronchial nodule or mass
    - ± calcified mediastinal lymph nodes
    - ± apical cavitary nodules
  - Rhinoscleroma
    - Endemic in Central America, Africa, and India
    - 95% have nasal polyps and soft tissue thickening
    - Paranasal sinuses spared
    - Concentric or nodular subglottic tracheal narrowing in 25%
    - Air-filled tracheal crypts nearly diagnostic
- **Wegener Granulomatosis**
  - 25% have airway involvement
    - Circumferential subglottic tracheal wall thickening
    - ± luminal narrowing
  - ± cavitary lung nodules
  - ± pan-sinus disease
  - Laboratory evidence of glomerulonephritis (microscopic hematuria, red cell casts, and proteinuria)
- **Fibrosing Mediastinitis**
  - Common associations
    - Histoplasmosis, tuberculosis, or sarcoidosis (unilateral)
    - Retroperitoneal fibrosis, drugs, or autoimmune disorders (bilateral)
  - Mediastinal fat replaced by fibrous tissue
  - Encases and narrows adjacent structures
    - Superior vena cava, mainstem bronchi, pulmonary artery, or esophagus
  - ± mediastinal or hilar lymph node calcification
- **Broncholith**
  - Irregularly shaped calcified material within airway arising from adjacent calcified lymph node
  - ± extraluminal air
  - Right middle and upper lobe bronchi
  - No contrast enhancement
- **Tracheobronchial Amyloidosis**
  - Most common presentation is multifocal nodular deposits throughout central airways
  - Single submucosal nodule is extremely rare

Mucus

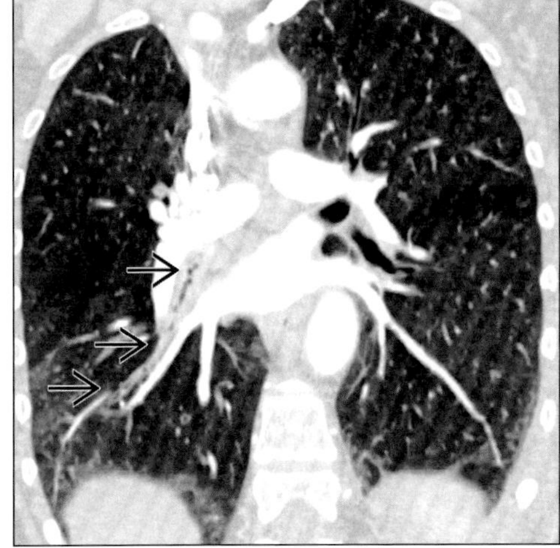

Coronal CECT shows mucus plugging in the bronchus intermedius ⇒ and right lower lobe segmental bronchi in this patient with chronic bronchitis secondary to smoking.

Mucus

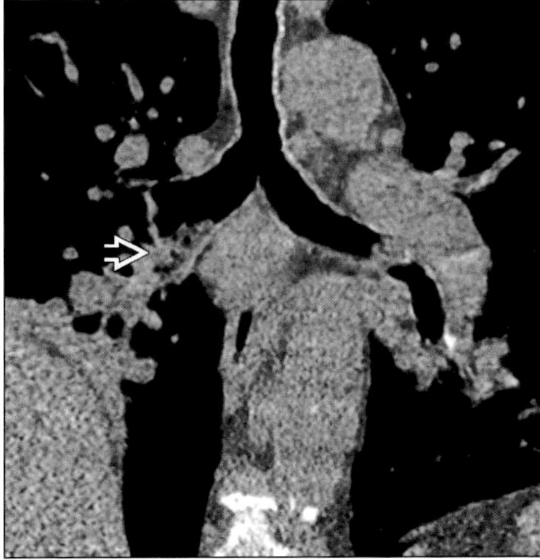

Coronal NECT shows a "bubbly" lesion within the dependent portion of the bronchus intermedius ⇒. The important distinguishing characteristic is portions of air seen within the lesion.

FOCAL TRACHEOBRONCHIAL WALL THICKENING

Bronchial Neoplasm

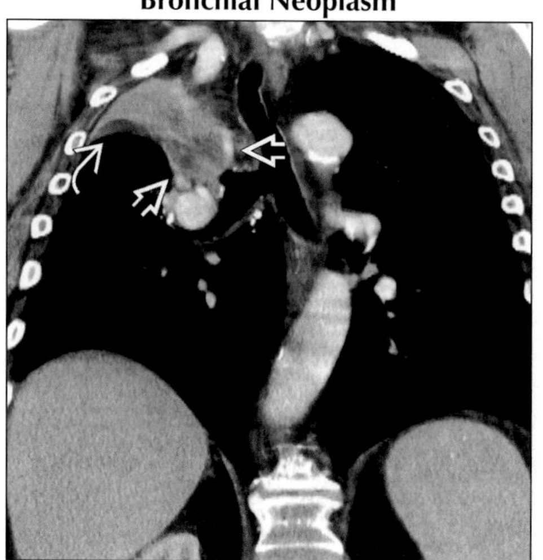

Bronchial Neoplasm

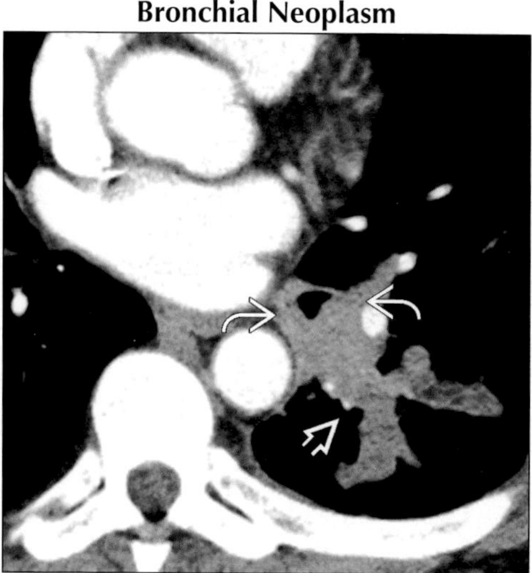

*(**Left**) Coronal CECT shows a collapsed right upper lobe with ipsilateral tracheal deviation and occlusion of the right upper lobe bronchus by tumor ➡, which has a lower density than atelectatic lung ➡. (**Right**) Axial CECT shows concentric asymmetric thickening of the left lower lobe bronchus ➡ in this patient with adenoid cystic carcinoma. Note partial collapse of a portion of the left lower lobe posterior segment ➡.*

Bronchial Neoplasm

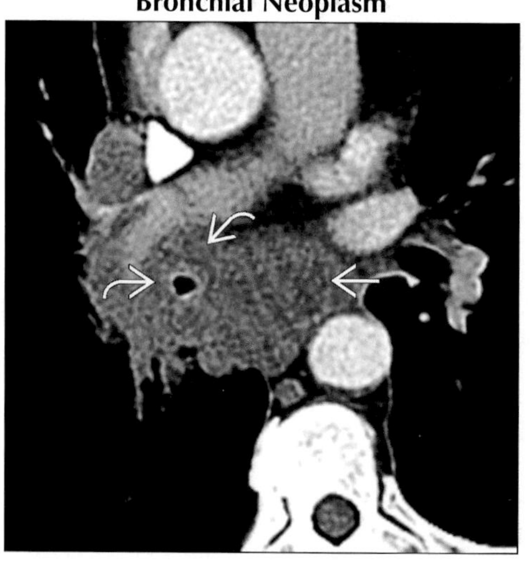

Bronchial Neoplasm

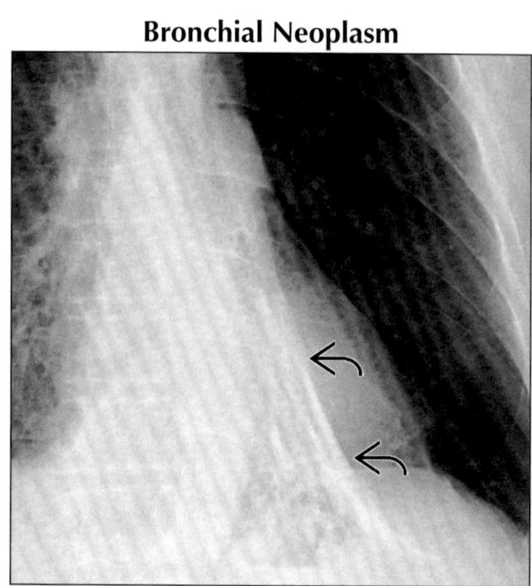

*(**Left**) Axial CECT shows concentric narrowing of the bronchus intermedius ➡ with associated subcarinal soft tissue mass ➡ in this patient with small cell lung carcinoma. (**Right**) Frontal radiograph shows left lower lobe collapse ➡ with hyperexpansion of the left upper lung in this patient with chronic obstruction secondary to an endobronchial hamartoma. CT showed characteristic fat and calcification associated with this lesion.*

Airway Stenosis

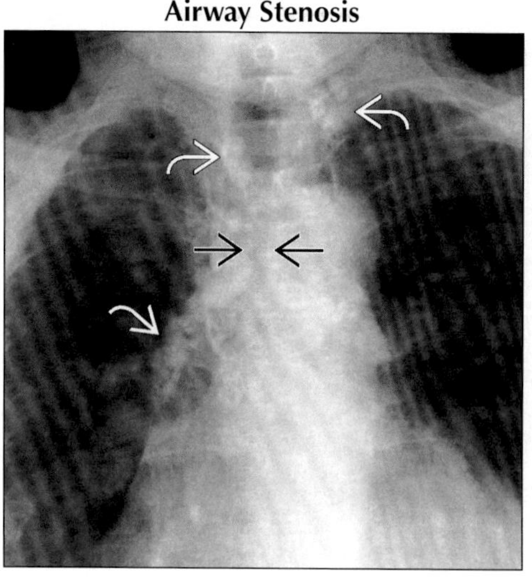

Airway Stenosis

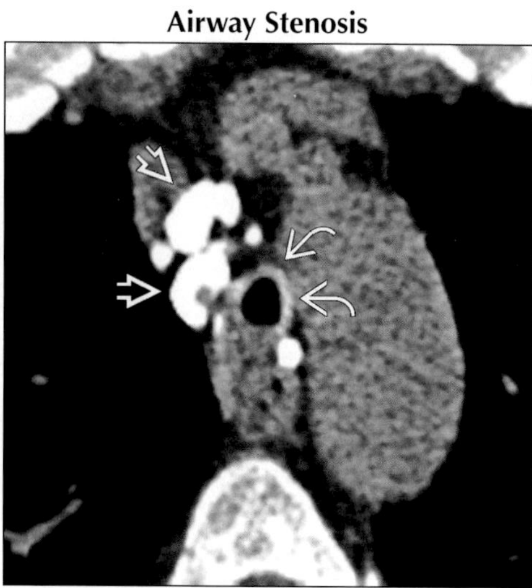

*(**Left**) Frontal radiograph shows extensive calcified mediastinal and hilar lymphadenopathy ➡ in this patient with sarcoidosis. Occasionally there is severe lymphadenopathy leading to tracheal stenosis ➡. (**Right**) Axial NECT in the same patient shows tracheal stenosis ➡ caused by calcified paratracheal lymphadenopathy ➡. Helpful clues to the diagnosis of sarcoidosis are symmetric lymphadenopathy and perilymphatic lung nodules (not shown).*

Airway Stenosis

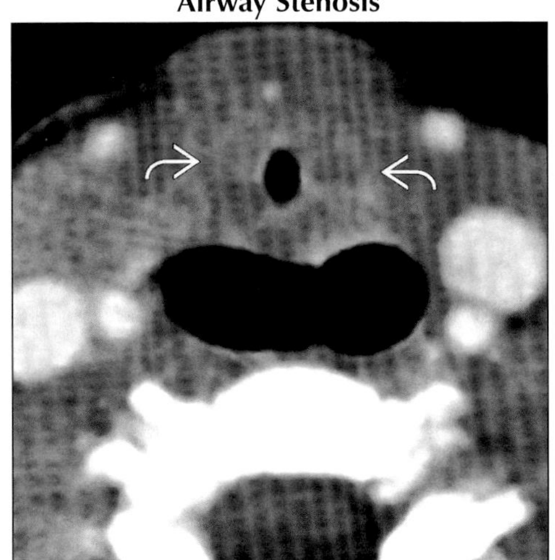

Airway Stenosis

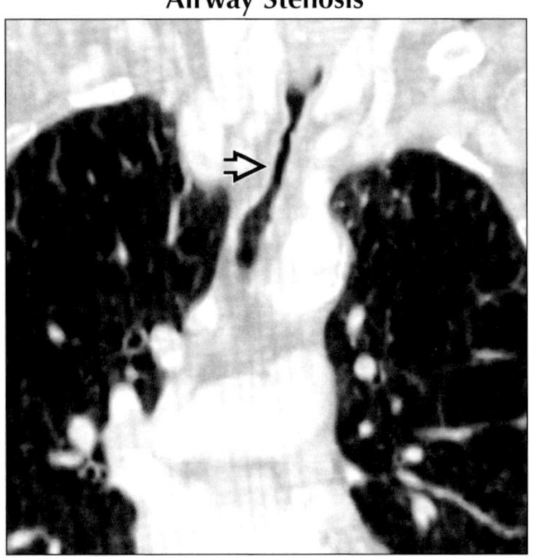

(Left) *Axial CECT shows concentric tracheal narrowing with circumferential wall thickening ➡. Clinical history of prolonged intubation and subglottic location are important clues to the diagnosis of post-intubation tracheal stenosis.* ***(Right)*** *Coronal CECT shows an hourglass narrowing of the upper intrathoracic trachea ⇨ in this patient with tracheal stenosis secondary to prior tracheostomy tube placement.*

Carcinoid

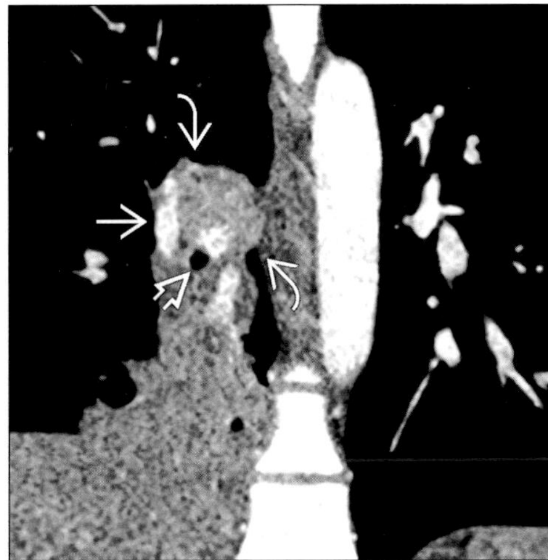

Carcinoid

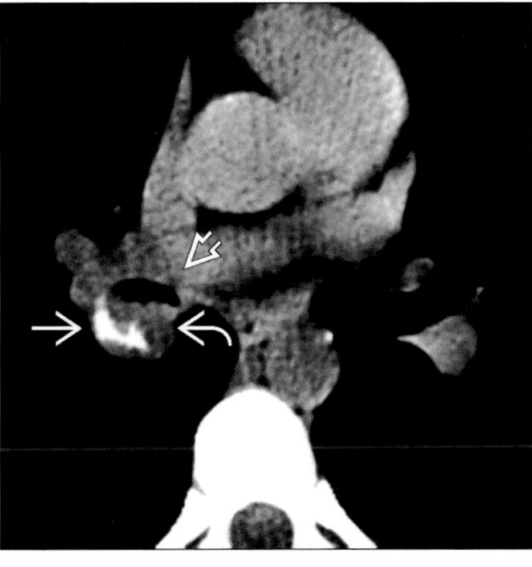

(Left) *Coronal CECT shows a round nodule ➡ narrowing the right lower lobe bronchus ➡. Note characteristic eccentric calcifications ➡, which are seen in approximately 25% of cases.* ***(Right)*** *Axial NECT shows a round nodule ➡ narrowing the bronchus intermedius ➡. Note calcification occupying the periphery of the nodule ➡. Most pulmonary carcinoids occur in patients between 30-60 years old and are in the main, lobar, or segmental bronchi.*

Metastasis

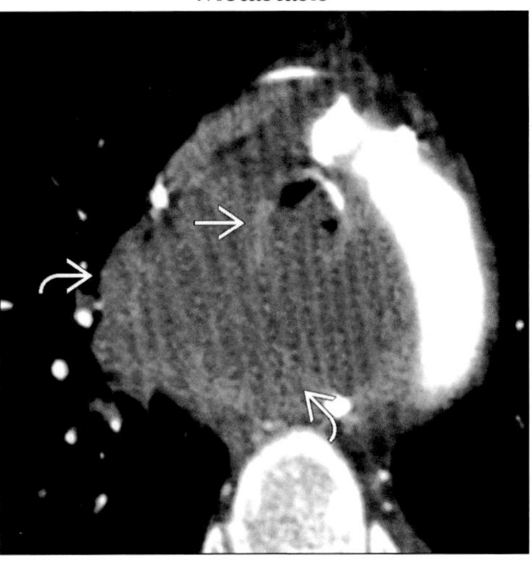

Metastasis

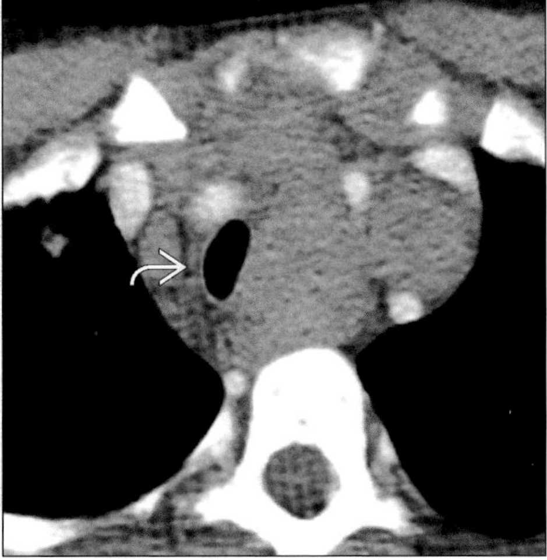

(Left) *Axial CECT shows a large homogeneous mass ➡ surrounding the trachea, corresponding to lymph node metastases in this patient with non-small cell lung carcinoma. Note corresponding soft tissue within the tracheal lumen ➡ proven to represent extension of carcinoma on bronchoscopy.* ***(Right)*** *Axial CECT shows external compression and displacement of the trachea ➡ secondary to confluent lymphadenopathy from lymphoma.*

FOCAL TRACHEOBRONCHIAL WALL THICKENING

*(**Left**) Coronal NECT shows a lobulated lesion ➔ that nearly completely occludes the tracheal lumen in this patient with metastatic disease from renal cell carcinoma. Primary squamous cell carcinoma or adenoid cystic carcinoma could have a similar appearance. (**Right**) Axial CECT shows a small, round, hyperdense lesion within the bronchus intermedius ➔. This was a small bag of cocaine at bronchoscopy.*

Metastasis

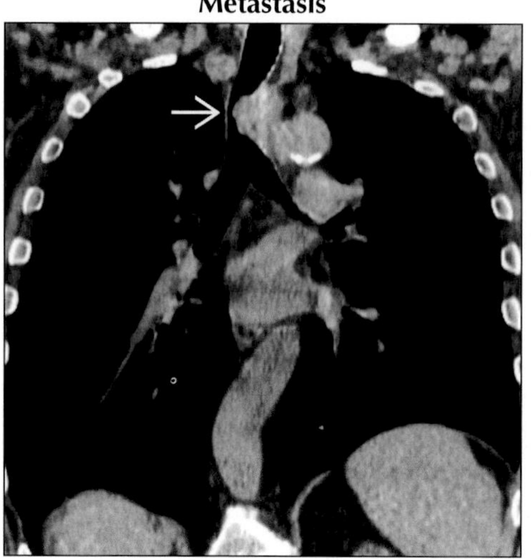

Foreign Body

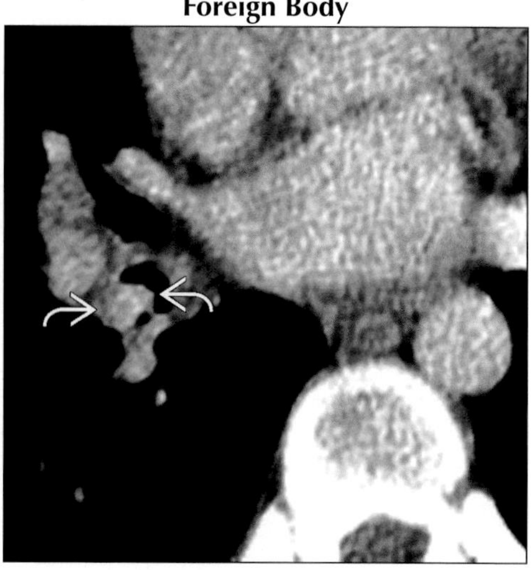

*(**Left**) Frontal radiograph shows a lobulated lesion along the left lateral tracheal wall ➔ proven to represent a primary tracheal squamous cell carcinoma. Differential considerations include metastatic disease and adenoid cystic carcinoma. (**Right**) Axial NECT in the same patient shows focal thickening of the left lateral tracheal wall ➔. Squamous cell carcinoma is the most common primary tracheal neoplasm.*

Tracheal Neoplasm

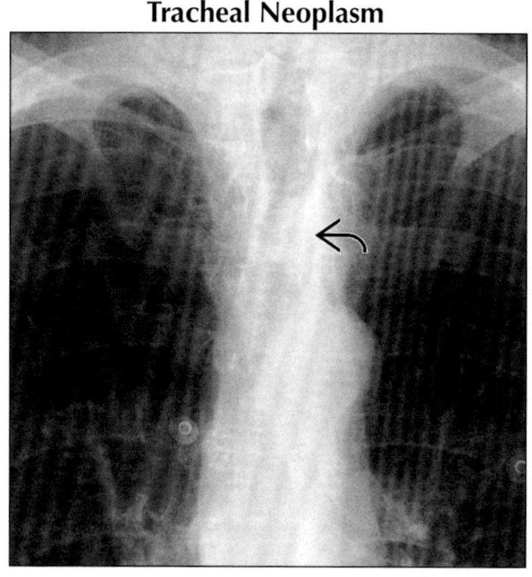

Tracheal Neoplasm

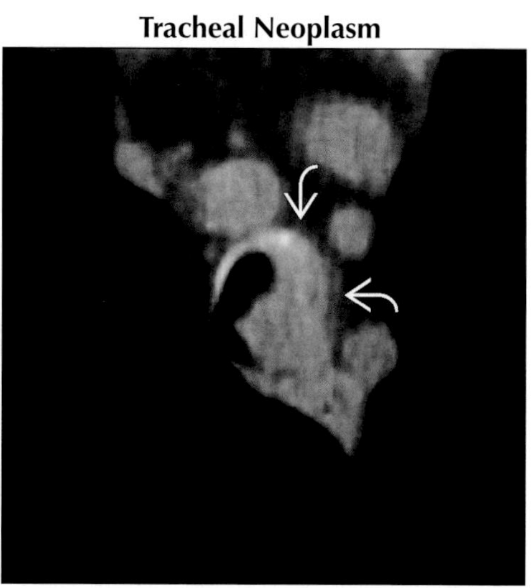

*(**Left**) Axial CECT shows an enhancing oval-shaped subglottic nodule ➔ representing a hemangioma, the most common soft tissue tracheal mass in children. Tracheal hemangiomas often have associated facial hemangiomas. (**Right**) Axial CECT shows circumferential subglottic narrowing containing crypt-like air spaces ➔. There was nodular thickening of nasal turbinates with a normal appearance to the maxillary sinuses (not shown) in this patient with rhinoscleroma.*

Tracheal Neoplasm

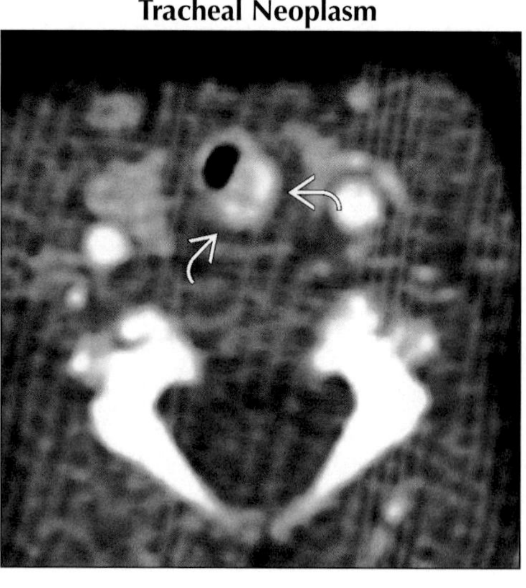

Infection

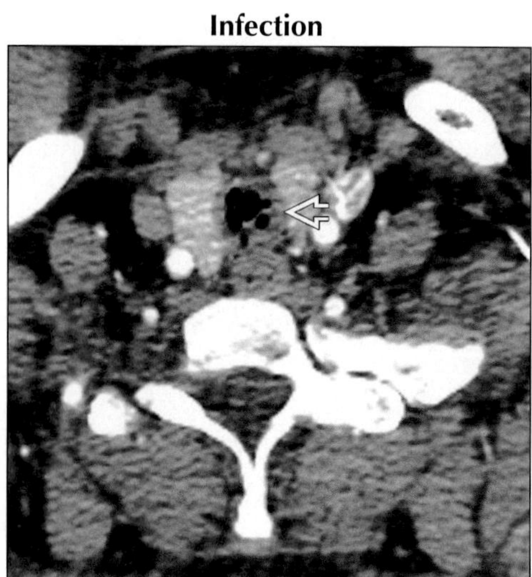

Infection

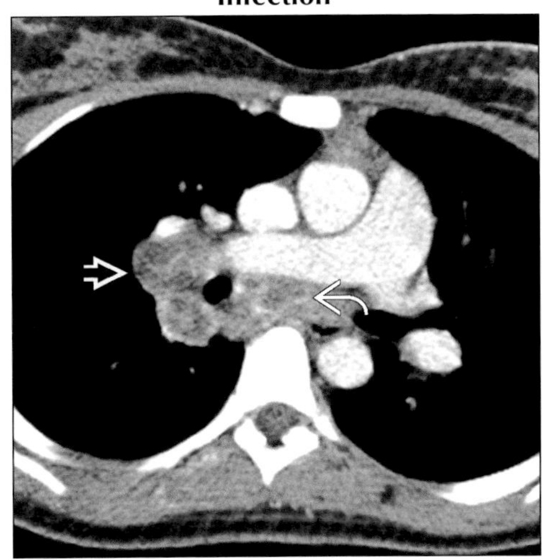

Wegener Granulomatosis

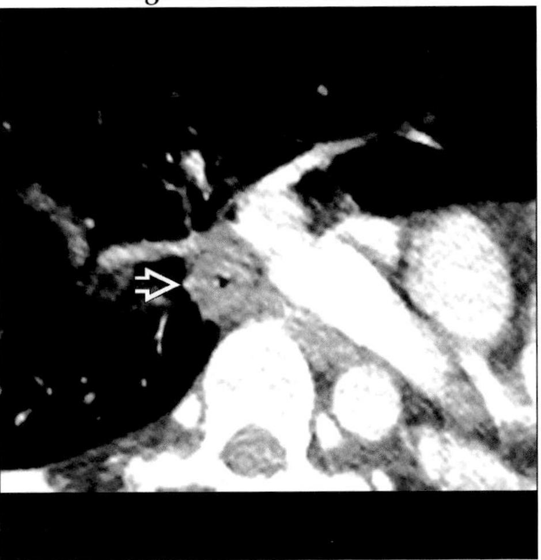

*(**Left**) Axial CECT shows multiple necrotic subcarinal ➔ and right hilar ➔ lymph nodes with focal narrowing of the bronchus intermedius. This case was due to primary tuberculosis infection. Differential considerations include endemic fungi, lymphoma, or metastatic disease. (**Right**) Axial CECT shows concentric thickening of the bronchus intermedius ➔. Cavitary lung nodules and pulmonary hemorrhage were seen in this patient with Wegener granulomatosis.*

Fibrosing Mediastinitis

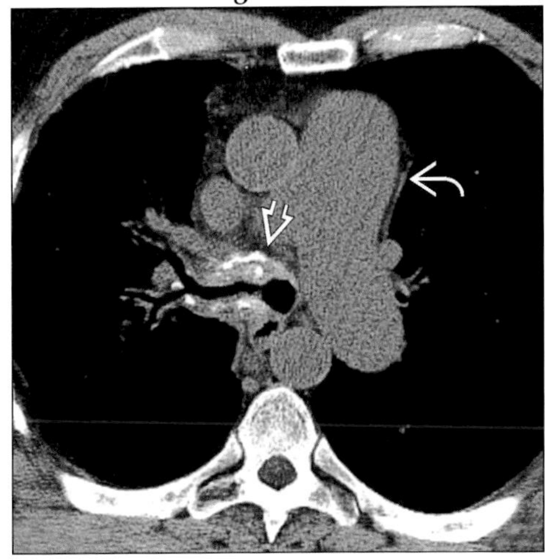

Fibrosing Mediastinitis

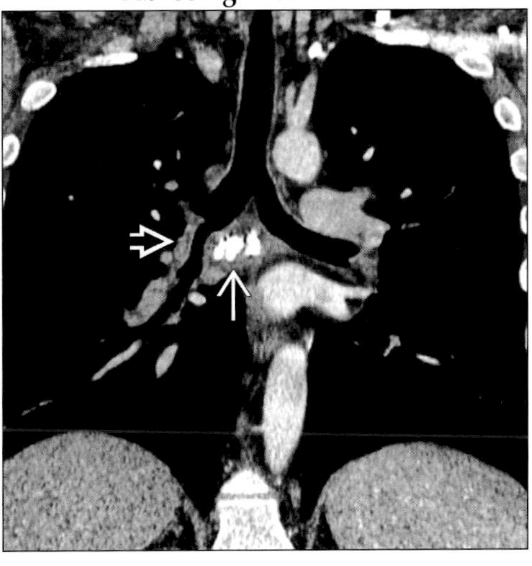

*(**Left**) Axial NECT shows a calcified subcarinal mass ➔ with narrowing of the right bronchi. Enlargement of the pulmonary artery ➔ indicates pulmonary arterial hypertension. (**Right**) Coronal CECT shows calcified subcarinal lymphadenopathy ➔ and narrowing of the bronchus intermedius ➔. This is most commonly seen with histoplasmosis infection. Calcified lymphadenopathy is an important distinguishing characteristic from tumor.*

Broncholith

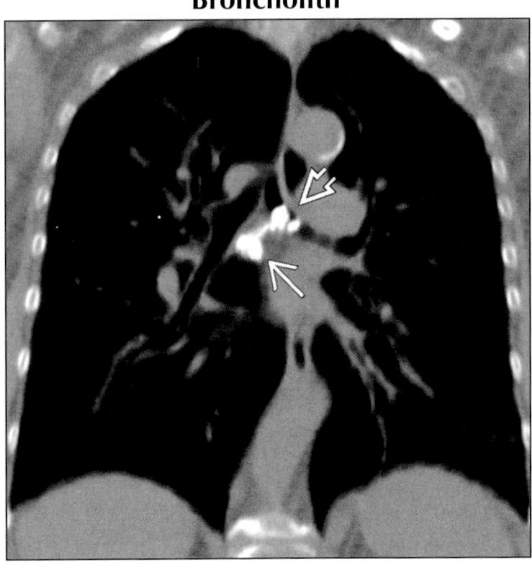

Tracheobronchial Amyloidosis

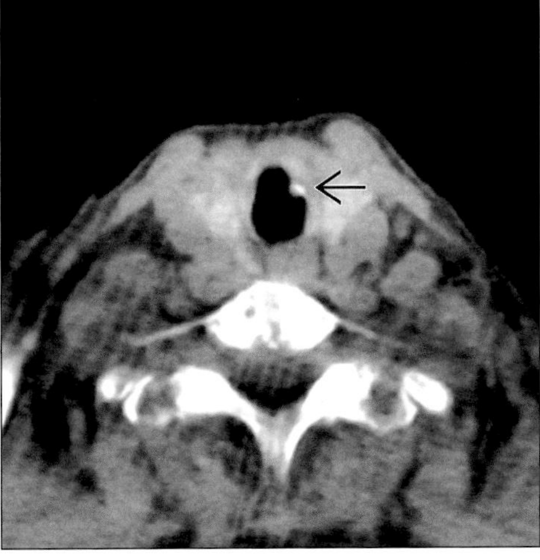

*(**Left**) Coronal NECT shows calcified subcarinal lymphadenopathy ➔ and broncholith ➔ in the left mainstem bronchus. (**Right**) Axial CECT shows a small calcified left tracheal nodule ➔, proven to represent an amyloid deposit. There were also calcified and noncalcified pulmonary nodules (not shown). Amyloidosis is typically multifocal when presenting in the central airways.*

DIFFUSE TRACHEOBRONCHIAL WALL THICKENING

DIFFERENTIAL DIAGNOSIS

Common
- Tracheal Neoplasms
- Acute Bronchitis
- Chronic Bronchitis

Less Common
- Relapsing Polychondritis
- Wegener Granulomatosis
- Amyloidosis
- Sarcoidosis

Rare but Important
- Laryngeal Papillomatosis
- Tracheopathia Osteochondroplastica
- Rhinoscleroma

ESSENTIAL INFORMATION

Key Differential Diagnosis Issues
- Diffuse or focal abnormality
- Involvement or sparing of posterior tracheal membrane
- Expiratory CT useful for detecting tracheomalacia

Helpful Clues for Common Diagnoses
- **Tracheal Neoplasms**
  - Uncommon
    - < 1% of all lower respiratory tract neoplasms
    - Squamous cell carcinoma and adenoid cystic carcinoma account for > 80%
    - Other tumor types rare
  - Polypoid intraluminal mass most common appearance
    - Squamous cell carcinomas often large at presentation (up to 4 cm)
  - Eccentric nodular wall thickening or diffuse tracheal wall infiltrating uncommon
  - Frequently extend into mediastinum and adjacent structures
    - Tracheoesophageal fistula in 15%
    - Main bronchial invasion in 25%
    - Regional lymph node metastases common
  - Adenoid cystic carcinomas most commonly occur near tracheal carina
- **Acute Bronchitis**
  - Viral most common cause
  - Bronchial wall thickening
    - Retained secretions
  - Patchy atelectasis
  - Peribronchial consolidation may indicate bronchopneumonia
  - Acute bacterial tracheitis
    - Most common in children
    - Less commonly immunocompromised adults
    - Diffuse tracheal wall edema
    - Edema of surrounding mediastinal tissues
- **Chronic Bronchitis**
  - Related to cigarette smoking
  - Clinical diagnosis
  - Tracheobronchial wall thickening
    - No significant stenosis
    - Retained secretions
  - Centrilobular pulmonary emphysema may be present

Helpful Clues for Less Common Diagnoses
- **Relapsing Polychondritis**
  - Involves only cartilaginous portions of trachea and main bronchi
  - Spares posterior membrane
  - Increased attenuation of tracheal wall
    - May become diffusely calcified
  - Smooth tracheal wall thickening
  - Tracheal stenosis
    - Occurs in 33-89% of patients
    - Diffuse or focal
    - Associated with bronchial narrowing
  - Tracheomalacia
    - Result of cartilaginous inflammation and destruction
    - Suggested by > 70% reduction of cross-sectional area on expiration
- **Wegener Granulomatosis**
  - Tracheal wall thickening in 15%
  - Bronchial wall thickening in 50-60%
  - Focal > diffuse
    - Subglottic narrowing most common
  - Tracheobronchial narrowing smooth or irregular
  - Associated lung findings may be present
    - Nodules and masses
    - Cavitary lesions
    - Consolidation
    - Ground-glass opacity
- **Amyloidosis**
  - Tracheobronchial tree most commonly affected

- Smooth or nodular calcification in up to 50%
- Circumferential tracheal or tracheobronchial wall thickening
- Associated lung findings (from airway obstruction)
  - Atelectasis or obstructive pneumonitis
  - Pulmonary amyloid
- **Sarcoidosis**
  - Tracheal involvement very uncommon
  - Larynx often affected
  - Stenosis smooth, irregular, nodular, or mass-like
  - Other typical findings usually present
    - Lymphadenopathy
    - Perilymphatic nodules

Helpful Clues for Rare Diagnoses

- **Laryngeal Papillomatosis**
  - Tracheobronchial involvement in 5-10%
  - Usually develops 10 years after laryngeal disease
  - May affect lungs
    - Nodules
    - Cavitary lesions
  - Degeneration into squamous cell carcinoma rare
- **Tracheopathia Osteochondroplastica**
  - Mild diffuse tracheobronchial stenosis with nodularity
  - Calcified nodules arising from tracheal cartilage protruding into lumen
    - Range in size from 3-8 mm
  - Lower trachea most commonly involved
  - May extend into bronchi to segmental level
    - Can cause atelectasis
  - Sparing of posterior tracheal membrane characteristic
  - Often associated with "saber-sheath" tracheal deformity
  - Slowly progressive
  - Older men with chronic obstructive lung disease most commonly affected
- **Rhinoscleroma**
  - Slowly progressive granulomatous infection caused by *Klebsiella rhinoscleromatis*
  - Endemic in tropical and subtropical regions
  - Upper respiratory tract most commonly involved
    - Especially nose, upper lip, hard palate, and maxillary sinuses
    - Trachea and proximal bronchi affected in up to 10%
  - Thickening of trachea and main bronchi with luminal stenosis
    - Stenoses usually concentric
    - Smooth or nodular
    - Diffuse uniform narrowing uncommon
    - Occasional mediastinal and hilar lymphadenopathy
    - Atelectasis and obstructive pneumonitis may develop

Tracheal Neoplasms

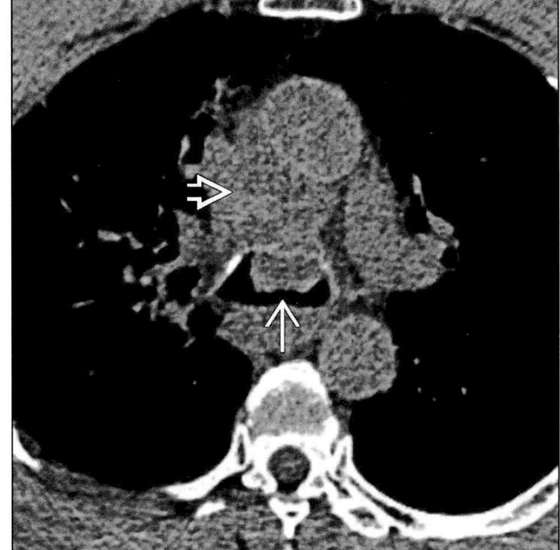

Axial NECT shows a polypoid carinal mass ➡ extending into the tracheal lumen at the carina. Note the extension into the mediastinum anteriorly ➡. Biopsy confirmed squamous cell carcinoma.

Tracheal Neoplasms

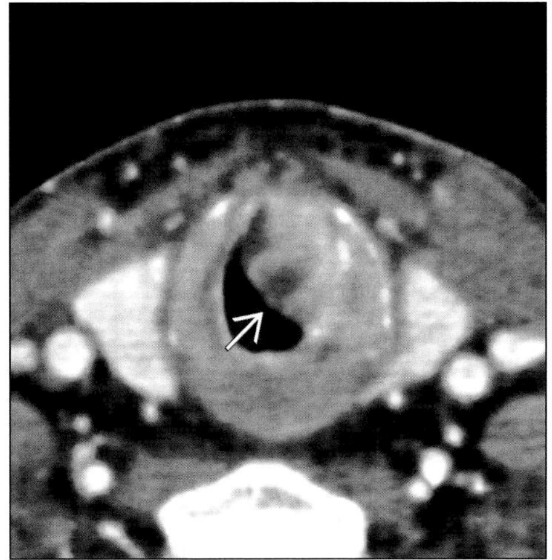

Axial CECT shows a heterogeneous mass ➡ protruding into the tracheal lumen at the level of the cricoid cartilage. Biopsy confirmed squamous cell carcinoma.

DIFFUSE TRACHEOBRONCHIAL WALL THICKENING

Tracheal Neoplasms

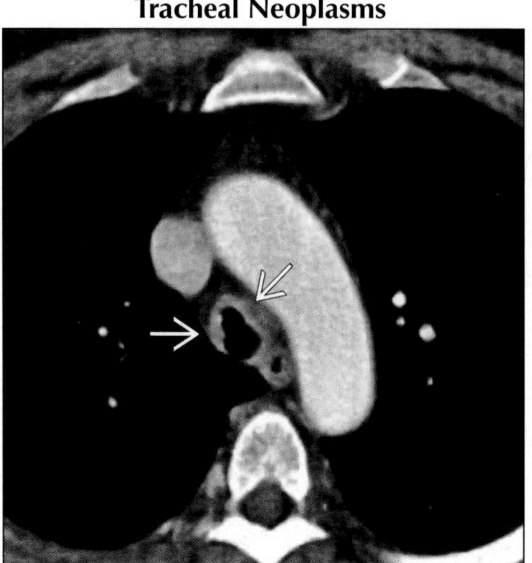

Tracheal Neoplasms

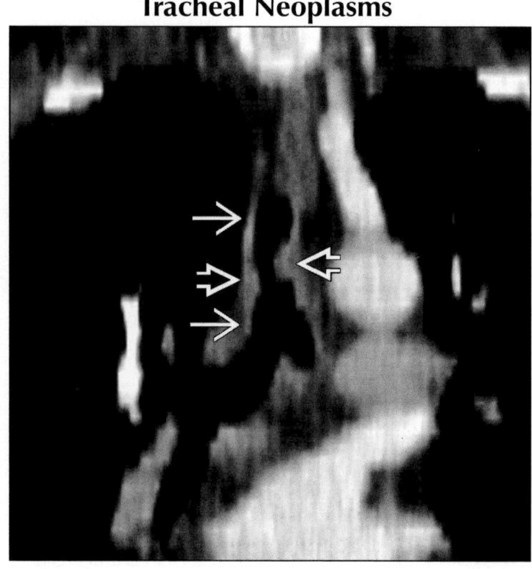

(Left) *Axial CECT shows nodular thickening of the tracheal wall ➔ in this patient with adenoid cystic carcinoma. Following resection, adenoid cystic carcinomas, while lower grade than squamous cell carcinoma, often recur because of submucosal growth.* ***(Right)*** *Coronal oblique CT reconstruction shows tracheal wall thickening ➔ with nodular protrusions into the tracheal lumen ➔ in this patient with adenoid cystic carcinoma.*

Acute Bronchitis

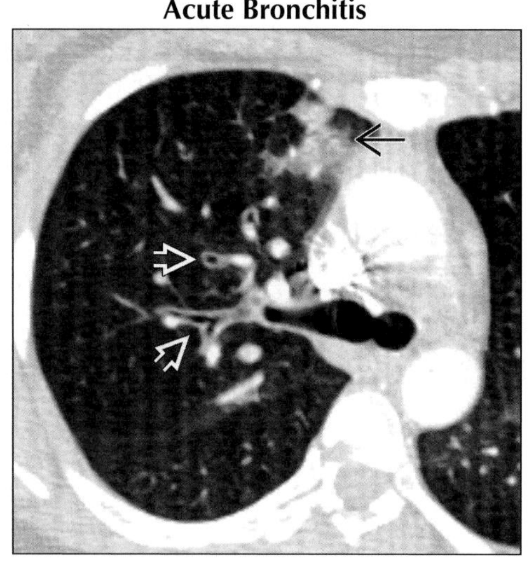

Chronic Bronchitis

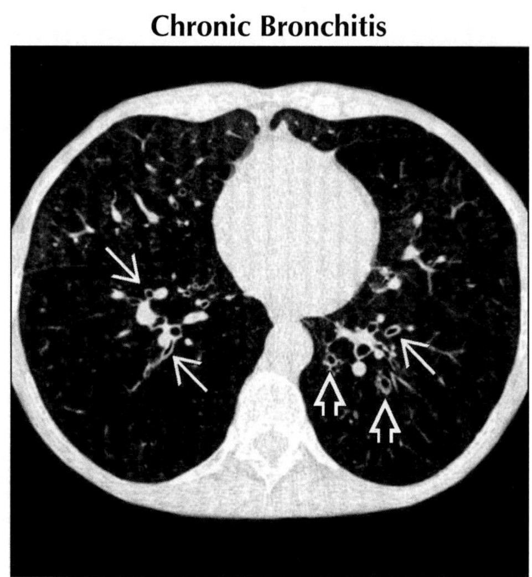

(Left) *Axial CECT shows bronchial wall thickening ➔ in a patient with acute bronchitis. The patchy ground-glass opacity in the right upper lobe ➔ reflects associated focal pneumonitis.* ***(Right)*** *Axial HRCT shows bronchial wall thickening and mild irregularity ➔ in the lower lobes. Mild bronchiectasis ➔ is in the left lower lobe. Extensive emphysema is present in both lungs.*

Relapsing Polychondritis

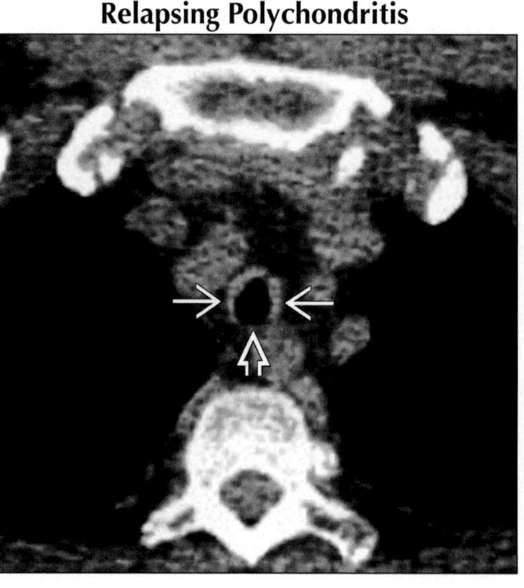

Relapsing Polychondritis

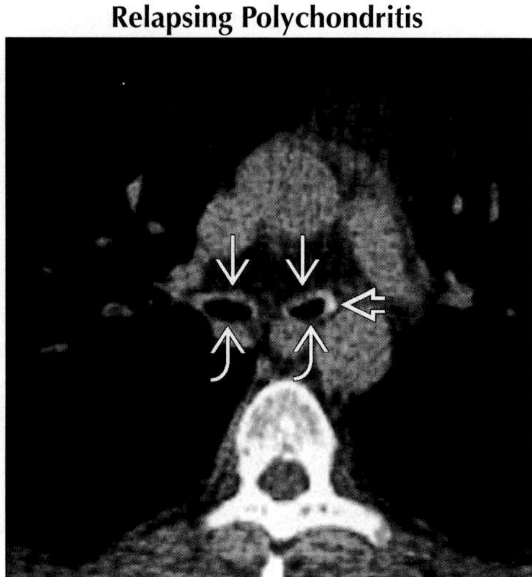

(Left) *Axial NECT shows thickening of the cartilaginous portion of the tracheal wall ➔ with characteristic sparing of the posterior tracheal membrane ➔ in this patient with relapsing polychondritis.* ***(Right)*** *Axial NECT shows thickening of the cartilaginous portions of the main bronchi with mild luminal stenosis ➔ and focal faint calcification of the left main bronchial wall ➔ with characteristic sparing of the posterior tracheal membrane ➔.*

Relapsing Polychondritis

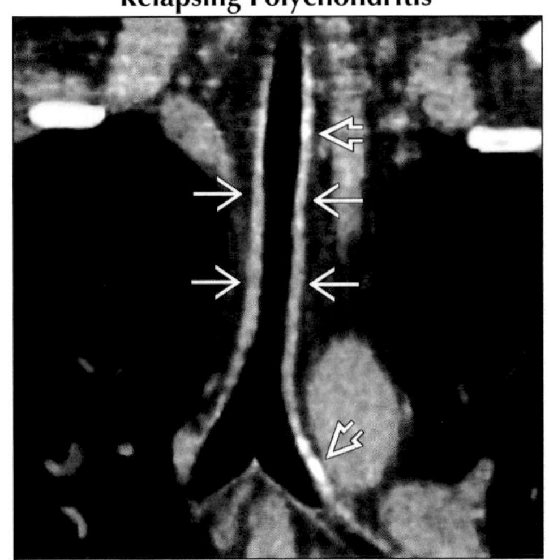

Relapsing Polychondritis

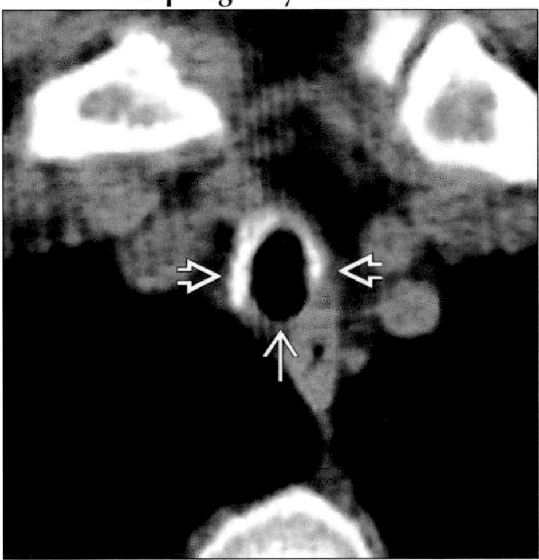

(Left) *Coronal oblique CT reconstruction shows diffuse tracheal wall thickening ➡ with foci of faint calcification ➡ and diffuse luminal narrowing. In contrast to age-related tracheal calcification, amyloidosis is associated with wall thickening.* ***(Right)*** *Axial NECT shows thickening of the cartilaginous portions of the tracheal wall with amorphous calcification ➡ and characteristic sparing of the posterior tracheal membrane ➡.*

Relapsing Polychondritis

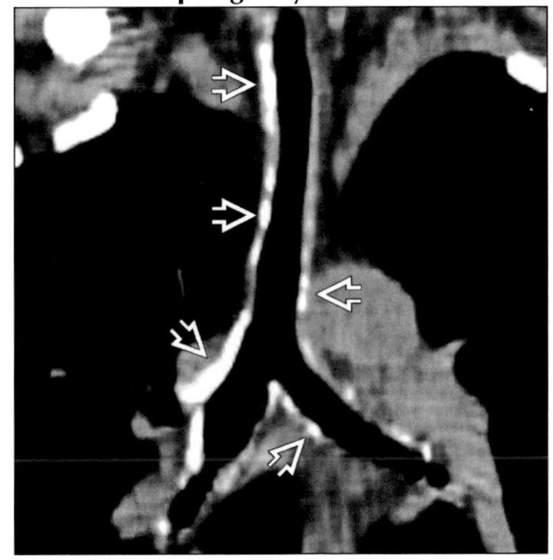

Wegener Granulomatosis

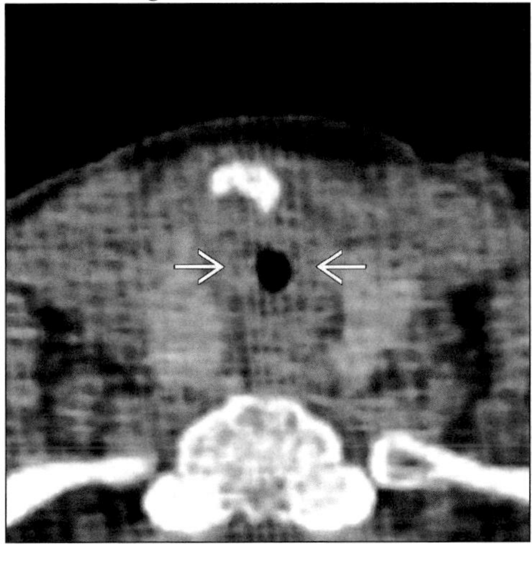

(Left) *Coronal oblique CT reconstruction shows diffuse tracheal and main bronchial wall thickening with thick, amorphous calcifications ➡ and diffuse mild tracheal stenosis. With progressive inflammation, the trachea and bronchi often lose their normal corrugated appearances and become smoother because of fibrosis.* ***(Right)*** *Axial NECT shows circumferential subglottic tracheal stenosis with diffuse wall thickening ➡, typical of Wegener granulomatosis.*

Wegener Granulomatosis

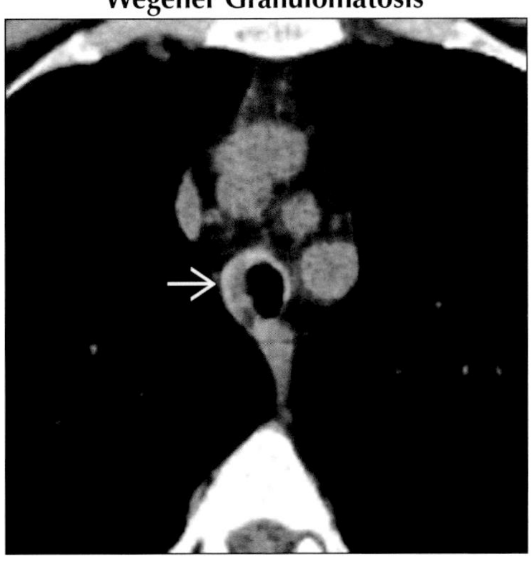

Wegener Granulomatosis

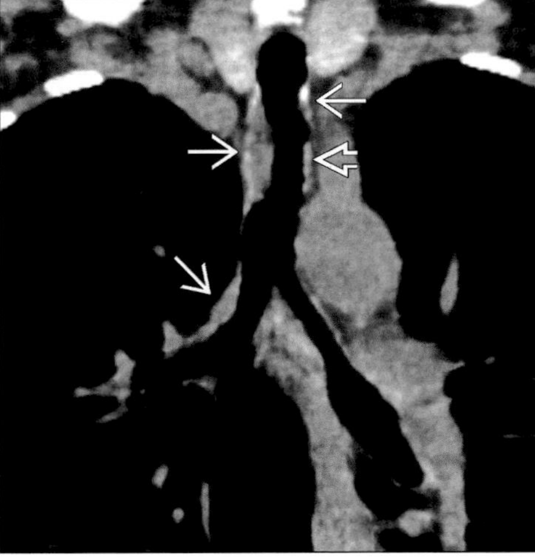

(Left) *Axial NECT shows eccentric tracheal wall thickening ➡ and mild luminal stenosis. Tracheal involvement in Wegener granulomatosis is often patchy with irregular wall thickening, nodularity, and stenosis. The subglottic trachea is most frequently involved.* ***(Right)*** *Coronal oblique CT reconstruction shows irregular tracheobronchial wall thickening ➡ with mild stenosis of the upper trachea ➡. Note the patchy distribution of disease.*

DIFFUSE TRACHEOBRONCHIAL WALL THICKENING

(Left) *Frontal radiograph shows smooth tracheal wall thickening ➡ and narrowing. Although not specific, the findings on the radiograph indicate a diffuse process affecting the trachea. CT frequently provides more specific information, and sometimes findings are characteristic of a particular diagnosis.* ***(Right)*** *Axial CECT shows circumferential tracheal wall thickening ➡ with mild luminal stenosis.*

Amyloidosis

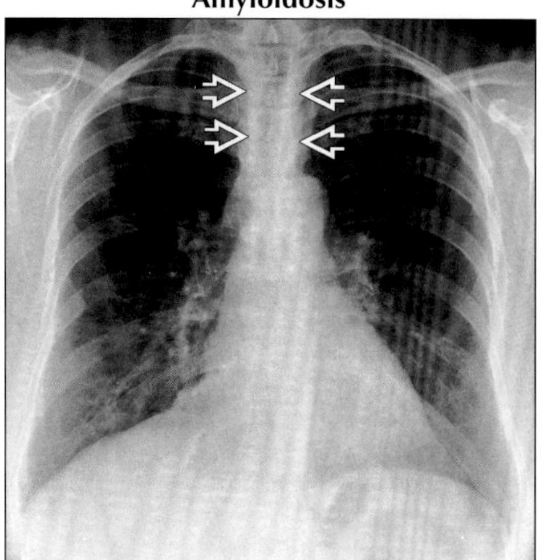

Amyloidosis

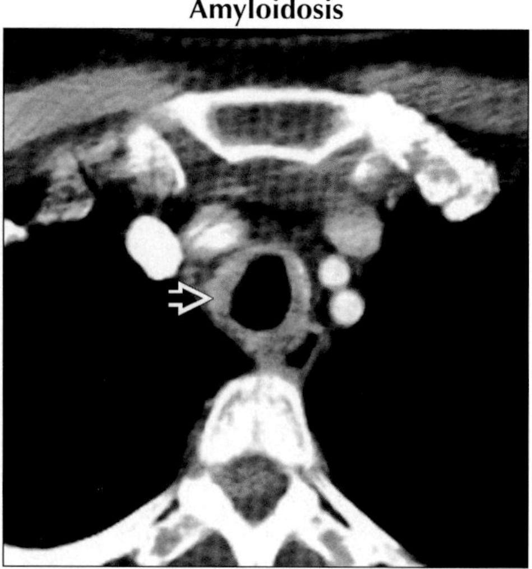

(Left) *Coronal oblique CT reconstruction shows diffuse tracheobronchial wall thickening ➡ with moderate stenosis of the left main bronchus ➡. Amyloidosis of the central airways is usually diffuse, helping narrow the differential diagnosis.* ***(Right)*** *Axial CECT shows circumferential tracheal wall thickening and nodularity ➡ with mild luminal stenosis. Right hilar lymphadenopathy ➡ and small pleural effusions ➡ are present.*

Amyloidosis

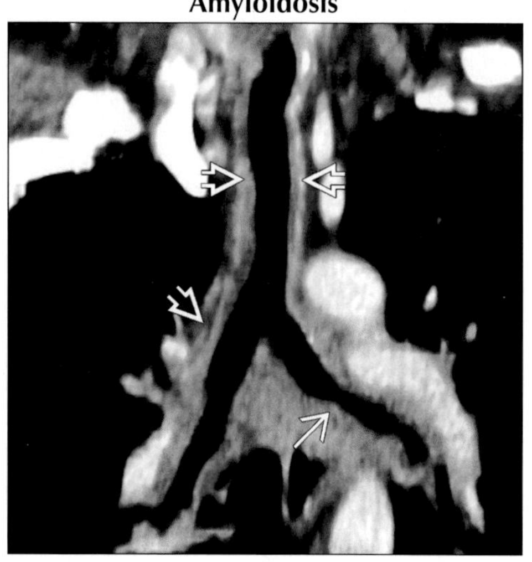

Sarcoidosis

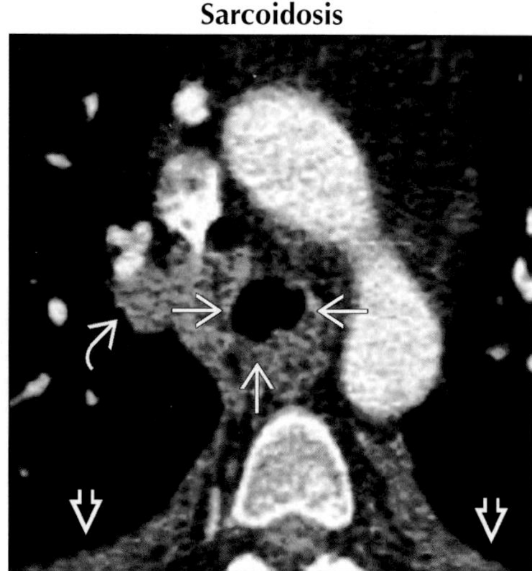

(Left) *Coronal oblique 3D reformation shows thickening of the distal tracheal wall ➡. Right hilar lymphadenopathy ➡ and calcified mediastinal lymph nodes ➡ are present. Tracheal involvement in sarcoidosis is uncommon but should be suspected in the setting of lung and bronchial involvement.* ***(Right)*** *Axial NECT shows soft tissue nodules ➡ protruding into the lumen of the trachea.*

Sarcoidosis

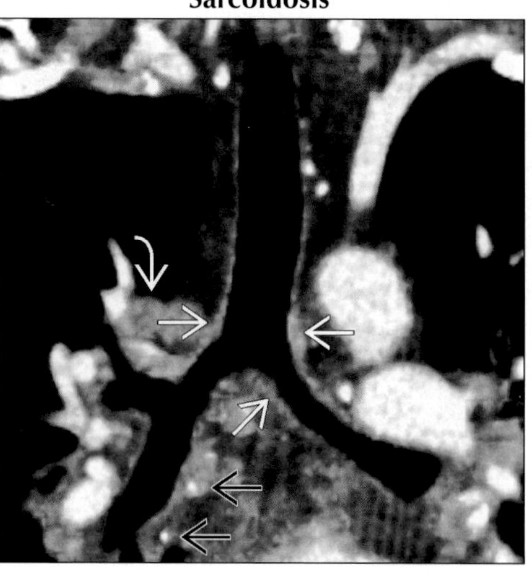

Laryngeal Papillomatosis

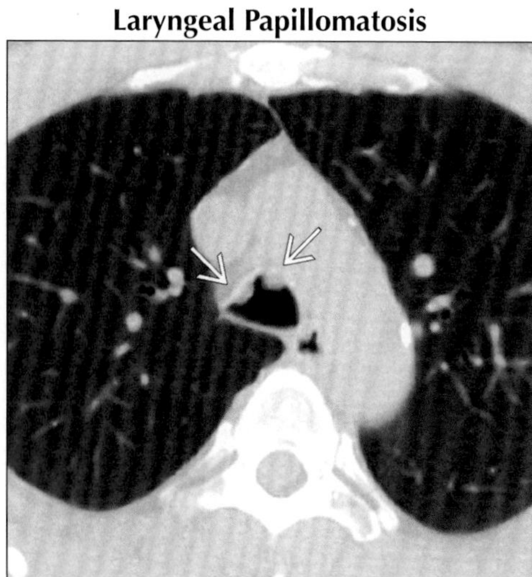

DIFFUSE TRACHEOBRONCHIAL WALL THICKENING

Laryngeal Papillomatosis

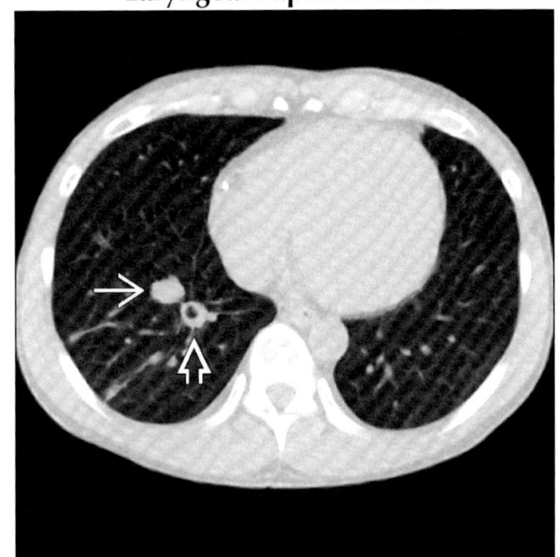

Laryngeal Papillomatosis

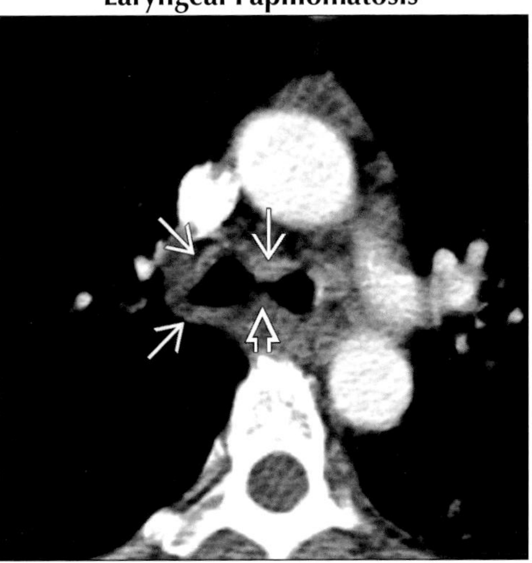

*(**Left**) Axial NECT shows 2 large nodules in the right lower lobe, 1 solid ➔ and 1 with central cavitation ➔. Involvement of the lungs is very uncommon in laryngeal papillomatosis. (**Right**) Axial CECT shows circumferential main bronchial wall thickening at the carina ➔ with a small nodule of soft tissue protruding into the airway lumen ➔.*

Laryngeal Papillomatosis

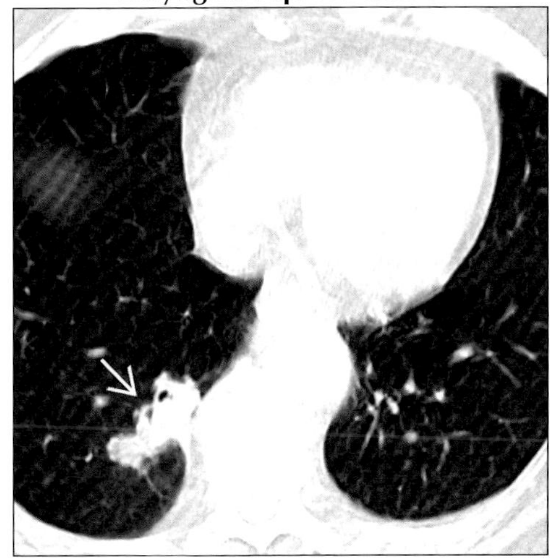

Tracheopathia Osteochondroplastica

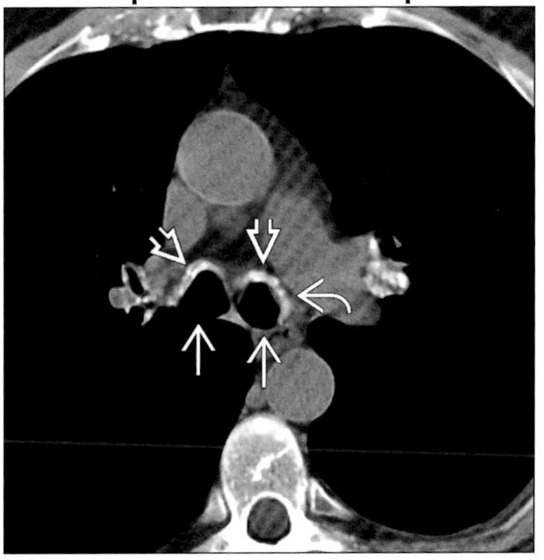

*(**Left**) Axial HRCT shows a lobulated mass ➔ in the right lower lobe, representing squamous cell carcinoma. Degeneration into squamous cell carcinoma is a rare occurrence in laryngeal papillomatosis. (**Right**) Axial NECT shows thickening and calcification ➔ of the main bronchial walls with luminal nodularity ➔ and characteristic sparing of the posterior bronchial wall membrane ➔.*

Tracheopathia Osteochondroplastica

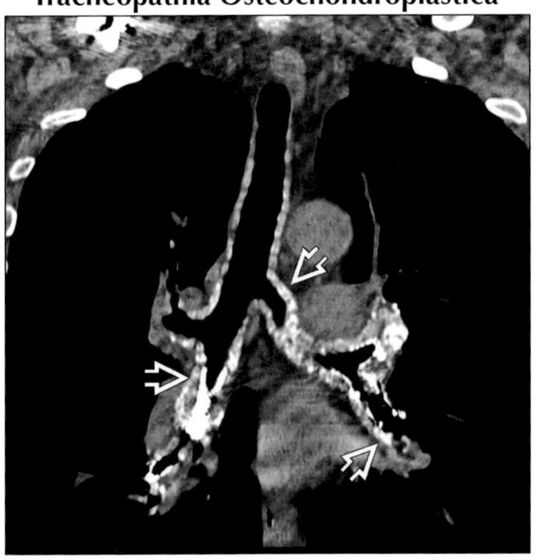

Rhinoscleroma

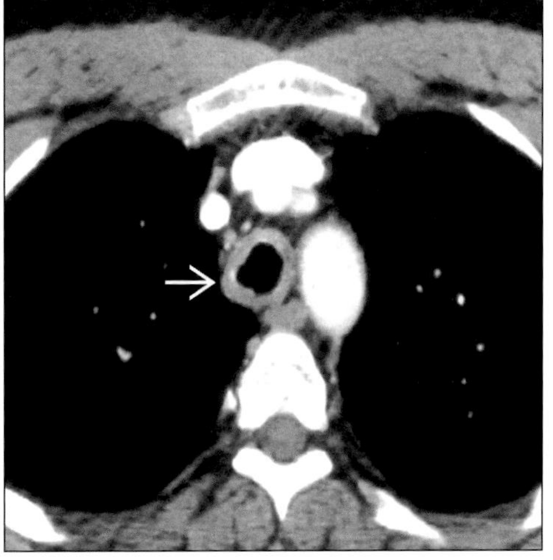

*(**Left**) Coronal CT reconstruction shows extensive nodular calcification of the trachea and central bronchi ➔. As in relapsing polychondritis, the posterior tracheal and bronchial membranes are spared in tracheobronchopathia osteochondroplastica, helping distinguish it from other causes of diffuse tracheobronchial wall thickening. (**Right**) Axial CECT shows smooth, circumferential tracheal wall thickening ➔.*

TRACHEAL MASS

DIFFERENTIAL DIAGNOSIS

Common
- Metastasis
- Primary Tracheal Neoplasms
  - Squamous Cell Carcinoma
  - Adenoid Cystic Carcinoma
- Mucus

Less Common
- Mucoepidermoid Carcinoma
- Tracheobronchopathia Osteochondroplastica (TBO)

Rare but Important
- Amyloidosis

ESSENTIAL INFORMATION

Key Differential Diagnosis Issues
- Malignant until proven otherwise
- Malignant features of tracheal mass include
  - Size more than 2 cm
  - Extraluminal component can be quite large
  - Invasion of surrounding structures

Helpful Clues for Common Diagnoses
- **Metastasis**
  - Direct invasion from adjacent tumors arising from lung, thyroid, and esophageal primary tumors
  - Metastasis from other distant primaries (e.g., melanoma) less common
- **Primary Tracheal Neoplasms**
  - **Squamous Cell Carcinoma**
    - Focal mass or diffuse nodular wall thickening
  - **Adenoid Cystic Carcinoma**
    - Common in young adults (age range: 30-56 years)
    - Extraluminal component is characteristic
    - Diffuse infiltration with submucosal extension
- **Mucus**
  - Generally not dense enough to be well seen on soft tissue window
  - Can demonstrate mobility with changing image position or coughing

Helpful Clues for Less Common Diagnoses
- **Mucoepidermoid Carcinoma**
  - Majority of patients are less than 30 years
  - Imaging features similar to other primary tracheal tumors
- **Tracheobronchopathia Osteochondroplastica (TBO)**
  - Men > 50 years
  - Cartilaginous and osseous nodules with "cobblestone" appearance
  - Spares posterior tracheal membrane

Helpful Clues for Rare Diagnoses
- **Amyloidosis**
  - Smooth, nodular, or tumoral wall thickening
  - Unlike TBO, involves posterior tracheal membrane
  - Can be soft tissue density ± calcified/ossified

Metastasis

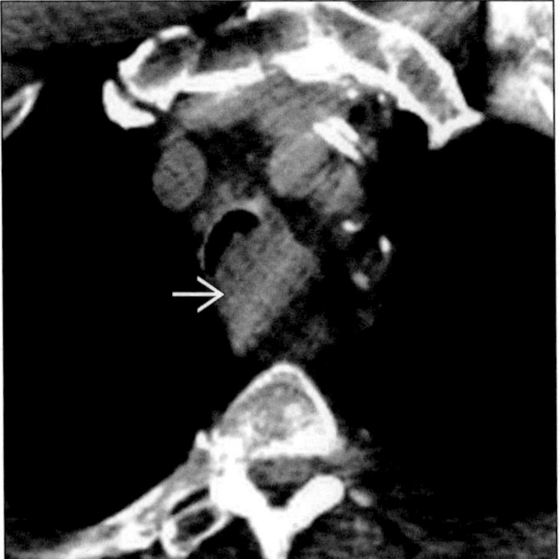

Axial NECT shows an iceberg lesion ➔ nearly completely occluding the tracheal lumen.

Squamous Cell Carcinoma

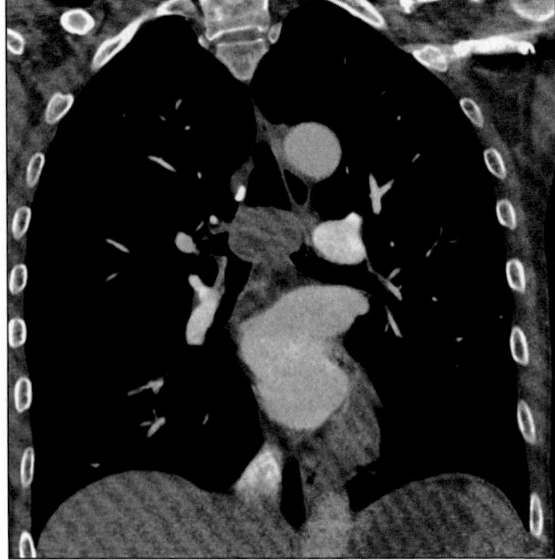

Coronal CECT in lung window shows the location and endoluminal polypoid component.

Squamous Cell Carcinoma

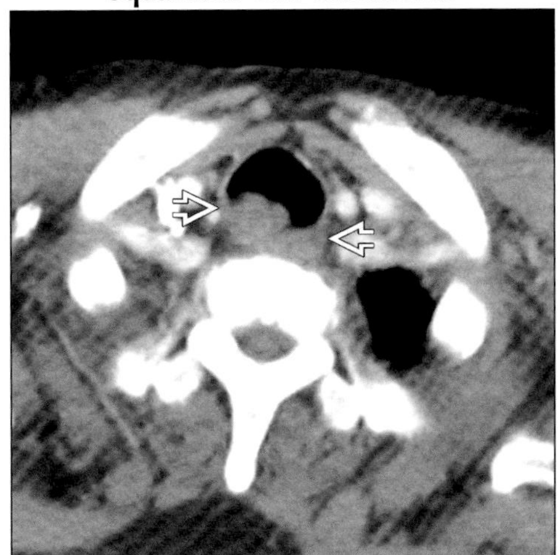

Adenoid Cystic Carcinoma

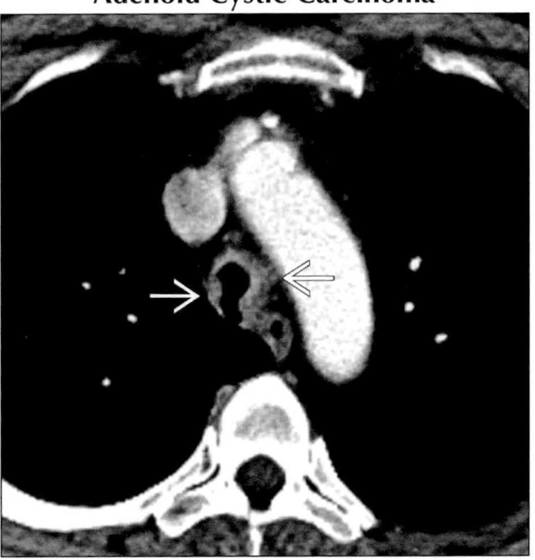

(Left) *Axial CECT shows a lobulated, homogeneous, eccentric soft tissue mass involving the posterior tracheal wall ⇨. There was no evident invasion of surrounding structures.* ***(Right)*** *Axial CECT shows nearly circumferential nodular soft tissue wall thickening of the trachea →. There is diffuse infiltration of the wall with narrowing of airway lumen. There was no invasion of surrounding structures evident.*

Mucus

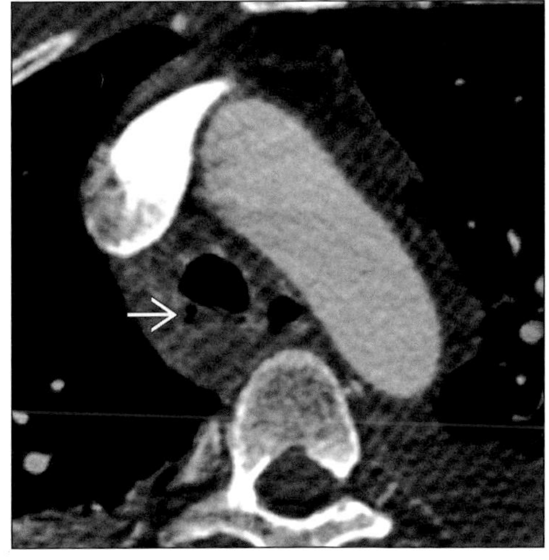

Mucoepidermoid Carcinoma

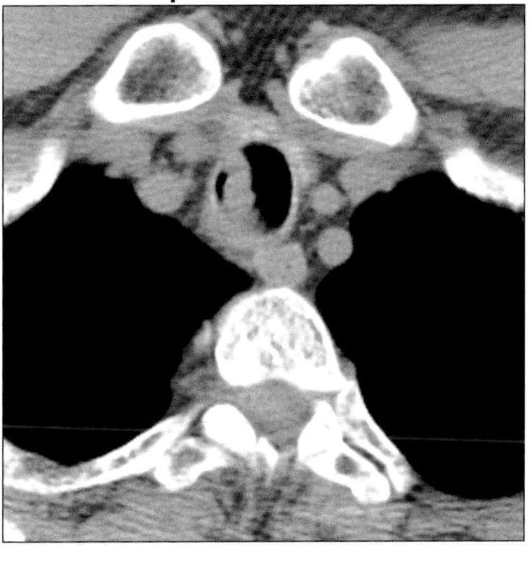

(Left) *Axial CECT shows an apparent soft tissue density in the tracheal lumen with intralesional gas →, a feature that is characteristic of mucus or mucoid material.* ***(Right)*** *Axial NECT from a different patient shows a large endoluminal "mass" at approximately the level of the thoracic inlet. This abnormality cleared on a subsequent scan.*

Tracheobronchopathia Osteochondroplastica (TBO)

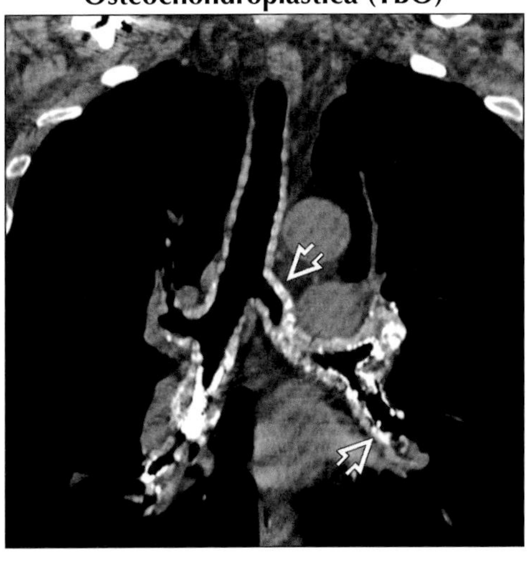

Amyloidosis

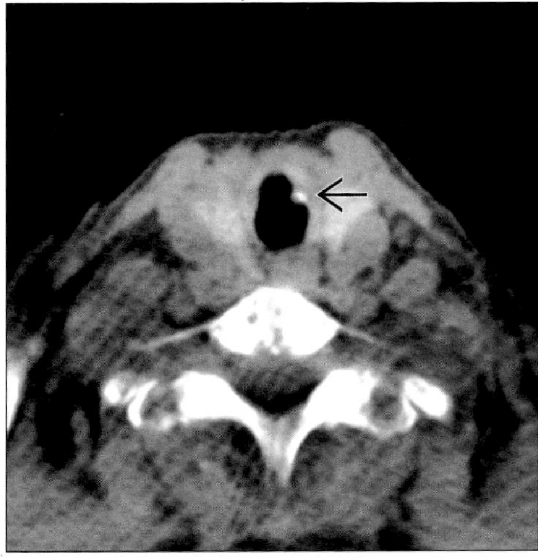

(Left) *Coronal NECT from an elderly man with cough shows extensive calcified nodular thickening of the airway walls with proliferation and protuberance of the tracheal cartilage rings ⇨.* ***(Right)*** *Axial CECT shows a focal calcified left tracheal wall nodule →, which represents a focal area of central airway amyloid deposition.*

ENDOBRONCHIAL MASS

DIFFERENTIAL DIAGNOSIS

Common
- Non-Small Cell Lung Cancer
- Small Cell Lung Cancer

Less Common
- Carcinoid
- Lung Metastases
- Other Malignant Endobronchial Tumors
- Aspiration

Rare but Important
- Bronchial Atresia
- Laryngeal Papillomatosis
- Hamartoma
- Broncholith

ESSENTIAL INFORMATION

Key Differential Diagnosis Issues
- Findings that suggest endobronchial lesion
  - Crescent of air around lesion
  - Lobar collapse or obstructive pneumonia
  - Recurrent pneumonia in same lobe
- Most neoplasms malignant
  - Vast majority non-small cell lung carcinoma
- CT has better sensitivity and specificity than chest radiography
- CT can serve as guide for bronchoscopic biopsy

Helpful Clues for Common Diagnoses
- **Non-Small Cell Lung Cancer**
  - Comprise more than 95% of malignant endobronchial tumors
  - Squamous cell most common cell type for endobronchial tumors
  - Often cause lobar or segmental atelectasis
    - Metastatic lymphadenopathy may extrinsically narrow bronchus
    - Obstructed airways may be dilated, impacted with secretions
  - Pulmonary artery and vein may be narrowed extrinsically by mass
- **Small Cell Lung Cancer**
  - 20% of all lung carcinomas
  - Usually peribronchial and invade into bronchial submucosa
    - May extend into bronchial lumen
  - Extensive metastatic lymphadenopathy common

Helpful Clues for Less Common Diagnoses
- **Carcinoid**
  - 1-2% of all pulmonary neoplasms
    - 80-90% typical carcinoids (low grade)
    - 10-20% atypical carcinoids (more aggressive)
  - Homogeneous endobronchial nodule on CT
    - 30% contain chunky calcification (apparent on radiographs in only 5%)
    - Hypervascular on contrast-enhanced imaging
  - Obstructive pneumonitis may be present
  - Lymphadenopathy from metastases
  - Reactive lymphoid hyperplasia
    - Recurrent or chronic obstructive pneumonia
- **Lung Metastases**
  - Less common than other primary sites
  - Breast, rectal, and renal carcinomas and melanoma most common
  - Can cause lobar or segmental atelectasis
  - Often enhance on CT (especially renal cell carcinoma and melanoma)
- **Other Malignant Endobronchial Tumors**
  - Adenoid cystic carcinoma
    - Vast majority arise from trachea or main bronchi
    - Lobulated or polypoid endoluminal lesion on CT
    - Associated airway wall thickening
    - May present as diffuse, irregular tracheobronchial wall thickening
  - Mucoepidermoid carcinoma
    - Most arise in segmental bronchi
    - Polypoid endoluminal lesion, usually aligned with long axis of airway
    - May extend outside of airway wall (more aggressive tumors)
  - Other cell types rare
- **Aspiration**
  - Foreign body
    - Most common in children (peak incidence between 1 and 2 years of age)
    - Food and broken teeth most frequent
    - Main bronchi most frequently affected
    - Pneumonia and atelectasis most common complications
    - Bronchiectasis may develop with prolonged retention of foreign body

- Chest radiograph shows aspirated foreign body in < 20% of patients
  - Air-trapping of affected lobe(s) important feature
  - Paired inspiratory and expiratory radiographs useful
  - Atelectasis or pneumonia in affected lobe(s)
- CT more sensitive

Helpful Clues for Rare Diagnoses

- **Bronchial Atresia**
  - Rare congenital abnormality
    - Short segment obliteration of bronchus at or near origin
    - Left upper lobe apicoposterior segmental bronchus most common
    - Lung distal to obstruction developmentally normal, may be hyperinflated
  - Most patients asymptomatic
  - Radiograph
    - Hyperlucent area of lung in ~ 90%
    - Hilar nodule or mass (bronchocele) in 80%
  - CT
    - Hyperinflated segment(s) with attenuated vessels
    - Mucoid impaction (bronchocele), finger in glove appearance
- **Laryngeal Papillomatosis**
  - Human papilloma virus mediated papillomatosis of upper aerodigestive tract
    - May progress to involve trachea, bronchi, and lungs
  - Endoluminal nodules in trachea or bronchi
  - Lung nodules
    - Often multiple, may cavitate
    - Rapid enlargement: Suspect malignant degeneration into squamous cell carcinoma
- **Hamartoma**
  - Comprise ~ 70% of benign endobronchial neoplasms
  - Approximately 5% of pulmonary hamartomas endobronchial
  - ~ 50% contain foci of fat attenuation
  - May contain "popcorn" calcification
- **Broncholith**
  - Endobronchial calcified or ossified material
    - Most caused by erosion of calcific material into airway, usually from adjacent calcified lymph node
    - Tuberculosis and histoplasmosis most common
  - Patients usually present with hemoptysis
  - Lithoptysis very uncommon; virtually diagnostic
  - Radiographs
    - Serial radiographs may show migration of calcified lesion
    - Atelectasis or obstructive pneumonitis
  - CT
    - May show bronchial distortion and better depict endoluminal calcium

Non-Small Cell Lung Cancer

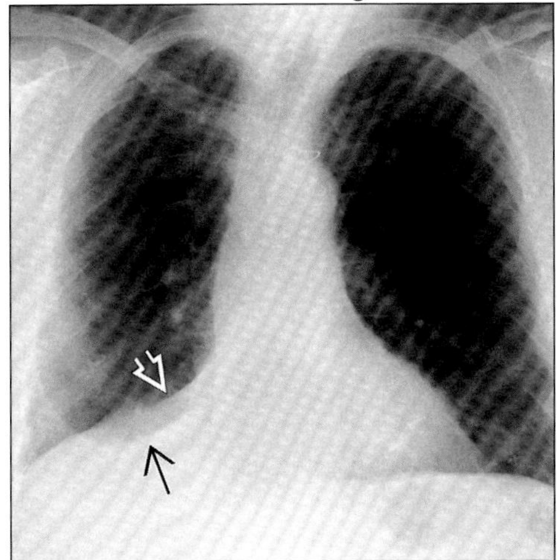

Frontal radiograph shows right middle and lower lobe collapse characterized by right lung volume loss and inferior displacement of the major ➡ and minor → fissures.

Non-Small Cell Lung Cancer

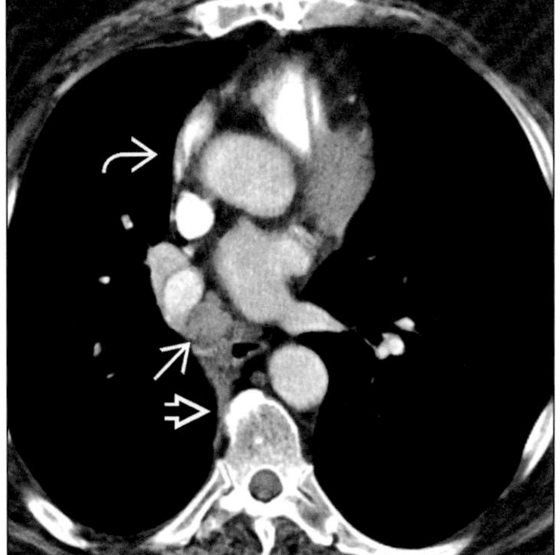

Axial CECT shows a mass filling the bronchus intermedius ➡. The right major fissure is displaced ➡, and there is mild rightward mediastinal shift ➡. Biopsy showed squamous cell carcinoma.

ENDOBRONCHIAL MASS

*(**Left**) Axial CECT shows collapsed left upper lobe ➩ that results from bronchial obstruction by heterogeneous endobronchial mass ➡ shown to be non-small cell lung carcinoma. Note the tubular mucus bronchograms. (**Right**) Axial CECT shows a small endoluminal lesion in distal left main bronchus ➩. Note bulky mediastinal and hilar metastatic lymphadenopathy ➡ and airway distortion, all common occurrences at presentation.*

Non-Small Cell Lung Cancer

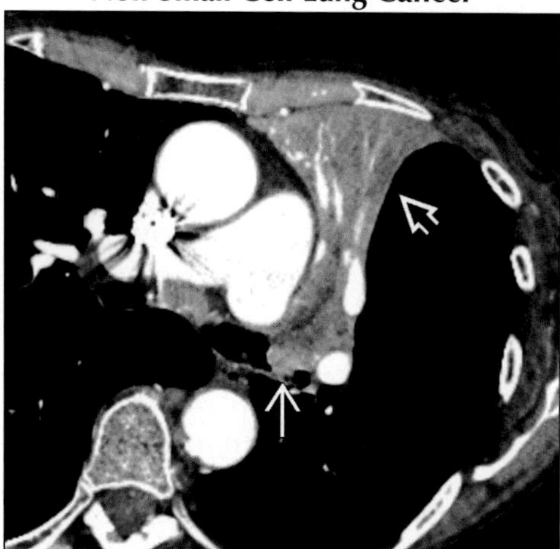

Small Cell Lung Cancer

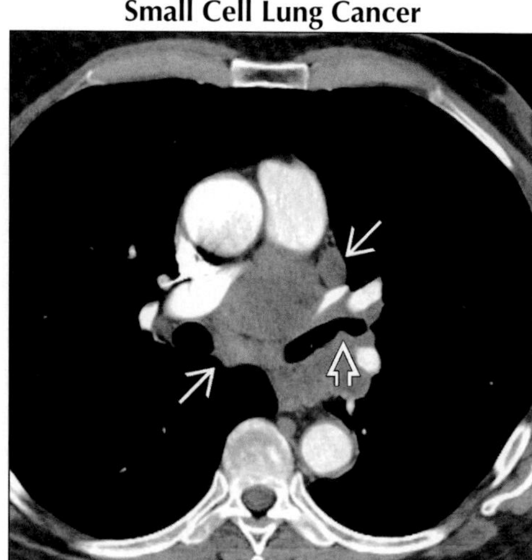

*(**Left**) Axial CECT shows an enhancing endoluminal nodule in right main bronchus ➡ shown to be a typical carcinoid on transbronchial biopsy. Lobar or pulmonary collapse can develop when an endobronchial neoplasm occludes the airway lumen. (**Right**) Sagittal CT reconstruction shows a left lower lobe nodule with smooth margins ➡ with a crescent of air along its superior margin ➩, indicating that it is endobronchial in location.*

Carcinoid

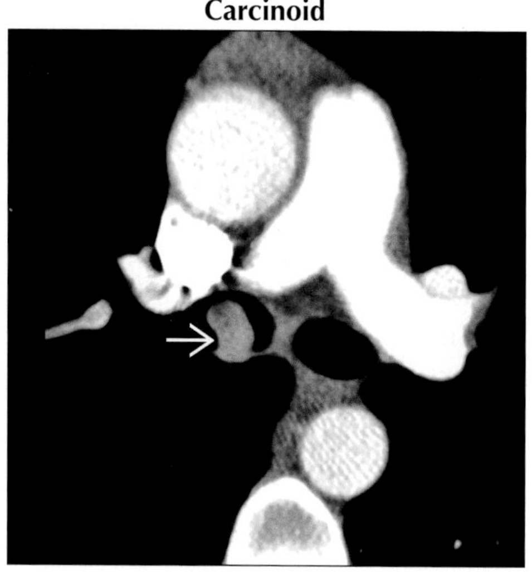

Carcinoid

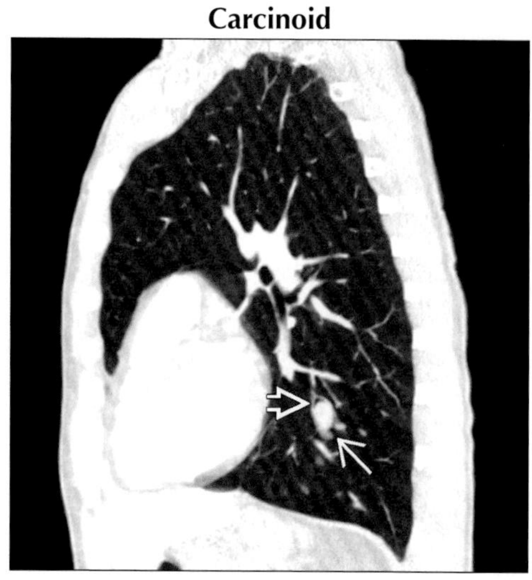

*(**Left**) Axial CECT shows a hypervascular nodule in the left upper lobe bronchus ➡ in this patient with metastatic renal cell carcinoma. Note mild obstructive atelectasis of the left upper lobe ➩. (**Right**) Coronal CT reconstruction shows round right lower lobe nodule ➡ with smooth margins extending into the lumen of the posterior basal segmental bronchus ➩. Biopsy showed mucoepidermoid carcinoma.*

Lung Metastases

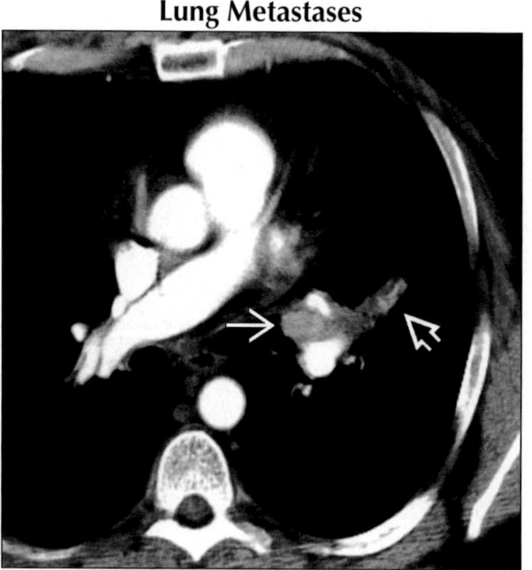

Other Malignant Endobronchial Tumors

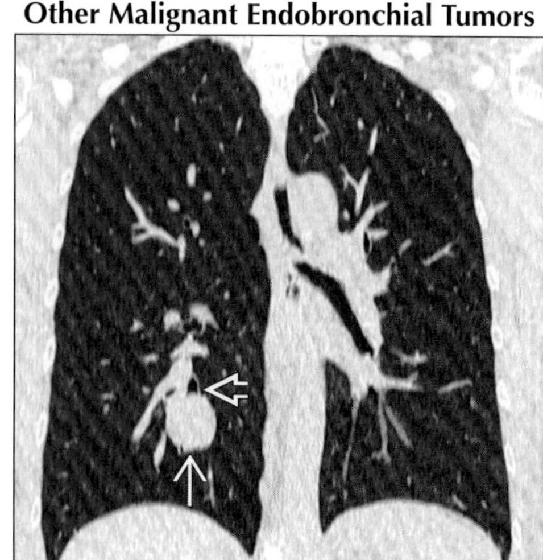

Aspiration

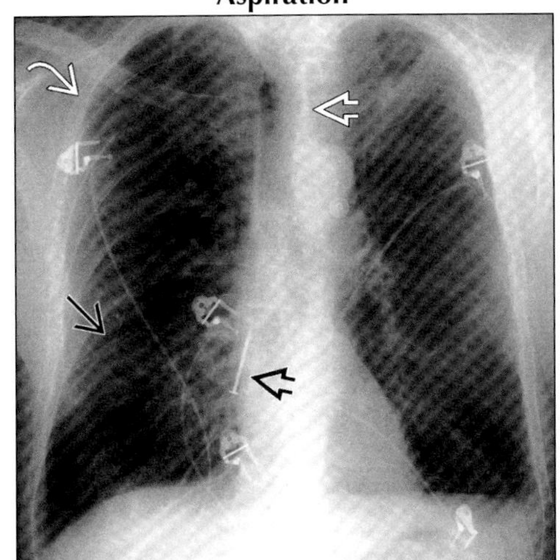

Bronchial Atresia

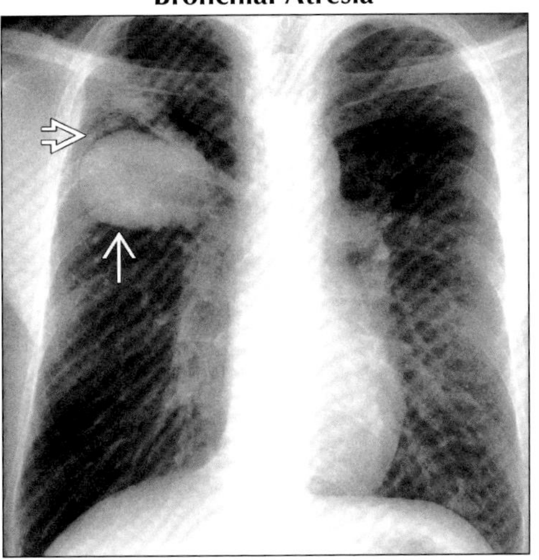

*(**Left**) Frontal radiograph shows a metallic nail projecting over the right lower lung ➲. Note relative hyperinflation of the right upper lobe ➨ and depression of the minor fissure ➔ secondary to right lower lobe atelectasis. The trachea is displaced slightly to the right at the thoracic inlet ➲. (**Right**) Frontal radiograph shows well-defined elliptical mass ➔ with peripheral air meniscus ➲ in the right upper lobe representing a bronchocele.*

Bronchial Atresia

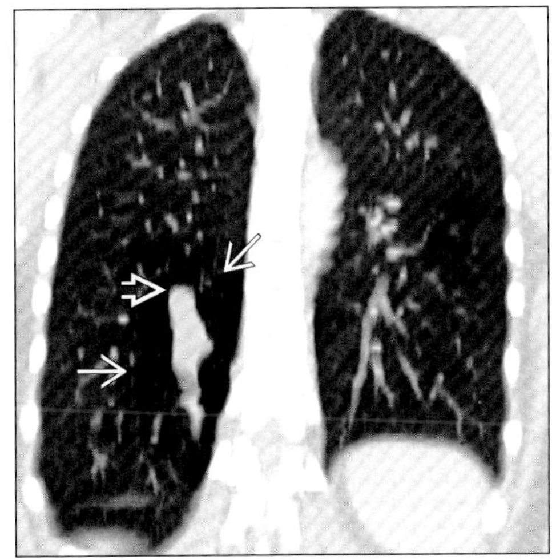

Laryngeal Papillomatosis

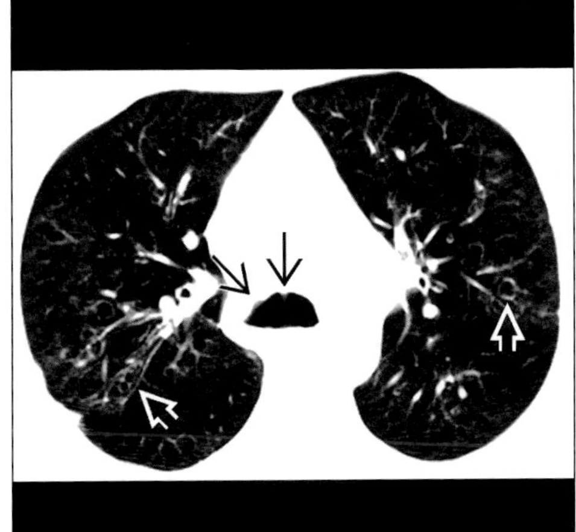

*(**Left**) Coronal CECT shows a tubular, fluid-filled structure representing a dilated bronchus ➲ in an area of low-attenuation, hyperinflated lung ➔. (**Right**) Axial NECT shows nodularity in the main bronchi at the carina ➔ in this patient with laryngotracheal papillomatosis. Note scattered cysts in the lungs ➲, characteristic of peripheral endobronchial papillomas. Rapid growth of a nodule is suspicious for malignant degeneration.*

Hamartoma

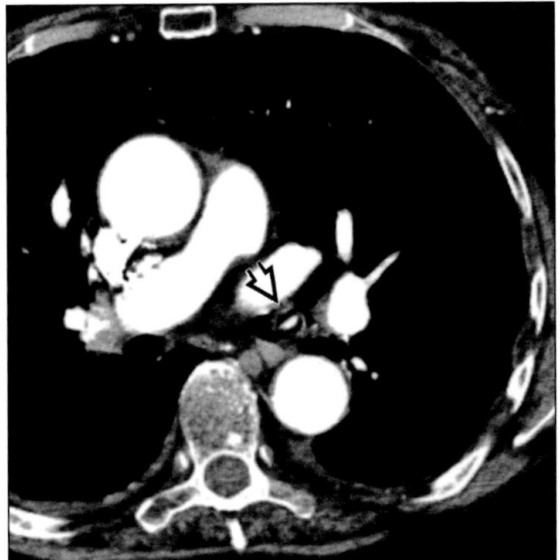

Broncholith

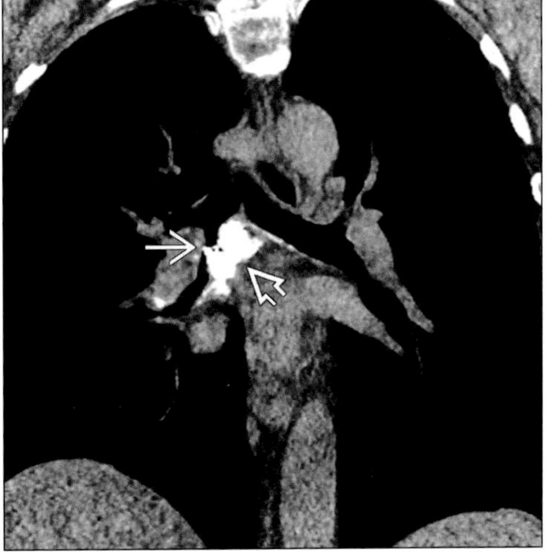

*(**Left**) Axial CECT shows endobronchial tumor in the distal left main bronchus with coarse calcification ➲. The presence of macroscopic fat within an endobronchial lesion is diagnostic of a hamartoma. (**Right**) Coronal CT reconstruction shows some large calcified subcarinal lymph nodes ➲ in a patient with remote histoplasmosis. Calcific material has eroded into the bronchus intermedius ➔. Hemoptysis from broncholiths can be severe and even fatal.*

RIGHT MIDDLE LOBE SYNDROME

DIFFERENTIAL DIAGNOSIS

Common

- Middle Lobe Syndrome
  - Central Obstruction
    - Extrinsic Obstruction by Lymph Nodes
    - Bronchostenosis
    - Endobronchial Mass (Tumor or Foreign Body)
  - Peripheral Obstruction
- Pneumonia (Mimic)
- Atelectasis (Mimic)

Less Common

- Pectus Excavatum (Mimic)

ESSENTIAL INFORMATION

Key Differential Diagnosis Issues

- Recurrent or chronic atelectasis of right middle lobe &/or lingula
- Due to extrinsic compression, central obstruction, or peripheral obstruction
  - Peripheral obstruction from lack of collateral ventilation due to complete fissures hampering clearance of secretions during coughing
- 60% benign etiology (e.g., tuberculous stricture, nodal compression)

Helpful Clues for Common Diagnoses

- **Middle Lobe Syndrome**
  - Chronic or recurrent volume loss in right middle lobe or lingula; often associated with bronchiectasis
  - Triangular opacity, which silhouettes right heart border on frontal chest radiograph
  - Wedge-shaped opacity overlying heart on lateral chest radiograph
  - CT may demonstrate endobronchial mass, lymph node, or broncholithiasis obstructing proximal bronchus
- **Pneumonia (Mimic)**
  - Ground-glass opacities to dense consolidation within right middle lobe or lingula
  - Reactive lymphadenopathy; very large lymph nodes unusual
  - Parapneumonic pleural effusion or empyema
- **Atelectasis (Mimic)**
  - Volume loss in right middle lobe or lingula
  - In acute setting, most often due to central mucous plugging or aspirated material
  - Similar imaging findings as in middle lobe syndrome
  - Mild reversible dilation of airways; not as severe as bronchiectasis in middle lobe syndrome

Helpful Clues for Less Common Diagnoses

- **Pectus Excavatum (Mimic)**
  - Sternum depressed posterior to anterior ribs
  - Right heart border obliterated as sternum displaces lung from right heart border
  - Cardiac displacement and rotation may give false appearance of cardiomegaly

Middle Lobe Syndrome

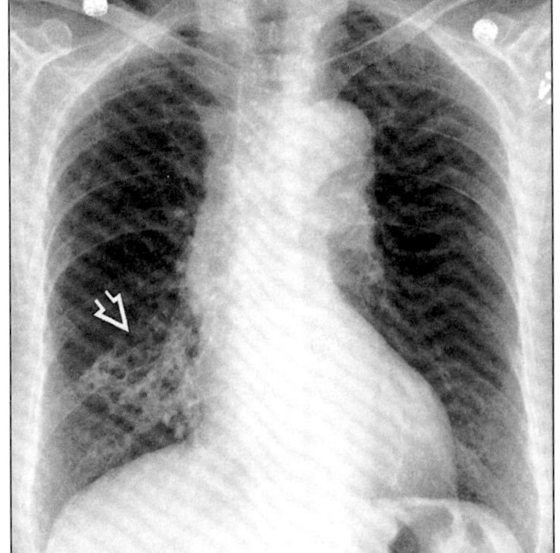

Frontal radiograph shows a triangular opacity ⇨ partially silhouetting the right heart border. There are internal cystic and tubular lucencies suggestive of bronchiectasis.

Middle Lobe Syndrome

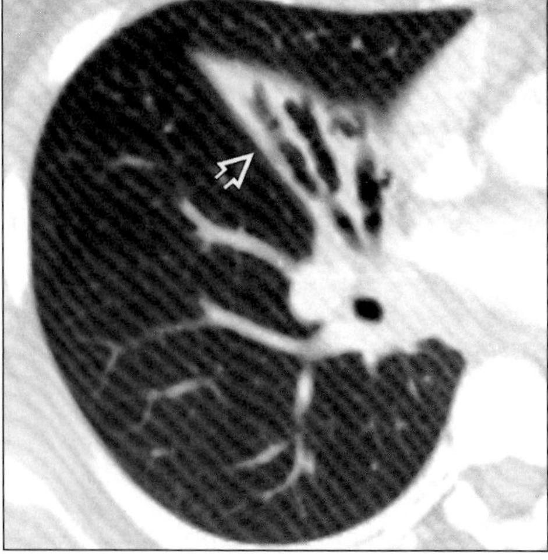

Axial CECT shows right middle lobe collapse ⇨ with associated bronchiectasis; the air-filled bronchi suggest absence of a central obstructing mass or nodule.

RIGHT MIDDLE LOBE SYNDROME

Middle Lobe Syndrome

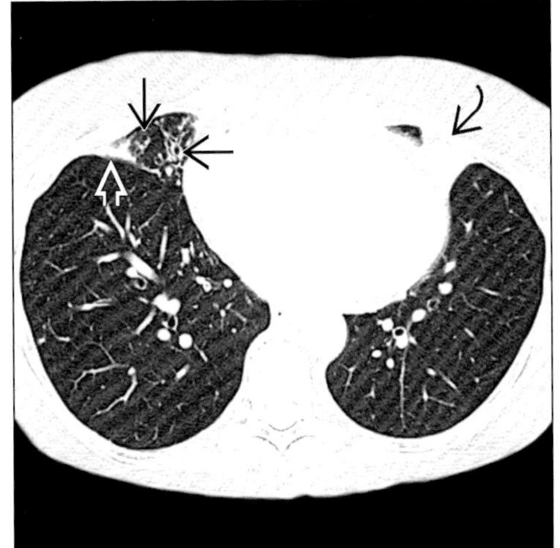

Pneumonia (Mimic)

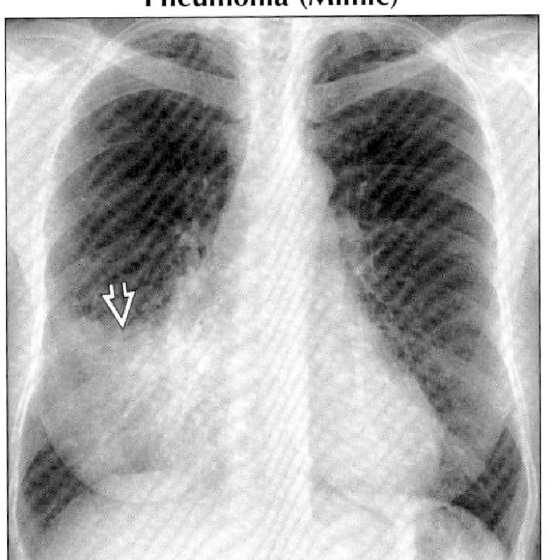

(Left) *Axial NECT shows mild cylindrical bronchiectasis ⇨ and atelectasis in the right middle lobe ➡ and lingula ⇗ related to infection with Mycobacterium avium-intracellulare.* ***(Right)*** *Frontal radiograph shows consolidation ➡ in the right middle lobe silhouetting the right heart border in this patient with fever and cough. Consolidation resolved on follow-up imaging.*

Atelectasis (Mimic)

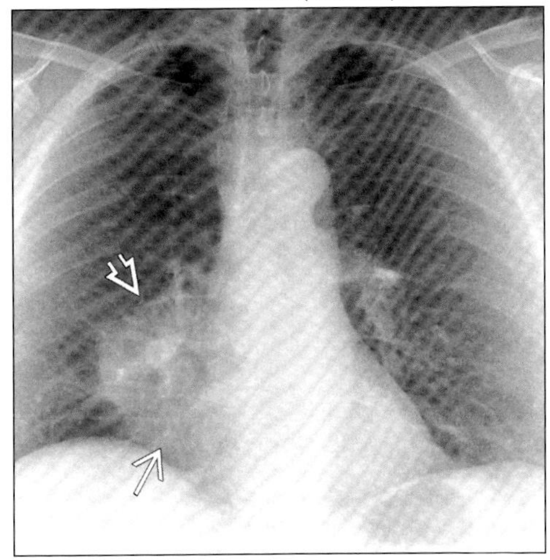

Atelectasis (Mimic)

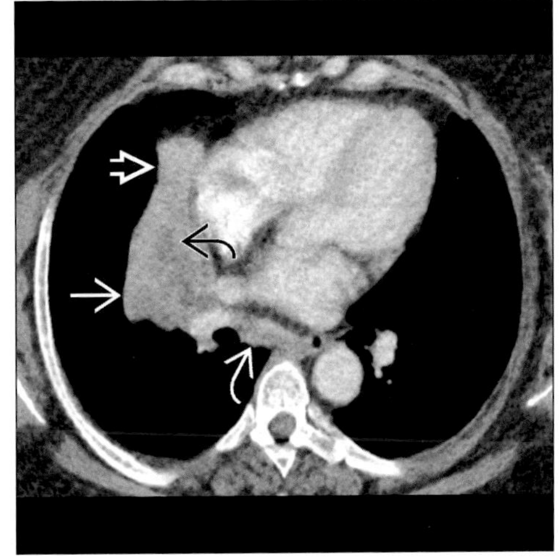

(Left) *Frontal radiograph shows a mass ➡ in the right middle lobe and postobstructive right middle lobe atelectasis ➡, which obscure the right heart border.* ***(Right)*** *Axial oblique CECT shows a low-density mass ➡ in the central aspect of the right middle lobe with postobstructive right middle lobe atelectasis ➡ and an enlarged periesophageal lymph node ➡. Note the mucus bronchograms ⇗.*

Pectus Excavatum (Mimic)

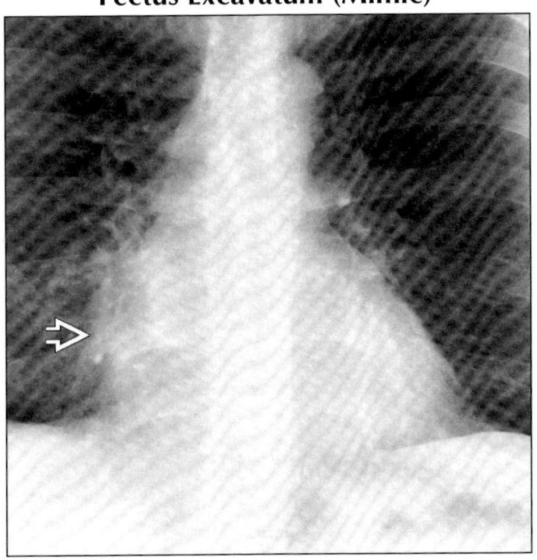

Pectus Excavatum (Mimic)

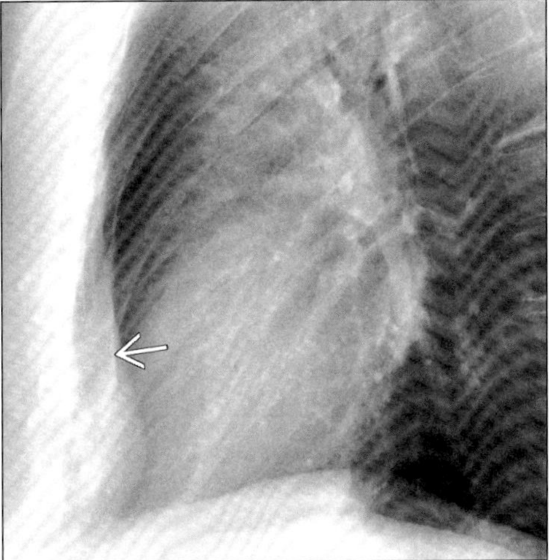

(Left) *Frontal radiograph shows loss of conspicuity ➡ of the right heart border in this patient without acute symptomatology.* ***(Right)*** *Lateral radiograph shows posterior displacement of the sternum ➡, diagnostic of pectus excavatum. Loss of the right heart border is a well-recognized manifestation of pectus excavatum, which can mimic right middle lobe syndrome or consolidation.*

BRONCHIECTASIS

DIFFERENTIAL DIAGNOSIS

Common

- Postinfectious
  - Mycobacterium Tuberculosis
  - Mycobacterial Avium Complex
  - Swyer-James (MacLeod) Syndrome
  - Aspiration (Recurrent)
- Postobstructive
  - Endobronchial Tumor
  - Lymphadenopathy
  - Foreign Body
- Traction Bronchiectasis
- Cystic Fibrosis
- Asthma

Less Common

- Allergic Bronchopulmonary Aspergillosis
- Immotile Cilia Syndrome
- Immunosuppression
  - Congenital
  - AIDS

Rare but Important

- Williams-Campbell Syndrome
- Tracheobronchomegaly (Mounier-Kuhn Syndrome)
- Young Syndrome
- Yellow-Nail Syndrome

ESSENTIAL INFORMATION

Key Differential Diagnosis Issues

- Definition: Pathologic, irreversible dilation of bronchi

Helpful Clues for Common Diagnoses

- **Postinfectious**
  - **Mycobacterium Tuberculosis**
    - Upper lung bronchiectasis
    - Signs of previous tuberculosis: Upper lung fibrocavitary disease, calcified lymph nodes, calcified granulomas
    - Low-attenuation lymphadenopathy, tree in bud or miliary nodules, or cavitary lung disease in active disease
  - **Mycobacterial Avium Complex**
    - Most common in older women
    - Cylindrical bronchiectasis most severe in middle lobe and lingula
    - Tree in bud nodules, larger random nodules (occasionally cavitate)
    - In minority of cases, mimics upper lung fibrocavitary disease of reactivation tuberculosis
  - **Swyer-James (MacLeod) Syndrome**
    - Due to childhood pneumonia (adenovirus, measles, *Mycoplasma*, pertussis)
    - Bilateral but asymmetric process; usually more involvement of 1 lung
    - Unilateral hyperlucency of more affected lung: Hypoplasia of pulmonary vasculature and constrictive bronchiolitis
    - Small to normal size of more affected lung
  - **Aspiration (Recurrent)**
    - Predisposition in patients with neuromuscular disorders or esophageal abnormalities
    - Dependent portions of lungs: Superior and basilar segments of lower lobes (right greater than left)
- **Postobstructive**
  - **Endobronchial Tumor**
    - Squamous cell carcinoma in older patients with history of smoking
    - Carcinoid tumor in young patients; often low activity on FDG PET
  - **Lymphadenopathy**
    - Chronic extrinsic compression of bronchi
    - A cause of middle lobe syndrome: Chronic atelectasis and bronchiectasis in middle lobe or lingula
  - **Foreign Body**
    - Abnormal fixed hyperinflation > atelectasis of lung or lobe even with expiration or lateral decubitus positioning
    - Direct visualization of foreign body (CT > radiographs)
- **Traction Bronchiectasis**
  - Concomitant end-stage lung disease or pulmonary fibrosis, radiation fibrosis
  - Reticular opacities, interlobular septal thickening, architectural distortion, honeycombing
- **Cystic Fibrosis**
  - Upper lung bronchiectasis; air-trapping; tree in bud opacities &/or centrilobular nodules
  - Fatty atrophy of pancreas

- **Asthma**
  - Mild cylindrical bronchiectasis with patchy regions of air-trapping and bronchial wall thickening

Helpful Clues for Less Common Diagnoses

- **Allergic Bronchopulmonary Aspergillosis**
  - Central cystic bronchiectasis and severe mucus plugging or air-fluid levels in asthmatic
- **Immotile Cilia Syndrome**
  - Middle and lower lobe bronchiectasis, situs inversus/dextrocardiac in 50%, paranasal sinusitis, male infertility
- **Immunosuppression**
  - **Congenital**
    - e.g., primary impaired cellular or humoral immunity, infantile X-linked agammaglobulinemia
    - Bronchiectasis secondary to recurrent infection
    - Hypogammaglobulinemia: Lower lung preponderance, severe bronchial wall thickening
    - Common variable immune deficiency syndrome: Concomitant reticular opacities
  - **AIDS**
    - Likely secondary to recurrent bacterial infection; lower lobe preponderance; air-trapping

Helpful Clues for Rare Diagnoses

- **Williams-Campbell Syndrome**
  - Defective cartilage in 4th to 6th order bronchi
  - Central cystic bronchiectasis; collapse with expiration and dilation with inspiration
- **Tracheobronchomegaly (Mounier-Kuhn Syndrome)**
  - Dilation of trachea and main bronchi; tracheal diverticula along posterior aspect of trachea; ± tracheomalacia
  - Central cystic bronchiectasis
- **Young Syndrome**
  - Resembles immotile cilia syndrome: Paranasal sinusitis, bronchiectasis, male infertility
- **Yellow-Nail Syndrome**
  - Bronchiectasis in setting of abnormally thick, discolored nails; exudative pleural effusions; lymphedema

Alternative Differential Approaches

- Unilateral bronchiectasis
  - Post-primary tuberculosis
  - Bronchial stenosis: Bronchial atresia, postinfectious, sarcoidosis
  - Obstructing endobronchial tumor
  - Foreign body
- Bilateral or diffuse bronchiectasis
  - Congenital: Cystic fibrosis, immotile cilia syndrome, congenital immunodeficiency
  - Infection: Recurrent aspiration, post-viral, allergic bronchopulmonary aspergillosis
  - Traction bronchiectasis

Mycobacterium Tuberculosis

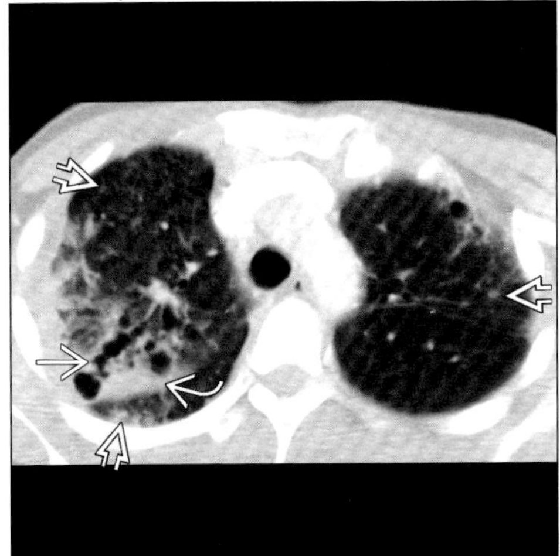

Axial CECT shows right upper lobe bronchiectasis ➡ with adjacent consolidation ➡ and bilateral small nodular opacities ➡ in this patient with active mycobacterial tuberculosis infection.

Mycobacterial Avium Complex

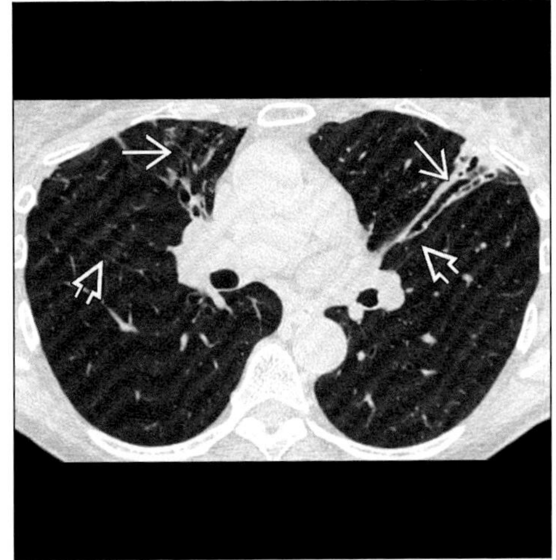

Axial NECT in this elderly woman shows mild bronchiectasis ➡ in the right middle lobe and lingula; there is associated volume loss suggested by anterior displacement of the major fissures ➡.

BRONCHIECTASIS

(**Left**) *Axial NECT shows bronchiectasis, paucity of vessels, and decreased density of the left lung, consistent with Swyer-James (MacLeod) syndrome. The patient had a history of a severe childhood respiratory infection.* (**Right**) *Axial NECT shows left lower lobe patchy centrilobular opacities and mild peribronchial thickening as well as left lower lobe mucus plugging within bronchiectatic airways in this patient with a history of chronic aspiration.*

Swyer-James (MacLeod) Syndrome

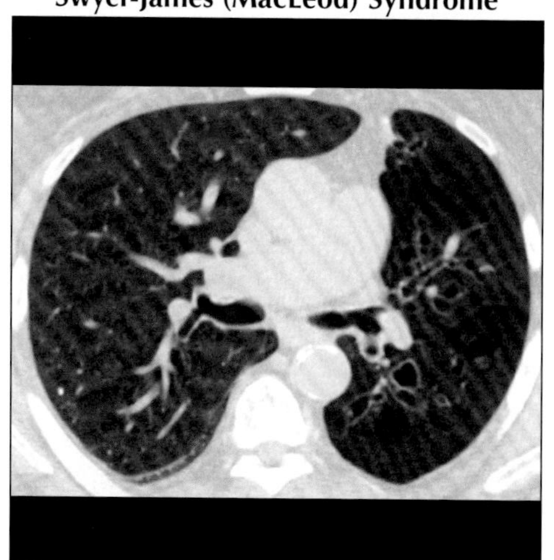

Aspiration (Recurrent)

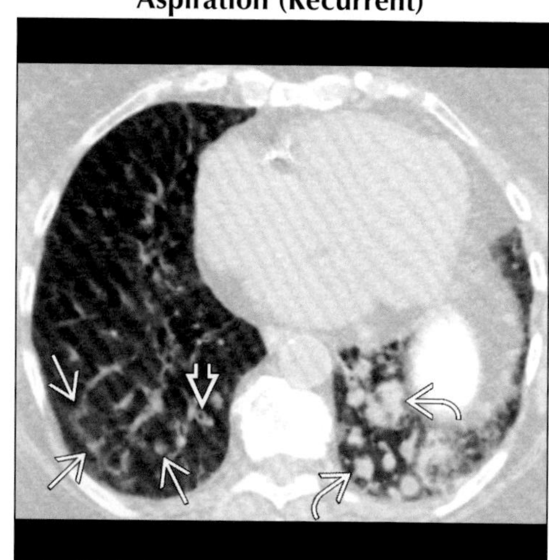

(**Left**) *Axial CECT in a young woman shows a partially calcified mass with posterior displacement of the major fissure. The patient's young age and calcification of the mass were consistent with the histological diagnosis of carcinoid tumor.* (**Right**) *Axial CECT more inferiorly shows partial right lower lobe atelectasis, postobstructive right lower lobe bronchiectasis (suggesting a longstanding process), and mucus plugging.*

Postobstructive

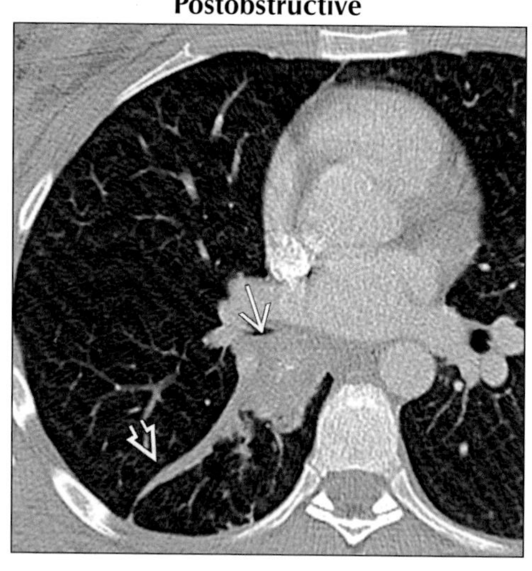

Postobstructive

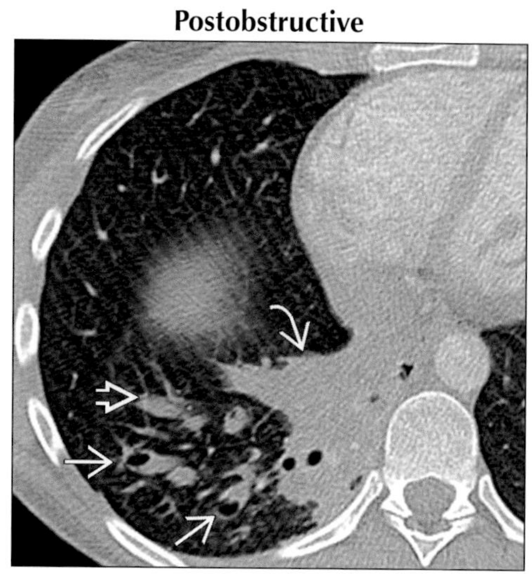

(**Left**) *Axial CECT shows a heterogeneously enhancing non-small cell lung cancer in the right lower lobe with a linear, low-density structure highly consistent with postobstructive bronchiectasis/mucus plugging.* (**Right**) *Axial CECT more inferiorly shows low-density branching structures emanating distally from the non-small cell lung cancer, highly suggestive of postobstructive bronchiectasis/mucus plugging.*

Postobstructive

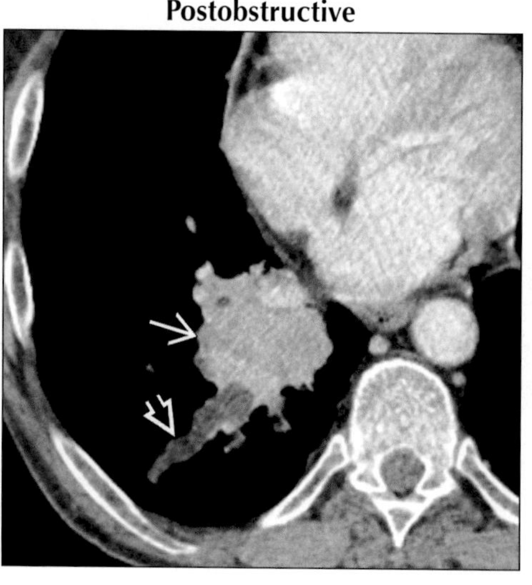

Postobstructive

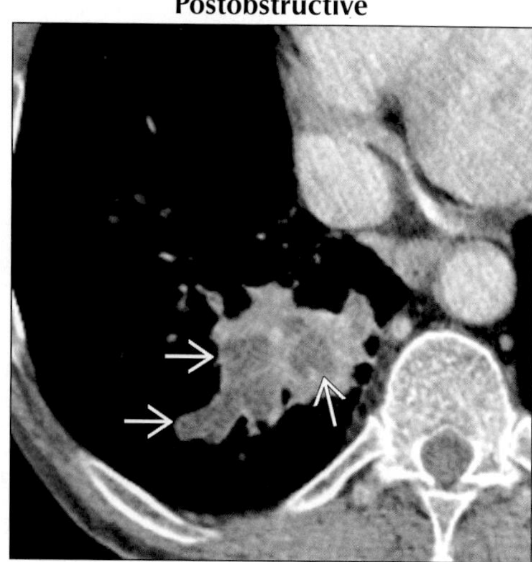

BRONCHIECTASIS

Traction Bronchiectasis

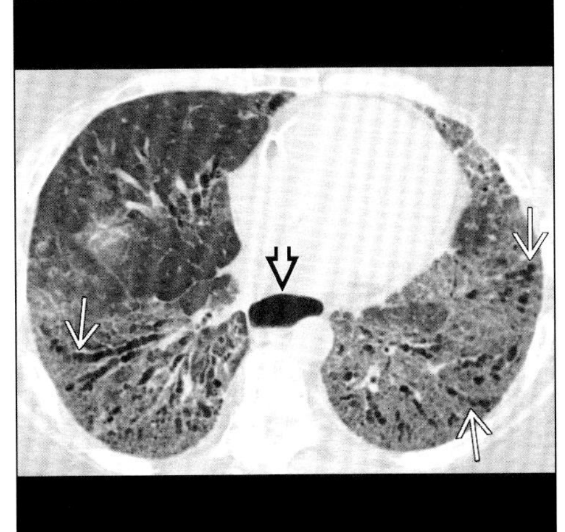

Traction Bronchiectasis

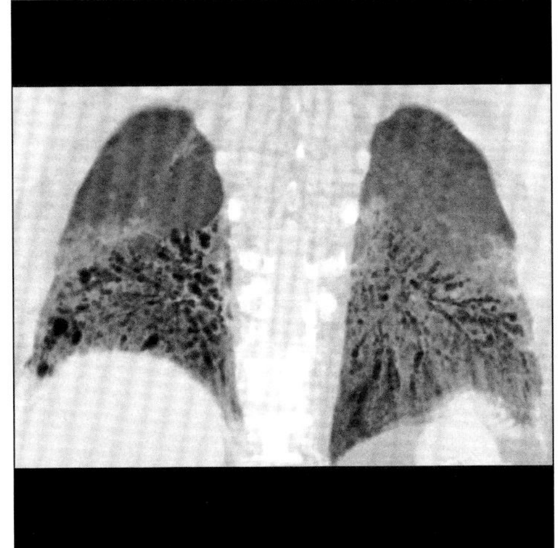

(Left) *Axial NECT shows diffuse pulmonary ground-glass opacity with less confluent involvement of the right middle and varicoid traction bronchiectasis ➡, highly suggestive of nonspecific interstitial pneumonitis. Concomitant esophageal dilation ⇨ is consistent with the patient's underlying diagnosis of scleroderma.* ***(Right)*** *Coronal NECT in the same patient shows symmetric, diffuse ground-glass opacity and traction bronchiectasis in the lower lobes.*

Traction Bronchiectasis

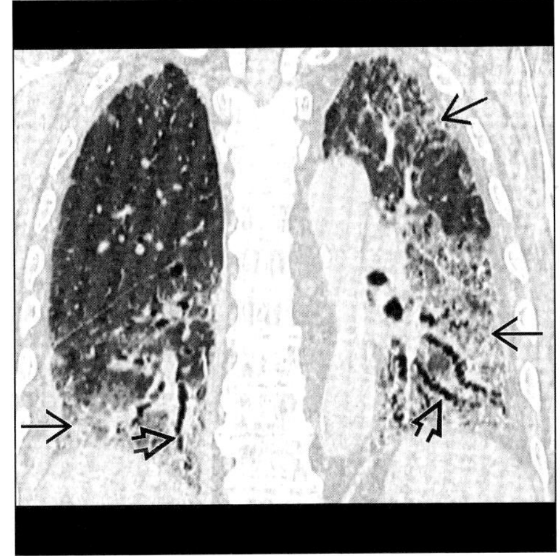

Cystic Fibrosis

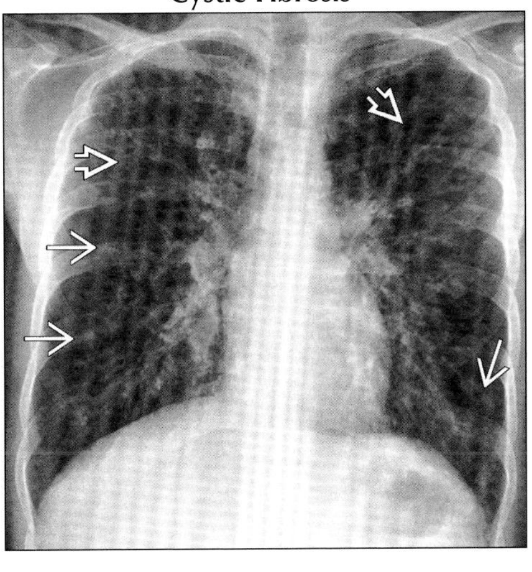

(Left) *Coronal NECT shows basilar and peripheral predominant ground-glass opacity → and lower lobe traction bronchiectasis ⇨ in this patient with fibrotic nonspecific interstitial pneumonitis.* ***(Right)*** *Frontal radiograph shows diffuse bronchiectasis ⇨ and mucus plugging ➡ in this patient with cystic fibrosis.*

Cystic Fibrosis

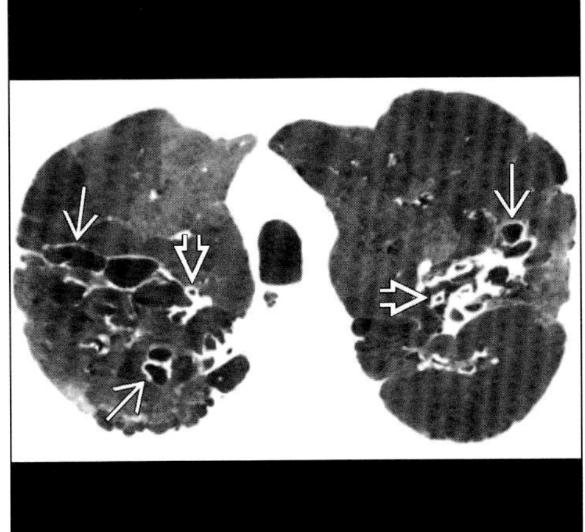

Cystic Fibrosis

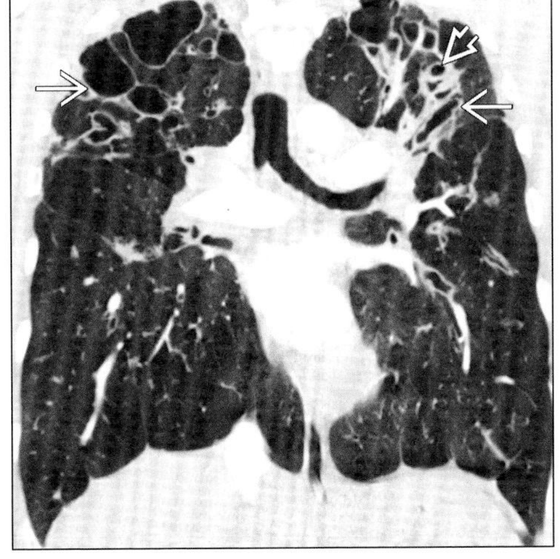

(Left) *Axial CECT minimum intensity projection image (minIP) shows bilateral bronchiectasis ➡ and peribronchial thickening ⇨ in this patient with cystic fibrosis. There is mosaic attenuation, consistent with air-trapping. MinIP images are an excellent method to display low-attenuation structures such as the airways.* ***(Right)*** *Coronal CECT shows severe biapical bronchiectasis ➡ with associated architectural distortion and peribronchial thickening ⇨.*

BRONCHIECTASIS

*(**Left**) Frontal radiograph shows central lung predominant bronchiectasis → and right upper lobe mucus plugging ↪. The so-called finger in glove sign can be seen in patients with allergic bronchopulmonary aspergillosis. (**Right**) Axial NECT shows bilateral varicoid bronchiectasis → and right upper lobe mucous plugging ↪ (finger in glove) in this patient with allergic bronchopulmonary aspergillosis.*

Allergic Bronchopulmonary Aspergillosis

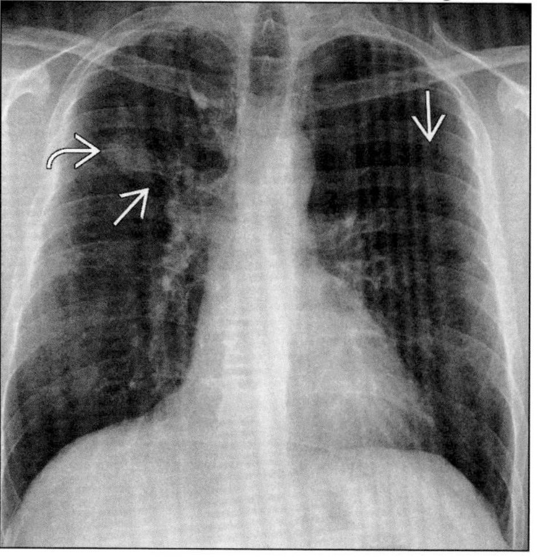

Allergic Bronchopulmonary Aspergillosis

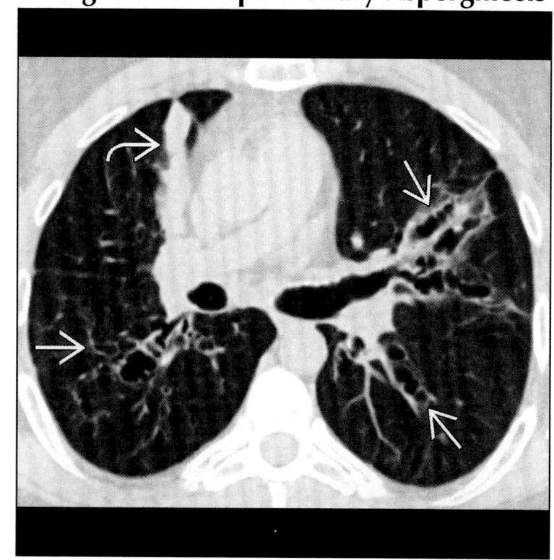

*(**Left**) Coronal NECT shows bilateral central predominant bronchiectasis → in this patient with asthma and allergic bronchopulmonary aspergillosis. Note the variation in severity, from mild cylindrical to varicoid to cystic bronchiectasis. (**Right**) Frontal radiograph shows dextrocardia ⇨, a right aortic arch →, and a right-sided stomach ⇨, consistent with situs inversus in this patient with immotile cilia syndrome.*

Allergic Bronchopulmonary Aspergillosis

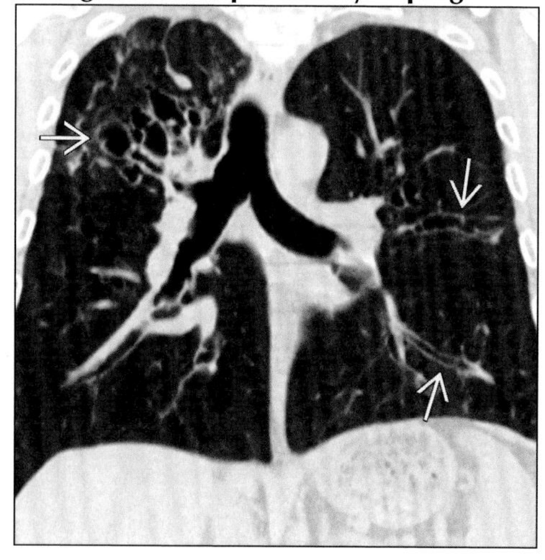

Immotile Cilia Syndrome

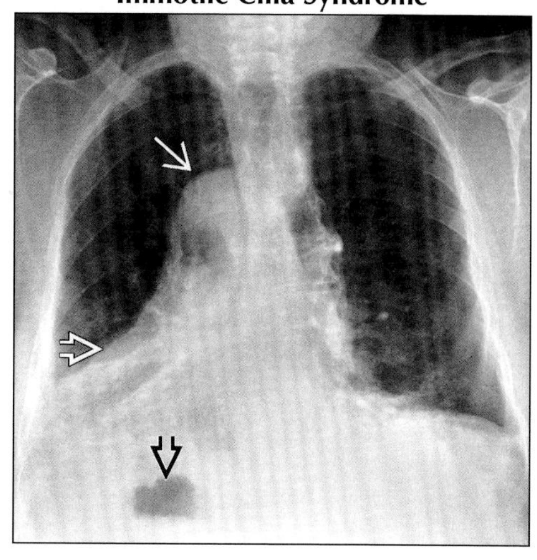

*(**Left**) Axial NECT shows bilateral bronchiectasis →, tree in bud opacities ↪, and dextrocardia highly suggestive of immotile cilia syndrome. The enlarged azygous vein → is due to azygous continuation of the IVC. (**Right**) Axial NECT shows dextrocardia and widespread lower lung bronchiectasis → with superimposed volume loss. The triad of bronchiectasis, situs inversus, and sinusitis is known as Kartagener syndrome.*

Immotile Cilia Syndrome

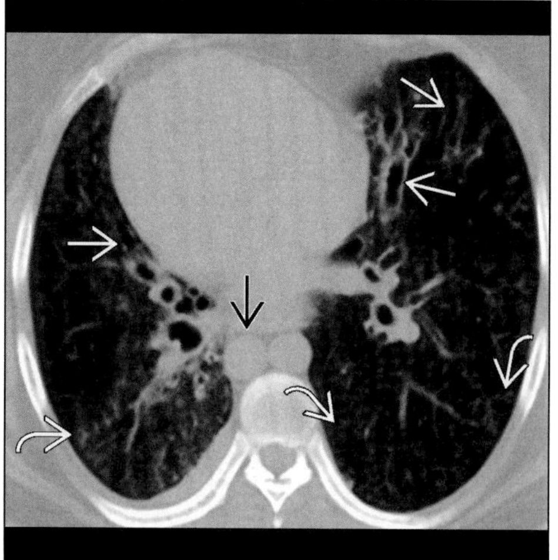

Immotile Cilia Syndrome

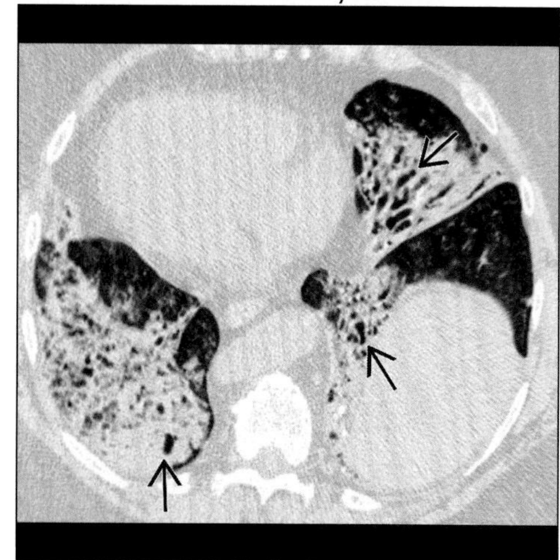

BRONCHIECTASIS

Immunosuppression

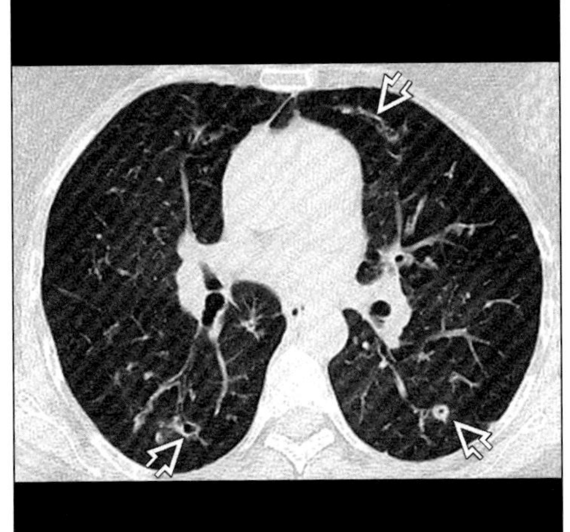

Williams-Campbell Syndrome

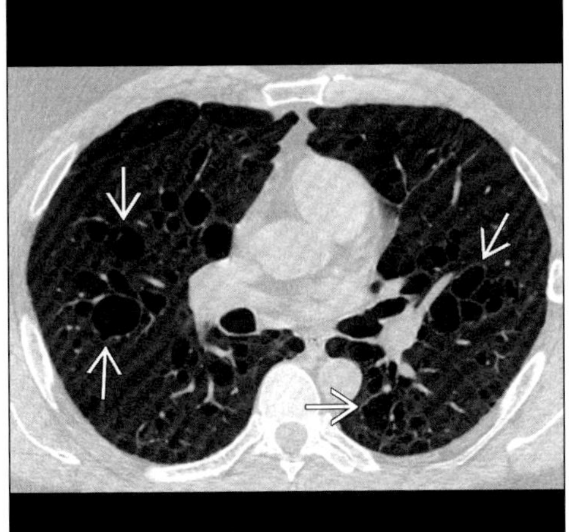

(Left) *Axial HRCT shows mild bilateral peripheral bronchiectasis ➔ from recurrent infection in this patient with common variable immunodeficiency syndrome.* ***(Right)*** *Axial NECT shows cystic bronchiectasis ➔ within the 4th to 6th order bronchi without dilation of central airways, diagnostic of Williams-Campbell syndrome. These findings can be easily confused for a cystic lung disease. MinIP reconstructions can be very helpful.*

Williams-Campbell Syndrome

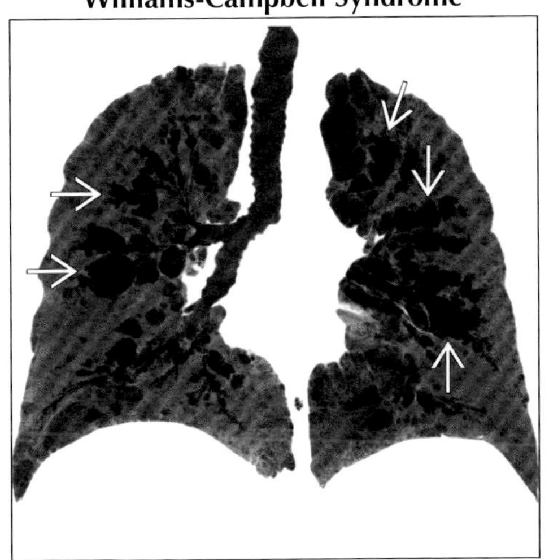

Tracheobronchomegaly (Mounier-Kuhn Syndrome)

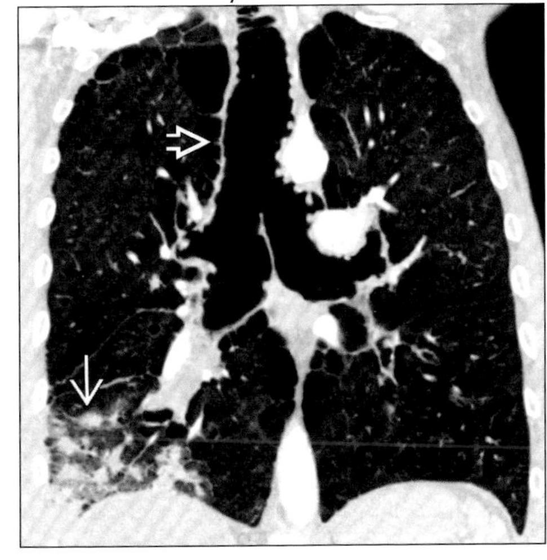

(Left) *Coronal NECT minIP image shows cystic bronchiectasis ➔ within the 4th to 6th order bronchi.* ***(Right)*** *Coronal CECT shows corrugated dilation of the central large airways ➔, essentially diagnostic of tracheobronchomegaly (also called Mounier-Kuhn syndrome). There is nodular right lower lobe pneumonia ➔; patients with tracheobronchomegaly are susceptible to recurrent pneumonia and bronchiectasis.*

Yellow-Nail Syndrome

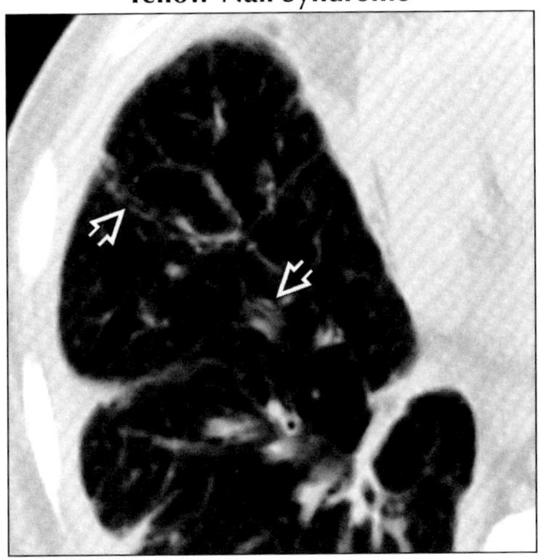

Yellow-Nail Syndrome

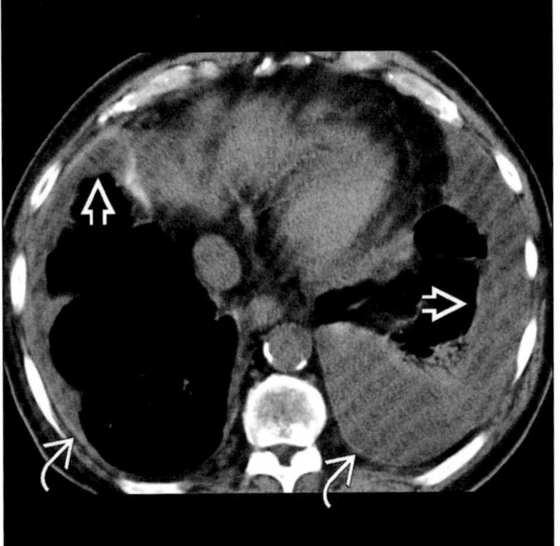

(Left) *Axial NECT shows mild cylindrical bronchiectasis ➔ in this patient with yellow-nail syndrome. Only 40% of patients with this syndrome have bronchiectasis.* ***(Right)*** *Axial NECT shows pleural thickening ➔ and loculated pleural effusion ➔ as manifestations of lymphedema in this patient with yellow-nail syndrome.*

FINGER IN GLOVE APPEARANCE

DIFFERENTIAL DIAGNOSIS

Common

- Allergic Bronchopulmonary Aspergillosis
- Congenital Bronchial Atresia

Less Common

- Cystic Fibrosis
- Obstructing Mass

ESSENTIAL INFORMATION

Key Differential Diagnosis Issues

- Finger in glove refers to mucoid impaction with dilation of large bronchi resulting in tubular or branching opacities
- Initially described in patients with allergic bronchopulmonary aspergillosis (ABPA)
- Tubular opacities seen on radiography may be bronchial or vascular in origin
- Can be confused with arteriovenous malformation on radiography
- CT reveals low-attenuation mucus in dilated central bronchi, thus differentiating from vascular causes

Helpful Clues for Common Diagnoses

- **Allergic Bronchopulmonary Aspergillosis**
  - Hypersensitivity reaction to *Aspergillus* antigens, usually *A. fumigatus*
  - Usually occurs in patients with asthma or cystic fibrosis
  - Associated with elevated IgE levels and peripheral eosinophilia
  - Usually affects upper lobes
  - Secretions may be hyperattenuating on CT due to presence of calcium oxalate
- **Congenital Bronchial Atresia**
  - Due to congenital atresia of segmental bronchus
  - Usually incidental finding but may cause recurrent infections in 20% of patients
  - Most common in apicoposterior segment of left upper lobe, followed by right upper lobe
  - CT reveals surrounding pulmonary hyperlucency due to air-trapping and oligemia

Helpful Clues for Less Common Diagnoses

- **Cystic Fibrosis**
  - Congenital disease caused by chloride channel mutation on chromosome 7
  - Recurrent infections lead to progressive bronchial wall injury
  - CT findings include bronchiectasis, mucoid impaction, peribronchial thickening, mosaic perfusion, and tree in bud opacities
- **Obstructing Mass**
  - Rare benign endobronchial tumors include lipoma, papilloma, and hamartoma
  - Malignant tumors are more common, including carcinoid, bronchogenic carcinoma, and endobronchial metastasis
  - Obstructing tumor may be directly visualized on CT

Allergic Bronchopulmonary Aspergillosis

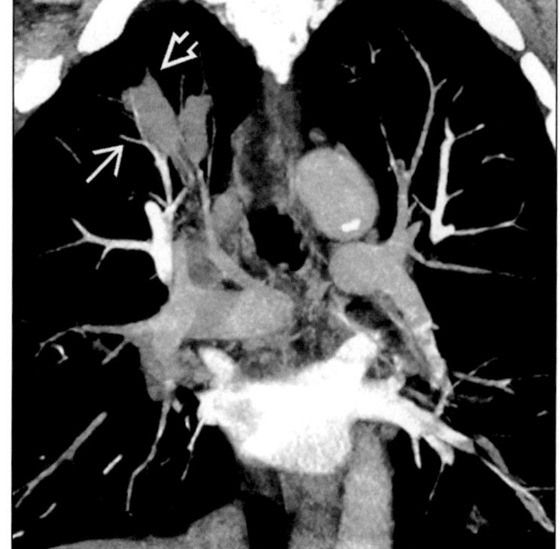

Coronal CECT MIP image shows finger in glove formation in the right upper lobe bronchi ➡. Notice how much larger the bronchi are than the adjacent pulmonary vessels ➡.

Allergic Bronchopulmonary Aspergillosis

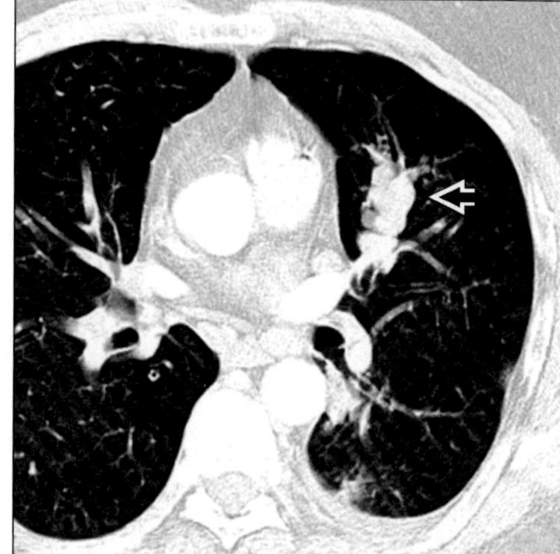

Axial CECT shows dilated, branching, and mucoid-impacted bronchi radiating from the hilum into the left upper lobe ➡ in this patient with allergic bronchopulmonary aspergillosis.

Allergic Bronchopulmonary Aspergillosis

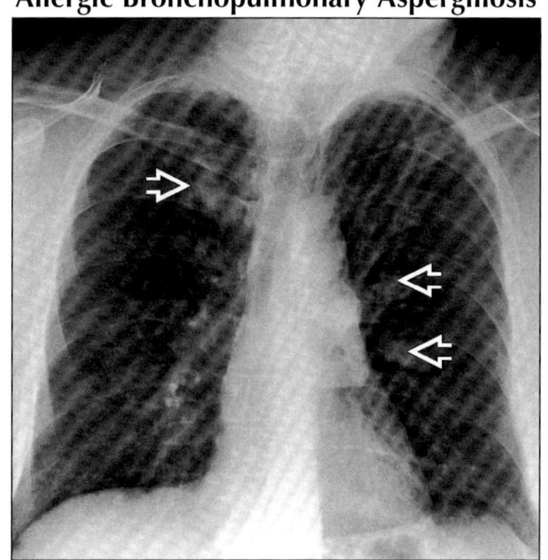

Allergic Bronchopulmonary Aspergillosis

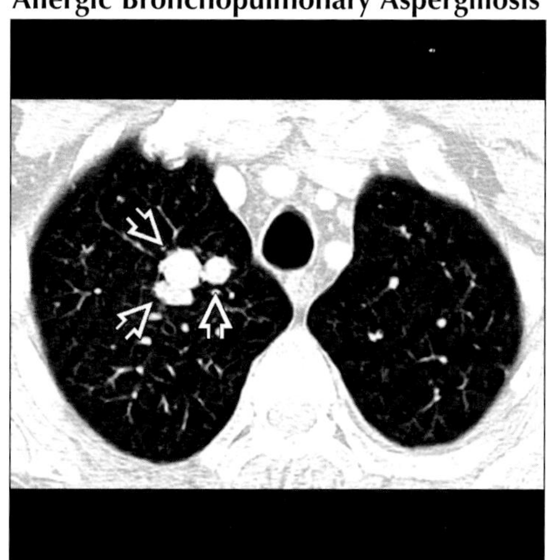

*(**Left**) Frontal radiograph shows multiple oval and tubular opacities bilaterally within the lungs ➡. (**Right**) Axial CECT in the same patient shows 3 dilated, mucoid-impacted bronchi in the right upper lobe ➡. This corresponds to the tubular opacities seen on the chest radiograph. This is a typical appearance of allergic bronchopulmonary aspergillosis.*

Allergic Bronchopulmonary Aspergillosis

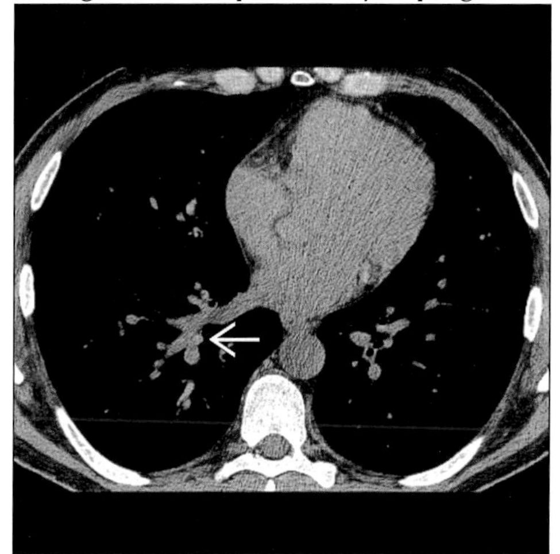

Congenital Bronchial Atresia

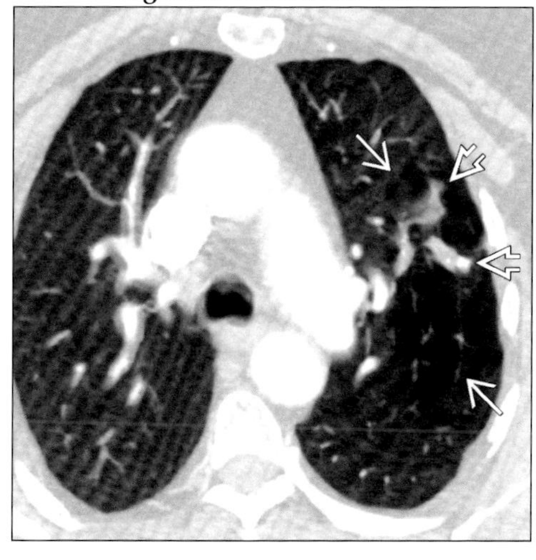

*(**Left**) Axial HRCT shows high-density mucoid impaction ➡ in this patient with allergic bronchopulmonary aspergillosis. This appearance of high-density material is caused by deposition of calcium oxalate and is suggestive of the diagnosis. (**Right**) Axial CECT shows dilated mucus-impacted bronchi in the left upper lobe ➡. There is hyperlucency of the surrounding pulmonary parenchyma ➡, typical of congenital bronchial atresia.*

Cystic Fibrosis

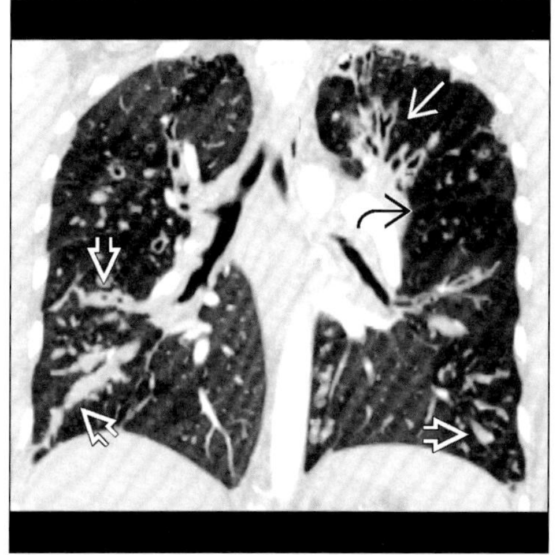

Obstructing Mass

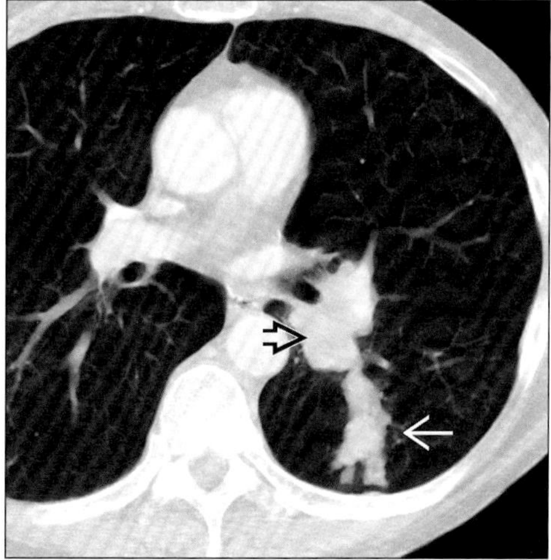

*(**Left**) Coronal CECT shows bronchiectasis with mucoid impaction ➡. Also notice diffuse bronchial wall thickening ➡ and patchy areas of air-trapping ➡. These findings are typical of cystic fibrosis. (**Right**) Axial CECT shows a central small cell carcinoma obstructing a left lower lobe bronchus ➡ with resultant dilation and mucoid impaction of the distal airways ➡.*

SECTION 3
Small Airways

MOSAIC PATTERN

DIFFERENTIAL DIAGNOSIS

Common
- Constrictive Bronchiolitis
- Hypersensitivity Pneumonitis
- Cystic Fibrosis
- Pulmonary Arterial Hypertension

Less Common
- Inflammatory Bronchiolitis

Rare but Important
- Chronic Pulmonary Thromboembolism

ESSENTIAL INFORMATION

Key Differential Diagnosis Issues
- Differentiating small airway disease from vascular disease-related mosaic pattern
  - Associated direct features of small airway disease, such as centrilobular nodules, bronchiolar wall thickening, bronchiolectasis, and bronchiectasis
  - Mosaic pattern from air-trapping shows diminished vascular caliber
  - Accentuation of mosaic pattern on expiratory scans
  - Pulmonary vascular diseases show markedly enlarged central pulmonary arteries as dominant feature
- "Head cheese" sign
  - Presence of ground-glass opacity, normal lung and air-trapping

Helpful Clues for Common Diagnoses
- **Constrictive Bronchiolitis**
  - Classic small airways disease associated with these clinical syndromes
    - Postinfectious: Patchy and bilateral
    - Swyer-James syndrome/McLeod syndrome: Classic description is unilateral disease but uncommon
    - Rheumatoid arthritis or other connective tissue diseases
    - Post lung transplant (bronchiolitis obliterans syndrome)
    - Chronic graft vs. host disease
- **Hypersensitivity Pneumonitis**
  - Poorly defined centrilobular opacities or nodules; "head cheese" sign
- **Cystic Fibrosis**
  - Extensive central and upper lung bronchiectasis and mucus plugging in younger patients
- **Pulmonary Arterial Hypertension**
  - Enlarged central pulmonary arteries

Helpful Clues for Less Common Diagnoses
- **Inflammatory Bronchiolitis**
  - Centrilobular nodules and tree in bud appearance are more common; acute or chronic airway infections most likely

Helpful Clues for Rare Diagnoses
- **Chronic Pulmonary Thromboembolism**
  - Presence of peripheral filling defects, intimal irregularities, bands and webs within pulmonary arteries

Constrictive Bronchiolitis

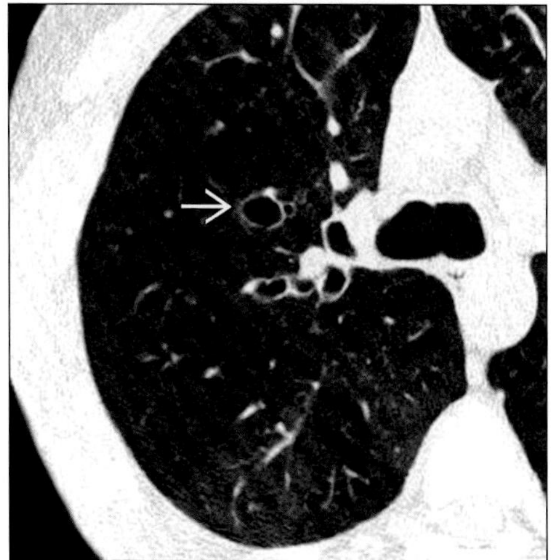

Axial NECT in inspiratory phase shows mosaic attenuation and bronchiectasis. There is a classic signet ring sign of bronchiectasis in the right upper lobe ➔.

Constrictive Bronchiolitis

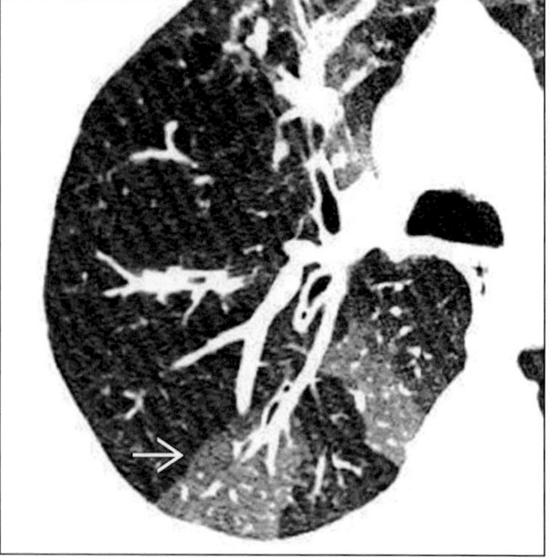

Axial NECT expiratory scan in the same patient shows increased density of normal lung ➔ and overall accentuation of mosaic attenuation. Note the collapse of the bronchiectatic airways.

MOSAIC PATTERN

Constrictive Bronchiolitis

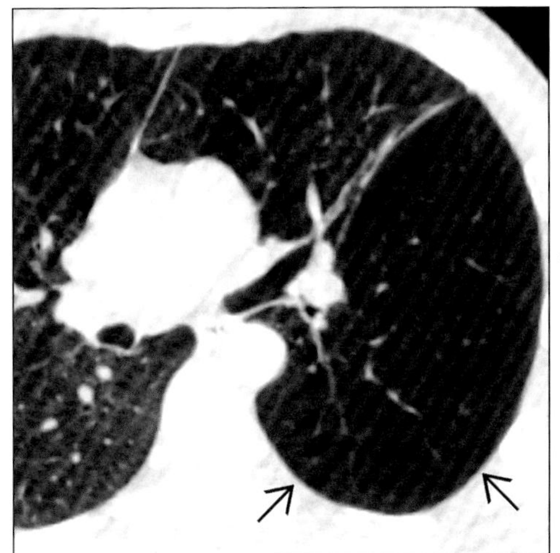

Hypersensitivity Pneumonitis

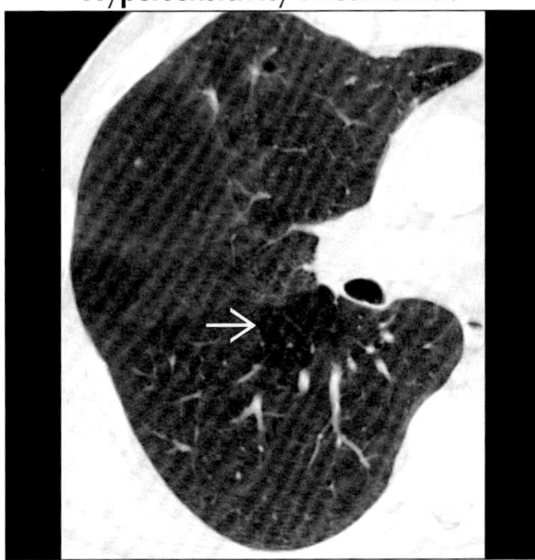

(Left) *Axial NECT shows focal hyperinflation and vascular attenuation in the left lower lobe ⇒ from constrictive bronchiolitis. Predominant involvement of 1 lobe or 1 lung is a subset of postinfectious constrictive bronchiolitis known as Swyer-James syndrome or Macleod syndrome.* ***(Right)*** *Axial HRCT shows typical CT features of hypersensitivity pneumonitis with faint centrilobular opacities and air-trapping ➡.*

Cystic Fibrosis

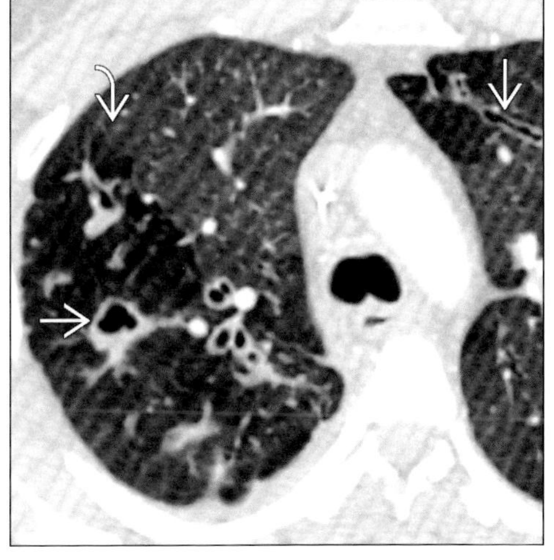

Pulmonary Arterial Hypertension

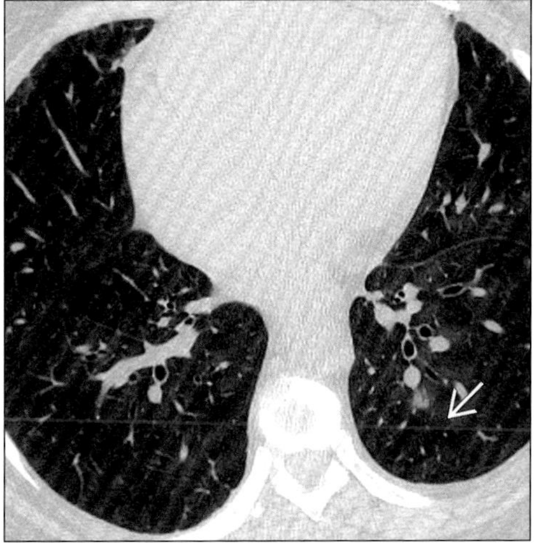

(Left) *Axial CECT shows bronchial wall thickening and bronchiectasis ➡. Note the mosaic pattern of attenuation indicating air-trapping ➡ in areas of lung subtended by the abnormal airways.* ***(Right)*** *Axial HRCT shows typical radiographic and CT features of mosaic attenuation ➡ from vascular disease. There is no associated bronchiectasis to suggest an airway etiology. Note the enlarged right heart.*

Pulmonary Arterial Hypertension

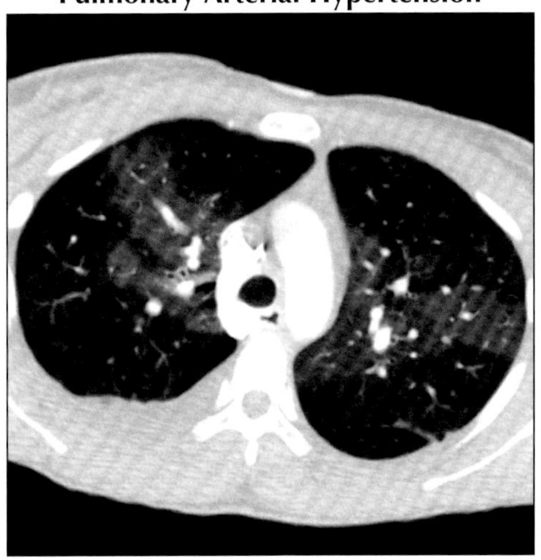

Inflammatory Bronchiolitis

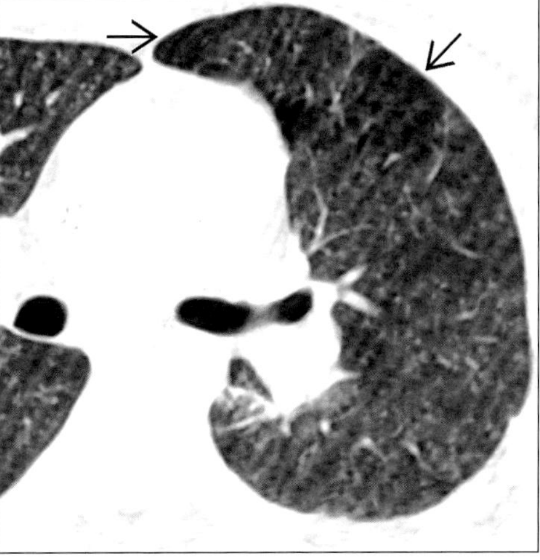

(Left) *Axial CECT from a patient with chronic pulmonary artery hypertension shows a mosaic perfusion pattern. Note the engorged pulmonary arteries in the denser areas of lung and the paucity of vascular markings in the more lucent areas of lung.* ***(Right)*** *Axial HRCT shows typical CT features of diffuse tree in bud opacities with resultant patchy mosaic attenuation from air-trapping ⇒.*

TREE IN BUD PATTERN

DIFFERENTIAL DIAGNOSIS

Common
- Infectious Bronchiolitis
  - Bacterial
    - Mycobacterial
  - Viral
  - Fungal
- Bronchiectasis
  - Cystic Fibrosis
  - Allergic Bronchopulmonary Aspergillosis
  - Immotile Cilia Syndrome
- Aspiration

Less Common
- Follicular Bronchiolitis
- Sarcoidosis

Rare but Important
- Diffuse Panbronchiolitis
- Laryngeal Papillomatosis
- Intravascular Metastases
- Illicit Drug Abuse, Cellulose Granulomatosis

ESSENTIAL INFORMATION

Key Differential Diagnosis Issues
- Definition of tree in bud (TIB) on CT
  - Fairly sharply circumscribed small centrilobular nodules or branching tubular structures (2-4 mm diameter) within secondary pulmonary lobules
  - Originally described in CT appearance of endobronchial spread of tuberculosis, now nonspecific
- Radiology-pathology correlation
  - Generally signifies bronchiolar disease; pattern produced by
    - Dilated, thickened, bronchiolar walls
    - Centrilobular bronchiolar luminal impaction filled with mucus, pus, fluid, or cells
    - Terminal tufts represent respiratory bronchioles and alveolar ducts; stems represent terminal bronchioles
- Secondary signs of airways disease
  - Mosaic attenuation from air-trapping
    - Supplementary exhalation CT scanning helpful to confirm air-trapping
  - Lobular ground-glass opacities or subsegmental consolidation or frank pneumonia
- Bronchiectasis or bronchial wall thickening proximal airways, consider
  - Mycobacterial disease, tuberculosis and avium complex (MAC)
  - Cystic fibrosis
  - Allergic bronchopulmonary aspergillosis
  - Chronic variable immunodeficiency syndromes
  - Immotile cilia syndrome
- Normal proximal airways, consider
  - Infectious bronchiolitis
  - Aspiration
  - Vascular tree in bud pattern from illicit drug abuse or intravascular/hematogenous metastases
- Distribution
  - Diffuse tree in bud, consider
    - Infections, especially viral
    - Diffuse panbronchiolitis
  - Basilar
    - Aspiration
    - Tuberculosis
  - Middle lobe and lingula together
    - Mycobacterium avium complex
    - Immotile cilia syndrome
- Associated sinus disease, consider
  - Diffuse panbronchiolitis, cystic fibrosis, immotile cilia syndrome, immune deficiency syndromes
- Situs inversus: Immotile cilia syndrome
- Age & gender
  - Elderly women
    - Lentil or psyllium aspiration
    - Mycobacterium avium complex (Lady Windermere syndrome)

Helpful Clues for Common Diagnoses
- **Infectious Bronchiolitis**
  - Overwhelmingly most common cause of TIB pattern
  - Not specific for any 1 infection; seen with
    - Mycobacterial pneumonia and atypical mycobacterial pneumonias
    - Mycoplasma pneumonia
    - Viral pneumonias, especially influenza
    - Wide spectrum of infections: Bacterial, viral, fungal, parasitic
  - Bronchoscopy and bronchoalveolar lavage (BAL) in TIB associated with high recovery rate of offending organism
- **Bronchiectasis**

- TIB minor component compared to bronchiectasis
- Mucoid impaction distally gives rise to TIB pattern

- **Aspiration**
  - Aspiration pattern, including TIB pattern, highly dependent on gravitational distribution of aspirate
  - Predisposing conditions
    - Unconsciousness, swallowing disorders, alcoholism
  - Endogenous: Spillage from preexisting cavity, typically *Mycobacterium tuberculosis*
    - Dorsal upper lobe cavitary disease in apical and posterior segment of upper lobe and superior segment of lower lobe
    - Cavities drain to basilar segments (pattern known as "upstairs-downstairs" lesion)
  - Exogenous: Location dependent on posture at time of event

Helpful Clues for Less Common Diagnoses

- **Follicular Bronchiolitis**
  - Proliferation of bronchus-associated lymphoid tissue (BALT)
    - Associated with immunologic conditions, such as rheumatoid arthritis and Sjögren syndrome
- **Sarcoidosis**
  - Subpleural or perilymphatic nodules and lymphadenopathy
  - Mid and upper lung distribution
  - Lymphadenopathy

Helpful Clues for Rare Diagnoses

- **Diffuse Panbronchiolitis**
  - Idiopathic; primarily seen in Asia (Japan, Korea, China)
  - Associated with sinusitis
- **Laryngeal Papillomatosis**
  - More commonly has solid and cystic nodules
  - Associated with airway nodules in trachea and main airways
  - Also tend to have gravity-dependent distribution in dorsal lung
- **Intravascular Metastases**
  - May have enlarged central pulmonary arteries from pulmonary arterial hypertension (especially illicit drug abuse)
  - Intravascular metastases are a rare cause of the tree in bud pattern
    - Angiosarcoma, renal cell carcinoma, hepatocellular carcinoma
- **Illicit Drug Abuse, Cellulose Granulomatosis**
  - Granulomatous reaction to injected crushed oral medications, cellulose often used as filler

Other Essential Information

- Tree in bud pattern: Direct sign of small-airways inflammatory disease

Infectious Bronchiolitis

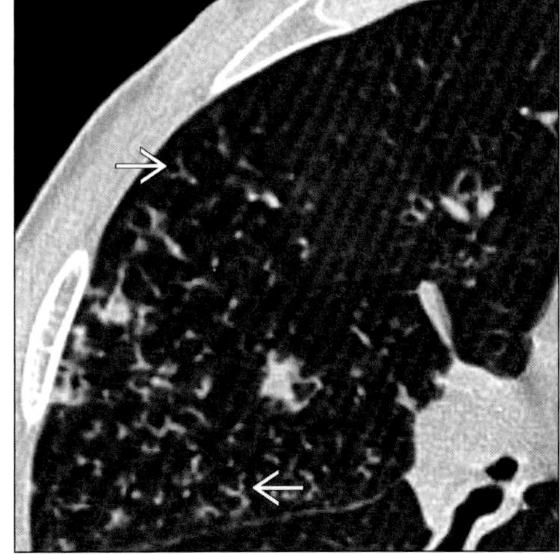

Axial HRCT shows tree in bud opacities ➔ in a patient with infectious bronchiolitis.

Infectious Bronchiolitis

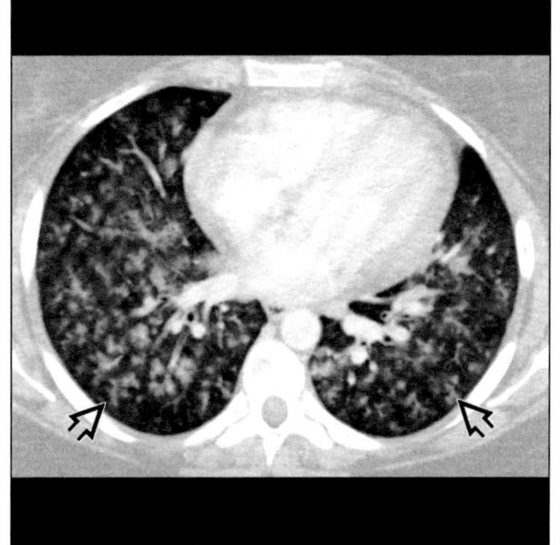

Axial CECT shows diffuse centrilobular tree in bud opacities ⇨ from infectious bronchiolitis, in this case, much more florid and extensive.

TREE IN BUD PATTERN

*(**Left**) Axial NECT shows the bronchogenic spread of post-primary tuberculosis. Note the tree in bud opacities ➡ in the left upper lobe. Such a patient should be isolated, especially if coughing. (**Right**) Axial HRCT shows tree in bud opacities ➡ in both lower lobes, in this case secondary to chronic infection with Mycobacterial avium complex.*

Mycobacterial

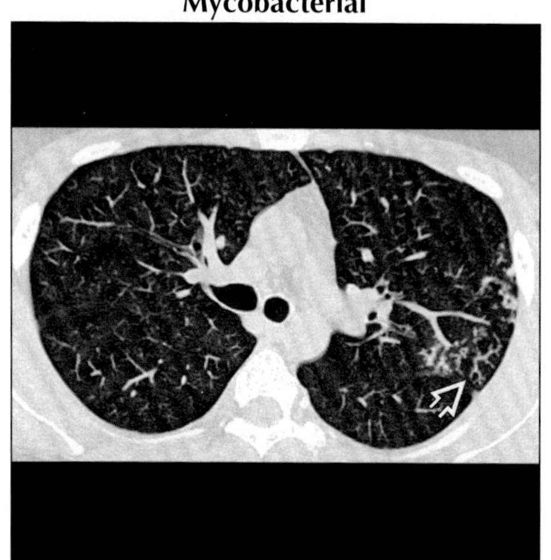

Mycobacterial

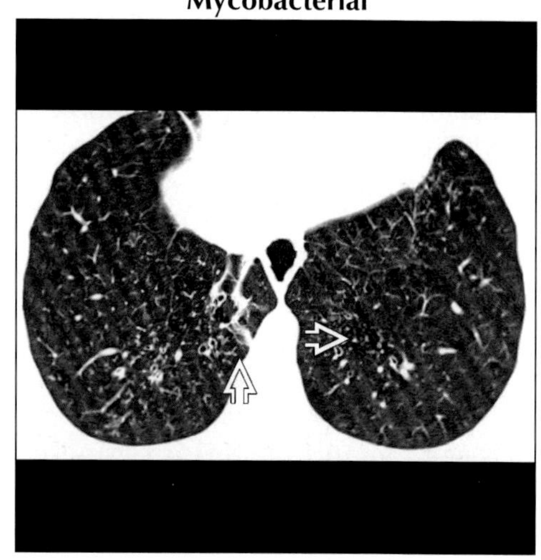

*(**Left**) Axial HRCT shows diffuse tree in bud opacities ➡ representing an acute inflammatory bronchiolitis, in this case secondary to infection with influenza A virus. (**Right**) Axial HRCT shows diffuse tree in bud opacities ➡ from diffuse panbronchiolitis. In this disease, the bronchiolitis is very extensive and chronic.*

Viral

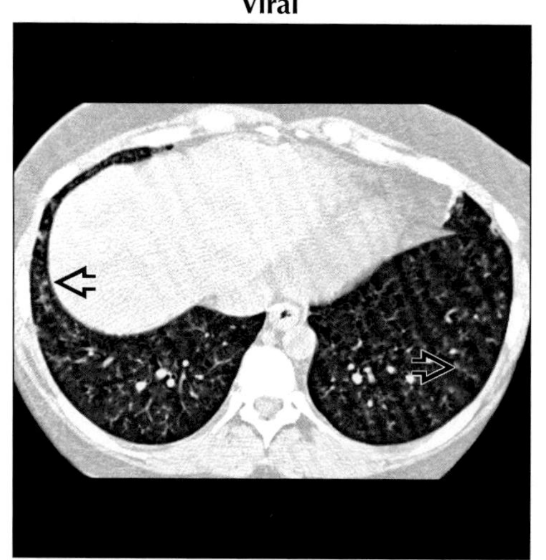

Diffuse Panbronchiolitis

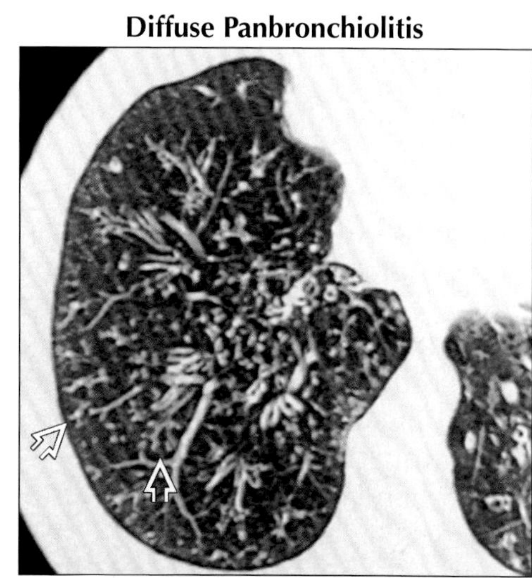

*(**Left**) Axial HRCT shows tree in bud opacities ➡ from aspiration in the basilar segments of the right lower lobe and lingula, which along with the right middle lobe and the superior segments of the lower lobes are a typical distribution for aspiration. (**Right**) Axial CECT shows tree in bud pattern in the right lower lobe ➡ from chronic aspiration in this patient with a hiatal hernia →.*

Aspiration

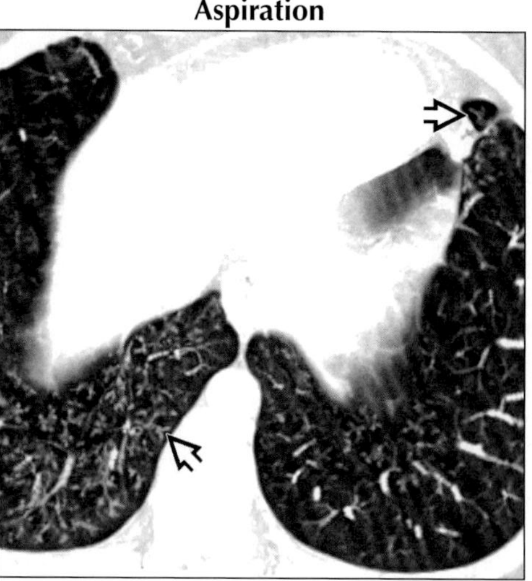

Aspiration

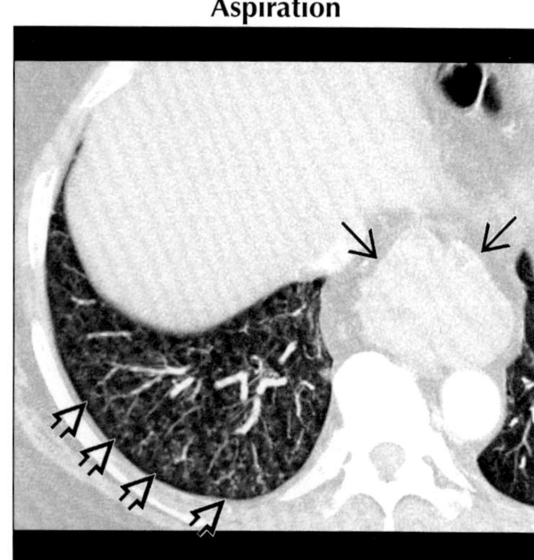

TREE IN BUD PATTERN

Aspiration

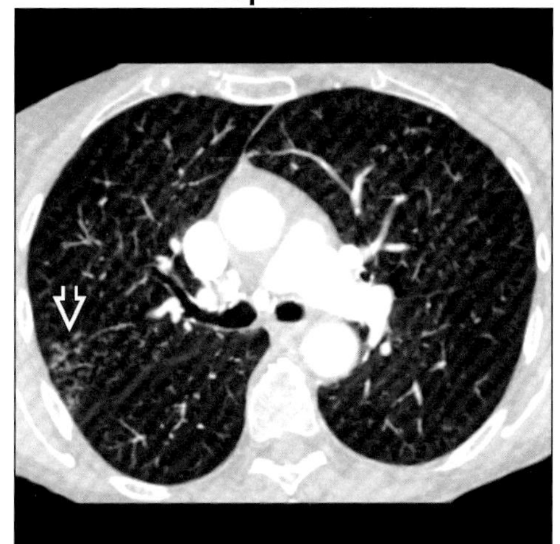

Follicular Bronchiolitis

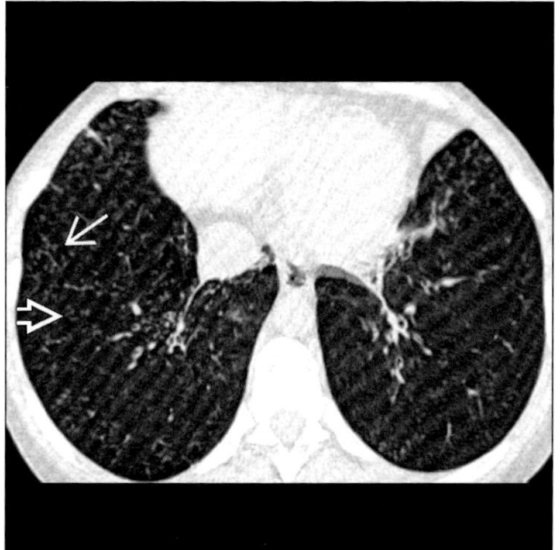

(Left) *Axial CECT shows the typical CT features of psyllium aspiration causing cellulose bronchiolitis and tree in bud opacities ➡. While the location is typical for aspiration, the appearance is indistinguishable from other forms of aspiration.* ***(Right)*** *Axial HRCT shows centrilobular nodules ➡ and tree in bud opacities ➡ from follicular bronchiolitis.*

Mycobacterial

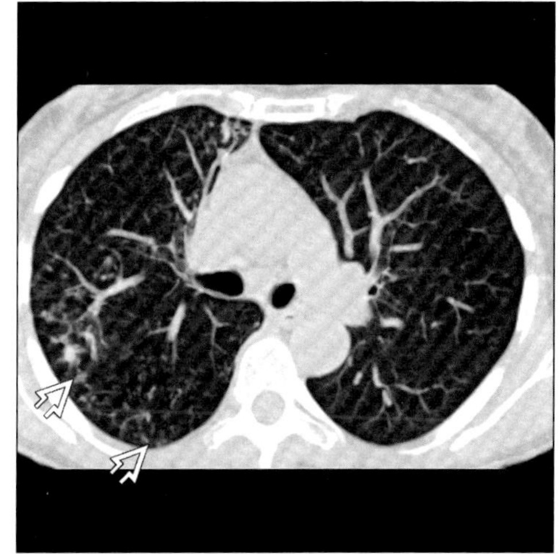

Immotile Cilia Syndrome

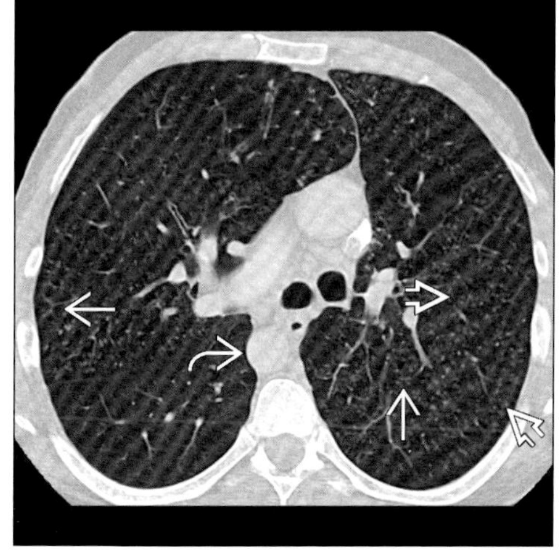

(Left) *Axial NECT shows tree in bud opacities ➡ in a patient with mycobacterial infection. Such findings, especially in patients with chronic cough and a cavity in another part of the lung, are suggestive of endobronchial tuberculosis.* ***(Right)*** *Axial HRCT shows tree in bud opacities ➡ and centrilobular nodules ➡ in a patient with bronchiectasis from Kartagener syndrome. Note the situs inversus (right descending thoracic aorta ➡).*

Intravascular Metastases

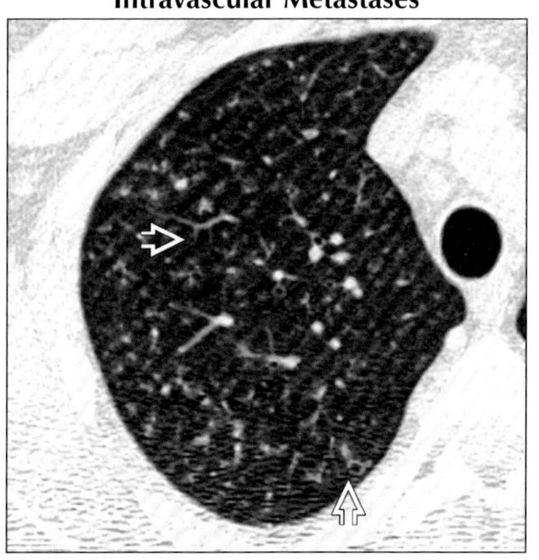

Intravascular Metastases

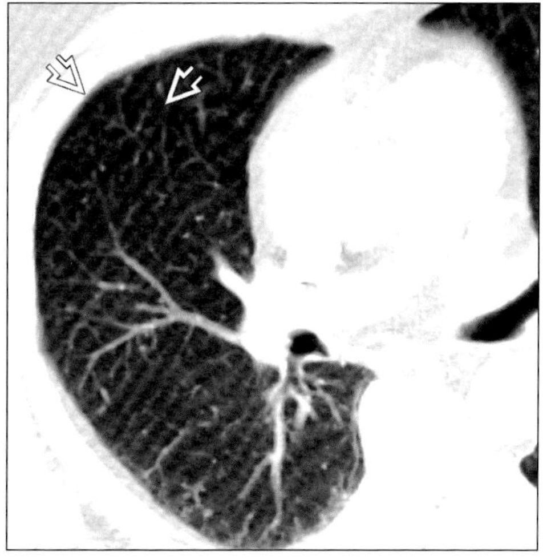

(Left) *Axial HRCT shows tree in bud opacities ➡ due to tumor emboli from cardiac rhabdomyosarcoma. Note the perpendicular vascular branching opacities, which distinguish this from more typical discrete hematogenous "miliary" metastases.* ***(Right)*** *Axial CECT shows tree in bud opacities ➡ due to tumor emboli from hepatoma.*

IMMUNE COMPROMISE

DIFFERENTIAL DIAGNOSIS

Common
- Pneumonia
  - Bacterial, Fungal, Viral, Mycobacterial, Protozoal
- Pulmonary Edema
- Pulmonary Hemorrhage
- Drug Toxicity

Less Common
- Pulmonary Emboli
- Septic Emboli

Rare but Important
- Nonspecific Interstitial Pneumonitis
- Organizing Pneumonia
- Tumor
  - Lung Cancer (HIV), AIDS-related Lymphoma, Kaposi Sarcoma, Post-transplant Lymphoproliferative Disease

ESSENTIAL INFORMATION

Key Differential Diagnosis Issues
- Immune compromise: Congenital or acquired conditions, which adversely affect immune system
  - Hematological malignancy, congenital immune deficiency, HIV
  - Stem cell transplantation, chemotherapy, corticosteroids, splenectomy
- Fever not always due to infection
  - Infection, drug toxicity, pulmonary hemorrhage, transfusion reaction, pulmonary emboli

Helpful Clues for Common Diagnoses
- **Pneumonia**
  - Often nonspecific clinical findings; fever, cough, chest pain, dyspnea
  - Different imaging findings for specific microbial agents
    - Nodular consolidation with ground-glass halo or cavitation: Invasive fungal pneumonia (especially in neutropenia)
    - Diffuse ground-glass opacity, ± interlobular septal thickening: PCP or viral pneumonia
    - Upper lung fibrocavitary consolidation and bronchiectasis: Mycobacterial pneumonia
  - Follow-up to resolution helpful to exclude malignancy
- **Pulmonary Edema**
  - History of left-sided heart failure, mitral valvular disease, or fluid overload
  - Central preponderant airspace opacities with superimposed interlobular septal thickening
    - Kerley A and B lines represent thickened interlobular septa
  - Rapid resolution with diuretics, inotropic agents, etc.
  - Bilateral pleural effusions
- **Pulmonary Hemorrhage**
  - Ground-glass opacities > consolidation; tendency to spare peripheral, apical, and costophrenic aspects of lungs
  - Increased interlobular and intralobular septal thickening over 1-2 days as blood products clear through lymphatics
  - Rapid resolution over course of days
- **Drug Toxicity**
  - Imaging appearance depends upon underlying histology
    - Diffuse alveolar damage, organizing pneumonia, NSIP, eosinophilic pneumonia, hemorrhage
    - Hypersensitivity pneumonitis (rarely)

Helpful Clues for Less Common Diagnoses
- **Pulmonary Emboli**
  - High relative risk of venous thrombosis in hematological malignancy
  - Filling defect in pulmonary artery
  - Subpleural and lower lung preponderant pulmonary infarct(s)
    - Infarcts resolve over months, shrink in size while retaining original shape
- **Septic Emboli**
  - Longstanding central venous catheters predispose to septic emboli
  - Multiple peripheral, basilar-predominant cavitary nodules/focal consolidation
  - Loculated empyema
  - Feeding vessel sign: Vessel leads directly into center of nodule or mass

Helpful Clues for Rare Diagnoses
- **Nonspecific Interstitial Pneumonitis**
  - Lower lung or diffuse ground-glass opacities; ± subpleural sparing
  - Extensive traction bronchiectasis
  - Reticular opacities (mild)

- Honeycombing not predominant CT pattern
- **Organizing Pneumonia**
  - Bilateral basilar predominant peripheral or peribronchovascular consolidation and ground-glass opacity
    - May be migratory or wax and wane
  - Atoll sign (a.k.a. reverse halo sign): Central ground-glass opacity surrounded by rim of consolidation
  - Perilobular opacities: Poorly marginated opacities outlining secondary pulmonary lobule
  - Linear band-like opacities superimposed on airspace opacities in setting of stem cell transplantation
- **Tumor**
  - Non-small cell lung cancer more common in HIV(+) patients
  - Kaposi sarcoma: Peribronchovascular, flame-shaped consolidation in AIDS
    - Usually associated mucocutaneous lesions
  - AIDS-related lymphoma: Extranodal disease common, multiple pulmonary nodules, mild lymphadenopathy
  - Post-transplant lymphoproliferative disease: Most common in solid organ transplant, multiple nodules or consolidation and lymphadenopathy

Alternative Differential Approaches

- HIV/AIDS
  - Infection (bacterial, mycobacterial, *Pneumocystis jiroveci* [other fungi], and viral pneumonias)
  - Pulmonary edema
  - Drug toxicity
  - Pulmonary hemorrhage
  - Tumor (AIDS-related lymphoma, Kaposi sarcoma, lung cancer)
  - Immune reconstitution inflammatory syndrome
    - After initiation of HAART; inflammatory response to latent subclinical infection
  - Interstitial lung disease (nonspecific interstitial pneumonia, lymphoid interstitial pneumonitis)
- Hematopoietic stem cell transplantation
  - 0-30 days (neutropenic phase)
    - Bacterial pneumonia or sepsis
    - Fungal pneumonia (aspergillosis or candidiasis)
    - Pulmonary edema
    - Pulmonary hemorrhage
    - Drug toxicity
  - 30-100 days (early phase)
    - Viral pneumonia (CMV most important)
    - Idiopathic pneumonia syndrome (diffuse alveolar damage histology)
    - Pulmonary venoocclusive disease
  - Greater than 100 days (late phase)
    - Pneumonia
    - Chronic graft-vs.-host disease (allogenic stem cell transplant only)
    - Constrictive bronchiolitis
    - Organizing pneumonia

Pneumonia

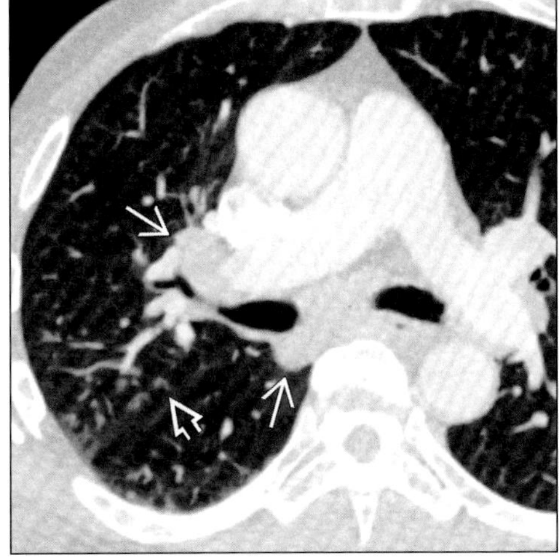

Axial CECT shows clustered centrilobular nodules ➡ in the right upper lobe, consistent with pneumonia; there is lymphomatous enlargement of mediastinal and hilar lymph nodes ➡.

Pneumonia

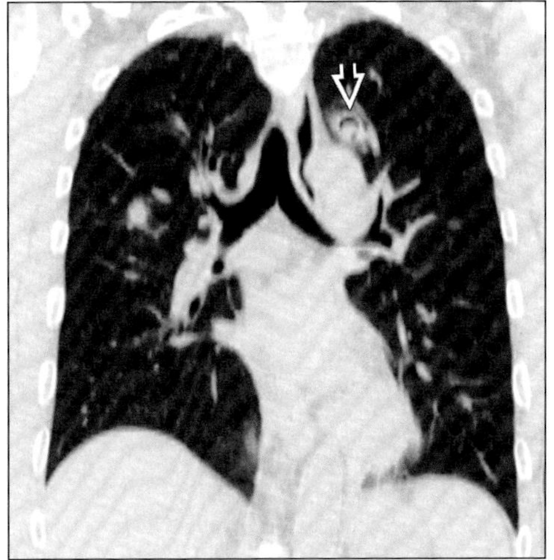

Coronal NECT shows bilateral lung nodules in this neutropenic patient. There is cavitation/air crescent sign within a left upper lobe nodule ➡, highly suggestive of invasive aspergillosis.

IMMUNE COMPROMISE

(Left) Frontal radiograph shows diffuse nodular perihilar consolidation ➡ in this AIDS patient with PCP. There is relative sparing of the costophrenic angles and no evidence of pleural effusions. **(Right)** Axial CECT in another patient shows diffuse ground-glass opacity with superimposed thin-walled cysts ➡ and regions of paraseptal emphysema ➡ in this AIDS patient with PCP. No pleural effusions are present. Thin-walled cysts predispose to pneumothorax.

Pneumonia

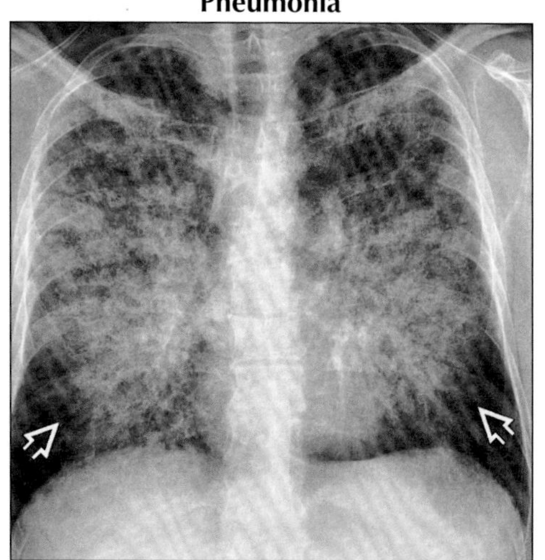

Pneumonia

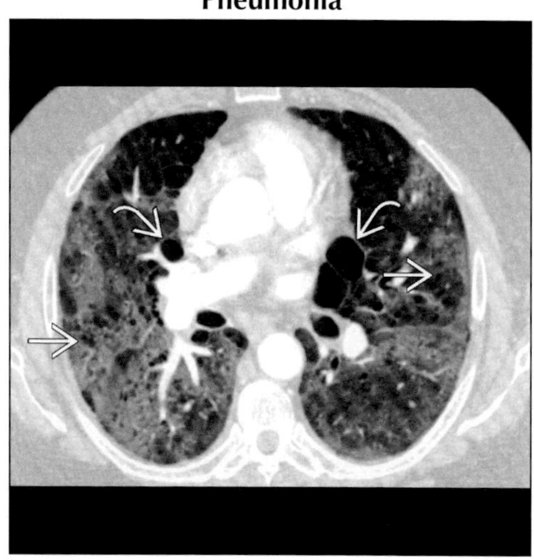

(Left) Frontal radiograph shows mild cardiomegaly and Kerley B lines ➡ (representing engorged lymphatics within the interlobular septa) from acute pulmonary edema. **(Right)** Axial NECT shows patchy ground-glass opacities in this patient with pulmonary hemorrhage in the setting of acute lymphocytic leukemia. Note superimposed reticular opacities ➡, which often develop 1-2 days after bleeding.

Pulmonary Edema

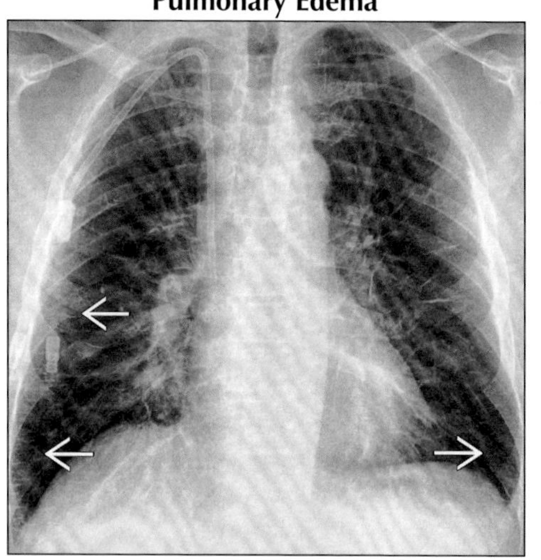

Pulmonary Hemorrhage

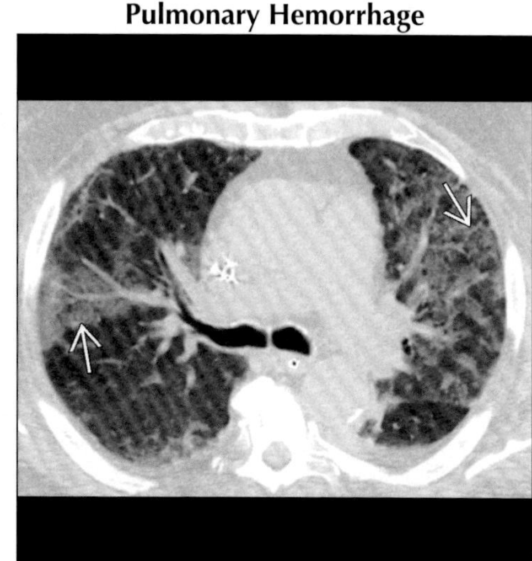

(Left) Coronal CECT shows diffuse ground-glass opacities with relative sparing of the lower lungs after a recent change in chemotherapy, consistent with drug reaction. No pleural effusions or reticular opacities are present. **(Right)** Axial CECT shows pulmonary emboli ➡ and a right pleural effusion ➡. Patients with hematological malignancy, lung cancer, and gastrointestinal cancers are susceptible to venous thrombosis and subsequent pulmonary embolism.

Drug Toxicity

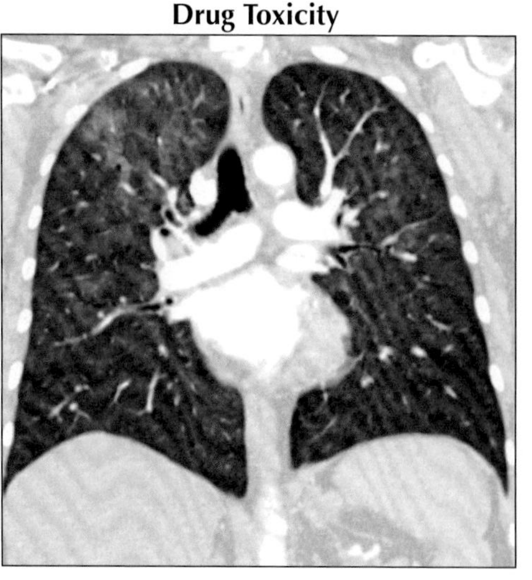

Pulmonary Emboli

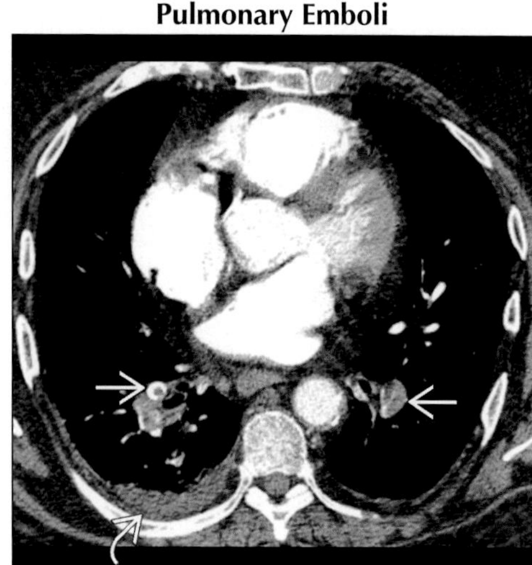

Septic Emboli

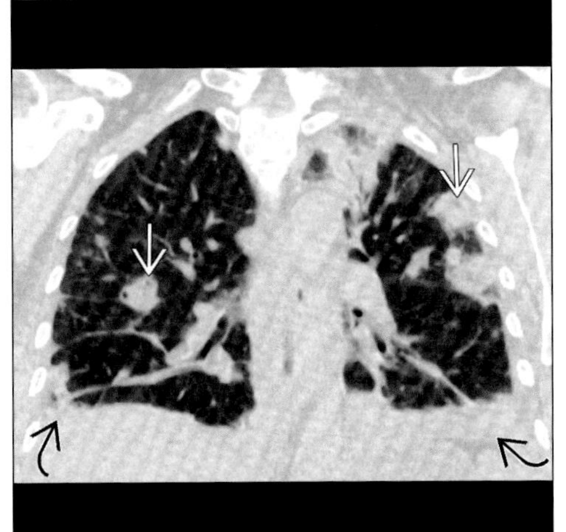

Nonspecific Interstitial Pneumonitis

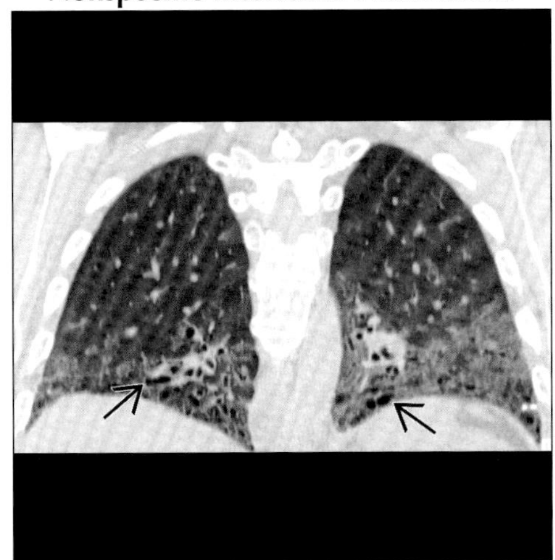

(Left) *Coronal NECT shows bilateral, nodular, peripheral preponderant consolidation (some demonstrating early cavitation ➔) and small pleural effusions ➔ in this patient with septic emboli.* ***(Right)*** *Coronal NECT shows lower lung preponderant ground-glass opacity with superimposed traction bronchiectasis ➔. There is no honeycombing. Findings are highly suggestive of nonspecific interstitial pneumonitis.*

Organizing Pneumonia

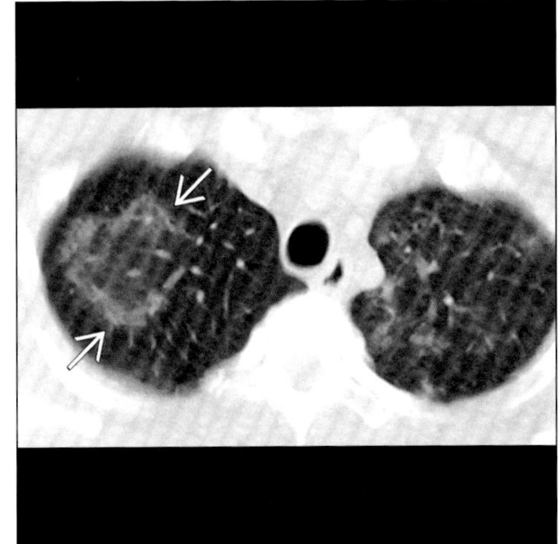

Tumor

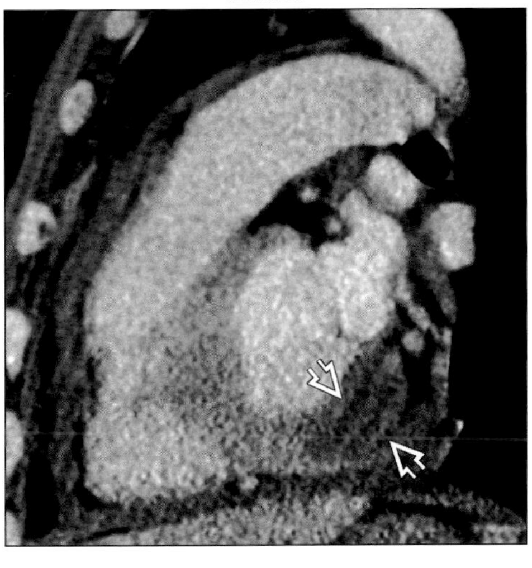

(Left) *Axial NECT shows patchy opacities in the upper lobes in this patient with organizing pneumonia. The right upper lobe opacity demonstrates a reverse halo configuration ➔ (central ground-glass opacity with surrounding rim of consolidation), which is associated with this diagnosis.* ***(Right)*** *Sagittal CECT shows lymphomatous infiltration ➔ of the basal inferior wall of the left ventricle in this AIDS patient. There is a small pericardial effusion.*

Tumor

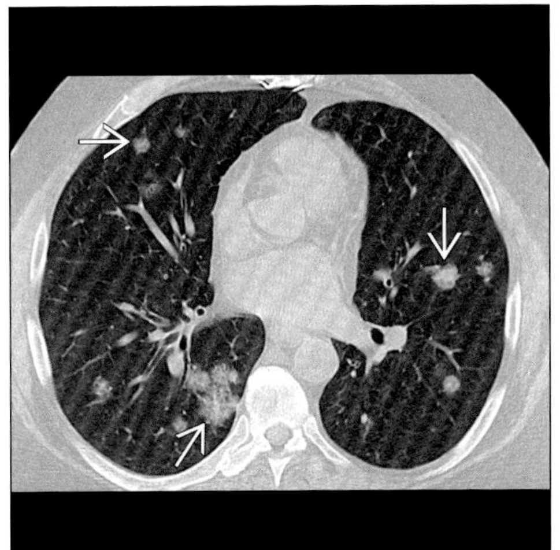

Tumor

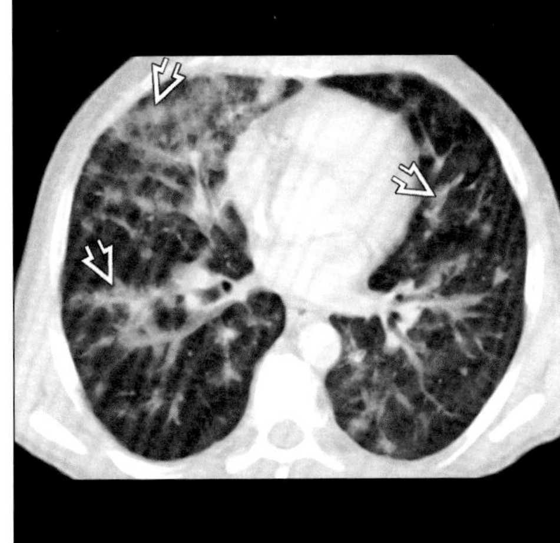

(Left) *Axial NECT shows bilateral pulmonary nodules ➔, representing post-transplant lymphoproliferative disease in this patient with a history of cardiac transplantation.* ***(Right)*** *Axial CECT shows flame-shaped, peribronchovascular pulmonary consolidation ➔ (right greater than left), highly suggestive of Kaposi sarcoma in the setting of AIDS. The patient had concomitant mucocutaneous lesions, which is often the case in Kaposi sarcoma.*

SECTION 4
Symptoms

HEMOPTYSIS

DIFFERENTIAL DIAGNOSIS

Common

- Bronchogenic Carcinoma
- Metastases
- Infection
  - Tuberculosis
  - Aspergilloma
  - Lung Abscess
- Bronchiectasis
- Bronchitis
- Pulmonary Emboli

Less Common

- Diffuse Alveolar Hemorrhage
- Cardiac Causes
  - Congestive Heart Failure
  - Mitral Stenosis

Rare but Important

- Pulmonary Artery Aneurysm
- Arteriovenous Malformation (AVM)
- Broncholithiasis
- Pseudosequestration
- Kaposi Sarcoma

ESSENTIAL INFORMATION

Key Differential Diagnosis Issues

- Hemoptysis definition
  - Expectoration of blood that originates from airways or lung
  - Massive hemoptysis: > 300 mL in 24 hours
  - Majority have identifiable etiology
    - Cryptogenic hemoptysis 3-15%
  - Bronchial arteries most common source of bleeding
- Bronchial artery anatomy
  - Orthotopic origin: Arises from descending aorta at level of 5th or 6th thoracic vertebra
  - CT location
    - Right bronchial artery at level of carina
    - Left bronchial artery(s) at level of proximal left main bronchus
  - Classic branching pattern
    - Type 1: 1 right intercostobronchial trunk and 2 left bronchial arteries (40%)
    - Type 2: 1 right intercostobronchial trunk and 1 left bronchial artery (20%)
    - Type 3: 1 intercostobronchial trunk, right bronchial artery, 2 left bronchial arteries (20%)
    - Type 4: 1 intercostobronchial trunk, right bronchial artery, 1 left bronchial artery (10%)
  - Ectopic origin: Bronchial arteries arise from other than expected site
  - Bronchial artery diameter > 2 mm abnormal

Helpful Clues for Common Diagnoses

- **Bronchogenic Carcinoma**
  - Hemoptysis usually seen in advanced cancers, accounts for up to 20% of cases of hemoptysis
  - Smokers > 40 years old with cryptogenic hemoptysis: 5% will develop lung cancer within 3 years
  - Carcinoid tumors
    - Often highly vascular, may enhance with intravenous contrast
- **Metastases**
  - Hemorrhagic metastases: Commonly from choriocarcinoma, renal cell carcinoma, melanoma, thyroid
  - CT: Multiple variable-sized nodules surrounded by ground-glass opacities
- **Tuberculosis**
  - Common cause of hemoptysis, generally seen in those with active cavitary disease
  - Rasmussen aneurysm: Pulmonary artery aneurysm arising adjacent to cavitary wall, hemoptysis may be massive
- **Aspergilloma**
  - Saprophytic mycelia growth in preexisting cavity
  - Hemoptysis may be massive
- **Lung Abscess**
  - Hemoptysis may be massive; foul-smelling sputum typical
- **Bronchiectasis**
  - Accounts for up to 25% of hemoptysis, may be massive
  - Distribution clue to etiology
    - Central bronchiectasis: Allergic bronchopulmonary aspergillosis, tracheobronchomegaly, Williams-Campbell syndrome
    - Upper lobe bronchiectasis: Cystic fibrosis, tuberculosis, allergic bronchopulmonary aspergillosis
    - Ventral bronchiectasis: *Mycobacterium avium complex*
    - Lower lobe: Postinfectious, aspiration

- **Bronchitis**
  - Accounts for 20% of cases of hemoptysis
  - Dieulafoy disease: Abnormal dilated submucosal vessels from chronic inflammation
  - CT usually normal; may have bronchial wall thickening; focal ground-glass opacities and consolidation suggest active hemorrhage
- **Pulmonary Emboli**
  - Hemoptysis from pulmonary infarcts
  - Infarcts in < 10% of embolic episodes
  - Infarcts are pleural-based, wedge-shaped, with no contrast enhancement

Helpful Clues for Less Common Diagnoses

- **Diffuse Alveolar Hemorrhage**
  - Inflammatory process involving blood vessels (large, medium, or small)
  - Spectrum includes Wegener granulomatosis, microscopic polyangiitis, Churg-Strauss syndrome
  - CT: Nonspecific lobular ground-glass opacities admixed with consolidation; crazy-paving pattern more common as hemorrhage resolves
  - Hemoptysis in 66%
- **Cardiac Causes**
  - Frothy blood sputum in congestive heart failure (accounts for 5% of cases of hemoptysis)
  - Patients with mitral stenosis may have repeated bouts of hemorrhage leading to hemosiderosis

Helpful Clues for Rare Diagnoses

- **Pulmonary Artery Aneurysm**
  - Causes: Swan-Ganz-induced pseudoaneurysm, Behçet syndrome
  - Swan-Ganz pseudoaneurysm: Mortality 45-65%
    - Usually lower lobe segmental artery in perihilar location
- **Arteriovenous Malformation (AVM)**
  - Epistaxis presenting features in hereditary hemorrhagic telangiectasis (HHT)
  - AVM vessels have thin walls, at risk for rupture
  - Rupture more common in pregnancy
- **Broncholithiasis**
  - Hemoptysis in 50%
  - Peribronchial calcified lymph node that distorts or narrows adjacent airway
- **Pseudosequestration**
  - Pure vascular pulmonary sequestration; lung and bronchi normal
  - Also refers to transpleural systemic-pulmonary artery anastomoses (most commonly seen with pulmonary artery stenosis)
- **Kaposi Sarcoma**
  - AIDS-related multicentric neoplasm involving skin, lymph nodes, GI tract, and lungs
  - Diffuse peribronchial nodules emanating from hilum

Bronchogenic Carcinoma

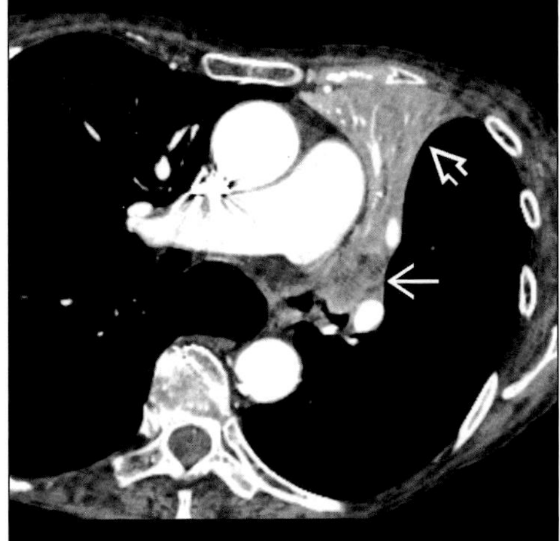

Axial CECT shows a collapsed LUL ⇒ from central obstructing carcinoma (squamous cell) ⇒.

Bronchogenic Carcinoma

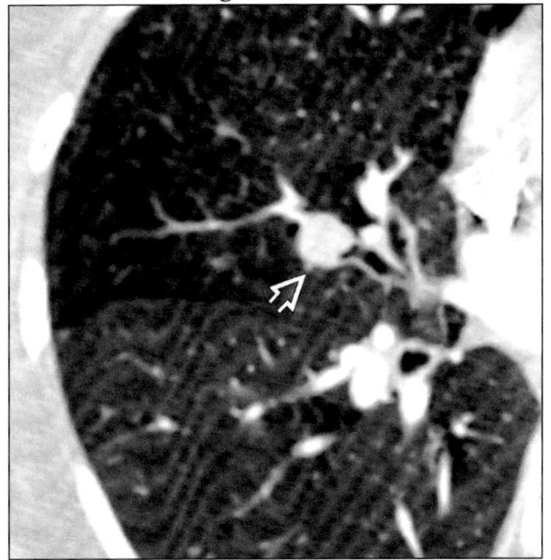

Axial CECT shows a small endobronchial carcinoid tumor ⇒. The tumor enhanced with contrast on mediastinal windows (not shown).

HEMOPTYSIS

Metastases

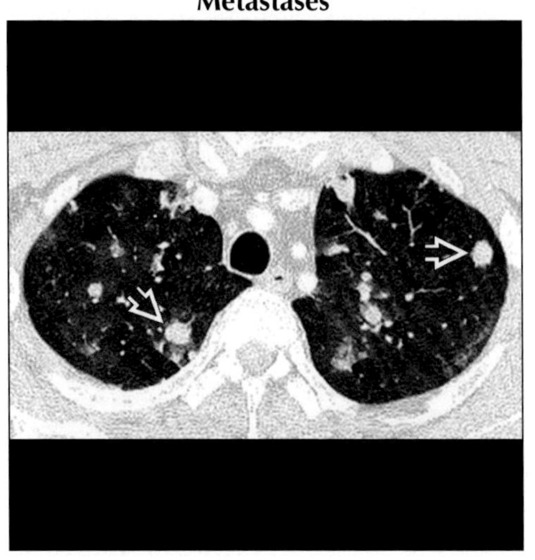

Metastases

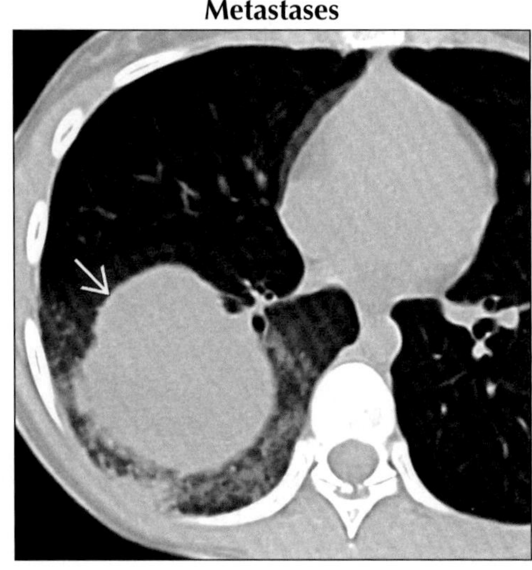

***(Left)** Axial CECT shows multiple pulmonary nodules ➡ and ground-glass opacities from hemorrhagic metastases in this young woman with choriocarcinoma. **(Right)** Axial NECT shows a large mass in the right lower lobe ➡ surrounded by ground-glass opacities from hemorrhage. The mass was a large melanoma metastasis.*

Tuberculosis

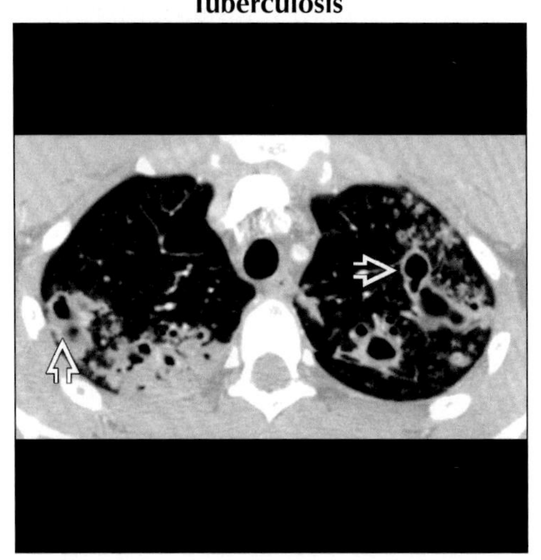

Aspergilloma

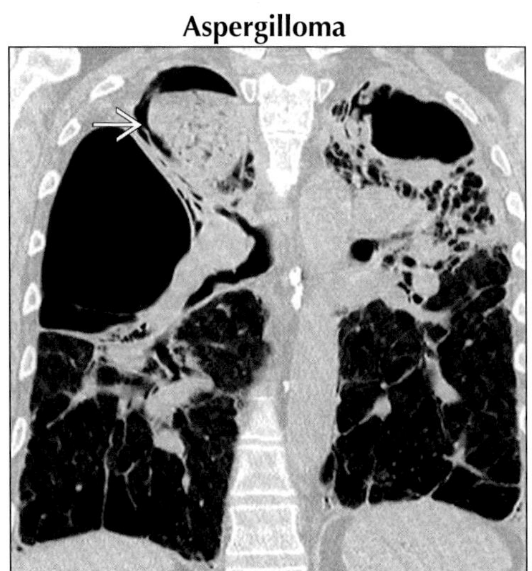

***(Left)** Axial CECT shows variable-sized and variable thickness cavities ➡ in the upper lobes from active tuberculosis. **(Right)** Coronal NECT shows endstage fibrosis and bullous disease from sarcoidosis. Cystic space was complicated by large aspergilloma ➡.*

Lung Abscess

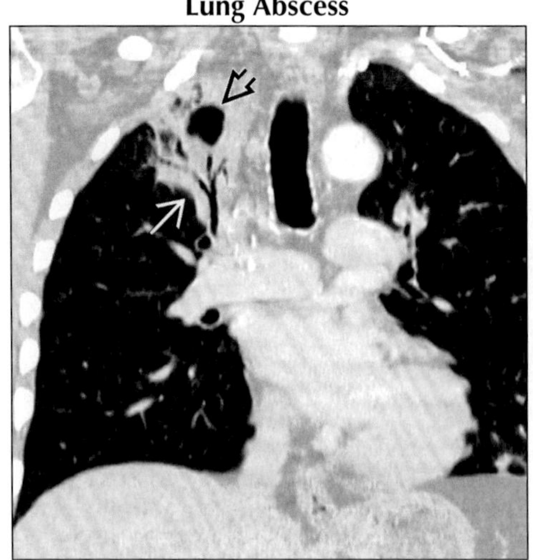

Bronchiectasis

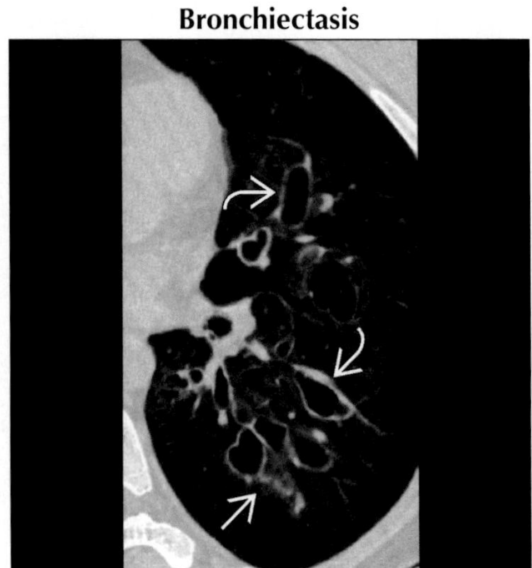

***(Left)** Coronal CECT reconstruction shows focal consolidation with air bronchograms ➡ in the right upper lobe in this patient with pneumonia complicated by lung abscess ➡. **(Right)** Axial CECT shows varicose bronchiectasis ➡. Ground-glass opacity ➡ may be due to hemorrhage or pneumonia. Etiology of bronchiectasis was post infection.*

HEMOPTYSIS

Bronchiectasis

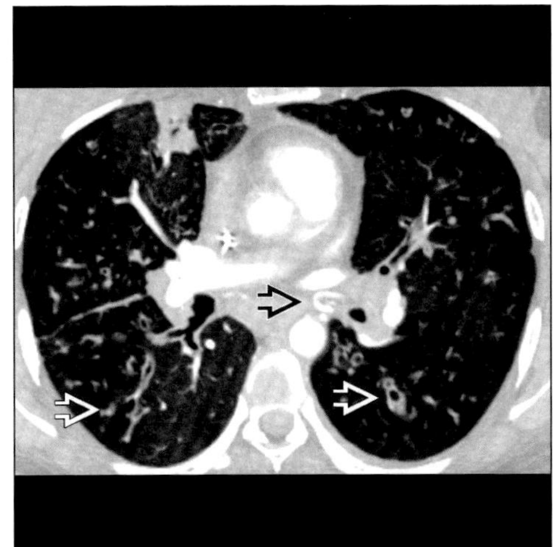

Bronchitis

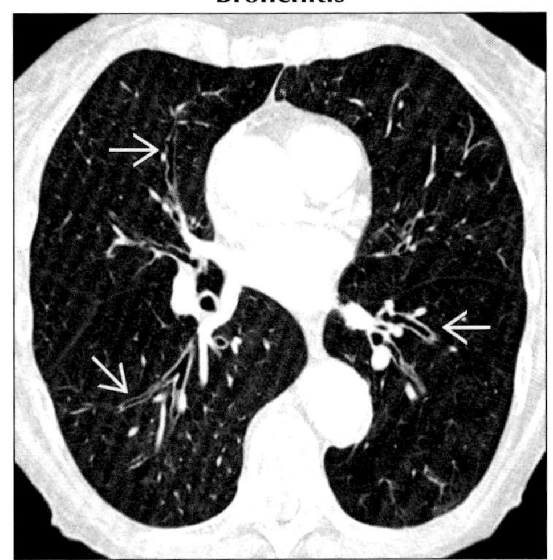

(Left) *Axial CECT shows bronchial wall thickening, bronchiectasis, and mucus plugging of both large and small airways in a patient with cystic fibrosis. Note the enlarged left bronchial artery.* ***(Right)*** *Axial CECT shows thickened and irregular bronchial walls with slight bronchial dilatation. This patient was a long-term smoker with chronic cough and hemoptysis.*

Pulmonary Emboli

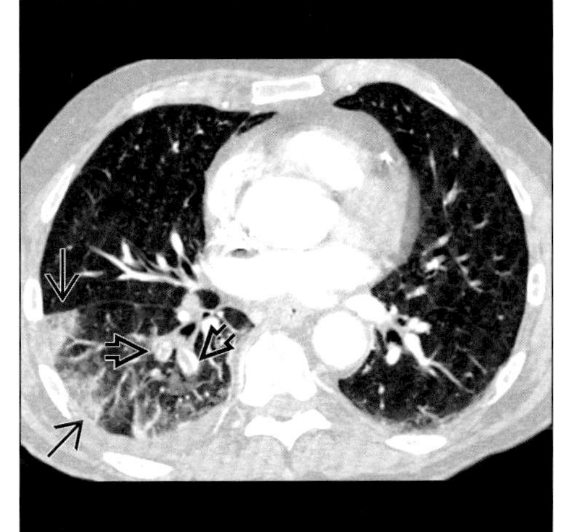

Pulmonary Emboli

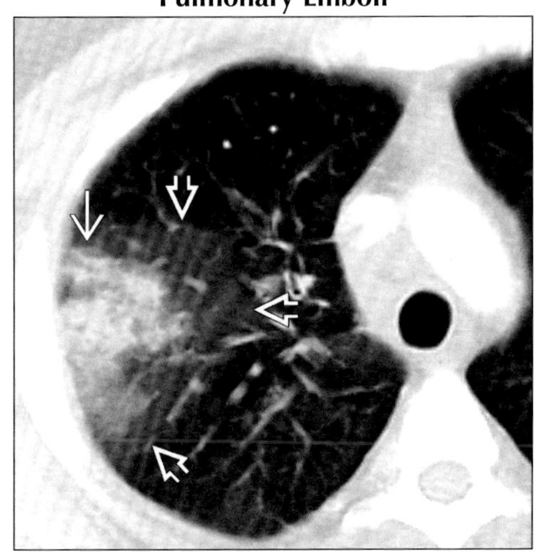

(Left) *Axial HRCT shows pulmonary infarcts in regions fed by embolized arteries.* ***(Right)*** *Axial CECT shows wedge-shaped consolidation in the right upper lobe. The central consolidation surrounded by ground-glass halo is due to a classic pulmonary infarct.*

Diffuse Alveolar Hemorrhage

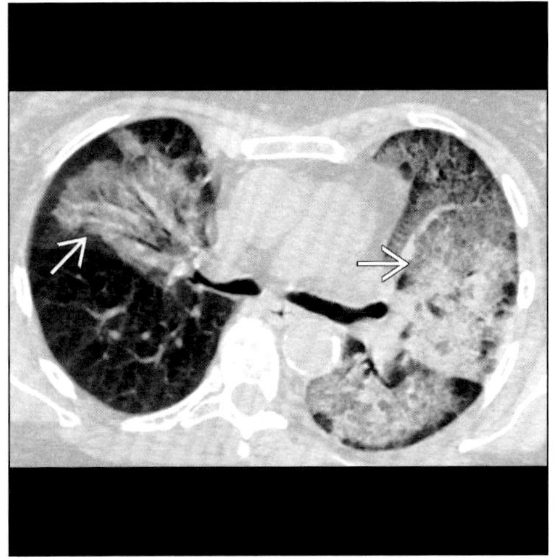

Diffuse Alveolar Hemorrhage

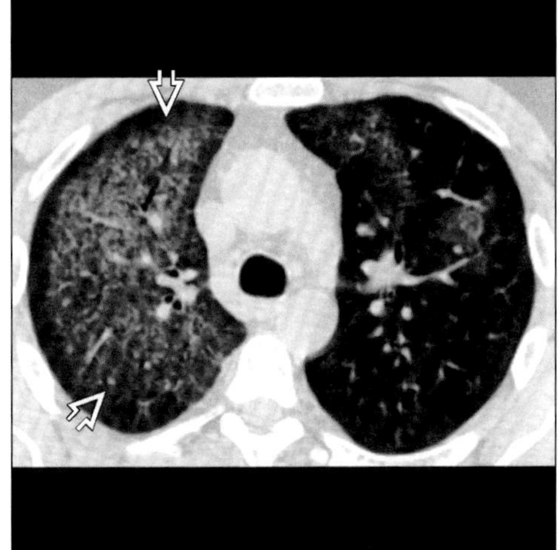

(Left) *Axial NECT shows asymmetric consolidation and ground-glass opacities from hemorrhage. Etiology was vasculitis.* ***(Right)*** *Axial CECT shows diffuse ground-glass opacities throughout the right lung with peripheral sparing and lobular involvement of the left lung. Renal biopsy showed Goodpasture syndrome.*

HEMOPTYSIS

*(**Left**) Frontal radiograph shows central "bat-wing" consolidation from acute pulmonary edema. Periphery of the lung was spared, and the heart size was normal. (**Right**) Frontal radiograph magnified view of the right lower lung shows nodules ➔ probably secondary to hemosiderosis in this patient with longstanding mitral stenosis.*

Congestive Heart Failure

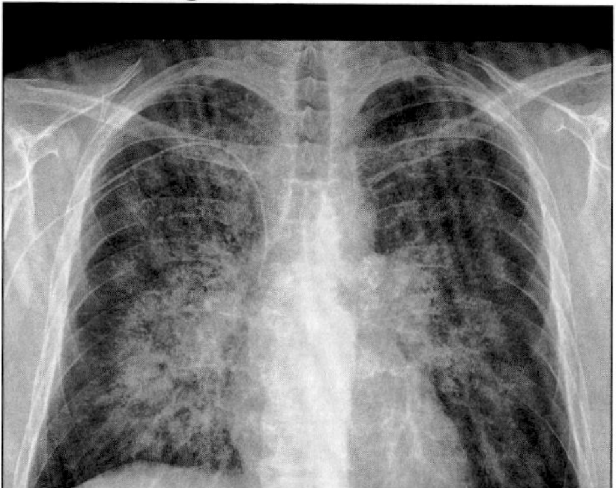

Mitral Stenosis

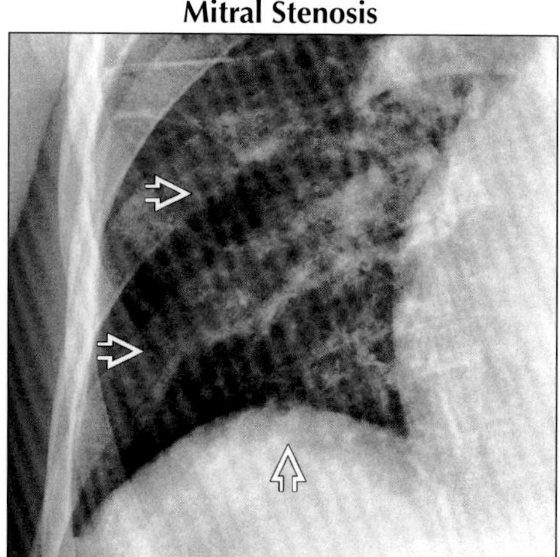

*(**Left**) Axial CECT shows contrast-enhancing pseudoaneurysm ➔ of the segmental artery in the right middle lobe in this patient with a pseudoaneurysm from Swan-Ganz catheter. (**Right**) Axial CECT on lung windows shows that the pseudoaneurysm is surrounded by ground-glass halo ➔ from hemorrhage. The patient died before treatment.*

Pulmonary Artery Aneurysm

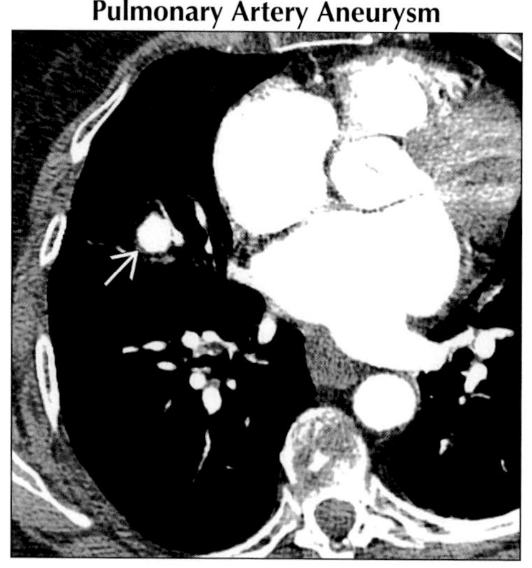

Pulmonary Artery Aneurysm

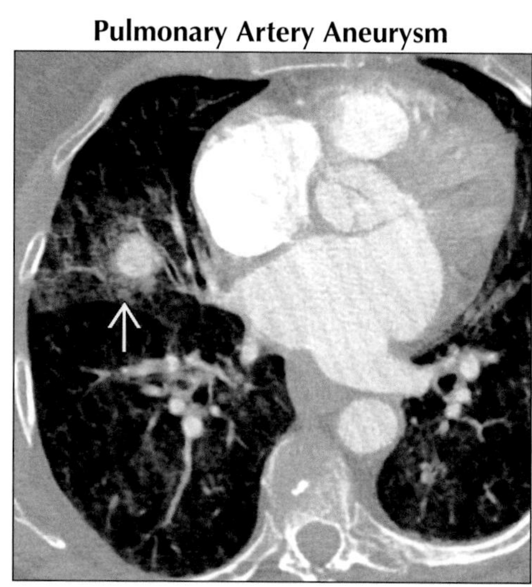

*(**Left**) Axial CECT MIP reconstruction shows multiple arteriovenous malformations ➔. Central pulmonary arteries are markedly enlarged ➔ due to pulmonary artery hypertension. (**Right**) Axial CECT MIP reconstruction in the same patient shows large wedge-shaped areas of hemorrhage with surrounding ground-glass opacities ➔.*

Arteriovenous Malformation (AVM)

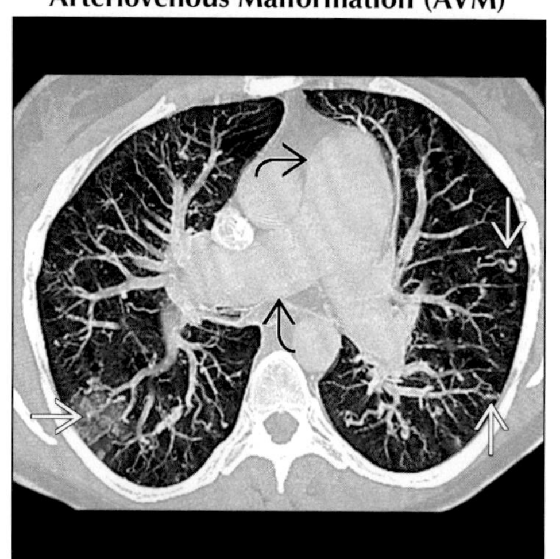

Arteriovenous Malformation (AVM)

Arteriovenous Malformation (AVM)

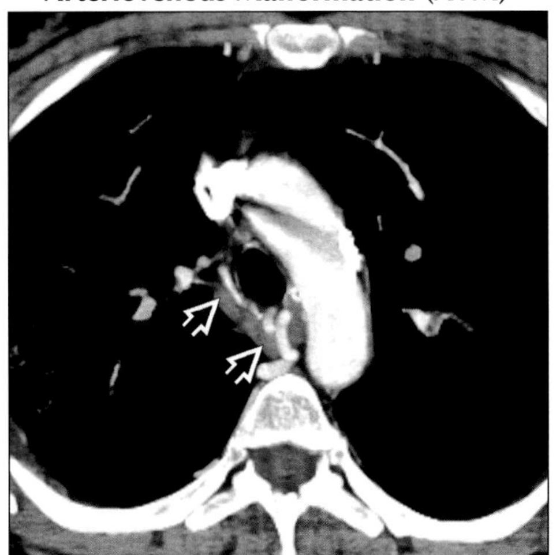

Arteriovenous Malformation (AVM)

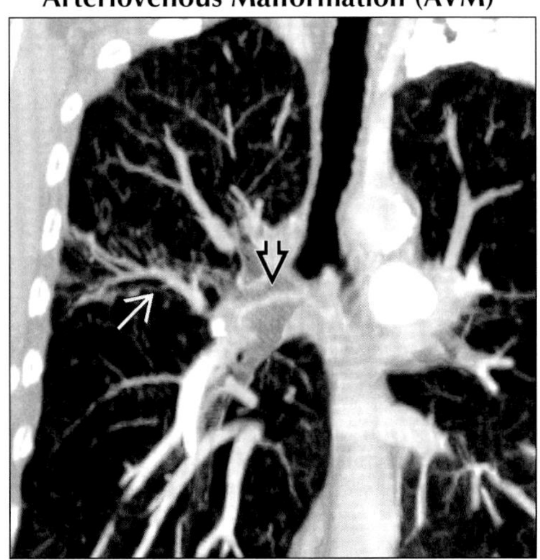

(Left) *Axial CECT shows enlarged bronchial arteries ➡, which measure more than 2 mm in diameter.* ***(Right)*** *Coronal CECT MIP reconstruction shows enlarged bronchial artery ➡ in communication with right upper lobe pulmonary veins ➡ in this patient with a rare bronchial artery arteriovenous malformation.*

Broncholithiasis

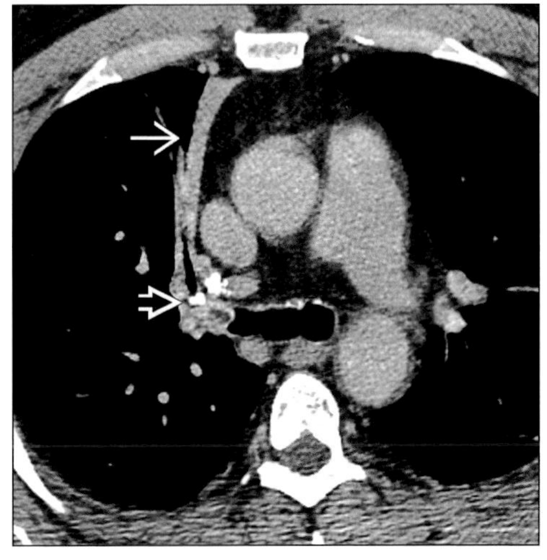

Pseudosequestration

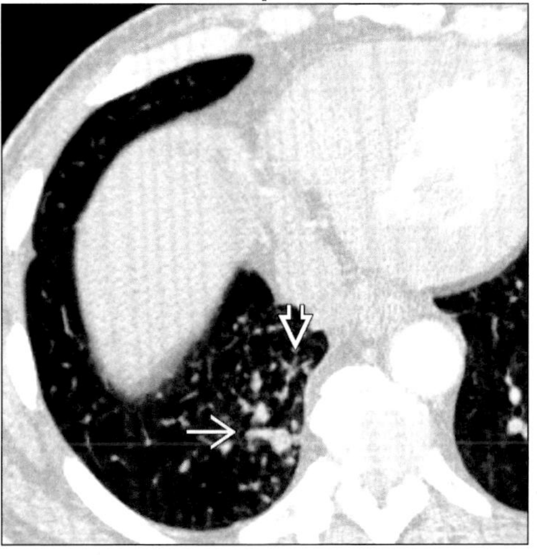

(Left) *Axial CECT shows partial atelectasis of the right upper lobe ➡. Right upper lobe bronchus is obstructed ➡ from calcified broncholith.* ***(Right)*** *Axial CECT on lung windows shows abnormal systemic vessels, both large ➡ and small ➡, feeding the right lower lobe. Systemic arteries arose from celiac axis (not shown).*

Kaposi Sarcoma

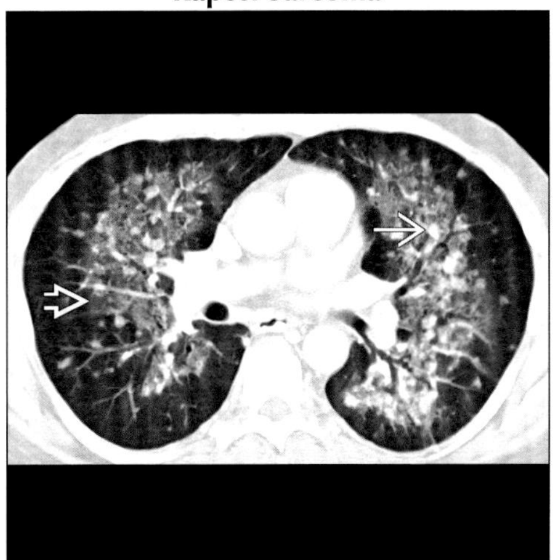

Kaposi Sarcoma

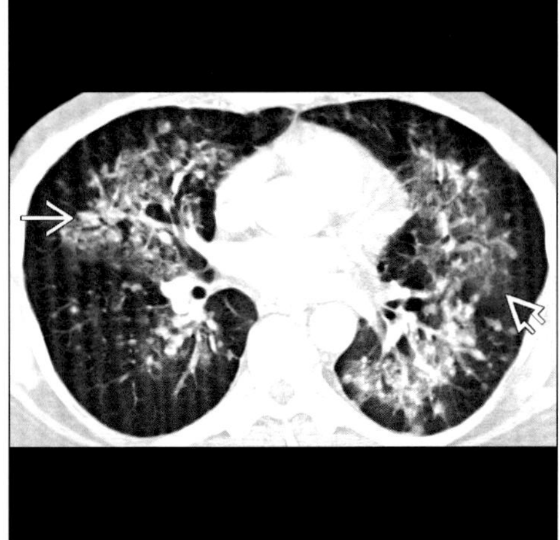

(Left) *Axial CECT shows uniform-sized peribronchial nodules ➡ superimposed on perihilar ground-glass opacities ➡ from hemorrhage.* ***(Right)*** *Axial CECT more inferiorly shows peribronchial nodules ➡ and ground-glass opacities ➡. Bronchoscopy showed red mucosal lesions that were growing into the lumen of the small airways.*

WHEEZING

DIFFERENTIAL DIAGNOSIS

Common
- Asthma
- Cardiogenic Pulmonary Edema
- Pulmonary Emboli
- Aspiration

Less Common
- Airway Obstruction
  - Extrinsic: Airway Compression
  - Intrinsic: Airway Narrowing
- Allergic Bronchopulmonary Aspergillosis
- Tracheobronchomalacia
- Churg-Strauss Syndrome
- Eosinophilic Pneumonia

Rare but Important
- Carcinoid
- Diffuse Neuroendocrine Hyperplasia
- Mastocytosis

ESSENTIAL INFORMATION

Key Differential Diagnosis Issues
- Wheezing: High-pitched adventitious sound superimposed on normal sounds of breathing; occurs when air flows rapidly through narrowed bronchi

Helpful Clues for Common Diagnoses
- **Asthma**
  - "All that wheezes is not asthma"
  - Primarily involves small to medium-sized bronchi
  - Bronchial wall (BW) thickened by edema, ↑ smooth muscle, ↑ size mucus glands
  - HRCT: BW thickening in 50-90%
  - Near-fatal asthma: Centrilobular nodules ↑, (seen in 100%) but not specific (seen in up to 1/3 of mild asthma)
  - Air-trapping (total volume > 1 segment) in 50%
  - Complications of asthmatic attacks
    - Pneumomediastinum (5%)
    - Pneumonia (2%)
    - Pneumothorax (0.3%)
    - Lobar atelectasis from mucus plugs (rare)
- **Cardiogenic Pulmonary Edema**
  - Interstitial edema thickens bronchial walls, narrowing their lumen
  - Associated findings: Cardiomegaly, pleural effusions, interstitial septal thickening
- **Pulmonary Emboli**
  - Acute emboli associated with reflex bronchoconstriction of embolized segment, leads to wheezing
  - Recurrent emboli may give rise to episodic wheezing and misdiagnosis of asthma
  - 10% of patients with acute pulmonary emboli have wheezing as predominant symptom
- **Aspiration**
  - Repeated episodes of aspiration may give rise to wheezing as aspirated material narrows airway lumen
  - Aspiration most common in dependent segments
    - Posterior segments of upper lobes and superior segments of lower lobes in recumbent position
    - Lower lobe basilar segments in upright position

Helpful Clues for Less Common Diagnoses
- **Airway Obstruction**
  - **Extrinsic: Airway Compression**
    - Most commonly goiters, vascular rings
  - **Intrinsic: Airway Narrowing**
    - Most commonly from neoplastic and nonneoplastic tumors, tuberculosis, or foreign bodies
  - Even with fixed obstruction, patient may have intermittent wheezing and be misdiagnosed with asthma for mths or yrs
- **Allergic Bronchopulmonary Aspergillosis**
  - Hypersensitivity reaction to *Aspergillus fumigatus*
  - Occurs in 1-2% of chronic asthmatics
  - HRCT: Central bronchiectasis with peripheral sparing, primarily involves upper lung zones
- **Tracheobronchomalacia**
  - Softening of airway cartilage
  - Excessive collapse (> 70%) of expected luminal area during expiratory CT scan
  - Typical morphology: Crescent, lunate, or "frown" sign
- **Churg-Strauss Syndrome**
  - Granulomatous small vessel vasculitis
  - Most present with peripheral neuropathy (mononeuritis multiplex)
  - Nearly 100% have asthma
  - Triad of allergic history, peripheral blood eosinophilia, and systemic vasculitis

- CT: Nonspecific but similar to chronic eosinophilic pneumonia with peripheral consolidation and ground-glass opacities
- Pleural effusions in 25% (extremely rare in eosinophilic pneumonia)

- **Eosinophilic Pneumonia**
  - Asthma seen in 50% of chronic eosinophilic pneumonia
  - Striking peripheral consolidation, primarily of upper lung zones

Helpful Clues for Rare Diagnoses

- **Carcinoid**
  - Carcinoid syndrome: Wheezing from excess serotonin and histamine
  - Carcinoid syndrome uncommon with pulmonary carcinoids, seen in 2-5% of patients, almost all of whom have hepatic metastases
  - Endobronchial component of carcinoid tumors may give rise to unilateral wheezing
  - Hemoptysis also common as tumors are vascular
- **Diffuse Neuroendocrine Hyperplasia**
  - Rare disorder of proliferation of carcinoid tumorlets (benign)
  - Primarily women; may also be more common in those living at high altitude
  - Multiple pulmonary nodules (< 5 mm diameter) + mosaic attenuation
  - Mosaicism may be related to endobronchial tumorlets or associated constrictive (obliterative) bronchiolitis
  - 1/3 have asthma
- **Mastocytosis**
  - Rare disorder with proliferation of mast cells in extracutaneous organs
  - Lung involvement shows centrilobular nodules and cysts (or emphysema)
  - Skeletal: Diffuse osteosclerosis from bone marrow infiltration
  - GI tract and spleen more often involved than lung
  - Asthma due to excess histamine

Other Essential Information

- Acute onset wheezing
  - Asthma
  - Congestive heart failure
  - Pneumonia
  - Pulmonary embolus
  - Aspiration syndromes
  - Foreign body
- Insidious onset wheezing
  - Endobronchial tumor
  - Congestive heart failure
  - Extrinsic airway narrowing
- Course of symptoms
  - Intermittent: Asthma, aspiration, pulmonary embolus, congestive heart failure, foreign bodies
  - Persistent: Asthma, extrinsic or intrinsic airway narrowing, Churg-Strauss vasculitis
  - Progressive: Asthma, tumors, eosinophilic pneumonia, Churg-Strauss vasculitis

Asthma

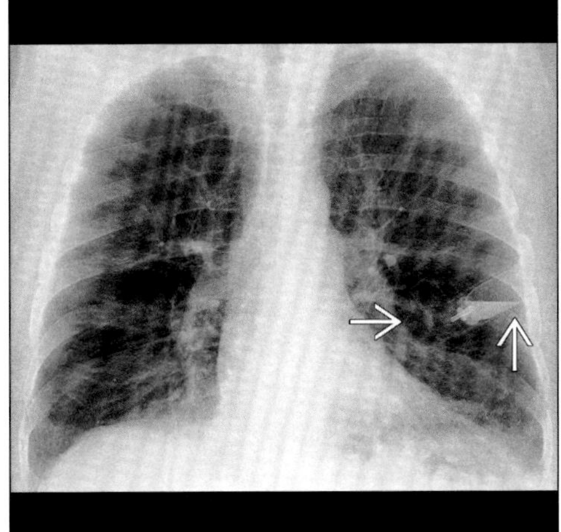

Frontal radiograph shows marked hyperinflation. Note the asthma inhaler ➔ left in shirt pocket. Radiographs have limited utility in asthma, as they may be normal even in patients with status asthmaticus.

Asthma

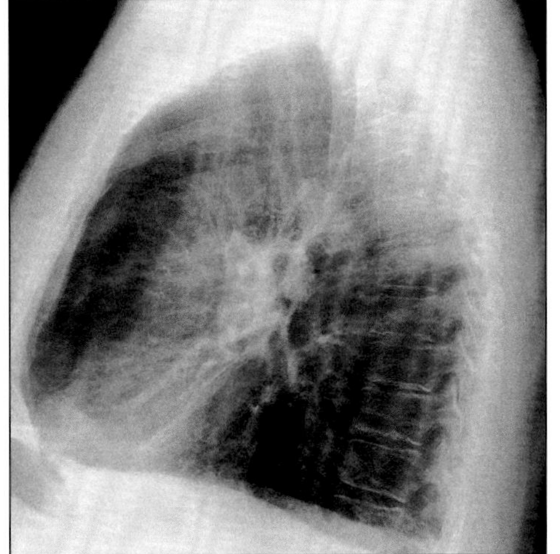

Lateral radiograph shows flattened hemidiaphragms and increased retrosternal lucency. Asthma complications include pneumomediastinum, pneumothorax, atelectasis from mucus plugging, and pneumonia.

WHEEZING

(Left) Axial HRCT shows bronchial wall thickening ➔; other airways are normal. Note that study was CTA for suspected pulmonary embolus. Some airways may be mildly dilated and may reflect bronchodilatation from uninvolved airways. (Right) Axial HRCT shows bronchial wall thickening ➔ and mucus plugs ➔. Mucus plug in this case is not associated with atelectasis. Note that bronchial wall thickening in asthma may be heterogeneous.

Asthma

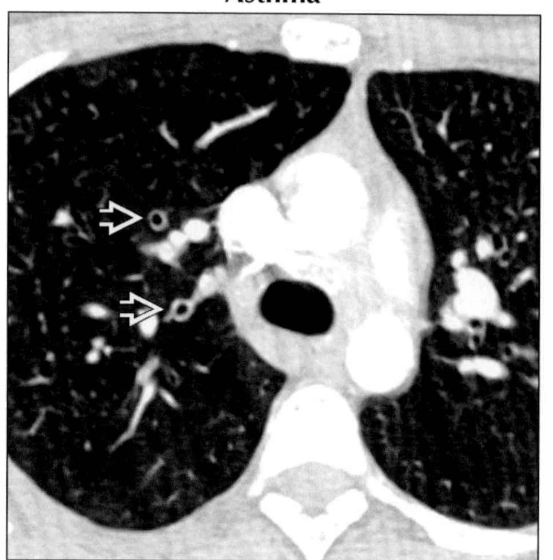

Asthma

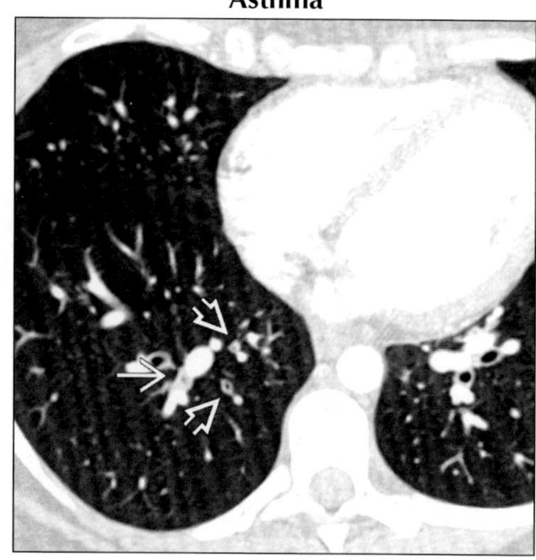

(Left) Coronal CECT shows basilar gradient in ground-glass opacities ➔, bronchial wall thickening ➔, and septal thickening ➔. (Right) Axial CECT shows mild diffuse smooth bronchial wall thickening ➔. Attacks of cardiac asthma usually occur at night in the recumbent position. Note that the left-sided airways are normal. This was positional; the patient was in the right decubitus position. Edema is gravitationally dependent, more severe in the right lung.

Cardiogenic Pulmonary Edema

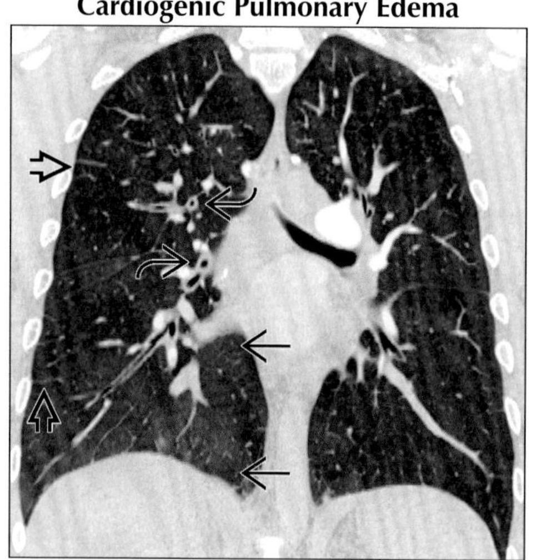

Cardiogenic Pulmonary Edema

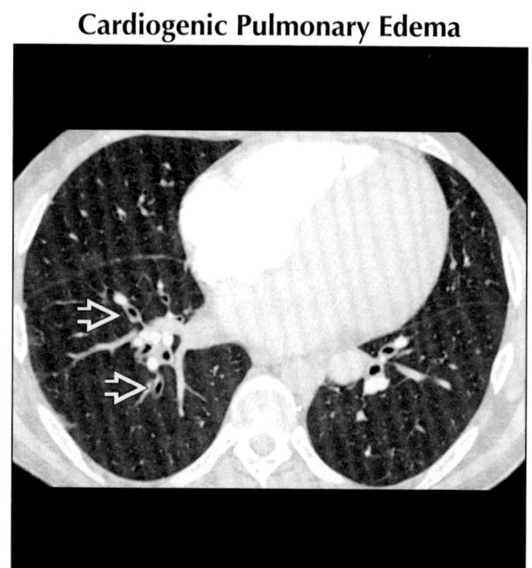

(Left) Longitudinal oblique CECT reconstruction shows chronic thromboembolus ➔ narrowing and filling the left lower lobe pulmonary artery. (Right) Axial CECT shows disparity in vessel size ➔ in the left lower lobe, better demonstrated with MIP reconstructions. Bronchial wall thickening ➔ narrows the airway lumen and leads to wheezing. Wheezing is the presenting symptom in 10% of patients with acute pulmonary embolus.

Pulmonary Emboli

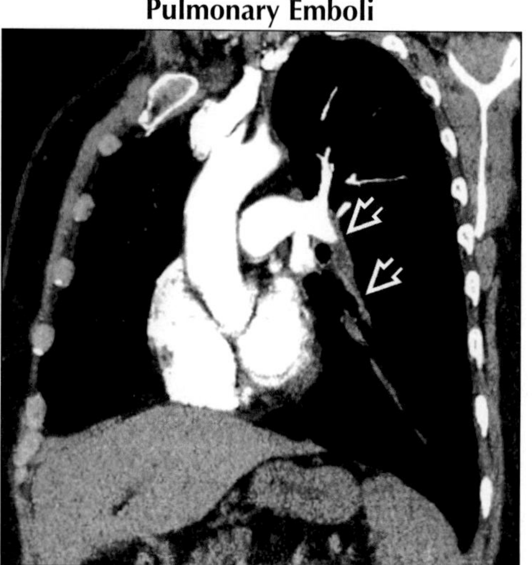

Pulmonary Emboli

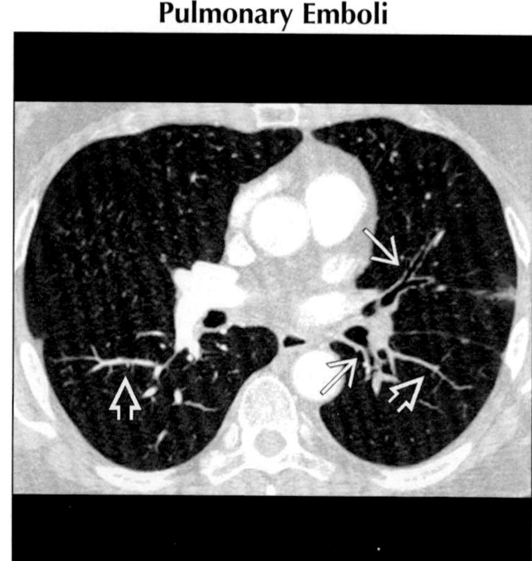

Aspiration

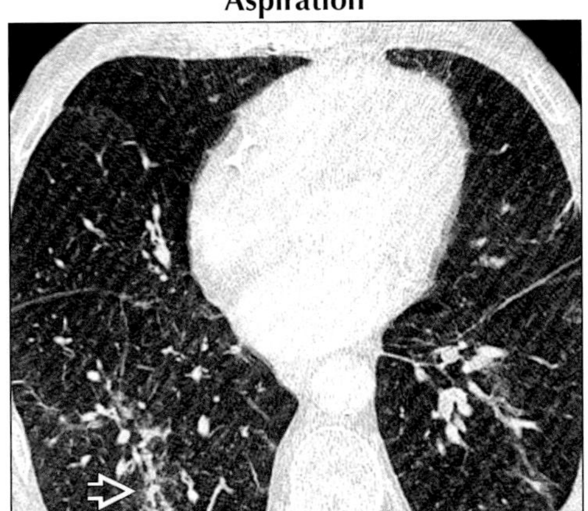

Aspiration

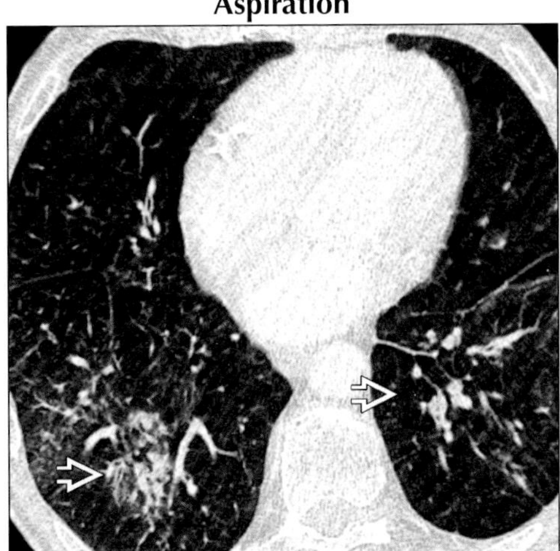

(Left) Axial CECT shows bibasilar peribronchovascular consolidation from aspiration. *(Right)* Axial CECT more inferiorly shows more extensive peribronchial consolidation. Aspiration is often asymmetric, primarily affects the dependent segments, and is more common in those with obtundation, esophageal reflux, or neuromuscular disease.

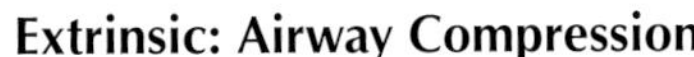

Extrinsic: Airway Compression

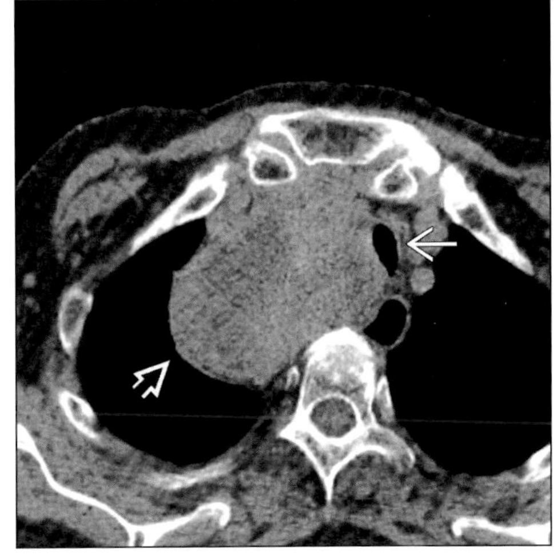

Extrinsic: Airway Compression

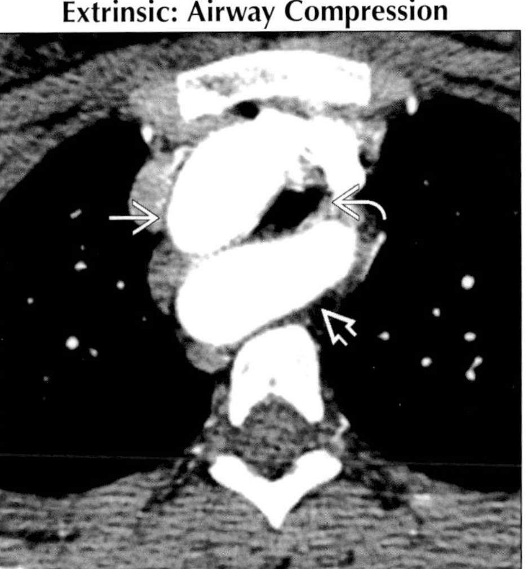

(Left) Axial NECT shows enlarged thyroid from goiter descending into the right paratracheal location. Trachea is deviated and narrowed. Symptoms generally occur when luminal area is decreased 50%. *(Right)* Axial CECT shows right cervical aortic arch, aberrant left subclavian artery, and tracheal compression. Long-term compression may result in tracheomalacia of compressed segment.

Intrinsic: Airway Narrowing

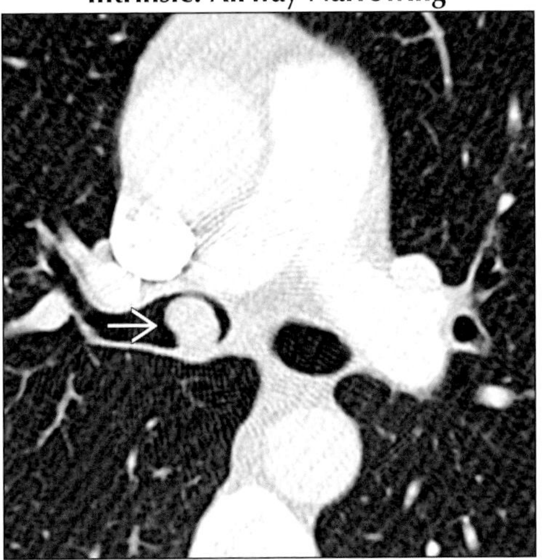

Intrinsic: Airway Narrowing

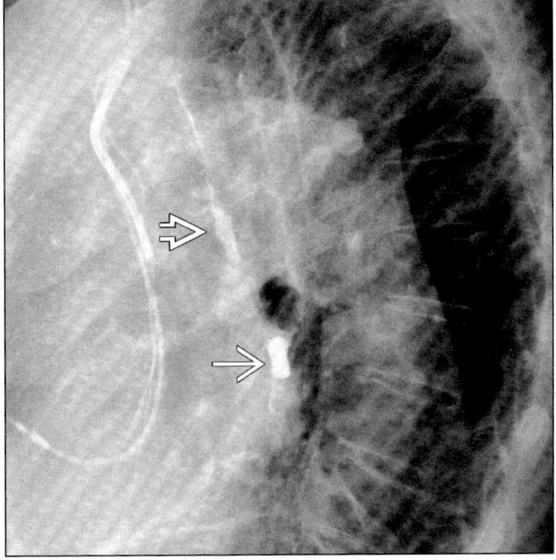

(Left) Axial CECT shows a solid, polypoid tumor arising from the posterior wall of the right mainstem bronchus due to a carcinoid tumor. Endobronchial narrowing may result in unilateral wheezing. *(Right)* Lateral radiograph shows a barium tablet in the bronchus intermedius. Liquid barium lines the anterior wall of the trachea. Foreign bodies may also give rise to wheezing. Up to 25% of adults with foreign bodies have no recollection of the event.

WHEEZING

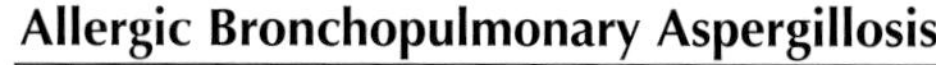

Allergic Bronchopulmonary Aspergillosis | **Allergic Bronchopulmonary Aspergillosis**

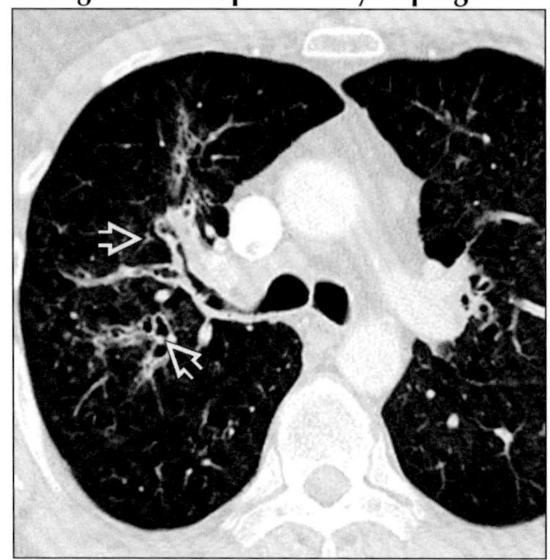

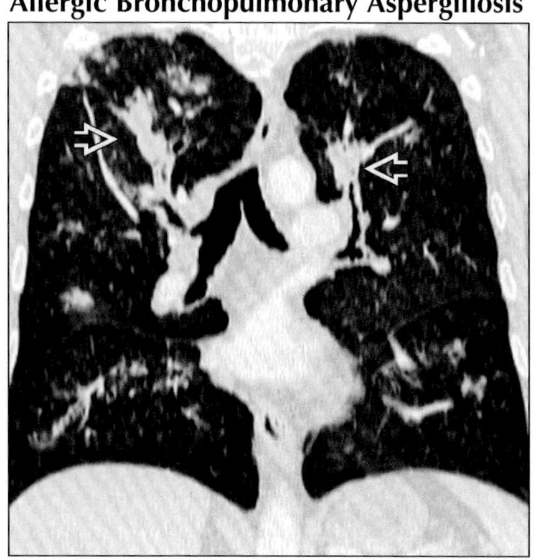

(Left) *Axial HRCT shows diffuse bronchiectasis ➡, mucoid impaction, and bronchial wall thickening.* ***(Right)*** *Coronal HRCT shows distribution of finger in glove opacities ➡ most severe in the upper lobes. Peripheral airways are often spared. Mild central bronchial dilatation is the earliest sign of allergic bronchopulmonary aspergillosis (ABPA) but is not specific, as dilatation may also be seen in 30% of asthmatics without ABPA.*

Tracheobronchomalacia | **Tracheobronchomalacia**

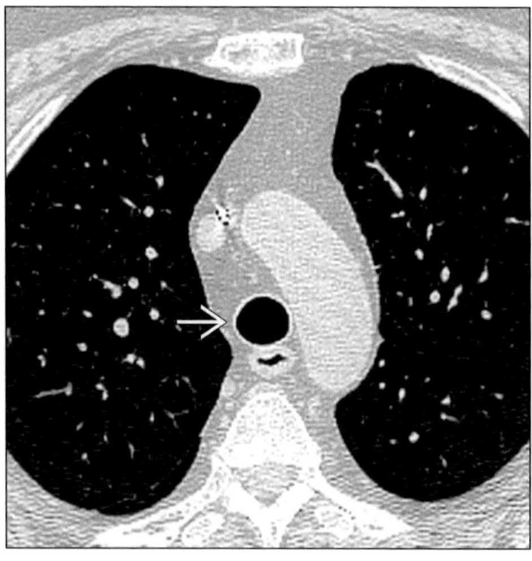

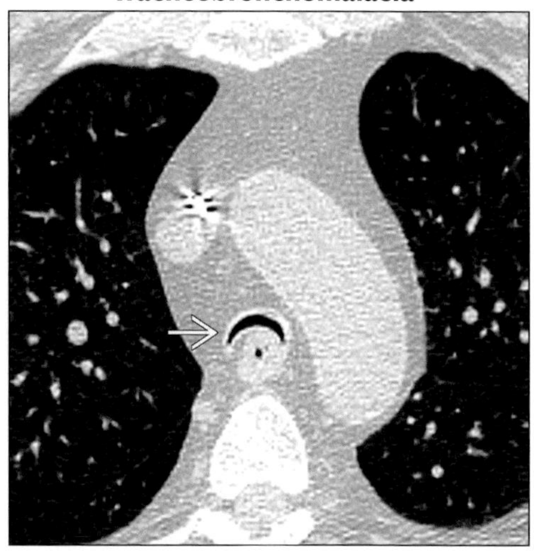

(Left) *Axial NECT shows the diameter and wall of the trachea and mainstem bronchi are normal ➡.* ***(Right)*** *Axial NECT in the same patient, at full expiration, shows more than 50% narrowing of the distal trachea ➡. Note the lunate morphology ("frown" sign). Patients with tracheomalacia may go for months or years misdiagnosed with asthma. Expiratory scanning is necessary for investigation of malacia.*

Churg-Strauss Syndrome | **Churg-Strauss Syndrome**

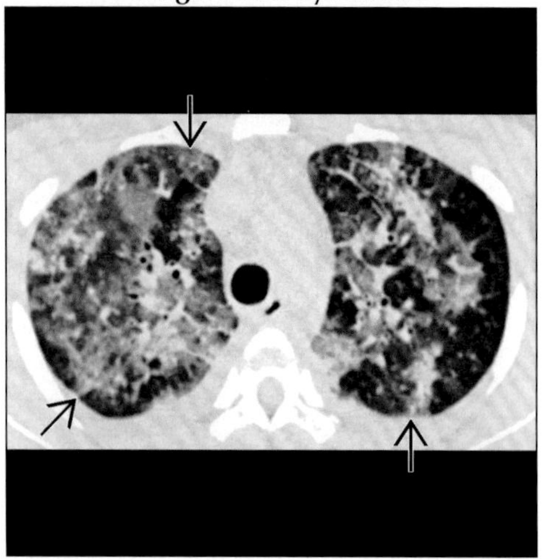

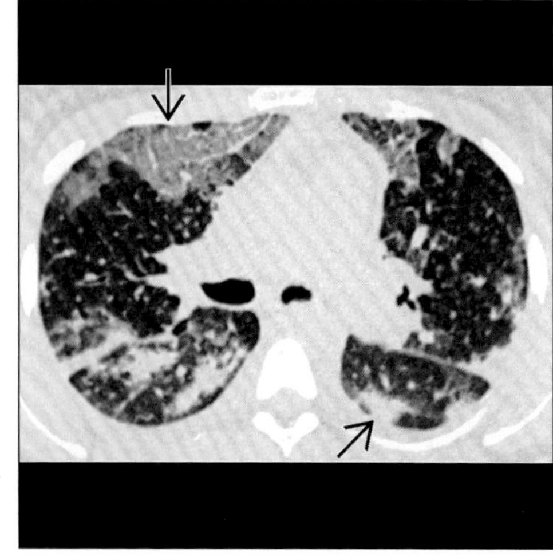

(Left) *Axial HRCT shows extensive ground-glass opacities and consolidation ➡ in the periphery of the upper lobes.* ***(Right)*** *Axial HRCT more inferiorly again shows findings of peripheral consolidation and ground-glass opacities ➡. These findings are similar to those with eosinophilic pneumonia (and may be fleeting). Pleural effusions may be seen with Churg-Strauss vasculitis and are uncommon in eosinophilic pneumonia.*

WHEEZING

Eosinophilic Pneumonia

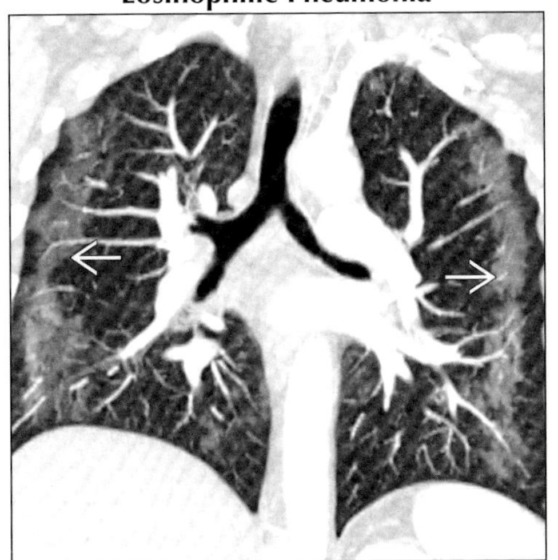

Carcinoid

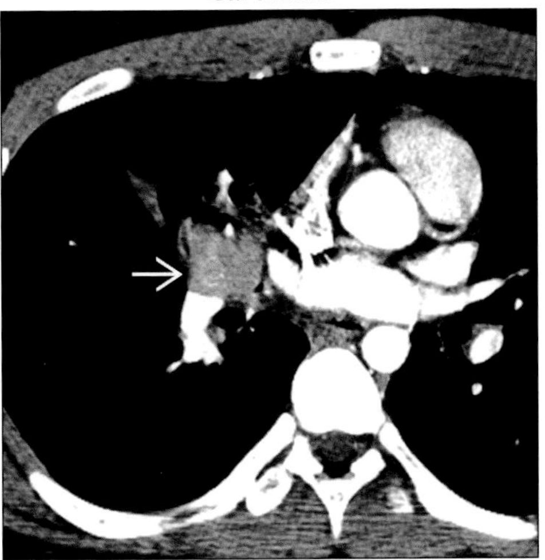

(Left) *Coronal CECT MIP reconstruction shows the distribution of peripheral consolidation from chronic eosinophilic pneumonia. Diffuse lung disease resolved 24 hours after administration of corticosteroids.* ***(Right)*** *Axial CECT shows a contrast-enhancing mass from carcinoid tumor. Carcinoid syndrome is uncommon unless the patient has liver metastases. Bone metastases are often osteosclerotic (similar to mastocytosis).*

Diffuse Neuroendocrine Hyperplasia

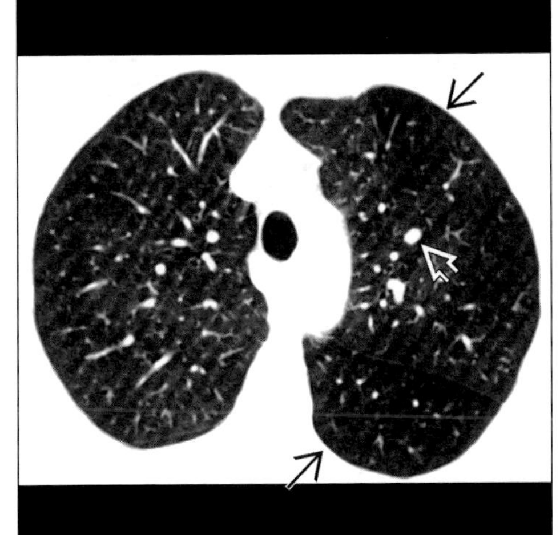

Diffuse Neuroendocrine Hyperplasia

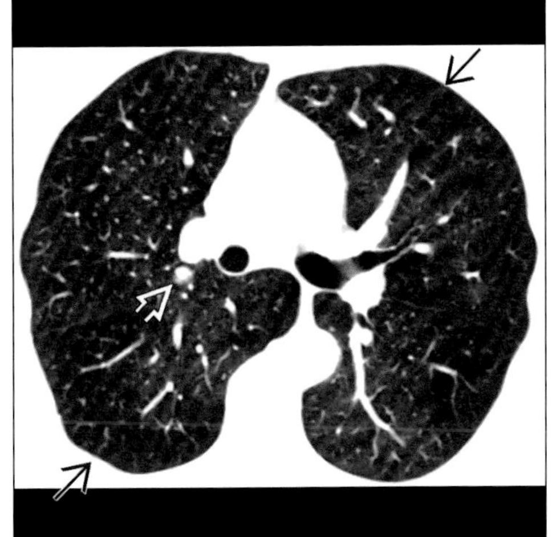

(Left) *Axial HRCT shows diffuse mosaic attenuation and a few scattered nodules.* ***(Right)*** *Axial HRCT more inferiorly shows the same findings of diffuse mosaic attenuation and a few scattered nodules. In some patients, nodules are the predominant finding leading to a work-up for possible metastatic disease.*

Mastocytosis

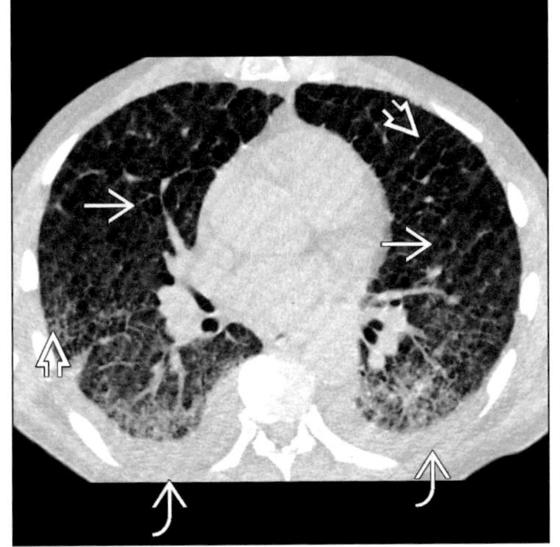

Mastocytosis

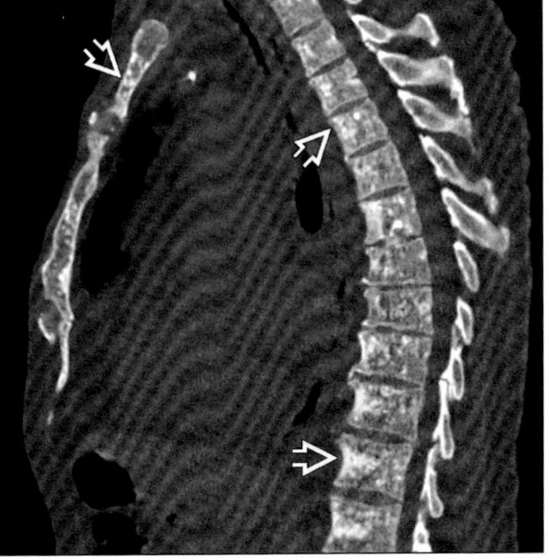

(Left) *Axial NECT shows cysts and septal thickening. Note the small bilateral pleural effusions.* ***(Right)*** *Sagittal NECT shows diffuse osteosclerosis, due to bone marrow infiltration. Other organs, particularly the spleen, may be involved. Splenic involvement may show generalized enlargement or enlargement from multiple focal masses. Wheezing is due to overproduction of histamine by mast cells.*

COUGH

DIFFERENTIAL DIAGNOSIS

Common

- Pneumonia
- Chronic Bronchitis
- Asthma
- Congestive Heart Failure
- Malignancy

Less Common

- Pulmonary Embolism
- Pneumothorax
- Mycobacterium Infection
- Cystic Fibrosis
- Sarcoidosis
- Bronchiectasis
- Smoking-Related Interstitial Lung Disease

Rare but Important

- Usual Interstitial Pneumonia
- Hypersensitivity Pneumonitis
- Pneumoconioses
- Langerhans Cell Histiocytosis
- Goodpasture Syndrome
- Bronchioloalveolar Cell Carcinoma
- Constrictive Bronchiolitis
- Pulmonary Alveolar Proteinosis
- Foreign Body
- Lipoid Pneumonia

ESSENTIAL INFORMATION

Key Differential Diagnosis Issues

- Over 1,000 conditions associated with cough
  - Review focuses on selected causes of cough identified on thoracic imaging
- Chronic cough defined by duration ≥ 3 weeks
  - Commonly secondary to post-nasal drip, asthma, GERD, chronic bronchitis, bronchiectasis, ACE inhibitor medications, and extrinsic tracheal compression
  - Most are radiographically occult

Helpful Clues for Common Diagnoses

- **Pneumonia**
  - Lobar or segmental lung consolidation
  - ± pleural effusion
- **Chronic Bronchitis**
  - ± bronchial wall thickening &/or mucus plugging
- **Asthma**
  - ± hyperinflation
  - ± bronchial wall thickening
  - Complications include pneumonia, pneumothorax, pneumomediastinum, or atelectasis
- **Congestive Heart Failure**
  - Cardiomegaly and pleural effusions
  - Kerley B lines
- **Malignancy**
  - Bronchogenic carcinoma
    - Spiculated lung nodule or mass
    - ± lymphadenopathy
  - Lymphangitic carcinomatosis
    - Smooth or nodular thickening of interlobular septa
    - ± pleural effusions and lymphadenopathy

Helpful Clues for Less Common Diagnoses

- **Pulmonary Embolism**
  - CTA: Filling defect diagnostic
    - "Railroad track" or "doughnut" signs
  - Document signs of right heart strain
    - RV/LV chamber size ≥ 1, leftward bowing of interventricular septum, or reflux of contrast into IVC
- **Pneumothorax**
  - Spontaneous
    - Young, tall, and thin male smokers
    - Also seen in emphysema, asthma, infection, lung fibrosis, or cystic lung disease
  - Traumatic or iatrogenic
- **Mycobacterium Infection**
  - *M. tuberculosis*
    - Upper lobe cavitary nodule
    - Tree in bud opacities indicates endobronchial spread of disease
  - *M. avium complex*
    - Older women
    - Middle lobe or lingular bronchiectasis
    - Tree in bud opacities
- **Cystic Fibrosis**
  - Hyperinflation with bronchiectasis
  - Early upper lobe involvement
- **Sarcoidosis**
  - Paratracheal and symmetric hilar lymphadenopathy
  - ± perilymphatic lung nodules (nodules along fissures, subpleural lung, and bronchovascular bundles)
- **Bronchiectasis**
  - Tram-tracking

- CT diagnostic
  - Bronchus ≥ in size than adjacent artery
- **Smoking-Related Interstitial Lung Disease**
  - Respiratory bronchiolitis associated interstitial lung disease
    - Symptomatic smoker
    - Upper lung predominant centrilobular nodules of ground-glass opacity
  - Desquamative interstitial pneumonia
    - Diffuse/patchy, lower lung predominant ground-glass opacity
    - ± cystic spaces and centrilobular emphysema

Helpful Clues for Rare Diagnoses

- **Usual Interstitial Pneumonia**
  - Basal and subpleural fibrosis with honeycombing
  - ± mediastinal lymphadenopathy
- **Hypersensitivity Pneumonitis**
  - Centrilobular nodules of ground-glass opacity
  - "Head-cheese" sign
    - Ground-glass opacity, air-trapping, and normal lung
- **Pneumoconioses**
  - Asbestosis
    - Posterobasal and subpleural lung
    - Bilateral pleural plaques
    - Reticular and dot-like opacities early
    - Fibrosis and distortion late
  - Silicosis/Coal worker's pneumoconiosis
    - Posterior and superior lung
    - Centrilobular and subpleural nodules
    - ± calcified lymphadenopathy
- **Langerhans Cell Histiocytosis**
  - Smokers, 20-40 years old
  - Centrilobular nodules and cavitary nodules
  - Spares costophrenic sulci
  - Round or bizarrely shaped cysts
  - ± pneumothorax
- **Goodpasture Syndrome**
  - Hemoptysis
  - Ground-glass opacity or consolidation
- **Bronchioloalveolar Cell Carcinoma**
  - Chronic ground-glass opacity with "pseudocavitation"
- **Constrictive Bronchiolitis**
  - Bronchiectasis, mosaic perfusion, and expiratory air-trapping
  - Causes include
    - Infection, toxic fume inhalation, collagen vascular diseases, and chronic lung transplant rejection
- **Pulmonary Alveolar Proteinosis**
  - Chronic crazy-paving
    - Geographic ground-glass opacity with superimposed interlobular septal thickening
- **Foreign Body**
  - History key to diagnosis
- **Lipoid Pneumonia**
  - Aspiration of oils used for laxatives
  - Lower lobe consolidation or mass
    - Central low attenuation areas (-80 to -30 HU)

Pneumonia

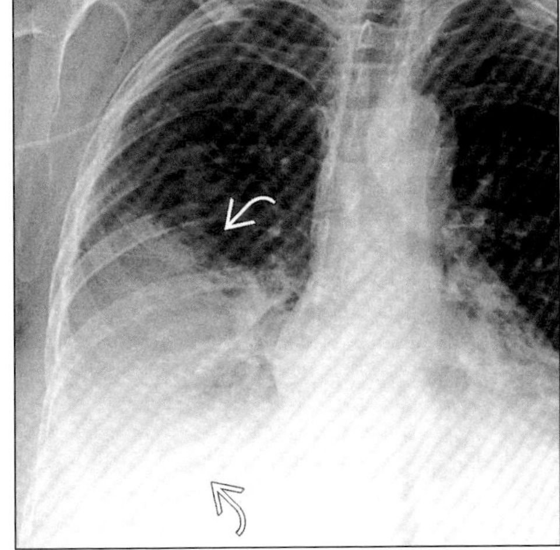

Frontal radiograph shows right lower lobe consolidation ➔ in this patient with high fevers, cough, and dyspnea. Clinical history of infection is key for making this diagnosis.

Pneumonia

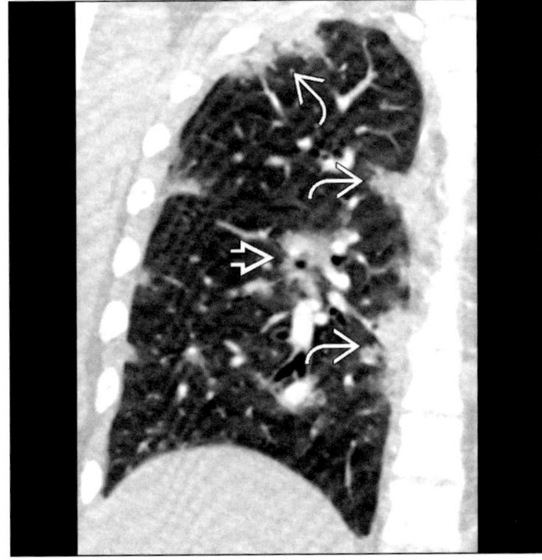

Coronal NECT shows peribronchial consolidation ➔ and peripheral subpleural consolidation ➔ reminiscent of organizing or eosinophilic pneumonia. This pattern is also described in H1N1 infection.

COUGH

(Left) Axial NECT shows thickening of the walls of the bronchus intermedius ➔. Other bronchial walls were thickened, helping to distinguish this from malignancy. Note centrilobular ➔ and paraseptal emphysema ➔. (Right) Frontal radiograph shows hyperinflated lungs and bilateral lower lung bronchial wall thickening ➔. Complications associated with an asthma attack include atelectasis, pneumonia, pneumothorax, or pneumomediastinum.

Chronic Bronchitis

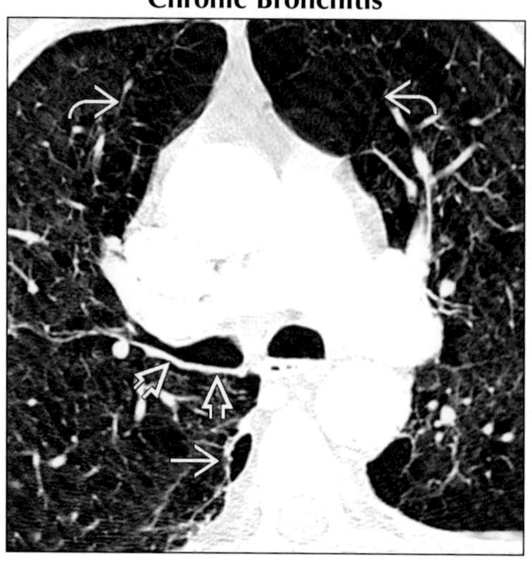

Asthma

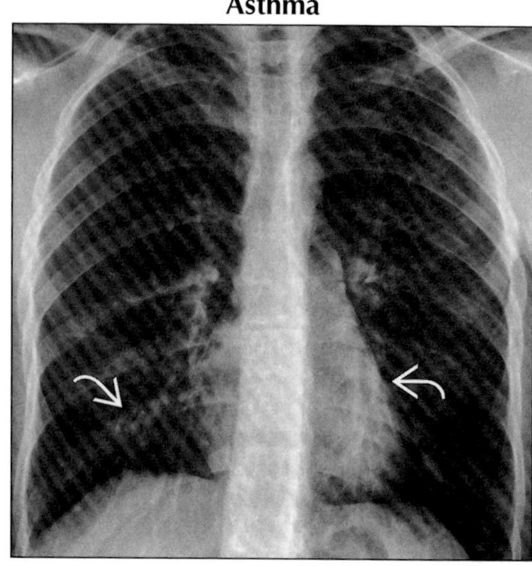

(Left) Frontal radiograph shows many Kerley B lines ➔ from acute pulmonary edema. Interlobular septal thickening caused by lymphangitic carcinomatosis is differentiated by a history of malignancy. (Right) Axial NECT shows variant CT features of smooth septal thickening ➔ in lymphangitic carcinomatosis in a patient with disseminated adenocarcinoma of unknown primary. Nodular thickening is more specific for metastases.

Congestive Heart Failure

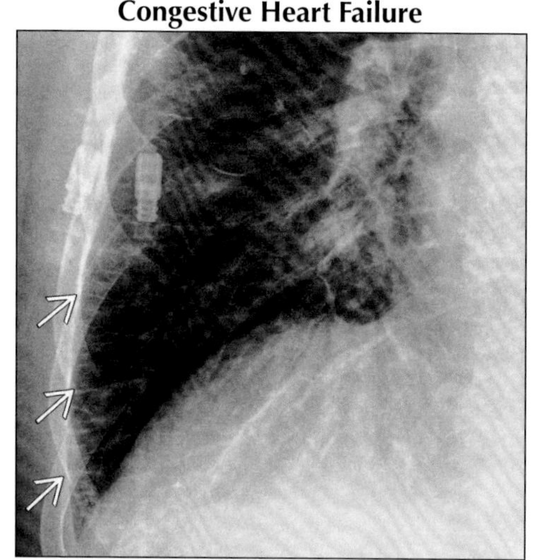

Malignancy

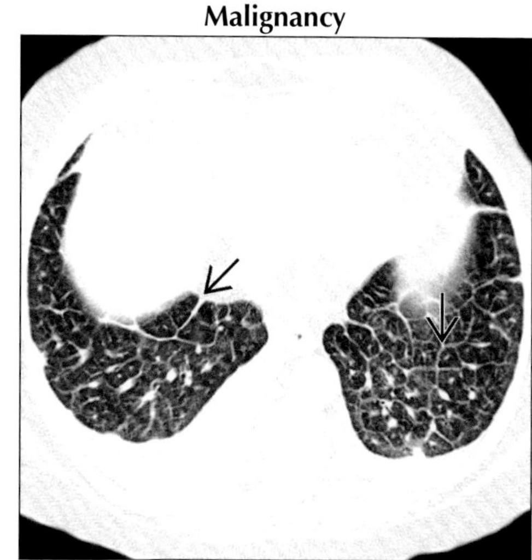

(Left) Frontal radiograph shows right upper lobe collapse with tracheal shift ➔, elevated minor fissure ➔, and elevated right hemidiaphragm ➔. Lobar collapse is highly concerning for a central obstructing malignancy in an outpatient. (Right) Axial CECT shows filling defects in the left descending pulmonary artery ➔ and segmental upper lobe pulmonary artery ➔. Document signs of right heart strain, including abnormal RV/LV ratio and IVC reflux.

Malignancy

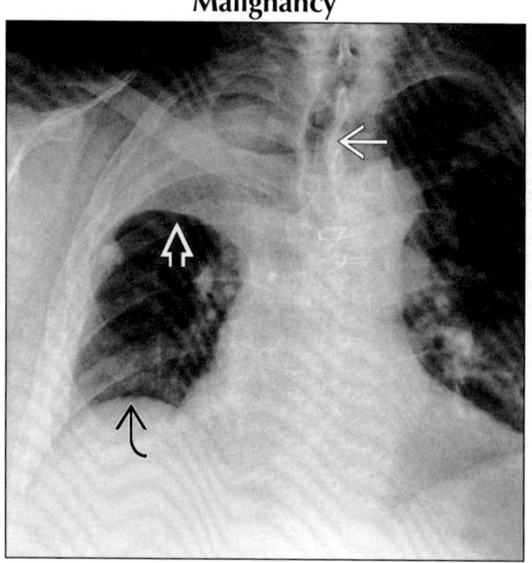

Pulmonary Embolism

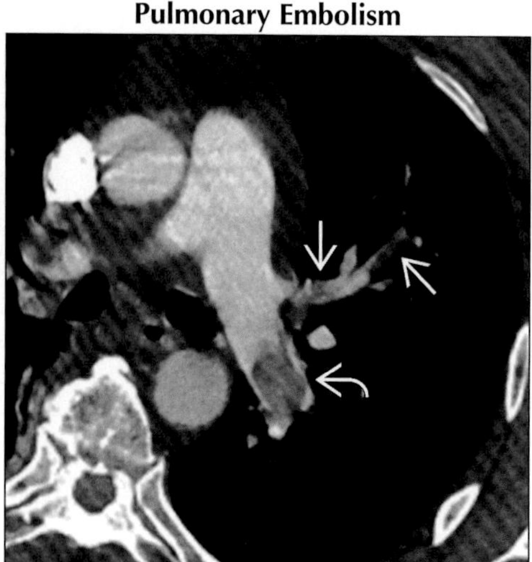

Pneumothorax

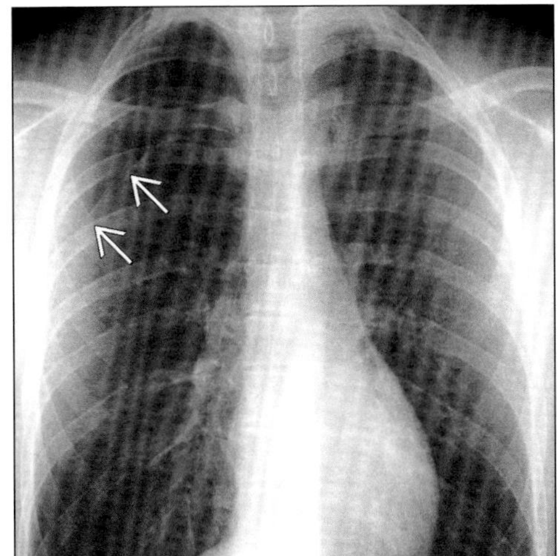

Mycobacterium Infection

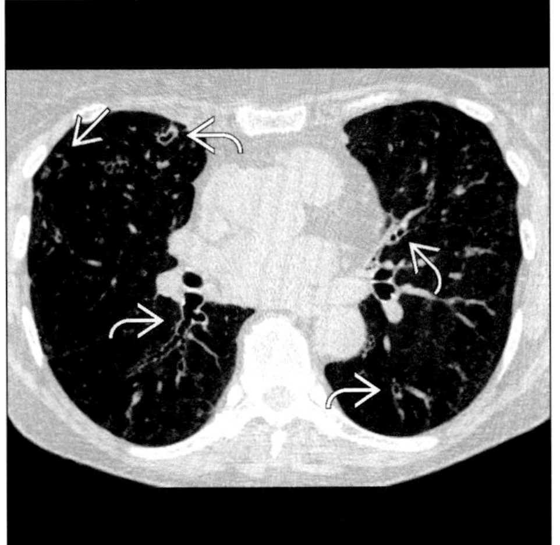

(Left) *Frontal radiograph shows spontaneous right pneumothorax ➡. This classically occurs in young, tall, and thin male smokers. Blebs or bullae at the pleural surface can rupture, creating a bronchopleural fistula.* ***(Right)*** *Axial NECT shows bronchiectasis involving the lower lobes, lingula, and middle lobe bronchi ↪. Note middle lobe opacities ➡ in this older woman with atypical mycobacterial infection.*

Mycobacterium Infection

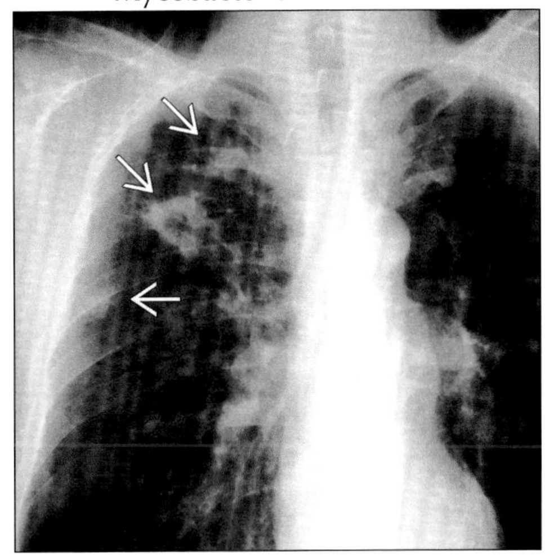

Cystic Fibrosis

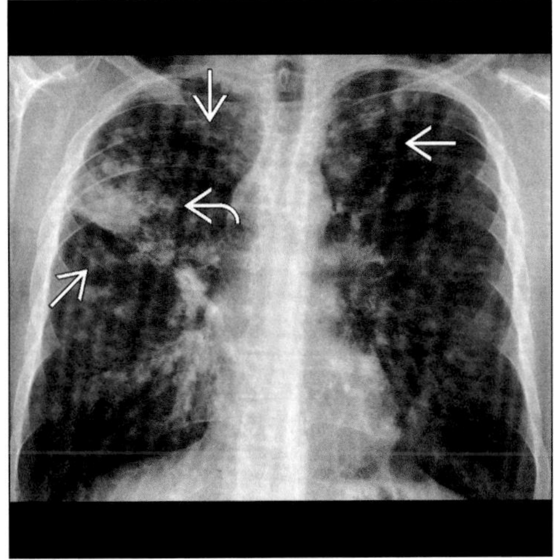

(Left) *Frontal radiograph shows right upper lobe multifocal irregular opacities with cavitation ➡. NECT (not shown) revealed variable thickness in cavity walls with irregular exterior and smooth inner margins in this case of postprimary tuberculosis infection.* ***(Right)*** *Frontal radiograph shows large lung volumes with upper lobe predominant bronchial wall thickening and bronchiectasis ➡. Right upper lobe consolidation ↪ was due to pneumonia.*

Sarcoidosis

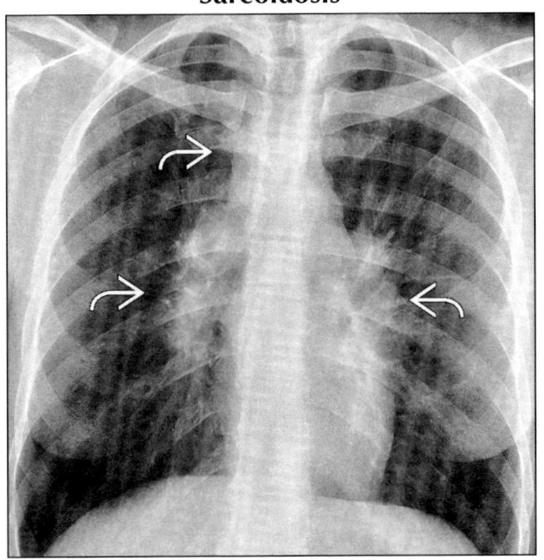

Bronchiectasis

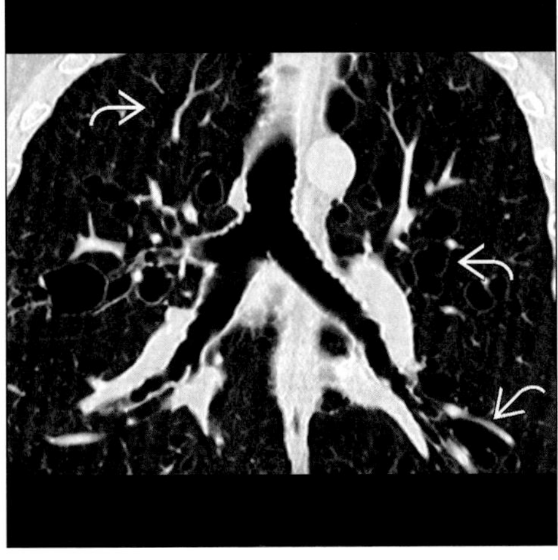

(Left) *Frontal radiograph shows right paratracheal and symmetric bilateral hilar lymphadenopathy ↪, representing Garland triad. Sarcoidosis commonly affects women 20-50 years old and often causes a dry cough and dyspnea.* ***(Right)*** *Coronal NECT shows bronchiectasis involving the 4th to 6th order bronchi ↪ secondary to defective cartilage in this patient with Williams-Campbell syndrome. Note the normal appearance of the central airways.*

COUGH

(Left) Axial NECT shows ill-defined centrilobular nodules of ground-glass opacity in this symptomatic smoker. Biopsy revealed respiratory bronchiolitis. This patient also had a dilated esophagus with manometry-proven achalasia. (Right) Axial HRCT shows extensive right lower lobe honeycombing, identified by multiple cysts stacked on each other. Note subpleural reticular opacities and traction bronchiectasis, indicating fibrosis.

Smoking-Related Interstitial Lung Disease

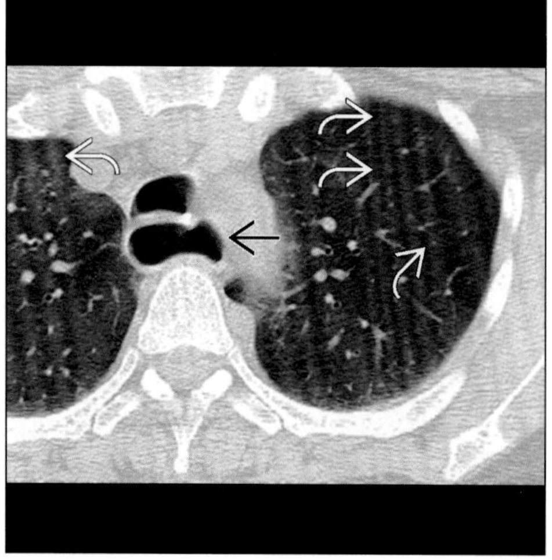

Usual Interstitial Pneumonia

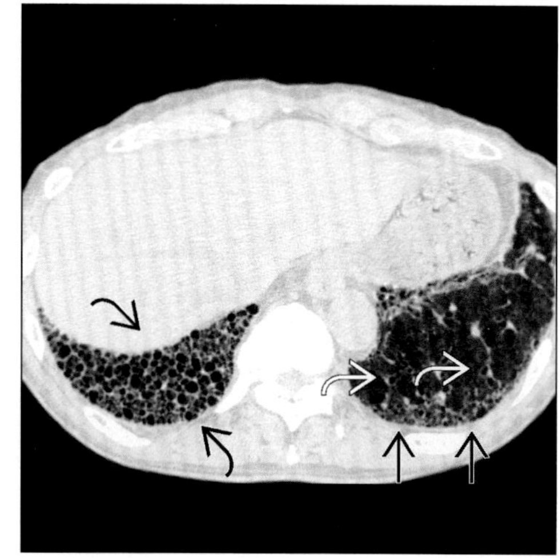

(Left) Axial NECT shows "head-cheese" sign with 3 different lung densities. Note ground-glass opacity, normal lung, and abnormally hyperlucent lung. Other common findings (not shown) in hypersensitivity pneumonitis are centrilobular nodules of ground-glass opacity. (Right) Axial HRCT shows reticular opacities and traction bronchiectasis from asbestosis. Note calcified pleural plaques, better seen on mediastinal windows.

Hypersensitivity Pneumonitis

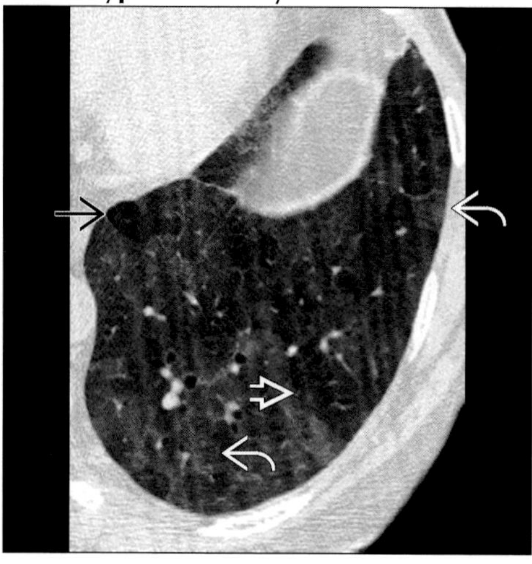

Pneumoconioses

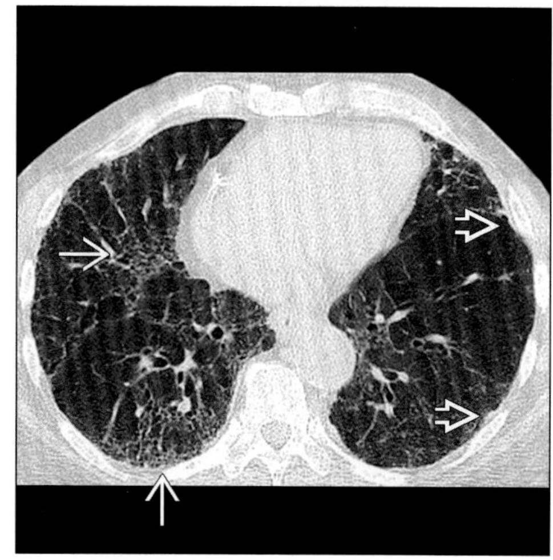

(Left) Frontal radiograph shows large upper lobe opacities with upward hilar retraction in this patient with progressive massive fibrosis from silicosis. The peripheral lung is emphysematous, and there are adjacent smaller nodules. (Right) Axial CECT shows multiple irregularly and bizarrely shaped lung cysts in endstage LCH. This is differentiated from centrilobular emphysema by definable walls and lack of centrilobular core structures.

Pneumoconioses

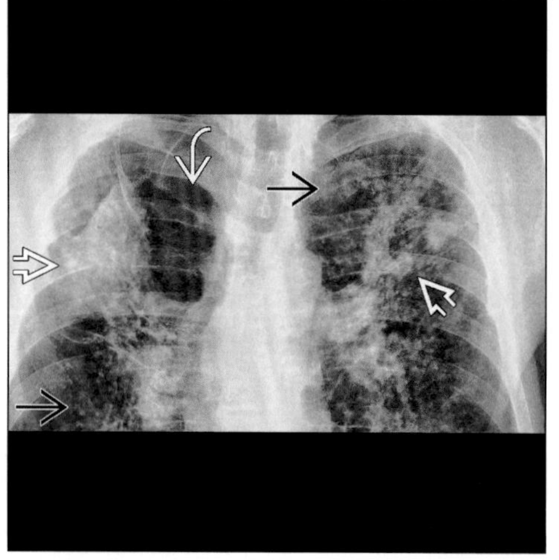

Langerhans Cell Histiocytosis

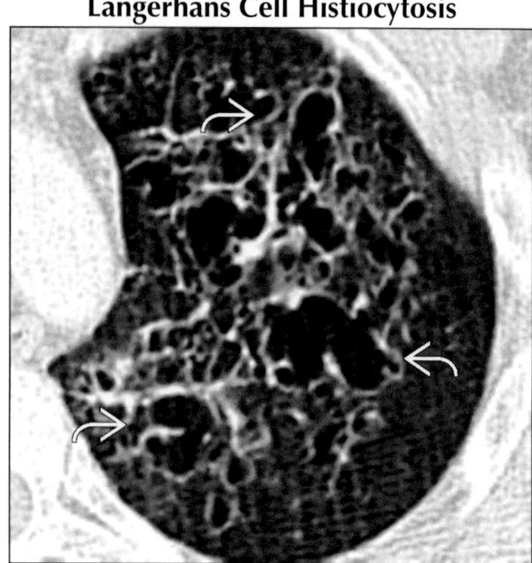

Goodpasture Syndrome

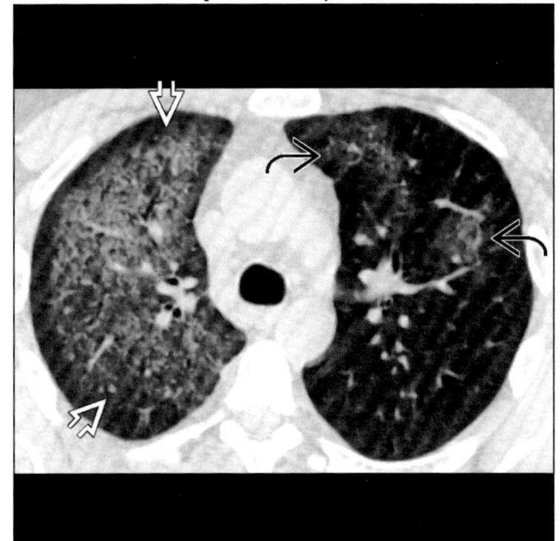

Bronchioloalveolar Cell Carcinoma

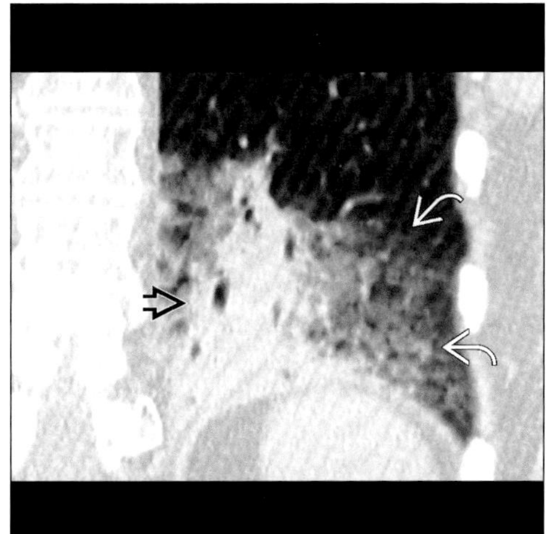

(Left) *Axial CECT shows diffuse ground-glass opacities throughout the right lung with peripheral subpleural sparing ➡ and lobular involvement of the left lung ↗. Edema or atypical infection could have a similar appearance.* ***(Right)*** *Coronal NECT shows consolidation ⇨ and surrounding ground-glass opacity ➡ unchanged over a 6-month period.*

Constrictive Bronchiolitis

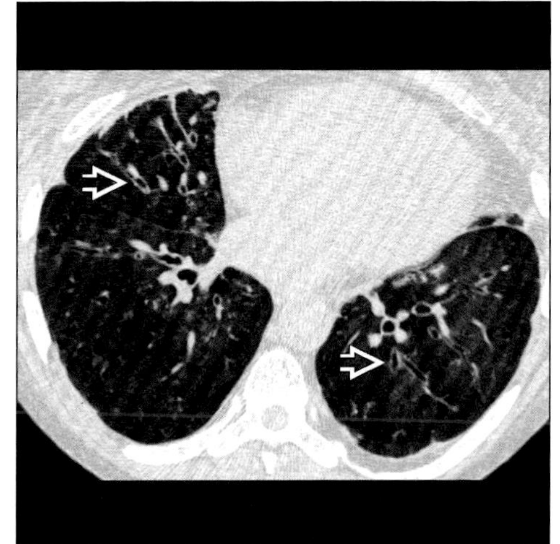

Pulmonary Alveolar Proteinosis

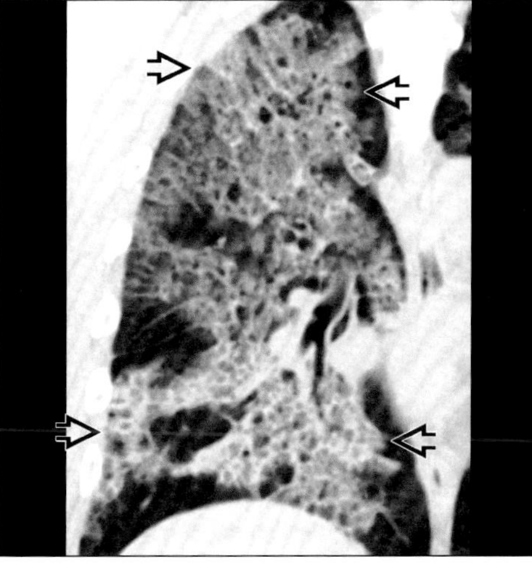

(Left) *Axial HRCT shows bronchiectasis ➡ and mosaic perfusion indicated by more lucent portions of lung with normal-appearing adjacent lung in this patient status post lung transplantation. This pattern is associated with constrictive bronchiolitis and chronic rejection.* ***(Right)*** *Coronal NECT shows geographic ground-glass opacity with superimposed interlobular septal thickening resulting in a crazy-paving pattern ⇨.*

Foreign Body

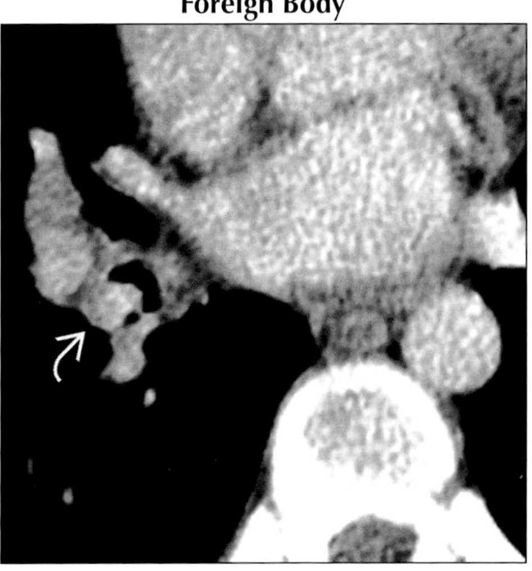

Lipoid Pneumonia

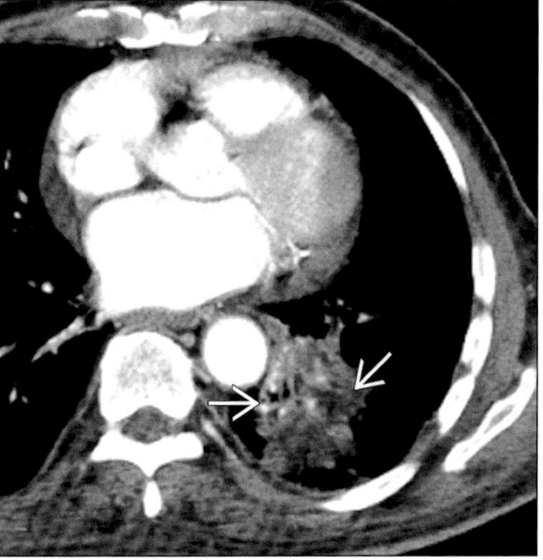

(Left) *Axial CECT shows a mildly hyperdense nodule ➡ within the bronchus intermedius. This represented a small bag of cocaine at bronchoscopy. An endobronchial carcinoma, carcinoid, or hamartoma could have a similar appearance.* ***(Right)*** *Axial CECT shows fat attenuation ➡ in a mass-like opacity located in the left lower lobe. This is associated with aspirated mineral oils occasionally used as laxatives.*

ACUTE DYSPNEA

DIFFERENTIAL DIAGNOSIS

Common
- Pneumonia
- Pulmonary Edema
- Pulmonary Embolism
- Pneumothorax
- Pleural Effusion
- Aspiration
- Asthma/COPD Exacerbation

Less Common
- Lobar Collapse
- Septic Embolism
- Pericardial Disease

Rare but Important
- Acute Interstitial Pneumonia
- Pulmonary Hemorrhage
- Fat Embolism
- Interstitial Lung Disease Exacerbation
- Acute Hypersensitivity Pneumonitis
- Acute Eosinophilic Pneumonia

ESSENTIAL INFORMATION

Key Differential Diagnosis Issues
- Review focuses on intrathoracic causes of dyspnea presenting within minutes to days

Helpful Clues for Common Diagnoses
- **Pneumonia**
  - Symptoms of infection
  - Lobar or segmental lung consolidation
  - ± pleural effusion
- **Pulmonary Edema**
  - Pulmonary venous hypertension with transudation of fluid
  - Radiographs and CT
    - Smooth interlobular septal thickening (Kerley B lines)
    - Fissural thickening
    - Dependent distribution
    - ± pleural effusions
- **Pulmonary Embolism**
  - CTA: Filling defect is diagnostic
    - "Railroad track" or "doughnut" signs
  - Document signs of right heart strain
    - RV/LV chamber size ≥ 1, reflux of contrast into IVC, or leftward bowing of interventricular septum
- **Pneumothorax**
  - Spontaneous
    - Rupture of apical bleb or bulla
    - Young, tall, and thin male smokers
    - Association with emphysema, asthma, infection, lung fibrosis, or cystic lung disease
    - Recurs in 50% of patients
  - Traumatic
    - Chest trauma or mechanical ventilation
- **Pleural Effusion**
  - Exudative effusions
    - Causes include infections, malignancy, connective tissue diseases, and asbestos exposure
    - Pleural thickening and enhancement seen in 60%
    - Ultrasound depicts septations and heterogeneous echotexture
  - Transudative effusions
    - Common in congestive heart failure, renal disease, and hypoalbuminemia
- **Aspiration**
  - Most common in right lower lobe
    - Secondary to more vertical orientation of right mainstem bronchus
  - Pleural effusion is uncommon
- **Asthma/COPD Exacerbation**
  - Flat diaphragms from lung hyperinflation
  - Exacerbation usually does not cause new radiographic findings
  - Associated complications
    - Pneumonia
    - Pneumothorax
    - Pneumomediastinum
    - Atelectasis

Helpful Clues for Less Common Diagnoses
- **Lobar Collapse**
  - Signs of volume loss
    - Mediastinal shift
    - Fissural displacement
    - Crowding of vessels
    - Diaphragmatic elevation
  - Occurs secondary to
    - Central obstructing mass or nodule in outpatients
    - Mucus plug in inpatients
- **Septic Embolism**
  - Multiple bilateral lower lobe predominant peripheral nodules
  - ± central cavitation
  - Most common in intravenous drug abusers
- **Pericardial Disease**

- Pericardial effusion
  - Rapid fluid accumulation secondary to malignancy or infection
- Acute pericarditis
  - Pericardial thickening ≥ 4 mm ± pericardial effusion
  - Contrast enhancement of thickened pericardium

Helpful Clues for Rare Diagnoses

- **Acute Interstitial Pneumonia**
  - Acute respiratory distress syndrome without identifiable cause
  - Viral respiratory syndrome followed by rapid respiratory decline
  - Bilateral patchy lung consolidation and ground-glass opacity
  - Most commonly affects dependent lung
  - 50% mortality
- **Pulmonary Hemorrhage**
  - Ground-glass opacity or patchy/diffuse consolidation
  - ± sparing of subpleural lung
  - Pleural effusions are rare
  - Important historical clue is presence of hemoptysis or anemia
  - Causes
    - Pulmonary-renal syndromes, vasculitis, anticoagulation, drug reactions, and collagen vascular disease
- **Fat Embolism**
  - Usually secondary to long bone fracture
  - Classic clinical triad
    - Petechial rash, altered mental status, and hypoxia
  - Small centrilobular and subpleural lung nodules
  - Nonspecific bilateral ground-glass opacity without zonal predominance
- **Interstitial Lung Disease Exacerbation**
  - Rapid deterioration in presence of known interstitial lung disease
  - Must exclude infection (*Pneumocystis*) and congestive heart failure
  - Ground-glass opacity or consolidation superimposed on interstitial lung disease pattern
- **Acute Hypersensitivity Pneumonitis**
  - Occurs with large inhaled antigen exposure
  - Middle and lower lung consolidation secondary to acute lung injury
  - ± centrilobular nodules of ground-glass opacity
  - ± mosaic perfusion and expiratory air-trapping
- **Acute Eosinophilic Pneumonia**
  - Fever with rapidly progressing respiratory distress
  - Eosinophils in serum and lavage fluid
  - Rapid response to steroids
  - Radiographic progression similar to pulmonary edema
    - Bilateral reticular opacities and Kerley B lines
    - Lower lobe consolidation, small pleural effusions

Pneumonia

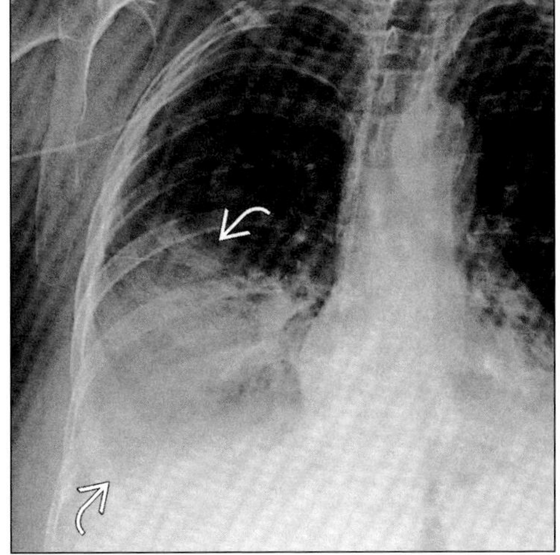

Frontal radiograph shows right mid and lower lung consolidation ➔ in this patient with a high fever and productive cough. Silhouetting of right hemidiaphragm indicates right lower lobe involvement.

Pneumonia

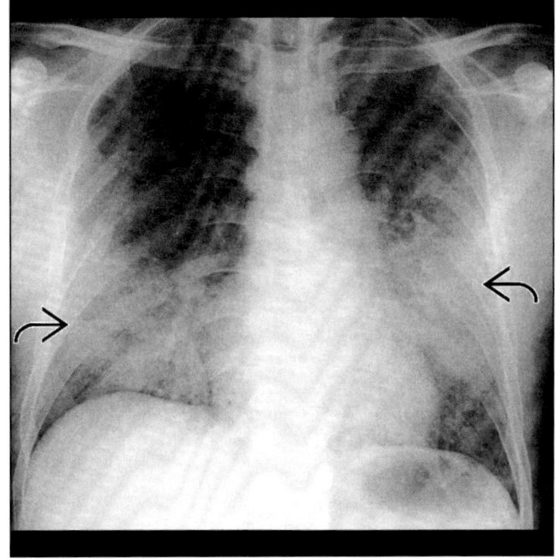

Frontal radiograph shows bilateral mid and lower lung consolidation ➔ in this patient presenting with severe hypoxia. Pneumocystis pneumonia and HIV were subsequently diagnosed.

ACUTE DYSPNEA

Pulmonary Edema

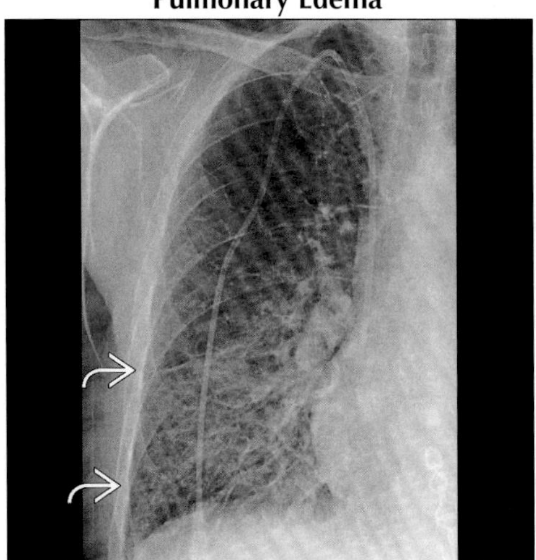

Pulmonary Edema

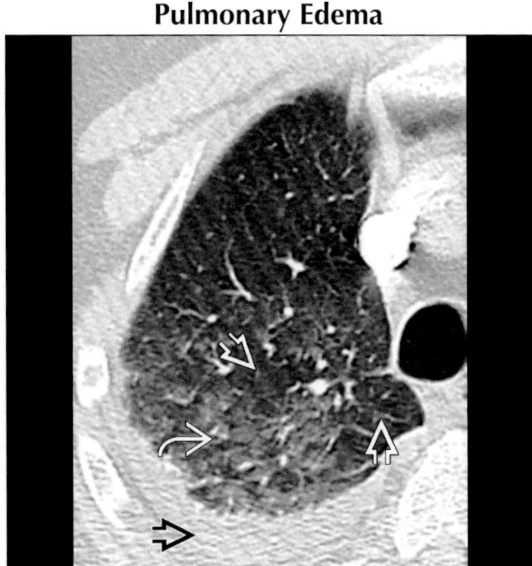

(Left) *Frontal radiograph shows multiple lower lobe septal lines or Kerley B lines ➔, which represent thickening of interlobular septa. Note vascular indistinctness without alveolar filling.* ***(Right)*** *Axial CECT shows dependent ground-glass opacity ➔ with lobular sparing ➔ secondary to differing lobular perfusion. Note right pleural effusion ➔. New onset edema is a presenting sign of myocardial infarction in 50% of patients, as in this case.*

Pulmonary Edema

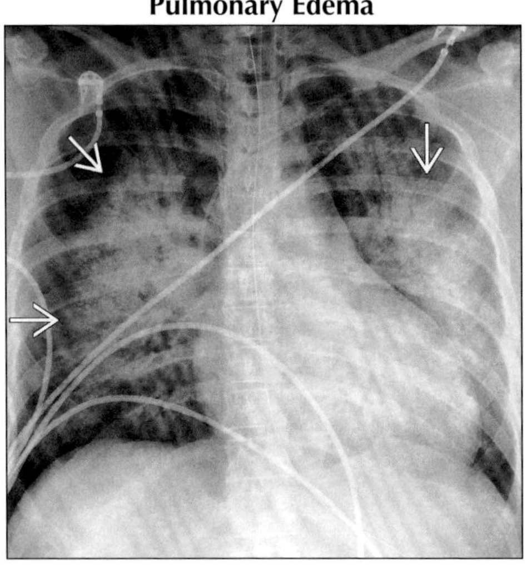

Pulmonary Embolism

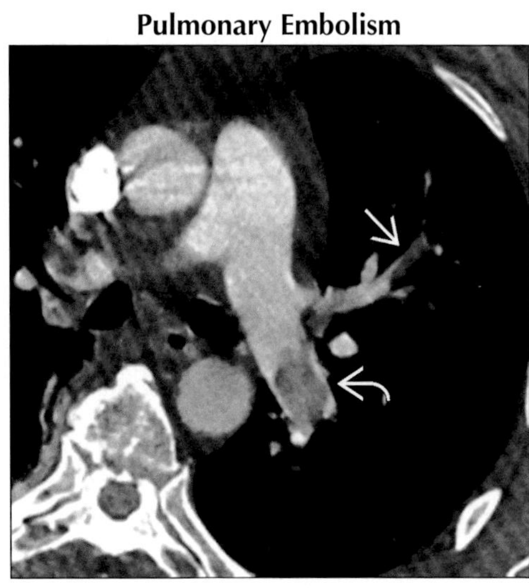

(Left) *Anteroposterior radiograph shows central pulmonary consolidation ➔ and moderate cardiomegaly. The patient was in acute congestive heart failure.* ***(Right)*** *Axial CECT shows a large filling defect within the left pulmonary artery with characteristic "railroad track" sign ➔. Note segmental pulmonary embolism to a left upper lobe pulmonary artery ➔. It is important to report signs of right heart strain, such as RV/LV > 1 and reflux into the IVC.*

Pulmonary Embolism

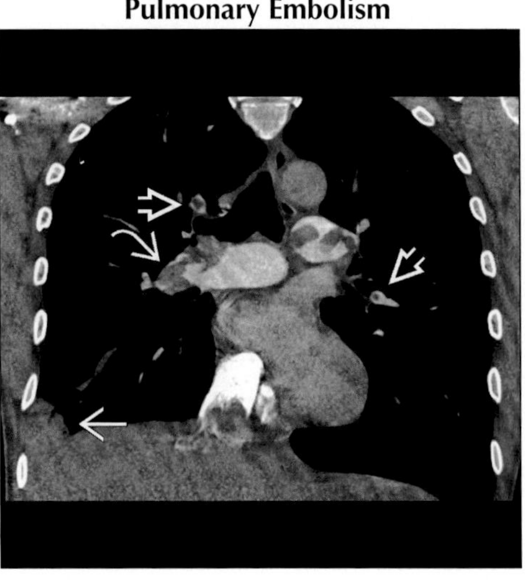

Pneumothorax

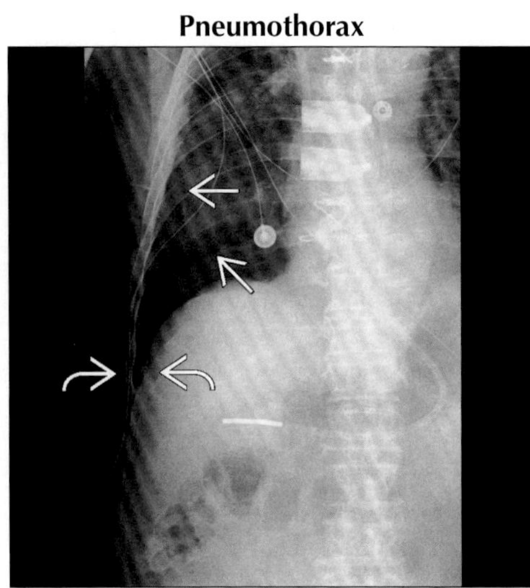

(Left) *Coronal CECT shows pulmonary embolism within the main and segmental pulmonary arteries with "doughnut" ➔ and "railroad track" signs ➔. Wedge-shaped right lower lobe opacity is a pulmonary infarct ➔.* ***(Right)*** *Frontal radiograph shows a right pneumothorax with deep sulcus sign ➔. Note pleural edge ➔ with no lung markings distal to this point. This finding was better seen on the abdominal radiograph, which is occasionally seen.*

ACUTE DYSPNEA

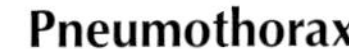

Pneumothorax

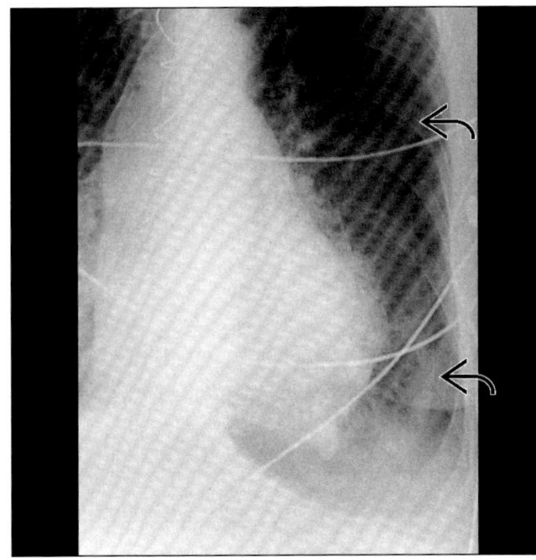

Pleural Effusion

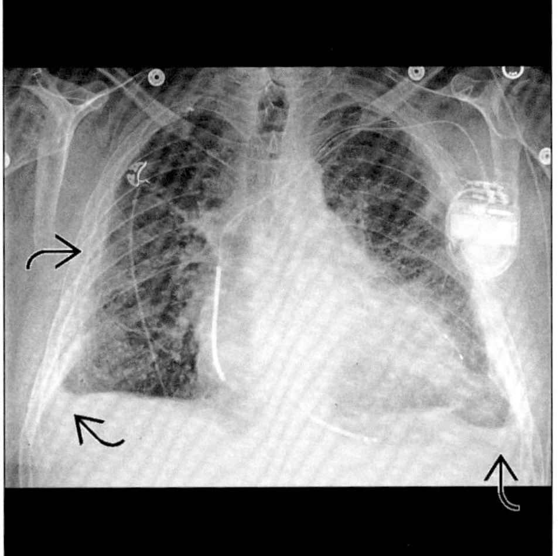

(Left) *Frontal radiograph shows a left pneumothorax → with ipsilateral hemidiaphragm depression. This patient died shortly after this radiograph secondary to hemodynamic compromise. Tension pneumothorax is a clinical diagnosis but must be suggested by the above radiographic presentation.* ***(Right)*** *Frontal radiograph shows cardiomegaly, bilateral pleural effusions →, and pulmonary edema in this patient with an elevated BNP and congestive heart failure.*

Aspiration

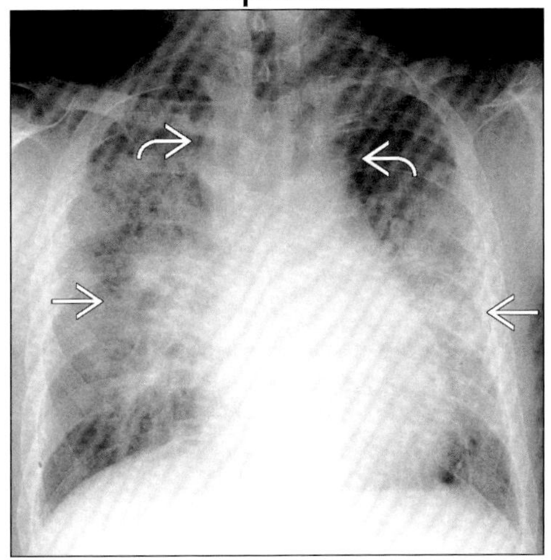

Asthma/COPD Exacerbation

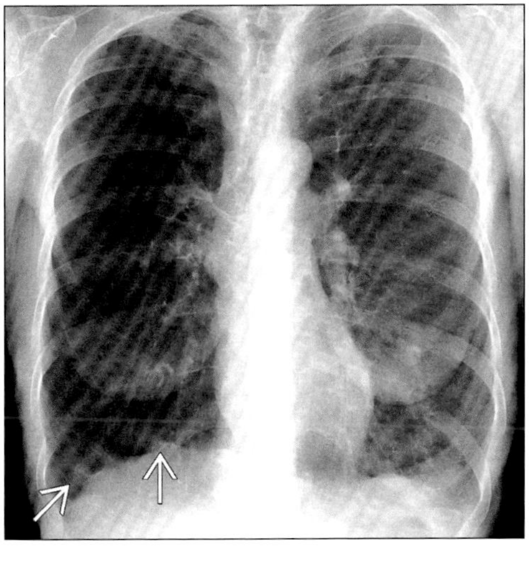

(Left) *Frontal radiograph shows central consolidation → from massive aspiration. Note mediastinal widening → from achalasia, the source of aspiration. Pulmonary edema or diffuse infection could also have this appearance.* ***(Right)*** *Frontal radiograph shows marked hyperinflation. Note flattened hemidiaphragms and diaphragmatic slips →. Peripheral vasculature is attenuated. No lung consolidation is identified to indicate superimposed pneumonia.*

Asthma/COPD Exacerbation

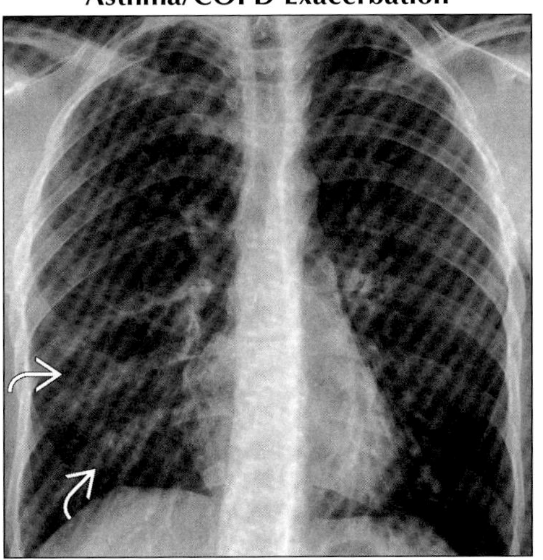

Lobar Collapse

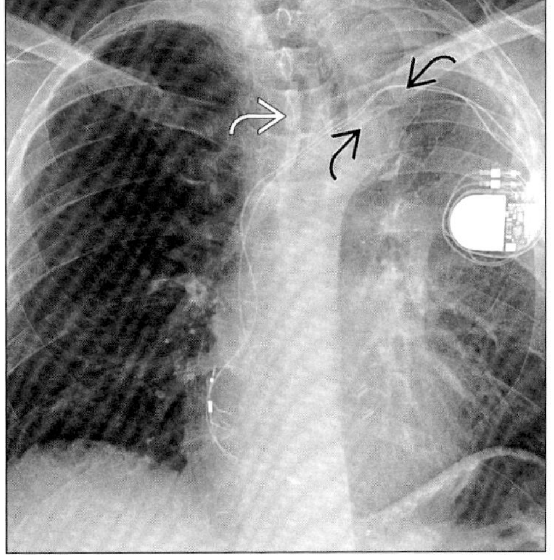

(Left) *Frontal radiograph shows hyperinflation with flattening of the diaphragm. There is right lower lung bronchial wall thickening → in this patient with an asthma exacerbation.* ***(Right)*** *Frontal radiograph shows classic left upper lobe collapse secondary to bronchial stenosis. Note ipsilateral tracheal shift → and loss of the left heart border. Luftsichel sign → is present from hyperinflation of the superior segment of the left lower lobe.*

ACUTE DYSPNEA

(Left) *Axial CECT shows multiple peripheral round areas of ground-glass opacity ➡. Multiple round nodules are also seen in various stages of cavitation ➡. This patient was a drug abuser with endocarditis, a common association.* **(Right)** *Axial CECT shows a pericardial effusion. Note abnormally enhancing parietal pericardium ➡, indicating pericarditis in this patient with endocarditis. Viral or malignant pericarditis could have a similar appearance.*

Septic Embolism

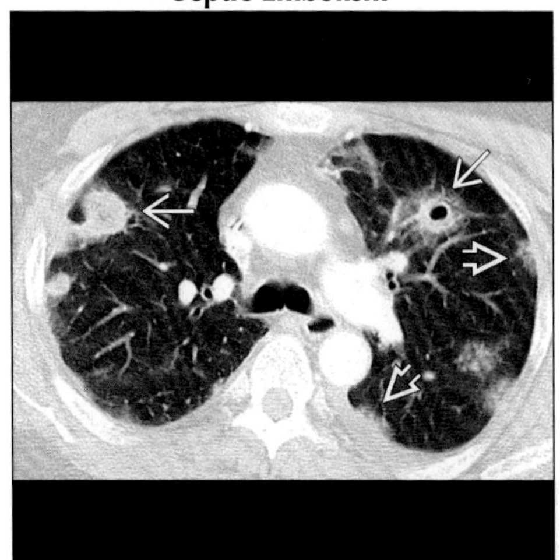

Pericardial Disease

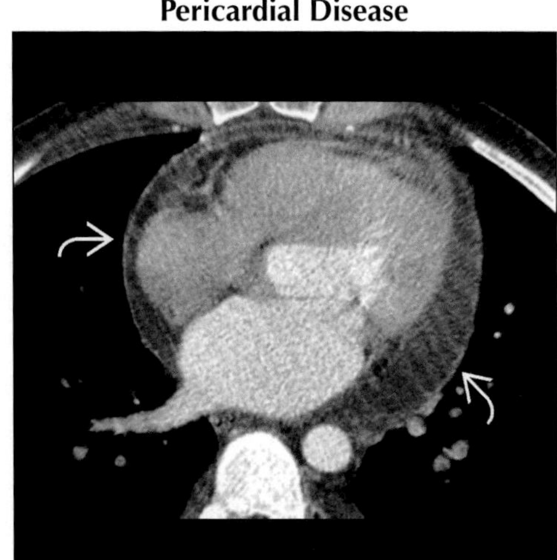

(Left) *Coronal CECT shows typical CT features of ground-glass opacities ➡ from acute interstitial pneumonia. Note sparing of the lower lung zones ➡. No etiology was discovered.* **(Right)** *Axial NECT shows a left pneumonectomy in a patient with Wegener granulomatosis. Note ground-glass opacity representing pulmonary hemorrhage ➡. Distal circumferential tracheal thickening ➡ was better demonstrated on mediastinal windows.*

Acute Interstitial Pneumonia

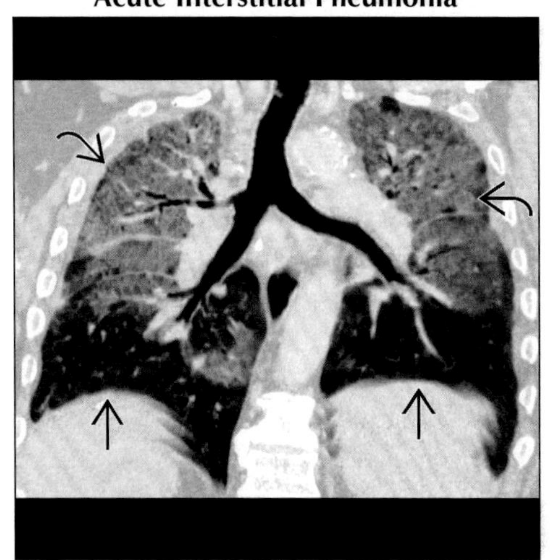

Pulmonary Hemorrhage

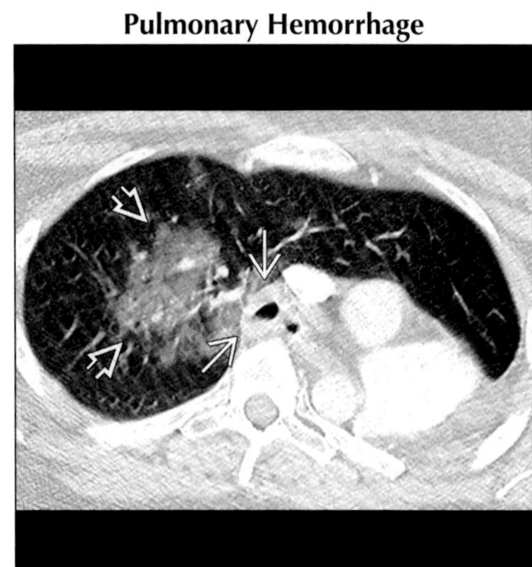

(Left) *Coronal CECT shows bilateral multifocal areas of ground-glass opacity ➡ in this patient with hemoptysis and Wegener granulomatosis.* **(Right)** *Axial NECT shows bilateral upper & left lower lobe ground-glass opacities ➡ in this patient with hemoptysis and Goodpasture syndrome. Renal biopsy showed linear IgG deposition along the glomerular basement membrane by immunofluorescence. Deposits may also be seen along alveolar septa.*

Pulmonary Hemorrhage

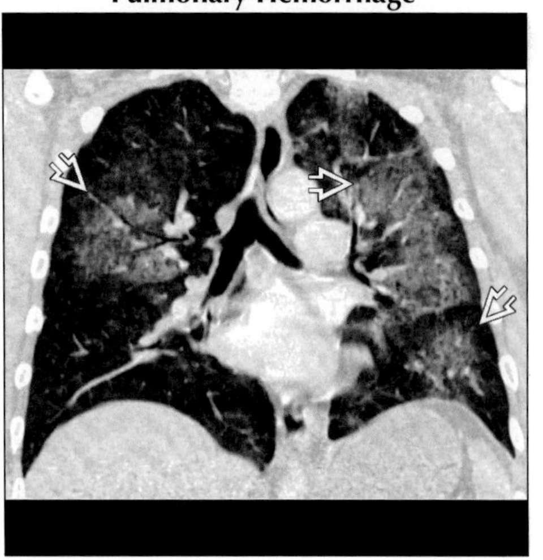

Pulmonary Hemorrhage

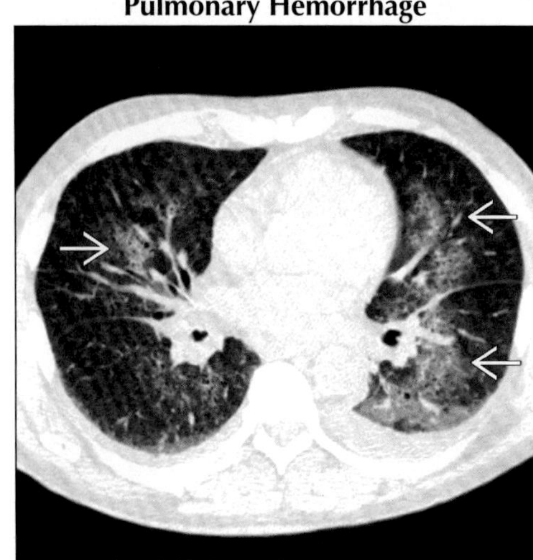

Fat Embolism

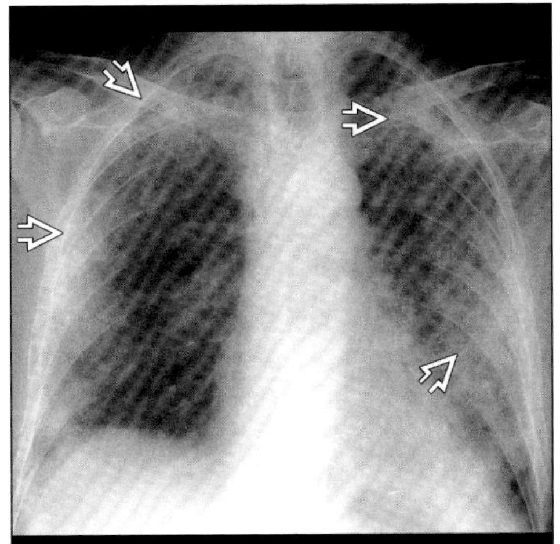

Fat Embolism

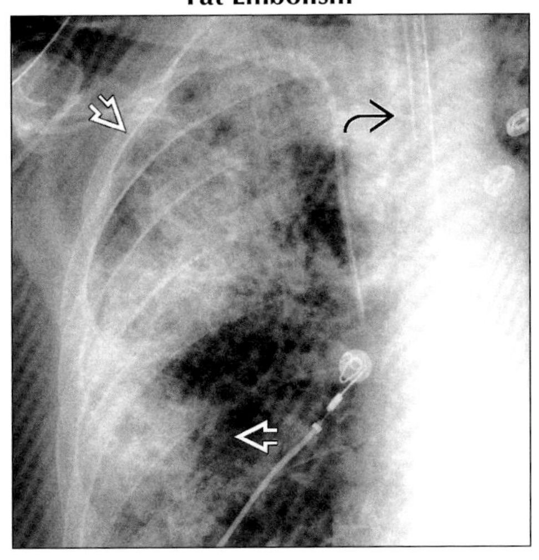

(Left) *Anteroposterior radiograph shows typical pulmonary consolidation, primarily in the lung periphery. This occurs most commonly in patients with recent long bone fracture. Common symptoms include petechial rash, altered mental status, and respiratory failure.* ***(Right)*** *Anteroposterior radiograph shows typical radiographic features of peripheral consolidation resulting from fat embolism. Note endotracheal tube, indicating respiratory compromise.*

Interstitial Lung Disease Exacerbation

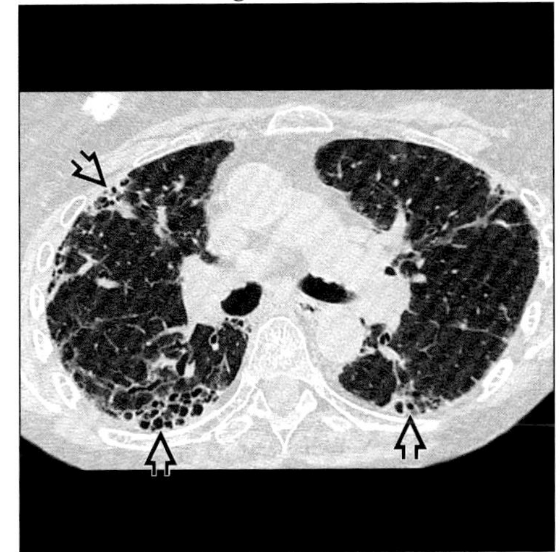

Interstitial Lung Disease Exacerbation

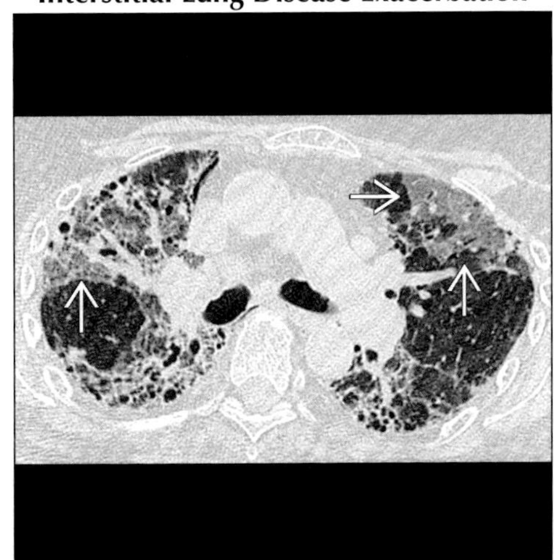

(Left) *Axial HRCT shows peripheral honeycombing from usual interstitial pneumonia in a patient with rheumatoid arthritis.* ***(Right)*** *Axial HRCT shows the same patient presenting with an acute exacerbation of usual interstitial pneumonia. Note superimposed ground-glass opacities. Underlying pneumonia, hemorrhage, or edema would be important differential considerations to exclude.*

Acute Hypersensitivity Pneumonitis

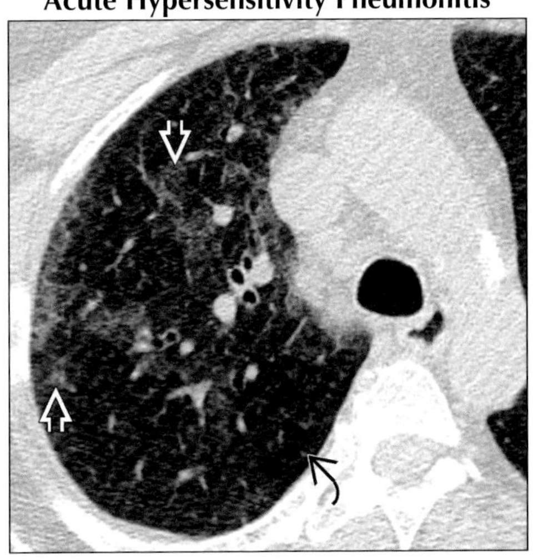

Acute Eosinophilic Pneumonia

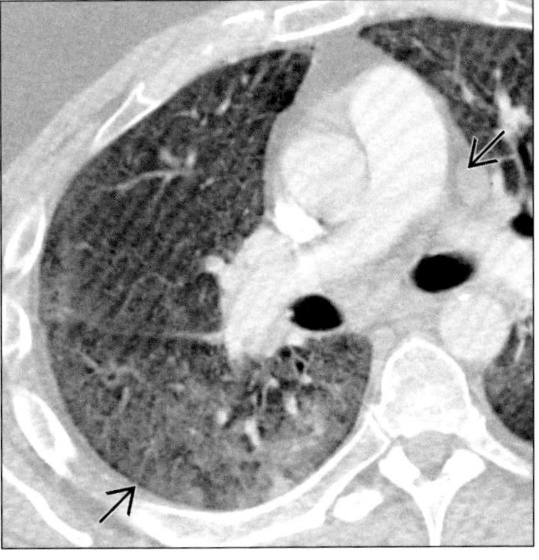

(Left) *Axial HRCT shows typical CT features of acute hypersensitivity pneumonitis. Note patchy ground-glass opacities and lobular hyperinflation, which accentuated on expiratory imaging in this patient with mold exposure.* ***(Right)*** *Axial CECT shows diffuse ground-glass opacities and interstitial thickening (crazy-paving pattern) in this patient with eosinophilia. Radiograph 4 days later showed clearing after initiation of corticosteroids.*

CHRONIC DYSPNEA

DIFFERENTIAL DIAGNOSIS

Common
- Pleural Effusion
- Emphysema
- Sarcoidosis
- Bronchogenic Carcinoma

Less Common
- Usual Interstitial Pneumonia
- Nonspecific Interstitial Pneumonia
- Respiratory Bronchiolitis-associated Interstitial Lung Disease
- Radiation Pneumonitis
- Mycobacterial Avium Complex
- Lymphangitic Carcinomatosis
- Pneumoconioses
- Left to Right Shunt

Rare but Important
- Bronchioloalveolar Cell Carcinoma
- Constrictive Bronchiolitis
- Lymphocytic Interstitial Pneumonia
- Pulmonary Alveolar Proteinosis
- Chronic Eosinophilic Pneumonia
- Organizing Pneumonia
- Lipoid Pneumonia
- Langerhans Cell Histiocytosis
- Lymphangiomyomatosis
- Hypersensitivity Pneumonitis
- Desquamative Interstitial Pneumonia

ESSENTIAL INFORMATION

Key Differential Diagnosis Issues
- Review focuses on adult intrathoracic causes of dyspnea lasting weeks to years

Helpful Clues for Common Diagnoses
- **Pleural Effusion**
  - Exudative effusions
    - Pleural thickening/enhancement in 60%
    - Infections, malignancy, connective tissue diseases, and asbestos exposure
- **Emphysema**
  - Flat diaphragm and increased retrosternal clear space
- **Sarcoidosis**
  - Symmetric right paratracheal, right hilar, and left hilar lymphadenopathy is called 1-2-3 sign or Garland triad
  - Perilymphatic lung nodules (nodules along fissures, subpleural lung, and bronchovascular bundles)
- **Bronchogenic Carcinoma**
  - Nodule or mass in current/former smoker

Helpful Clues for Less Common Diagnoses
- **Usual Interstitial Pneumonia**
  - Basal and subpleural fibrosis with honeycombing
  - ± mediastinal lymphadenopathy
  - Most common cause is idiopathic pulmonary fibrosis
- **Nonspecific Interstitial Pneumonia**
  - Associated with collagen vascular diseases
  - Lower lobe and peripheral ground-glass opacity
  - ± subpleural sparing
  - Honeycombing rare
- **Respiratory Bronchiolitis-associated Interstitial Lung Disease**
  - Symptomatic smoker
  - Upper lung centrilobular nodules of ground-glass opacity
- **Radiation Pneumonitis**
  - 1-4 months following radiation therapy
  - Ground-glass opacity with sharp borders
    - Disobeys anatomic boundaries
- **Mycobacterium Avium Complex**
  - Older women
  - Middle lobe and lingular bronchiectasis
  - Tree in bud centrilobular opacities
- **Lymphangitic Carcinomatosis**
  - Smooth or nodular thickening of interlobular septa
  - ± hilar or mediastinal lymphadenopathy
  - ± pleural effusion
- **Pneumoconioses**
  - Asbestosis
    - Posterobasal and subpleural lung
    - Bilateral pleural plaques
    - Honeycombing and thickened septa late
  - Silicosis and coal worker's pneumoconiosis
    - Posterior upper lung predominant
    - Centrilobular and subpleural nodules
    - Nodules may coalesce to form progressive massive fibrosis
- **Left to Right Shunt**
  - ASD and partial anomalous pulmonary venous return are most common etiologies in adults

Helpful Clues for Rare Diagnoses

- **Bronchioloalveolar Cell Carcinoma**
  - Most common presentation
    - Solitary pulmonary nodule
  - Chronic ground-glass opacity
    - ± "pseudocavitation" with cystic spaces
- **Constrictive Bronchiolitis**
  - Synonyms
    - Bronchiolitis obliterans or obliterative bronchiolitis
  - Causes include
    - Infection, toxic fume inhalation, collagen vascular diseases, and chronic rejection
  - Bronchiectasis, mosaic perfusion, and expiratory air-trapping
- **Lymphocytic Interstitial Pneumonia**
  - Strong association with Sjögren syndrome
  - AIDS defining in children
  - Ground-glass opacity and nodules ± isolated or diffuse lung cysts
- **Pulmonary Alveolar Proteinosis**
  - Crazy-paving pattern
    - Geographic bilateral ground-glass opacities with interlobular septal thickening
  - Idiopathic or seen with silicosis, malignancy, and chemotherapeutic medications
  - Exclude acute causes of crazy-paving, such as ARDS by history
- **Chronic Eosinophilic Pneumonia**
  - Peripheral upper lung consolidation
  - Blood eosinophilia
- **Organizing Pneumonia**
  - Idiopathic, collagen vascular diseases, and infections
  - Lower lobe and peripheral ground-glass opacity, small nodules, or focal consolidation
  - "Atoll" or "reverse halo" sign
- **Lipoid Pneumonia**
  - Aspiration of oils used for laxatives
  - Lower lobe consolidation or mass
    - Central low-attenuation areas (-80 to -30 HU)
- **Langerhans Cell Histiocytosis**
  - Centrilobular nodules ± central cavitation
  - Costophrenic angles spared
  - Round or bizarrely shaped cysts in upper lungs
- **Lymphangiomyomatosis**
  - Women of childbearing age
  - Large lung volumes with chylous effusions and pneumothoraces
  - Numerous diffuse round lung cysts
- **Hypersensitivity Pneumonitis**
  - Centrilobular nodules of ground-glass opacity
  - "Head-cheese" sign: Ground-glass opacity, decreased lung attenuation, and normal lung
- **Desquamative Interstitial Pneumonia**
  - Diffuse/patchy ground-glass opacity
  - ± cystic lesions or centrilobular emphysema
  - ± lower lobe predominance

Pleural Effusion

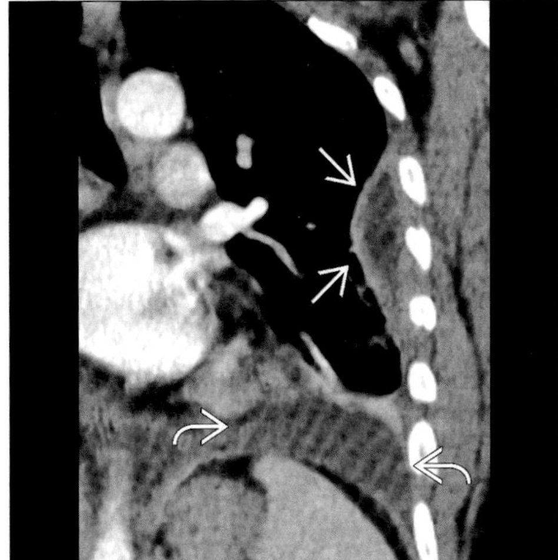

Coronal CECT shows a chronic pleural effusion ➡ in this patient with lupus. Note separate loculated fluid collection ➡ with an enhancing pleural lining indicating its exudative nature.

Pleural Effusion

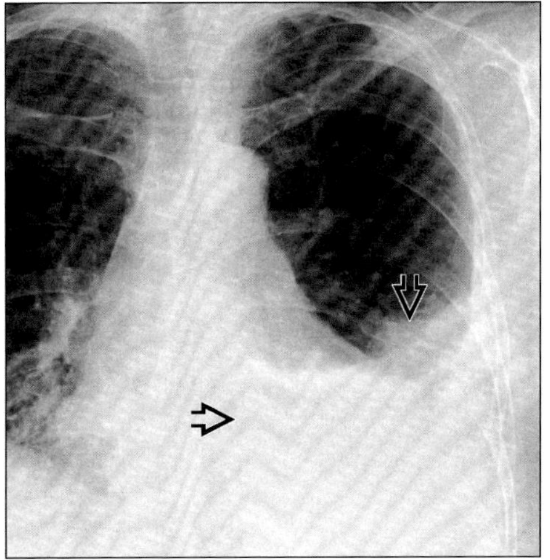

Frontal radiograph shows a left-sided pleural fluid collection ⇨ that was unchanged over months. Pleural effusion/thickening is the most common thoracic manifestation seen in patients with lupus.

CHRONIC DYSPNEA

*(**Left**) Axial CECT shows severe centrilobular emphysema with near complete destruction of the secondary pulmonary lobule. Note preservation of centrilobular core structures ➔ and lack of definable walls. (**Right**) Coronal NECT shows small perilymphatic lung nodules typically seen in sarcoidosis. Note the beaded major fissure ➔, subpleural nodularity ⇨, and lobular mosaic perfusion ➔ secondary to sarcoid granulomas involving small airways.*

Emphysema

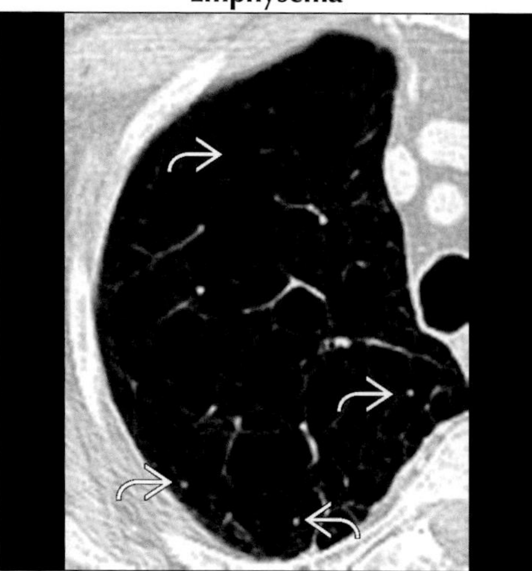

Sarcoidosis

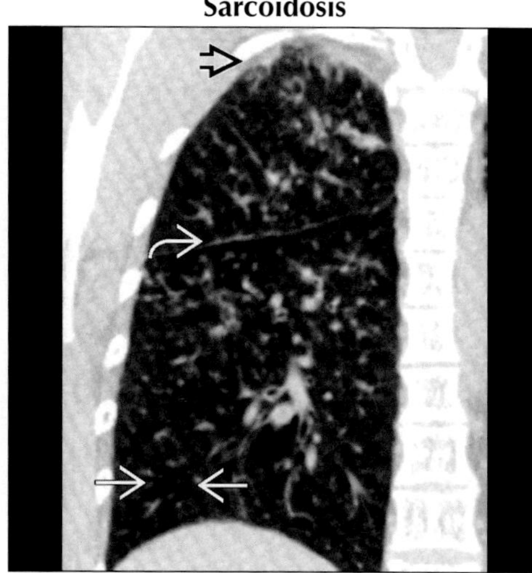

*(**Left**) Axial CECT shows a large lobulated mass ➔, which contacts the left and main pulmonary artery over a large distance. This patient presented with chest pain and dyspnea and had metastatic disease to bone and adrenal glands. (**Right**) Axial HRCT shows extensive right greater than left lower lobe honeycombing ➔ as evidenced by multiple cysts stacked on top of each other. Note traction bronchiectasis ➔ from lung fibrosis.*

Bronchogenic Carcinoma

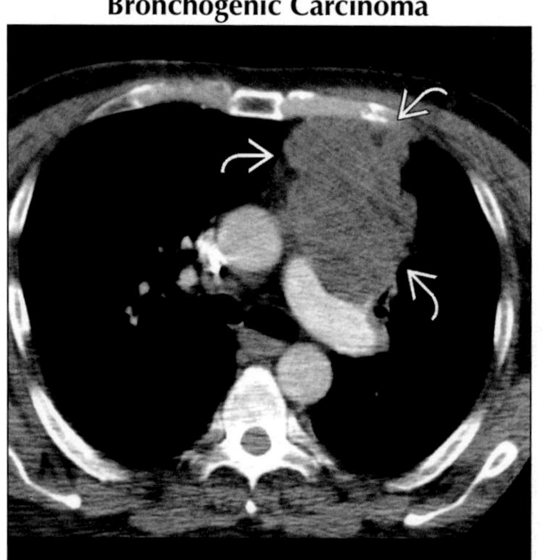

Usual Interstitial Pneumonia

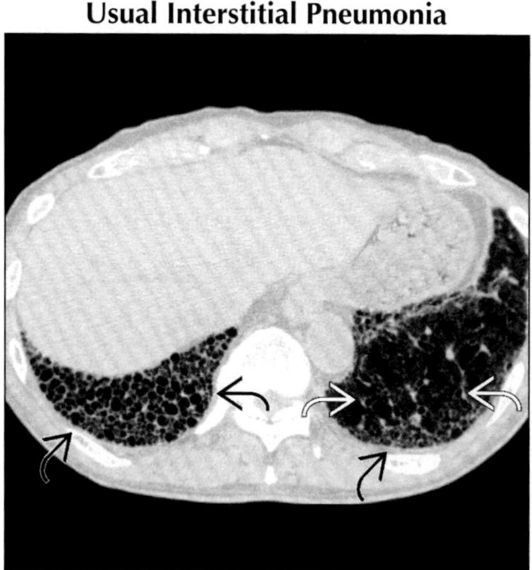

*(**Left**) Axial HRCT shows ground-glass opacities ➔ in the lower lungs. Note absence of honeycombing, an important distinction from UIP. NSIP most commonly occurs with connective tissue diseases, drug toxicity, or hypersensitivity pneumonitis. (**Right**) Axial NECT shows a dilated esophagus in primary proven achalasia ➔. Note ill-defined centrilobular nodules of ground-glass opacity in this symptomatic smoker with respiratory bronchiolitis ➔.*

Nonspecific Interstitial Pneumonia

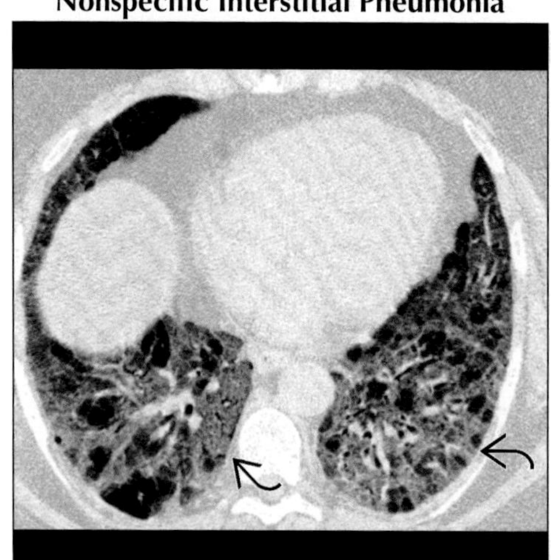

Respiratory Bronchiolitis-associated Interstitial Lung Disease

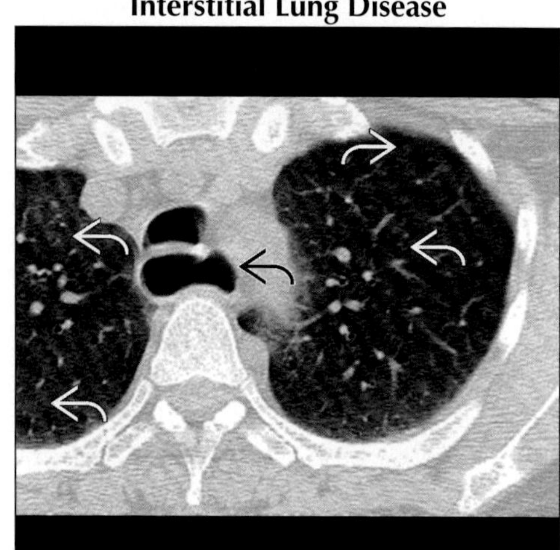

Radiation Pneumonitis

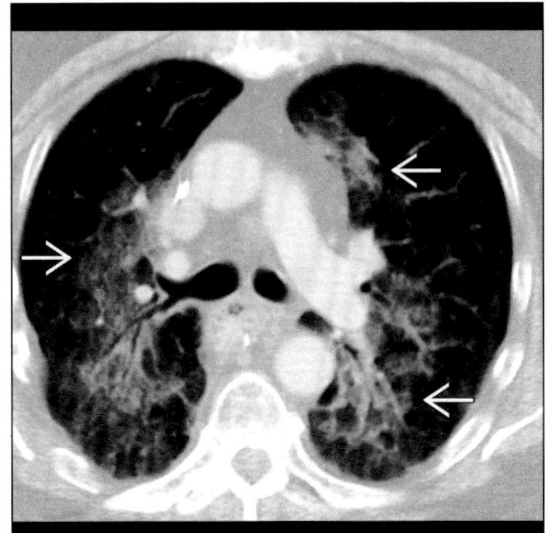

Mycobacterial Avium Complex

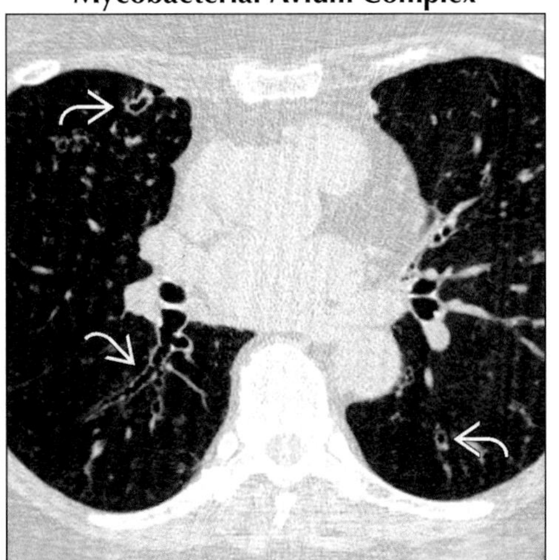

(Left) *Axial CECT shows perihilar ground-glass opacity and consolidation paralleling the mediastinum ➔. The patient was treated with radiation for lymphoma. The most important distinguishing characteristic is sharp demarcation disobeying normal lung boundaries (fissures).* ***(Right)*** *Axial NECT shows middle & lower lobe bronchiectasis with bronchial wall thickening ➔ in this case of MAC infection. This was an older woman with a cough and dyspnea.*

Lymphangitic Carcinomatosis

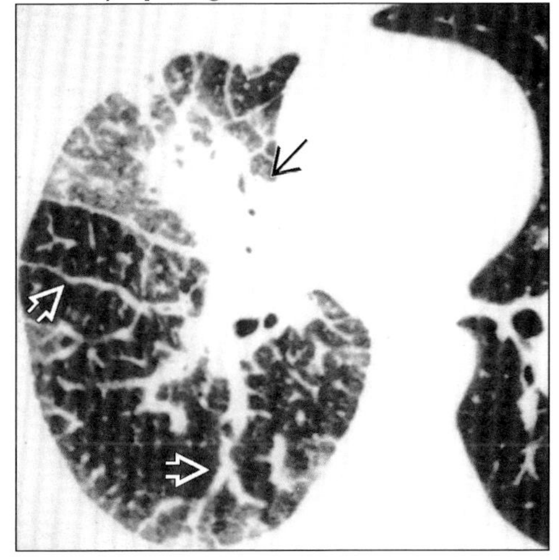

Pneumoconioses

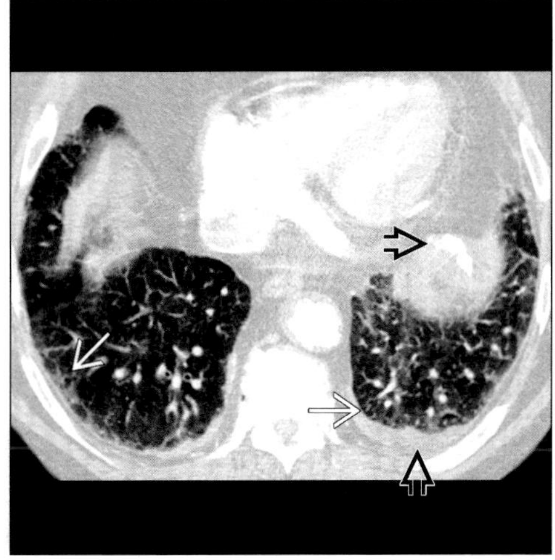

(Left) *Axial HRCT shows diffuse nodular and irregular bronchovascular interstitial and interlobular septal thickening ➔ from adenocarcinoma of the lung ➔. The left lung is normal. Unilateral disease is most commonly due to lung carcinoma.* ***(Right)*** *Axial NECT shows reticular interstitial thickening ➔ and pleural plaques ➔. Asbestosis typically predominates in the lower lungs, occurs 20-30 years after exposure, and leads to usual interstitial pneumonia.*

Left to Right Shunt

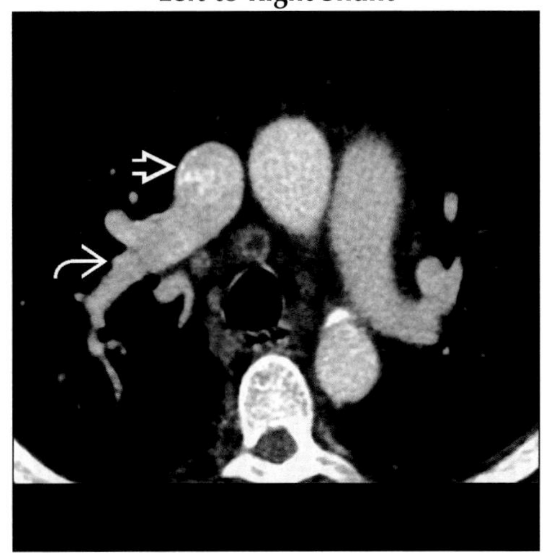

Bronchioloalveolar Cell Carcinoma

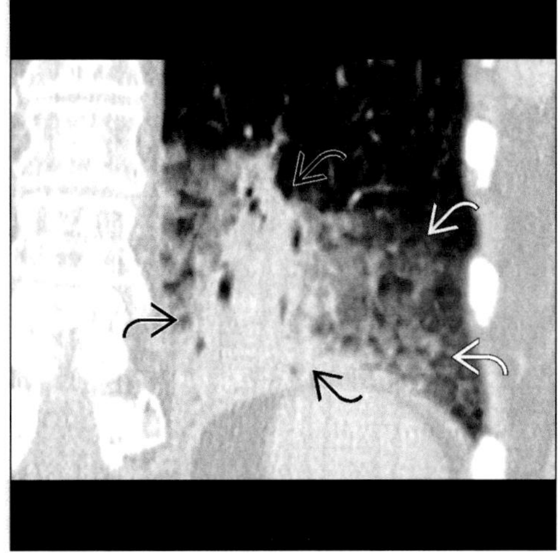

(Left) *Axial CECT shows a right upper lobe pulmonary vein ➔ draining directly into the superior vena cava ➔ in this case of partial anomalous pulmonary venous return. Sinus venosus-type atrial septal defect is commonly associated with this anomaly.* ***(Right)*** *Coronal NECT shows left lower lobe consolidation ➔ and surrounding ground-glass opacity ➔. This did not respond to antibiotic therapy and enlarged on subsequent radiographs and CT.*

CHRONIC DYSPNEA

*(**Left**) Axial HRCT shows extensive bronchiectasis → and mosaic perfusion → reflecting small airways disease. This was accentuated on expiratory imaging, indicating air-trapping. This is a form of chronic rejection following lung transplantation. (**Right**) Axial CECT shows multiple thin-walled, variable-sized cysts → and a lung nodule →. The most common association is Sjögren syndrome in adults and AIDS in children.*

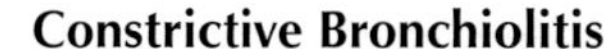

Constrictive Bronchiolitis

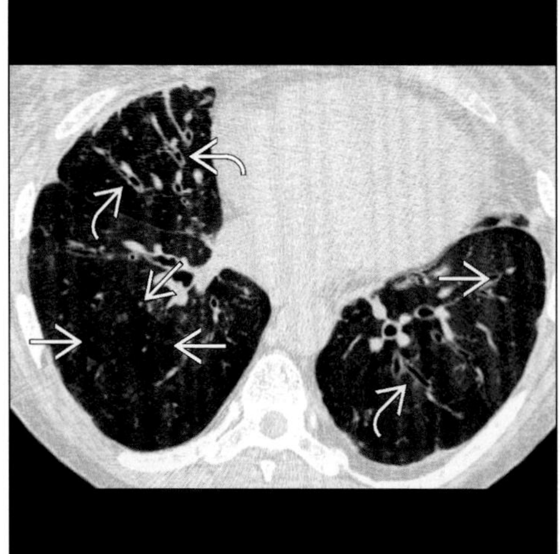

Lymphocytic Interstitial Pneumonia

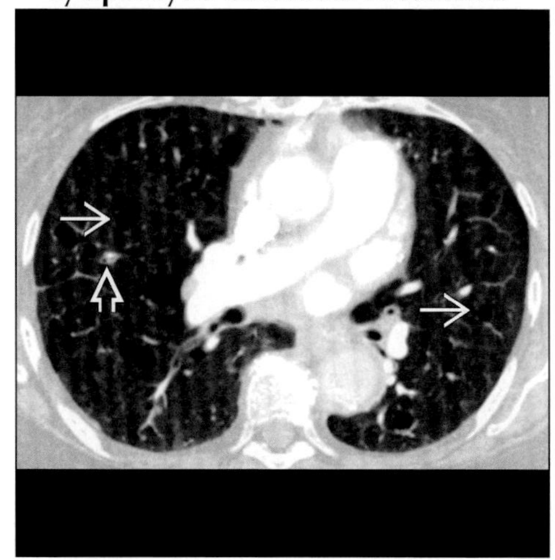

*(**Left**) Frontal radiograph shows bilateral consolidation → with relative sparing of the lung bases. This was unchanged in appearance over 6 months, and the patient was complaining of mild dyspnea. (**Right**) Axial NECT shows peripheral consolidation predominantly located in the upper lobes →, a common finding in chronic eosinophilic pneumonia. Peripheral blood eosinophilia is often present and a distinguishing point from cryptogenic organizing pneumonia.*

Pulmonary Alveolar Proteinosis

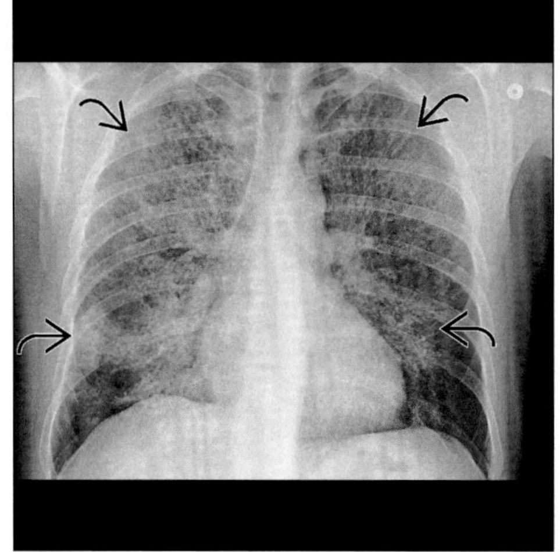

Chronic Eosinophilic Pneumonia

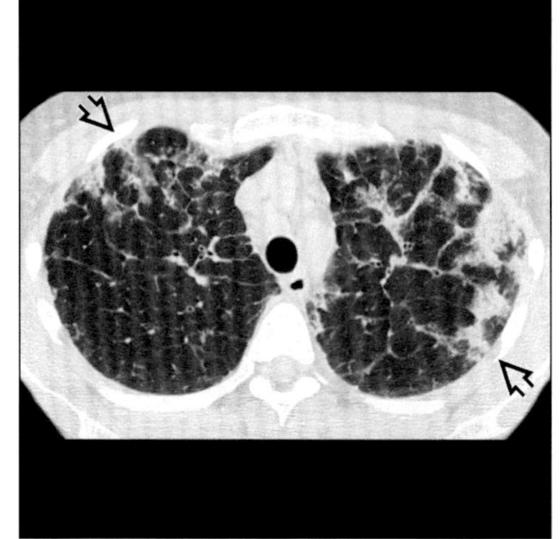

*(**Left**) Axial CECT shows chronic peripheral consolidation predominating in the lower lungs →. Patients typically respond well to corticosteroids and have a good prognosis. (**Right**) Axial CECT shows multifocal consolidation, particularly in the right middle lobe and lower lobes. Consolidated lung is of fat density → in this case of mineral oil aspiration. Note descending thoracic aortic aneurysm with dissection →.*

Organizing Pneumonia

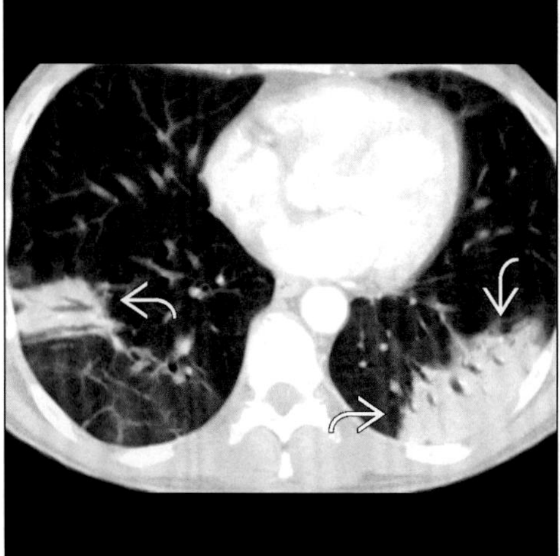

Lipoid Pneumonia

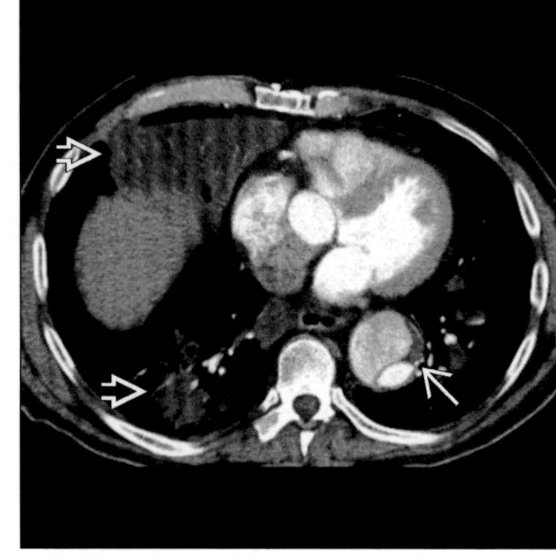

Langerhans Cell Histiocytosis

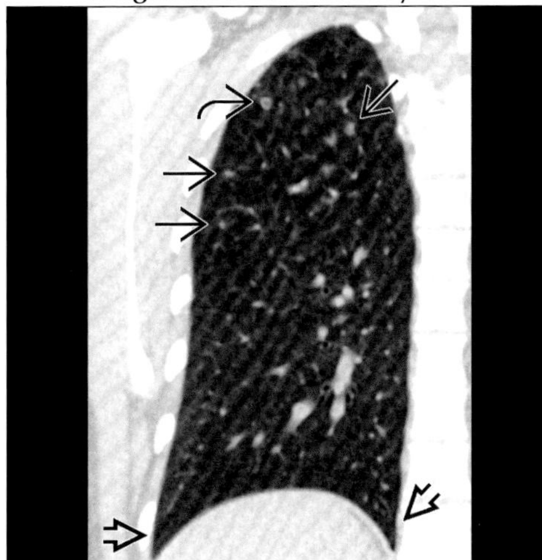

Langerhans Cell Histiocytosis

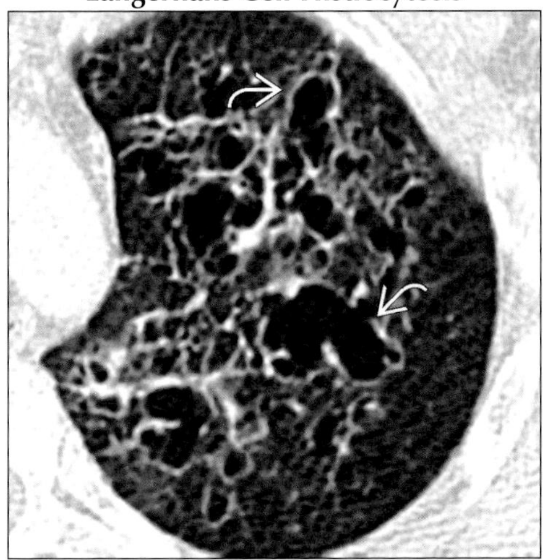

(Left) *Coronal HRCT shows a small cavitary right upper lobe lung nodule. Note noncavitary upper lobe lung nodules and characteristic sparing of the costophrenic sulci. This patient was a heavy smoker, a common association with Langerhans cell histiocytosis.* ***(Right)*** *Axial HRCT shows end-stage LCH with innumerable bizarrely shaped cysts. This is differentiated from severe centrilobular emphysema by thick walls and lack of centrilobular core structures.*

Lymphangiomyomatosis

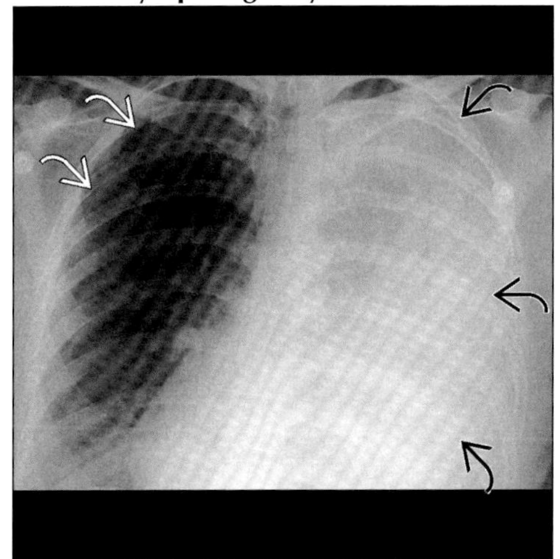

Hypersensitivity Pneumonitis

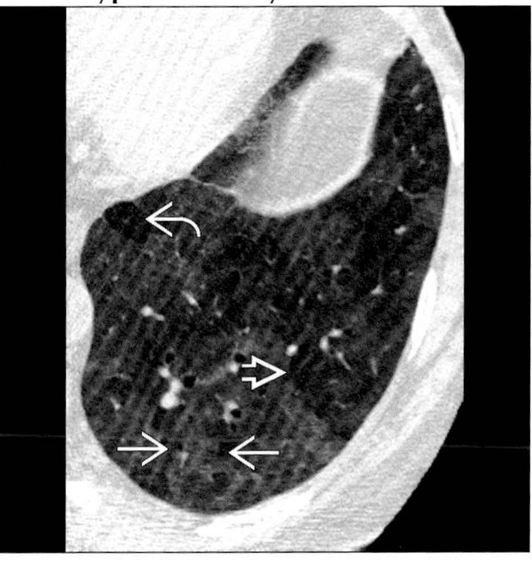

(Left) *Frontal radiograph shows left hemithorax opacification with contralateral mediastinal shift occurring secondary to a large chylous pleural effusion. Note small right pneumothorax. This constellation of findings in a woman of child-bearing age is consistent with LAM.* ***(Right)*** *Axial HRCT shows typical "head-cheese" sign with ground-glass opacity, normal lung, and hyperlucent lung from mosaic perfusion.*

Hypersensitivity Pneumonitis

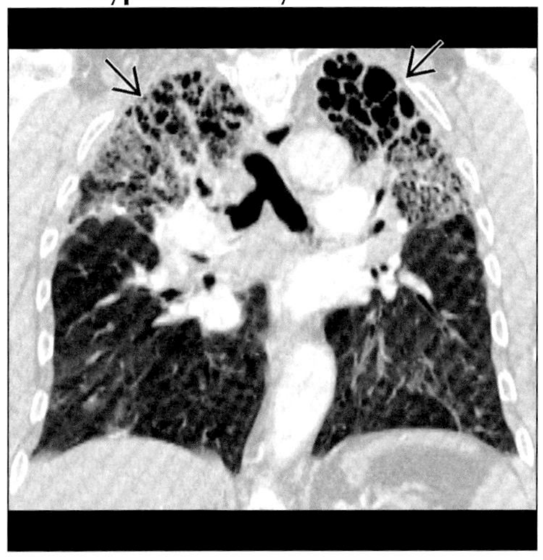

Desquamative Interstitial Pneumonia

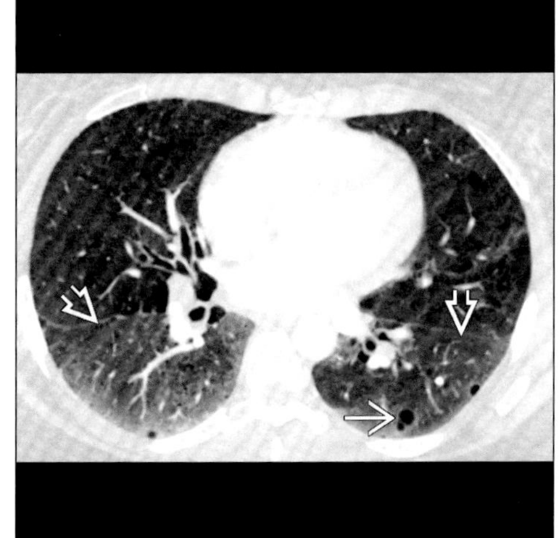

(Left) *Coronal CECT shows extensive upper lung predominant honeycombing in this patient with chronic mold exposure. Important clues to this diagnosis include distribution of disease, mosaic perfusion, and expiratory air-trapping.* ***(Right)*** *Axial HRCT shows ground-glass opacities and round lucent lesions representing emphysema or cysts. Cysts, lower lobe ground-glass opacities, and smoking history are commonly present in this condition.*

CHEST PAIN

DIFFERENTIAL DIAGNOSIS

Common
- Acute Myocardial Infarction
- Pulmonary Embolism
- Pneumothorax
- Rib Fracture
- Pneumonia
- Bronchitis

Less Common
- Acute Aortic Syndrome
- Pleural Effusion
- Diffuse Esophageal Spasm
- Gastrointestinal Abnormalities
- Aortic Stenosis
- Pericardial Disease
- Metastatic Disease
- Sickle Cell Anemia
- Sarcoidosis

Rare but Important
- Esophageal Tear
- Mediastinitis
- Chest Wall Mass
- Chest Wall Infection

ESSENTIAL INFORMATION

Key Differential Diagnosis Issues
- Chest pain presenting to primary care physician is usually benign
  - Usually no radiographic abnormalities
- Chest radiograph is initial radiographic examination in emergency department
  - Helps to exclude conditions that may mimic acute coronary syndrome

Helpful Clues for Common Diagnoses
- **Acute Myocardial Infarction**
  - Chest radiograph normal in 50%
  - Pulmonary edema without cardiomegaly in 50%
- **Pulmonary Embolism**
  - Chest radiograph abnormal in most patients
    - Cardiomegaly is most common finding
    - Hampton hump and Westermark sign infrequently seen
  - CTA: Intraluminal filling defect surrounded by contrast is diagnostic
    - "Doughnut" or "railroad track" sign
  - Signs of right heart strain
    - RV/LV chamber size ≥ 1, leftward bowing of interventricular septum, and reflux into inferior vena cava
- **Pneumothorax**
  - Spontaneous
    - Rupture of apical bleb or bulla
    - Young, tall, and thin male smokers
    - Association with emphysema, cystic lung disease, asthma, infection, or lung fibrosis
    - Recurrence is common
  - Traumatic pneumothorax due to
    - Chest trauma or mechanical ventilation
- **Rib Fracture**
  - ACR states rib radiography not recommended for diagnosis
- **Pneumonia**
  - Symptoms of infection
  - Lobar or segmental lung consolidation
- **Bronchitis**
  - Radiograph usually normal
  - ± bronchial wall thickening and mucus plugging

Helpful Clues for Less Common Diagnoses
- **Acute Aortic Syndrome**
  - Sudden onset of severe chest/back pain
  - Predisposing factors
    - Hypertension, bicuspid aortic valve, and connective tissue disorders
  - All 3 conditions have similar classification
    - Stanford type A involves ascending aorta and is treated surgically
    - Stanford type B occurs distal to left subclavian artery and is treated medically
  - Life-threatening complications of type A aortic dissection
    - Pericardial tamponade, myocardial infarction, acute aortic insufficiency, and stroke
  - Intramural hematoma
    - Diagnose with noncontrast CT
    - Crescent-shaped, high-density thickening of aortic wall
  - Penetrating aortic ulcer
    - Atherosclerotic plaque rupture with focal contrast collection within media
    - Common in descending thoracic aorta
    - May propagate and lead to dissection
- **Pleural Effusion**
  - Pain usually indicates pleuritis
- **Diffuse Esophageal Spasm**

- Reproduction of pain with tertiary contractions on esophagram
- **Gastrointestinal Abnormalities**
  - Occasionally present with chest pain
  - Normal chest radiograph or basal atelectasis
  - Chest CT may detect unsuspected intraabdominal abnormality
- **Aortic Stenosis**
  - Radiograph shows
    - ± aortic valvular calcifications
    - Enlarged ascending aorta with normal heart size
- **Pericardial Disease**
  - Pain with pericarditis, pericardial effusion, or metastatic disease
  - Pericarditis
    - Thickening and enhancement of pericardium
    - Pericardial fluid
- **Metastatic Disease**
  - Bone or lung metastases can cause pain
  - Multiple well-circumscribed lung nodules in random distribution
  - Lytic or blastic bony lesions
- **Sickle Cell Anemia**
  - Acute chest syndrome
    - Vasoocclusive crisis with new lung opacity, ± fever, chest pain, and respiratory symptoms
    - Secondary to infection, infarction, pain episode, or fat embolism
    - Predisposes to pulmonary arterial hypertension through lung fibrosis
  - H-shaped vertebral bodies, avascular necrosis of humeral heads, and expanded ribs
  - ± posterior mediastinal extramedullary hematopoiesis
- **Sarcoidosis**
  - Bilateral hilar and right paratracheal lymphadenopathy
  - Perilymphatic distribution of lung nodules (nodules along fissures, subpleural lung, and bronchovascular bundles)

Helpful Clues for Rare Diagnoses

- **Esophageal Tear**
  - Occurs with trauma, retching, or iatrogenic injury
  - Pneumomediastinum, extravasated oral contrast, and periesophageal fluid collections
- **Mediastinitis**
  - Associated with sternotomy, esophageal perforation, or spread of adjacent infection
  - Postoperative fluid collections normally resolve in 2-3 weeks
  - CT findings
    - Diffuse mediastinal fat stranding and fluid collections
    - Pneumomediastinum
- **Chest Wall Mass**
  - Pain occurs with Pancoast tumor and numerous sarcomas
- **Chest Wall Infection**
  - Rib sclerosis or periosteal reaction indicates osteomyelitis

Acute Myocardial Infarction

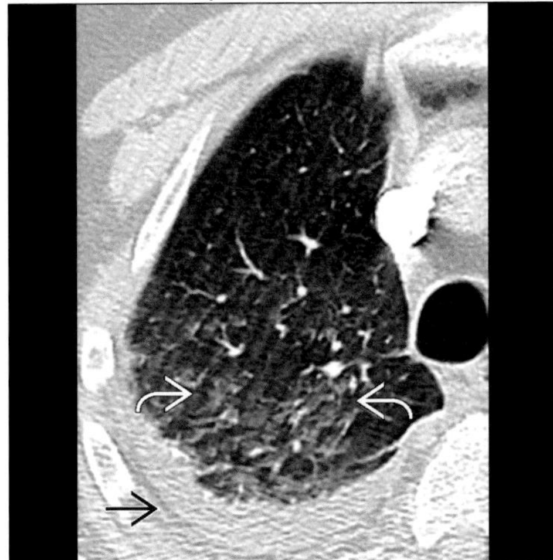

Axial CECT shows dependent ground-glass opacity ➔ with characteristic spared pulmonary lobules. Note right pleural effusion →. Patient had a NSTEMI and 3 vessel disease at angiography.

Acute Myocardial Infarction

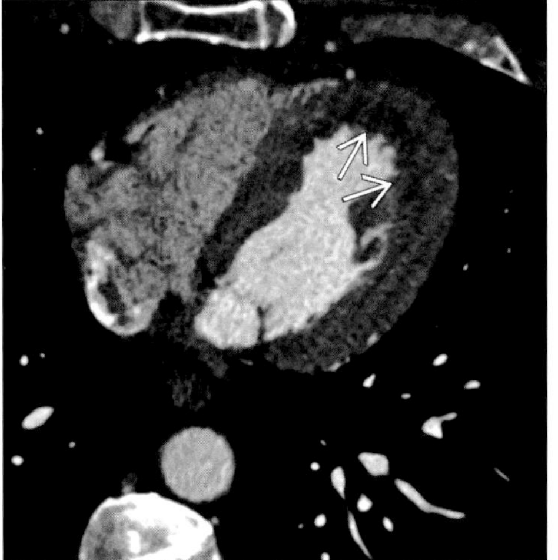

Axial cardiac CT shows normal wall thickness with subendocardial low-attenuation perfusion defect ➔ occupying less than 50% diameter of the myocardium.

CHEST PAIN

Pulmonary Embolism

Pulmonary Embolism

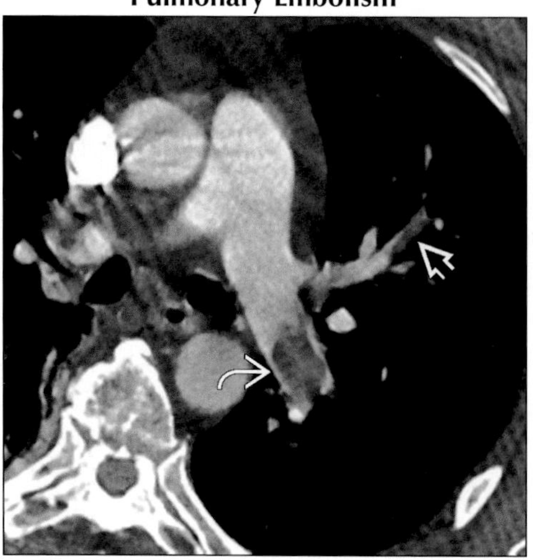

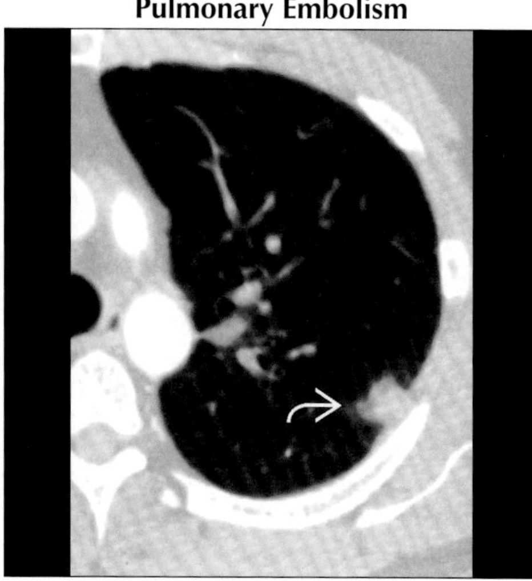

(Left) *Axial CECT shows large pulmonary embolism in the left pulmonary artery ➔ with typical "railroad track" sign. Smaller embolism is noted in a segmental left upper lobe pulmonary artery ➔. It is important to report signs of right heart strain in the setting of pulmonary embolism as it has prognostic implications.* ***(Right)*** *Axial CECT shows a peripheral infarct in the same patient ➔.*

Pulmonary Embolism

Pneumothorax

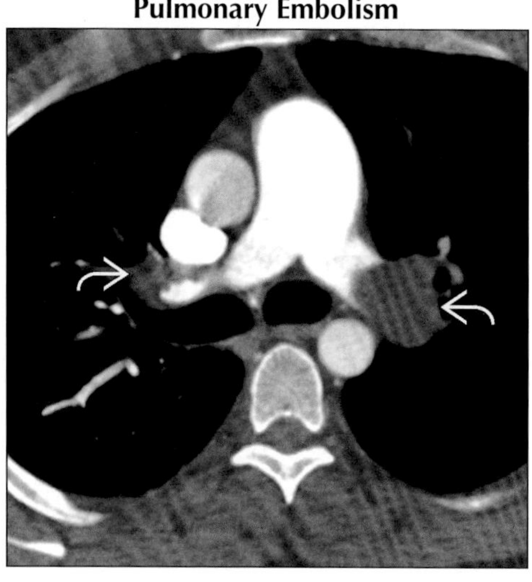

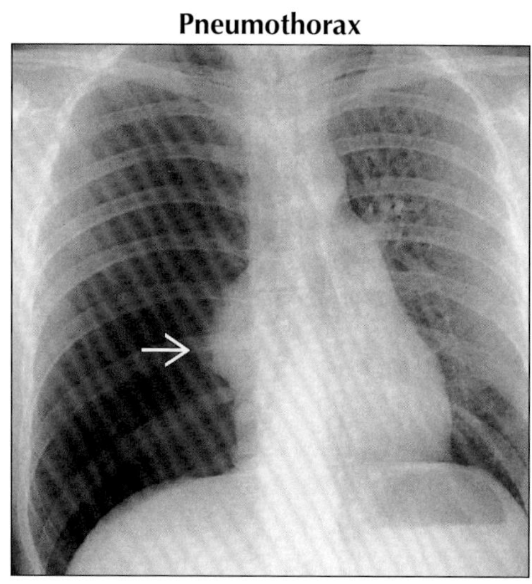

(Left) *Axial CECT shows bilateral main pulmonary artery embolism ➔.* ***(Right)*** *Frontal radiograph shows lucent right hemithorax and collapsed right lung ➔ as well as leftward mediastinal shift. Right hemidiaphragm is depressed, and the right rib interspaces are larger than the left. Findings are suggestive but not diagnostic of tension pneumothorax, as this is a clinical diagnosis.*

Rib Fracture

Pneumonia

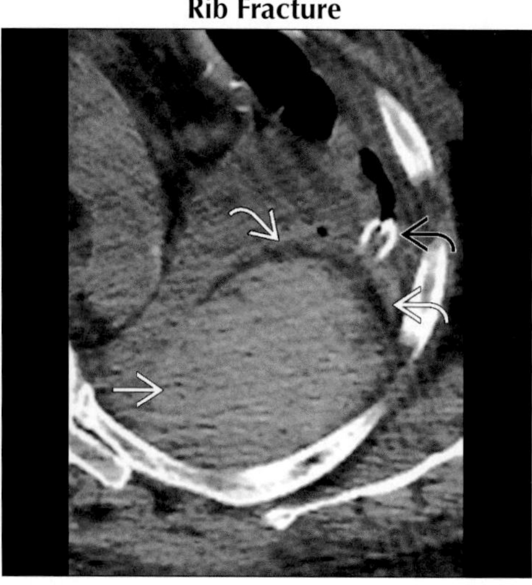

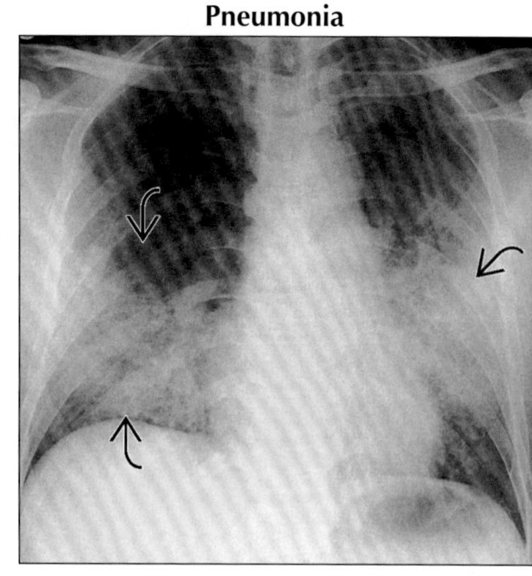

(Left) *Axial NECT shows large extrapleural hematoma ➔ indicated by displaced extrapleural fat ➔. Displaced rib fracture was present on lower sections. Note anteriorly displaced chest tube ➔ within the pleural space.* ***(Right)*** *Frontal radiograph shows bilateral perihilar and lower lung consolidation ➔. The patient was severely hypoxic and received a new diagnosis of HIV and Pneumocystis pneumonia.*

Pneumonia

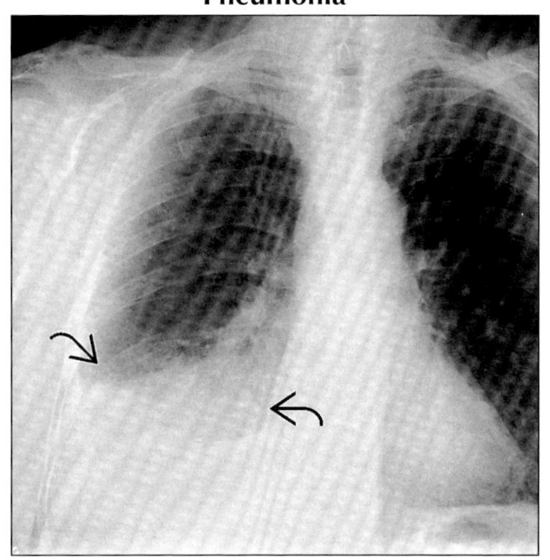

Bronchitis

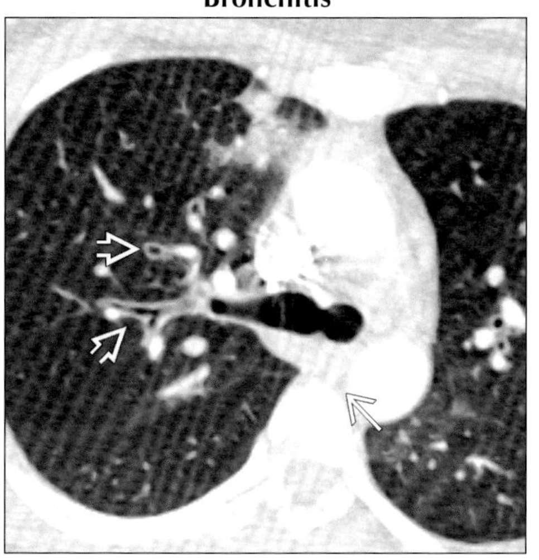

(Left) *Frontal radiograph shows right lower lobe consolidation ➔ with silhouetting of the right hemidiaphragm in this patient with productive cough and high fevers. Note preservation of the right heart border, indicating the medial segment of the right middle lobe is not involved.* ***(Right)*** *Axial CECT shows bronchial wall thickening ➔ and patchy ground-glass opacities ➔.*

Acute Aortic Syndrome

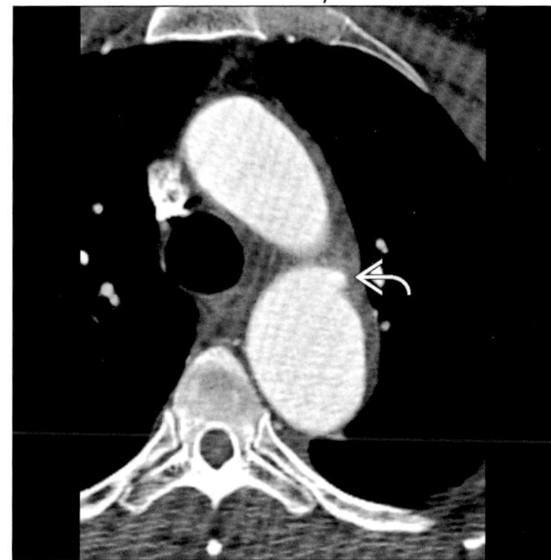

Acute Aortic Syndrome

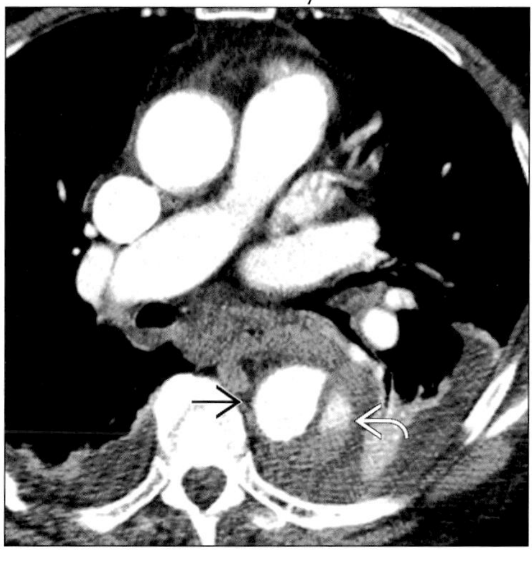

(Left) *Axial CECT shows a penetrating aortic ulcer ➔ originating distal to the left subclavian artery origin, making this penetrating ulcer Stanford type B. Treatment depends on the patient's symptoms.* ***(Right)*** *Axial CTA shows a type B aortic dissection with true lumen located anteromedially ➔ and false lumen posterior and laterally ➔. The true lumen contains dense contrast. There are bilateral pleural effusions.*

Acute Aortic Syndrome

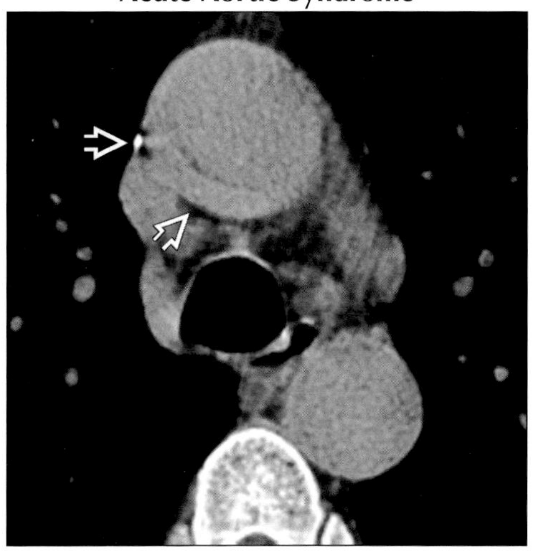

Pleural Effusion

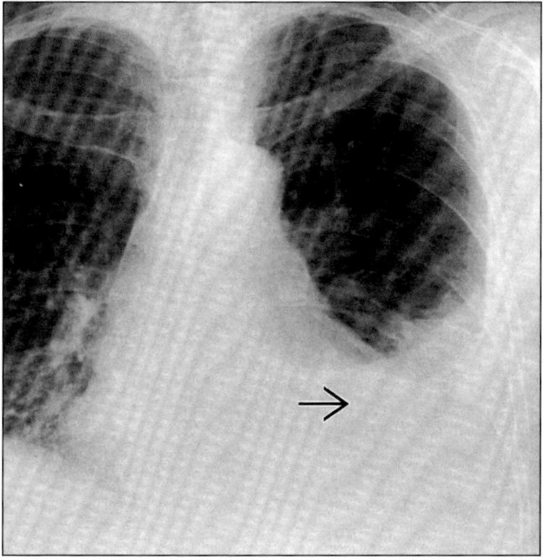

(Left) *Axial NECT shows mildly hyperdense type A intramural hematoma ➔. This illustrates the importance of a noncontrast examination in the setting of suspected aortic pathology.* ***(Right)*** *Frontal radiograph shows a left pleural effusion ➔ in this patient with lupus and chest pain. Presence of an isolated pleural effusion with pain usually indicates pleuritis. Effusion without pleuritis usually causes only dyspnea.*

CHEST PAIN

*(**Left**) Frontal esophagram shows tertiary contractions ➢. Patient's pain was reproduced with these contractions. (**Right**) Axial CECT shows a large heterogeneous subcapsular splenic hematoma ➢. Note compression of the spleen ➢. Blood was also visible within the pelvis (not shown). Patient presented with severe left shoulder and chest pain.*

Diffuse Esophageal Spasm

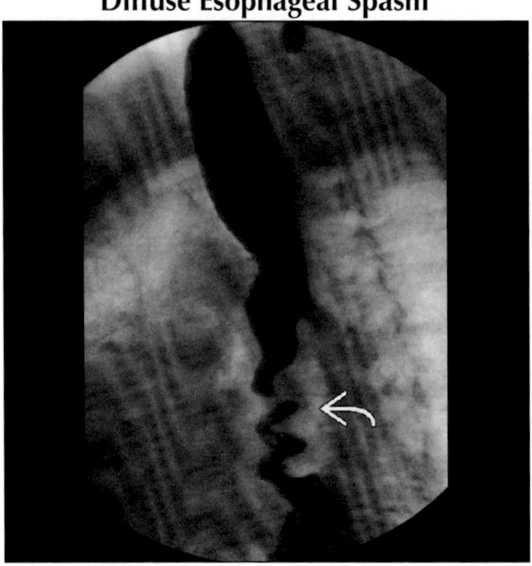

Gastrointestinal Abnormalities

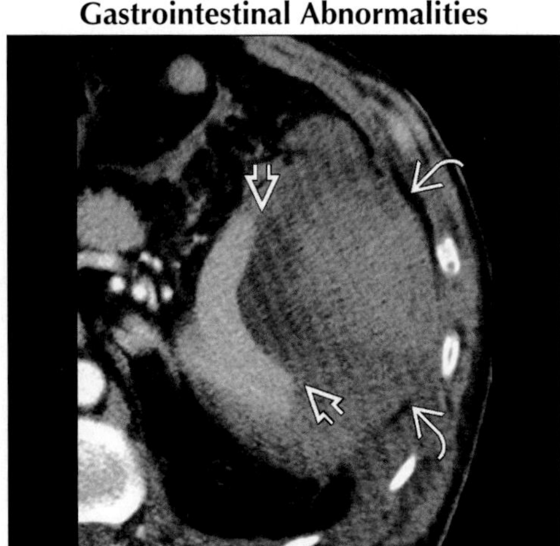

*(**Left**) Lateral radiograph shows a calcified aortic valve ➢. Presence of calcification on chest radiography usually indicates severe hemodynamic aortic stenosis. (**Right**) Axial CTA shows type A dissection flap within the ascending aorta ➢ and high-density hemopericardium ➢. Reflux into the inferior vena cava and azygous vein were also present (not shown). Patient was hemodynamically unstable and was diagnosed with pericardial tamponade.*

Aortic Stenosis

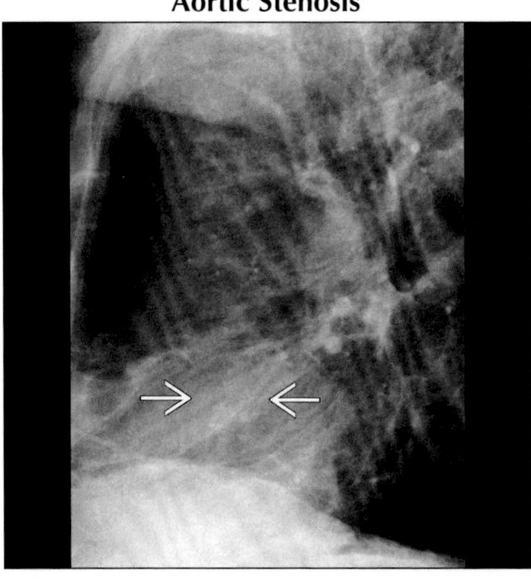

Pericardial Disease

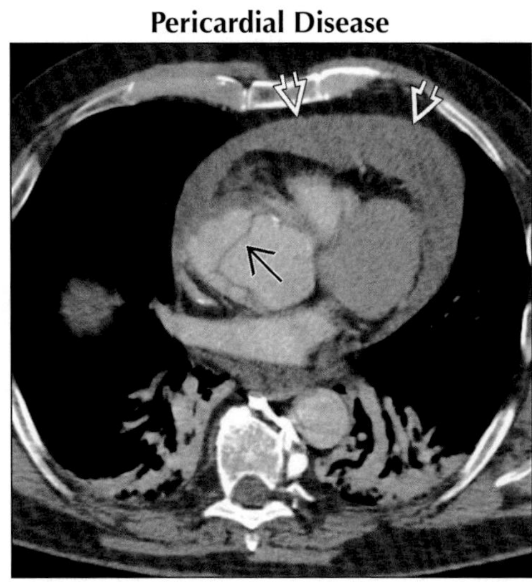

*(**Left**) Axial CECT shows multiple pericardial masses ➢ and pericardial effusion from metastatic breast cancer. Pericardial masses are most common from metastatic disease. (**Right**) Axial CECT shows a large enhancing soft tissue mass causing destruction of a left posterior rib ➢. Multiple lung metastases ➢ were better seen on lung windows. There is a right hepatic lobe ring-enhancing metastasis ➢ in this patient with renal cell carcinoma.*

Pericardial Disease

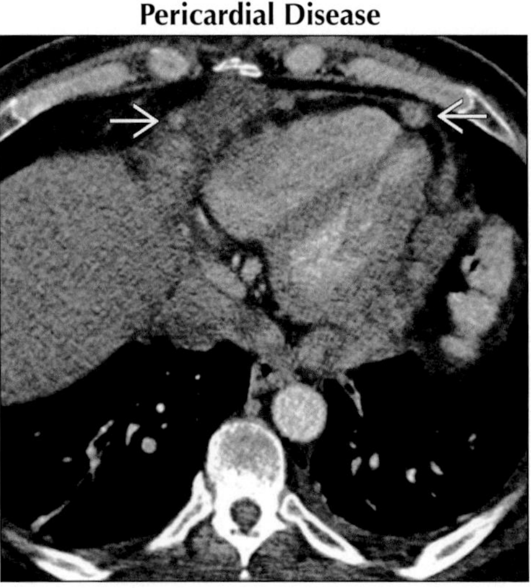

Metastatic Disease

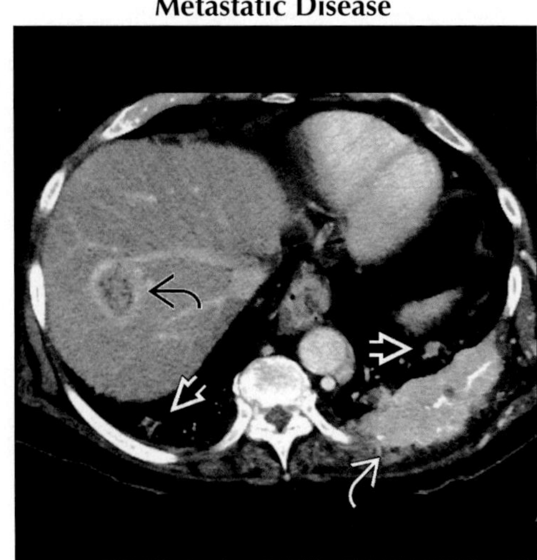

Sickle Cell Anemia

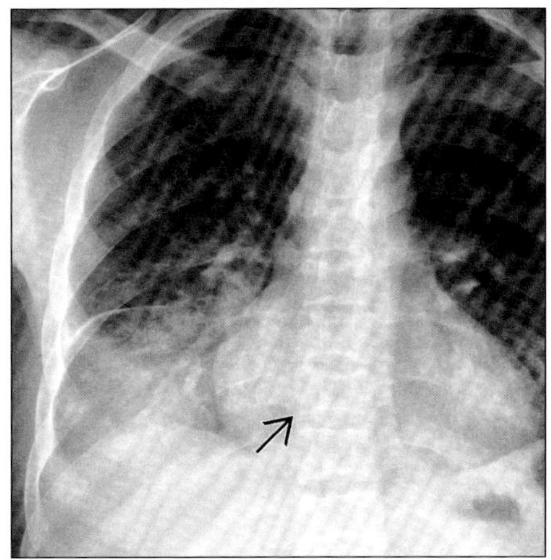

Sarcoidosis

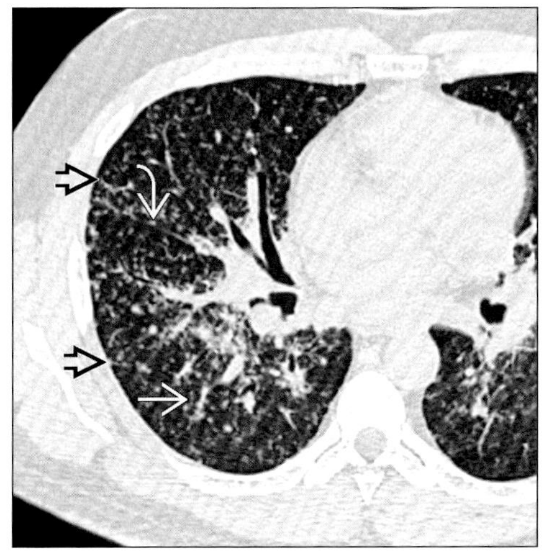

(Left) *Frontal radiograph shows right greater than left lower lobe consolidation in this patient with pneumonia. Note preservation of the heart borders. H-shaped vertebral bodies ➔ are also seen and are characteristic of sickle cell anemia.* ***(Right)*** *Axial HRCT shows perilymphatic distribution of nodules on the interlobular septa ➔, right major fissure ➔, and bronchovascular bundles ➔.*

Esophageal Tear

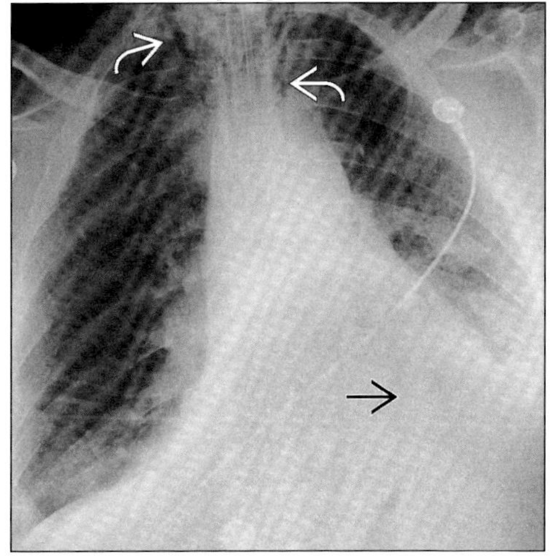

Esophageal Tear

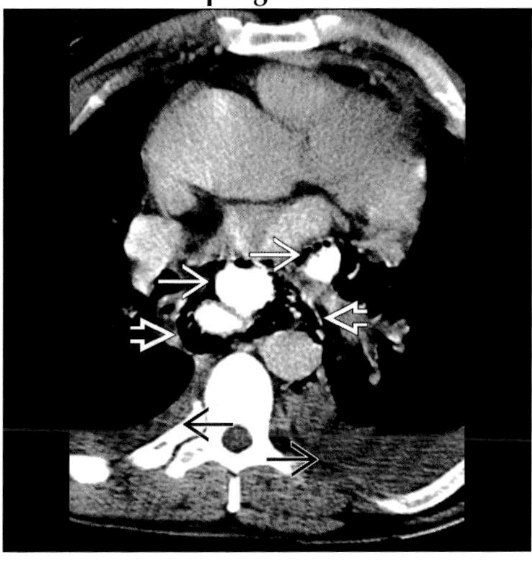

(Left) *Frontal radiograph shows pneumomediastinum extending into the neck ➔ and left pleural effusion ➔ in this patient with recurrent dry heaves and hematemesis. Esophagram revealed an esophageal tear, and the patient was diagnosed with Boerhaave syndrome.* ***(Right)*** *Axial CECT shows a large amount of pneumomediastinum ➔, bilateral pleural effusions ➔, and extravasated oral contrast ➔.*

Mediastinitis

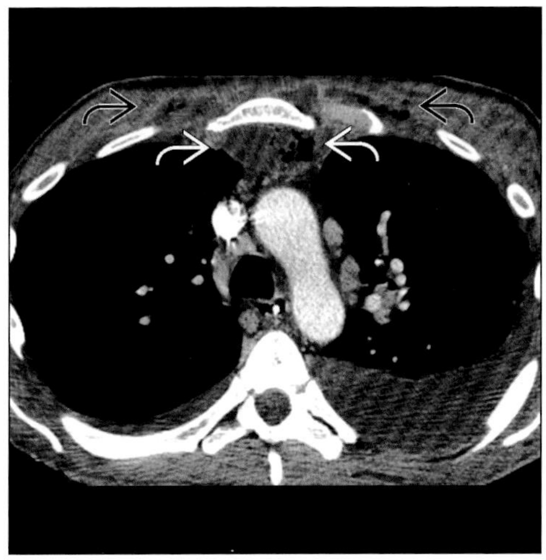

Chest Wall Mass

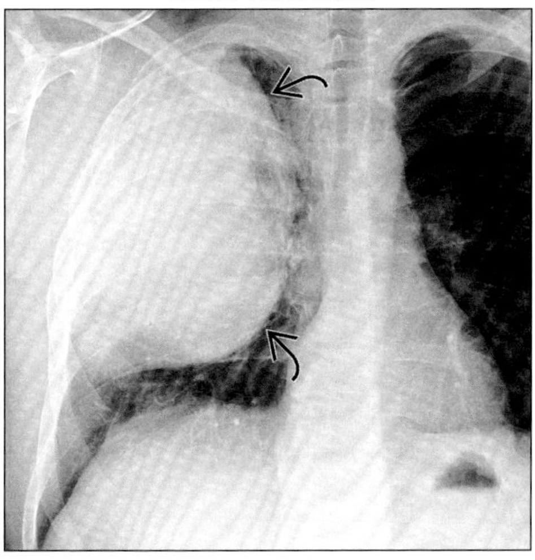

(Left) *Axial CECT shows a fluid and gas collection posterior to the sternum ➔ in this patient with mediastinitis secondary to group A Streptococcus infection. Note bilateral left greater than right pleural effusions and gas and fluid in the subcutaneous chest wall ➔.* ***(Right)*** *Frontal radiograph shows large right chest wall mass ➔ in this patient with Ewing sarcoma. Rib origin was noted on CECT.*

STRIDOR

DIFFERENTIAL DIAGNOSIS

Common
- Tracheobronchomalacia
- Saber-Sheath Trachea
- Laryngeal/Pharyngeal Tumor
- Thyroid Mass

Less Common
- Trauma
- Tracheal Stenosis
- Foreign Body
- Wegener Granulomatosis

Rare but Important
- Tracheopathia Osteochondroplastica
- Infection
- Tracheal Neoplasm
- Tracheobronchial Amyloidosis
- Relapsing Polychondritis

ESSENTIAL INFORMATION

Key Differential Diagnosis Issues
- Review focuses on stridor in adults
- Stridor
  - High pitched sound secondary to turbulent flow in upper airway
  - Indicates pathology in trachea or larynx
- Radiography and CT
  - Primary imaging modalities used in directing differential diagnosis
- Final diagnosis may require bronchoscopy with biopsy

Helpful Clues for Common Diagnoses
- **Tracheobronchomalacia**
  - Abnormal tracheal or bronchial cartilage
    - ≥ 50% decrease in cross-sectional area with expiration
    - Trachea may appear normal on inspiratory images
  - Congenital or acquired causes secondary to
    - Intubation, external mass or vessel causing compression, infections, or COPD
- **Saber-Sheath Trachea**
  - Strong association with COPD
  - Cartilage damage through repeated coughing
  - Coronal tracheal diameter ≤ 2/3 sagittal diameter
  - Normal tracheal wall thickness
- **Laryngeal/Pharyngeal Tumor**
  - Squamous cell carcinoma most common etiology
  - Document extent of disease, as it influences surgical and therapeutic plan
- **Thyroid Mass**
  - Goiter or malignancy may externally compress trachea

Helpful Clues for Less Common Diagnoses
- **Trauma**
  - Hematoma compressing airway
  - Secondary tracheal stenosis from remote trauma
- **Tracheal Stenosis**
  - Focal stricture with circumferential wall thickening
  - ± cartilage damage with resulting tracheomalacia
  - Prolonged endotracheal intubation
    - Subglottic tracheal stenosis at cuff site
    - Reduced incidence with low-pressure balloon cuffs
  - Tracheostomy tube placement
    - Stenosis at stoma site
  - Other etiologies
    - Complete cartilaginous tracheal ring and sarcoidosis
  - Treat with mechanical dilation or stenting
- **Foreign Body**
  - History essential for diagnosis
  - Foreign body rarely radiopaque
- **Wegener Granulomatosis**
  - Circumferential subglottic tracheal wall thickening with luminal narrowing
  - ± cavitary lung nodules
  - ± pansinus disease
  - Laboratory evidence of glomerulonephritis (microscopic hematuria and proteinuria)

Helpful Clues for Rare Diagnoses
- **Tracheopathia Osteochondroplastica**
  - Benign disease occurring in older men
  - Often incidental at bronchoscopy
  - Rarely leads to symptoms
  - Small and irregularly shaped calcified nodules arising from cartilage
  - Spares noncartilaginous posterior tracheal membrane
- **Infection**
  - Tuberculosis
    - Circumferential wall thickening with tracheal narrowing

  - Mediastinal lymphadenopathy
- Epiglottitis
  - More indolent than pediatric epiglottitis, secondary to larger hypopharynx
- Rhinoscleroma
  - Chronic granulomatous infection by *Klebsiella rhinoscleromatis*
  - Central America, Africa, and India
  - Nasal cavity involved in 95% with polyps and soft tissue thickening
  - Spares paranasal sinuses
  - 25% have subglottic tracheal involvement with concentric or nodular narrowing
  - Air-filled crypts in tracheal lumen nearly diagnostic

- **Tracheal Neoplasm**
  - 3 different forms
    - Primary malignant, metastatic disease, and primary benign tumors
  - 3 growth patterns
    - Sessile, polypoid, and circumferential growth
  - CT documents extent of disease and trachea distal to lesion
  - Squamous cell carcinoma
    - Most common primary malignant disease of trachea
    - Strong association with smoking
    - 10% multifocal at presentation
  - Adenoid cystic carcinoma
    - Posterolateral tracheal wall
    - ± growth along airways
  - Metastatic disease
    - Invasion or compression from bronchogenic or esophageal carcinoma
    - Hematogenous metastases from melanoma, breast, colon, and renal cell carcinoma
    - ± single or multiple endotracheal lesions
  - Tracheobronchial papillomatosis
    - HPV infection of tracheal and bronchial tree
    - Small well-circumscribed noncalcified tracheal nodules
    - ± cystic lung lesions
- **Tracheobronchial Amyloidosis**
  - Nodular or concentric wall thickening of trachea and mainstem bronchi
    - ± nodular calcification
  - ± atelectasis or lobar collapse
  - Usually no lung nodules
  - Treatment with stenting or resection
- **Relapsing Polychondritis**
  - Systemic disorder associated with repeated bouts of cartilaginous inflammation
  - Trachea and bronchi affected late in disease course
  - Also affects cartilage of
    - Ears, nose, and joints
  - CT shows
    - Tracheobronchial wall thickening with sparing of noncartilaginous posterior wall
    - Severe disease may affect posterior wall
  - Stenosis leads to recurrent pneumonia
  - Treat with stents and corticosteroids

Tracheobronchomalacia

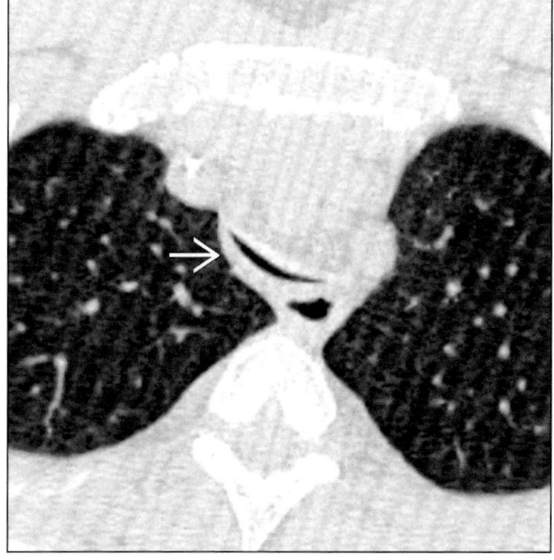

Axial NECT shows diffuse intrathoracic tracheal narrowing ➔ with more than 50% reduction in cross-sectional area when compared to inspiratory images, which is diagnostic of tracheomalacia.

Tracheobronchomalacia

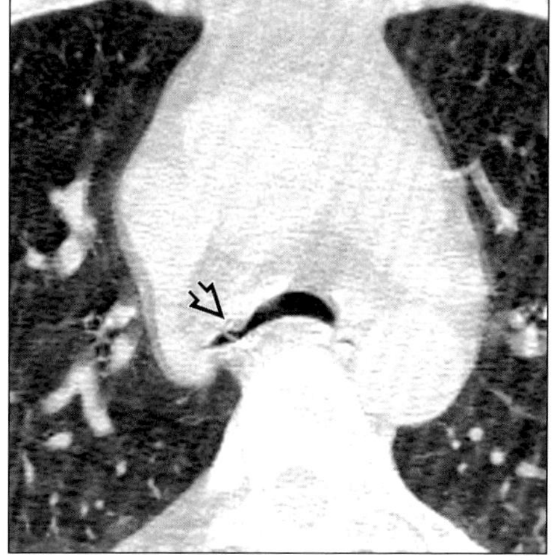

Axial HRCT shows collapse of the bronchus intermedius and right upper lobe bronchus ⇨ from tracheobronchomalacia. Patient required stenting secondary to persistent respiratory symptoms.

STRIDOR

(Left) Sagittal CECT shows tracheal compression by an aberrant left subclavian artery with right aortic arch. In this patient with cervical arch, the vascular structures crowded into a narrow thoracic inlet causing compression and resultant tracheomalacia. *(Right)* Axial CECT shows saber-sheath intrathoracic trachea with the sagittal diameter greater than the coronal diameter. There is severe centrilobular emphysema, a common association.

Tracheobronchomalacia

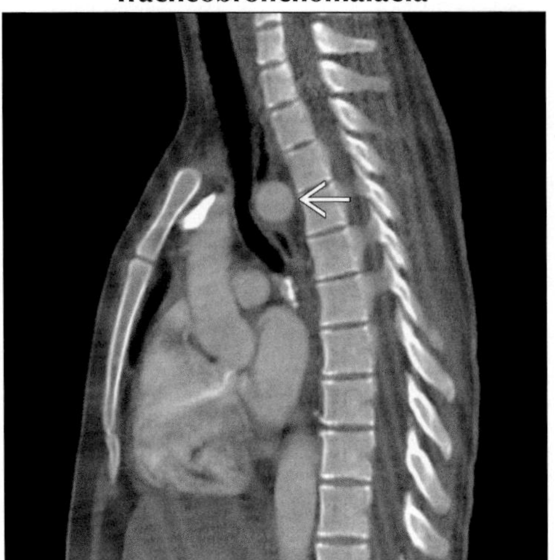

Saber-Sheath Trachea

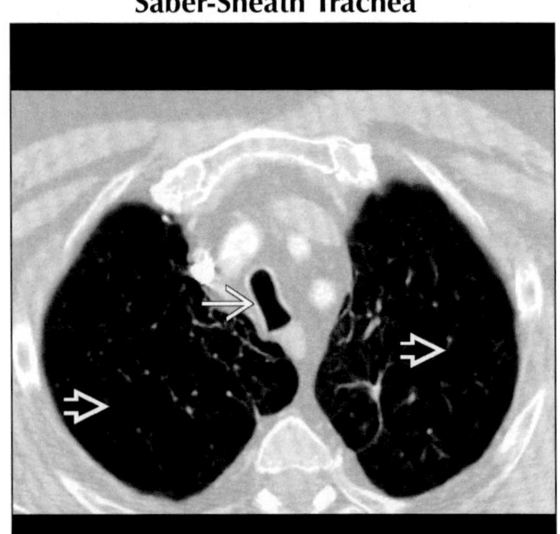

(Left) Axial NECT shows a mass located superior to the left true vocal cord. This proved to represent a squamous cell carcinoma. The vocal cord was not involved on lower sections, an important finding to report as this influences surgical therapy. *(Right)* Axial PET/CT fusion image shows hypermetabolism in a left supraglottic mass. This proved to be a primary squamous cell carcinoma on resection.

Laryngeal/Pharyngeal Tumor

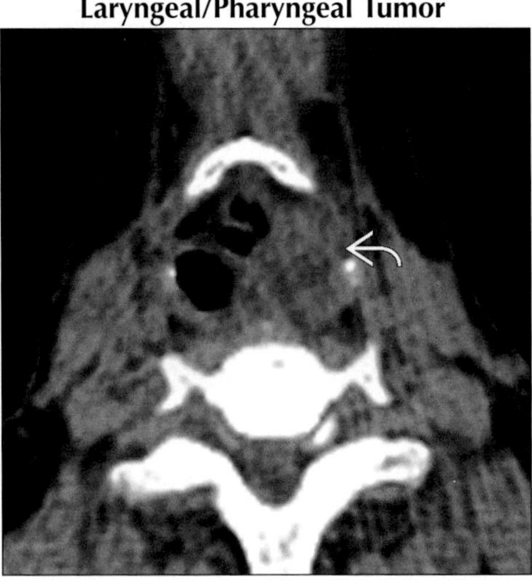

Laryngeal/Pharyngeal Tumor

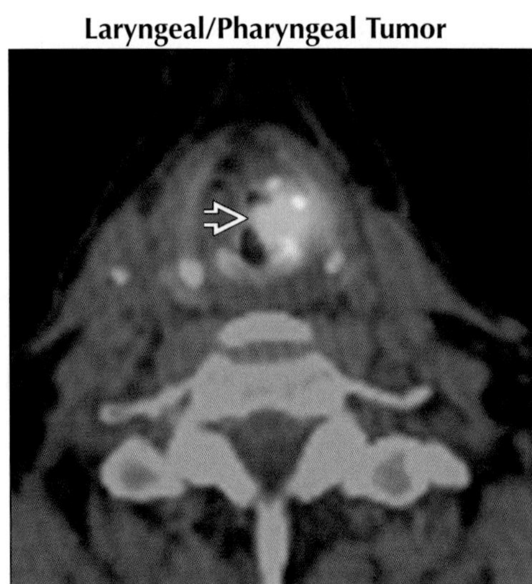

(Left) Frontal radiograph shows a large right paratracheal mass with narrowing and leftward displacement of the trachea. This was a large substernal goiter without malignancy. *(Right)* Coronal CECT shows a high-density heterogeneously enhancing mass in the thoracic inlet deviating the trachea to the right. There is associated tracheal narrowing. This proved to be a thyroid goiter, and connection to the thyroid was revealed on axial sections.

Thyroid Mass

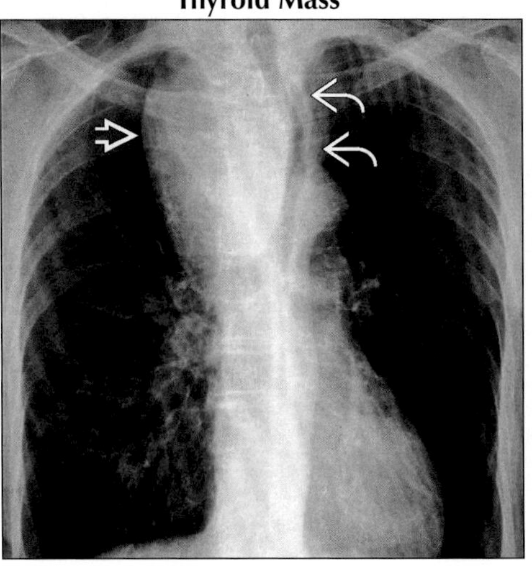

Thyroid Mass

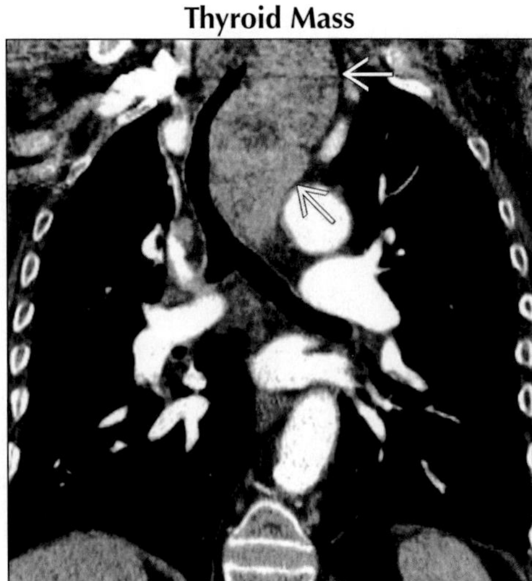

STRIDOR

Tracheal Stenosis

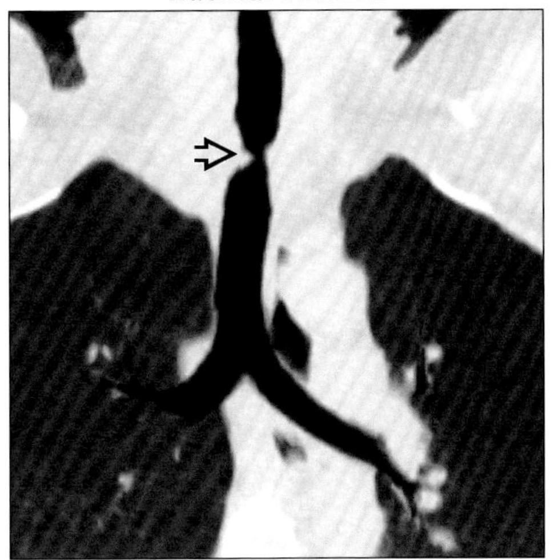

Tracheal Stenosis

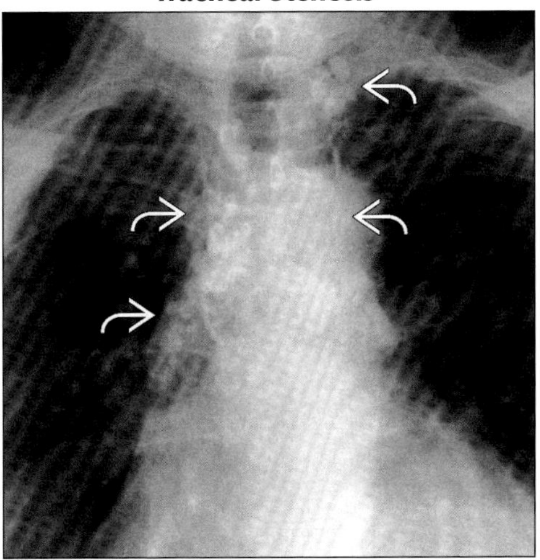

(Left) Coronal NECT demonstrates short segment tracheal narrowing ➲ at the level of the thoracic inlet in this patient with post-intubation stenosis. *(Right)* Frontal radiograph shows extensive calcified bilateral hilar, paratracheal, and cervical lymph nodes ➦. Note external compression of the trachea caused by lymphadenopathy in this patient with sarcoidosis. This required treatment with stenting.

Tracheal Stenosis

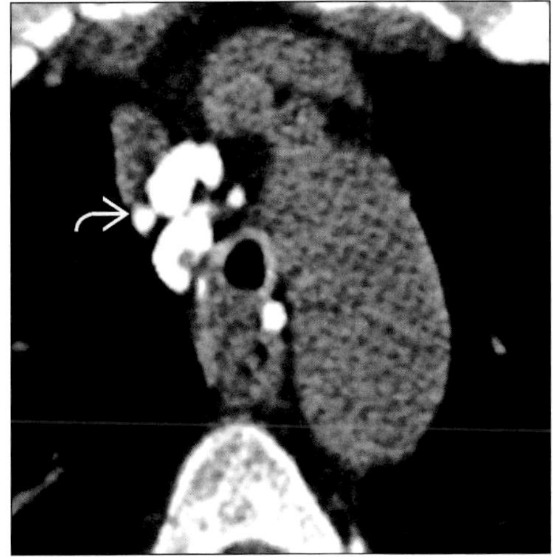

Foreign Body

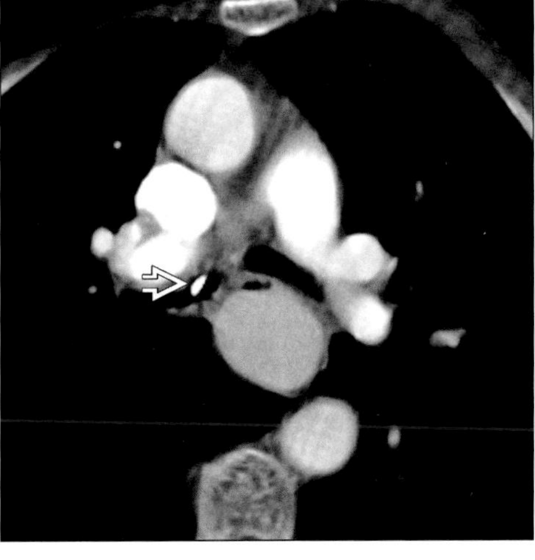

(Left) Axial NECT shows multiple calcified paratracheal lymph nodes ➦ with extrinsic tracheal stenosis secondary to sarcoidosis. Tracheal stenosis from sarcoidosis can be from extrinsic compression, as in this case, or intrinsic compression secondary to luminal granulomas. *(Right)* Axial CECT shows an aspirated wire in the bronchus intermedius ➲. Lung windows (not shown) revealed tree in bud opacities from postobstructive pneumonia.

Wegener Granulomatosis

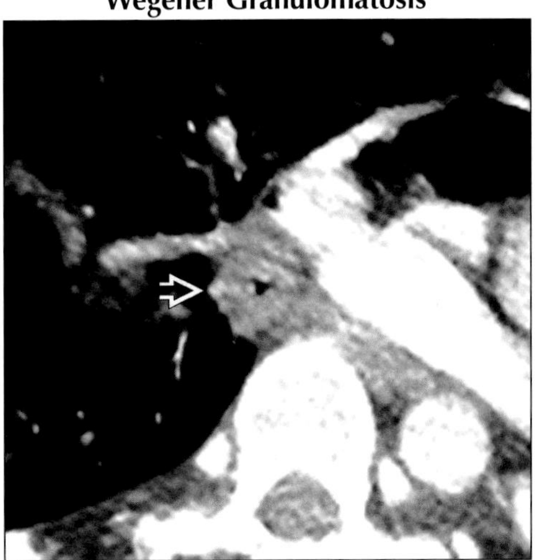

Tracheopathia Osteochondroplastica

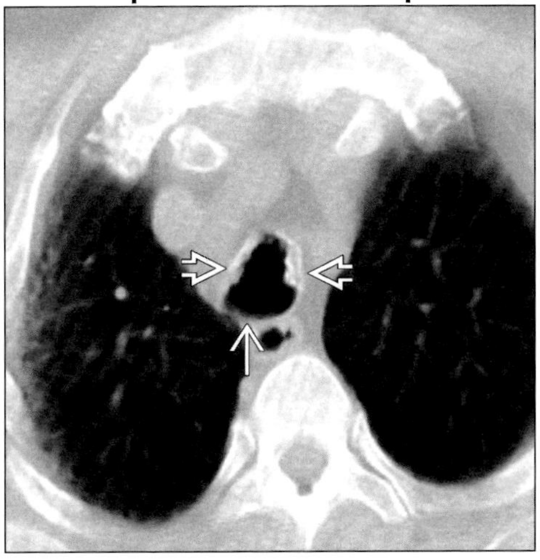

(Left) Axial CECT shows severe circumferential tracheal narrowing with near complete obliteration of the lumen ➲. Patient had a left pneumonectomy for complications related to Wegener granulomatosis. *(Right)* Axial NECT shows calcified nodules along the anterior and lateral wall of the trachea ➲. Nodules arise from cartilage; the posterior tracheal wall is thus spared ➔, as it does not contain cartilage.

STRIDOR

*(**Left**) Coronal NECT shows multiple nodular mucosal protrusions that extend into the mainstem bronchi. There is associated tracheal narrowing. Soft tissue windows demonstrated the nodules were calcified. Note bilateral apical blebs/bullae . (**Right**) Axial CECT shows typical CT features of circumferential subglottic narrowing from rhinoscleroma. Note typical crypt-like air spaces .*

Tracheopathia Osteochondroplastica

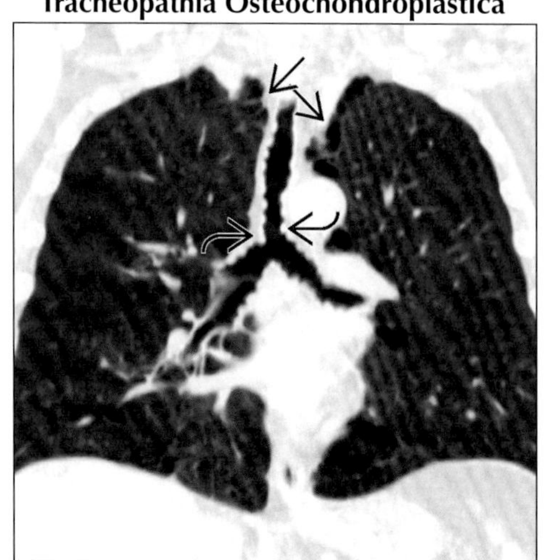

Infection

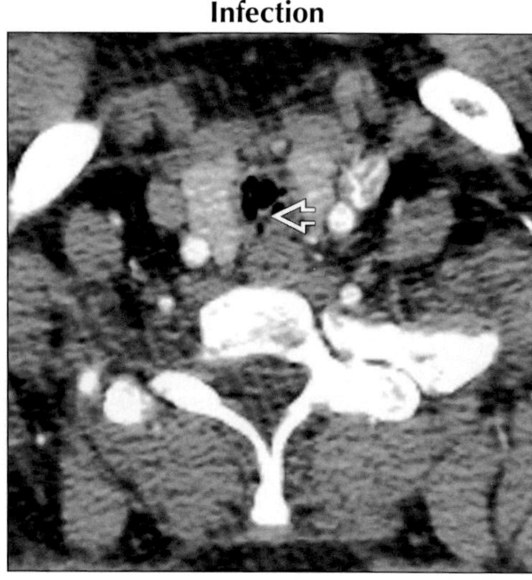

*(**Left**) Frontal radiograph shows a left-sided tracheal nodule , proven to represent a primary tracheal squamous cell carcinoma. (**Right**) Axial NECT shows typical CT features of laryngotracheal papillomatosis. Note discrete tracheal nodules involving the lateral and posterior walls . Mediastinal windows (not shown) showed that the nodules were not calcified, characteristic of this disorder.*

Tracheal Neoplasm

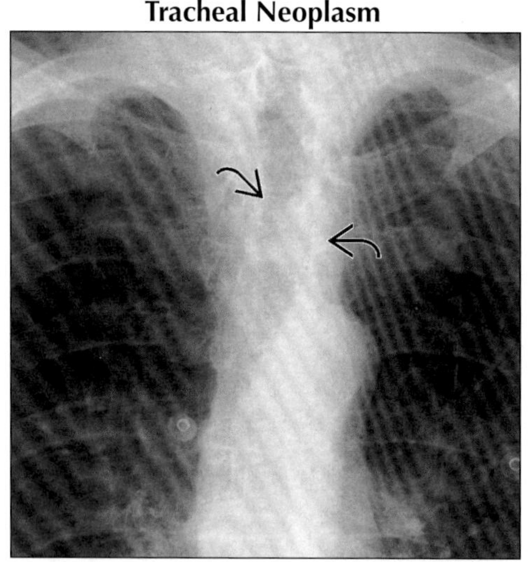

Tracheal Neoplasm

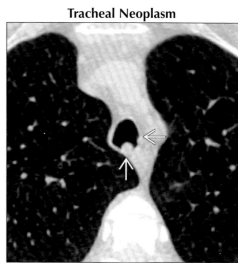

*(**Left**) Coronal CECT shows typical CT features of diffuse tracheal wall thickening from adenoid cystic carcinoma. Note the characteristic extent of the tumor growing along the length of the trachea . (**Right**) Axial NECT shows thickening and nodularity of the anterior and left side of the trachea . This proved to represent a primary squamous cell carcinoma of the trachea.*

Tracheal Neoplasm

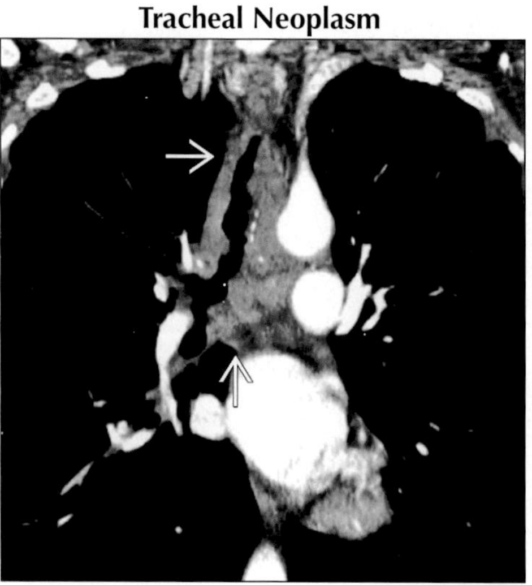

Tracheal Neoplasm

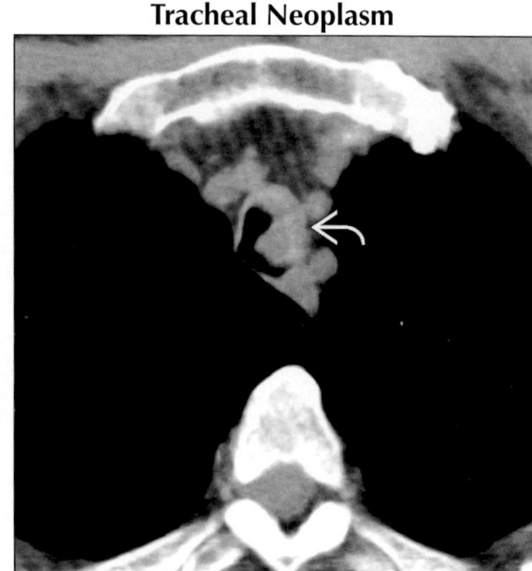

STRIDOR

Tracheal Neoplasm

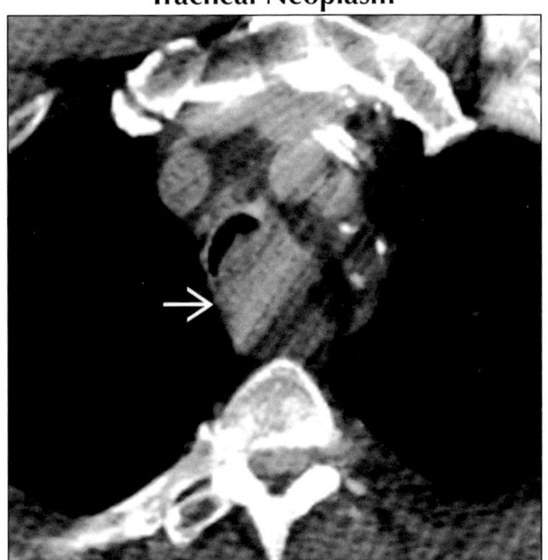

Tracheal Neoplasm

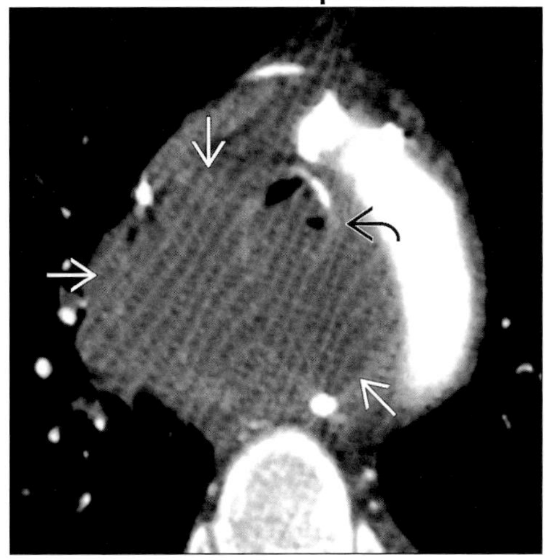

(Left) *Axial NECT shows typical radiographic and CT features of tracheal metastasis from renal cell carcinoma. Note large lesion nearly completely occluding the tracheal lumen* ➔. ***(Right)*** *Axial CECT shows a large homogeneous-appearing mass growing around the trachea* ➔. *This proved to represent a bronchogenic carcinoma. The tumor has grown into the tracheal lumen causing near complete occlusion* ↪.

Tracheobronchial Amyloidosis

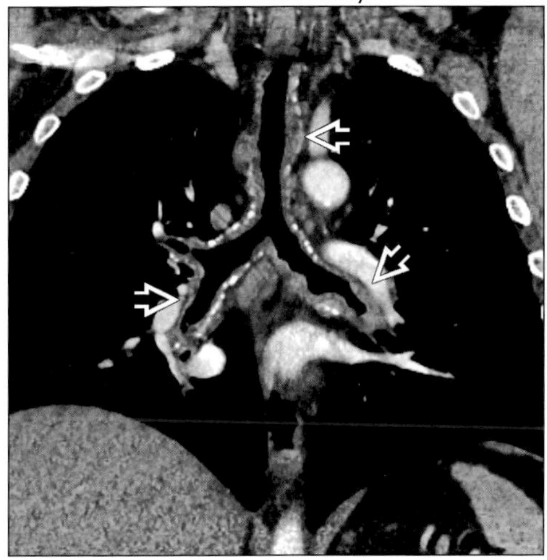

Relapsing Polychondritis

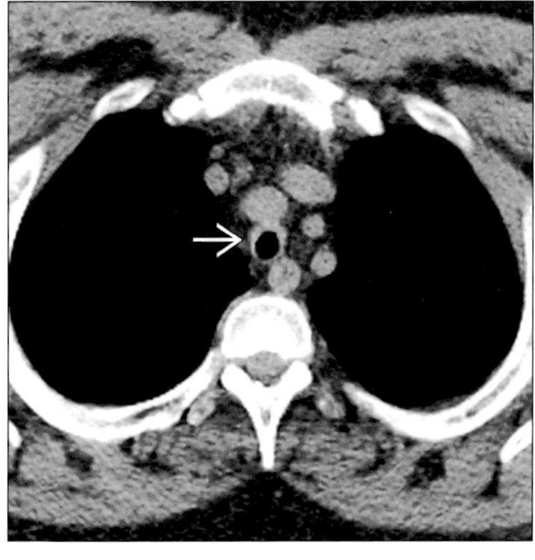

(Left) *Coronal CECT shows diffuse thickening of the trachea and main and lobar bronchi* ⇨. *Some of the nodules are calcified. Involvement of the posterior tracheal membrane was demonstrated on axial images.* ***(Right)*** *Axial NECT shows typical CT features of a small trachea from relapsing polychondritis. Note tracheal wall thickening* ➔ *that spares the posterior noncartilaginous tracheal wall. The tracheal diameter was 8 mm.*

Relapsing Polychondritis

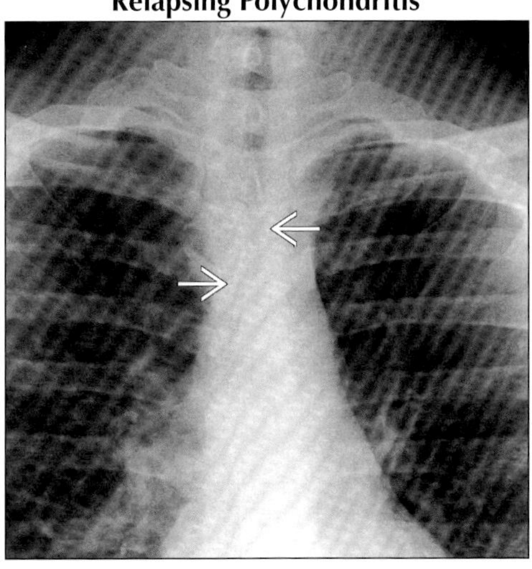

Relapsing Polychondritis

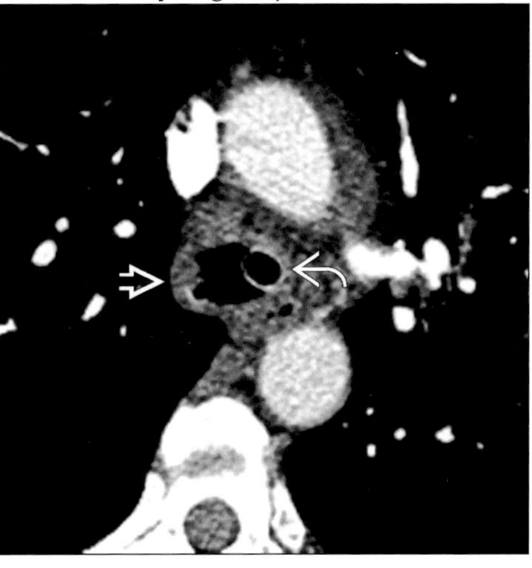

(Left) *Frontal radiograph shows a diffusely narrowed trachea* ➔. *CT revealed characteristic sparing of the posterior tracheal wall. Patient also had other cartilaginous involvement with deformity of the pinna of the ear.* ***(Right)*** *Axial CECT shows diffuse circumferential tracheal wall thickening* ⇨. *The posterior tracheal membrane is involved in this case, secondary to severe inflammation. Endotracheal tube* ↪ *was needed for respiratory support.*

SECTION 5
Airspace

CENTRAL DISTRIBUTION (BAT-WING)

DIFFERENTIAL DIAGNOSIS

Common
- Hydrostatic Pulmonary Edema
- Pneumonia

Less Common
- Lung Injury
- Pulmonary Hemorrhage

Rare but Important
- Pulmonary Alveolar Proteinosis
- Acute Interstitial Pneumonia

ESSENTIAL INFORMATION

Key Differential Diagnosis Issues
- Classically described on frontal radiograph, though can be seen on CT
- Bilateral perihilar opacities with relative sparing of peripheral lung tissue
- Clinical information is key to diagnosis

Helpful Clues for Common Diagnoses
- **Hydrostatic Pulmonary Edema**
  - Usually caused by increased pulmonary venous pressure
  - Most common etiologies include left-sided heart failure and volume overload
  - Interstitial edema: Kerley lines, peribronchial cuffing, perihilar haze
  - Airspace edema: Patchy or diffuse airspace opacities, may present as bat-wing edema
  - Central distribution may be due to rapid onset of edema and better lymphatic clearance of lung periphery
- **Pneumonia**
  - Seen with bacterial and atypical pathogens
  - Dense consolidation
  - May see air bronchograms

Helpful Clues for Less Common Diagnoses
- **Lung Injury**
  - Caused by illicit drugs (crack cocaine), near drowning, smoke inhalation, sepsis, etc.
  - Disruption of alveolar-capillary interface leads to noncardiogenic pulmonary edema
  - Diffuse alveolar damage
- **Pulmonary Hemorrhage**
  - Numerous causes that may present similarly by radiograph
  - Patchy or diffuse ground-glass opacities or consolidation, often with central distribution
  - Can present as ill-defined centrilobular nodules, especially on CT

Helpful Clues for Rare Diagnoses
- **Pulmonary Alveolar Proteinosis**
  - Most cases are idiopathic
  - Airspaces filled with proteinaceous material; interstitium thickened
  - Crazy-paving pattern on HRCT
- **Acute Interstitial Pneumonia**
  - Idiopathic disease resulting in diffuse alveolar damage
  - Associated with viral prodrome
  - Also known as Hamman-Rich syndrome
  - Bilateral airspace consolidation that may be patchy or diffuse

Hydrostatic Pulmonary Edema

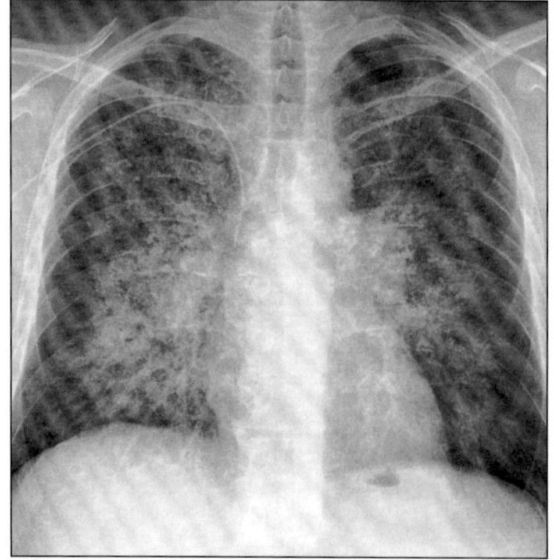

Frontal radiograph shows typical radiographic features of acute pulmonary edema presenting with bat-wing consolidation. This was caused by acute left-sided congestive heart failure.

Pneumonia

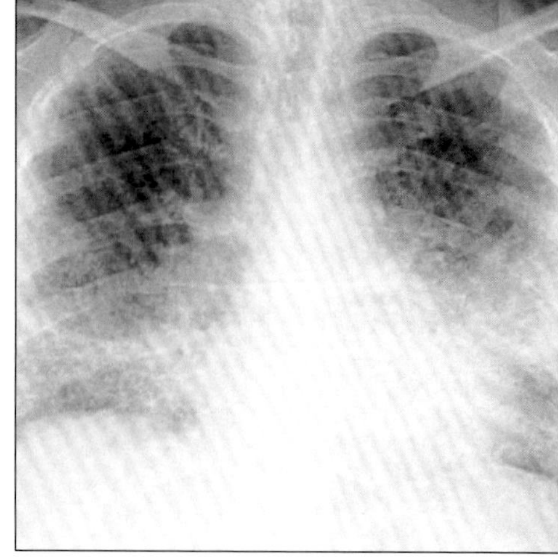

Frontal radiograph shows central bilateral lung consolidation, worse on the left. This proved to be Pneumocystis pneumonia in this immunocompromised patient.

CENTRAL DISTRIBUTION (BAT-WING)

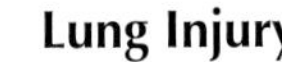

Lung Injury

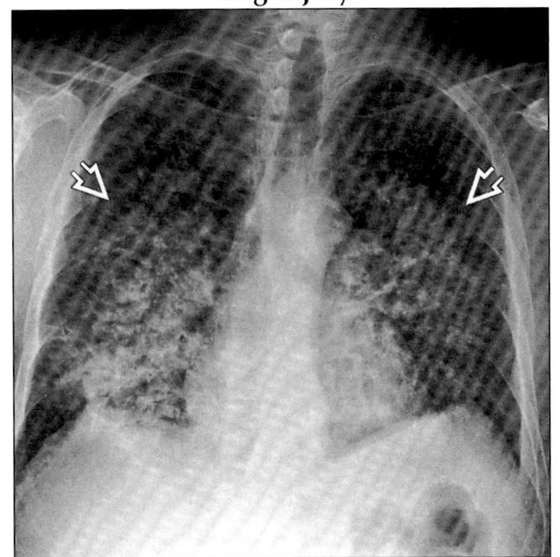

Lung Injury

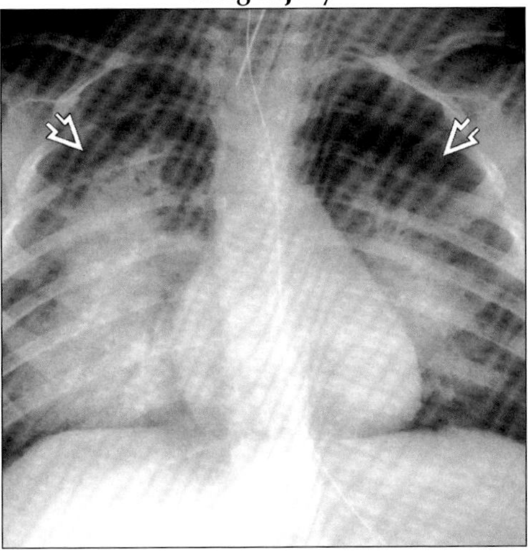

(Left) *Frontal radiograph shows bilateral central pulmonary edema in a bat-wing distribution → caused by inhalation of crack cocaine.* ***(Right)*** *Frontal radiograph shows bilateral central consolidation → in this patient with a history of near-drowning. Injury to the lungs results in noncardiogenic pulmonary edema. Note that this is similar to other causes of central consolidation, emphasizing the importance of clinical history.*

Pulmonary Hemorrhage

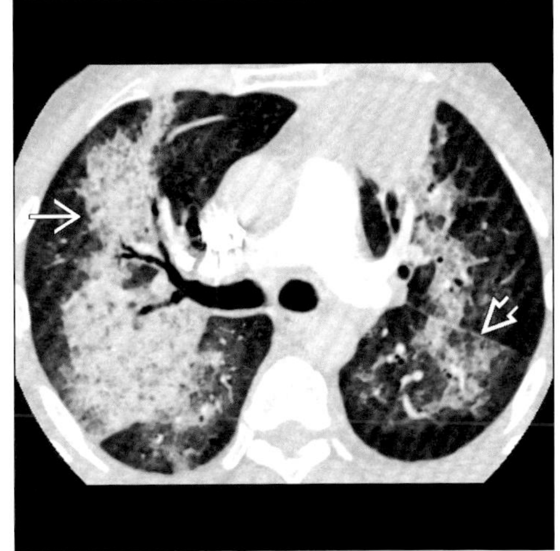

Pulmonary Hemorrhage

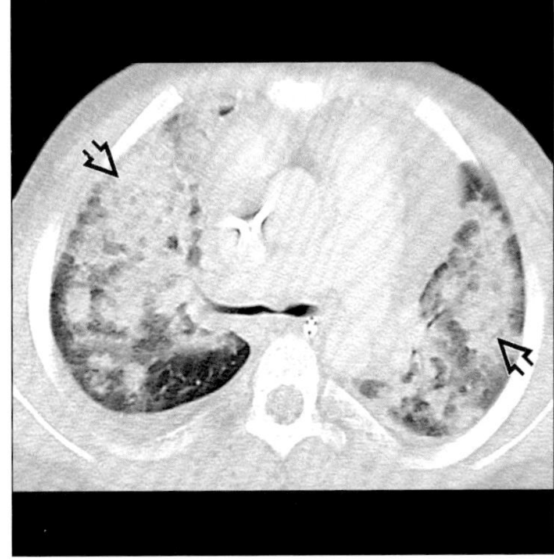

(Left) *Axial CECT shows a variant presentation of Wegener granulomatosis with bilateral pulmonary hemorrhage in a bat-wing distribution →. Notice also the crazy-paving pattern in the left lower lobe →.* ***(Right)*** *Axial NECT shows dense bilateral central consolidation → in this patient with pulmonary hemorrhage. Blood was being aspirated from the endotracheal tube, an important clue to the diagnosis.*

Pulmonary Alveolar Proteinosis

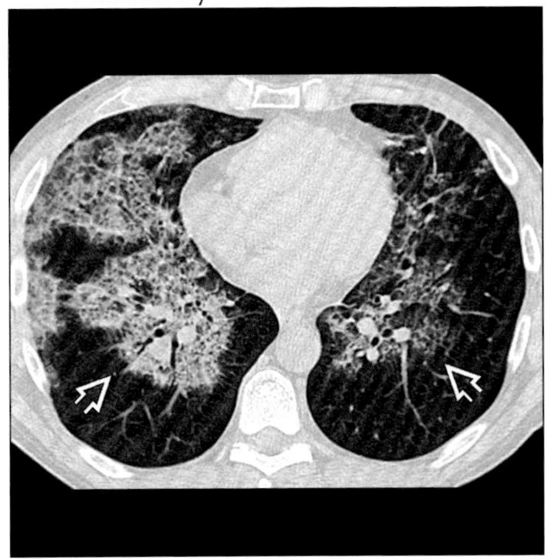

Acute Interstitial Pneumonia

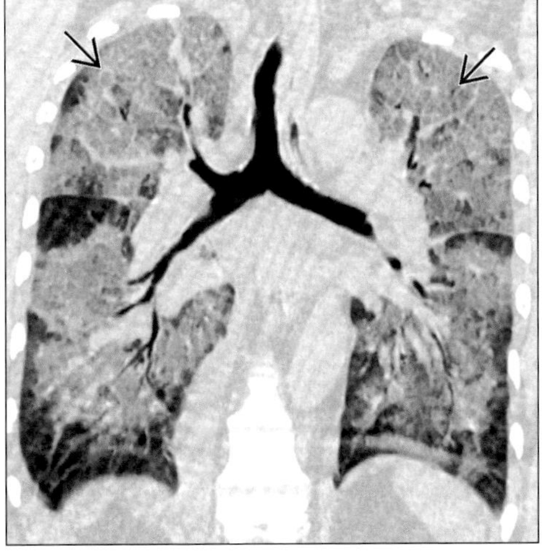

(Left) *Axial NECT shows bilateral ground-glass opacity with interstitial septal thickening, known as crazy-paving. Notice the predominantly central distribution →. While this is nonspecific, in the appropriate clinical setting it is consistent with pulmonary alveolar proteinosis.* ***(Right)*** *Coronal NECT shows extensive bilateral ground-glass opacities → with geographic areas of sparing at the periphery. This is typical of acute interstitial pneumonia.*

PERIPHERAL DISTRIBUTION (REVERSE BAT-WING)

DIFFERENTIAL DIAGNOSIS

Common

- Contusion

Less Common

- Eosinophilic Lung Disease
- Cryptogenic Organizing Pneumonia
- Pulmonary Infarct
- Acute Respiratory Distress Syndrome
- Radiation Pneumonitis

Rare but Important

- Collagen Vascular Disease
- Fat Embolism Syndrome

ESSENTIAL INFORMATION

Key Differential Diagnosis Issues

- Spares perihilar regions
- Initially described on chest radiography
- CT is more sensitive for detection of peripheral consolidation
- Clinical history is essential

Helpful Clues for Common Diagnoses

- **Contusion**
  - Interstitial and alveolar hemorrhage due to blunt thoracic injury
  - Occurs adjacent to site of chest wall trauma
  - Contrecoup contusions can occur, but rare
  - Not confined by fissural or segmental anatomic boundaries
  - Usually resolves within a few days
  - Persistence of opacities beyond a few days suggests alternate diagnosis, such as superimposed infection or aspiration

Helpful Clues for Less Common Diagnoses

- **Eosinophilic Lung Disease**
  - Accumulation of eosinophils within distal airways and interstitium
  - Several forms of disease exist
  - Loeffler syndrome is most common form
  - Peripheral opacities are typical findings with these forms
    - Loeffler syndrome: Idiopathic peripheral consolidation that clears within 1 month (fleeting); also known as simple eosinophilic pneumonia
    - Chronic eosinophilic pneumonia: Peripheral consolidation associated with severe respiratory symptoms lasting at least 3 months, often with upper lobe predominance
    - Churg-Strauss syndrome: Middle-aged patient with allergies; lung disease resembles simple or chronic eosinophilic lung disease
  - Peripheral opacities are less commonly associated with these forms
    - Acute eosinophilic pneumonia: Acute respiratory failure with rapid response to steroids; appearance resembles more typical pulmonary edema
    - Hypereosinophilic syndrome: Multiorgan infiltration of eosinophils; usually presents with bilateral pulmonary nodules
- **Cryptogenic Organizing Pneumonia**
  - Formerly known as idiopathic bronchiolitis obliterans organizing pneumonia (BOOP)
  - Accumulation of foamy macrophages and fibrosis in distal airways
  - Restrictive lung disease with chronic cough, shortness of breath, low-grade fever
  - Patchy areas of airspace consolidation or ground-glass opacities
  - Airspace disease is often in peripheral distribution
  - Tends to be peribronchovascular; can be unilateral or bilateral
  - More common in lower lungs
  - Other CT findings include
    - Peribronchial and centrilobular nodules
    - Atoll or reverse halo sign: Crescentic opacity with central ground-glass opacity
- **Pulmonary Infarct**
  - Usually due to pulmonary artery emboli
  - Also associated with central bronchogenic carcinoma
  - More common in patients with poor cardiopulmonary reserve, impaired bronchial circulation
  - Subpleural pulmonary parenchymal consolidation, often wedge-shaped
  - Hampton hump: Wedge-shaped peripheral opacity with medial border oriented toward hilum

- Central "bubbly" lucencies within peripheral consolidation is suggestive of diagnosis
- **Acute Respiratory Distress Syndrome**
  - Damage to capillaries allows for loss of fluid into lung interstitium and alveolar spaces
  - Numerous causes: Trauma, infection, toxin exposure, emboli, DIC, drugs, pancreatitis, etc.
  - Idiopathic ARDS is known as acute interstitial pneumonia (AIP)
  - Often follows predictable time course
    - 1st 12-24 hours: Normal radiographic appearance
    - Several days: Bilateral scattered areas of consolidation; begins peripherally and then becomes confluent
    - Weeks: Slow resolution of lung consolidation
    - Months: May progress to lung fibrosis, often with anterior predominance
- **Radiation Pneumonitis**
  - Occurs 1-3 months after radiation therapy
  - Occurs in approximately 40% of patients
  - Associated with diffuse alveolar damage within irradiated tissue
  - Ground-glass opacity &/or consolidation within lung tissue corresponding to location of radiation port
  - Does not respect fissural and segmental boundaries
  - Often asymptomatic
  - May resolve or progress to radiation fibrosis
  - Persistence > 9 months post radiation suggests presence of radiation fibrosis

Helpful Clues for Rare Diagnoses

- **Collagen Vascular Disease**
  - Heterogeneous group of diseases
    - Systemic lupus erythematosus
    - Dermatomyositis/polymyositis
    - Scleroderma
    - Rheumatoid arthritis
  - Interstitial lung disease is most common pulmonary complication
  - May see peripheral ground-glass opacity and reticulation
- **Fat Embolism Syndrome**
  - Usually caused by trauma to long bone or pelvis
  - Fat droplets are deposited within small vascular spaces
  - Symptoms develop 1-3 days after blunt trauma
  - Radiography is nonspecific but may reveal ARDS pattern, often with peripheral consolidation
  - Radiography may be normal initially
  - Diagnosis is clinical
    - Respiratory symptoms
    - Neurological changes due to cerebral disease
    - Hematological changes, such as anemia
    - Petechial rash

Contusion

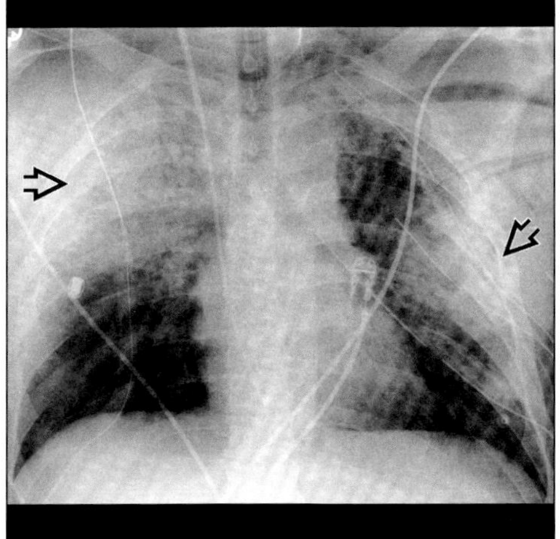

Anteroposterior radiograph shows bilateral peripheral lung consolidation ⇨ caused by lung contusions in this patient with blunt thoracic injury. Notice the relative perihilar sparing.

Contusion

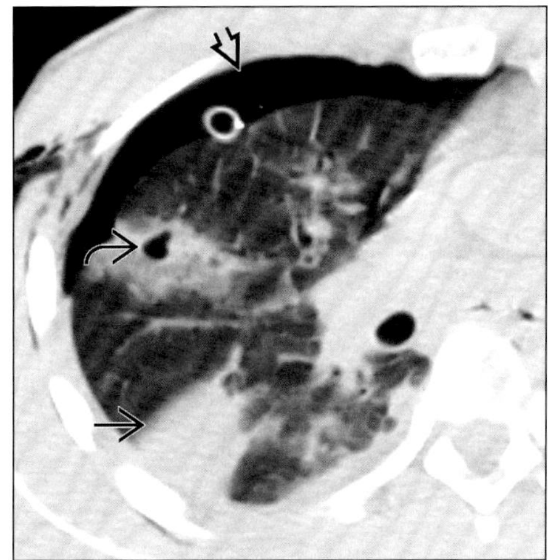

Axial NECT shows a pulmonary contusion in the peripheral right lung →. Also notice the lung laceration with surrounding contusion ↷ and pneumothorax ⇨.

PERIPHERAL DISTRIBUTION (REVERSE BAT-WING)

*(**Left**) Frontal radiograph shows bilateral peripheral consolidation in the lower lungs → in this patient with a several month history of shortness of breath. (**Right**) Axial NECT in the same patient confirms the findings seen on the radiograph. There are bilateral peripheral ground-glass opacities → and consolidation →. These are typical findings of chronic eosinophilic pneumonia. This patient also had peripheral blood eosinophilia.*

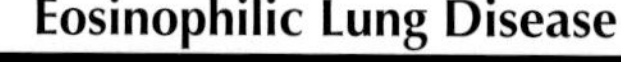

Eosinophilic Lung Disease

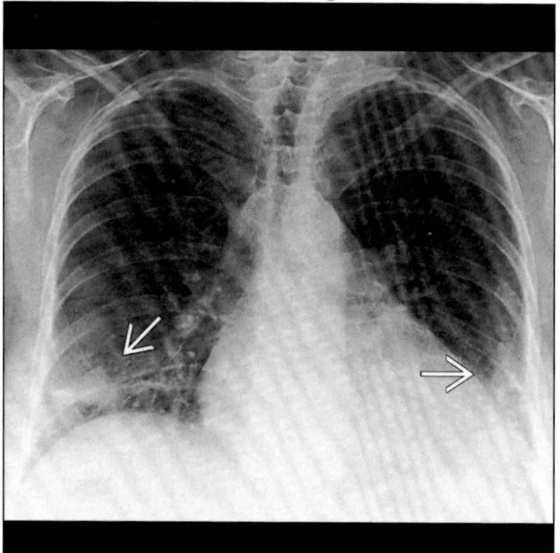

Eosinophilic Lung Disease

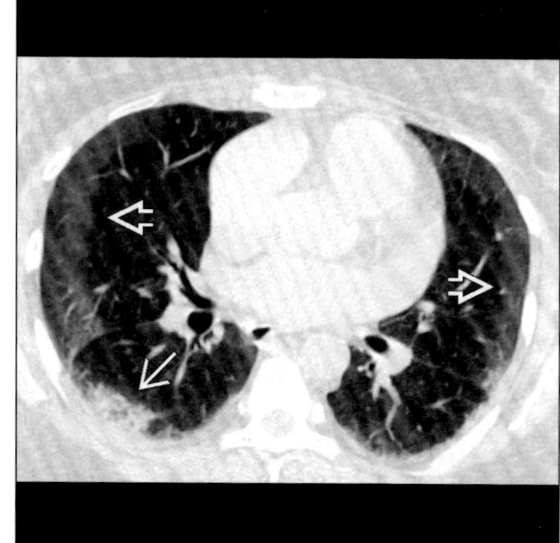

*(**Left**) Axial CECT shows peripheral bands of consolidation and ground-glass opacity → in this patient with chronic eosinophilic pneumonia. Blood eosinophilia, chronic respiratory symptoms, and resolution with steroid therapy are associated findings. (**Right**) Axial HRCT shows subpleural consolidation → due to vasculitis in this patient with Churg-Strauss disease. The patient also had asthma, a common coexisting condition.*

Eosinophilic Lung Disease

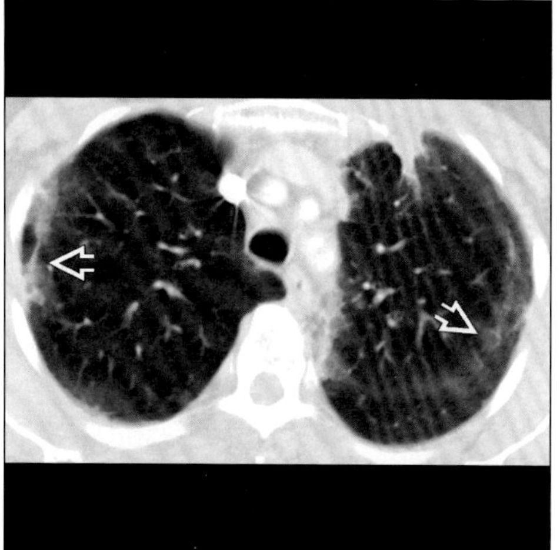

Eosinophilic Lung Disease

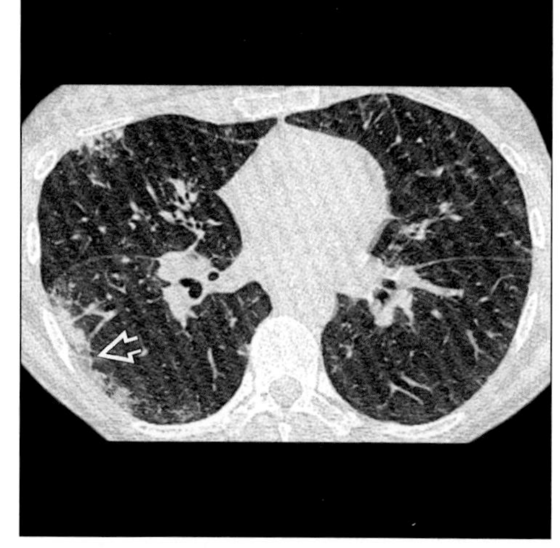

*(**Left**) Axial NECT shows bilateral peripheral airspace consolidation →, especially within the posterior lungs. Notice the sparing of the central lungs. This is a typical appearance of cryptogenic organizing pneumonia. (**Right**) Axial HRCT shows peripheral consolidation in the right upper lobe → and peribronchial consolidation →. These are typical findings in cryptogenic organizing pneumonia.*

Cryptogenic Organizing Pneumonia

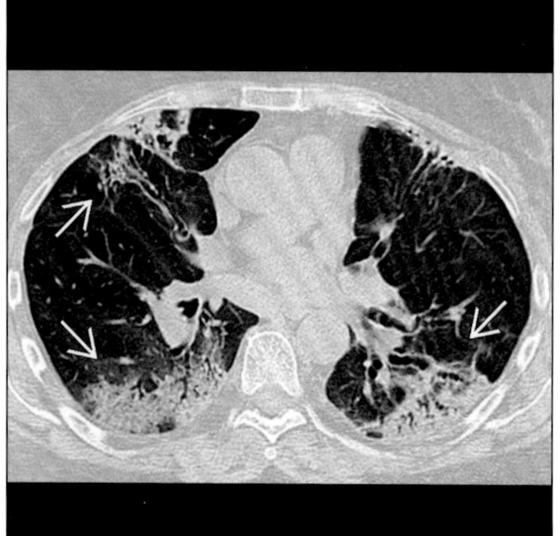

Cryptogenic Organizing Pneumonia

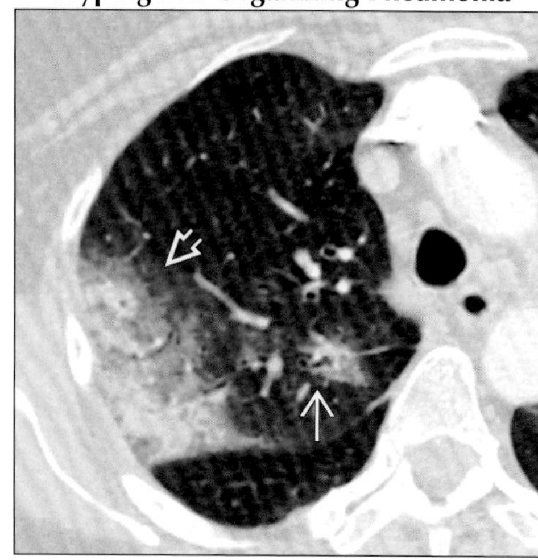

PERIPHERAL DISTRIBUTION (REVERSE BAT-WING)

Pulmonary Infarct

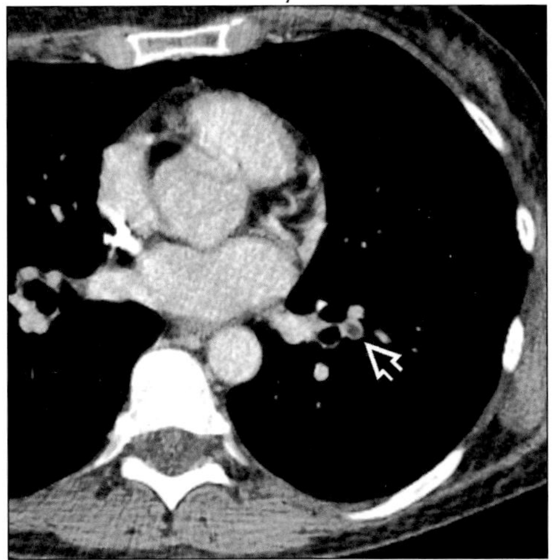

Pulmonary Infarct

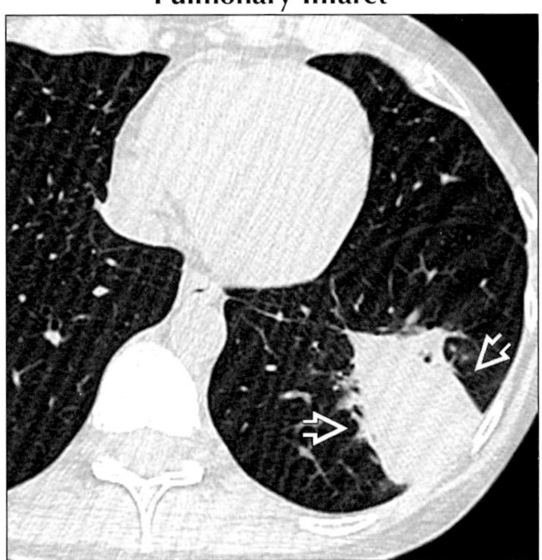

(Left) Axial CECT shows a round filling defect ➡ in a left lower lobe pulmonary artery, consistent with a pulmonary embolus. ***(Right)*** Axial NECT obtained 14 days later because of worsening chest pain reveals a peripheral wedge-shaped area of consolidation distal to the pulmonary embolus ➡. This is a typical appearance of a pulmonary infarct.

Acute Respiratory Distress Syndrome

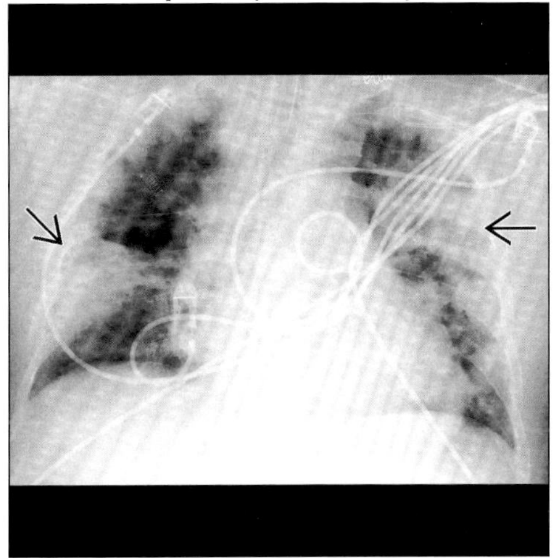

Radiation Pneumonitis

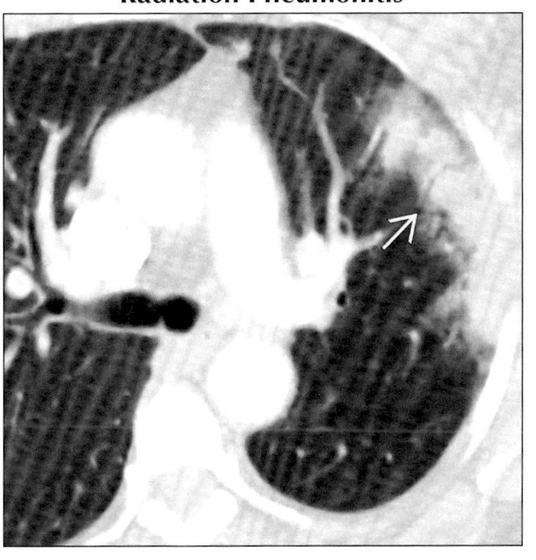

(Left) *Anteroposterior radiograph shows typical radiographic features of peripheral consolidation* → *from acute respiratory distress syndrome (ARDS). Early ARDS may present differently from cardiogenic pulmonary edema, which is often central in distribution.* ***(Right)*** *Axial CECT shows peripheral lung consolidation in the left upper lobe* ➡. *This lung tissue was in the radiation port and may progress to radiation fibrosis over the next several months.*

Collagen Vascular Disease

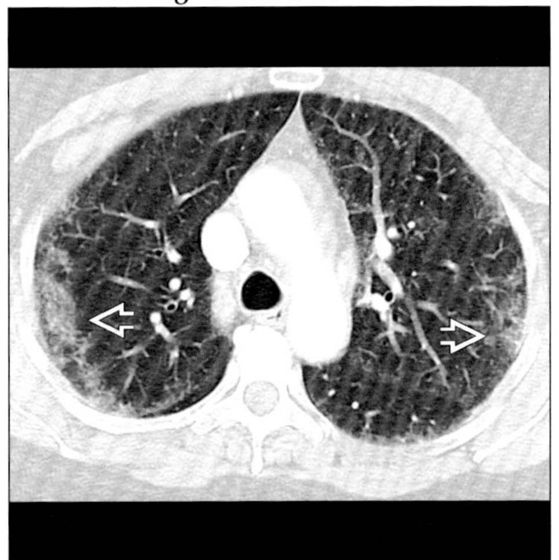

Fat Embolism Syndrome

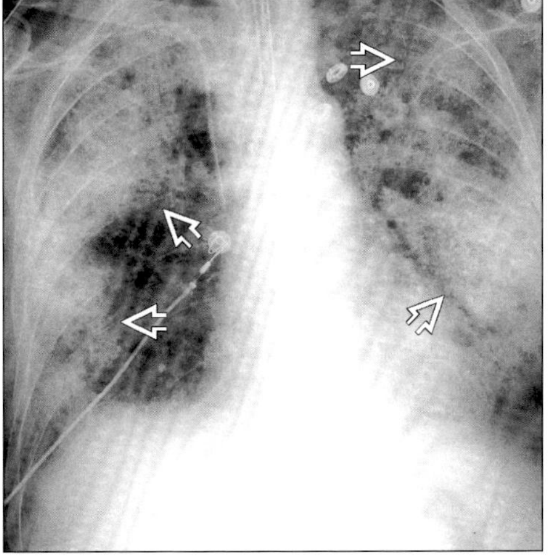

(Left) *Axial NECT shows bilateral peripheral ground-glass opacities* ➡ *in this patient with dermatomyositis.* ***(Right)*** *Anteroposterior radiograph shows typical radiographic features of peripheral consolidation from fat embolism syndrome* ➡. *This syndrome most commonly follows blunt trauma to a long bone or the pelvis, and the diagnosis is clinical.*

MIGRATORY DISTRIBUTION

DIFFERENTIAL DIAGNOSIS

Common
- Asthma
- Recurrent Aspiration
- Atelectasis
- Pulmonary Infarct

Less Common
- Septic Emboli
- Organizing Pneumonia
- Cystic Fibrosis
- Allergic Bronchopulmonary Aspergillosis
- Eosinophilic Pneumonia

Rare but Important
- Pulmonary Vasculitis

ESSENTIAL INFORMATION

Key Differential Diagnosis Issues
- Migratory pulmonary opacities more suggestive of infectious or inflammatory abnormalities rather than malignancy

Helpful Clues for Common Diagnoses
- **Asthma**
  - Airway inflammation resulting in reversible airflow obstruction
  - Imaging for complications: Pneumomediastinum, pneumonia, pneumothorax
  - Patchy distribution
  - Bronchial wall thickening and bronchial dilation
  - Air-trapping or mosaic attenuation
  - Mucus plugging, subsegmental to lobar atelectasis
  - Occasional bronchiectasis
- **Recurrent Aspiration**
  - Consolidation in gravity-dependent portions of lungs
  - Predisposed patients (i.e., those with alcoholism, epilepsy, hiatal hernia, esophageal dysmotility or obstruction, neuromuscular disorders)
  - Supine: Superior segments of lower lobes and posterior segments of upper lobes
  - Upright: Basilar segments of lower lobes
  - Centrilobular or tree in bud opacities common
  - May progress to necrotizing pneumonia or pulmonary abscess without treatment
  - Bland aspiration clears quickly (within hours)
- **Atelectasis**
  - Recurrent mucus plugging can result in fleeting or migratory atelectasis
    - Subsegmental to lobar in distribution
    - Low-density material visible in airways
  - Recurrent atelectasis or pneumonitis due to incomplete obstruction of airway by aspirated foreign body or endobronchial lesion
- **Pulmonary Infarct**
  - Lower lung predominant, peripheral/subpleural, wedge-shaped consolidation
  - Acute pulmonary arterial thromboembolism
  - CT: Reverse halo configuration common (central ground-glass opacity and peripheral rim of consolidation)
    - Also central lucencies and absence of air bronchograms
  - Often in setting of superimposed cardiac dysfunction (cardiomyopathy, congestive heart failure)
    - Both pulmonary and bronchial arterial supply to lung reduced
  - May be migratory: Recurrent emboli lead to new pulmonary infarcts as old infarcts resolve

Helpful Clues for Less Common Diagnoses
- **Septic Emboli**
  - Multiple, peripheral, and basilar consolidation or nodules with early cavitation
  - Feeding artery sign: Pulmonary artery branches extend to nodules, implying hematogenous spread
  - Loculated pleural effusion common
  - Risk factors: Indwelling intravenous catheter or right heart endocarditis
  - Migratory appearance from recurrent septic embolic events
- **Organizing Pneumonia**
  - Bilateral basal-predominant peripheral and peribronchovascular consolidation
  - Scattered areas of ground-glass opacities and nodules
  - Atoll sign (a.k.a. reverse halo sign): Central ground-glass opacity surrounded by rim of consolidation

- Perilobular opacities: Ill-defined opacities outlining interlobular septa of secondary pulmonary lobule
- Opacities may wax and wane
- Waxing and waning pulmonary opacities in breast cancer following radiation therapy
  - Not isolated to irradiated portion of lungs

- **Cystic Fibrosis**
  - Diffuse, upper lung preponderant bronchiectasis and bronchial wall thickening
  - Mucus plugging in airways: Centrilobular or tree in bud opacities
  - Air-trapping or mosaic lung attenuation
  - Hyperinflation
  - Recurrent areas of consolidation: Pneumonia or atelectasis distal to secretions in airways
  - Fatty atrophy of pancreas in combination with above findings highly suggestive
- **Allergic Bronchopulmonary Aspergillosis**
  - Occurs in patients with cystic fibrosis and asthma
  - Central bronchiectasis in multiple lobes; often severe (cystic or varicoid)
  - Mucus-filled bronchi; may have gas-fluid levels
  - Centrilobular nodules
  - Fleeting pulmonary opacities and atelectasis
- **Eosinophilic Pneumonia**
  - Simple eosinophilic pneumonia
    - Usually asymptomatic
    - Patchy mid and upper lung consolidation
    - Migratory; changes rapidly; spontaneous regression
  - Chronic eosinophilic pneumonia
    - Photographic negative of pulmonary edema: Upper and peripheral preponderant consolidation
    - May shift in distribution
    - Most peripheral portions resolve 1st in response to steroids
    - Tendency to recur in same locations

Helpful Clues for Rare Diagnoses

- **Pulmonary Vasculitis**
  - Diffuse alveolar hemorrhage
    - Ground-glass opacities > consolidation; may be diffuse, patchy, lobular, or centrilobular
    - Tendency to spare peripheral, apical, and costophrenic aspects of lungs
    - Increased interlobular and intralobular septal thickening over 1-2 days
    - Resolution in days; not as rapid as in cardiogenic pulmonary edema or bland aspiration
  - Large, medium, and small vessel vasculitides
    - Takayasu arteritis, Behçet disease, Churg-Strauss syndrome, microscopic polyangiitis, Goodpasture disease, Wegener granulomatosis

Asthma

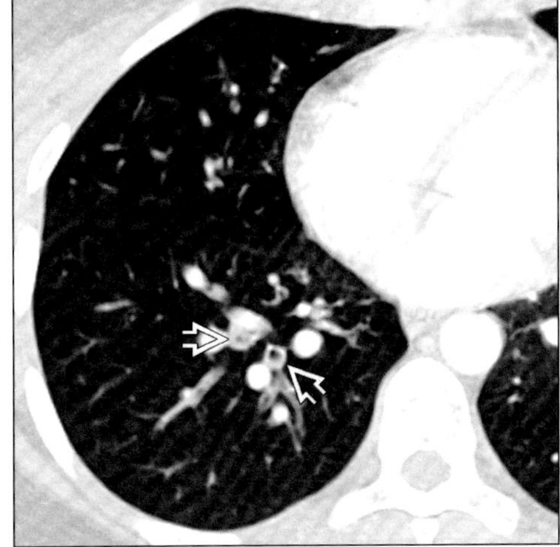

Axial CECT shows mucus plugs ➡ and narrowing of segmental and subsegmental airways, consistent with acute exacerbation of asthma.

Recurrent Aspiration

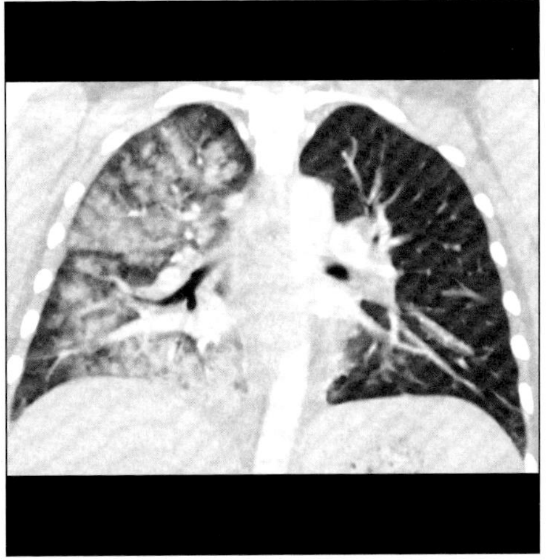

Coronal CECT shows right lung preponderant centrilobular opacities from massive aspiration after seizure while laying on right side. Opacities resolved rapidly, consistent with bland aspiration.

MIGRATORY DISTRIBUTION

*(**Left**) Frontal radiograph shows dense left lower lobe opacity ➡ and a small left pleural effusion. (**Right**) Coronal CECT in the same patient shows partial left lower lobe opacification ➡ and inferior displacement of the left major fissure ➡, consistent with partial left lower lobe atelectasis. Subtle ground-glass opacities ➡ in the contralateral lung are most consistent with aspiration in this trauma patient. Note right major fissure ➡.*

Atelectasis

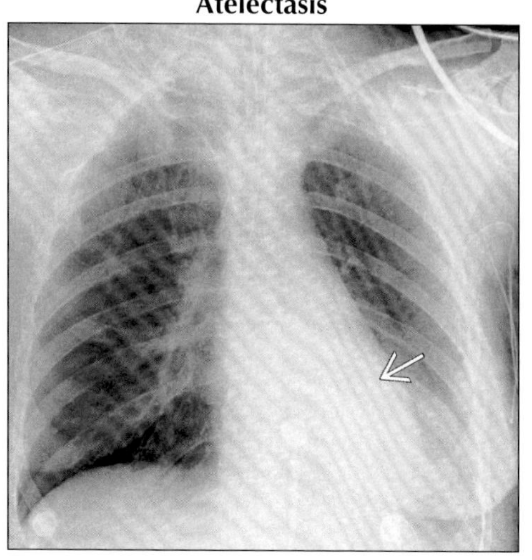

Atelectasis

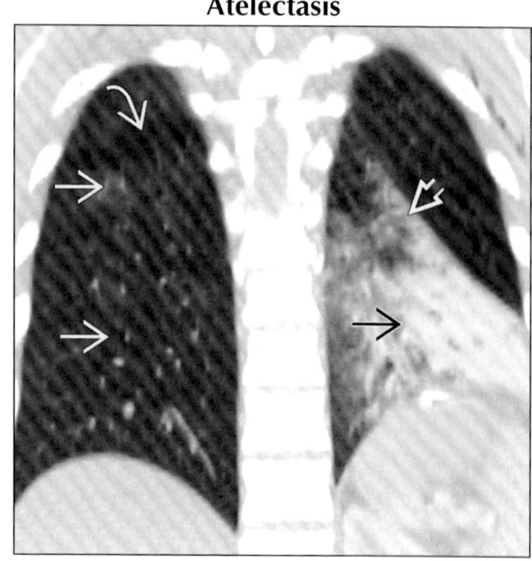

*(**Left**) Coronal CECT MIP image shows an acute pulmonary embolus ➡ in a right lower lobe pulmonary artery and subpleural mixed ground-glass opacity and consolidation ➡ with central lucencies, suggestive of pulmonary infarct. (**Right**) Axial NECT shows bilateral peripheral pulmonary nodules ➡ (some of which are cavitary), highly suggestive of septic emboli in this patient with sepsis. Bilateral pleural effusions are worrisome for parapneumonic effusions.*

Pulmonary Infarct

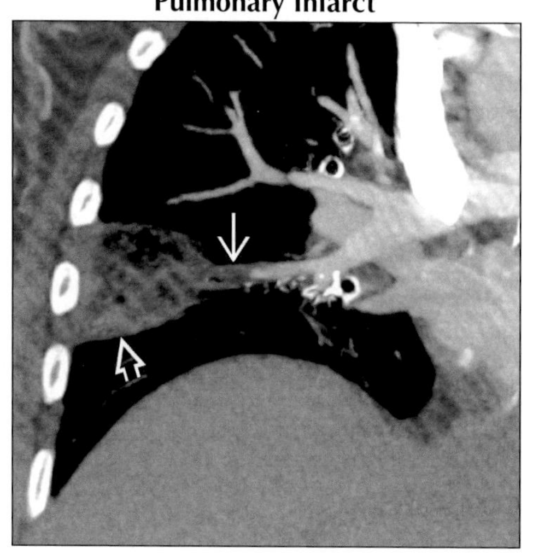

Septic Emboli

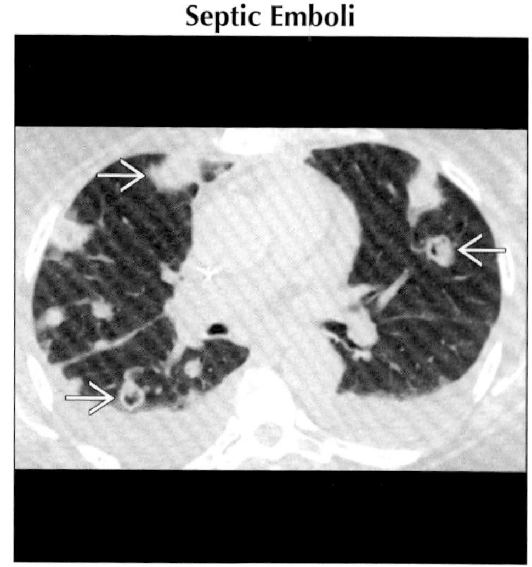

*(**Left**) Axial HRCT shows multifocal areas of consolidation centered on bronchi with peripheral ground-glass opacities ➡ in this patient with organizing pneumonia. These findings can be quite nonspecific. (**Right**) Axial NECT shows bilateral peripheral ➡ and peribronchial ➡ consolidation, consistent with organizing pneumonia. There is a suggestion of the reverse halo sign ➡ in the left lung.*

Organizing Pneumonia

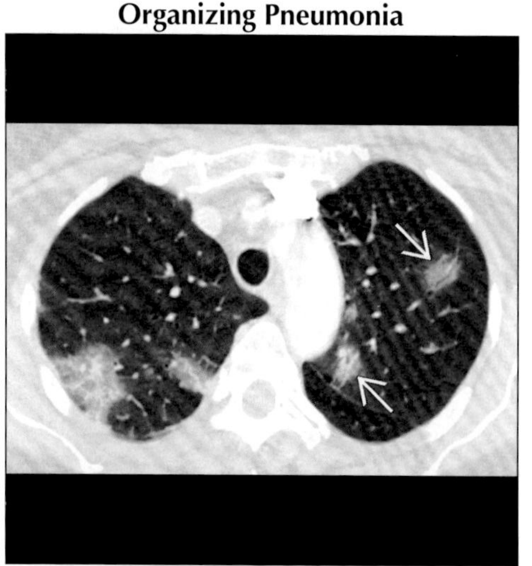

Organizing Pneumonia

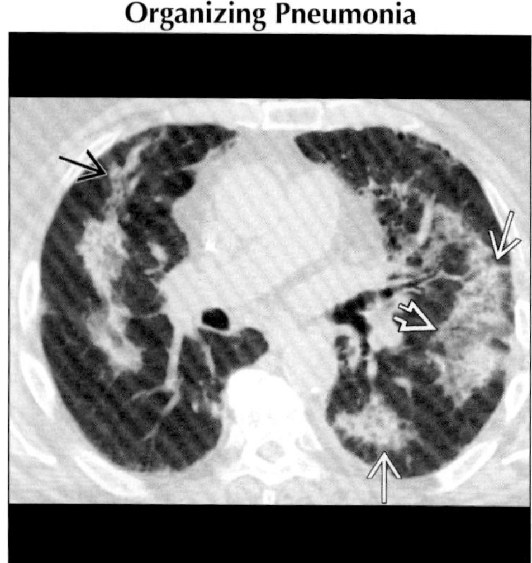

MIGRATORY DISTRIBUTION

Cystic Fibrosis

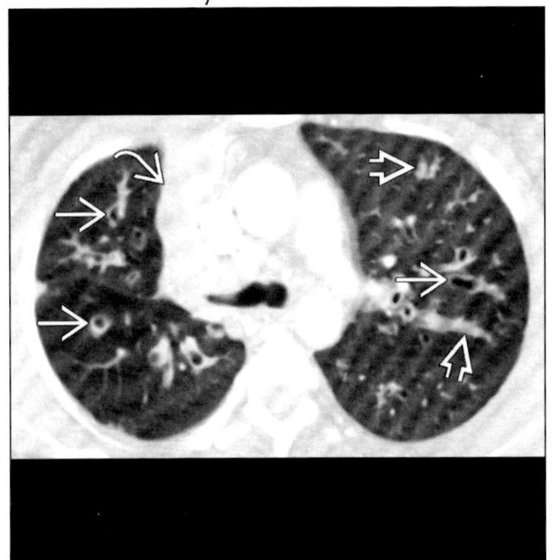

Cystic Fibrosis

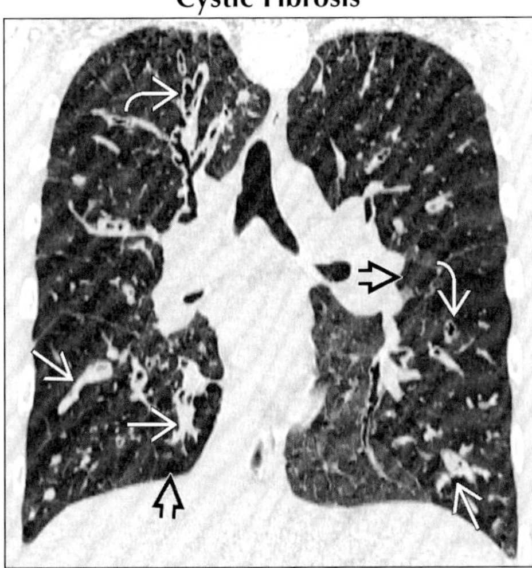

(Left) *Axial CECT shows bilateral bronchiectasis ➡, mucus plugging ➡, and right upper lobe collapse ➡. Right upper lobe collapse from proximal mucus plugging resolved with aggressive respiratory therapy.* ***(Right)*** *Coronal HRCT shows patchy bronchiectasis ➡ and mosaic attenuation ⇨. Mucus plugging ➡ is present in the lower lobes. Mucus plugging often shifts rapidly in patients with cystic fibrosis.*

Allergic Bronchopulmonary Aspergillosis

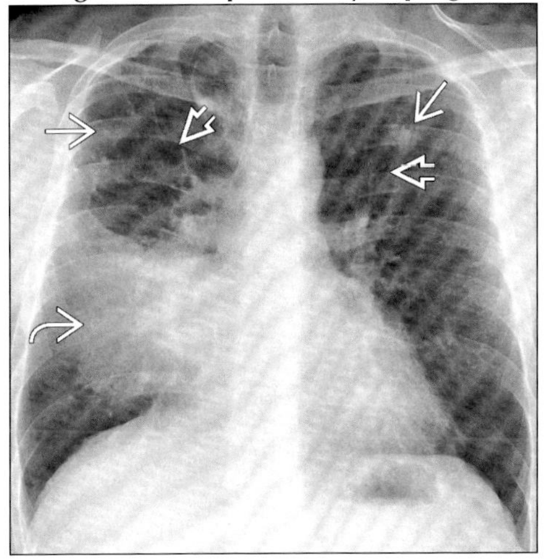

Allergic Bronchopulmonary Aspergillosis

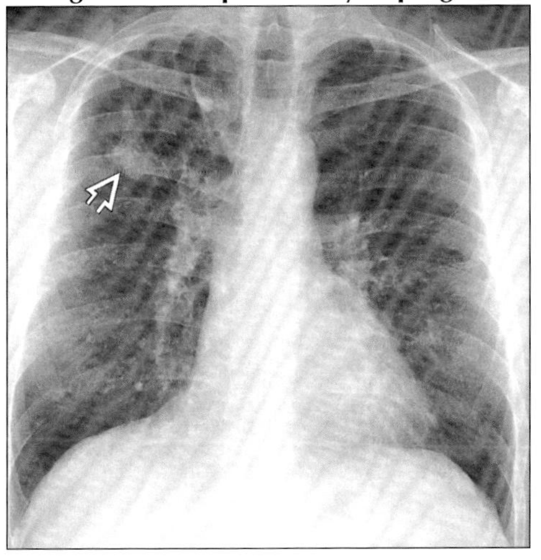

(Left) *Frontal radiograph shows right middle lobe consolidation ➡ (which silhouettes the right heart border), nodular upper lung opacities ➡, and central preponderant bronchiectasis ➡.* ***(Right)*** *Frontal radiograph 2 weeks after the previous chest radiograph shows resolution of the right middle lobe and upper lung opacities with development of mucoid impaction ➡ in a bronchiectatic right upper lobe bronchus.*

Eosinophilic Pneumonia

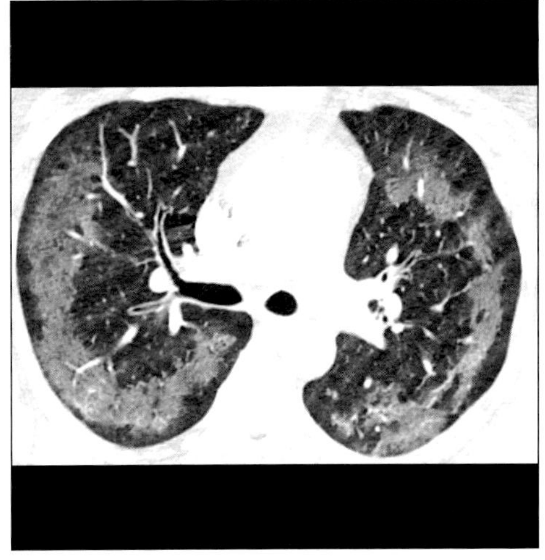

Pulmonary Vasculitis

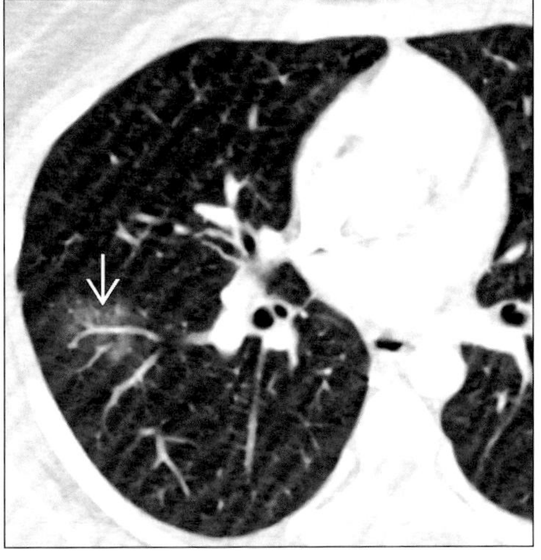

(Left) *Axial CECT shows diffuse peripheral ground-glass opacities with subpleural sparing, consistent with chronic eosinophilic pneumonia. Subpleural sparing is typical of healing chronic eosinophilic pneumonia. Nonspecific interstitial pneumonitis and organizing pneumonia may also demonstrate peripheral sparing.* ***(Right)*** *Axial CECT shows ground-glass opacity ➡ centered on a pulmonary vessel, a typical pattern for pulmonary vasculitis.*

SOLITARY PULMONARY NODULE

DIFFERENTIAL DIAGNOSIS

Common
- Granuloma
- Lung Cancer
- Intrapulmonary Lymph Node

Less Common
- Carcinoid
- Solitary Metastasis
- Nodule Mimics (Pseudonodules)
  - Nipple
  - Skeletal Lesions
- Infectious/Inflammatory Process

Rare but Important
- Hamartoma
- Pulmonary Arteriovenous Malformation

ESSENTIAL INFORMATION

Key Differential Diagnosis Issues
- Solitary pulmonary nodule (SPN): Single, focal-rounded, or ovoid opacity ≤ 3 cm
- SPN detection
  - Radiography
    - SPN found in up to 2% of chest radiographs
    - SPNs measuring < 9 mm are likely calcified granulomas
    - Dual energy or tomosynthesis are promising techniques to increase sensitivity for detecting SPNs
  - CT: Superior detection/characterization
    - Multiplanar reconstructions, maximum intensity projections (MIPs) increase confidence
- Risk factors for malignancy in SPN
  - Exposure to cigarette smoke or other carcinogens
  - History of malignancy (pulmonary or extrapulmonary)
  - History of pulmonary fibrosis
  - Age > 40 years
- SPN imaging assessment
  - Characterization
    - Benign SPN: No follow-up required
    - Indeterminate SPN: Imaging follow-up to document growth or stability
    - Possibly malignant SPN: Further imaging assessment ± biopsy

Helpful Clues for Common Diagnoses
- **Granuloma**
  - Solid, rounded SPN, stable in size
  - Satellite nodules
  - Benign patterns of calcification include solid, laminar, or concentric
    - Complete or diffuse (pitfall, metastatic osteosarcoma)
    - Central, > 10% of SPN cross section (pitfall, calcified carcinoid tumor)
  - Most common: Histoplasmosis, tuberculosis, coccidioidomycosis
- **Lung Cancer**
  - Upper lobes most common, but peripheral and basilar in patients with preexisting pulmonary fibrosis
  - Increased risk of cancer in nodules > 1 cm
  - Doubling times typically between 1-18 months; average: 100 days
  - Irregular, spiculated, or lobular borders
  - Calcification in 13%, usually eccentric, stippled
- **Intrapulmonary Lymph Node**
  - Common normal finding on multidetector CT
  - Elongate morphology, fissural location; typically located within 20 mm of pleura

Helpful Clues for Less Common Diagnoses
- **Carcinoid**
  - Well-defined lobular borders
  - Contrast enhancement, vascularity
  - Multifocal or coarse calcification
    - Calcification more common with lesions adjacent to central airways
- **Solitary Metastasis**
  - Typically from sarcomas, melanomas, testicular cancers
  - Peripheral location
- **Nodule Mimics (Pseudonodules)**
  - **Nipple**
    - Bilaterally symmetric rounded opacities, mid to inferior hemithorax, midaxillary line
  - **Skeletal Lesions**
    - 1st costochondral junction: Contiguity with anterior 1st rib; often asymmetric
    - Rib fracture callus, bone island: CT, tomosynthesis, or shallow oblique radiography to determine location
- **Infectious/Inflammatory Process**
  - Air bronchograms

- More likely in younger patients (< 40 yrs)
- Rapid changes in size

Helpful Clues for Rare Diagnoses

- **Hamartoma**
  - Slow growing with well-defined lobular or notched borders
  - Fat (33%) or popcorn calcification (25%) in 50% (pitfall, metastatic chondrosarcoma)
  - If multiple, consider Carney triad or Cowden syndrome
- **Pulmonary Arteriovenous Malformation**
  - Peripheral lower lobe location
  - Typically 1-5 cm in diameter, with feeding and draining vessel(s)
  - Vascular enhancement
  - Single in 2/3; when multiple, usually 2-8

Alternative Differential Approaches

- SPN features
  - Size: 90% of nodules < 2 cm are benign
  - Growth pattern
    - 2-year stability implies benignity, but rare indolent lung cancers occur, especially in screening studies
    - Doubling time < 30 days or > 465 days favors benignity
  - Morphology and border characteristics
    - Spiculation: Highly suggestive of malignancy
    - Pleural tags in 60-80% of peripheral lung cancers
    - Lobulation (histologic heterogeneity) seen in 40% of malignant nodules
    - Round, more characteristic of benign lesions
  - Attenuation
    - Solid (soft tissue): Most lung cancers but less likely malignant than part-solid or nonsolid SPNs
    - Part-solid (soft tissue and ground-glass): 40-50% of part-solid SPNs < 1.5 cm are malignant; risk increases with size
    - Nonsolid (ground-glass): 34% are malignant; particularly if > 1.5 cm
    - Air bronchograms/bronchiolograms more common in malignant SPNs
    - Cavitation: Irregular walls > 16 mm thick suggest malignancy
    - Fat seen with hamartomas and lipomas
    - Benign patterns of calcification include solid, laminar, concentric, popcorn
  - Enhancement on dynamic CT
    - Enhancement < 15 HU strongly indicative of benignity
    - Enhancement > 15 HU sensitive but not specific for malignancy
  - Metabolic activity: F18 PET
    - 90% likelihood of malignancy for PET-positive SPNs in patients > 60 years
    - False-negatives: Indolent and low-grade malignancies (carcinoid, bronchioalveolar cell carcinoma) and malignant SPNs < 1 cm
    - False-positives: Infectious/inflammatory SPNs

Granuloma

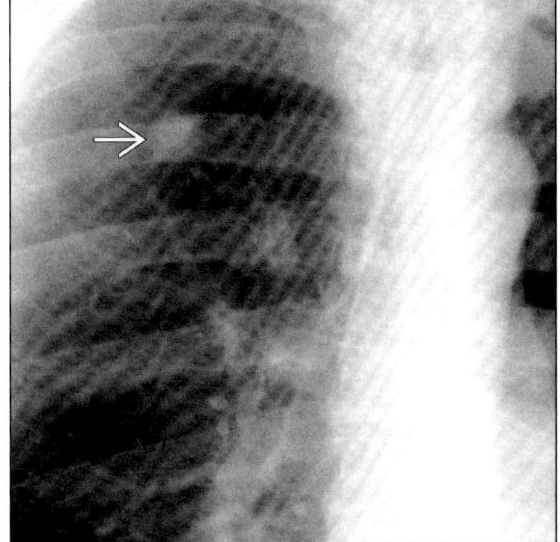

Frontal radiograph shows a right upper lobe ovoid nodule ➡ with intrinsic central calcification that occupies the majority of the visualized SPN area.

Granuloma

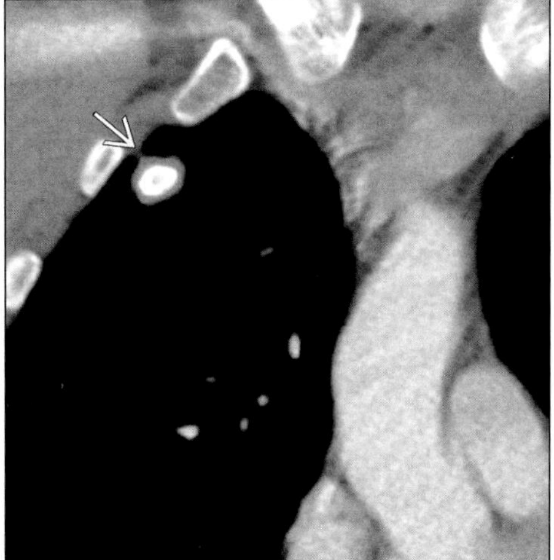

Coronal CECT (soft tissue window) confirms dense laminar calcification within the nodule, surrounded by a thin soft tissue rim and a small pleural tag ➡. The findings are diagnostic of granuloma.

SOLITARY PULMONARY NODULE

*(**Left**) Axial NECT (soft tissue window) shows a completely calcified solitary nodule ➔. Bone window image demonstrates the concentric or laminar nature of the calcification ➔. (**Right**) Axial NECT (soft tissue window) shows laminar calcification in a right lower lobe SPN ➔. The left lower lobe SPN displays central high attenuation rounded calcification ➔. The CT findings are diagnostic of granuloma.*

Granuloma

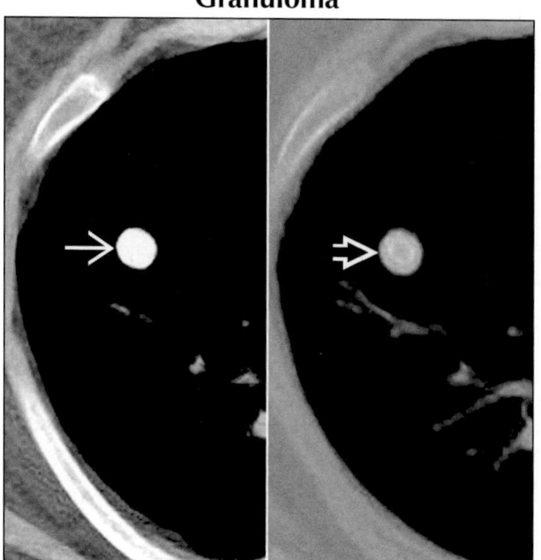

Granuloma

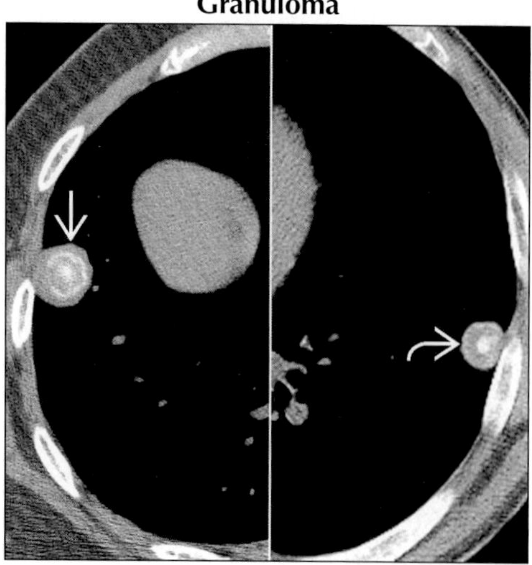

*(**Left**) Coronal CECT (lung window) shows a solid right upper lobe SPN with spiculated borders and a pleural tag ➔. Note the mild upper lobe predominant centrilobular emphysema. The SPN morphology is characteristic of lung cancer. (**Right**) Axial CECT (lung window) shows a left upper lobe part-solid SPN with predominant ground-glass opacity and intrinsic small nodular soft tissue ➔ components. The CT features are highly suspicious for lung cancer.*

Lung Cancer

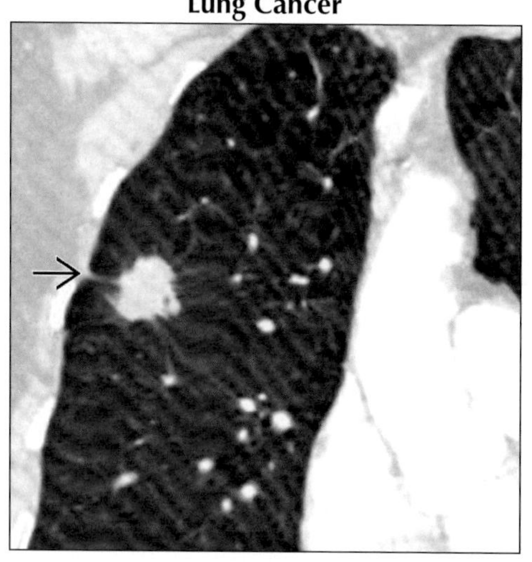

Lung Cancer

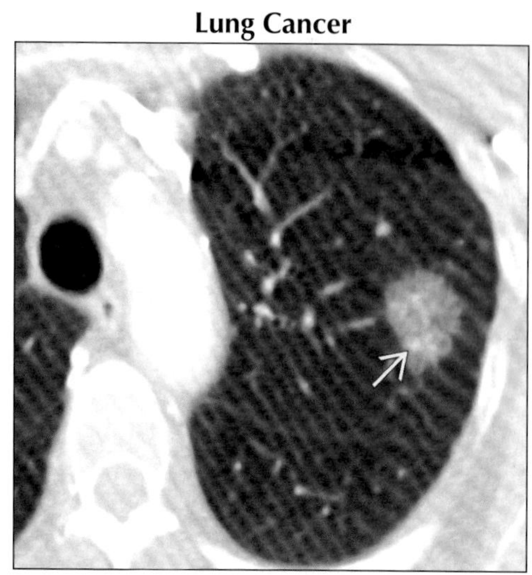

*(**Left**) Axial NECT (lung window) shows nonsolid or ground-glass SPN in left upper lobe. Underlying pulmonary architecture and normal anatomic structures are visible in nodule. Lesion represented bronchioloalveolar carcinoma. (**Right**) Axial CECT (lung window) shows a tiny SPN near minor fissure ➔. HRCT through SPN ➔ shows triangular morphology and orientation along fissure, characteristic of intrapulmonary lymphoid tissue.*

Lung Cancer

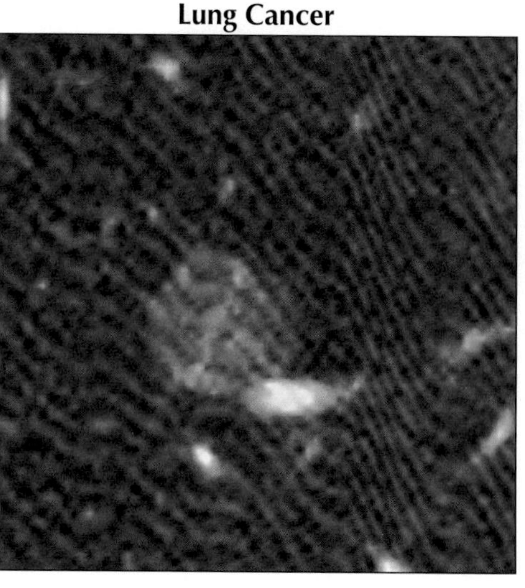

Intrapulmonary Lymph Node

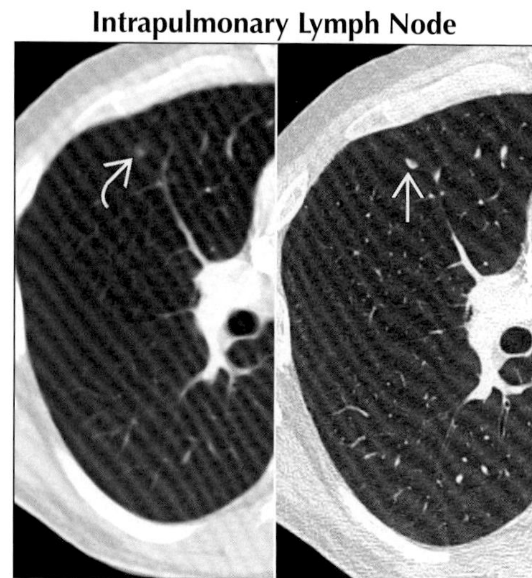

SOLITARY PULMONARY NODULE

Carcinoid

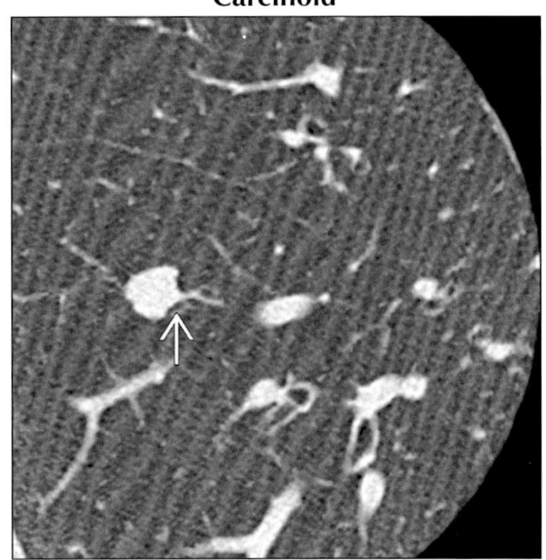

Solitary Metastasis

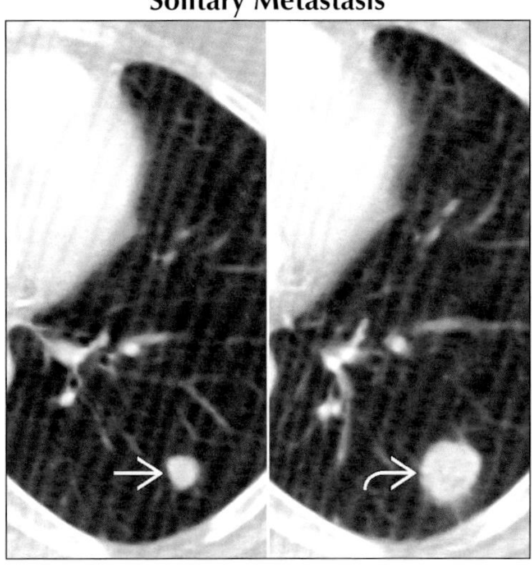

(Left) *Axial HRCT (lung window) shows a small pulmonary nodule with well-defined lobular margins. The nodule is intimately related to adjacent airways ➔, characteristic of carcinoid tumor.* ***(Right)*** *Axial CECT (lung window) shows a left lower lobe SPN ➔. Axial CECT 3 months later shows interval growth of the SPN, new spiculated borders ➔, and at least 1 pleural tag. Although this lesion was a solitary metastasis, primary lung cancer cannot be excluded.*

Nodule Mimics (Pseudonodules)

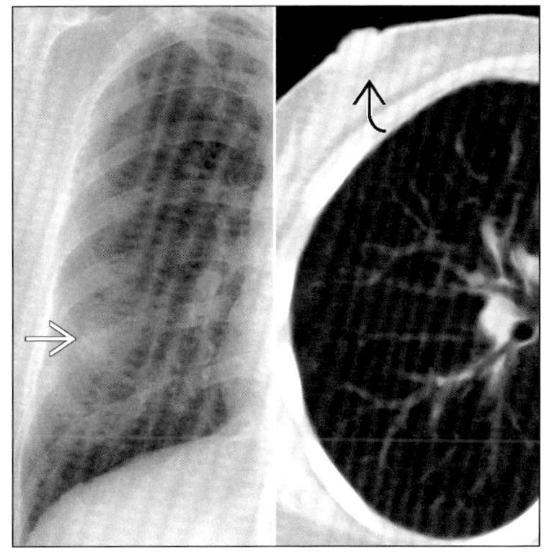

Skeletal Lesions

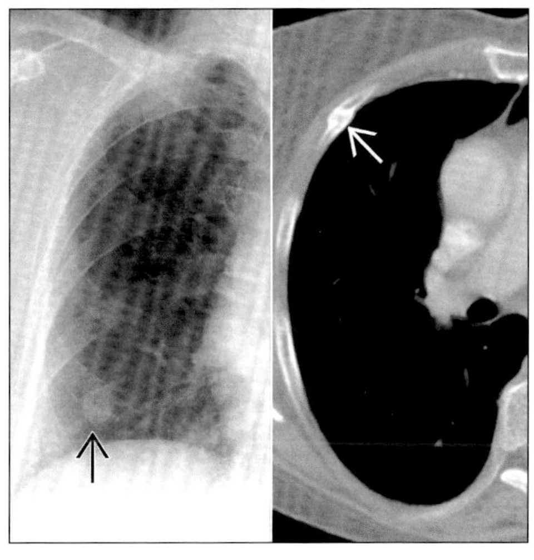

(Left) *Frontal radiograph shows a nodular opacity ➔ with a sharp outer margin and an indistinct inner margin. These features are characteristic of a nipple shadow ➔, confirmed on CT.* ***(Right)*** *Frontal radiograph shows a nodular opacity ➔ projecting over the inferior aspect of the right anterior 4th rib. The lesion corresponds to a minimally displaced healed rib fracture ➔ on axial CECT (bone window).*

Hamartoma

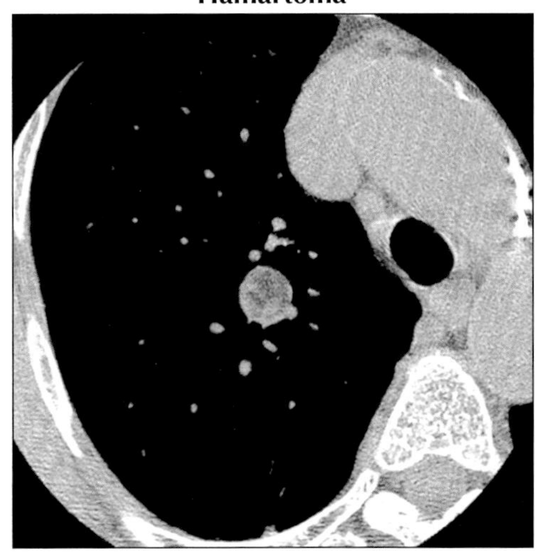

Pulmonary Arteriovenous Malformation

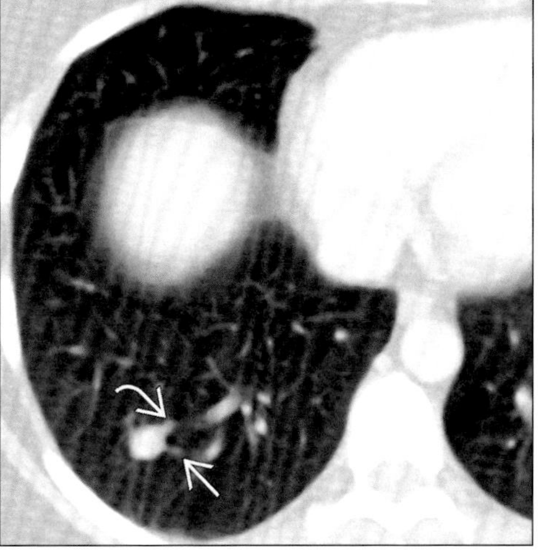

(Left) *Axial NECT (soft tissue window) shows a right upper lobe SPN with well-defined borders and intrinsic fat and soft tissue attenuation. The CT features are diagnostic of pulmonary hamartoma.* ***(Right)*** *Axial CECT shows a right lower lobe enhancing nodule with 2 associated tubular opacities that represent a feeding artery ➔ and a draining vein ➔. The CT findings are diagnostic of pulmonary arteriovenous malformation.*

MULTIPLE WELL-DEFINED NODULES

DIFFERENTIAL DIAGNOSIS

Common
- Metastasis
- Granulomatous Infection
- Septic Emboli
- Wegener Granulomatosis

Less Common
- Pulmonary Langerhans Cell Histiocytosis
- Varicella Pneumonia
- Sarcoidosis
- Lymphoma

Rare but Important
- Rheumatoid Nodules

ESSENTIAL INFORMATION

Key Differential Diagnosis Issues
- Nodules of variable size indicate lesions growing at different rates (metastasis) or are temporally heterogeneous (septic emboli)
- Cavitary nodules indicate metastasis, septic emboli, or Wegener granulomatosis
- Calcified nodules indicate healed varicella or sequela of histoplasmosis or TB

Helpful Clues for Common Diagnoses
- **Metastasis**
  - Nodules of varying size
  - Known primary
- **Granulomatous Infection**
  - Histoplasmosis: Calcified nodules, splenic granulomas
  - Coccidioidomycosis and cryptococcosis: Noncalcified nodules
  - Tuberculosis: Travel history; history of recent immigration
- **Septic Emboli**
  - Nodules may evolve into cavitary nodules and could be temporally heterogeneous
- **Wegener Granulomatosis**
  - Tracheal involvement with diffuse wall thickening in addition to lung nodules
  - C-ANCA positive
  - Renal and paranasal sinus involvement

Helpful Clues for Less Common Diagnoses
- **Pulmonary Langerhans Cell Histiocytosis**
  - Almost always in cigarette smokers
  - Combination of nodules and irregular lung cysts with upper lung predominance
- **Varicella Pneumonia**
  - Multiple small, randomly distributed, calcified nodules
- **Sarcoidosis**
  - Presence of enlarged calcified or noncalcified mediastinal and hilar lymph nodes
- **Lymphoma**
  - Associated mediastinal lymphadenopathy
  - Risk factors such as Sjögren syndrome, immunosuppression, solid organ transplantation

Helpful Clues for Rare Diagnoses
- **Rheumatoid Nodules**
  - History of rheumatoid arthritis

Metastasis

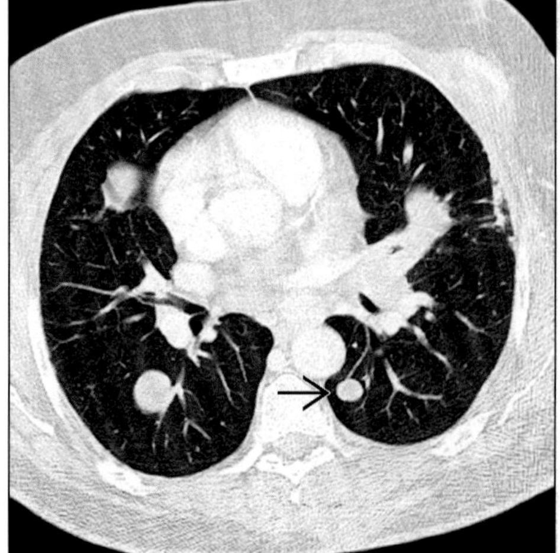

Axial CECT shows multiple lung nodules ⇨ indicating metastasis from a primary melanoma malignancy. Nodules of varying size favor this diagnosis.

Granulomatous Infection

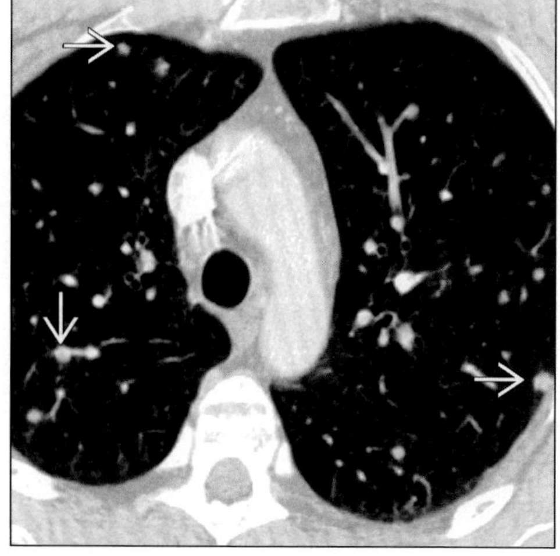

Axial CECT shows multiple random nodules ➡ from histoplasmosis. Presence of microabscesses (active) or calcified foci (old) in the spleen are helpful clues.

MULTIPLE WELL-DEFINED NODULES

Granulomatous Infection

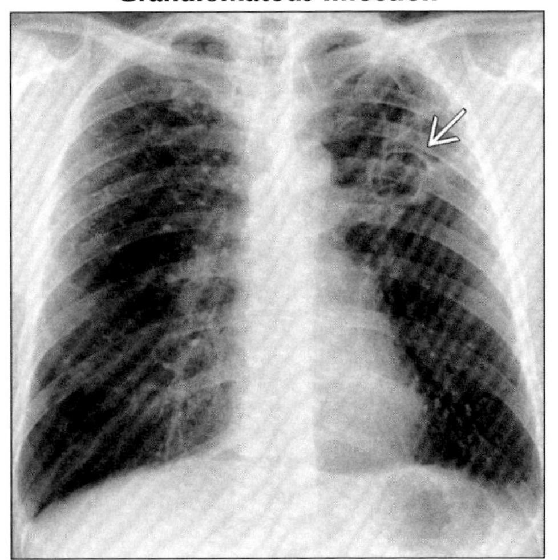

Septic Emboli

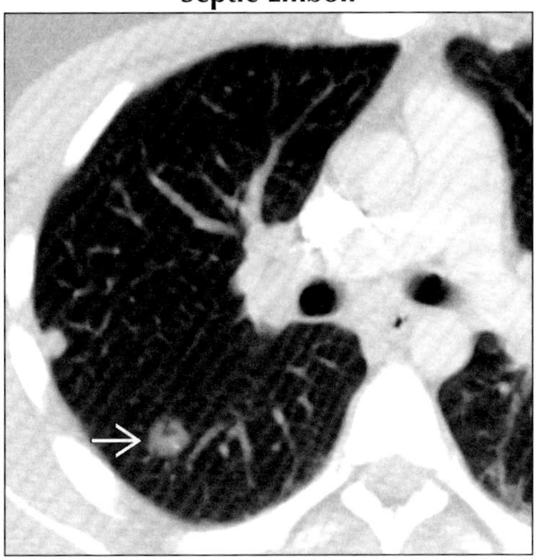

(Left) *Frontal radiograph from a patient with tuberculosis shows multiple calcified nodules scattered in the lungs bilaterally. In addition, there are thin-walled cavities in the left upper lobe ➡.* ***(Right)*** *Axial CECT shows 2 peripheral pulmonary nodules with 1 showing cavitation ➡ from septic emboli. There were several other nodules (not shown) in various stages of cavitation.*

Wegener Granulomatosis

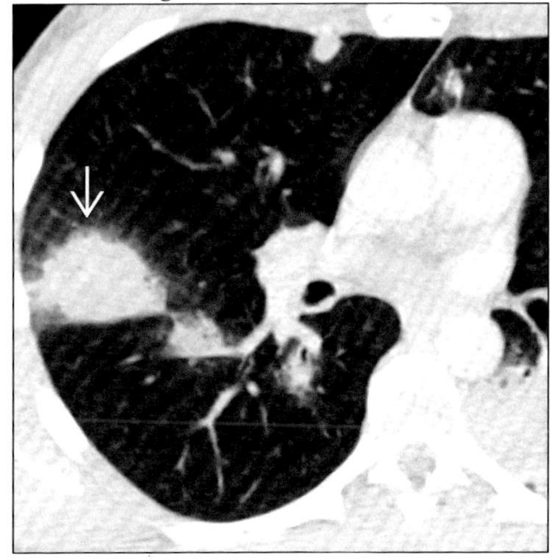

Pulmonary Langerhans Cell Histiocytosis

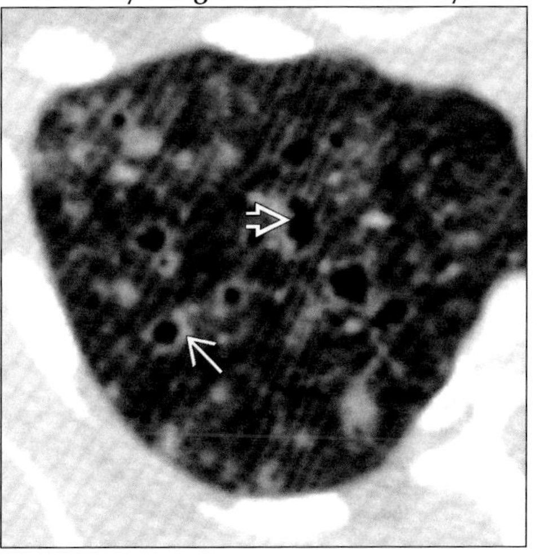

(Left) *Axial CECT in this young man shows multiple nodules and masses of varying sizes with some showing surrounding halo ➡. C-ANCA was strongly positive.* ***(Right)*** *Axial NECT shows typical CT features of nodules and cysts in the upper lobes (right upper lobe shown here). Cysts are initially regular ➡ and later may evolve to be irregularly ➡ shaped.*

Lymphoma

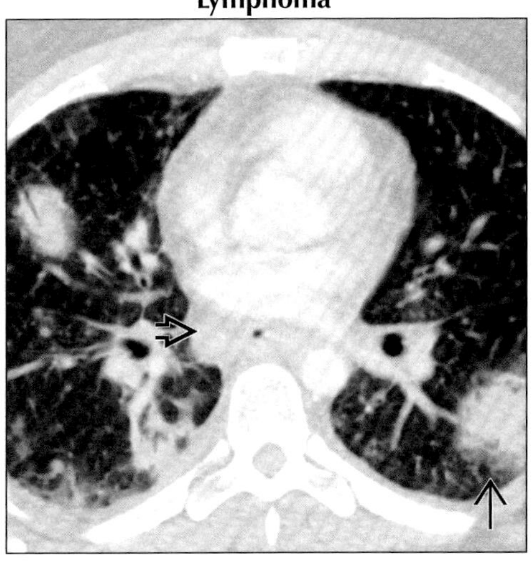

Rheumatoid Nodules

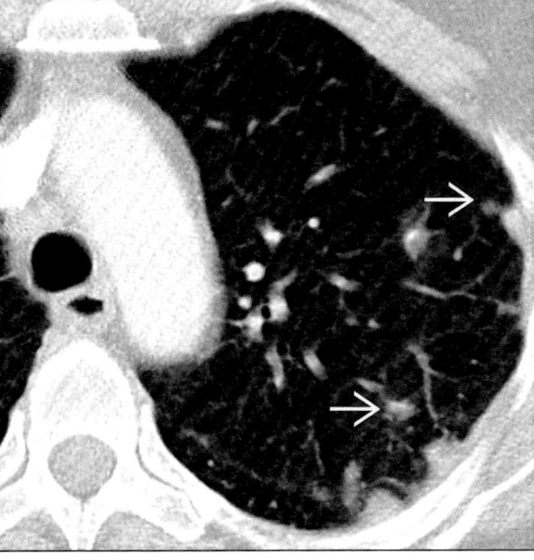

(Left) *Axial CECT shows typical CT features of nodular/mass-like consolidation ➡ and generalized mediastinal adenopathy ➡ from non-Hodgkin lymphoma.* ***(Right)*** *Axial CECT shows multiple, mostly peripheral pulmonary nodules ➡. There are no specific characteristics that distinguish rheumatoid nodules from nodules of other causes, except for the clinical history of rheumatoid arthritis.*

MULTIPLE ILL-DEFINED NODULES

DIFFERENTIAL DIAGNOSIS

Common

- Pneumonia
  - Mycobacterial
  - Fungal
  - Bacterial
- Metastases (Typically Hemorrhagic)
- Bronchoalveolar Cell Carcinoma
- Septic Emboli
- Hypersensitivity Pneumonitis

Less Common

- Wegener Granulomatosis
- Silicosis/Coal Worker's Pneumoconiosis
- Pulmonary Langerhans Cell Histiocytosis
- Pulmonary Infarcts
- Kaposi Sarcoma
- Sarcoidosis (Alveolar Type)

Rare but Important

- Rheumatoid Nodules
- Lymphoma

ESSENTIAL INFORMATION

Key Differential Diagnosis Issues

- Clinical correlation paramount given large overlap of imaging manifestations

Helpful Clues for Common Diagnoses

- **Pneumonia**
  - Acute clinical presentation in most cases: Fever, chills, malaise
  - Mycobacterial or fungal pneumonia may be indolent
  - Angioinvasive fungal pneumonia in immunosuppressed patients, often with neutropenia
  - Reactive lymphadenopathy common
  - Cavitary lung nodules and central low-attenuation lymphadenopathy: Tuberculous or fungal pneumonia
- **Metastases (Typically Hemorrhagic)**
  - Variable-sized pulmonary nodules preferentially in peripheral and lower lungs
  - Ill-defined metastases on radiographs usually hemorrhagic
    - Choriocarcinoma, renal cell carcinoma, melanoma
  - CT often shows solid central nodule surrounded by halo of ground-glass opacity
  - Feeding artery sign: Pulmonary artery branches extend to nodules, implying hematogenous spread
- **Bronchoalveolar Cell Carcinoma**
  - Subtype of adenocarcinoma with good prognosis relative to other types of lung cancer
  - Focal or multifocal ground-glass, mixed, or solid pulmonary nodules
    - Internal air bronchograms, cystic lucencies, or pseudocavitation
  - Chronic consolidation or ground-glass opacity, which mimics pneumonia; may be multifocal
- **Septic Emboli**
  - Multiple, peripheral, and basilar consolidation or nodules with early cavitation
  - Feeding artery sign: Pulmonary artery branches extend to nodules, implying hematogenous spread
  - Loculated pleural effusion common
- **Hypersensitivity Pneumonitis**
  - Allergic reaction to inhaled organic dust or chemicals
  - Geographic or centrilobular ground-glass opacities in all patients; air-trapping common
  - "Head-cheese" sign: Geographic regions of air-trapping, ground-glass opacities, and normal lung

Helpful Clues for Less Common Diagnoses

- **Wegener Granulomatosis**
  - Multiple bilateral nodules that can coalesce into masses; may cavitate
  - Associated with upper airway and renal abnormalities
  - Halo sign: Ground-glass opacities surrounding nodules/masses
  - Large airway stenosis: Most often subglottic trachea
- **Silicosis/Coal Worker's Pneumoconiosis**
  - Small, upper lobe preponderant centrilobular and perilymphatic nodules with appropriate exposure history
  - Progressive massive fibrosis: Small nodules coalesce into elliptical upper lobe masses with adjacent emphysema

- Superimposed mediastinal and hilar lymphadenopathy; ± eggshell calcification
- **Pulmonary Langerhans Cell Histiocytosis**
  - Multiple upper and mid lung subcentimeter pulmonary nodules in smoker
    - Typically centrilobular, ill defined, spares costophrenic angles
  - Multiple cysts; thin or thick walled; may be bizarre in shape
  - Other concomitant smoking-related conditions
    - Centrilobular emphysema, respiratory bronchiolitis, lung cancer, desquamative interstitial pneumonitis
- **Pulmonary Infarcts**
  - Most often from pulmonary arterial embolism
  - Often in setting of superimposed cardiac dysfunction (cardiomyopathy, congestive heart failure)
  - Lower lung predominant, peripheral/subpleural, wedge-shaped consolidation
  - Reverse halo configuration (central ground-glass opacity with surrounding rim of consolidation) not uncommon
  - Resolves over months, retaining its original shape, rather than patchy resolution as in pneumonia
- **Kaposi Sarcoma**
  - Peribronchovascular or perihilar, ill-defined, flame-shaped consolidation or nodules in patients with AIDS
  - Vast majority with pulmonary disease have cutaneous involvement
  - Mediastinal and hilar lymphadenopathy with avid contrast enhancement
- **Sarcoidosis (Alveolar Type)**
  - Symmetric hilar and mediastinal lymphadenopathy; ± calcification
  - Perilymphatic nodules; interlobular septal thickening
  - Nodules may coalesce into focal nodular consolidation or foci of ground-glass opacity
    - Galaxy sign: Fine nodular opacities present along margins of focal consolidation or ground-glass opacity

Helpful Clues for Rare Diagnoses

- **Rheumatoid Nodules**
  - Rare manifestation of rheumatoid arthritis; nodules may cavitate
  - Pleural effusion or thickening most common thoracic manifestation of rheumatoid arthritis
  - Interstitial lung disease in up to 40% of patients (UIP, NSIP, or OP)
- **Lymphoma**
  - Multiple ill-defined nodules that may cavitate
  - May occur in association with nodal disease or primarily in lungs

Pneumonia

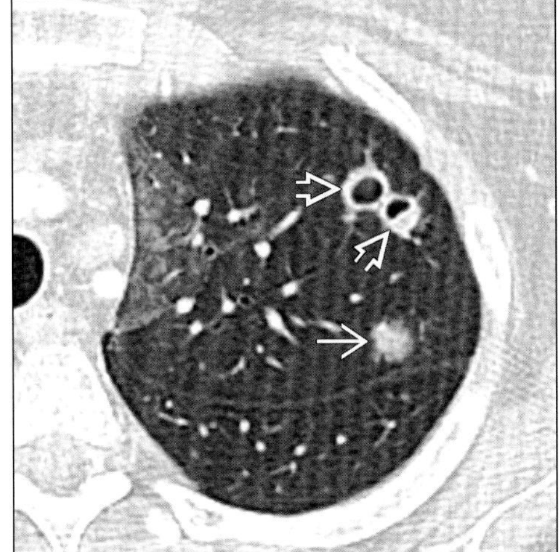

Axial CECT shows cavitary ➔ and ground-glass ➔ nodules in the left upper lobe; a focal region of ground-glass opacity is also present medially in this patient with invasive aspergillosis.

Metastases (Typically Hemorrhagic)

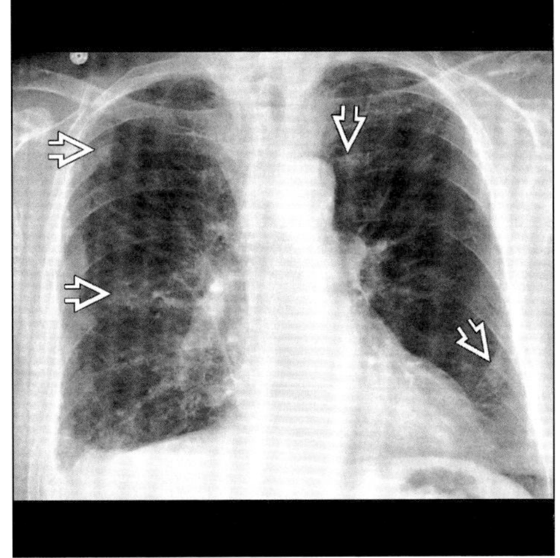

Frontal radiograph shows bilateral ill-defined nodules ➔ in this patient with a history of renal cell carcinoma.

MULTIPLE ILL-DEFINED NODULES

*(**Left**) Axial CECT shows peripheral pulmonary nodules ➔ with poorly marginated borders, consistent with metastases from renal cell carcinoma. There is a small right pleural effusion. (**Right**) Coronal CECT shows poorly marginated, mixed density nodules in the right apex representing bronchoalveolar carcinoma. An air bronchogram ➔ is present in one of the nodules. Presumed focal adenomatous hyperplasia ➔ is present in the left apex.*

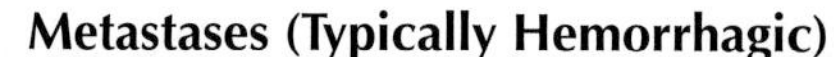

Metastases (Typically Hemorrhagic)

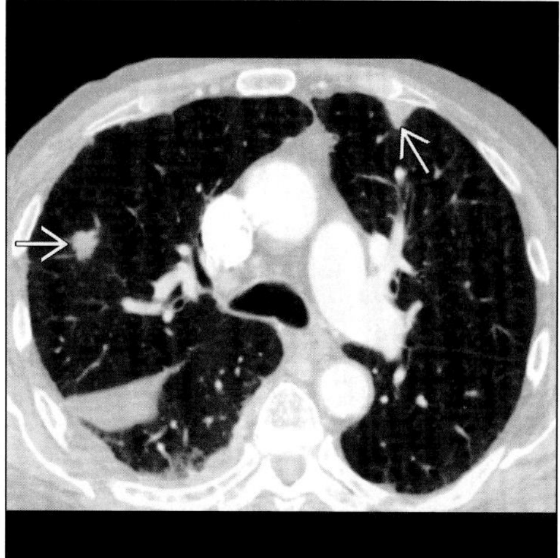

Bronchoalveolar Cell Carcinoma

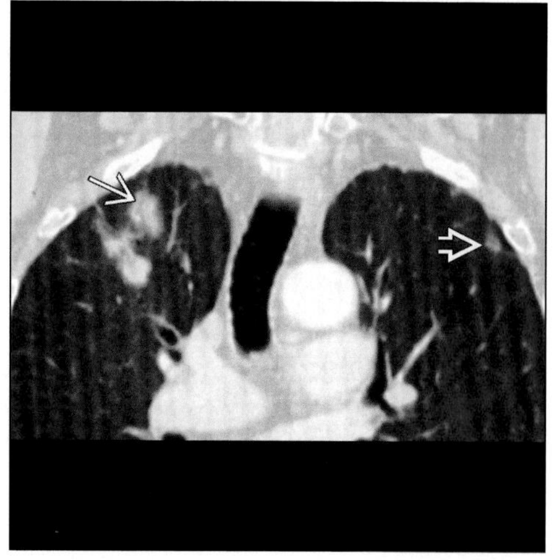

*(**Left**) Coronal NECT shows bilateral peripheral nodules → with cavitation ➔ in a left upper lobe nodule in this patient with bacteremia. There are also bilateral pleural effusions & left lower lobe atelectasis. (**Right**) Axial NECT minIP image shows innumerable bilateral centrilobular ground-glass pulmonary nodules, highly suggestive of hypersensitivity pneumonitis in this nonsmoking bird owner. In a patient with smoking history, respiratory bronchiolitis should be considered.*

Septic Emboli

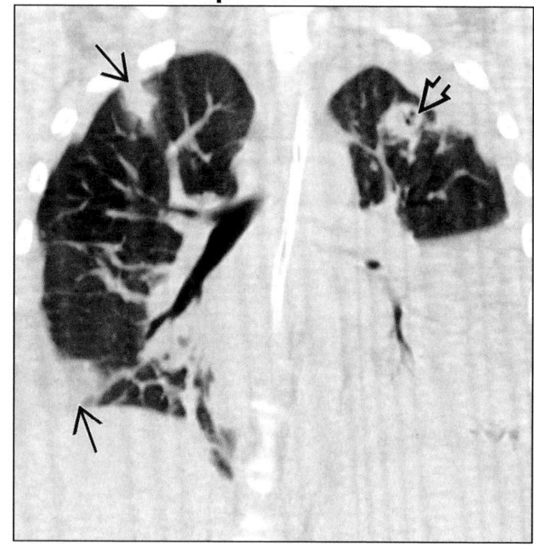

Hypersensitivity Pneumonitis

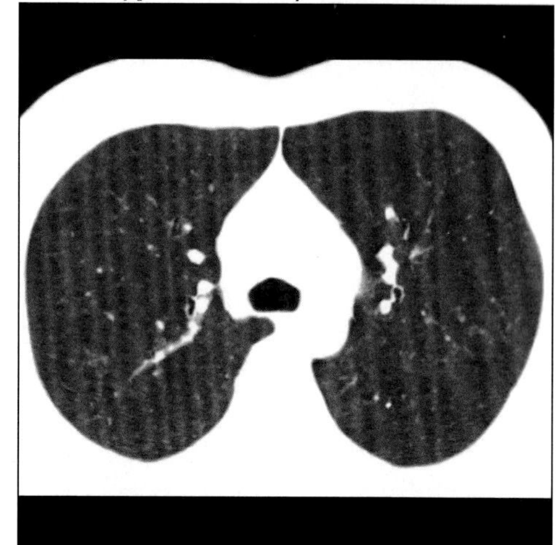

*(**Left**) Axial CECT shows an irregularly marginated, cavitary nodule ➔ in the right upper lobe with adjacent ground-glass attenuation and pleural tags ➔. (**Right**) Coronal CECT minIP image shows narrowing ➔ of the superior aspect of the trachea due to Wegener granulomatosis. As in this case, the subglottic region is most commonly affected.*

Wegener Granulomatosis

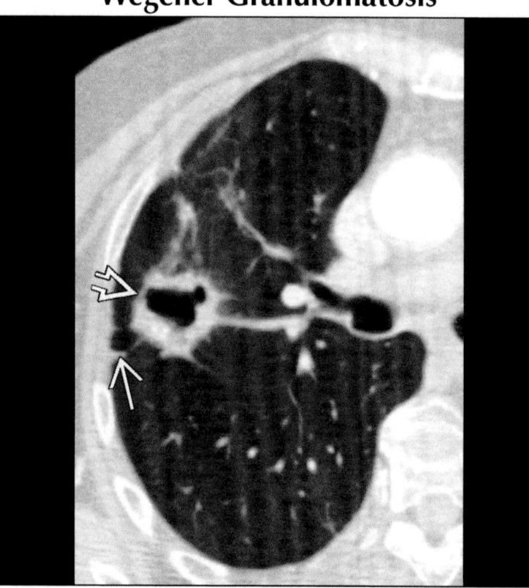

Wegener Granulomatosis

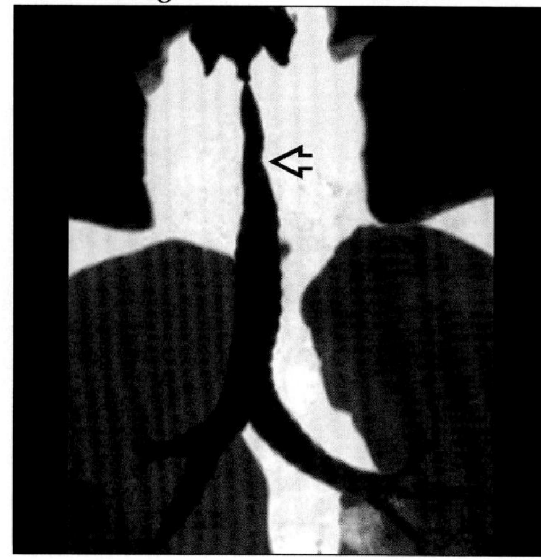

MULTIPLE ILL-DEFINED NODULES

Silicosis/Coal Worker's Pneumoconiosis

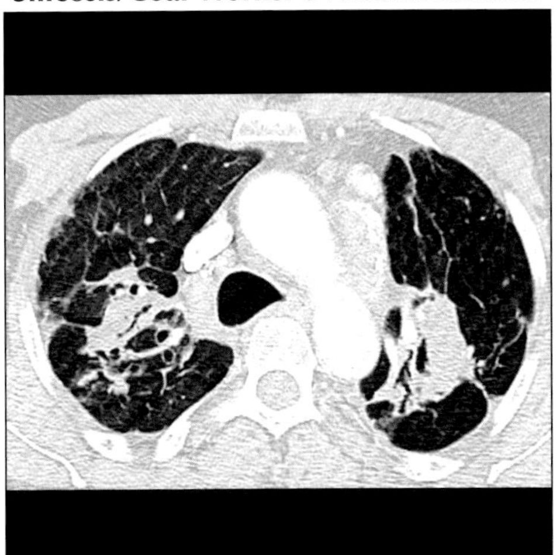

Pulmonary Langerhans Cell Histiocytosis

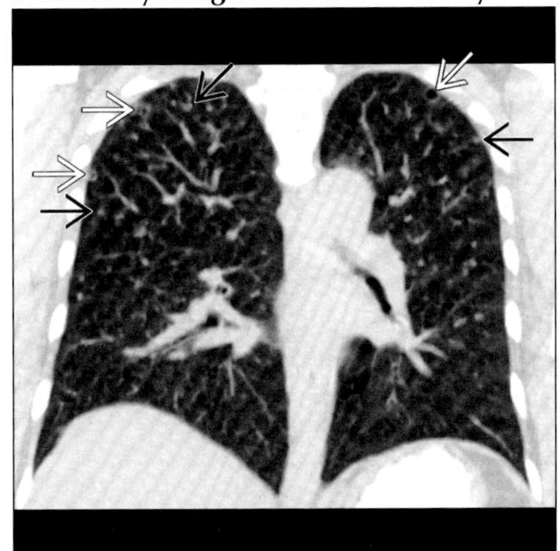

(Left) *Axial CECT shows symmetric upper lobe mass-like consolidation with adjacent architectural distortion, highly suggestive of progressive massive fibrosis in this patient with history of silica exposure.* ***(Right)*** *Coronal NECT shows multiple subcentimeter pulmonary nodules ⇨ and cysts ➡ sparing the lower lungs in this long-time smoker. Other smoking related conditions must be excluded (emphysema, lung cancer, etc.).*

Kaposi Sarcoma

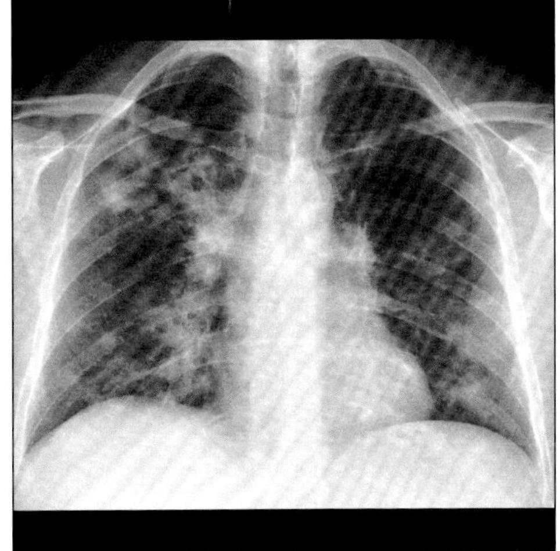

Kaposi Sarcoma

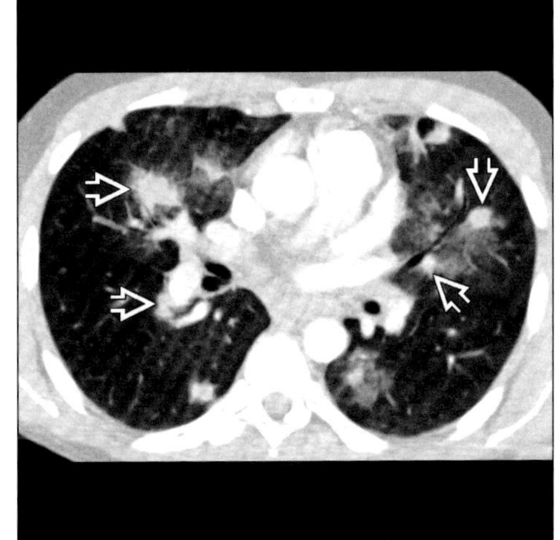

(Left) *Frontal radiograph shows multiple bilateral, poorly marginated pulmonary nodules in this patient with AIDS.* ***(Right)*** *Axial CECT shows multiple pulmonary nodules ➡ with surrounding ground-glass opacities primarily in the central aspect of the lungs, highly suggestive of Kaposi sarcoma in this man with AIDS and cutaneous lesions.*

Sarcoidosis (Alveolar Type)

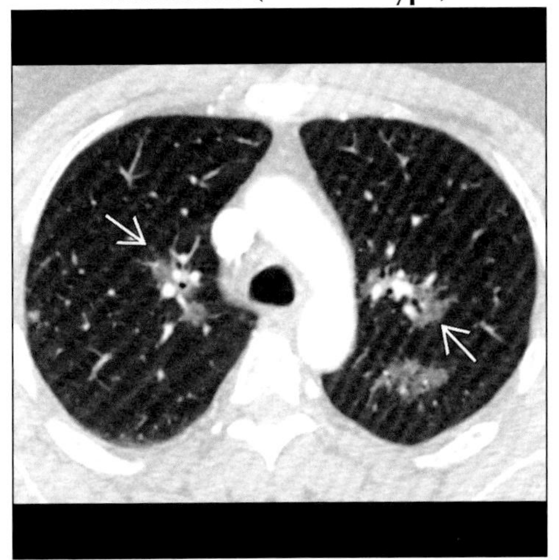

Lymphoma

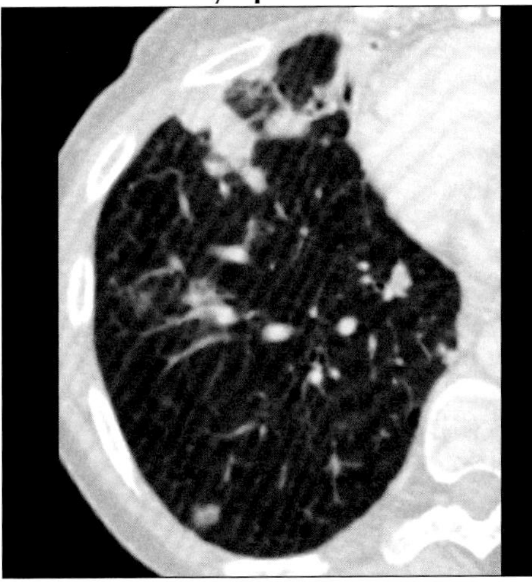

(Left) *Axial CECT shows multiple foci of ground-glass with subtle peripheral nodularity ➡, suggestive of alveolar sarcoidosis. Soft tissue window (not shown) showed moderate lymphadenopathy supporting the patient's histological diagnosis of sarcoidosis.* ***(Right)*** *Axial NECT shows multiple nonspecific pulmonary nodules in the right lung; biopsy was diagnostic for extranodal lymphoma.*

TUBULAR MASS

DIFFERENTIAL DIAGNOSIS

Common

- Bronchiectasis (with Mucous Plugging)
  - Cystic Fibrosis
  - Allergic Bronchopulmonary Aspergillosis
- Endobronchial Tumor (with Distal Mucous Plugging)
- Pulmonary Laceration

Less Common

- Pulmonary AVM

Rare but Important

- Scimitar Vein
- Bronchial Atresia

ESSENTIAL INFORMATION

Helpful Clues for Common Diagnoses

- **Cystic Fibrosis**
  - Diffuse, upper lung preponderant bronchiectasis, bronchial wall thickening
  - Mucous plugging in medium and large airways
  - Mosaic lung attenuation
- **Allergic Bronchopulmonary Aspergillosis**
  - Occurs in cystic fibrosis and asthma
  - Central bronchiectasis in multiple lobes
  - Mucous-filled bronchi; may have gas-fluid level
- **Endobronchial Tumor (with Distal Mucous Plugging)**
  - Slow-growing tumor, aspirated foreign body, broncholithiasis
  - Results in distal bronchiectasis ± mucous plugging, air-trapping
- **Pulmonary Laceration**
  - Tubular lacerations more common with penetrating injuries (e.g., knife, bullets)
  - Laceration initially blood-filled (hematoma)
  - May have oblong or tubular configuration

Helpful Clues for Less Common Diagnoses

- **Pulmonary AVM**
  - Single or multiple nodules with feeding artery or arteries and draining vein
  - Lower lung and medial lungs
  - History of hereditary hemorrhagic telangiectasia

Helpful Clues for Rare Diagnoses

- **Scimitar Vein**
  - Anomalous pulmonary vein from right lung; drains into IVC
  - Hypoplastic right lung; systemic arterial supply common; ± hypoplastic pulmonary artery
  - Bronchial anomalies common: Bilobed right lung, bronchial diverticula, horseshoe lung
- **Bronchial Atresia**
  - Congenital atresia of segmental bronchus
  - Left upper lobe (most common), right upper lobe, lower lobes
  - Bronchocele: Mucoid impaction in obstructed bronchus
  - Hyperlucency and paucity of vessels within affected segment

Cystic Fibrosis

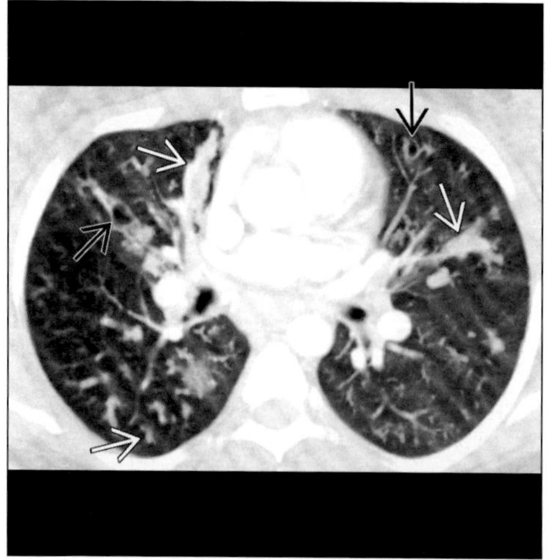

Axial CECT shows tubular mucous plugging ➡ and bronchiectasis ⇨ in the lungs consistent with cystic fibrosis.

Allergic Bronchopulmonary Aspergillosis

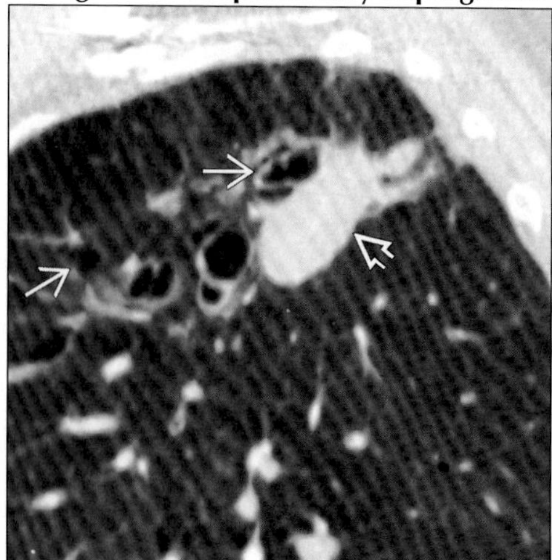

Sagittal NECT demonstrates varicoid bronchiectasis ➡ in the lung apex; there is focal tubular mucous plugging ➡ posteriorly in this patient with allergic bronchopulmonary aspergillosis.

Endobronchial Tumor (with Distal Mucous Plugging)

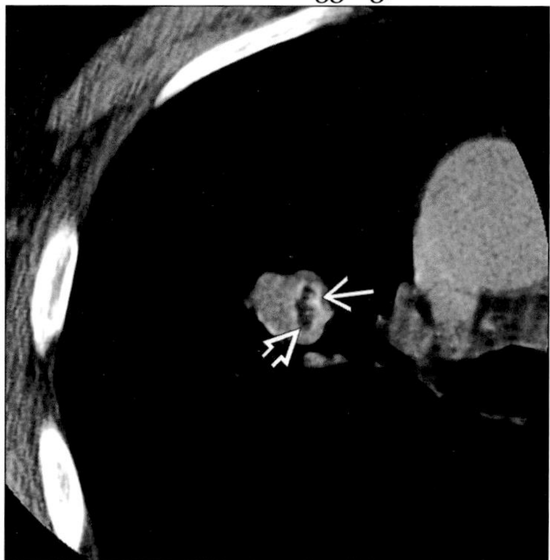

Endobronchial Tumor (with Distal Mucous Plugging)

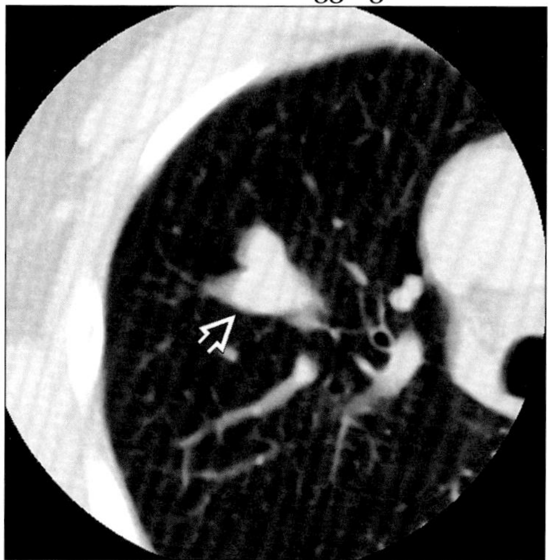

*(**Left**) Axial NECT shows a solid nodule arising within a right upper lobe bronchus with regions of fat ➲ and calcium ➔, essentially diagnostic of a pulmonary hamartoma. No other abnormalities are present. (**Right**) Axial NECT shows branching mucoid impaction ➲ distal to the obstructing endobronchial hamartoma. In this case, there is no distal air-trapping, suggesting good collateral ventilation.*

Pulmonary Laceration

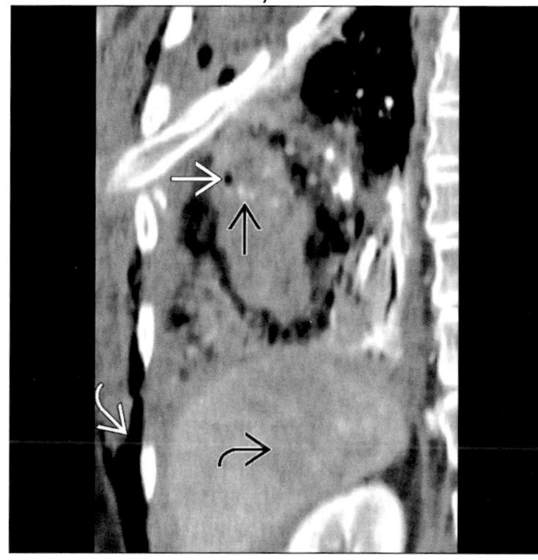

Pulmonary AVM

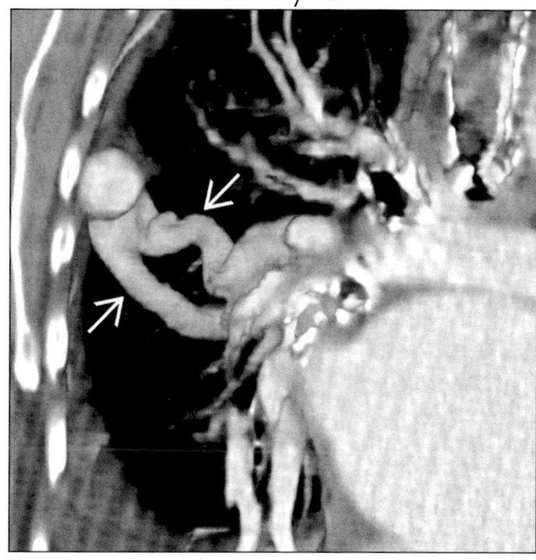

*(**Left**) Coronal CECT shows an oblong right pulmonary opacity with a focal pocket of gas ➔ and nodular contrast extravasation →. Other sequelae of blunt trauma are also present, including splenic laceration ↷, hemothorax, hemoperitoneum, and subcutaneous gas ➚. (**Right**) Coronal oblique CECT VR image shows an AVM in the lateral aspect of the right lung with a feeding artery and draining vein ➔; other scattered pulmonary AVMs were also present.*

Scimitar Vein

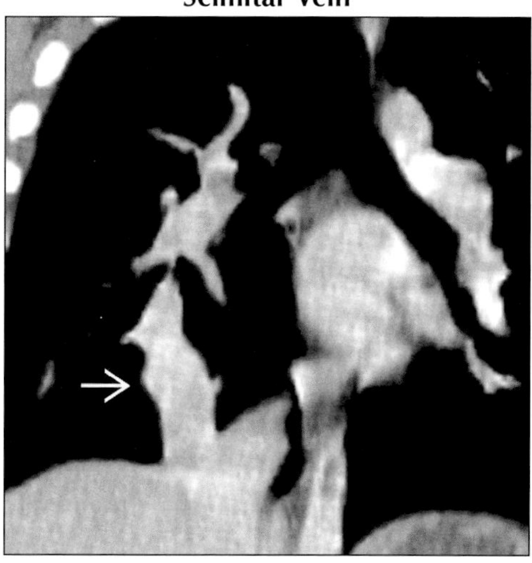

Bronchial Atresia

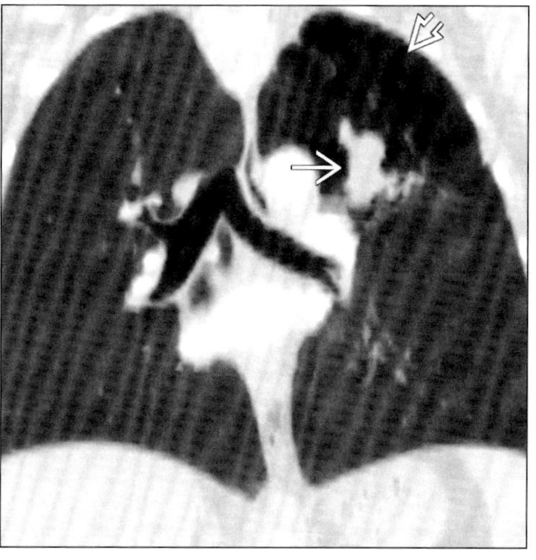

*(**Left**) Coronal CECT shows partial anomalous pulmonary venous drainage ➔ of the right lower lobe to the IVC in this patient with scimitar syndrome. (**Right**) Coronal CECT shows a tubular opacity ➔ in the left upper lobe consistent with a bronchocele from segmental bronchial atresia. There is associated air-trapping ➲ in the left upper lung.*

APICAL MASS

DIFFERENTIAL DIAGNOSIS

Common
- Apical Pleural Thickening
- Extrapleural Fat
- Pleural Effusion
- Post-primary Tuberculosis
- Pancoast Tumor
- Chronic Fungal Infection
- Radiation-Induced Lung Disease

Less Common
- Sarcoidosis
- Progressive Massive Fibrosis
- Mediastinal Hematoma
- Pleural Metastases

Rare but Important
- Nerve Sheath Tumors
- Mesothelioma
- Lymphoma

ESSENTIAL INFORMATION

Key Differential Diagnosis Issues
- Apical masses: Pulmonary and extrapulmonary (pleural, extrapleural, or mediastinal) etiologies

Helpful Clues for Common Diagnoses
- **Apical Pleural Thickening**
  - Benign bilateral or unilateral apical soft tissue thickening on radiographs; usually < 5 mm thick
  - Increased incidence with age
  - Lower border usually sharply marginated; no adjacent bony destruction
  - Apical lung scarring, visceral pleural thickening, and hypertrophy of extrapleural fat on CT
- **Extrapleural Fat**
  - Normal variant that can be confused with other diseases
  - Bilaterally symmetric apical extrapleural soft tissue thickening on radiographs
  - Hypertrophy of extrapleural fat apparent on CT
- **Pleural Effusion**
  - In supine position or loculated effusion
  - Other signs of pleural effusion on supine view
    - Increased density of hemithorax without silhouetting of pulmonary vasculature
    - Blunting of costophrenic angle, subtle blurring of hemidiaphragm, &/or thickening of minor fissure
- **Post-primary Tuberculosis**
  - Upper lung fibrocavitary consolidation; often associated calcification and bronchiectasis
  - Large or small airway stenosis
  - In contrast to primary tuberculosis, pleural effusions and lymphadenopathy uncommon
  - CT commonly shows extensive extrapleural fatty hyperplasia as result of chronic inflammation
- **Pancoast Tumor**
  - Ipsilateral arm and shoulder pain; ± Horner syndrome (ipsilateral miosis, ptosis, and anhydrosis)
  - Slow growth of asymmetric apical pleuropulmonary thickening highly suggestive
  - Associated rib or vertebral destruction; invasion of adjacent vessels or nerves
- **Chronic Fungal Infection**
  - Chronic endemic fungal pneumonia closely resembles fibrocavitary, post-primary tuberculosis
    - Upper lobe preponderance; often bilateral
    - Mediastinal or hilar lymphadenopathy unusual in chronic infection
    - Most often histoplasmosis; also chronic progressive pulmonary coccidioidomycosis or chronic blastomycosis
- **Radiation-Induced Lung Disease**
  - Pulmonary opacities corresponding to radiation ports
  - Time course important
    - Pulmonary ground-glass opacities and consolidation (radiation pneumonitis) 6-8 weeks after initial treatment
    - Radiation pneumonitis peaks 3 months after end of treatment
    - Evolution of pulmonary opacities into lung fibrosis from 3-18 months after end of treatment
    - From 18 months after end of treatment and onward, stable lung fibrosis

Helpful Clues for Less Common Diagnoses
- **Sarcoidosis**

- Upper lung mass-like fibrosis, ± cavitation
- Associated perilymphatic micronodules (< 4 mm): Subpleural, centrilobular, peribronchovascular, along interlobular septa
- Interlobular septal thickening
- Symmetric hilar and mediastinal lymphadenopathy, ± calcification

- **Progressive Massive Fibrosis**
  - Nodules from silicosis or coal worker's pneumoconiosis coalesce into biapical mass-like consolidation, ± cavitation
  - Lateral margin parallels chest wall, sharply defined
  - Tendency to migrate centrally; peripheral lung becomes emphysematous
  - Hilar and mediastinal lymphadenopathy, ± eggshell calcification
- **Mediastinal Hematoma**
  - So-called "apical cap"
  - Arterial or venous hemorrhage, most often from blunt or penetrating trauma
  - History/signs of blunt or penetrating trauma
  - Active contrast extravasation suggests significant vascular injury
- **Pleural Metastases**
  - Most common primary tumors: Lung cancer, breast cancer, lymphoma
  - Associated ipsilateral moderate to large pleural effusion
  - Other areas of nodularity in pleura or interlobar fissures

Helpful Clues for Rare Diagnoses

- **Nerve Sheath Tumors**
  - Smoothly marginated, extrapleural nodule or mass
  - Paravertebral tumors may extend into neuroforamina; local remodeling of bone
  - Most often solitary; multiplicity characteristic of neurofibromatosis type 1 (von Recklinghausen disease)
  - Characteristically, hyperintense on T2 with central low signal; variable enhancement
- **Mesothelioma**
  - Irregular, nodular mass in patient with history of asbestos exposure
  - Circumferential pleural thickening, mediastinal pleural involvement, or thickness > 1 cm suggestive of malignant pleural disease
  - Associated pleural effusion, pleural thickening, &/or pleural plaques (± calcification)
  - Decreased size of ipsilateral hemithorax
- **Lymphoma**
  - Nonspecific appearance; pleural or extrapleural nodules or masses with associated mediastinal lymphadenopathy and pleural effusion

Apical Pleural Thickening

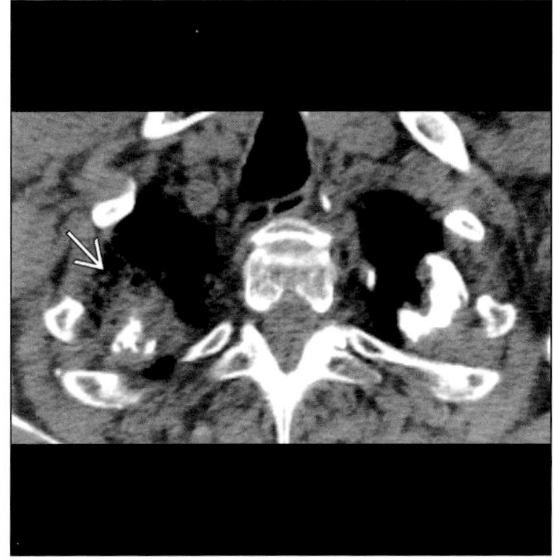

Axial NECT shows partially calcified pleural thickening above the lung apices from previous granulomatous infection; scarring ➔ of the right lung apex is also present.

Pleural Effusion

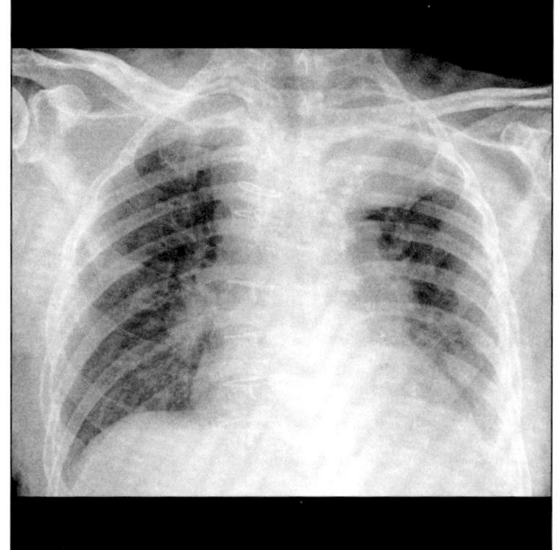

Frontal radiograph shows a large opacity in the left upper hemithorax without associated air bronchograms, representative of loculated left apical pleural effusion.

APICAL MASS

*(**Left**) Axial CECT shows thick-walled, cavitary, mass-like consolidation in the right apex. Multiple small nodules ➡ are also present within the left upper lobe in this patient with active post-primary tuberculosis. (**Right**) Axial CECT shows a large right apical mass with heterogeneous enhancement highly suggestive of a primary bronchogenic carcinoma. There is invasion of the extrapleural space ➡ and leftward deviation of the mediastinum.*

Post-primary Tuberculosis

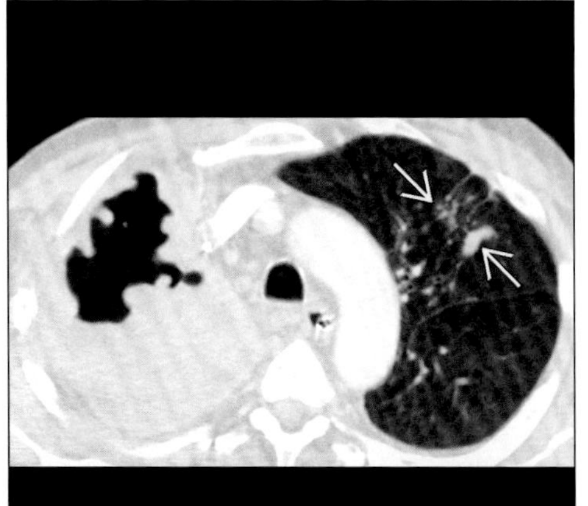

Pancoast Tumor

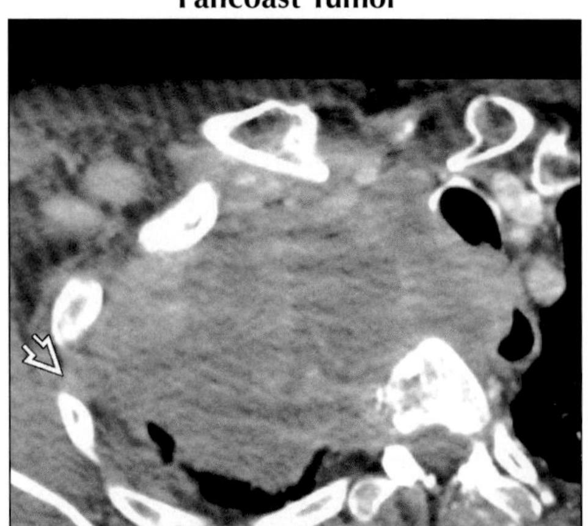

*(**Left**) Coronal CECT shows a bronchogenic carcinoma arising from the right apex. Fat stranding and nodularity in the right axillary and supraclavicular fat suggests extension into the chest wall. The superior vena cava ➡ is nearly completely obliterated. (**Right**) Axial NECT shows geographic ground-glass opacity and reticular opacities ➡ in the medial aspect of the right lung apex, highly suggestive of radiation fibrosis in the setting of remote radiation treatment.*

Pancoast Tumor

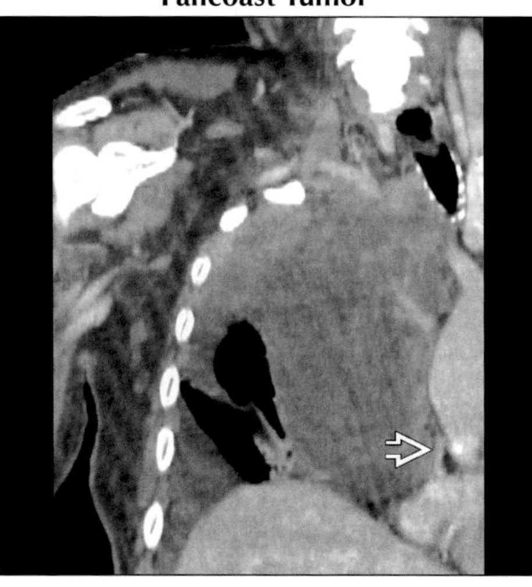

Radiation-Induced Lung Disease

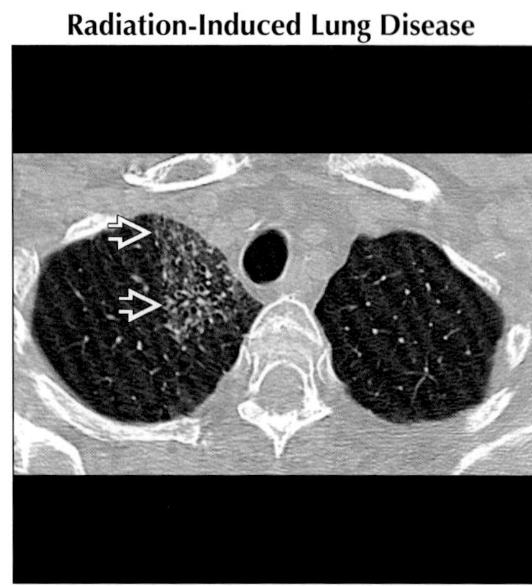

*(**Left**) Axial NECT shows upper lobe nodular consolidation with traction bronchiectasis ➡, architectural distortion, and scattered pleural tags. Small micronodules ➡ and interlobular septal thickening ➡ are also present. (**Right**) Coronal CECT shows bilateral upper lobe masses with architectural distortion, parenchymal bands ➡, traction bronchiectasis ➡, and calcified hilar lymph nodes ➡, consistent with progressive massive fibrosis from silicosis.*

Sarcoidosis

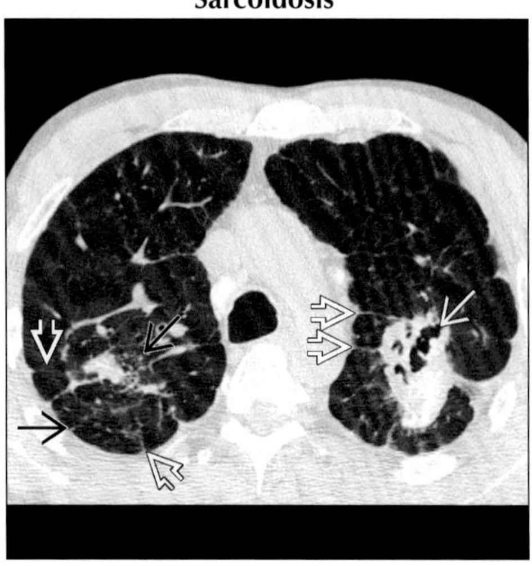

Progressive Massive Fibrosis

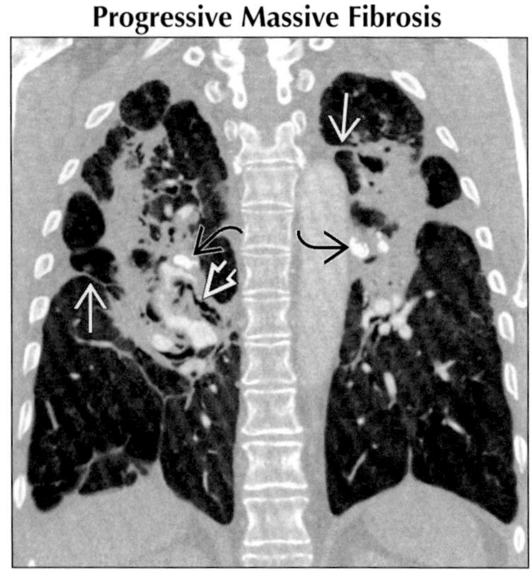

APICAL MASS

Mediastinal Hematoma

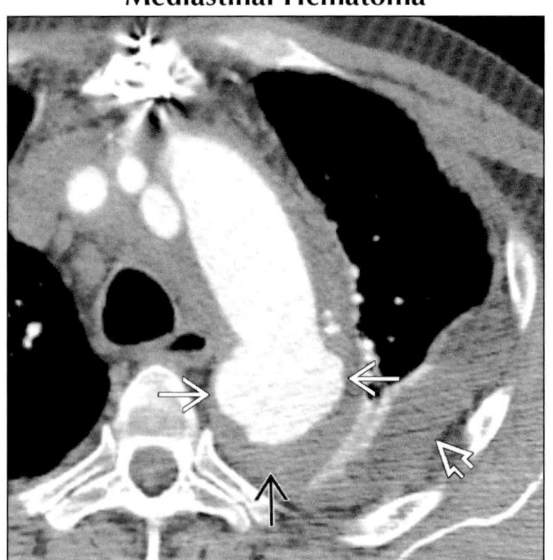

Mediastinal Hematoma

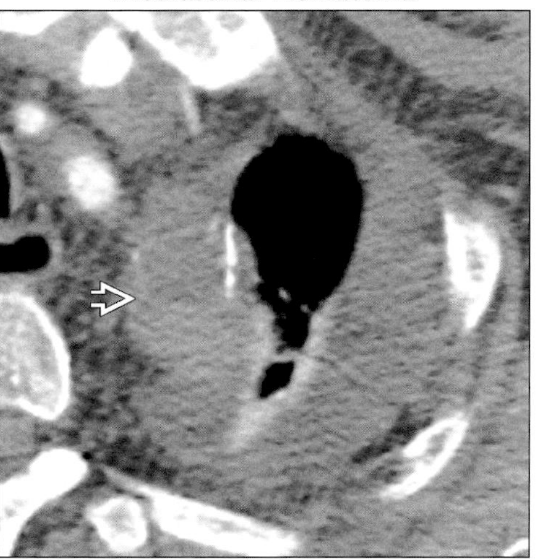

*(**Left**) Axial CECT shows dilation and contour irregularity of the distal aortic arch ➡ consistent with acute traumatic aortic injury. Note adjacent hyperdense mediastinal hematoma ➡ and left posterior hemothorax ➡. (**Right**) Axial CECT shows a hyperdense mediastinal hematoma ➡ with adjacent left apical hemothorax extending cephalad from an aortic rupture.*

Pleural Metastases

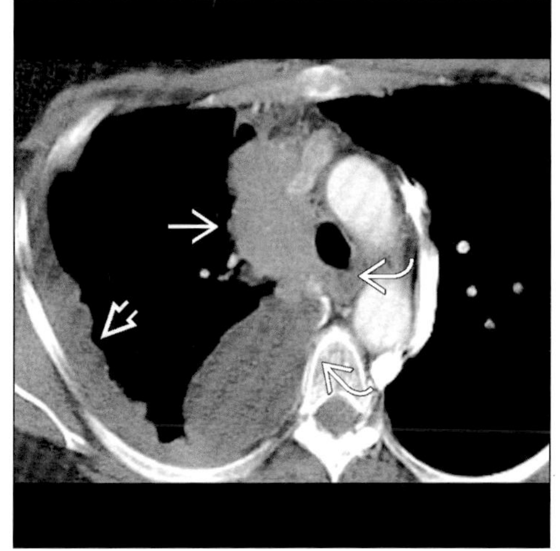

Nerve Sheath Tumors

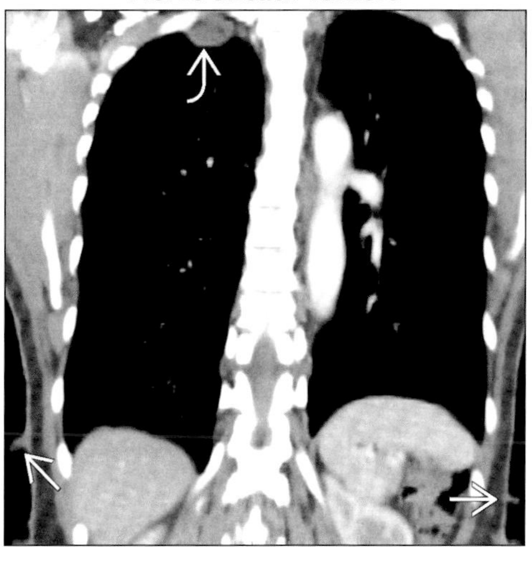

*(**Left**) Axial CECT shows invasive thymoma obliterating the superior vena cava ➡ and pleural metastases ➡. Dilated collateral veins ➡ bypassing the superior vena cava are present. (**Right**) Coronal CECT shows an extrapleural nodule ➡ in the right apex and multiple bilateral cutaneous nodules ➡, consistent with neurofibromas in this patient with neurofibromatosis type 1.*

Mesothelioma

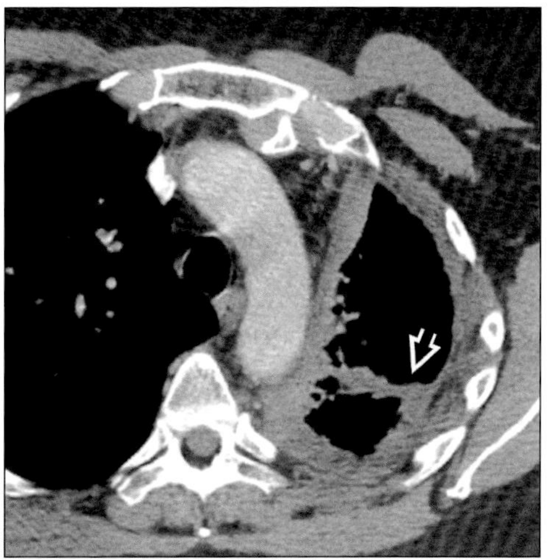

Lymphoma

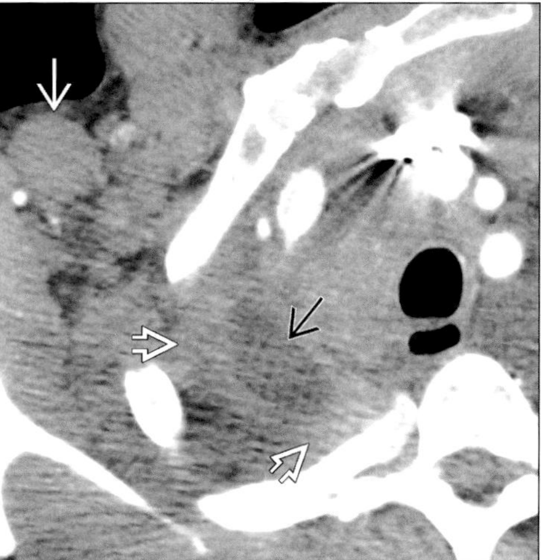

*(**Left**) Axial CECT shows irregular pleural soft tissue thickening extending into the left major fissure ➡ with contraction of the left hemithorax in this patient with previous asbestos exposure. (**Right**) Axial CECT shows extrapulmonary right apical soft tissue attenuation ➡ with a central region of low density ➡ and a markedly enlarged right axillary lymph node ➡.*

CAVITATING MASS

DIFFERENTIAL DIAGNOSIS

Common
- Non-Small Cell Lung Cancer
- Lung Metastases
- Lung Abscess
- Mycobacterial Pneumonia
- Fungal Pneumonia
- Pulmonary Septic Emboli
- Pulmonary Laceration

Less Common
- Progressive Massive Fibrosis
- Wegener Granulomatosis
- Lymphoma
- Cystic Adenomatoid Malformation
- Sequestration

Rare but Important
- Hydatid (Echinococcal) Cyst
- Amebic Lung Abscess
- Lymphomatoid Granulomatosis

ESSENTIAL INFORMATION

Key Differential Diagnosis Issues
- Cavity
  - Air-containing lesion, walls thicker than 4 mm, surrounding consolidation or mass
- Cyst
  - Air-containing lesion, walls thinner than or equal to 4 mm, no surrounding consolidation or mass
- Time course: Acute vs. chronic
  - Acute time course suggestive of infectious or inflammatory diseases
- Thickness of cavity wall
  - Thickest portion of cavity thinner than 4 mm, highly suggestive of benign etiology
  - Thickest portion of cavity thicker than 15 mm, highly suggestive of malignant etiology
- Nodularity of cavity wall
  - Smooth wall more often benign
  - Nodular wall more often malignant

Helpful Clues for Common Diagnoses
- **Non-Small Cell Lung Cancer**
  - Most likely diagnosis for solitary nodule or opacity in smoker
  - Thick and nodular cavity wall, spiculated nodule or mass; most common in upper lobes
  - Very large lymph nodes (> 2 cm in short axis) suggestive of malignant etiology
  - Cavitation most common in squamous subtype
- **Lung Metastases**
  - History of malignancy, particularly squamous cell carcinoma, transitional cell carcinoma, or sarcoma
  - Lower lung preponderance due to increased blood flow
- **Lung Abscess**
  - Round, thick-walled cavity with smooth inner margins within consolidated lung
  - Often related to aspiration pneumonia; usually gravitationally dependent location
  - Slow resolution even with appropriate antimicrobial treatment
- **Mycobacterial Pneumonia**
  - Usually post-primary tuberculosis
  - 90% in apical segment of upper lobes or superior segment of lower lobes
  - Centrilobular or tree in bud nodules suggest endobronchial spread
  - Large airway stenosis
  - In contradistinction to primary tuberculosis, pleural effusions and lymphadenopathy uncommon
- **Fungal Pneumonia**
  - Chronic endemic fungal pneumonia closely resembles fibrocavitary, post-primary tuberculosis
    - Upper lobe preponderance; often bilateral
    - Mediastinal or hilar lymphadenopathy unusual in chronic infection
    - Most often histoplasmosis; also chronic progressive pulmonary coccidioidomycosis or chronic blastomycosis
  - Persistent pulmonary coccidioidomycosis: Lower lung predominant, ill-defined nodules with cavitation
- **Pulmonary Septic Emboli**
  - Frequently multiple, peripheral, basilar, and bilateral
  - Early cavitation
  - "Feeding vessel" sign: Vessel leads directly into nodule or mass
  - Loculated pleural effusion common
- **Pulmonary Laceration**

- History or other imaging findings suggestive of trauma
- Pneumatocele or gas-fluid level

Helpful Clues for Less Common Diagnoses

- **Progressive Massive Fibrosis**
  - Nodules from simple silicosis or coal worker's pneumoconiosis coalesce into biapical mass-like consolidation
  - Lateral margin parallels chest wall, sharply defined
  - Medial inner edge less defined
  - Tendency to migrate centrally; peripheral lung becomes emphysematous
- **Wegener Granulomatosis**
  - Bilateral, multiple nodules that can coalesce into masses; may cavitate
  - Associated with upper airway and renal abnormalities
  - Halo sign: Ground-glass opacities surrounding nodules/masses
  - Large airway stenosis: Most often subglottic trachea
- **Lymphoma**
  - Cavitation unusual
  - Associated mediastinal lymphadenopathy with predilection for anterior mediastinum and thymus
- **Cystic Adenomatoid Malformation**
  - Multicystic pulmonary lesion
  - May contain gas, fluid, or combination of gas and fluid
  - Normal interspersed lung parenchyma
- **Sequestration**
  - Nonfunctioning lung without normal connection with functioning lung
  - Complex mass (solid, fluid, &/or cystic) in either lower lobe with systemic arterial supply

Helpful Clues for Rare Diagnoses

- **Hydatid (Echinococcal) Cyst**
  - Endemic to Mediterranean, Africa, and Australia
  - "Meniscus" sign: Crescent of gas around endocyst
  - "Water lily" sign: Collapse of hydatid cyst; endocyst membrane floating in intact pericyst
  - Cumbo or "onion peel" sign: Gas outlines both sides of collapsed endocyst membrane
  - Hepatic cystic lesions; right hepatic lobe > left hepatic lobe
- **Amebic Lung Abscess**
  - Right lower lobe consolidation with pleural effusion
  - Associated with abscess in right hepatic lobe
  - Expectoration of "anchovy paste" or "chocolate sauce" sputum
- **Lymphomatoid Granulomatosis**
  - Poorly responsive B-cell mediated extranodal lymphoproliferative disorder
  - Multiple nodules or masses most common
  - Central necrosis/cavitation and peripheral enhancement
  - Halo sign and air bronchogram sign

Non-Small Cell Lung Cancer

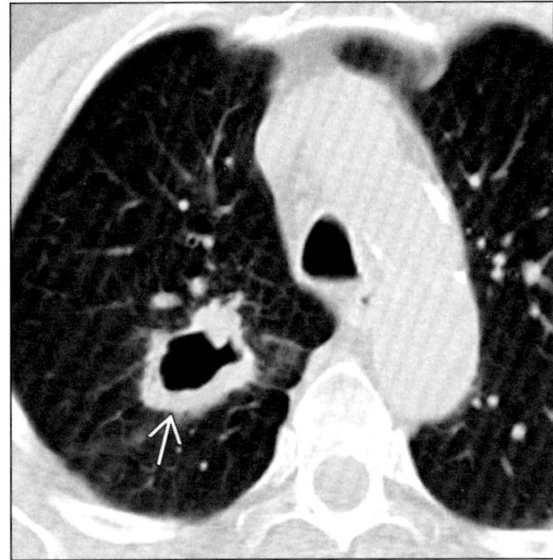

Axial CECT shows a thick-walled, cavitary mass ➡ in the posterior segment of the right upper lobe, highly suggestive of bronchogenic carcinoma.

Lung Metastases

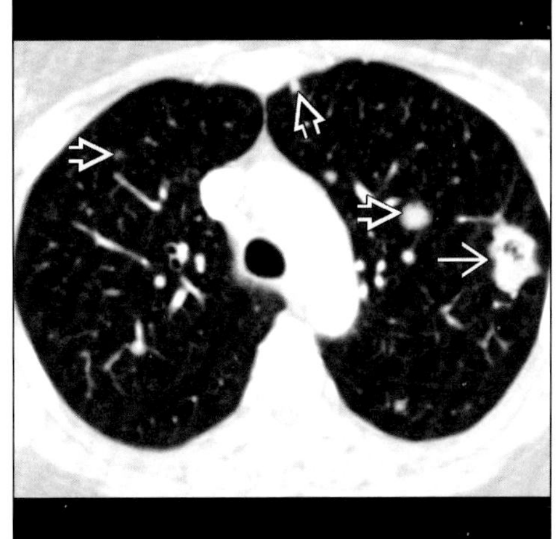

Axial CECT shows a lobulated, cavitary mass ➡ in the left upper lobe and scattered pulmonary nodules ⇨ within the lungs in this patient with metastatic colon adenocarcinoma.

CAVITATING MASS

*(**Left**) Axial CECT shows cavitary, mass-like consolidation ➔ in the superior segment of the right lower lobe, most consistent with pulmonary abscess from aspiration related to esophageal carcinoma ➔. (**Right**) Axial CECT shows a lobulated, cavitary mass ➔ in the posterior segment of the right upper lobe with patchy adjacent ground-glass opacities. Ill-defined, centrilobular, ground-glass nodules ➔ suggest endobronchial spread of infection.*

Lung Abscess

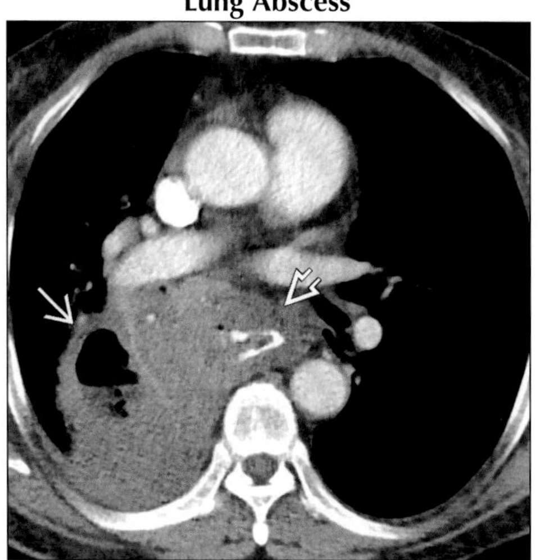

Mycobacterial Pneumonia

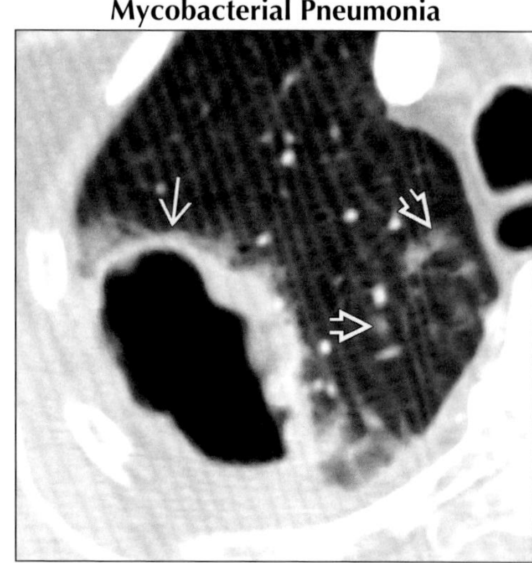

*(**Left**) Coned-in view of the right lung base shows a thick-walled, cavitary mass ➔ in the right lower lobe in this patient with persistent pulmonary coccidioidomycosis. (**Right**) Axial CECT shows a peripheral, cavitary mass ➔ in the apicoposterior segment of the left upper lobe, as well as peripheral, cavitary nodules and reactive prevascular lymphadenopathy ➔. A partially loculated left pleural effusion is also present.*

Fungal Pneumonia

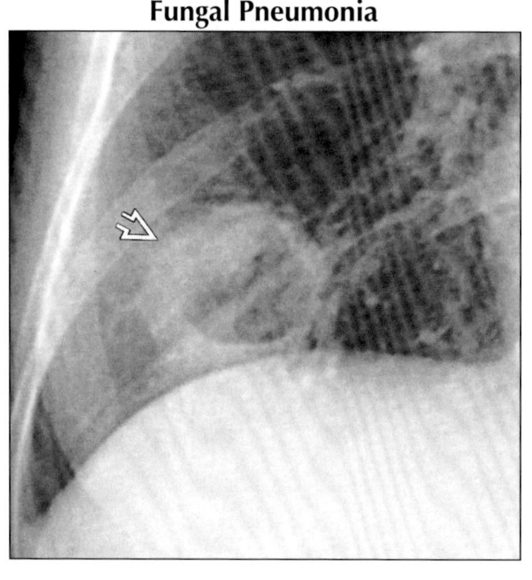

Pulmonary Septic Emboli

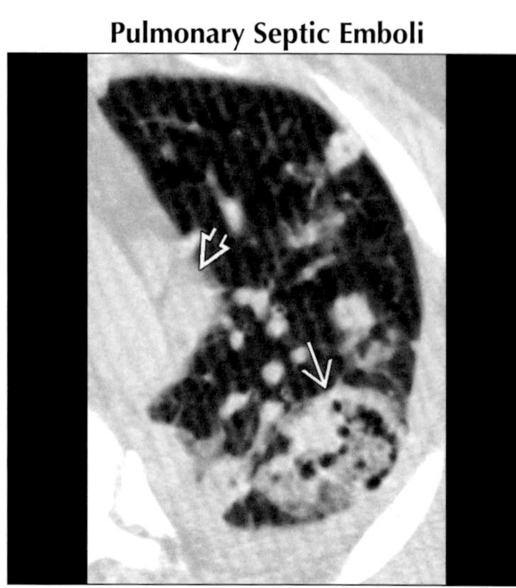

*(**Left**) Axial CECT shows small gas pockets ➔ within a right lower lobe pulmonary laceration/hematoma. Adjacent consolidation and ground-glass opacities represent pulmonary hemorrhage and contusion. Traumatic right lateral rib fracture ➔, right pneumothorax, and subcutaneous emphysema are also present. (**Right**) Axial CECT shows biapical, cavitary, mass-like fibrosis ➔ and architectural distortion in this patient with complicated silicosis.*

Pulmonary Laceration

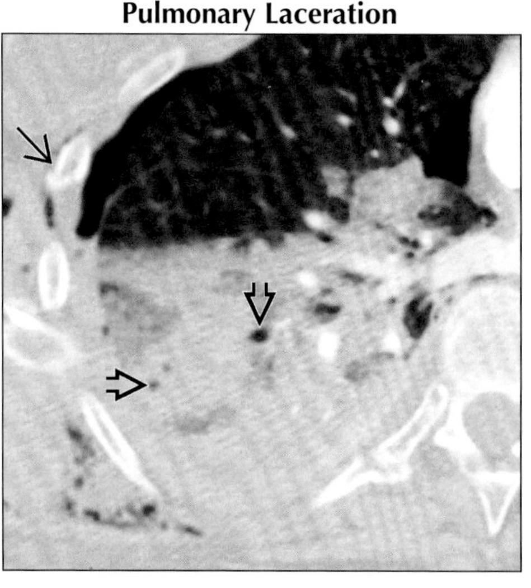

Progressive Massive Fibrosis

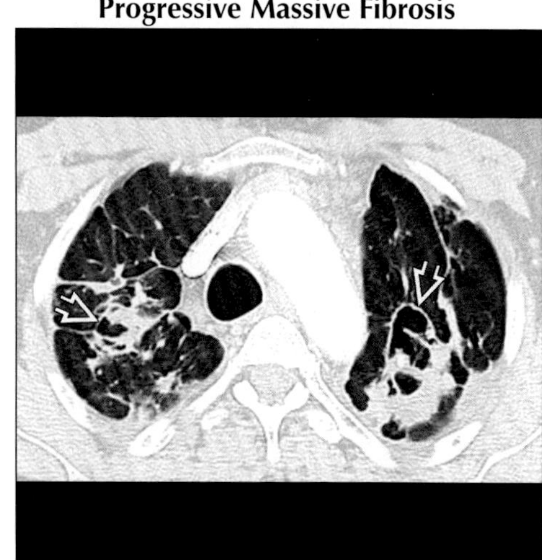

CAVITATING MASS

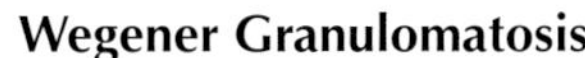

Wegener Granulomatosis

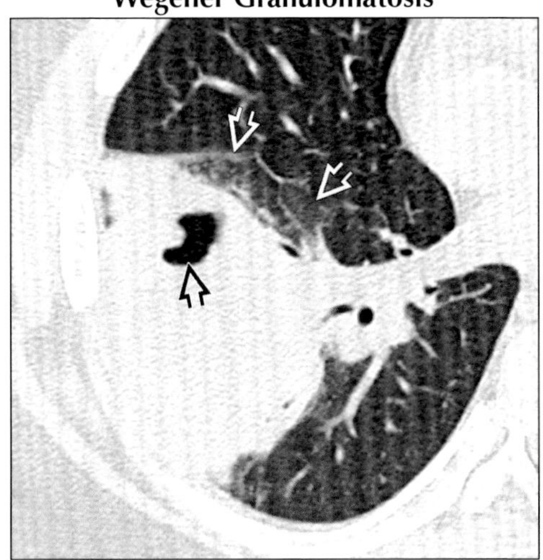

Cystic Adenomatoid Malformation

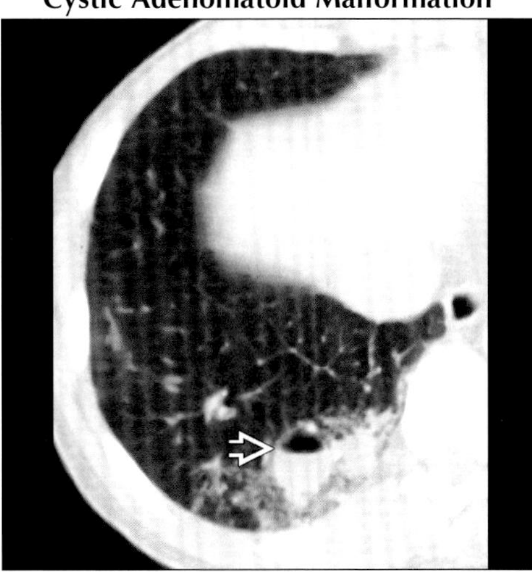

(Left) *Axial NECT shows a large mass with a focus of thick-walled cavitation ⇨ in the right lower lobe. Adjacent ground-glass opacities ➡ may represent focal edema, pneumonitis, or hemorrhage.* ***(Right)*** *Axial CECT shows a gas-fluid level ➡ in a complex mass in the posterior basilar segment of the right lower lobe, representing infection of a cystic adenomatoid malformation.*

Sequestration

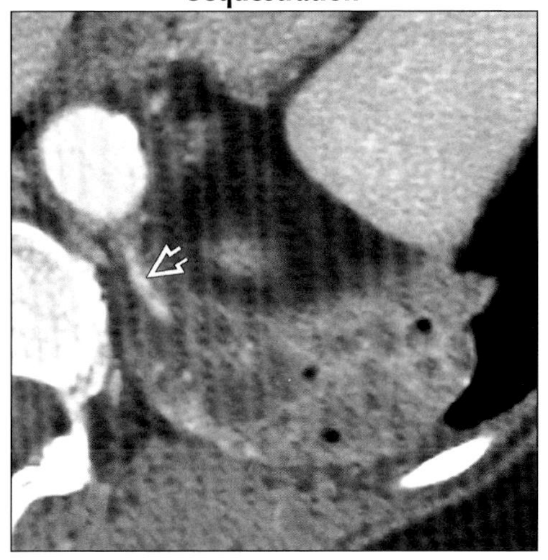

Hydatid (Echinococcal) Cyst

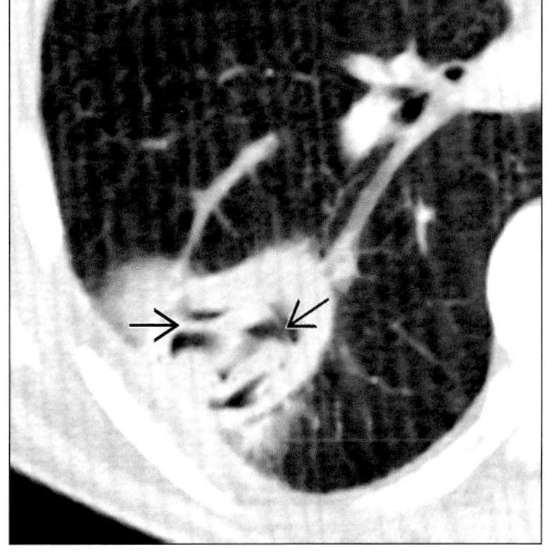

(Left) *Axial CECT shows a systemic artery ➡ supplying a complex solid, fluid, and cystic mass in the posterior basilar segment of the left lower lobe, diagnostic of a sequestration.* ***(Right)*** *Axial CECT shows gas outlining both sides of the endocyst membrane →, diagnostic of a hydatid cyst. Adjacent ground-glass opacities are also present.*

Lymphomatoid Granulomatosis

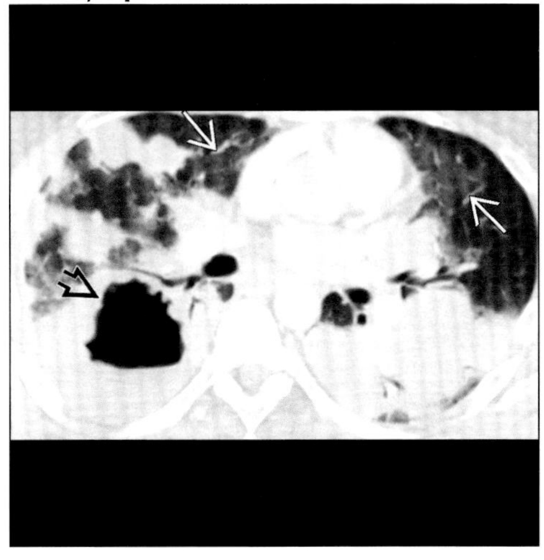

Lymphomatoid Granulomatosis

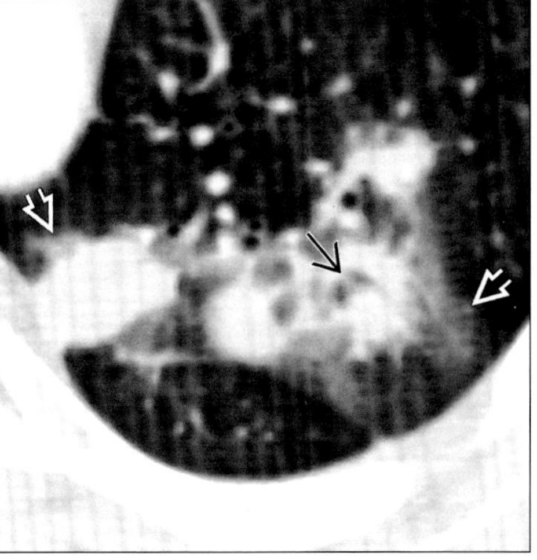

(Left) *Axial CECT shows multiple, bilateral pulmonary nodules and masses; the largest mass in the right lower lobe has cavitated ⇨. There are scattered ground-glass opacities ➡.* ***(Right)*** *Axial CECT shows a branching bronchus → within a pulmonary nodule (air bronchogram sign) and ground-glass opacities ➡ adjacent to multiple pulmonary nodules (halo sign) in the apicoposterior segment of the left upper lobe.*

PNEUMATOCELE

DIFFERENTIAL DIAGNOSIS

Common
- Traumatic Pneumatocele
- Postinfectious Pneumatocele
- Bullous Emphysema
- Paraseptal Emphysema
- Tuberculosis

Less Common
- Lung Abscess

Rare but Important
- Hydrocarbon Aspiration

ESSENTIAL INFORMATION

Key Differential Diagnosis Issues
- Proper history of trauma or prior infection is paramount

Helpful Clues for Common Diagnoses
- **Traumatic Pneumatocele**
  - Result from laceration of lung tissue
  - Penetrating injury; stab wound, gunshot wound
  - Blunt injury
    - Small, peripheral lacerations from overlying rib fractures
    - Paravertebral lacerations from shearing injury
    - Central lacerations from compression rupture; larger and more irregular in shape
  - Often initially obscured by surrounding pulmonary contusion/hemorrhage
  - Can initially present filled with blood (hematoma); fills with air as blood clears
  - Resolve/heal without treatment over 1-2 weeks
- **Postinfectious Pneumatocele**
  - Common after *Staphylococcus* and *Coccidioides* infections
  - Thin walled
  - Pneumatocele can persist for years
- **Bullous Emphysema**
  - Underlying centrilobular emphysema
  - Emphysematous spaces > 1 cm
- **Paraseptal Emphysema**
  - Peripheral lung along fissures and sharp pleural reflections
- **Tuberculosis**
  - Other features of nodular scarring, bronchiectasis, volume loss, ipsilateral tracheal deviation
  - Typically unilateral, upper lobe/apical

Helpful Clues for Less Common Diagnoses
- **Lung Abscess**
  - Patients more acutely ill; fever, cough, chest pain
  - Ill-defined walls
  - Air-fluid levels common

Helpful Clues for Rare Diagnoses
- **Hydrocarbon Aspiration**
  - Rare complication of unintended hydrocarbon inhalation or aspiration
  - Pneumatoceles are rare sequelae of initial inflammatory pneumonitis

Traumatic Pneumatocele

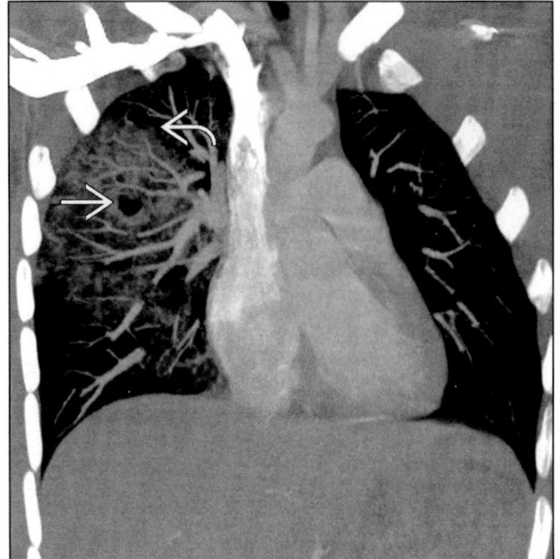

Coronal CECT shows right upper lobe laceration ➡ with extensive surrounding pulmonary hemorrhage and contusion ➡. This results from rapid compression of the lung against a closed glottis.

Traumatic Pneumatocele

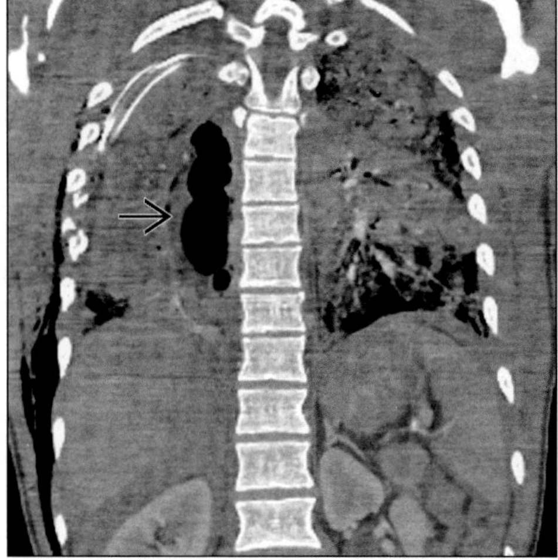

Coronal CECT after a high speed motor vehicle crash shows a large paravertebral pulmonary laceration ➡. This typically occurs from shearing of the lung over the spine during a rapid compression of the chest wall.

PNEUMATOCELE

Postinfectious Pneumatocele

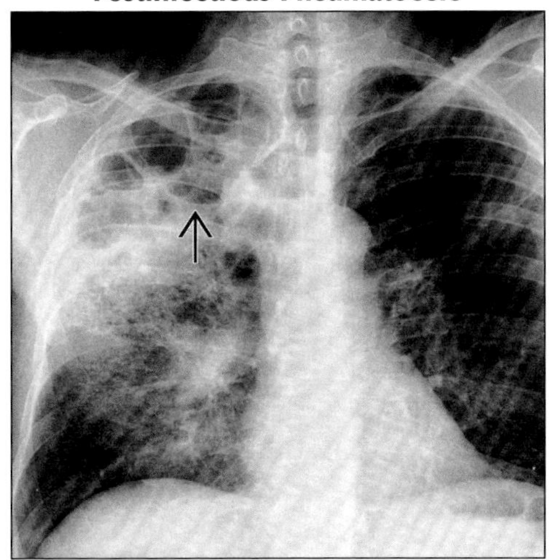

Bullous Emphysema

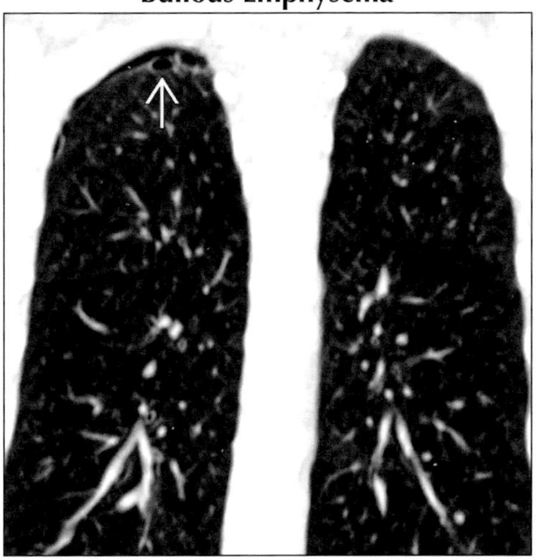

(Left) *Frontal radiograph from a patient recovering from a severe Staphylococcus pneumonia shows extensive pneumatocele formation in the right upper lobe. Note that some of these pneumatoceles have air-fluid levels ➙.* ***(Right)*** *Coronal NECT shows several small right apical bulla ➙. These were detected after the patient presented with sudden chest pain and a spontaneous pneumothorax, still evident.*

Paraseptal Emphysema

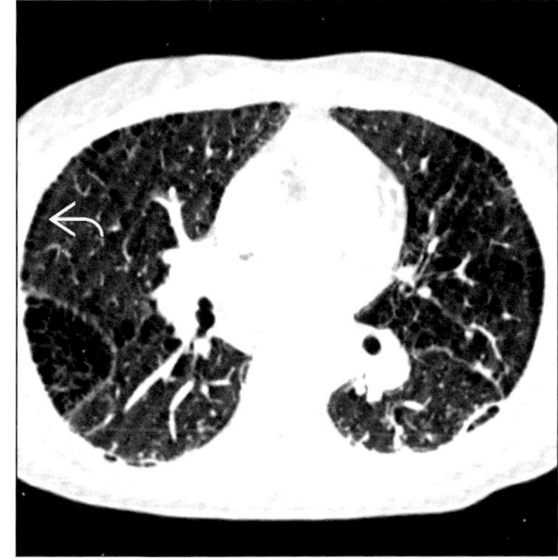

Tuberculosis

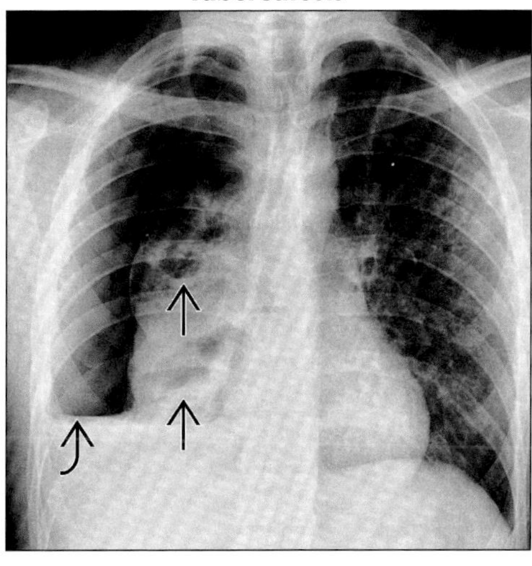

(Left) *Axial CECT shows extensive paraseptal pulmonary emphysema, notably around the lung periphery, within the pulmonary fissures ➙. This type of emphysema is not associated with cigarette smoking.* ***(Right)*** *Frontal radiograph from a patient with extensive reactivation tuberculosis infection shows multiple cavity formation within the right lung ➙. Also note the right hydropneumothorax ➙ suggesting bronchopleural fistula.*

Lung Abscess

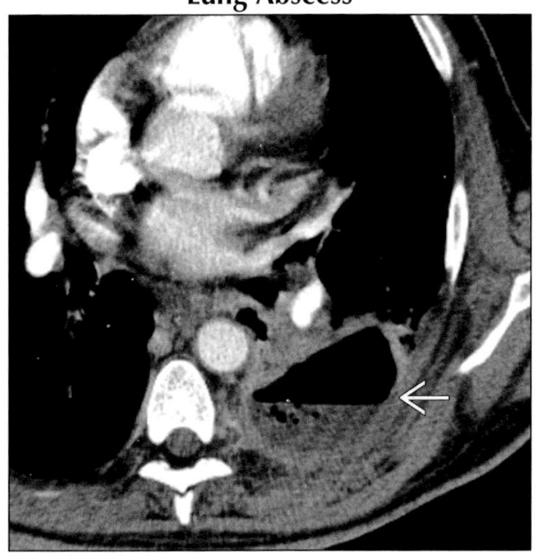

Hydrocarbon Aspiration

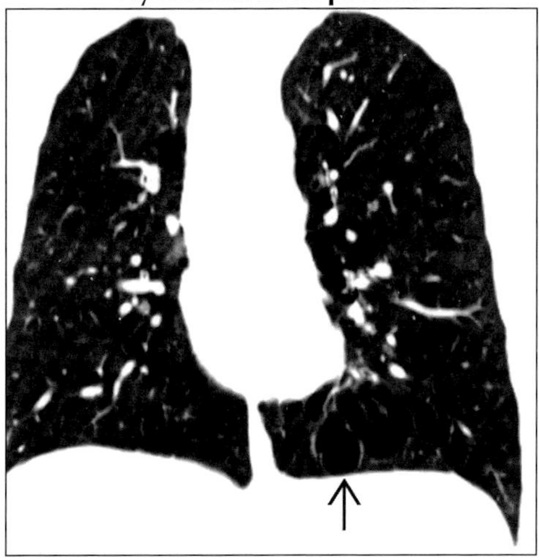

(Left) *Axial CECT shows a large, left lower lobe, thick-walled lung abscess ➙. Note the air-fluid level and associated pleural thickening secondary to the extensive inflammation.* ***(Right)*** *Coronal CECT shows several thin-walled pneumatoceles ➙ in the left lower lobe. These resulted from accidental hydrocarbon (gasoline) aspiration that occurred 40 years prior to this presentation.*

FOCAL LUNG OPACITY

DIFFERENTIAL DIAGNOSIS

Common
- Pneumonia
- Aspiration
- Pulmonary Abscess
- Subsegmental Atelectasis
- Lung Cancer
- Metastatic Disease

Less Common
- Pulmonary Hemorrhage
- Radiation Pneumonitis
- Progressive Massive Fibrosis
- Sarcoidosis
- Pulmonary Infarct
- Pulmonary AVM

Rare but Important
- Lymphoma
- Lipoid Pneumonia

ESSENTIAL INFORMATION

Helpful Clues for Common Diagnoses
- **Pneumonia**
  - Airspace opacities: Ground-glass opacity to dense consolidation
  - Reactive lymphadenopathy; very large lymph nodes unusual
  - Parapneumonic pleural effusion or empyema
  - Correlation with sputum, WBC count, and clinical presentation paramount
  - Consider fungal agents and PCP in the correct clinical setting
- **Aspiration**
  - Consolidation in gravity-dependent portions of lungs
  - Predisposed patients (alcoholism, epilepsy, hiatal hernia, esophageal dysmotility or obstruction, neuromuscular disorders)
  - Supine: Superior segments of lower lobes and posterior segments of upper lobes
  - Upright: Basilar segments of lower lobes
  - Centrilobular or tree in bud opacities common on CT
  - May progress to necrotizing pneumonia or pulmonary abscess without treatment
- **Pulmonary Abscess**
  - Gas-filled cavity arising from focal pneumonia (usually due to aspiration)
  - Abscess 1-2 weeks after development of pneumonia
  - Gas-fluid level or smaller foci of gas
  - Empyema and bronchopleural fistula
  - May be difficult to differentiate from empyema
    - Abscess: Round, thick walls, acute margins with chest wall
    - Empyema: Elliptical, thin walls, obtuse margins with chest wall; atelectasis of adjacent lung
- **Subsegmental Atelectasis**
  - Discoid or plate-shaped
  - Usually in dependent aspects of lower lobes or in basilar aspects of right middle lobe or lingula
  - Crosses pulmonary segments
  - Often touches visceral pleura
- **Lung Cancer**
  - Most common in upper lung zone (2/3 of primary lung cancers)
  - Spiculated or irregular margins; pleural tail
  - Thick-walled or nodular cavitation
  - Large hilar &/or mediastinal lymphadenopathy (> 2 cm)
  - Concomitant emphysema and smoking history
- **Metastatic Disease**
  - Variable-sized, well-marginated pulmonary nodules preferentially in peripheral and lower lungs
  - Feeding artery sign: Pulmonary artery branches extend to nodules, implying hematogenous spread
  - Solitary metastasis: Renal cell carcinoma, colon cancer, breast cancer, sarcomas, melanoma

Helpful Clues for Less Common Diagnoses
- **Pulmonary Hemorrhage**
  - Ground-glass opacities > consolidation; may be diffuse, patchy, lobular, or centrilobular
  - Increased interlobular and intralobular septal thickening over 1-2 days
  - Rapid resolution in days; not as rapid as in cardiogenic pulmonary edema or bland aspiration
- **Radiation Pneumonitis**
  - Pulmonary opacities corresponding to radiation ports

- Pulmonary ground-glass opacities and consolidation (radiation pneumonitis) appears 6-8 weeks after initial treatment
- Radiation pneumonitis peaks 3 months after end of treatment
- Evolution of pulmonary opacities into lung fibrosis from 3-18 months after end of treatment
- From 18 months after end of treatment and onward lung fibrosis stable

- **Progressive Massive Fibrosis**
  - Nodules from silicosis or coal worker's pneumoconiosis coalesce into biapical mass-like consolidation, ± cavitation
  - Lateral margin parallels chest wall, sharply defined
  - Hilar and mediastinal lymphadenopathy, ± eggshell calcification
- **Sarcoidosis**
  - Perilymphatic nodules with symmetric mediastinal and hilar lymphadenopathy
  - Small nodules may coalesce into focal opacity (alveolar sarcoidosis)
  - Tiny nodules around a larger dominant nodule (galaxy sign)
  - Interlobular septal thickening
- **Pulmonary Infarct**
  - Lower lung predominant, peripheral/subpleural, wedge-shaped consolidation
  - In setting of acute pulmonary arterial thromboembolism
  - Reverse halo configuration (central ground-glass opacity and peripheral rim of consolidation)
  - Often in setting of superimposed cardiac dysfunction (cardiomyopathy, congestive heart failure)
    - Both pulmonary and bronchial arterial supply to lung reduced
- **Pulmonary AVM**
  - Single or multiple nodules with feeding artery and vein
  - Lower and medial lungs
  - History of hereditary hemorrhagic telangiectasia

Helpful Clues for Rare Diagnoses

- **Lymphoma**
  - Multiple ill-defined nodules that may cavitate
  - May occur in association with nodal disease or primarily in lungs
- **Lipoid Pneumonia**
  - Exogenous aspiration of fatty material
  - Nodular or mass-like consolidation often with fatty CT attenuation
  - Fat density may not be evident because of inflammation and scarring
  - Irregular margins, may mimic bronchogenic carcinoma
  - Gravity-dependent portions of lungs
    - Supine: Superior segments of lower lobes and posterior segments of upper lobes
    - Upright: Basilar segments of lower lobes

Pneumonia

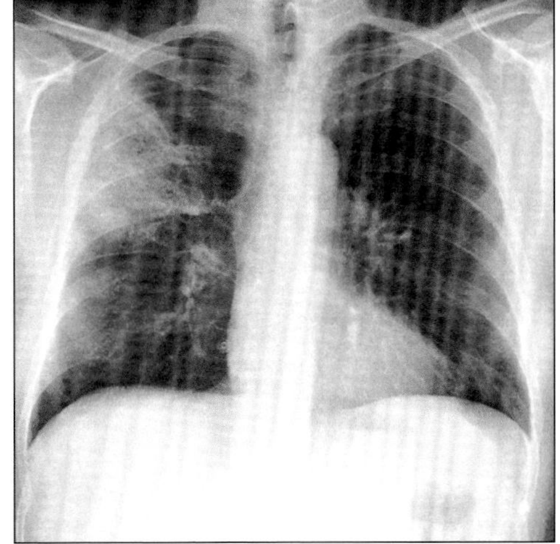

Frontal radiograph shows focal consolidation in the right upper lobe due to bacterial pneumonia.

Aspiration

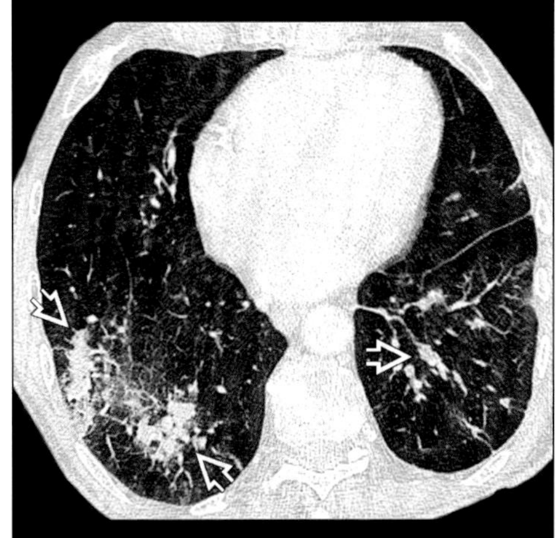

Axial CECT shows bilateral basilar peribronchovascular consolidation ➔ with a typical distribution for aspiration in this patient with a history of a Zenker diverticulum.

FOCAL LUNG OPACITY

(Left) Coronal CECT shows a typical sliding-type hiatal hernia ➡, which puts this patient at risk for aspiration. *(Right)* Axial CECT shows diffuse low density ➡ within the atelectatic left lower lobe compared to the normally enhancing atelectatic right lower lobe in this patient with left lower lobe aspiration pneumonia. Tubular regions of low density ➡ in the right lower lobe may represent aspirated material or retained secretions.

Aspiration

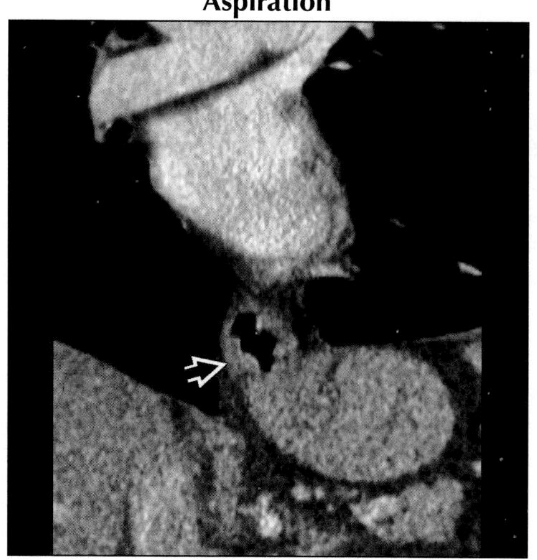

Aspiration

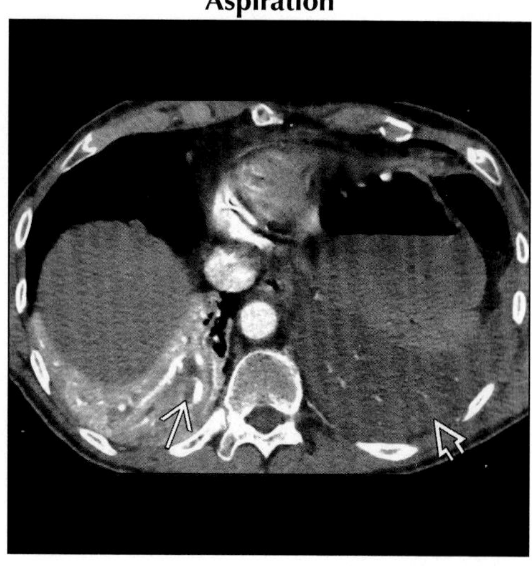

(Left) Axial CECT shows focal consolidation in the superior segment of the left lower lobe with central cavitation due to pulmonary abscess in this patient with history of aspiration. *(Right)* Axial CECT shows cavitary, mass-like consolidation ➡ in the superior segment of the right lower lobe, most consistent with pulmonary abscess from aspiration related to esophageal carcinoma ➡.

Pulmonary Abscess

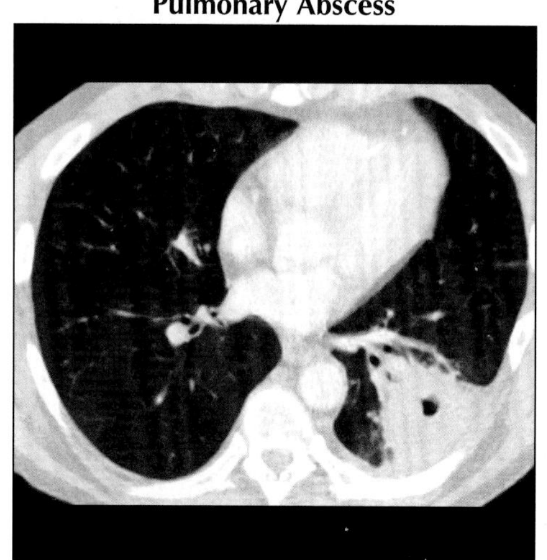

Pulmonary Abscess

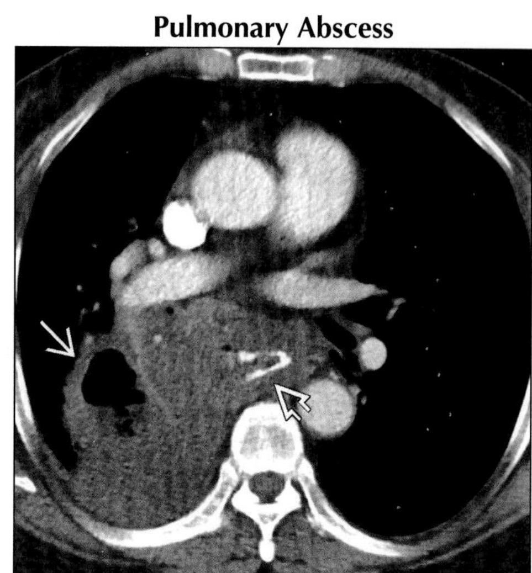

(Left) Frontal radiograph shows a thin, band-like opacity ➡ in the left lung base with dense left lower lobe atelectasis (ivory heart sign) ➡. *(Right)* Axial CECT in the same patient shows subsegmental, plate-like atelectasis ➡ in the lingula with complete atelectasis ➡ of the left lower lobe.

Subsegmental Atelectasis

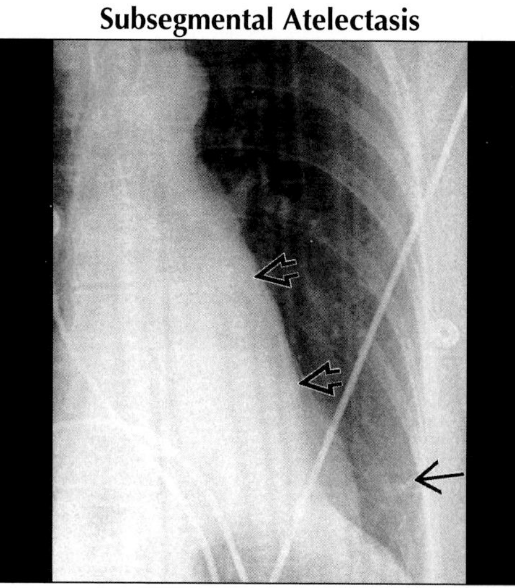

Subsegmental Atelectasis

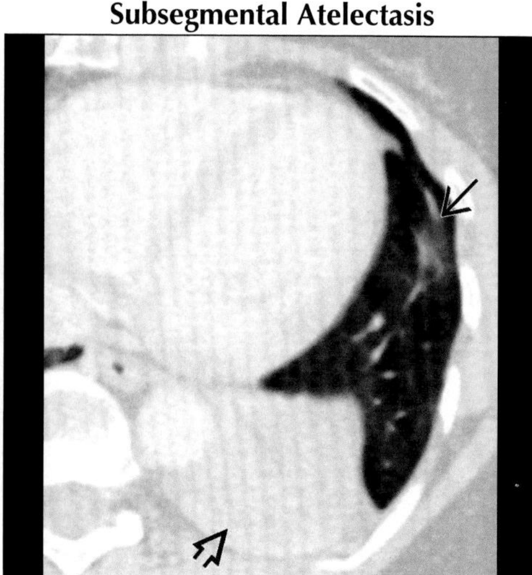

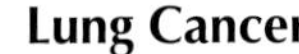

Lung Cancer

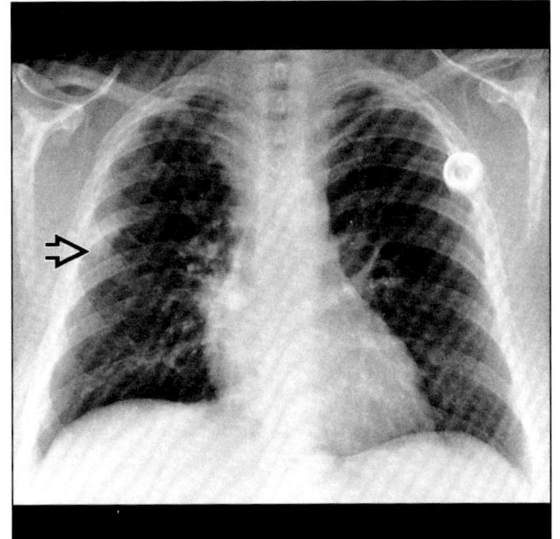

Lung Cancer

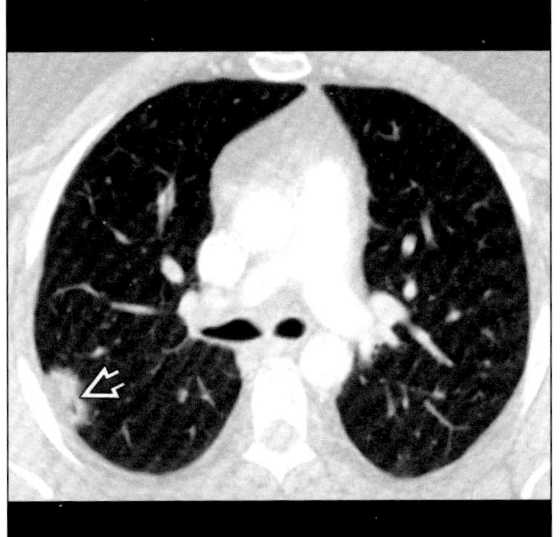

(Left) *Frontal radiograph shows a subtle focal opacity ⇨ in the lateral aspect of the right lung partially obscured by overlying ribs.* ***(Right)*** *Axial CECT shows a subpleural nodule ⇨ with irregular margins in the right lower lobe due to bronchogenic carcinoma.*

Lung Cancer

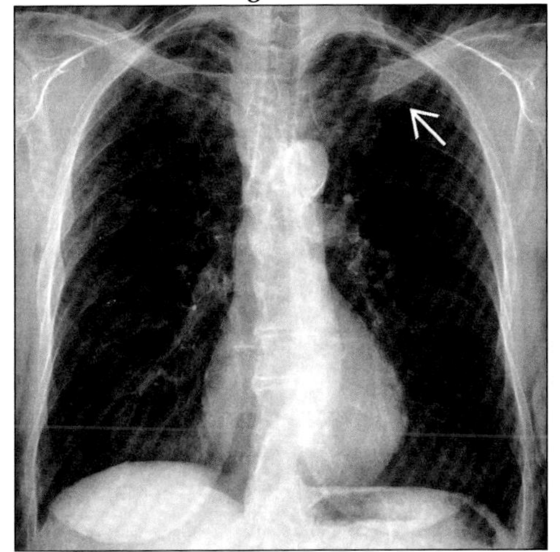

Lung Cancer

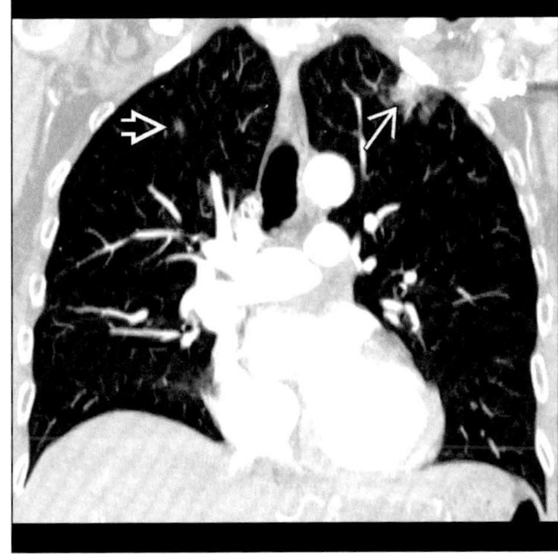

(Left) *Frontal radiograph shows a subtle focal opacity in the left apex ➡ obscured by overlying ribs and the left clavicle. This is a common "blind" spot on chest radiographs.* ***(Right)*** *Coronal CECT MIP image shows mixed solid and ground-glass opacity in the left upper lobe ➡ due to bronchoalveolar carcinoma. Note a right upper lobe focal ground-glass opacity ⇨ concerning for a 2nd primary tumor or bronchogenic spread.*

Metastatic Disease

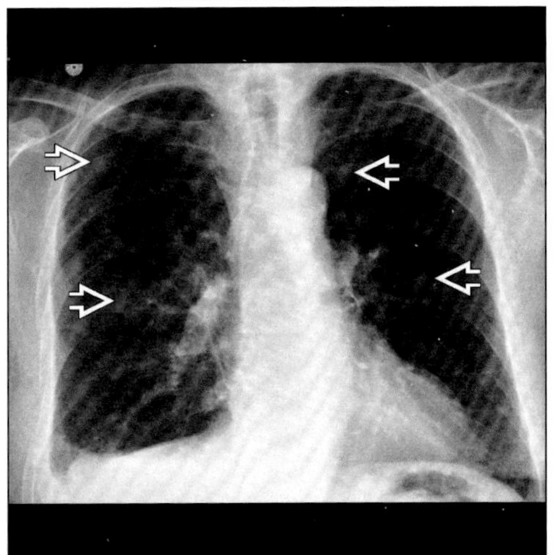

Metastatic Disease

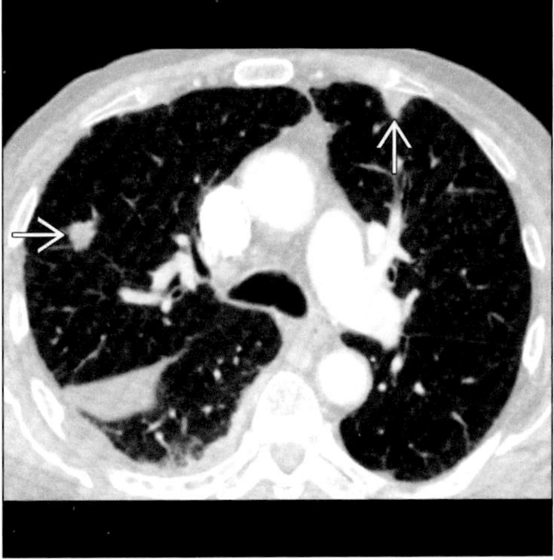

(Left) *Frontal radiograph shows bilateral ill-defined nodules ⇨ in this patient with history of renal cell carcinoma.* ***(Right)*** *Axial CECT shows peripheral pulmonary nodules ➡ due to metastases from renal cell carcinoma. There is a small right pleural effusion. Though well-defined margins are the hallmark of hematogenous metastases, hemorrhagic metastases (renal cell carcinoma, melanoma, choriocarcinoma) often have poorly marginated borders.*

FOCAL LUNG OPACITY

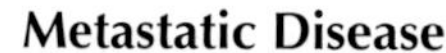

(**Left**) *Axial CECT shows soft tissue nodules within the subcutaneous fat →, ribs →, and lungs → due to metastatic melanoma.* (**Right**) *Axial NECT shows patchy opacities in the lungs highly suggestive of pulmonary hemorrhage given history of hemoptysis and dropping hematocrit.*

Metastatic Disease

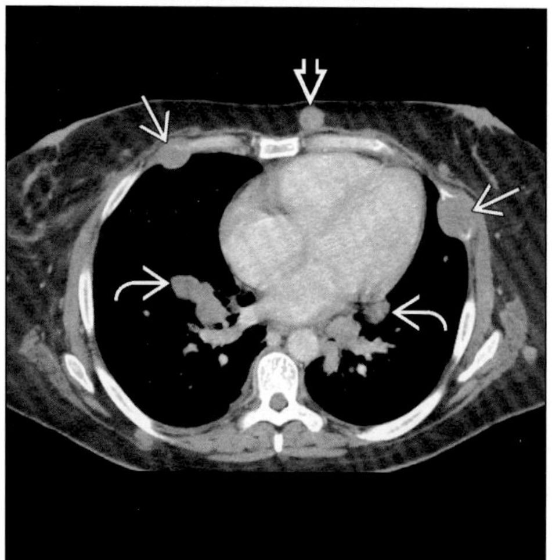

Pulmonary Hemorrhage

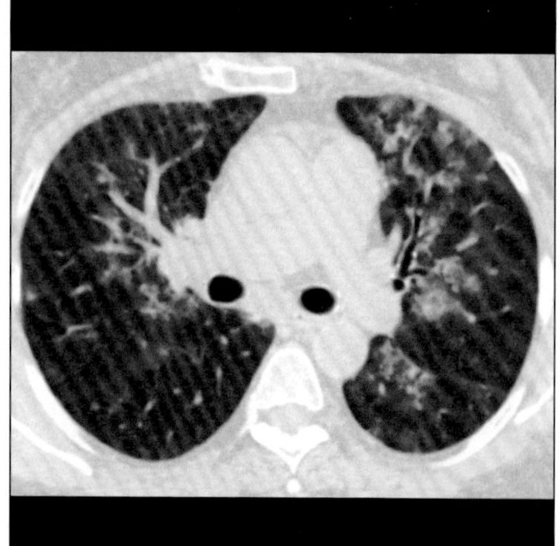

(**Left**) *Frontal radiograph shows subtle opacity in the medial aspect of the right lung apex →. The right hilum → is superiorly displaced suggesting volume loss in the right upper lung. The left hilum is almost always higher than the right hilum.* (**Right**) *Axial NECT shows geographic ground-glass and reticular opacities → in the medial aspect of the right lung apex, highly suggestive of radiation fibrosis from remote radiation therapy.*

Radiation Pneumonitis

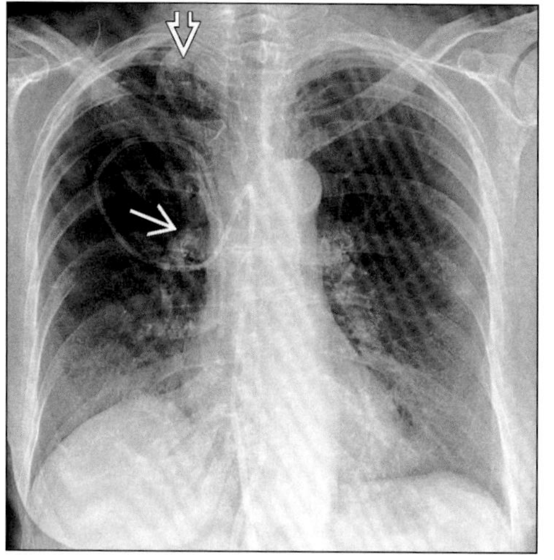

Radiation Pneumonitis

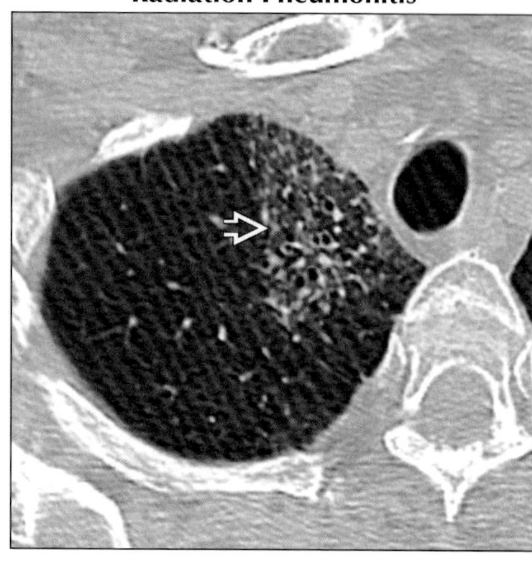

(**Left**) *Axial NECT shows bilateral upper lobe masses with architectural distortion, parenchymal bands →, and scattered subcentimeter nodules → consistent with progressive massive fibrosis from silicosis.* (**Right**) *Axial CECT shows focal ground-glass opacities in the subpleural lung → and surrounding the pulmonary bronchovasculature → due to alveolar sarcoidosis.*

Progressive Massive Fibrosis

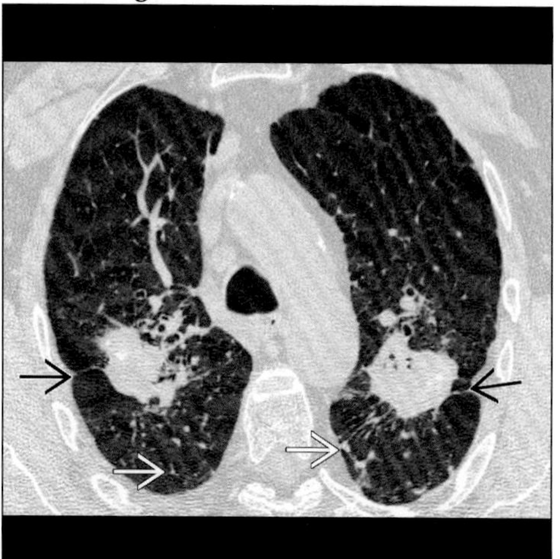

Sarcoidosis

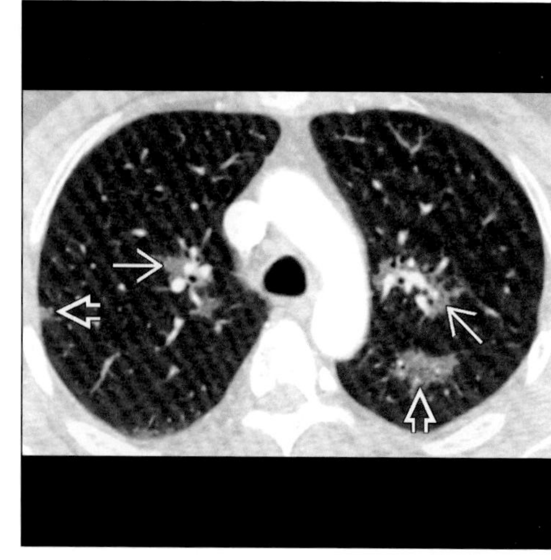

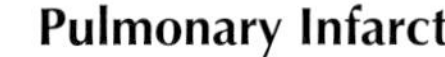

Pulmonary Infarct

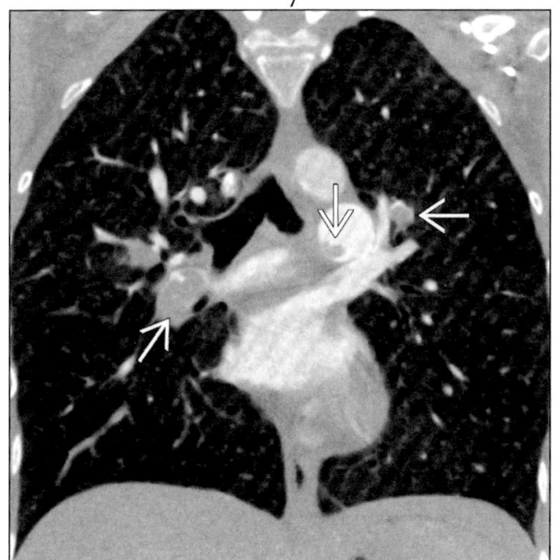

Pulmonary Infarct

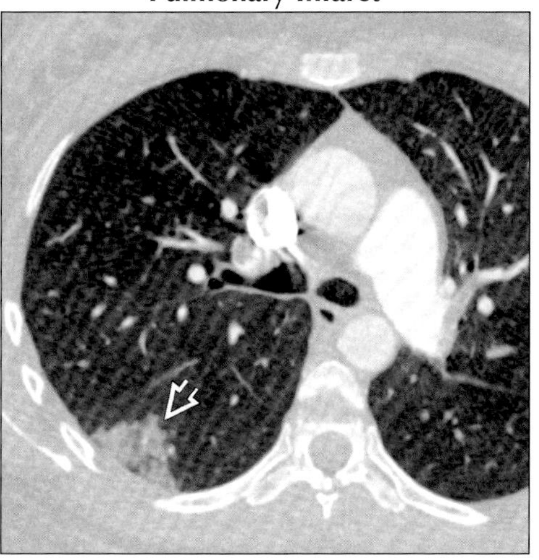

(Left) *Coronal CECT shows filling defects → within the pulmonary arteries due to extensive central pulmonary arterial thromboembolism.* ***(Right)*** *Axial CECT in the same patient shows subpleural consolidation → with internal lucencies highly suggestive of pulmonary infarct. Pulmonary infarcts often demonstrate internal regions of lower density, sometimes in a reverse halo configuration.*

Pulmonary AVM

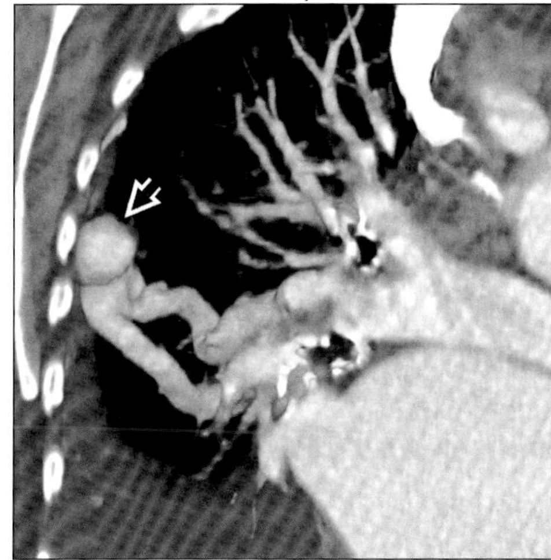

Lymphoma

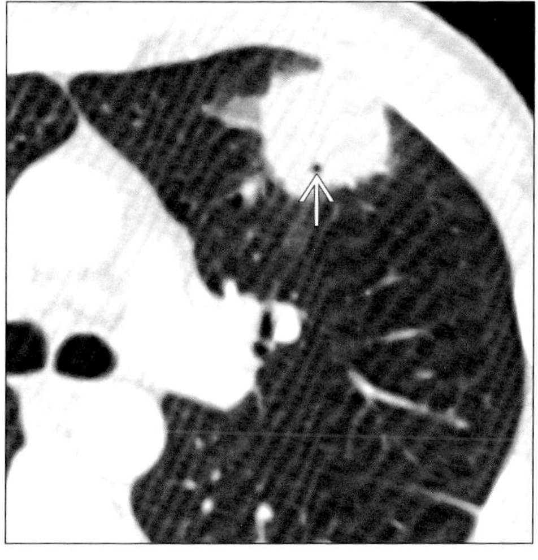

(Left) *Coronal oblique CECT volume rendered image shows a peripheral nodule → in the mid aspect of the right lung with a feeding artery and vein diagnostic of a pulmonary AVM.* ***(Right)*** *Axial CECT shows a nodule with early cavitation → and adjacent areas of ground-glass opacity in the left upper lobe; biopsy demonstrated features suggestive of B-cell lymphoma.*

Lipoid Pneumonia

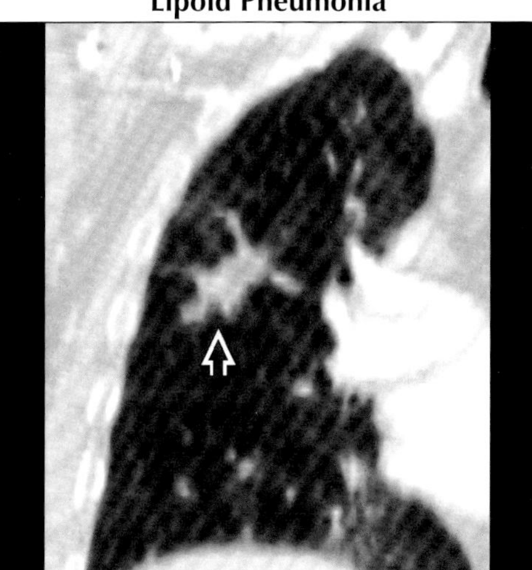

Lipoid Pneumonia

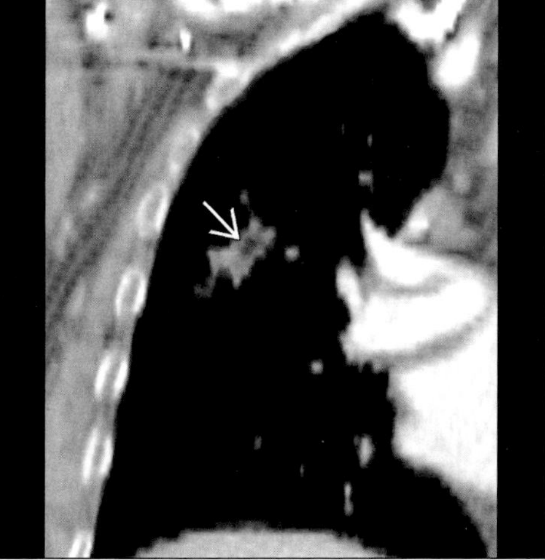

(Left) *Coronal CECT in lung window shows an irregularly marginated opacity → in the right upper lobe worrisome for primary bronchogenic carcinoma.* ***(Right)*** *Coronal CECT in soft tissue window from the same patient shows fatty density → within the focal opacity, highly suggestive of lipoid pneumonia rather than bronchogenic carcinoma.*

LUNG MASS > 3 CM

DIFFERENTIAL DIAGNOSIS

Common
- Lung Cancer
- Lung Metastases
- Pneumonia
  - Mycobacterial Pneumonia
  - Fungal Pneumonia
  - Lung Abscess
- Pseudotumor
- Rounded Atelectasis

Less Common
- Pulmonary Arteriovenous Malformation
- Hematoma
- Bronchogenic Cyst
- Sequestration
- Cystic Adenomatoid Malformation

Rare but Important
- Pulmonary Vein Varix
- Hydatid Cyst (Echinococcal Disease)

ESSENTIAL INFORMATION

Key Differential Diagnosis Issues
- High likelihood of malignancy in pulmonary lesions > 3 cm
- Margins
  - Benign lesions: Smooth margins
  - Malignant lesions: Multilobular, spiculated margins (corona radiata), or pleural tail
- Clinical history essential in suggesting correct radiological diagnosis
  - History of smoking, asbestos exposure, or pulmonary fibrosis: Primary lung cancer
  - Previous malignancy: Metastatic disease
  - Appropriate exposure history: Endemic fungal/mycobacterial/parasitic infection

Helpful Clues for Common Diagnoses
- **Lung Cancer**
  - Most common malignant cause of death
  - Adenocarcinoma most common
  - Most common in upper lung zone (2/3 of primary lung cancers)
  - Spiculated margins, pleural tail, thick-walled cavitation
  - Hilar and mediastinal lymphadenopathy
- **Lung Metastases**
  - Metastases more common in lower lung zones due to increased blood flow
  - Usually multiple, variable sizes, and well marginated
  - Large single metastasis to lungs: Colon cancer, sarcomas, breast cancer, renal cell carcinoma, melanoma
  - Large metastases also in testicular cancer, ovarian cancer, and head and neck cancers, though usually multiple
- **Mycobacterial Pneumonia**
  - Most cases in adults post primary, upper lung consolidation, which may cavitate
  - Tuberculoma
- **Fungal Pneumonia**
  - Immunosuppressed patients susceptible to invasive aspergillosis
  - Endemic fungi: *Histoplasma* and *Blastomyces* in Ohio and Mississippi River valleys, *Coccidioides* in desert southwestern USA
- **Lung Abscess**
  - Irregular, thick-walled cavity; air-fluid level; gravity-dependent portions of lungs secondary to aspiration
- **Pseudotumor**
  - Loculated pleural effusion in pulmonary fissure
  - Common among patients with congestive heart failure
  - Lenticular opacity in fissure
  - Most commonly in minor fissure
  - Margins of pseudotumor taper along course of pulmonary fissure
  - Can be multiple
- **Rounded Atelectasis**
  - Definitive diagnosis on CT requires 4 findings
    - Pleural abnormality: Pleural thickening, pleural effusion, or pleural plaque
    - Broad-based attachment of mass-like consolidation to pleural abnormality
    - Volume loss
    - Comet tail (or hurricane) sign: Swirling of bronchovasculature into mass-like consolidation

Helpful Clues for Less Common Diagnoses
- **Pulmonary Arteriovenous Malformation**
  - Lobulated nodule with feeding artery and vein diagnostic
  - Lower lung predominance

- Associated with Osler-Weber-Rendu syndrome (hereditary hemorrhagic telangiectasis)
- Embolization or surgery considered if feeding artery ≥ 3 mm in diameter

- **Hematoma**
  - Blood filling pulmonary laceration secondary to blunt or penetrating trauma
  - More common in younger patients
  - In blunt trauma, often initially obscured by adjacent contusion on radiographs; readily evident on CT
- **Bronchogenic Cyst**
  - Pulmonary bronchogenic cysts less common than mediastinal bronchogenic cysts
  - Usually medial lower lobes
  - Fluid density, round and well defined
  - Usually asymptomatic and incidental
  - Infection of bronchogenic cysts: Rapid increase in size, development of air or air-fluid levels
- **Sequestration**
  - Nonfunctioning lung, which does not have normal connection with functioning lung
  - Complex mass (solid, &/or cystic) in either of lower lobes with systemic arterial supply
  - Intralobar sequestration
    - 75% of sequestrations
    - Presentation: Recurrent infection in young adults
    - Often pulmonary venous drainage
    - Shares visceral pleura with normal lung
    - Air-trapping
  - Extralobar sequestration
    - 25% of sequestrations
    - Presentation: Respiratory distress in neonates
    - Often systemic venous drainage
    - Isolated visceral pleura
- **Cystic Adenomatoid Malformation**
  - Multicystic lesion in lobe
  - Can contain gas, fluid, or combination

Helpful Clues for Rare Diagnoses

- **Pulmonary Vein Varix**
  - Isolated dilation of pulmonary vein usually in right lower lobe
  - Often associated with mitral stenosis or mitral regurgitation
- **Hydatid Cyst (Echinococcal Disease)**
  - Endemic to Mediterranean, Africa, and Australia: Most commonly in sheep- and cattle-raising areas
  - Meniscus sign: Crescent of gas around endocyst
  - Cyst rupture: Air around or within endocyst, crumpled membranes float in fluid
    - Variety of descriptive terms, e.g., meniscus/crescent sign, "water lily" sign, "rising sun," "serpent" sign, "whirl" sign, "onion peel" sign, and "cumbo" sign
  - Hepatic cystic lesions; right hepatic lobe > left hepatic lobe

Lung Cancer

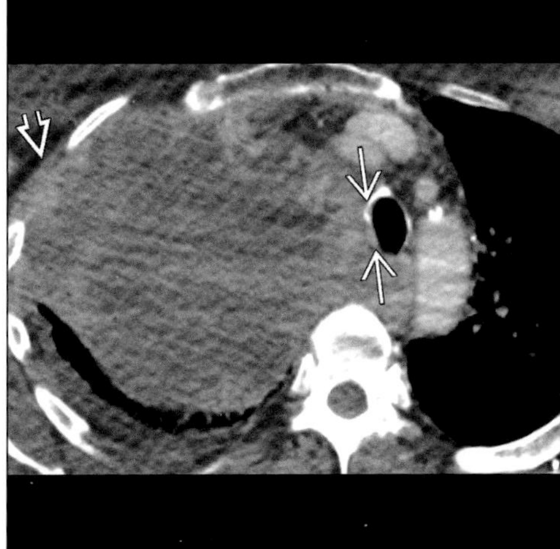

Axial CECT shows a large mass in right upper lobe with leftward mediastinal shift & extrapleural extension ➡. Fat plane between mass and trachea has been obliterated ➡, suggesting possible tracheal invasion.

Lung Metastases

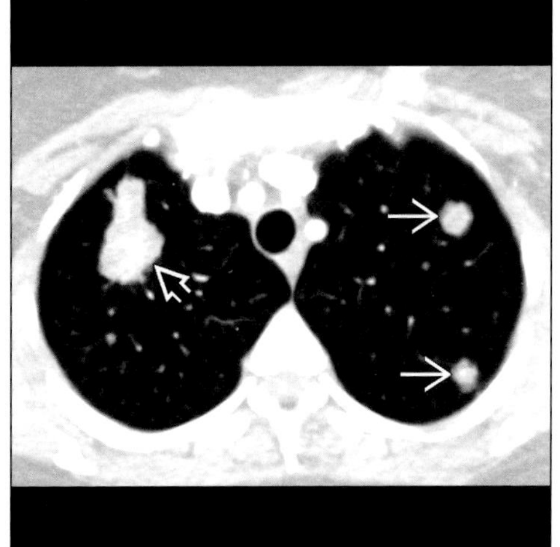

Axial CECT shows a right apical pulmonary mass ➡ and 2 left apical pulmonary nodules ➡. The multiplicity of pulmonary lesions argues against primary pulmonary neoplasms.

LUNG MASS > 3 CM

(Left) *Axial CECT shows a large right apical cavitary mass-like area of consolidation. Clustered nodules with associated pleural tags are present in the left upper lobe in this patient with active post-primary tuberculosis.* **(Right)** *Axial CECT shows focal mass-like consolidation in the posterior segment of the right upper lobe with central low attenuation ➔ suggesting necrosis.*

Mycobacterial Pneumonia

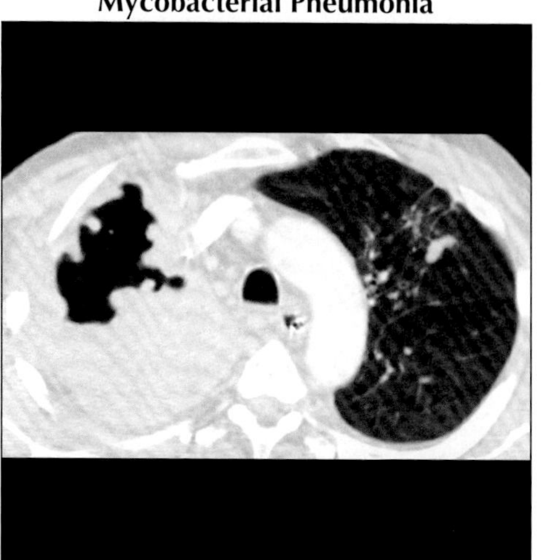

Lung Abscess

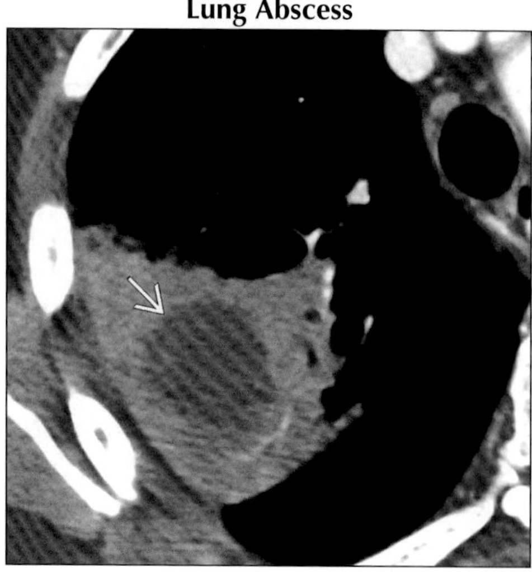

(Left) *Frontal radiograph shows an oval mass ➔ in the peripheral mid right lung in this patient with cardiomegaly and a history of heart failure.* **(Right)** *Lateral radiograph shows that the mass is located along the minor fissure and has tapered anterior and posterior margins (best seen anteriorly ➔). Findings are most consistent with a loculated pleural fluid collection.*

Pseudotumor

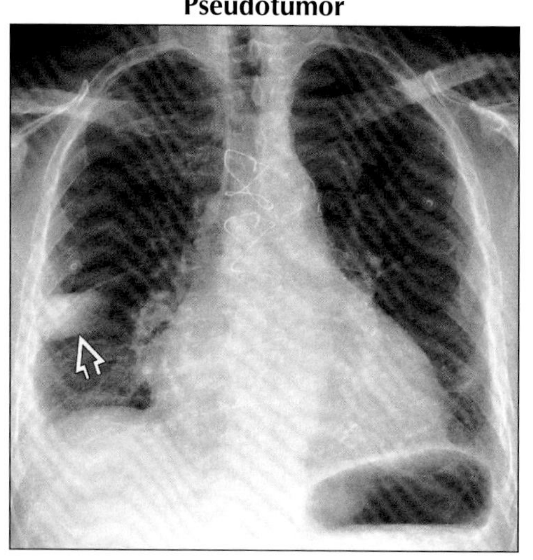

Pseudotumor

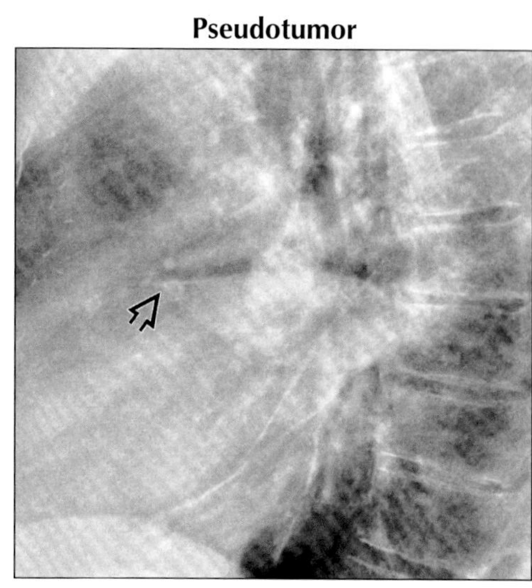

(Left) *Axial NECT shows a rounded mass in the right lower lobe with broad-based attachment to calcified pleural thickening. There is characteristic swirling of the bronchovasculature into the mass-like consolidation ➔ (the comet tail sign).* **(Right)** *Axial CECT shows a serpiginous cluster of vessels ➔ in the right lower lobe, highly suggestive of a pulmonary arteriovenous malformation. Bilateral pleural effusions and dilation of the right heart are also present.*

Rounded Atelectasis

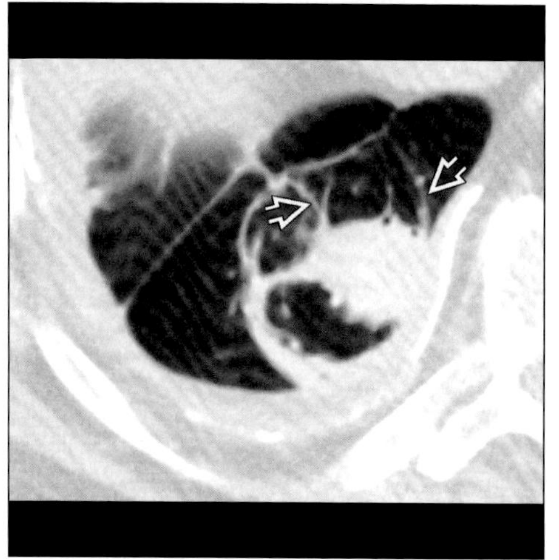

Pulmonary Arteriovenous Malformation

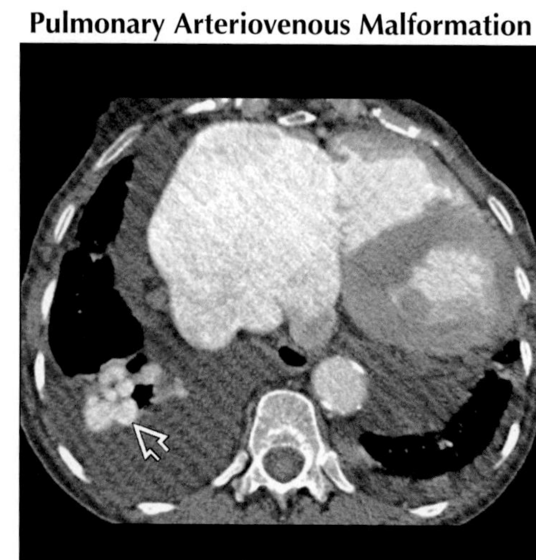

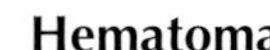

Hematoma

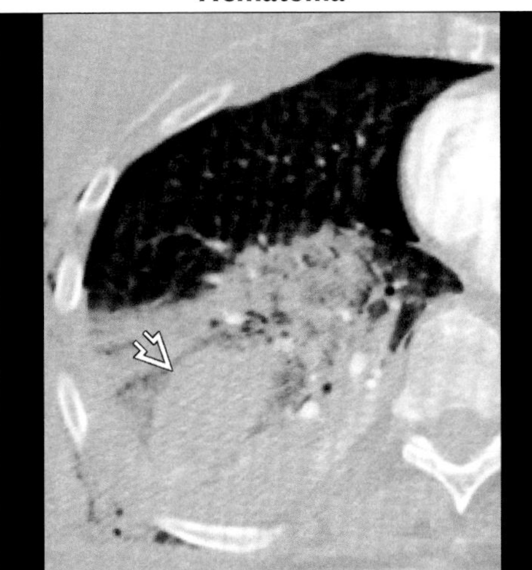

Sequestration

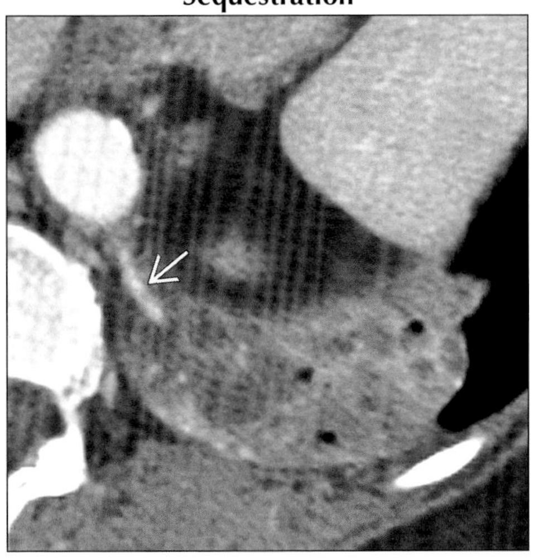

(Left) *Axial CECT shows a right lower lobe pulmonary hematoma ➔. Adjacent consolidation and ground-glass opacities represent pulmonary hemorrhage and contusion. Right pneumothorax and subcutaneous emphysema are also present.* ***(Right)*** *Axial CECT shows a complex mass ➔ in the left lower lobe with systemic arterial supply, diagnostic of a sequestration.*

Cystic Adenomatoid Malformation

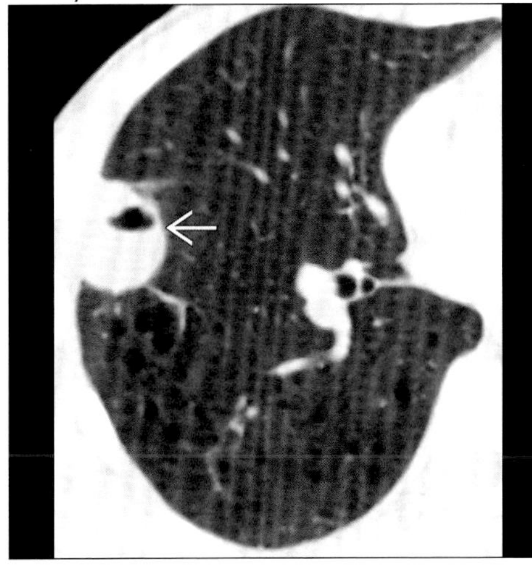

Hydatid Cyst (Echinococcal Disease)

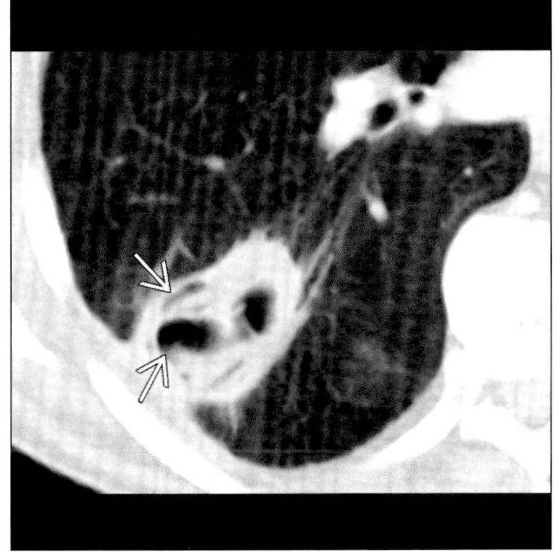

(Left) *Axial CECT shows a complex, predominantly cystic mass ➔ in the right lower lobe; no systemic arterial supply is present. The gas-fluid level present within the lateral aspect of the mass represents superinfection of the mass.* ***(Right)*** *Axial CECT shows gas outlining both sides of the endocyst membrane ➔, diagnostic of a hydatid cyst. There is adjacent postinflammatory pleural thickening.*

Pulmonary Vein Varix

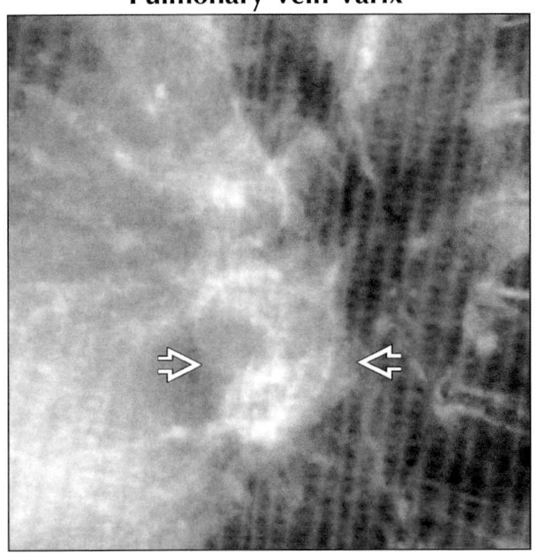

Pulmonary Vein Varix

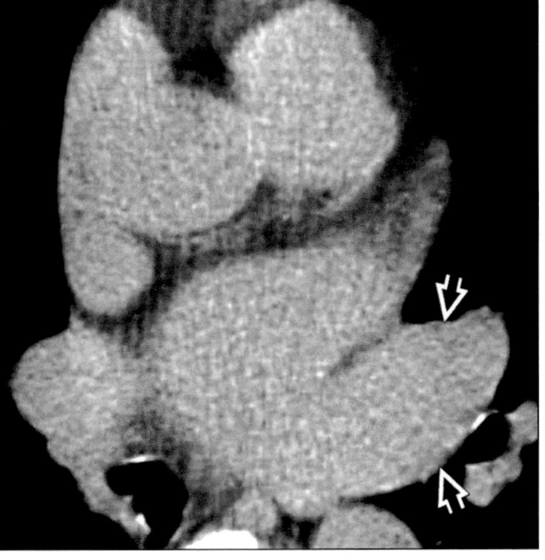

(Left) *Lateral radiograph shows a round mass ➔ overlying the posterior aspect of the heart.* ***(Right)*** *Axial NECT shows that the mass on lateral chest radiograph represents a large left-sided pulmonary vein varix ➔.*

ACUTE PULMONARY CONSOLIDATION

DIFFERENTIAL DIAGNOSIS

Common

- Pneumonia
- Cardiogenic Pulmonary Edema
- Atelectasis
- Aspiration
- Pulmonary Contusion
- Pulmonary Hemorrhage

Less Common

- Hypersensitivity Pneumonitis (Acute)
- Diffuse Alveolar Damage
- Pulmonary Infarct

Rare but Important

- Acute Eosinophilic Pneumonia
- "Crack Lung"

ESSENTIAL INFORMATION

Helpful Clues for Common Diagnoses

- **Pneumonia**
  - Airspace opacities: Ground-glass to dense consolidation
  - Reactive lymphadenopathy; very large lymph nodes unusual
  - Parapneumonic pleural effusion or empyema
  - Correlation with sputum, WBC count, and clinical presentation paramount
- **Cardiogenic Pulmonary Edema**
  - Due to imbalances in Starling forces: Usually due to increased pulmonary venous pressure
    - Left-sided heart failure (myocardial infarct or ischemic cardiomyopathy)
    - Fluid overload or renal failure
    - Mitral valve disease
  - Interlobular septal thickening: Kerley-B and Kerley-A lines on chest radiograph
  - Diffuse, hazy airspace opacities
    - Characteristically central-predominant due to higher concentration of lymphatics in peripheral aspect of lungs
  - Cardiomegaly frequently noted
  - Signs of coronary artery disease (coronary artery calcification, CABG, coronary artery stents, subendocardial fatty metaplasia)
- **Atelectasis**
  - Subsegmental
    - Discoid or linear opacity most often in mid and lower lungs
    - Hypoventilation or decreased diaphragmatic excursion (splinting, neuromuscular abnormality, subdiaphragmatic mass effect)
    - Small airways disease (secretions leading to resorptive atelectasis, asthma, viral bronchiolitis)
    - Decreased surfactant production (pulmonary embolism)
    - Compression (mass effect from adjacent pathology)
  - Lobar
    - Lobar volume loss: Displacement of pulmonary fissures, ipsilateral shift of mediastinum and hilum toward affected lobe, superior shift of diaphragm
    - Increased opacity of affected lobe
    - Combined right middle and lower lobe atelectasis from bronchus intermedius obstruction; mimics pleural effusion
    - In acute setting, most often due to obstruction of bronchus due to mucous plugging or foreign body
- **Aspiration**
  - Consolidation in gravity-dependent portions of lungs
  - Predisposed patients (e.g., those with alcoholism, epilepsy, hiatal hernia, esophageal dysmotility or obstruction, neuromuscular disorders)
  - Supine: Superior segments of lower lobes and posterior segments of upper lobes
  - Upright: Basilar segments of lower lobes
  - Centrilobular or tree in bud opacities common on CT
  - Can progress to necrotizing pneumonia or pulmonary abscess without treatment
- **Pulmonary Contusion**
  - Acute blunt trauma; appears at time of injury and resolves in 3-5 days
  - Peripheral, under point of blunt kinetic energy absorption
    - Often lateral portions of lung away from overlying musculature
    - Overlying rib fractures; but can occur without rib fractures in children and young adults
- **Pulmonary Hemorrhage**
  - Widespread
    - Vasculitis, anticoagulation, idiopathic pulmonary hemosiderosis

- Focal
  - Mass, aspiration, bronchiectasis, trauma
- Ground-glass opacities > consolidation; may be diffuse, patchy, lobular, or centrilobular
- Tendency to spare peripheral, apical, and costophrenic aspects of lungs
- Increased interlobular and intralobular septal thickening over 1-2 days
- Rapid resolution in days, though not as rapid as in cardiogenic pulmonary edema or bland aspiration
- In recurrent hemorrhage, may result in lung fibrosis

Helpful Clues for Less Common Diagnoses

- **Hypersensitivity Pneumonitis (Acute)**
  - Allergic reaction to airborne organic particles
  - Diffuse or centrilobular ground-glass opacities; lobular air-trapping
- **Diffuse Alveolar Damage**
  - Noncardiogenic pulmonary edema
  - Clinical correlate is acute respiratory distress syndrome
  - Heterogeneous, diffuse ground-glass opacities and consolidation
  - Often with anterior-posterior and superior-inferior gradient
  - Large pleural effusions and severe interlobular septal thickening uncommon
  - Varicoid bronchiectasis, reticular opacities, and honeycombing common 2-3 weeks after onset of respiratory distress
- **Pulmonary Infarct**
  - Most often from pulmonary arterial embolism
  - Often in setting of superimposed cardiac dysfunction (cardiomyopathy, congestive heart failure)
  - Lower lung predominant, peripheral/subpleural, wedge-shaped consolidation: Hampton hump sign
  - Resolves over months; retains its original shape rather than patchy resolution as in pneumonia

Helpful Clues for Rare Diagnoses

- **Acute Eosinophilic Pneumonia**
  - Probable hypersensitivity reaction to inhaled agents; possible association with smoking
  - Imaging mimics pulmonary edema
    - Ground-glass opacities > consolidation
    - Interlobular septal thickening
    - Pleural effusions
  - Acute high fever, profound dyspnea, myalgia, pleuritic chest pain
  - Responds rapidly to steroids
- **"Crack Lung"**
  - "Crack" = smoked form of cocaine
  - Hypersensitivity reaction, pulmonary hemorrhage, pulmonary edema (cardiogenic and noncardiogenic)
  - Noncardiogenic pulmonary edema may be peripheral and bilateral as opposed to cardiogenic edema
  - Pneumomediastinum or pneumothorax

Pneumonia

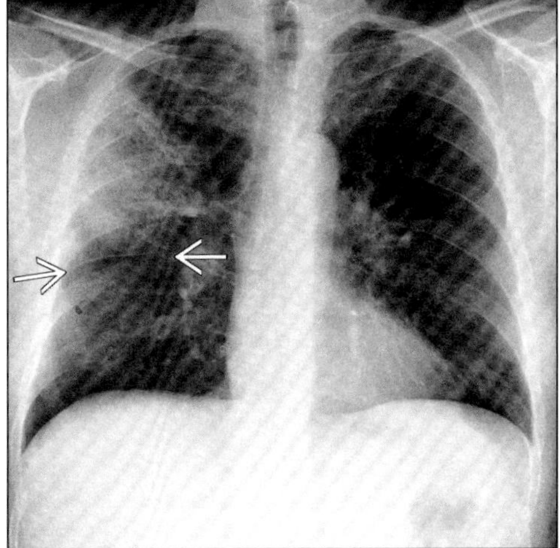

Frontal radiograph shows consolidation in the right upper lobe, marginated inferiorly by the minor fissure ➡, highly suggestive of pneumonia in this patient with cough and fever.

Pneumonia

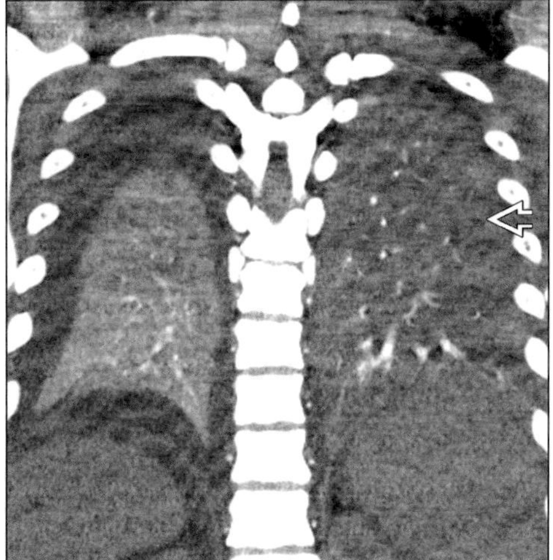

Coronal CECT shows consolidation of both lower lobes. The lower attenuation of the left lower lobe ➡ suggests superimposed pneumonia or aspiration, while the denser right lower lobe suggests atelectasis.

ACUTE PULMONARY CONSOLIDATION

(Left) *Frontal radiograph shows cardiomegaly and prominence of interstitial markings suggestive of cardiogenic pulmonary edema.* **(Right)** *Axial CECT in the same patient shows thickening of the interlobular septa* → *and increased prominence of the centrilobular aspect* ➡ *of the secondary pulmonary lobules, highly suggestive of cardiogenic pulmonary edema.*

Cardiogenic Pulmonary Edema

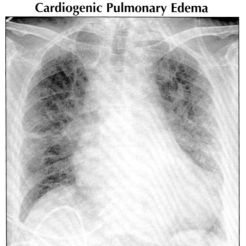

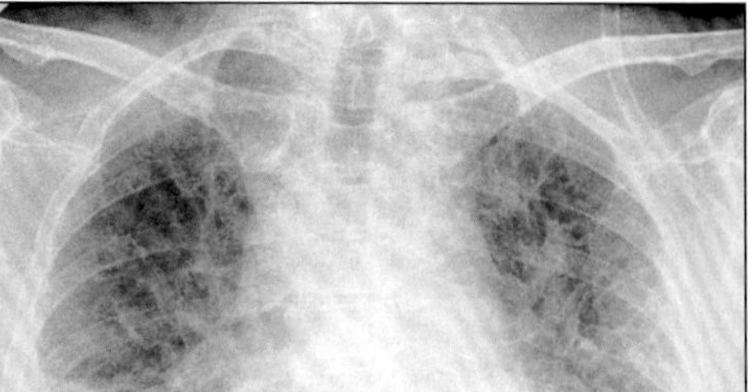

Cardiogenic Pulmonary Edema

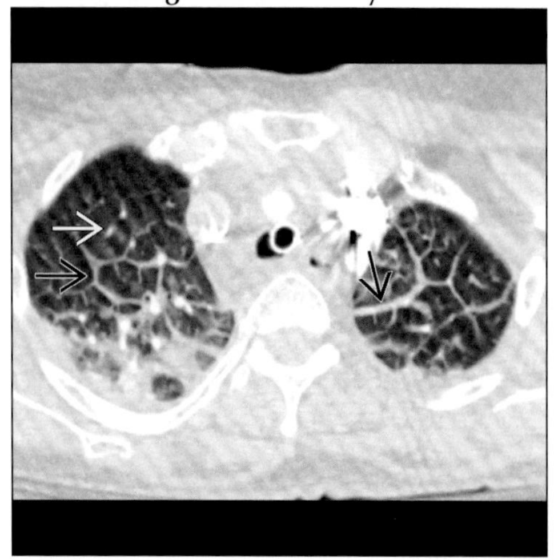

(Left) *Axial CECT in this vasculopathic patient shows cardiomegaly, interlobular septal thickening* ➡*, and small pleural effusions highly consistent with cardiogenic pulmonary edema.* **(Right)** *Frontal radiograph shows diffuse pulmonary opacities most consistent with pulmonary edema, though diffuse alveolar damage, diffuse pneumonia, aspiration, or diffuse pulmonary hemorrhage could also have this appearance in the acute setting.*

Cardiogenic Pulmonary Edema

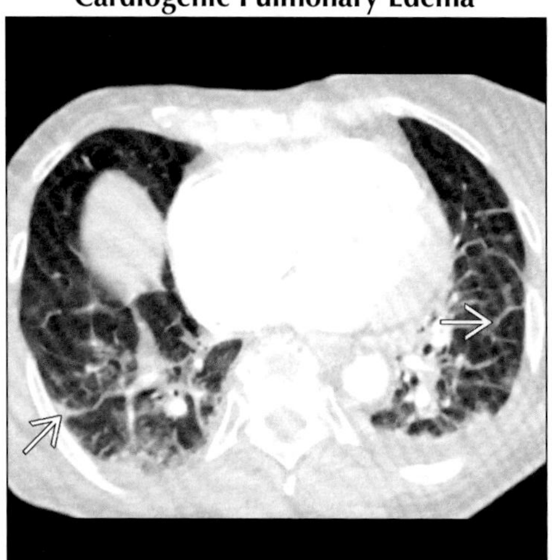

Cardiogenic Pulmonary Edema

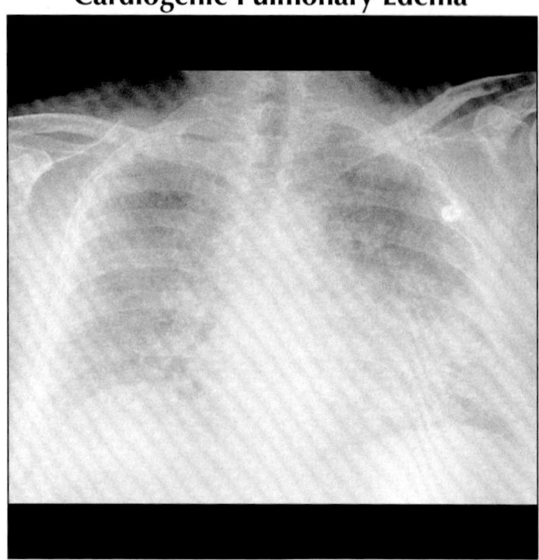

(Left) *Coronal CECT shows diffuse ground-glass opacities throughout the lungs with thickening of the interlobular septa* ➡ *suggestive of cardiogenic pulmonary edema. Pulmonary abnormalities cleared rapidly with diuresis.* **(Right)** *Frontal radiograph shows diffuse hazy opacity sparing the paraaortic* ➡ *aspect of the left lung (luftsichel sign) and silhouetting the left heart border. There is a juxtaphrenic peak* ➡*. Findings are diagnostic of left upper lobe atelectasis.*

Cardiogenic Pulmonary Edema

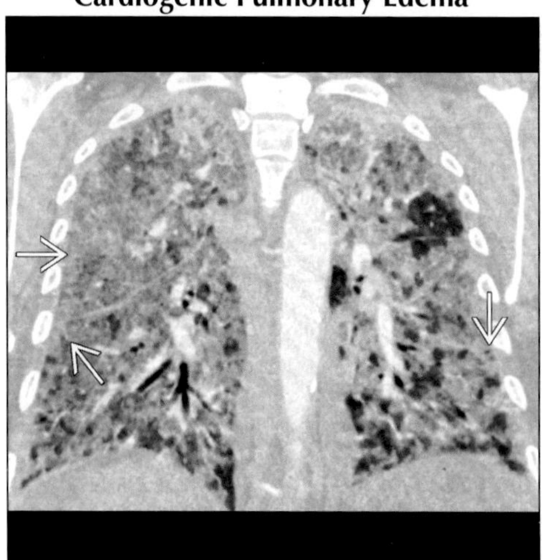

Atelectasis

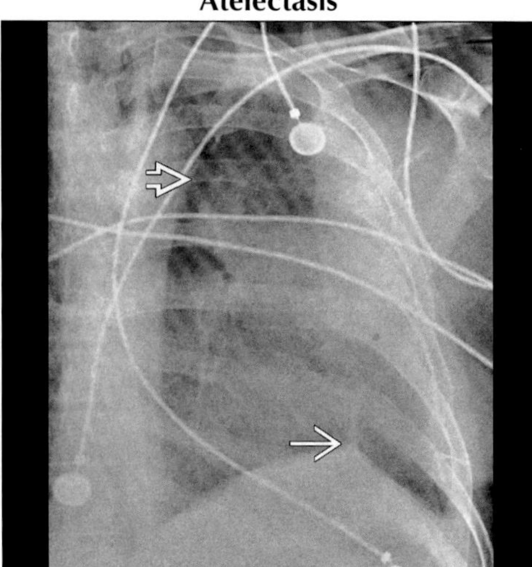

ACUTE PULMONARY CONSOLIDATION

Atelectasis

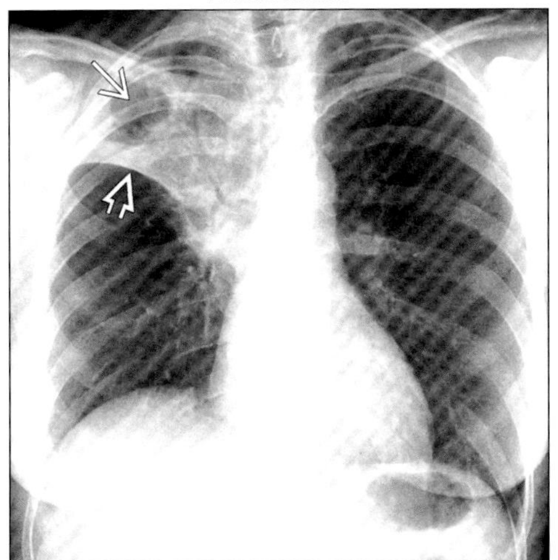

Atelectasis

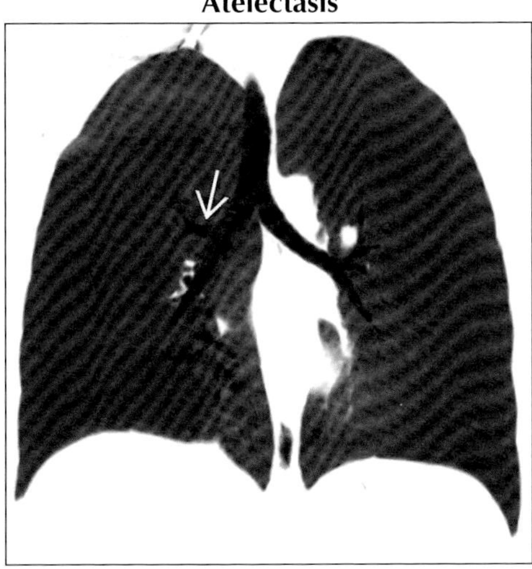

(Left) *Frontal radiograph shows partial right upper lobe atelectasis with superior displacement of the minor fissure ➡. There is persistent aeration of the right apex ➡.* ***(Right)*** *Coronal NECT minIP image from the same patient shows re-expansion of the right upper lobe without underlying endobronchial or central lung lesion. The transient right upper lobe atelectasis was thought to be most likely due to mucous plugging. Note the right upper lobe bronchus ➡.*

Aspiration

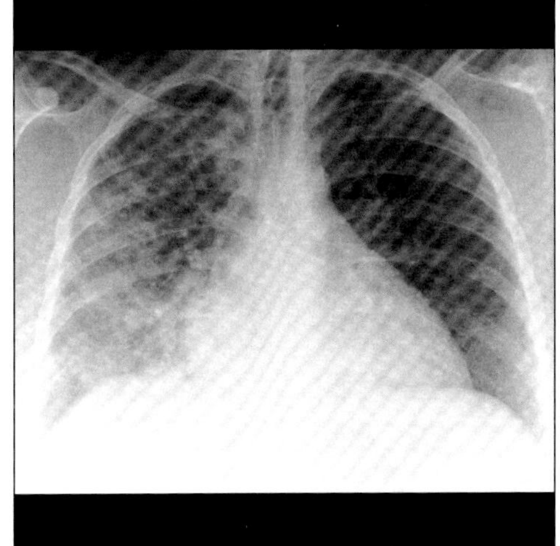

Aspiration

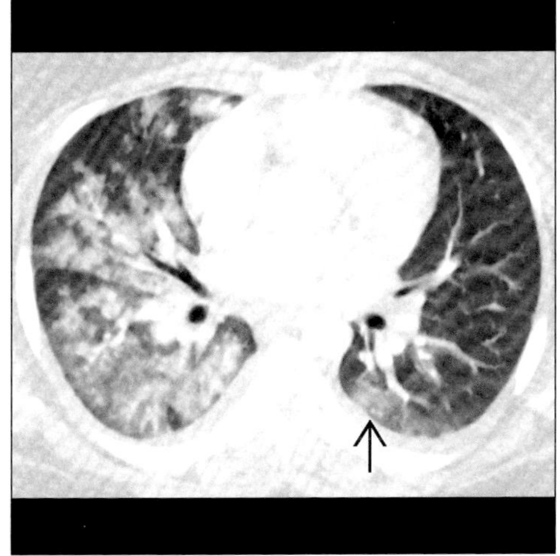

(Left) *Frontal radiograph shows patchy airspace opacities throughout the right lung and in the retrocardiac aspect of the left lower lobe.* ***(Right)*** *Axial CECT shows patchy consolidation and ground-glass opacities throughout the right lung and in the medial aspect ➡ of the left lower lobe. Findings were thought most likely to represent aspiration, given that the patient slept on her right side and had a recent seizure.*

Aspiration

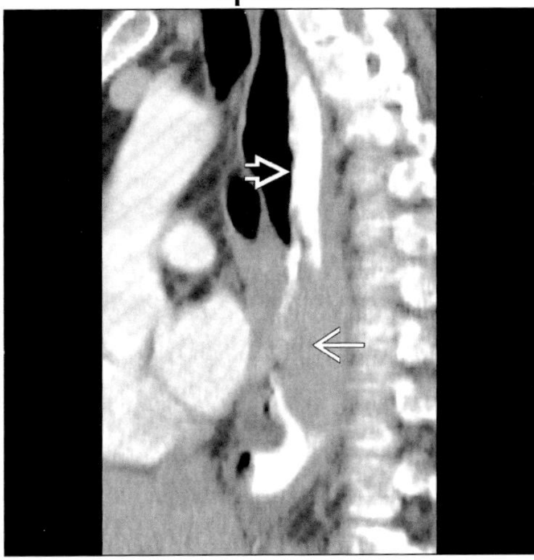

Aspiration

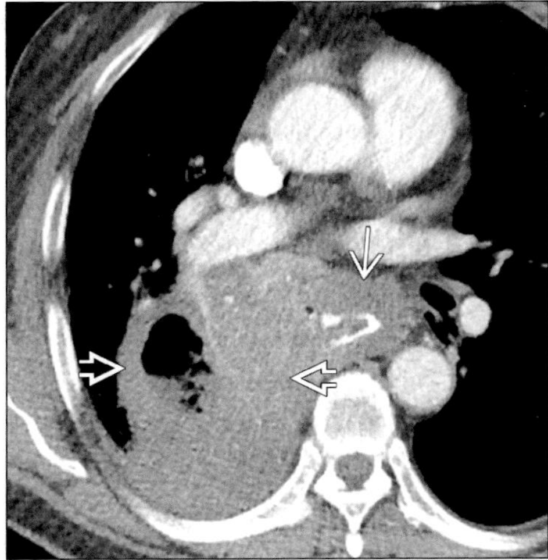

(Left) *Sagittal CECT shows a nodular cancer in the distal esophagus ➡ with proximal esophageal dilation and a gas-contrast level ➡, which puts the patient at risk for aspiration.* ***(Right)*** *Axial CECT in the same patient shows cavitary consolidation ➡ in the right lung highly consistent with a pulmonary abscess given the patient's aspiration risk. The distal esophageal cancer ➡ is again shown.*

ACUTE PULMONARY CONSOLIDATION

(Left) Axial CECT shows airspace opacities in the right lower lobe likely representing a combination of contusion, hematoma, and atelectasis. The rib fracture ➔, pneumothorax ➔, and subcutaneous emphysema resulted from recent blunt trauma. (Right) Coronal NECT shows patchy ground-glass opacities ➔ consistent with pulmonary hemorrhage given this patient's history of hemoptysis and dropping hematocrit.

Pulmonary Contusion

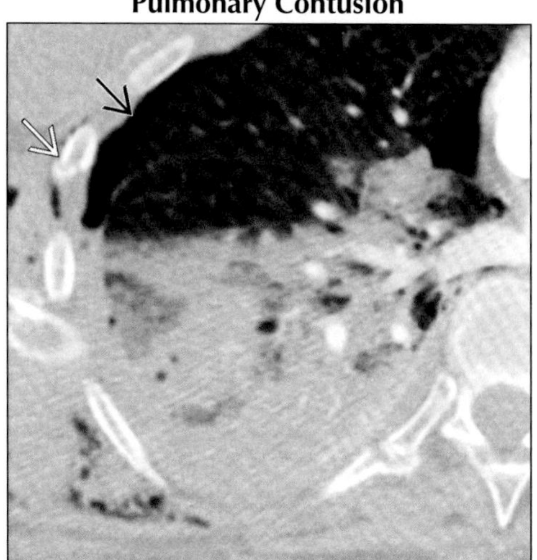

Pulmonary Hemorrhage

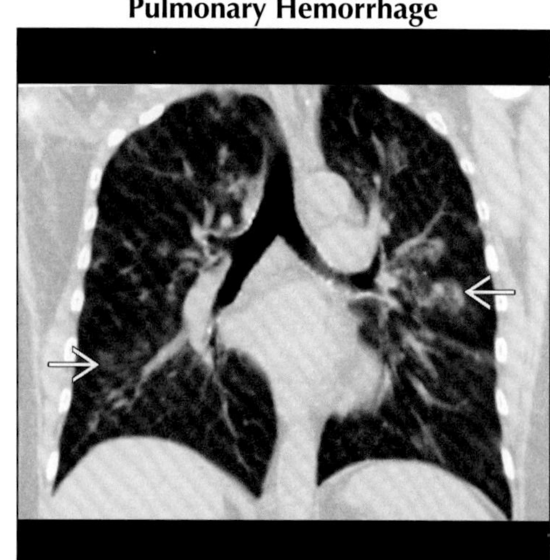

(Left) Axial NECT in the same patient shows patchy opacities ➔ in the lungs. The differential diagnosis is broad without correlation with history of hemoptysis and dropping hematocrit. (Right) Axial HRCT shows diffuse ground-glass opacities with focal lobular regions of sparing ➔, suggesting air-trapping, consistent with hypersensitivity pneumonitis.

Pulmonary Hemorrhage

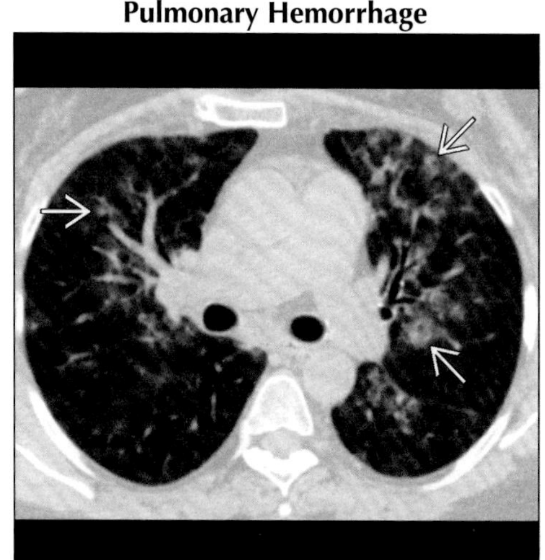

Hypersensitivity Pneumonitis (Acute)

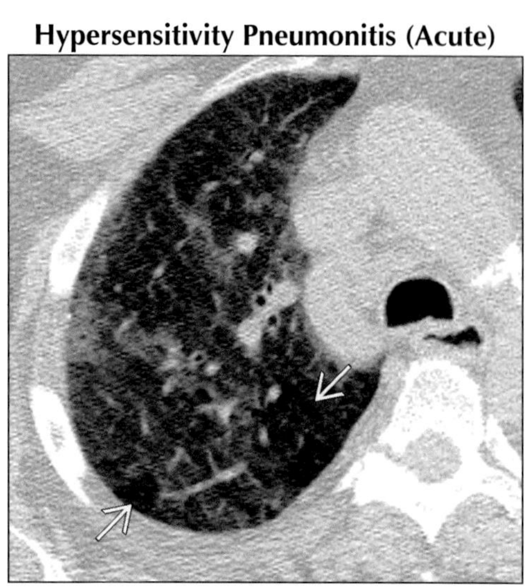

(Left) Axial HRCT in the same patient shows denser regions of ground-glass opacity and patchy foci of probable lobular air-trapping ➔ consistent with hypersensitivity pneumonitis (head cheese sign). (Right) Axial CECT shows diffuse airspace opacities with a dependent gradient (more consolidative in the dependent aspect of the lungs) consistent with diffuse alveolar damage in this patient with acute respiratory distress syndrome. Small left pleural effusion is present.

Hypersensitivity Pneumonitis (Acute)

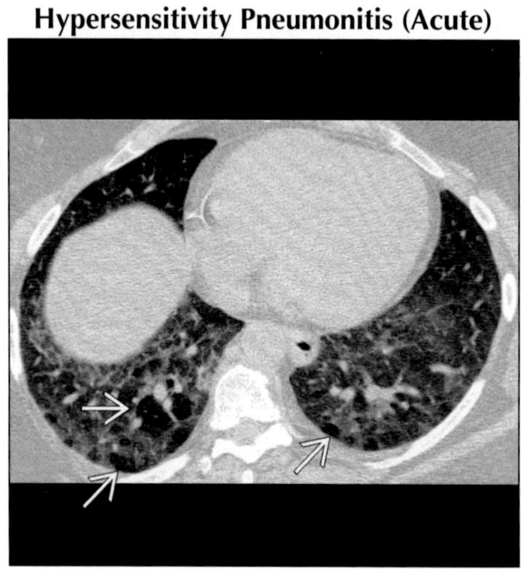

Diffuse Alveolar Damage

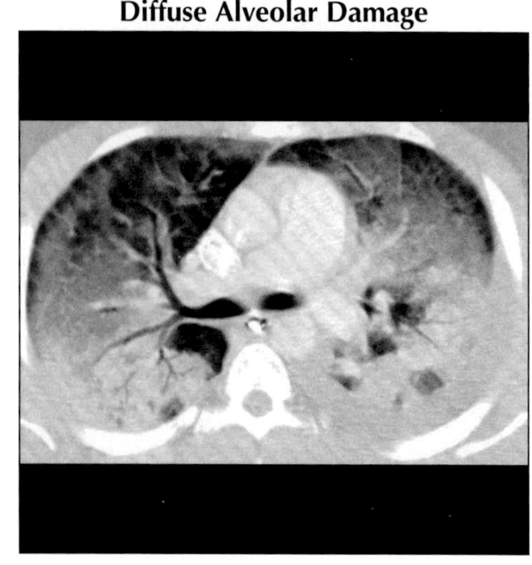

Diffuse Alveolar Damage

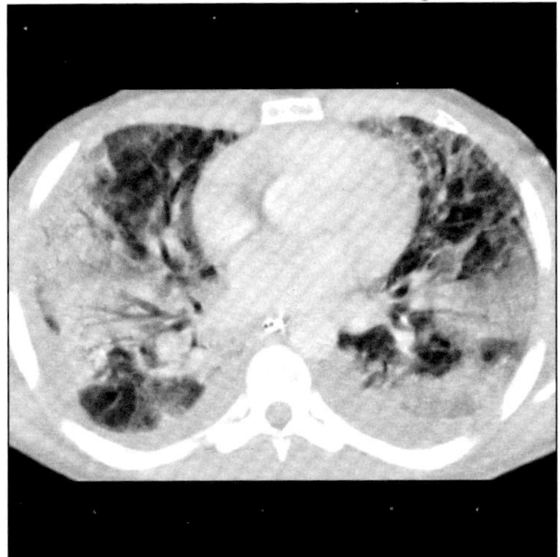

Diffuse Alveolar Damage

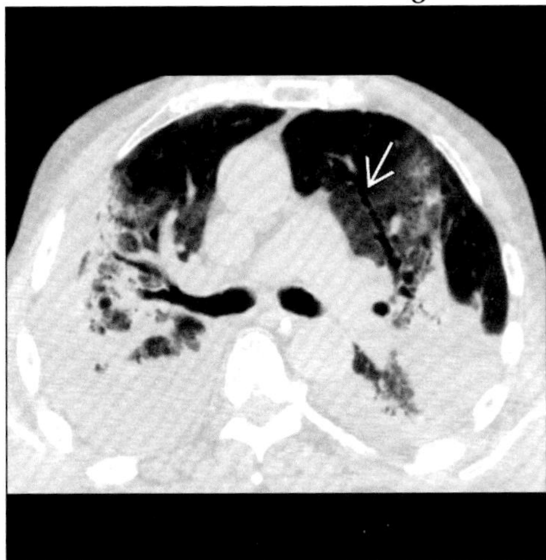

*(**Left**) Axial NECT shows diffuse, heterogeneous airspace opacities and small pleural effusions suggestive of diffuse alveolar damage in this patient with sepsis. (**Right**) Axial NECT shows dependent ground-glass opacities and consolidation with mild varicoid bronchiectasis ➔ in the left upper lobe suggestive of diffuse alveolar damage. Findings consistent with pulmonary fibrosis often occur within weeks of onset of diffuse alveolar damage.*

Pulmonary Infarct

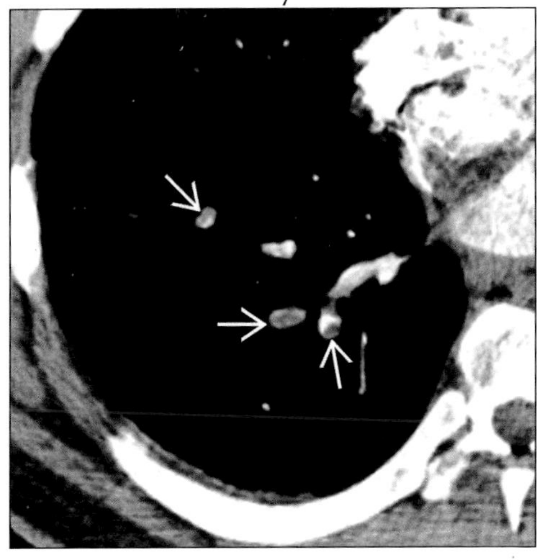

Pulmonary Infarct

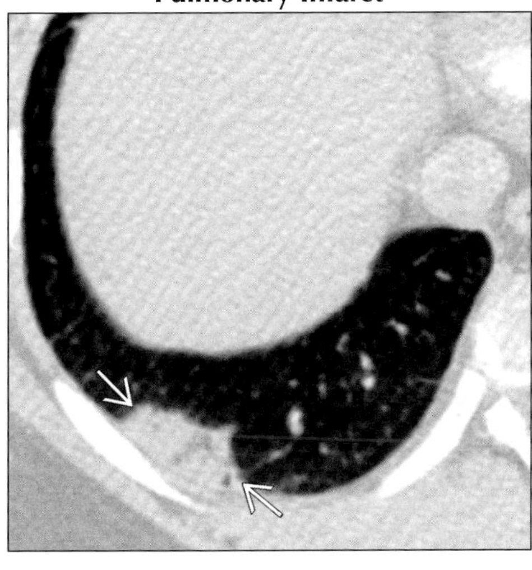

*(**Left**) Axial CECT shows small filling defects ➔ in the right lower lobe pulmonary arteries, diagnostic of pulmonary emboli in this patient with chest pain and shortness of breath. (**Right**) Axial CECT in the same patient shows subpleural, wedge-shaped consolidation ➔ in the right lower lobe, highly suggestive of pulmonary infarct given concomitant pulmonary emboli. The patient had a history of reduced left ventricular ejection fraction.*

Acute Eosinophilic Pneumonia

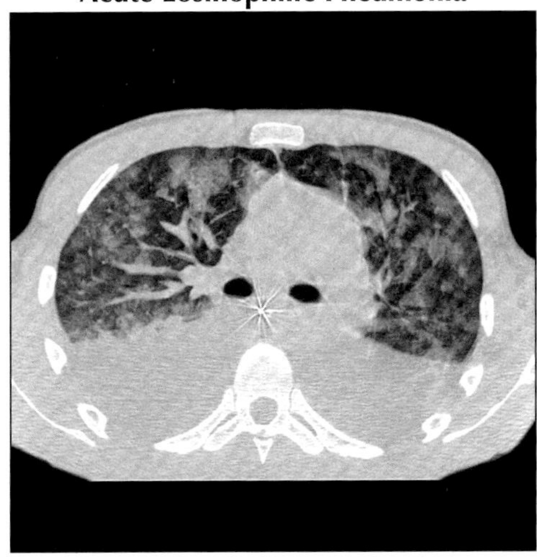

"Crack Lung"

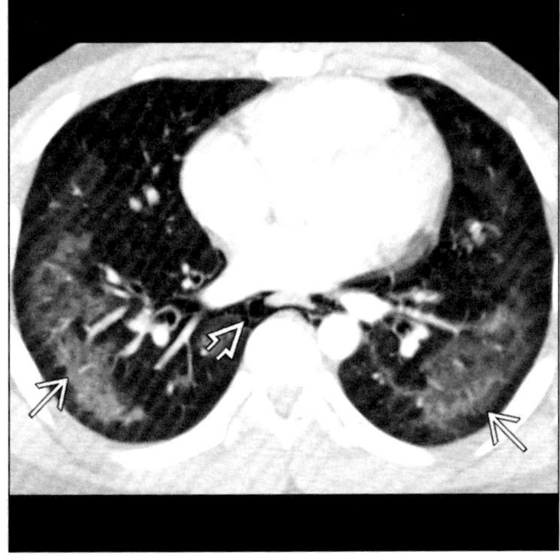

*(**Left**) Axial HRCT shows diffuse, multifocal ground-glass opacities with patchy areas of lobular sparing and large bilateral pleural effusions in this patient with acute eosinophilic pneumonia. Imaging findings in this condition mimic pulmonary edema. (**Right**) Axial CECT shows ground-glass opacity ➔ in the peripheral lungs with subpleural sparing and pneumomediastinum ➲; this patient admitted to recent heavy use of "crack" cocaine.*

CHRONIC PULMONARY CONSOLIDATION

DIFFERENTIAL DIAGNOSIS

Common
- Endobronchial Tumor
- Aspiration
- Bronchioloalveolar Carcinoma

Less Common
- Coccidioidomycosis
- Blastomycosis
- Cryptogenic Organizing Pneumonia
- Lymphoma
- Chronic Eosinophilic Pneumonia

Rare but Important
- Sarcoidosis
- Lipoid Pneumonia
- Churg-Strauss Syndrome
- Pulmonary Alveolar Proteinosis

ESSENTIAL INFORMATION

Key Differential Diagnosis Issues
- Acute vs. chronic

Helpful Clues for Common Diagnoses
- **Endobronchial Tumor**
  - Endobronchial soft tissue mass or broncholith obstructing bronchus
  - Air bronchograms often absent within consolidation
    - CT may show fluid attenuation filling bronchi
  - Signs of volume loss, such as fissural or hilar displacement
  - Consider broncholith in presence of calcified lung nodules and calcified lymph nodes
- **Aspiration**
  - Basal predominant consolidation, often bilateral
  - CT shows peribronchial consolidation with bronchial wall thickening and tree in bud opacities
    - Debris and fluid in central airways
    - Bronchiectasis suggests chronicity
  - Findings of esophageal dysmotility such as retained fluid and debris
- **Bronchioloalveolar Carcinoma**
  - Slowly progressive lung consolidation
    - May increase in both size and density
  - CT often shows mixed consolidation and ground-glass opacity
    - Crazy-paving and septal thickening less common
    - Dilated airways within consolidation: "Pseudocavitation"

Helpful Clues for Less Common Diagnoses
- **Coccidioidomycosis**
  - Endemic in desert regions of southwestern USA
  - Single or multiple foci of lung consolidation
  - Nodules less common, may cavitate
  - Lymphadenopathy in 20% of patients
  - Pleural effusion in 10-20% of patients
- **Blastomycosis**
  - Endemic in central and eastern USA along major rivers and around the Great Lakes
  - Single or multiple foci of lung consolidation
    - Slow to resolve or respond to therapy
  - Nodules and masses; cavitate in 1/3 of patients
  - Lymphadenopathy uncommon
  - Pleural effusion in 20% of patients
- **Cryptogenic Organizing Pneumonia**
  - Subpleural, peribronchial, or perilobular consolidation or ground-glass opacity
    - Often has basal predominance
    - May wax and wane without treatment
  - Atoll or reverse halo sign: Focus of ground-glass opacity surrounded by ring-like or crescentic consolidation (20% of patients)
    - May also occur with infection, hemorrhage, and vasculitis
  - Responds to steroids
- **Lymphoma**
  - Multiple nodules or foci of consolidation with associated lymphadenopathy
  - Primary pulmonary lymphoma far less common than secondary involvement
    - May present as solitary lung nodule or mass
- **Chronic Eosinophilic Pneumonia**
  - Mid and upper lung predominant peripheral consolidation
  - "Reverse bat-wing" or "photographic negative of pulmonary edema" pattern on radiography
  - Responsive to steroid therapy

Helpful Clues for Rare Diagnoses
- **Sarcoidosis**

- Chronic lung consolidation uncommon manifestation
  - Upper lung predominance with air bronchograms
  - HRCT may show cluster of tiny nodules "galaxy" sign
  - Other features of sarcoidosis often present (e.g., lymphadenopathy)
- **Lipoid Pneumonia**
  - Chronic mass-like consolidation and ground-glass opacity
    - Basal predominance (similar distribution to other causes of aspiration)
    - Fat attenuation of consolidation on CT virtually diagnostic
  - Mineral oil aspiration most common cause (exogenous)
  - Endogenous lipoid pneumonia from impaired surfactant metabolism
    - Chronic amiodarone therapy
- **Churg-Strauss Syndrome**
  - Transient pulmonary consolidation or ground-glass opacity in peripheral or random distribution
  - Associated with eosinophilic vasculitis and asthma
- **Pulmonary Alveolar Proteinosis**
  - Accumulation of periodic-Schiff (PAS) positive material in alveolar spaces
  - Primary (idiopathic): Middle-aged men most commonly affected
  - Secondary: Related to blood stem cell transplant or hematologic malignancy
  - Imaging abnormalities out of proportion to clinical signs and symptoms
    - Chest radiograph: Diffuse or patchy consolidation and ground-glass opacity
    - CT: Crazy-paving in geographic distribution with interspersed areas of normal lung
  - Bronchoalveolar lavage is both diagnostic and therapeutic
    - Clinical improvement promptly after therapeutic lavage
    - Radiographic improvement may lag behind clinical improvement

Alternative Differential Approaches

- Unilateral consolidation
  - Obstructive pneumonia
  - Bronchioloalveolar carcinoma
- Bilateral
  - Aspiration, especially if basilar
  - Cryptogenic organizing pneumonia
  - Chronic eosinophilic pneumonia
  - Alveolar proteinosis
- Multifocal peripheral consolidation
  - Lymphoma in setting of systemic lymphoma
  - Chronic eosinophilic pneumonia: Upper lung zone predominance and peripheral blood eosinophilia
  - Cryptogenic organizing pneumonia: Migratory opacities or basilar predominance
  - Sarcoidosis: Other findings of sarcoidosis (e.g., lymphadenopathy)

Endobronchial Tumor

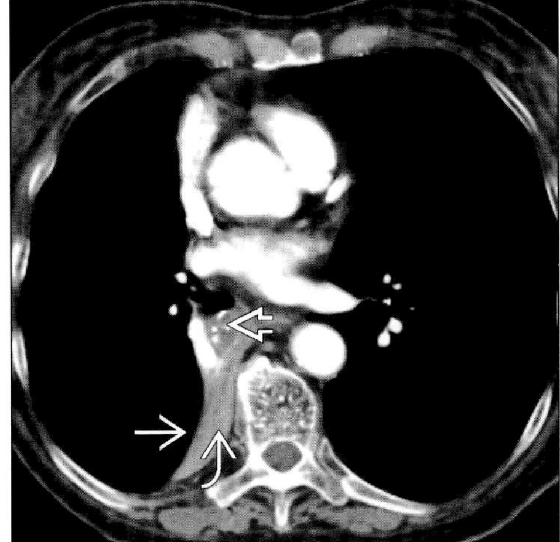

Axial CECT shows collapse of the right lower lobe ➡ with posteromedial displacement of the major fissure ➡ secondary to an obstructing lung carcinoma ➡ in the right lower lobe bronchus.

Aspiration

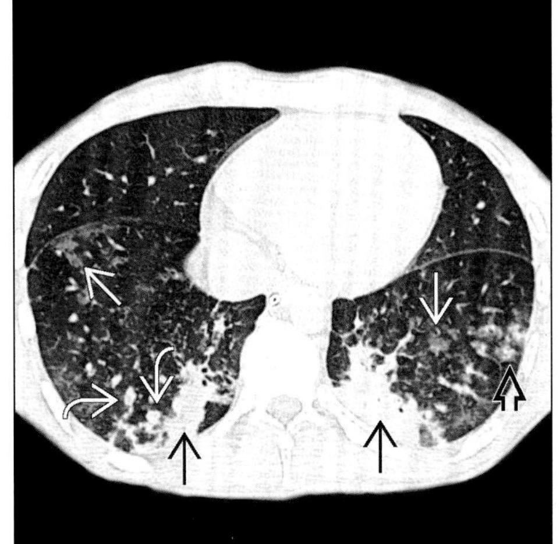

Axial HRCT shows peribronchial consolidation ➡ in the dependent lower lobes with foci of bronchial filling ➡ and scattered ground-glass nodules ➡, as well as more well-defined nodules ➡.

CHRONIC PULMONARY CONSOLIDATION

(**Left**) *Axial NECT shows dense consolidation → in the left upper lobe with peripheral ground-glass opacity →. Note mixed consolidation and ground-glass opacity → in the right upper lobe with foci of pseudocavitation →. A few nodules with central lucencies → are also present.* (**Right**) *Axial NECT shows focal mass-like consolidation → in the right mid-lung, surrounded by clusters of centrilobular nodules →.*

Bronchioloalveolar Carcinoma

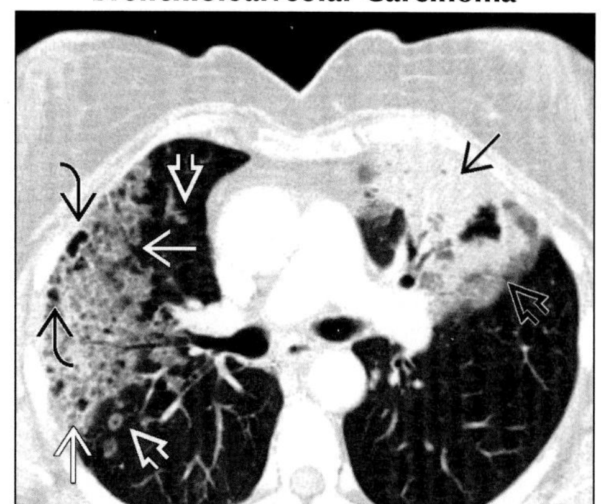

Coccidioidomycosis

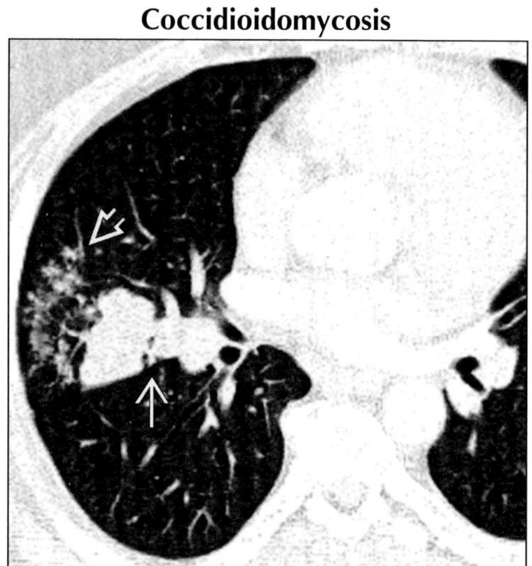

(**Left**) *Axial NECT shows focal right upper lobe consolidation → with an adjacent focus of ground-glass opacity →. Note central cavitation →. Pulmonary blastomycosis can mimic other forms of community acquired pneumonia.* (**Right**) *Axial HRCT shows multiple foci of peribronchial consolidation → with air bronchograms in both lungs. A few foci of peripheral ground-glass opacity → are also present.*

Blastomycosis

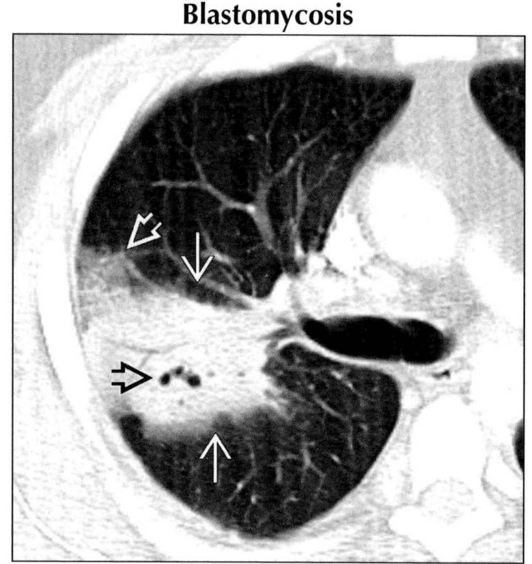

Cryptogenic Organizing Pneumonia

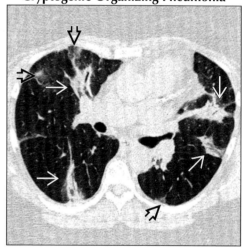

(**Left**) *Axial HRCT shows multiple foci of peripheral → and peribronchial → lung consolidation primarily involving the left lower lobe. Air bronchograms → are usually present within foci of consolidation.* (**Right**) *Axial NECT shows mass-like consolidation → in the right middle lobe containing air bronchograms →. Note surrounding ground-glass opacity → and small adjacent lung nodules →.*

Cryptogenic Organizing Pneumonia

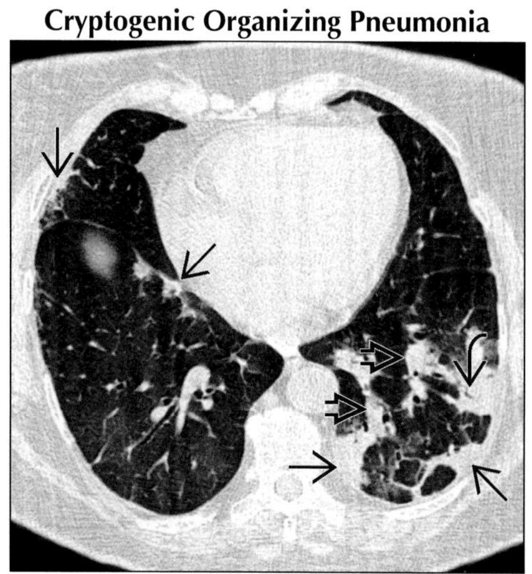

Lymphoma

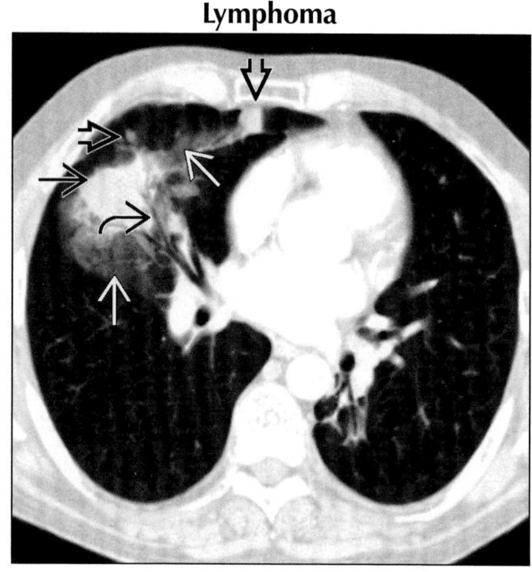

CHRONIC PULMONARY CONSOLIDATION

Chronic Eosinophilic Pneumonia

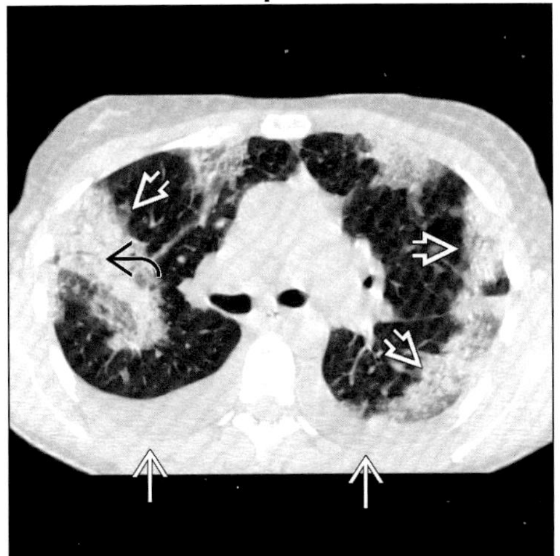

Sarcoidosis

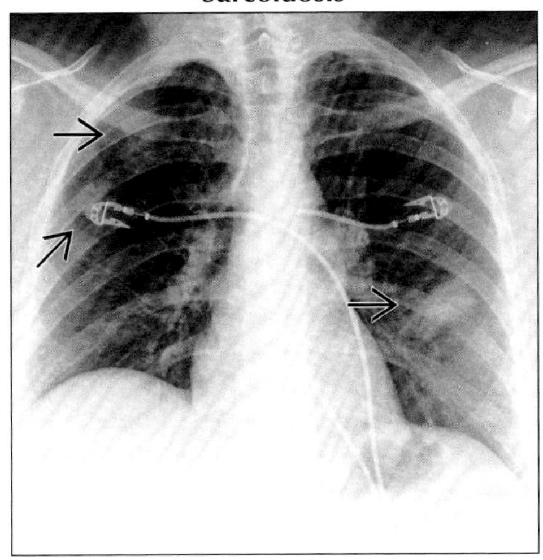

*(**Left**) Axial NECT shows extensive peripheral lung consolidation ➡ with air bronchograms ➡. Small pleural effusions ➡ are also present. An upper lung and peripheral distribution is characteristic of chronic eosinophilic pneumonia. (**Right**) Frontal radiograph shows multiple round opacities ➡ in both lungs in this patient with known sarcoidosis.*

Sarcoidosis

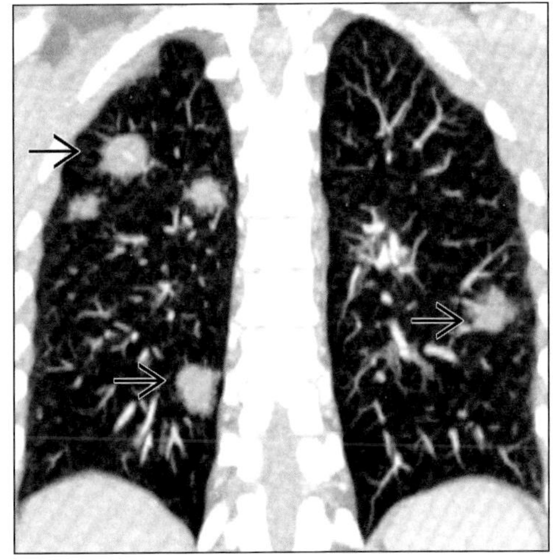

Lipoid Pneumonia

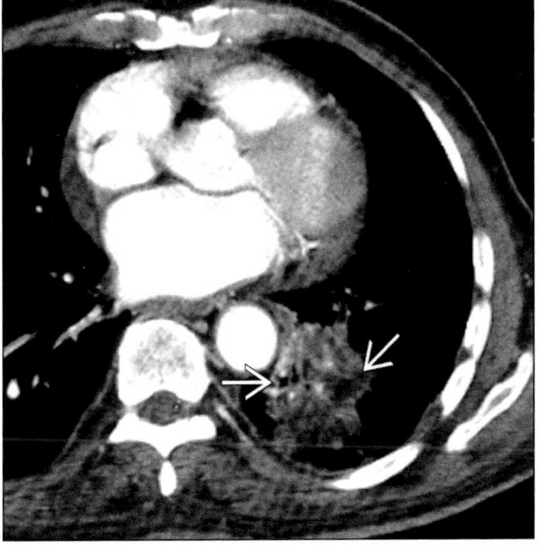

*(**Left**) Coronal CT reconstruction shows multiple well-defined nodules ➡ in this patient with known sarcoidosis. This appearance is uncommon and mimics infections, such as fungal pneumonia. Other features of sarcoidosis, such as lymphadenopathy, may be helpful but are also nonspecific. (**Right**) Axial CECT shows mass-like consolidation ➡ in the left lower lobe. The presence of fat attenuation within area of consolidation is indicative of lipoid pneumonia.*

Churg-Strauss Syndrome

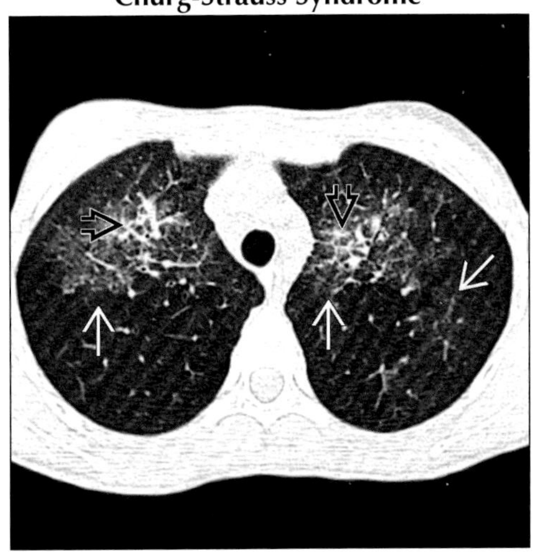

Pulmonary Alveolar Proteinosis

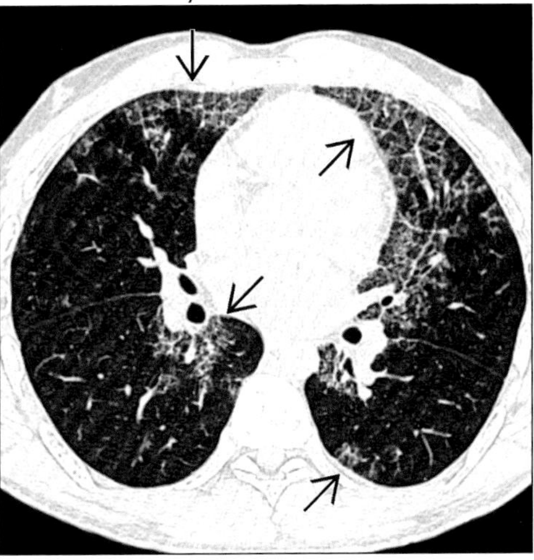

*(**Left**) Axial NECT shows patchy ground-glass opacity ➡ in both lungs with mild consolidation ➡ around several bronchovascular bundles centrally. Although CT findings of Churg-Strauss syndrome are nonspecific, the diagnosis should be considered in patients with asthma and signs of vasculitis. (**Right**) Axial HRCT shows a geographic distribution of crazy-paving ➡, which is characterized by ground-glass opacity and superimposed septal thickening.*

UNILATERAL PULMONARY CONSOLIDATION

DIFFERENTIAL DIAGNOSIS

Common
- Community Acquired Pneumonia
- Bronchioloalveolar Carcinoma
- Lung Contusion
- Endobronchial Tumor

Less Common
- Coccidioidomycosis
- Blastomycosis
- Diffuse Alveolar Hemorrhage
- Eosinophilic Pneumonia
- Pulmonary Emboli

Rare but Important
- Lymphoma
- Lipoid Pneumonia
- Lobar Torsion, Lung

ESSENTIAL INFORMATION

Helpful Clues for Common Diagnoses
- **Community Acquired Pneumonia**
    - Lobar
        - Bacterial: *Streptococcus pneumoniae*, *H. influenzae*, TB, and *Legionella*
    - Bronchopneumonia
        - Peribronchial, often multifocal consolidation
        - Possible endobronchial spread
        - *Staphylococcus*, *Haemophilus*, *Pseudomonas*, TB
- **Bronchioloalveolar Carcinoma**
    - Slowly progressive lung consolidation
        - May increase in both size and density
        - Patients often treated for recurrent pneumonia in same lobe
    - CT often shows mixed consolidation and ground-glass opacity
        - Crazy-paving and septal thickening less common
        - Dilated airways within consolidation: "Pseudocavitation"
- **Lung Contusion**
    - Most common lung injury from blunt trauma
    - Hemorrhage into parenchyma and air spaces
    - Marker of high-energy trauma
    - Radiography and CT
        - Nonanatomic distribution of consolidation and ground-glass opacity
        - Usually present on initial imaging
        - Should clear within 7 days
- **Endobronchial Tumor**
    - Endobronchial soft tissue mass or broncholith obstructing bronchus
        - Primary lung carcinoma
        - Metastases: Melanoma, breast, renal cell, colon
    - Air bronchograms often absent within consolidation
        - CT may show fluid attenuation filling bronchi
    - Signs of volume loss, such as fissural or hilar displacement
    - Consider broncholith in presence of calcified lung nodules and calcified lymph nodes

Helpful Clues for Less Common Diagnoses
- **Coccidioidomycosis**
    - Endemic in desert regions of southwestern USA
    - Single or multiple foci of lung consolidation
    - Nodules less common, may cavitate
    - Lymphadenopathy in 20% of patients
    - Pleural effusion in 10-20% of patients
- **Blastomycosis**
    - Endemic in central and eastern USA along major rivers and around the Great Lakes
    - Single or multiple foci of lung consolidation
        - Slow to resolve or respond to therapy
    - Nodules and masses cavitate in 1/3 of patients
    - Lymphadenopathy uncommon
    - Pleural effusion in 20% of patients
- **Diffuse Alveolar Hemorrhage**
    - Usually related to capillaritis
        - Wegener granulomatosis
        - Microscopic polyangiitis
        - Systemic lupus erythematosus
        - Drug toxicity
    - Unilateral less common than bilateral
    - Lung periphery often spared
    - Elevated diffusing capacity (DLCO)
    - Bronchoalveolar lavage diagnostic
- **Eosinophilic Pneumonia**
    - Löffler syndrome
        - Simple pulmonary eosinophilia
        - Patients asymptomatic or present with fever and cough; spontaneously resolves

- Transient or migratory solitary or multiple foci of lung consolidation
  - Other forms of eosinophilic pneumonia usually bilateral
- **Pulmonary Emboli**
  - Consolidation from infarction, atelectasis, or hemorrhage
  - Solitary or multiple
  - Small pleural effusion may be present
  - Infarct on chest radiograph: Hampton hump
  - Infarct on CT: Peripheral wedge-shaped, unenhancing focus of consolidation with central lucencies
    - Resolves from periphery to center

Helpful Clues for Rare Diagnoses

- **Lymphoma**
  - 4% of lung malignancies
  - Non-Hodgkin lymphoma
    - More common than Hodgkin lymphoma
    - 30% lung involvement
  - Unifocal or multifocal consolidation or nodules
  - Air bronchograms often present
- **Lipoid Pneumonia**
  - Chronic mass-like consolidation and ground-glass opacity
    - Basal predominance (similar distribution to other causes of aspiration), unilateral or bilateral
    - Fat attenuation of consolidation on CT virtually diagnostic
  - Mineral oil aspiration most common cause (exogenous)
- **Lobar Torsion, Lung**
  - Rare, usually occurs after lobectomy or transplant
  - Progressive lobar consolidation on imaging
  - Contrast-enhanced CT: Dense lobar consolidation with narrowing of airways and vessels
    - Derangement of normal bronchovascular configuration
  - Prompt identification and treatment required to prevent ischemic necrosis

Alternative Differential Approaches

- Acute (< 2 weeks)
  - Community acquired pneumonia
  - Lung contusion
  - Fungal infection
  - Diffuse alveolar hemorrhage
  - Eosinophilic pneumonia
    - Löffler syndrome
  - Pulmonary emboli
    - Infarcts, atelectasis, and hemorrhage
  - Lobar torsion
- Chronic (> 4 weeks)
  - Bronchioloalveolar carcinoma
  - Endobronchial tumor
  - Fungal infection
    - May be slow to resolve or respond
  - Lymphoma
  - Lipoid pneumonia

Community Acquired Pneumonia

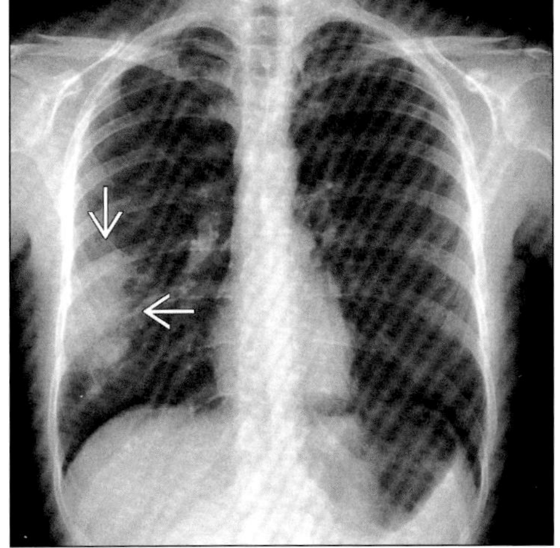

Frontal radiograph shows focal consolidation ➡ in the mid right lung in this patient with S. pneumoniae infection.

Community Acquired Pneumonia

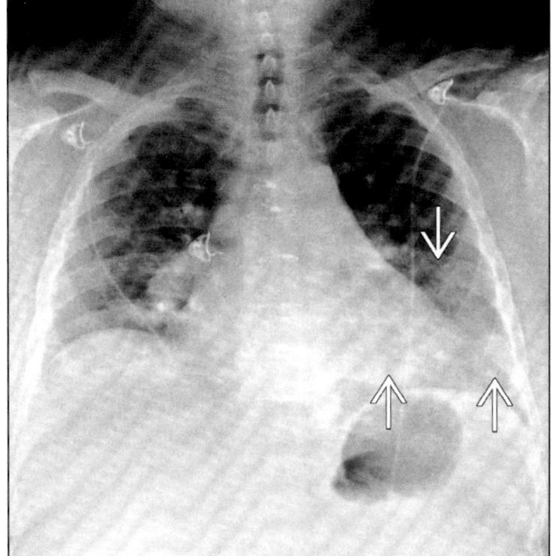

Frontal radiograph shows patchy consolidation ➡ in the mid and basal left lung in this patient with Legionella pneumophila pneumonia.

UNILATERAL PULMONARY CONSOLIDATION

(Left) Frontal radiograph shows a focus of well-defined consolidation ➡ in the right lower lobe. No findings of volume loss are present. *(Right)* Axial CECT shows dense consolidation ➡ containing air bronchograms ⇨ in the right lower lobe. This patient's radiographs (not shown) revealed slow progression of right lower lobe consolidation. This form of bronchioloalveolar carcinoma can be mistaken for recurrent or chronic pneumonia.

Bronchioloalveolar Carcinoma

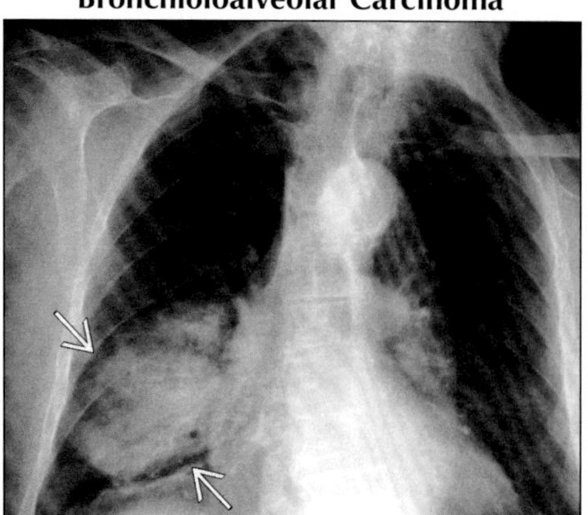

Bronchioloalveolar Carcinoma

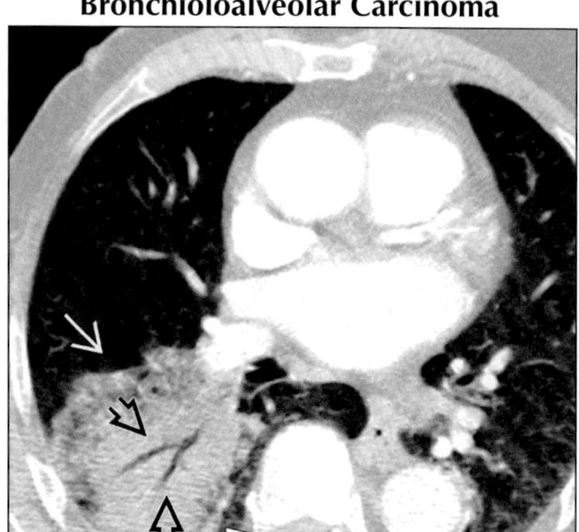

(Left) Anteroposterior radiograph shows homogeneous consolidation in the right upper lung ➡. Adjacent chest wall fractures are also present ➡. Pulmonary contusion is usually apparent on the initial chest radiograph and will gradually resolve over 1 week. *(Right)* Axial CECT shows a round solid mass lesion ⇨ in the left upper lobe bronchus resulting in collapse of the left upper lobe. Note anteromedial displacement of the left major fissure ➡.

Lung Contusion

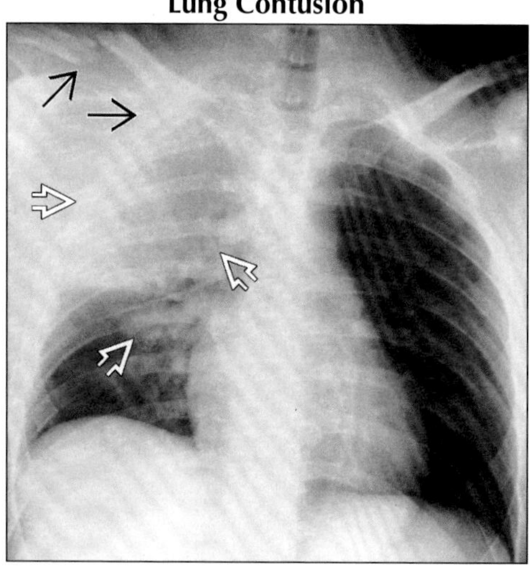

Endobronchial Tumor

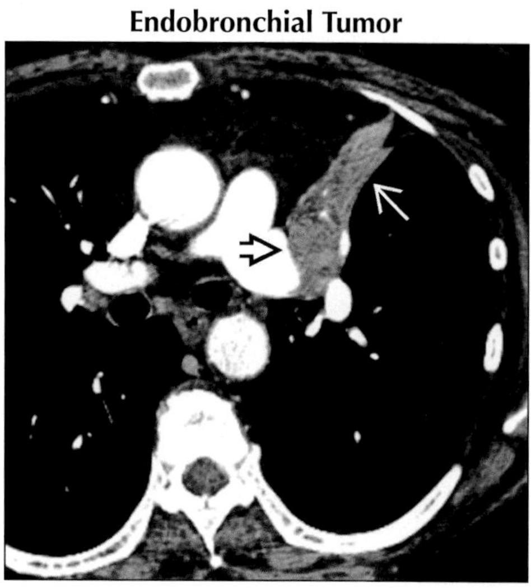

(Left) Coronal CT reconstruction shows peribronchial mass-like consolidation ➡ in the mid right lung. Coccidioidomycosis can also manifest as single or multiple lung nodules without or with cavitation. *(Right)* Axial CECT shows dense right upper lobe consolidation ➡ containing small air bronchograms ⇨. Other common sites of involvement in blastomycosis include the skin and bones.

Coccidioidomycosis

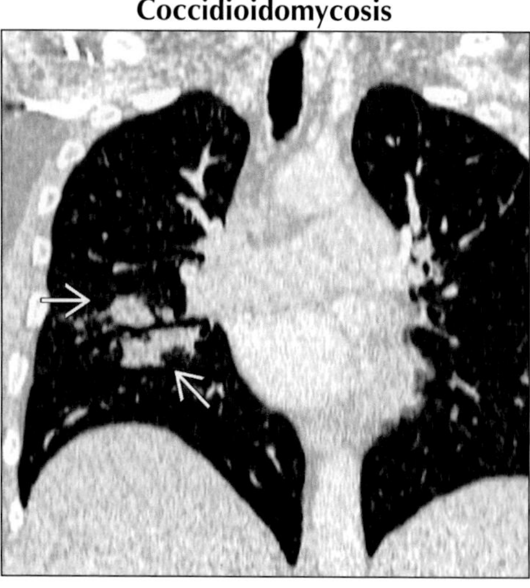

Blastomycosis

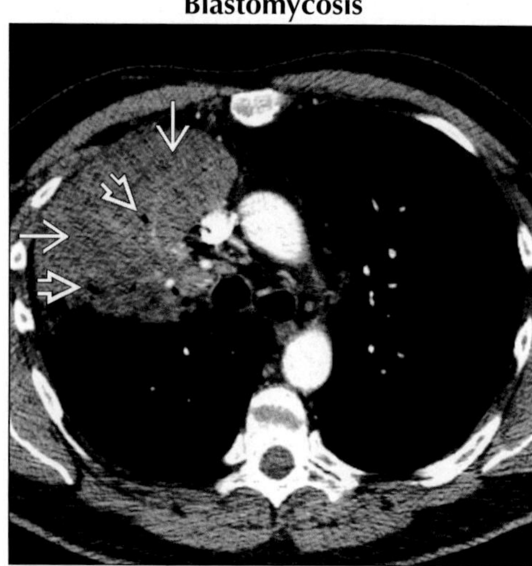

UNILATERAL PULMONARY CONSOLIDATION

Diffuse Alveolar Hemorrhage

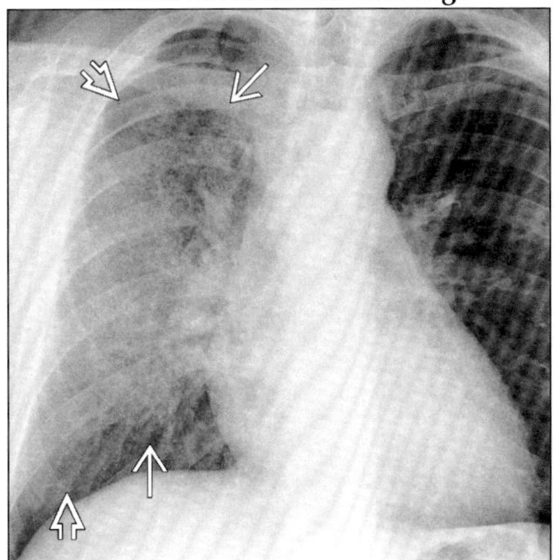

Eosinophilic Pneumonia

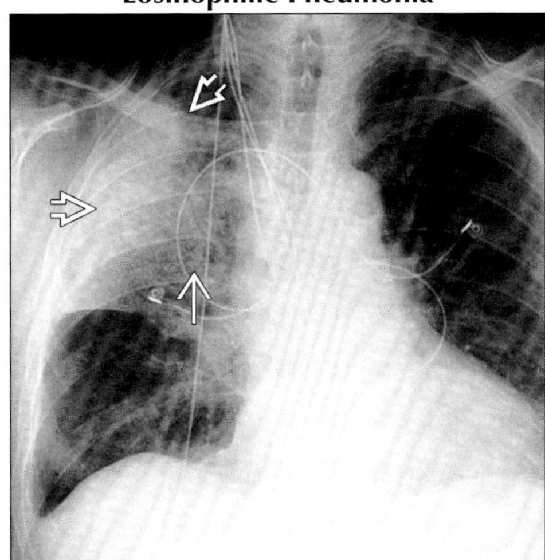

*(**Left**) Frontal radiograph shows diffuse hazy opacity ➡ in the right lung in this patient with Goodpasture syndrome. Note relative peripheral sparing ➡. Alveolar hemorrhage is usually bilateral but can be strikingly asymmetric. (**Right**) Frontal radiograph shows dense peripheral consolidation ➡ in the right upper lobe with ground-glass attenuation ➡ located more centrally. Radiographic findings of acute and chronic eosinophilic pneumonia often overlap.*

Pulmonary Emboli

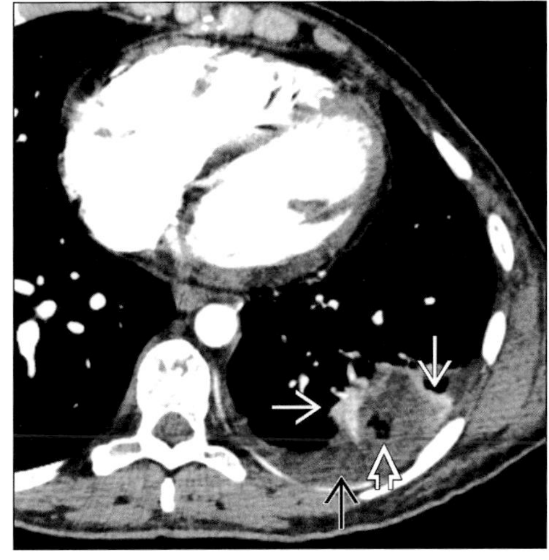

Lymphoma

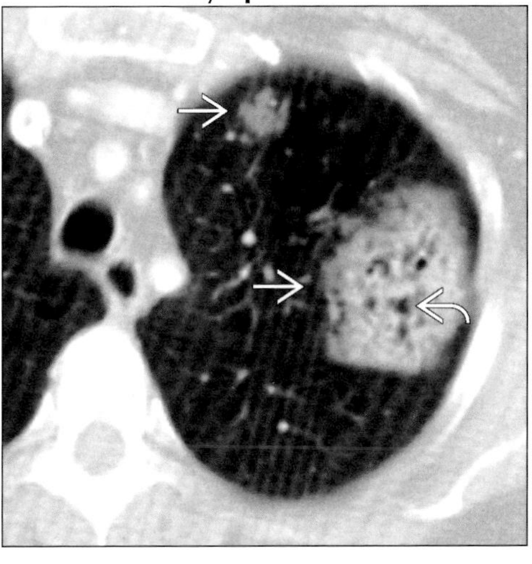

*(**Left**) Axial CECT shows a wedge-shaped focus of low attenuation with central lucency ➡ representing an infarct in this patient with acute pulmonary emboli (not shown). Note the surrounding enhancing atelectatic lung ➡. A small pleural effusion ➡ is also present. (**Right**) Axial CECT shows 2 mass-like foci of lung consolidation ➡ proven to be pulmonary lymphoma. Note the air bronchograms ➡ within the large focus of consolidation.*

Lipoid Pneumonia

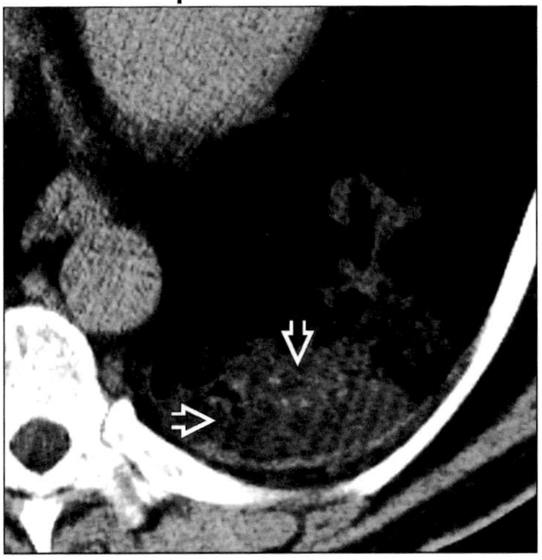

Lobar Torsion, Lung

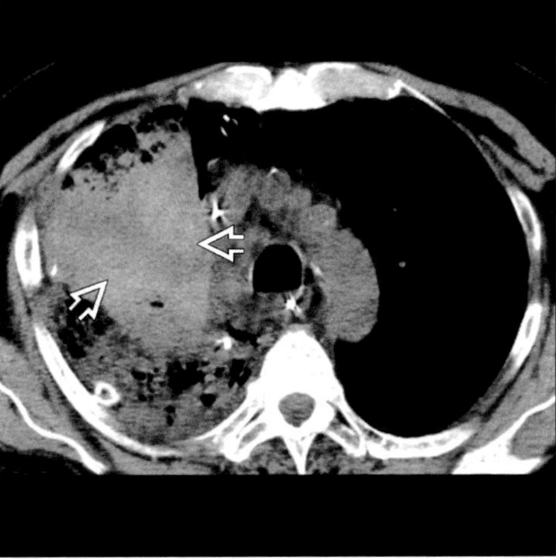

*(**Left**) Axial NECT shows dense, low-attenuation consolidation ➡ in the left lower lobe in this patient who used oil-based nose drops to relieve symptoms related to treatment of head and neck cancer. Fat attenuation consolidation is almost pathognomonic for lipoid pneumonia. (**Right**) Axial NECT shows dense consolidation representing hemorrhage ➡ in the torsed right middle lobe following upper lobectomy for lung carcinoma.*

CAVITATION

DIFFERENTIAL DIAGNOSIS

Common

- Tuberculosis (TB)
- Lung Cancer
- Wegener Granulomatosis
- Septic Emboli
- Pneumatocele
- Lung Abscess

Less Common

- Cavitary Lung Metastasis
- Fungal Infections
  - Angioinvasive Aspergillosis
  - Blastomycosis
  - Coccidioidomycosis
  - Paracoccidioidomycosis
  - Pneumocystis Pneumonia

Rare but Important

- Recurrent Respiratory Papillomatosis
- Intralobar Sequestration with Superinfection
- Hydatid Cyst (Echinococcus)

ESSENTIAL INFORMATION

Key Differential Diagnosis Issues

- Features of cavity to consider in differential diagnosis
  - Wall thickness of cavity can be thick or thin
    - Thick wall usually indicates neoplastic disease
    - Thin walls favor benignity
  - Nodularity of internal wall is associated with neoplastic etiology
  - Solitary cavities: Primary lung cancer, lung abscess (except when part of septic emboli), intralobar sequestration, and tuberculosis
  - Multiple cavities: Wegener granulomatosis, septic emboli, metastasis, fungal infection, and recurrent respiratory papillomatosis
  - Associated airway wall (tracheal) thickening: Wegener granulomatosis, sarcoidosis, and recurrent respiratory papillomatosis
  - Location of abnormalities: Left lower lobe for intralobar sequestration, lower and peripheral lungs are favored by septic emboli, and posterior upper lobes are favorite site for TB

Helpful Clues for Common Diagnoses

- **Tuberculosis (TB)**
  - Imaging clues
    - Thick- or thin-walled cavity in posterior upper lobe
    - Associated findings, such as consolidation or nodules in airway distribution (tree in bud pattern)
    - Typically in posterior upper lobes
  - Clinical clues
    - Patients present with cough, low-grade fever, night sweats
    - Purified protein derivative (PPD) skin test shows induration above 10 mm, except in anergic conditions, (e.g., HIV infection)
- **Lung Cancer**
  - Solitary mass with central necrosis
  - Thick-walled cavity with nodularity of inner wall
  - Cavitation is typically seen in lung cancers of squamous cell histopathology
- **Wegener Granulomatosis**
  - Imaging clues
    - Combination of nodules, nodules with cavitation, and airway wall thickening is characteristic
    - In most cases, not all features are present at same time
    - Pulmonary hemorrhage presenting as diffuse airspace disease, sometimes with sparing of peripheral lung
  - Clinical clues
    - Antineutrophil cytoplasmic antibodies (c-ANCA) test carries high sensitivity (90%) and specificity (70%)
    - Renal and sinus involvement is seen in majority
- **Septic Emboli**
  - Imaging clues
    - Multiple peripheral lung nodules or nodules with cavitation that appear and evolve rapidly
    - Lower and peripheral lungs are typically involved
  - Clinical clues
    - Longstanding indwelling venous catheter
    - IV drug use (abuse)
    - Right-sided (tricuspid or pulmonic valve) endocarditis

- Recent dental/periodontal disease or procedure
- **Pneumatocele**
  - Thin-walled air-filled cavity that may result from either prior trauma or necrotizing lung infection
  - Can completely resolve or persist indefinitely
- **Lung Abscess**
  - Imaging clues
    - Lung consolidation with nonenhancing center indicating necrosis
    - Cavitation and air-fluid level (suggestive of communication with airway) with surrounding lung consolidation
    - Usually solitary, except when associated with septic embolism, where there are usually multiple abscesses
  - Clinical clues
    - Aspiration, poor dental hygiene, esophageal dysmotility, low level of consciousness are some predisposing factors
    - Mixed anaerobic infection, *Staphylococcus aureus*, and *Pseudomonas aeruginosa* are some commonly involved organisms

Helpful Clues for Less Common Diagnoses

- **Cavitary Lung Metastasis**
  - Thick or thin walled, may have internal nodularity, and are often multiple
  - Head and neck cancers, transitional cell carcinoma of urinary bladder, high-grade sarcomas
- **Fungal Infections**
  - **Angioinvasive Aspergillosis**
    - Radiographs often show solitary or multifocal lung consolidation or ill-defined nodules
    - CT often shows rapid evolution of ill-defined nodule with surrounding halo (halo sign) into cavity with centrally sequestered lung "air crescent" sign
    - Always in immunocompromised host, (e.g., HIV infection, solid organ transplant, etc.)
  - **Pneumocystis Pneumonia**
    - Upper lobe thin-walled cysts surrounded by extensive ground-glass opacities

Helpful Clues for Rare Diagnoses

- **Recurrent Respiratory Papillomatosis**
  - Caused by birth canal infection from human papillomavirus (HPV)
  - Lung involvement is rare, but when present it is almost always preceded by longstanding laryngeo-tracheal involvement
- **Intralobar Sequestration with Superinfection**
  - Posterior left lower lobe location most common, absent bronchial communication
  - Systemic arterial supply, often directly from aorta

Tuberculosis (TB)

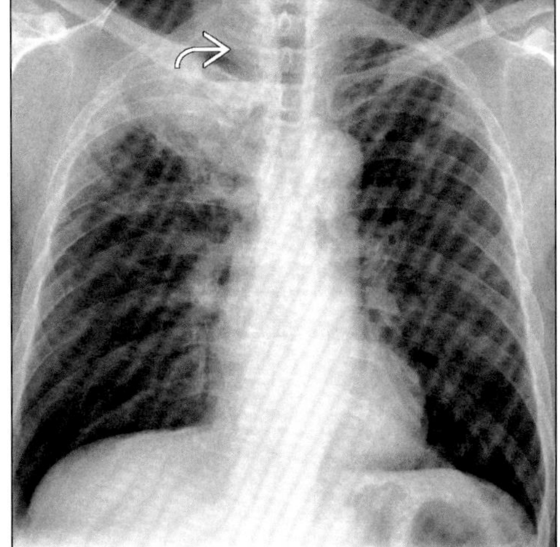

Frontal radiograph in a patient with reactivation tuberculosis shows dense right upper lobe consolidation and cavitation ➡. There are also lesser patchy opacities in the left upper lobe.

Tuberculosis (TB)

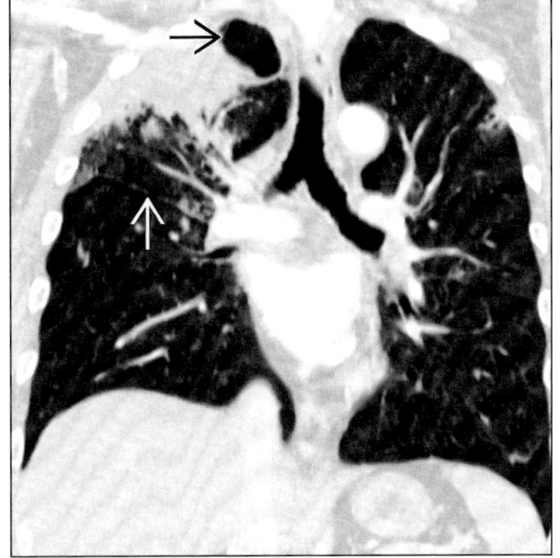

Coronal CT reconstruction from the same patient shows right upper lobe consolidation and cavitation ➡ with associated volume loss. Note the elevation of the minor fissure ➡.

CAVITATION

*(**Left**) Axial CECT shows typical CT features of Wegener granulomatosis with a combination of multiple bilateral, large, somewhat lobulated nodules and cavitary nodules ➡. (**Right**) Axial CECT shows typical features of airway involvement from Wegener granulomatosis. Note circumferential thickening and narrowing of the left main bronchus ➡ with postobstructive pneumonia.*

Wegener Granulomatosis

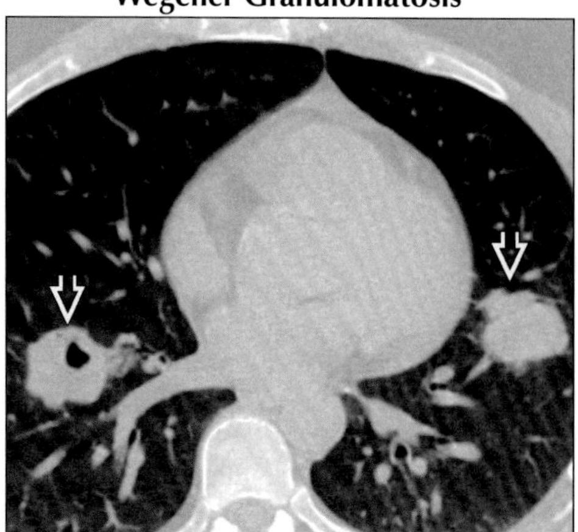

Wegener Granulomatosis

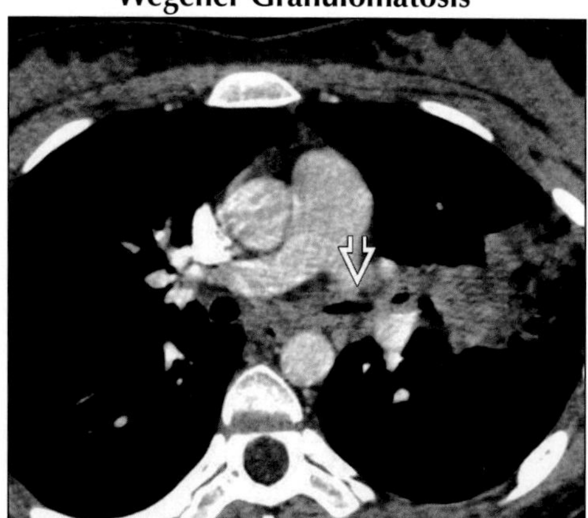

*(**Left**) Coronal CT reconstruction from a patient with squamous cell carcinoma shows a right lower lobe superior segment thick-walled cavitary mass with inner wall nodularity, abutting the major fissure ➡. (**Right**) Anteroposterior radiograph shows typical radiographic features of pneumatoceles in a patient with Staphylococcal pneumonia. Note the consolidation and multiple pneumatoceles ➡.*

Lung Cancer

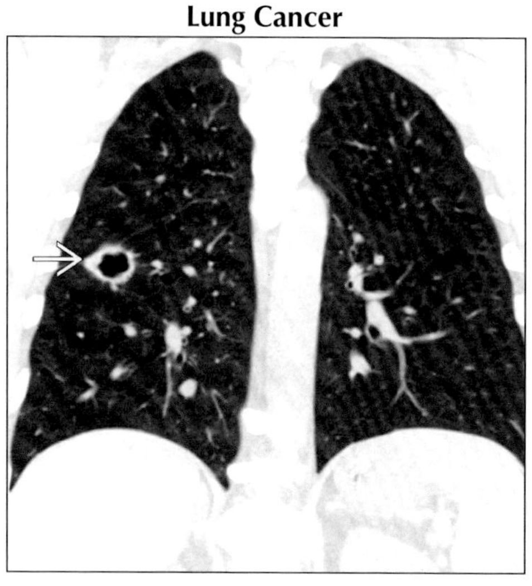

Pneumatocele

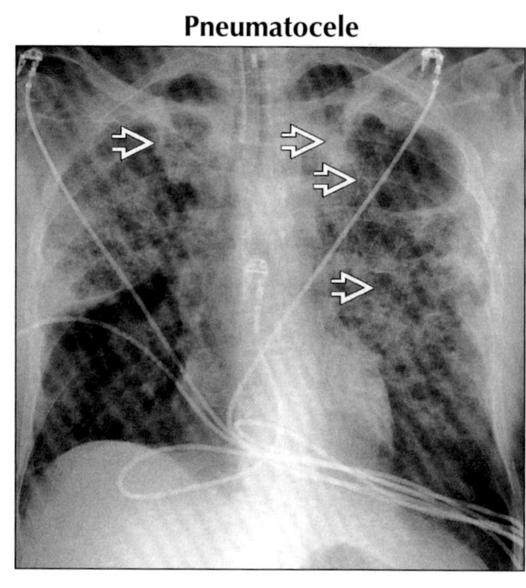

*(**Left**) Axial CECT of the neck shows retropharyngeal hypoattenuating abnormality on the right ➡, possible abscess, and external jugular vein thrombosis ➡ indicating Lemierre syndrome. (**Right**) Axial CECT from this patient with Lemierre syndrome shows 2 peripheral left lower lobe nodules, one with cavitation → indicating multiple septic emboli. Lower lobes are the most common location for septic emboli because of the physiologically greater blood flow.*

Septic Emboli

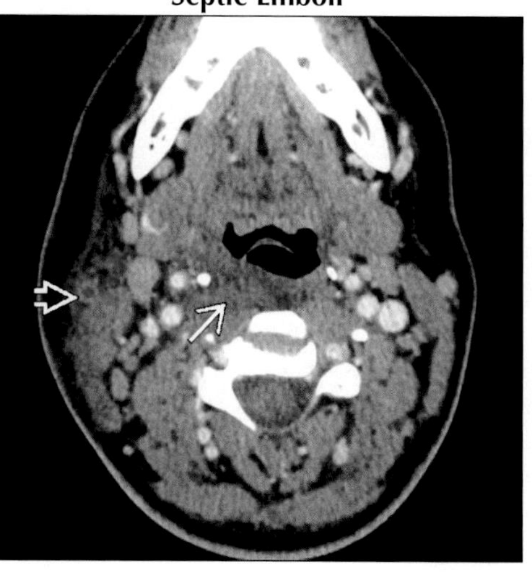

Septic Emboli

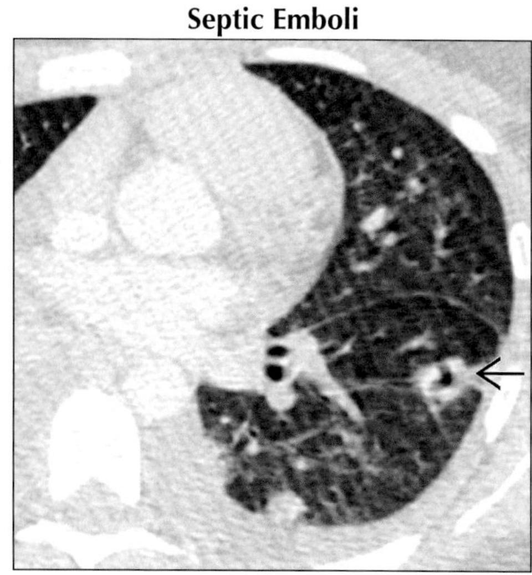

CAVITATION

Lung Abscess

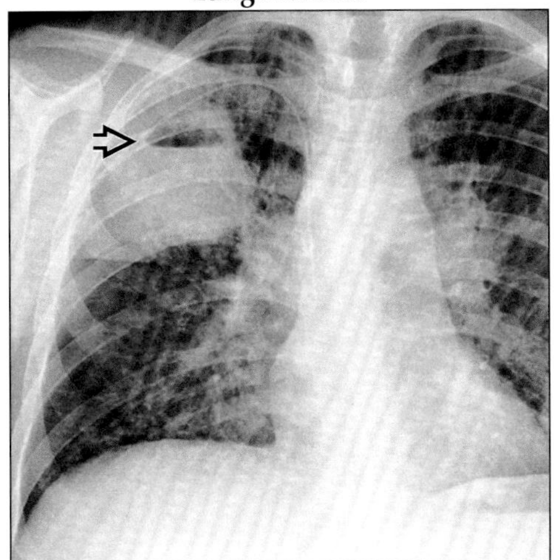

Lung Abscess

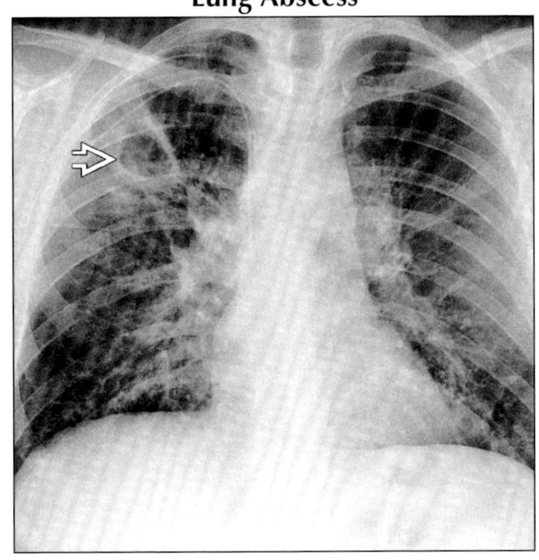

(Left) *Frontal radiograph shows variant features of the evolution of lung abscess in this patient with underlying cystic fibrosis. A large right upper lobe consolidation with an air-fluid level ⇨ and bronchiectasis due to known cystic fibrosis are evident.* ***(Right)*** *Frontal radiograph of the same patient, 4 weeks later, shows evolution of the abscess into a thin-walled cavity ➡ indicating response to treatment.*

Cavitary Lung Metastasis

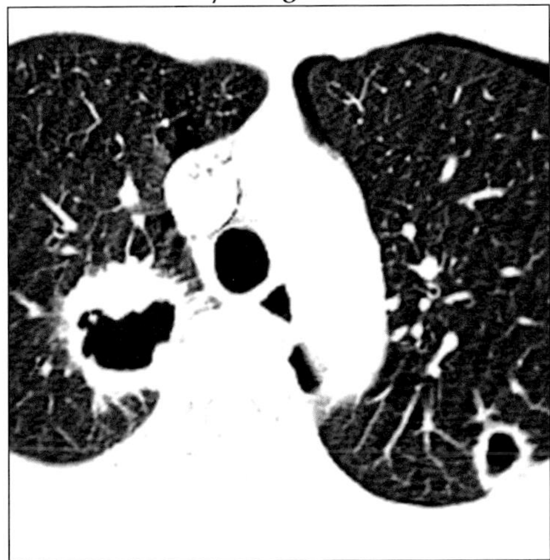

Intralobar Sequestration with Superinfection

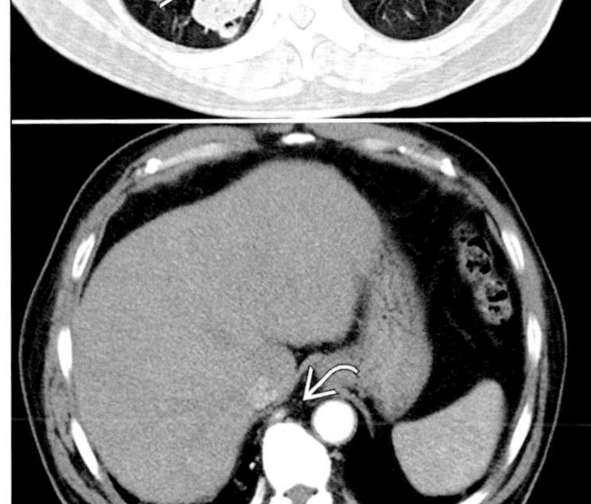

(Left) *Axial CECT from a patient with squamous cell head and neck primary shows 2 thick-walled cavitary metastases in each upper lobe. Note internal nodularity of the right upper lobe lesion and left-sided pneumothorax.* ***(Right)*** *Axial CECT lung window (top) shows posterior right lower lobe cavity with an air-fluid level ➡, and the soft tissue window (bottom) shows a systemic arterial supply ➡. (Courtesy J.D. Godwin, MD.)*

Fungal Infections

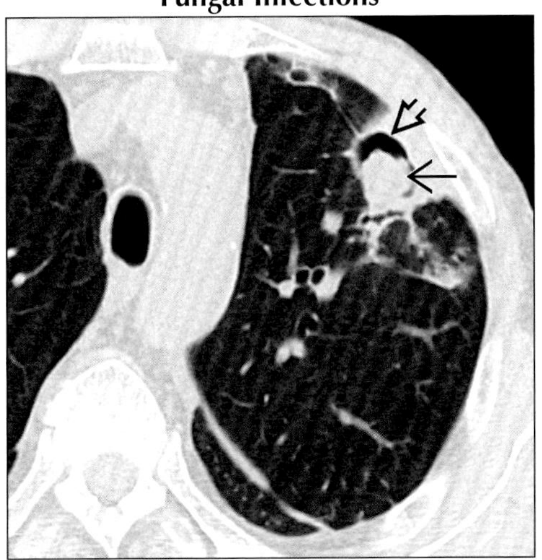

Fungal Infections

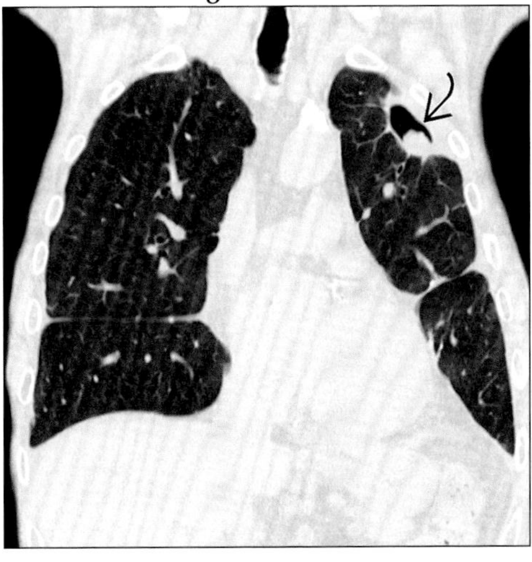

(Left) *Transverse HRCT shows CT features of air crescent sign in aspergillosis from a patient with immunosuppression. NECT shows a thick-walled peripheral lung cavity ⇨ with a mass → within the cavity.* ***(Right)*** *Coronal HRCT in the same patient with aspergillosis shows the fungus ball within the cranio-caudal location of the cavity ↗. This was an isolated finding.*

AIR-CRESCENT SIGN

DIFFERENTIAL DIAGNOSIS

Common
- Angioinvasive Aspergillosis
- Mycetoma

Less Common
- Bronchogenic Carcinoma

Rare but Important
- Echinococcosis

ESSENTIAL INFORMATION

Key Differential Diagnosis Issues
- Air-crescent sign: Air outlining edge of mass in sickle shape

Helpful Clues for Common Diagnoses
- **Angioinvasive Aspergillosis**
  - Occurs in immunocompromised patients
  - Invades small arteries and often causes lung infarction
  - Begins as single or multiple lung nodules or areas of focal consolidation, often with associated halo sign
  - Cavitation occurs approximately 2 weeks later and is due to tissue necrosis
  - Necrotic tissue retracts and forms air crescent
  - Air-crescent sign is good clinical prognostic indicator as it indicates immune recovery phase
- **Mycetoma**
  - Occurs in immunologically competent patients
  - Also called aspergilloma
  - Fungal ball usually caused by *Aspergillus*, as saprophyte
  - Forms within preexisting lung cavity or cyst
  - Inflammation can cause hemorrhage and hemoptysis
    - Rarely hematoma in cavity mimics mycetoma
  - Mass may shift with changes in position
  - Monod sign: Shifting of air crescent with changes in position, pathognomonic for mobile mass

Helpful Clues for Less Common Diagnoses
- **Bronchogenic Carcinoma**
  - 2 mechanisms of air crescent formation
    - Tumor may arise within preexisting cyst or cavity
    - Tumor itself may cavitate, forming crescent at margin
  - Not typical presentation

Helpful Clues for Rare Diagnoses
- **Echinococcosis**
  - Caused by canine tapeworm
  - Pericyst: Compressed lung and fibrotic tissue
  - Ectocyst and endocyst: Layers of parasite
  - Pericyst rupture allows air between pericyst and ectocyst, forming air-crescent sign
  - Water lily sign: Floating endocyst caused by ectocyst rupture

Angioinvasive Aspergillosis

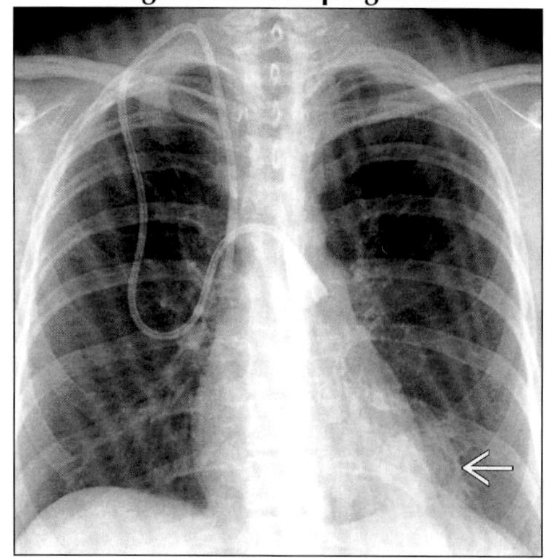

Frontal radiograph shows a large mass in the left lower lung with a peripheral air-crescent sign ➔. In this immunocompromised patient, this is highly suggestive of angioinvasive aspergillosis.

Angioinvasive Aspergillosis

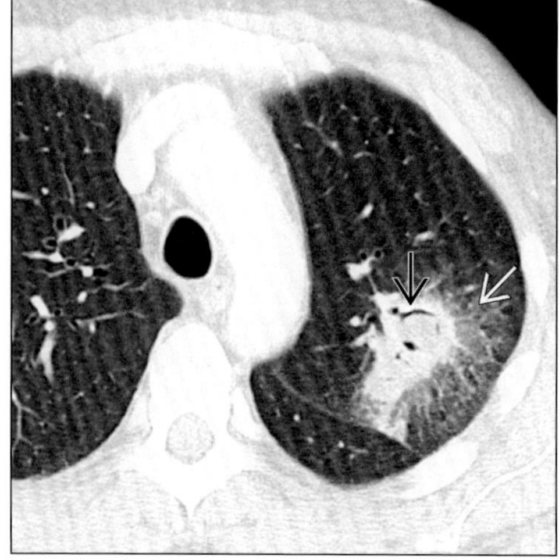

Transverse CECT shows typical CT features of angioinvasive aspergillosis. Notice the halo sign surrounding the lesion ➔ and the air-crescent sign ⇨ caused by tissue necrosis and retraction.

AIR-CRESCENT SIGN

Angioinvasive Aspergillosis

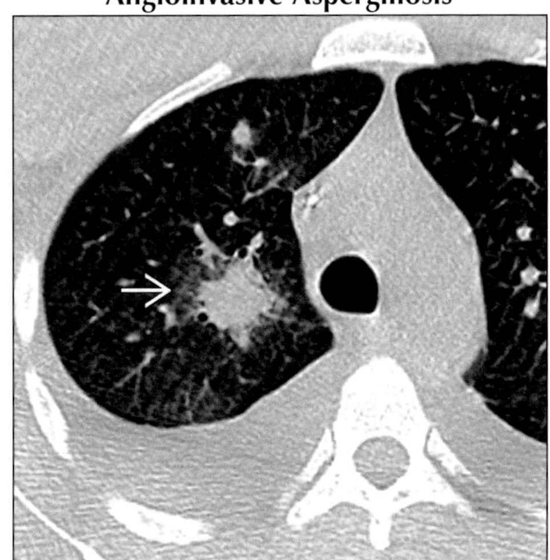

Angioinvasive Aspergillosis

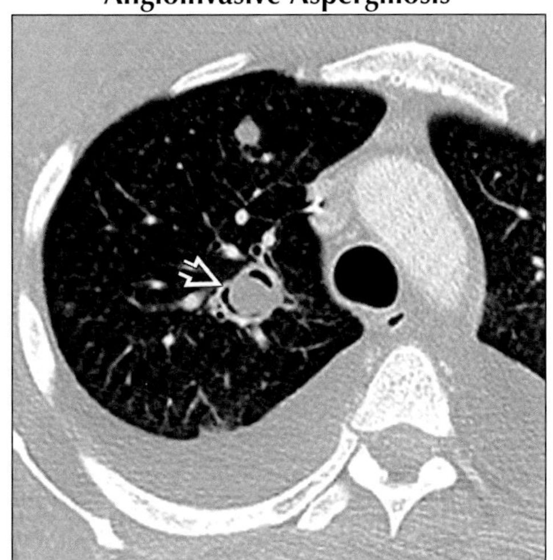

(Left) *Axial NECT shows a nodule in the right upper lobe with a surrounding rim of ground-glass opacity ➔ in this immunocompromised patient.* ***(Right)*** *Axial CECT obtained a few weeks later in the same patient shows resolution of the halo sign with progression to an air-crescent sign ➔, which is caused by lung necrosis and retraction. This is a good prognostic sign in this patient with angioinvasive aspergillosis.*

Mycetoma

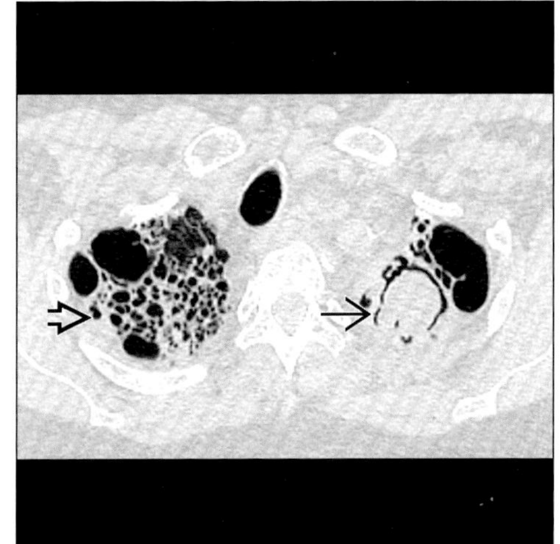

Mycetoma

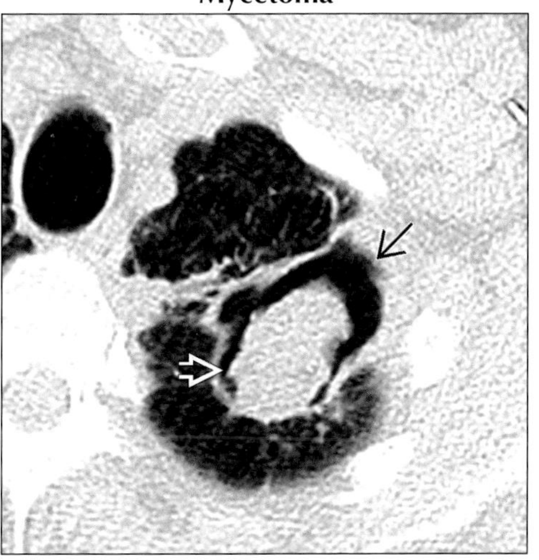

(Left) *Axial HRCT shows severe traction bronchiectasis and honeycombing in the upper lobes ➔ as a consequence of sarcoidosis. A mycetoma has formed within a cystic space in the left upper lobe ➔.* ***(Right)*** *Axial NECT shows a large cavity in the left upper lobe, caused by prior tuberculosis. There is a dependent mass within this cavity ➔ with a surrounding air crescent ➔. This is a typical appearance of mycetoma.*

Mycetoma

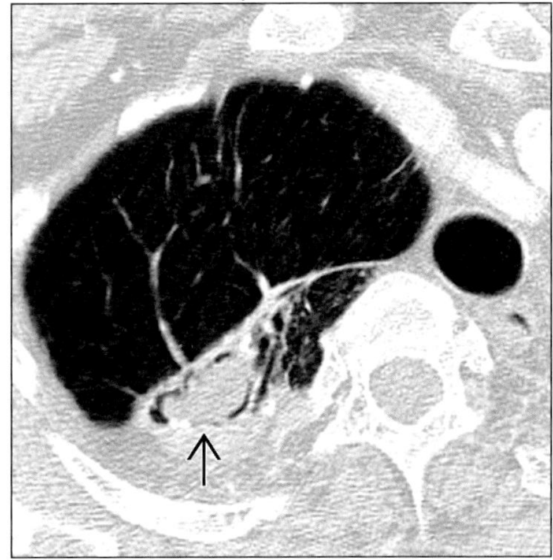

Bronchogenic Carcinoma

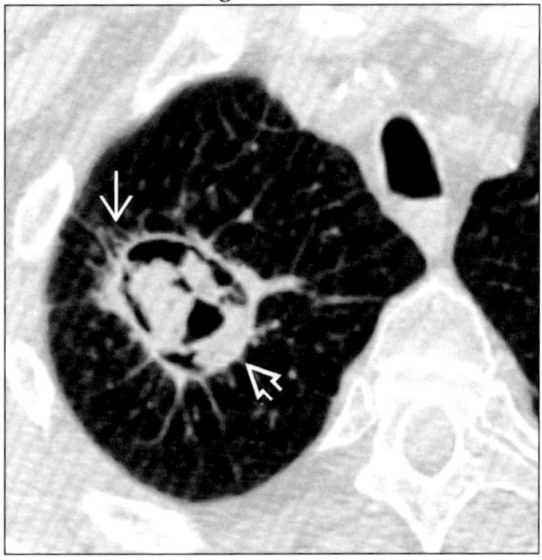

(Left) *Axial CECT shows a mass within a cavity ➔ in this patient with a history of upper lobe tuberculosis. Notice the thin air crescent surrounding the mass. This is a typical appearance of mycetoma.* ***(Right)*** *Axial NECT shows shows a cavitary mass ➔ in the right upper lobe with an air-crescent sign caused by necrosis in this bronchogenic carcinoma mimicking angioinvasive aspergillosis. Notice the spiculations formed at the edge of the lesion ➔.*

PULMONARY CALCIFICATION

DIFFERENTIAL DIAGNOSIS

Common
- Mycobacterial Pneumonia
- Fungal, Histoplasmosis

Less Common
- Hamartoma
- Silicosis/Coal Worker's Pneumoconiosis
- Carcinoid
- Lung Metastases

Rare but Important
- Amyloidosis
- Metastatic Pulmonary Calcification
- Lung Ossification
- Alveolar Microlithiasis

ESSENTIAL INFORMATION

Key Differential Diagnosis Issues
- Nodules
  - Diffuse, central, lamellated, or "popcorn" pattern calcification in lung nodule usually reflects benign etiology
  - Eccentric or stippled calcification in lung nodule is indeterminate

Helpful Clues for Common Diagnoses
- **Mycobacterial Pneumonia**
  - Most common cause of granulomatous infection worldwide
  - Calcified lung nodule indicates healed disease with fibrosis and dystrophic calcification
  - Calcifications in ipsilateral hilar and mediastinal lymph nodes frequent
- **Fungal, Histoplasmosis**
  - Endemic fungus commonly encountered in Ohio and Mississippi river valleys
  - Calcified lung nodule indicates healed disease with fibrosis and dystrophic calcification
    - Indistinguishable on imaging from healed mycobacterial infection
  - Splenic calcifications more common and more numerous with histoplasmosis than mycobacterial disease

Helpful Clues for Less Common Diagnoses
- **Hamartoma**
  - Most common benign lung neoplasm
    - 8% of all primary lung tumors
  - Vast majority (~ 95%) occur in lung parenchyma
  - ~ 5% hamartomas endobronchial
  - Chest radiograph
    - Well-circumscribed lung nodule with smooth margins
    - Calcification apparent in 10%
    - Most < 4 cm in diameter
  - CT
    - Approximately 2/3 contain focal fat attenuation, which is diagnostic
    - Coarse "popcorn" calcification in nodule suggestive but uncommon
    - Endobronchial hamartomas usually associated with obstructive pneumonia or atelectasis
- **Silicosis/Coal Worker's Pneumoconiosis**
  - Exposure to free silica (silicosis) or coal dust (CWP)
  - Usually develops after 20 years of exposure
  - Silicosis and CWP indistinguishable radiographically
  - Chest radiograph and CT
    - Small (3-6 mm) round, well-defined calcified or noncalcified nodules
    - Upper lobe, posterior predominance
    - Perilymphatic distribution (CT)
    - Mediastinal and hilar lymphadenopathy in up to 40% (~ 50% with calcification)
- **Carcinoid**
  - 1-2% of all pulmonary neoplasms
  - < 5% have visible calcification on chest radiograph
  - Calcification present in ~ 30% on CT
    - More common with central than peripheral carcinoid tumors
    - Pattern of calcification is variable
    - Can diffusely calcify and mimic a broncholith
- **Lung Metastases**
  - Sarcomas (most common), especially chondrosarcoma, osteosarcoma, and synovial cell sarcoma
  - Mucinous adenocarcinomas (digestive tract, breast, ovarian)
  - Medullary thyroid carcinoma (uncommon)

Helpful Clues for Rare Diagnoses
- **Amyloidosis**
  - Accumulation of insoluble protein in extracellular space

- Can be limited to lungs (most common) or part of systemic disease, such as multiple myeloma
- Nodular parenchymal most common pattern of pulmonary amyloidosis
  - Solitary nodule more common than multiple nodules
  - Nodules usually range from 5-50 mm in diameter
  - Occasional large mass
  - Calcification rarely apparent on chest radiograph
  - Up to 50% have calcification on CT

- **Metastatic Pulmonary Calcification**
  - Occurs from hypercalcemia, most frequently from chronic renal failure
  - Chest radiograph usually normal but may show fluffy nodule or patchy lung consolidation
    - Upper lobes mainly affected
  - CT findings include poorly defined, centrilobular nodules with upper lobe predominance
    - 3-10 mm in diameter
    - Calcification may be diffuse, stippled, or circumferential
    - Calcification may not be apparent on CT
  - Lung parenchyma may take up radiotracer on bone scan
- **Lung Ossification**
  - Characterized by metaplastic bone formation in lung parenchyma
  - 2 patterns: Nodular and dendriform
    - Nodular pattern most common with longstanding mitral valve stenosis
    - Dendriform pattern associated with chronic inflammation and interstitial fibrosis
    - CT shows calcification better than chest radiography
  - Can be confused with metastatic calcification
- **Alveolar Microlithiasis**
  - Characterized by accumulation of innumerable tiny calcifications in alveolar lumen
  - Most commonly occurs in adults 20-50 years old
  - Approximately 1/3 of patients have family history of alveolar microlithiasis
  - Chest radiograph
    - Diffuse fine micronodules with relative mid and lower zone predominance
    - Apical bullae may be present
    - Zone of sparing between lung and ribs ("black pleural line") may be evident
  - CT
    - Innumerable tiny (< 1 mm) calcified nodules with posterior predominance
    - Associated findings include ground-glass opacity, calcified and thickened interlobular septa, and paraseptal emphysema
  - Bone scan
    - Diffuse pulmonary uptake of technetium-99m methylene diphosphonate (Tc-99m-MDP)

Mycobacterial Pneumonia

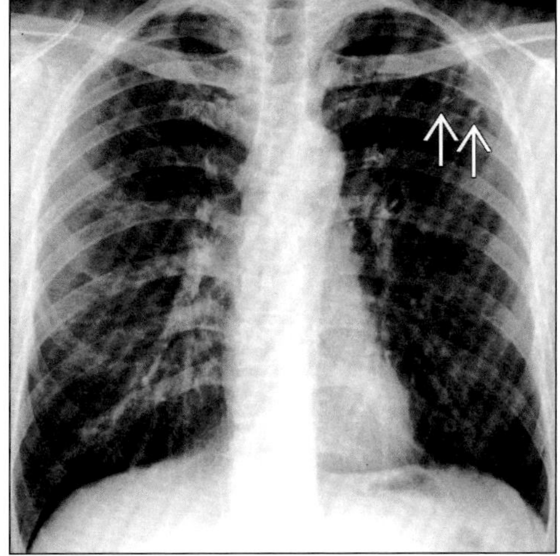

Frontal radiograph shows fibrocalcific scar ➔ in the left lung apex, typical of old tuberculosis. Calcified ipsilateral hilar and mediastinal lymph nodes are sometimes evident on chest radiographs.

Fungal, Histoplasmosis

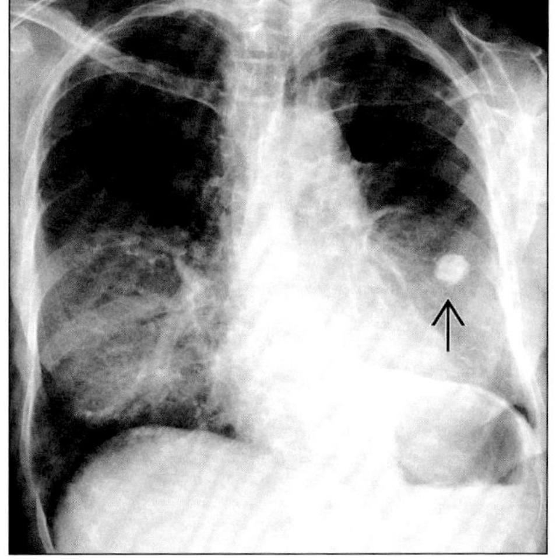

Frontal radiograph shows a large calcified nodule in the mid left lung ➔ representing the sequela of remote histoplasmosis. Histoplasmosis is endemic in the Ohio and Mississippi river valleys.

PULMONARY CALCIFICATION

(Left) *Frontal radiograph shows a solitary nodule with smooth margins in the mid right lung ➔ containing coarse "popcorn" calcifications, typical of a hamartoma. Fat attenuation in pulmonary hamartomas is only apparent on CT.* **(Right)** *Axial CECT shows a large nodule with margins and coarse "popcorn" calcifications in the right middle lobe ➔, typical of a hamartoma. However, "popcorn" calcifications are not present in most pulmonary hamartomas.*

Hamartoma

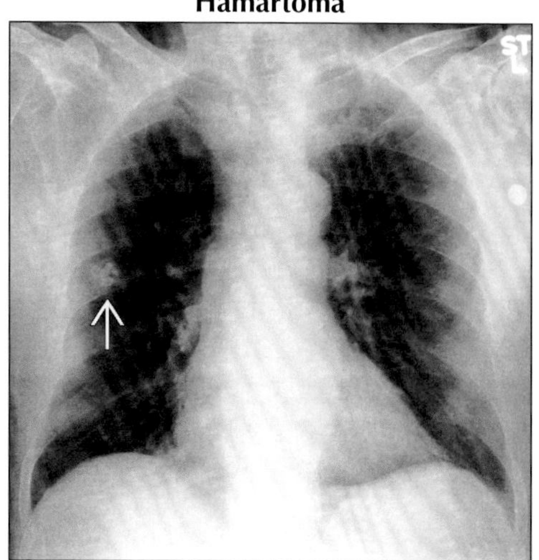

Hamartoma

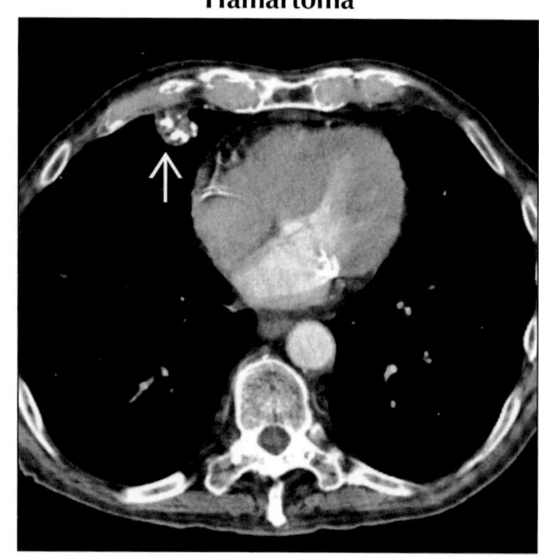

(Left) *Axial HRCT shows small nodules with central calcifications in both lungs ➔ adjacent to bilateral cavitary large masses ➔ representing progressive massive fibrosis in this patient with coal worker's pneumoconiosis.* **(Right)** *Frontal radiograph shows numerous small, well-defined nodules, many of which are calcified, predominating in the upper lobes ➔ in this patient with simple silicosis. Coalescence of subpleural nodules ➔ forms pseudoplaques.*

Silicosis/Coal Worker's Pneumoconiosis

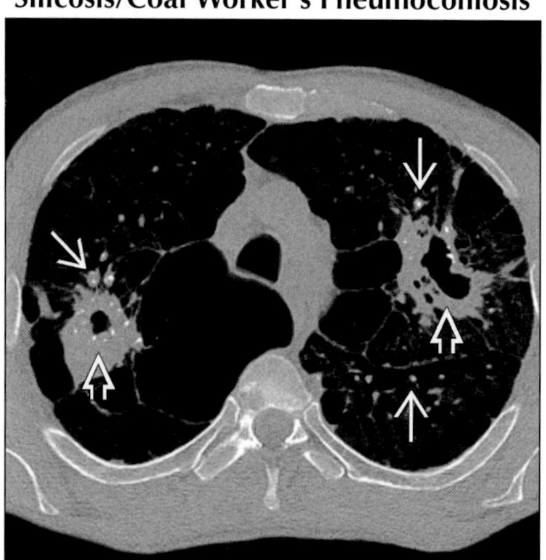

Silicosis/Coal Worker's Pneumoconiosis

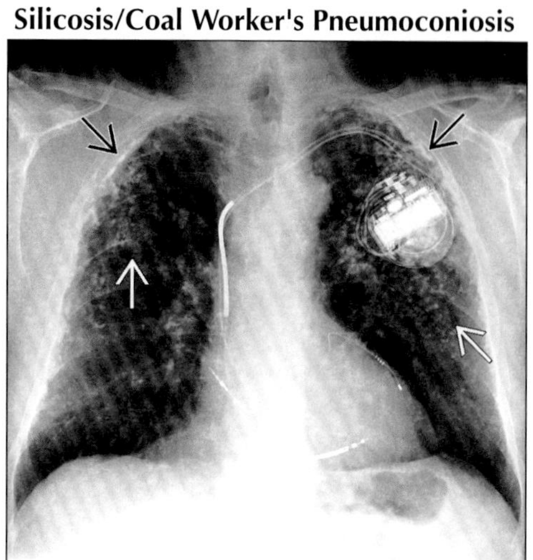

(Left) *Axial HRCT shows numerous well-defined nodules, many of which are calcified ➔, in the upper lung zones in this patient with simple silicosis. Note the pseudoplaques formed from coalescence of subpleural nodules ➔. A small right paratracheal lymph node is also calcified ➔.* **(Right)** *Axial CECT shows a heterogeneous left perihilar mass ➔ containing a slightly eccentric calcification ➔. Biopsy showed a typical carcinoid.*

Silicosis/Coal Worker's Pneumoconiosis

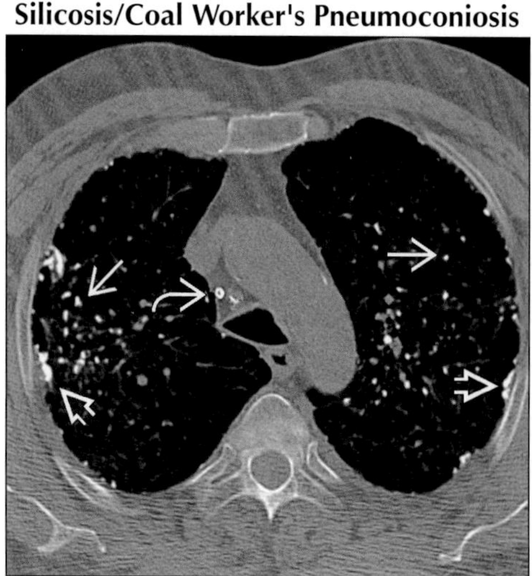

Carcinoid

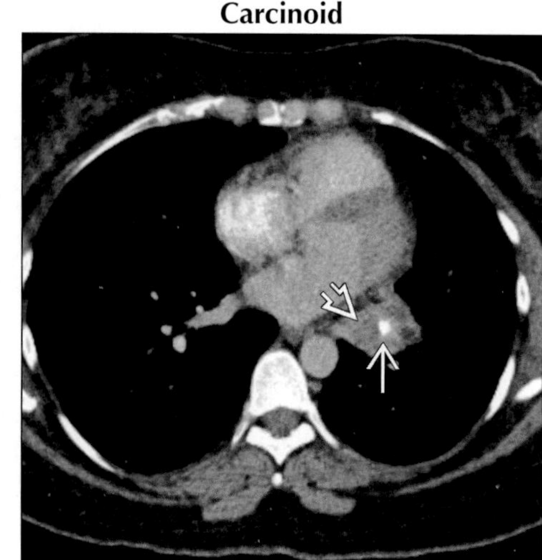

PULMONARY CALCIFICATION

Lung Metastases

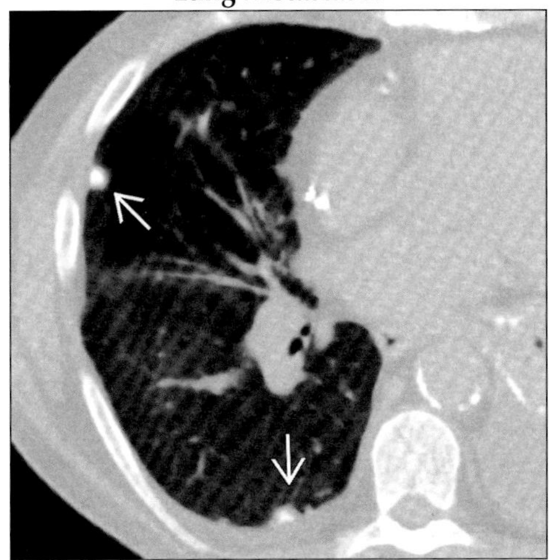

Amyloidosis

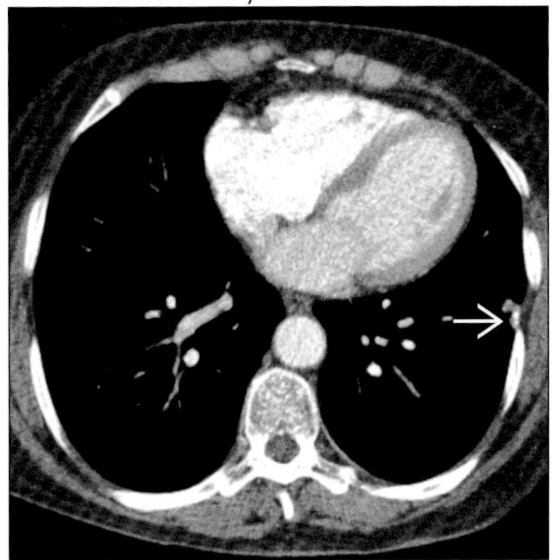

(Left) *Axial oblique shows 2 centrally calcified subpleural nodules in the right lung ➡ in this patient with metastatic chondrosarcoma. Sarcomas have a propensity to metastasize to the lungs, and chondrosarcomas and osteosarcomas are the most common causes of calcified lung metastases.* ***(Right)*** *Axial CECT demonstrates a bilobed nodule containing small calcifications ➡ shown to represent focal parenchymal nodular amyloidosis.*

Metastatic Pulmonary Calcification

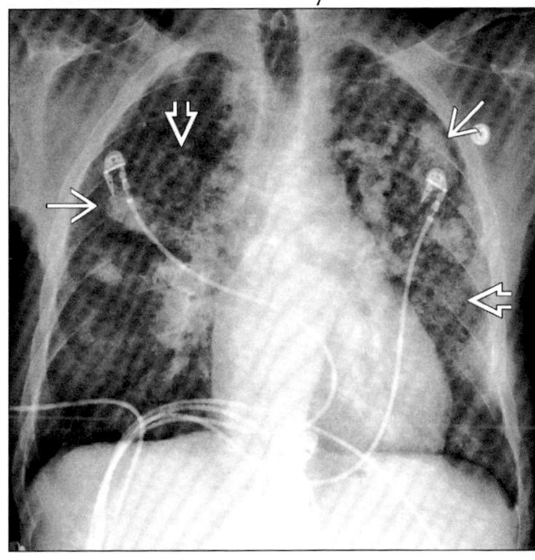

Metastatic Pulmonary Calcification

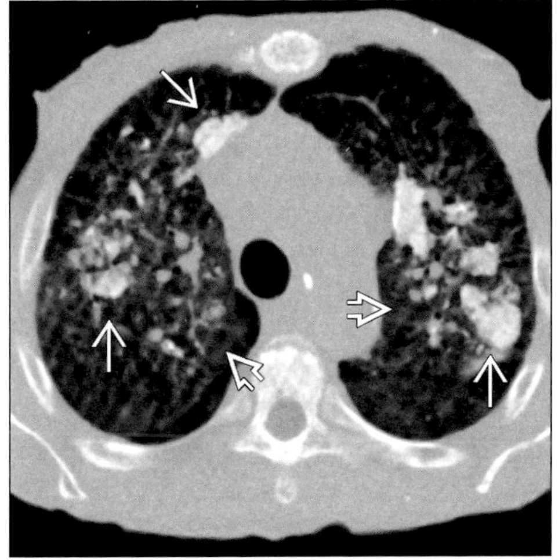

(Left) *Frontal radiograph shows diffuse tiny nodules in both lungs ➡ and larger high-attenuation nodules ➡ bilaterally in this patient with longstanding chronic renal insufficiency. Hypercalcemia of any cause can lead to metastatic pulmonary calcification; hemodialysis-dependent renal failure is the most common.* ***(Right)*** *Axial NECT shows high-attenuation nodules in both lungs ➡ and fluffy ground-glass attenuation ➡.*

Lung Ossification

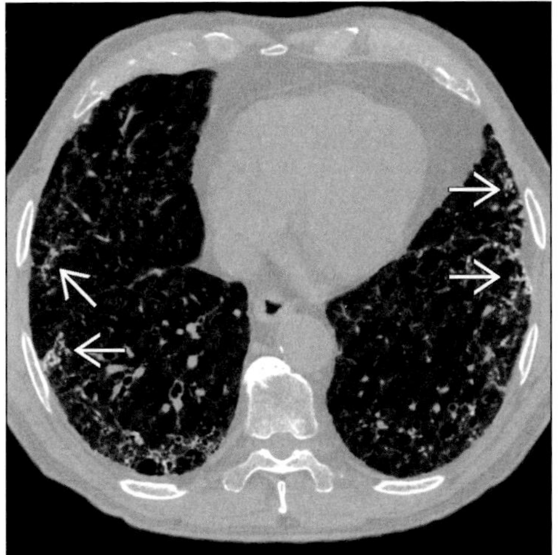

Alveolar Microlithiasis

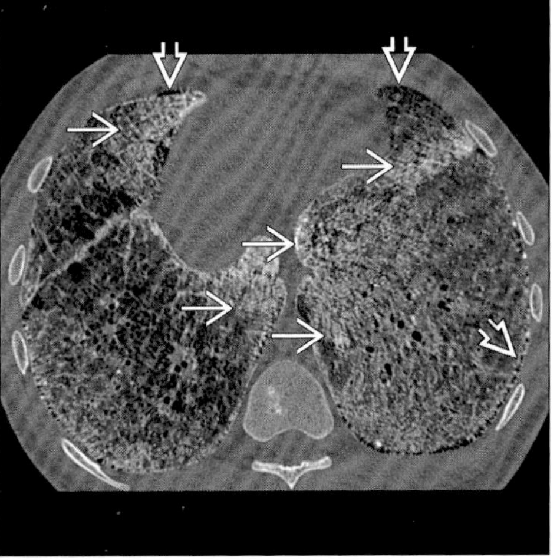

(Left) *Axial HRCT shows punctate calcification predominantly along alveolar septa ➡ representing pulmonary ossification in this patient with chronic interstitial fibrosis. Pulmonary ossification is frequently an incidental finding on HRCT and biopsy specimens.* ***(Right)*** *Axial HRCT shows diffuse, confluent micronodules ➡. Band-like subpleural sparing is the result of paraseptal emphysema ➡ and known as "black pleural stripe" sign.*

HALO SIGN

DIFFERENTIAL DIAGNOSIS

Common
- Angioinvasive Aspergillosis

Less Common
- Pulmonary Metastasis
- Kaposi Sarcoma
- Wegener Granulomatosis

Rare but Important
- Bronchioloalveolar Carcinoma
- Atypical Infection

ESSENTIAL INFORMATION

Key Differential Diagnosis Issues
- Halo sign refers to ring of ground-glass opacity surrounding pulmonary mass or nodule on CT
- Ground-glass opacity usually represents alveolar hemorrhage

Helpful Clues for Common Diagnoses
- **Angioinvasive Aspergillosis**
  - Occurs in immunocompromised patients, especially AIDS, organ transplant, and chemotherapy
  - Fungal invasion with occlusion of small- and medium-sized pulmonary arteries
  - Results in tissue infarction, necrosis, and hemorrhage

Helpful Clues for Less Common Diagnoses
- **Pulmonary Metastasis**
  - Central nodule represents metastatic lesion
  - Halo surrounding nodule represents hemorrhage
  - May be seen uncommonly with numerous malignancies, including melanoma, choriocarcinoma, and angiosarcoma
- **Kaposi Sarcoma**
  - Usually occurs in patients with AIDS
  - Commonly preceded by appearance of mucocutaneous lesions
  - Ill-defined nodules in peribronchovascular distribution
  - Some nodules produce halo sign due to surrounding hemorrhage
- **Wegener Granulomatosis**
  - Bilateral nodules and masses usually > 2 cm in size with no predilection for specific lung region
  - Approximately 50% of cases show cavitation
  - Look for associated tracheal involvement

Helpful Clues for Rare Diagnoses
- **Bronchioloalveolar Carcinoma**
  - Lepidic growth: Growth along alveolar and bronchiolar walls and septa without stromal invasion
  - Halo sign is caused by infiltration of tumor cells growing in lepidic fashion
  - May have internal bubbly lucencies referred to as pseudocavitation
- **Atypical Infection**
  - Has been described with tuberculosis, MAI, CMV, HSV, *Mucor,* candidiasis, coccidioidomycosis, pseudomonas

Angioinvasive Aspergillosis

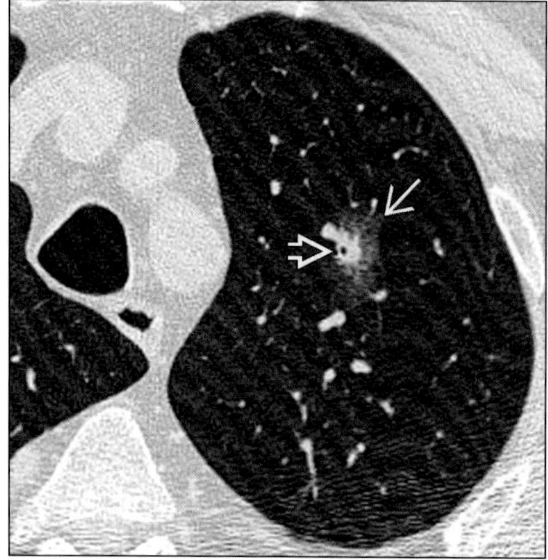

Axial NECT shows a pulmonary nodule in the left upper lobe ⮚, which is partially surrounded by a rim of ground-glass opacity ➔. This halo was caused by angioinvasive aspergillosis.

Angioinvasive Aspergillosis

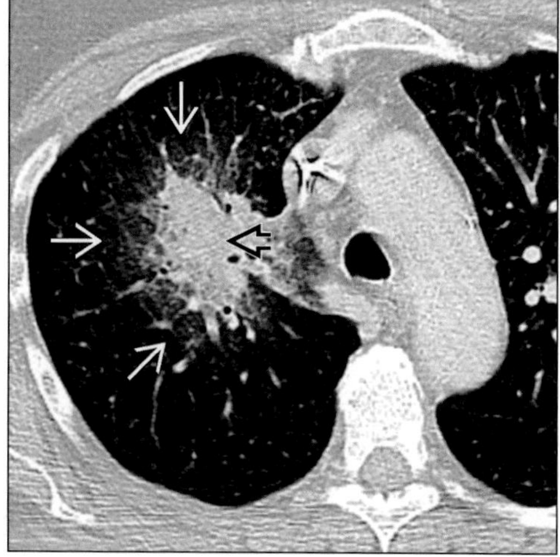

Axial NECT shows a large mass in the right upper lobe ⮚, which is surrounded by a rim of ground-glass density ➔. This patient was immunosuppressed due to chemotherapy.

HALO SIGN

Angioinvasive Aspergillosis

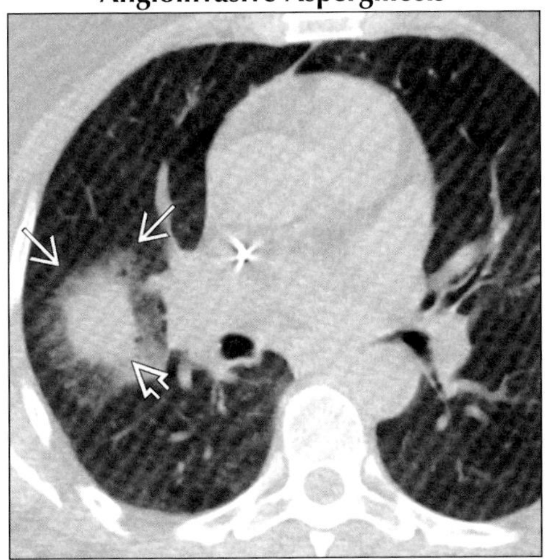

Pulmonary Metastasis

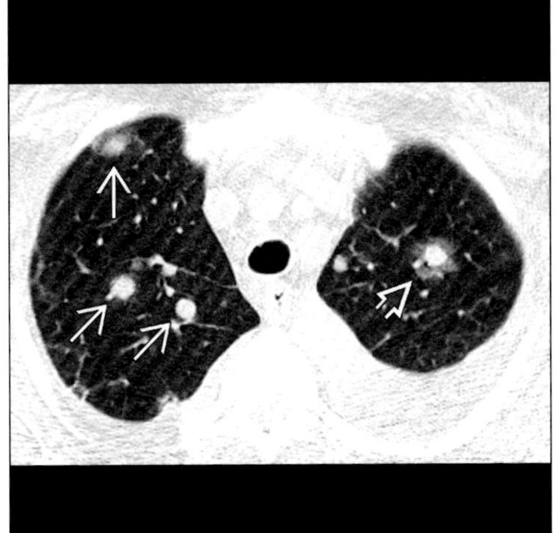

*(**Left**) Axial NECT shows a large mass in the right lung ➡ with a surrounding ground-glass halo ➡. In an immunocompromised patient, this is highly suggestive of angioinvasive aspergillosis. (**Right**) Axial NECT shows a nodule in the left upper lobe with a halo sign ➡. Several other nodules are present ➡. These findings are caused by metastatic melanoma, a vascular lesion that may produce surrounding hemorrhage.*

Kaposi Sarcoma

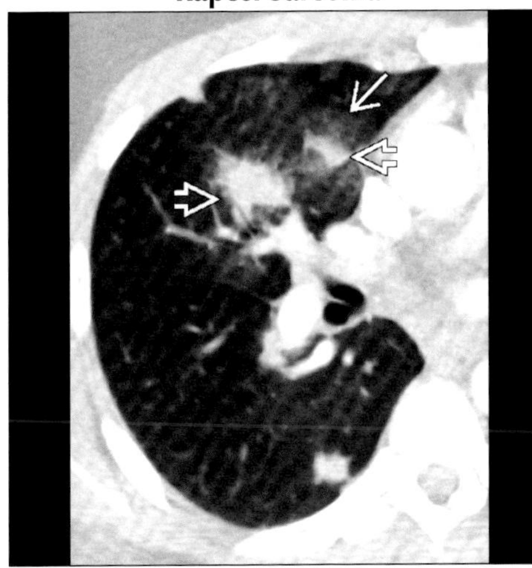

Wegener Granulomatosis

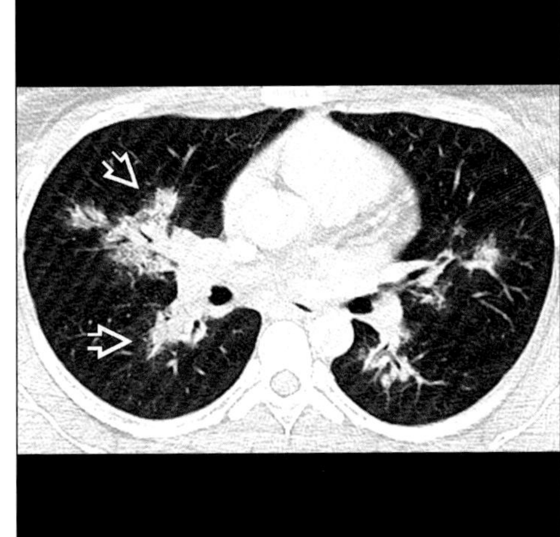

*(**Left**) Axial CECT shows flame-shaped nodules ➡ in this patient with AIDS. Notice the surrounding ground-glass halo ➡. This is typical of Kaposi sarcoma, especially if there is concurrent cutaneous disease. (**Right**) Axial NECT shows numerous bilateral nodules in a peribronchovascular distribution. There is faint ground-glass density surrounding some of the lesions ➡. These findings are caused by Wegener granulomatosis.*

Bronchioloalveolar Carcinoma

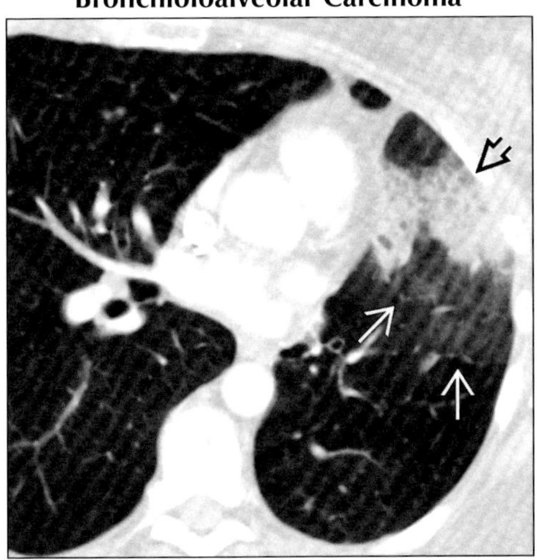

Atypical Infection

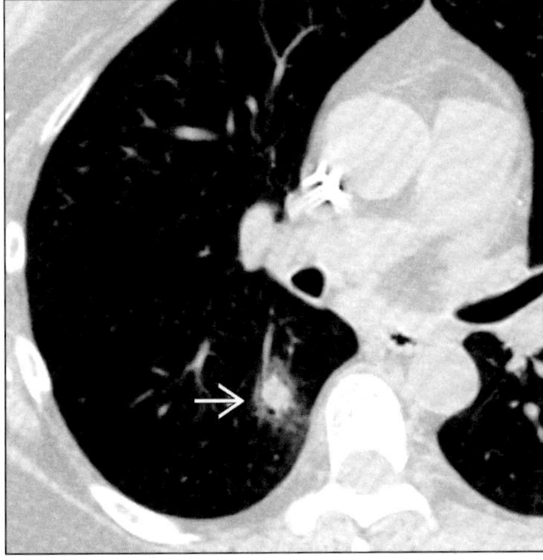

*(**Left**) Axial CECT shows a mass in the left lung, which contains internal pseudocavitation ➡. A halo sign is formed by surrounding ground-glass density ➡. This is a typical appearance of bronchioloalveolar carcinoma. (**Right**) Axial NECT shows a typical halo sign in the superior segment of the right lower lobe ➡. This was caused by pseudomonas pneumonia in an immunosuppressed patient.*

REVERSE HALO SIGN

DIFFERENTIAL DIAGNOSIS

Common
- Cryptogenic Organizing Pneumonia
- Fungal Pneumonia
  - Invasive Fungal Pneumonia (Aspergillosis, Mucormycosis)
  - Paracoccidioidomycosis
- Bacterial Pneumonia

Less Common
- Wegener Granulomatosis
- Pulmonary Infarct
- Primary Tuberculosis
- Sarcoidosis
- Tumor

Rare but Important
- Lymphomatoid Granulomatosis

ESSENTIAL INFORMATION

Key Differential Diagnosis Issues
- Reverse halo: Central ground-glass opacity surrounded by rim of consolidation

Helpful Clues for Common Diagnoses
- **Cryptogenic Organizing Pneumonia**
  - Subacute to chronic pulmonary opacities; may be migratory
  - Mid and lower lung zone, peripheral or peribronchovascular consolidation
- **Fungal Pneumonia**
  - **Invasive Fungal Pneumonia (Aspergillosis, Mucormycosis)**
    - Immunocompromised patients
    - Voriconazole prophylaxis and history of diabetes suggestive of mucormycosis
    - Multiple nodular or mass-like areas of consolidation; halo or air crescent sign
  - **Paracoccidioidomycosis**
    - Endemic to South America
    - Ground-glass opacities, parenchymal bands, centrilobular nodules ± cavitation

Helpful Clues for Less Common Diagnoses
- **Wegener Granulomatosis**
  - Pulmonary nodules, ± cavitation; subglottic tracheal stenosis
- **Pulmonary Infarct**
  - Pulmonary emboli; lower lung and peripheral opacities
- **Primary Tuberculosis**
  - Consolidation, hilar and mediastinal lymphadenopathy, pleural effusion
- **Sarcoidosis**
  - Mediastinal and hilar lymphadenopathy; perilymphatic pulmonary nodules
- **Tumor**
  - Chronic pulmonary abnormality with slow growth
  - Lung cancer: Smoking history, irregular margins, ipsilateral lymphadenopathy
  - Metastases: Multiple inferior preponderant pulmonary nodules of differing sizes

Helpful Clues for Rare Diagnoses
- **Lymphomatoid Granulomatosis**
  - Multiple lung nodules or masses with air bronchogram or halo sign, ± cavitation, ± peripheral enhancement

Cryptogenic Organizing Pneumonia

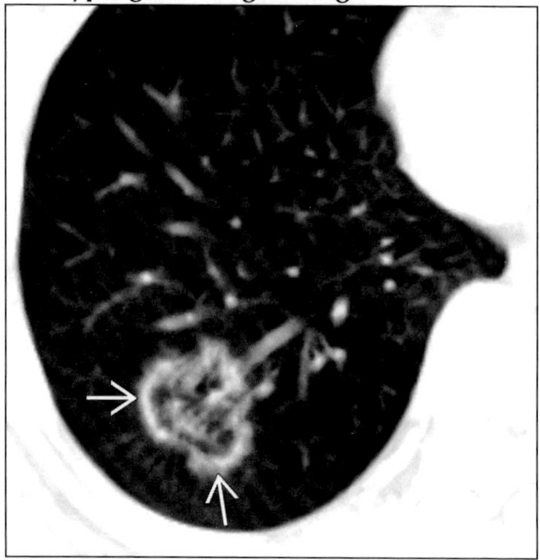

Axial NECT shows a thin rim of consolidation ➔ surrounding a focus of ground-glass opacity consistent with cryptogenic organizing pneumonia.

Cryptogenic Organizing Pneumonia

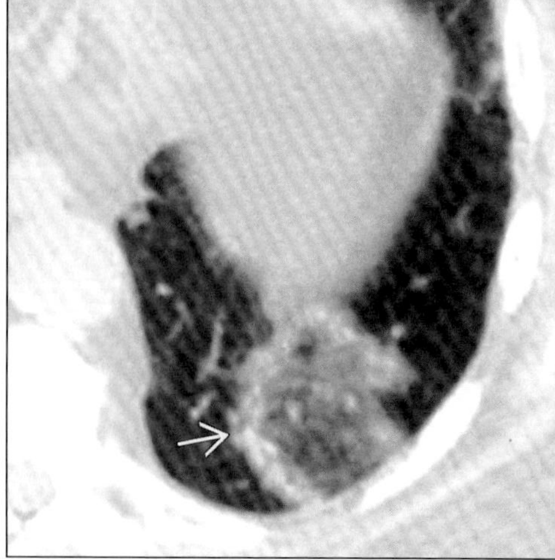

Axial NECT shows a focus of central ground-glass opacity with surrounding halo of consolidation ➔ in the left lower lobe.

REVERSE HALO SIGN

Fungal Pneumonia

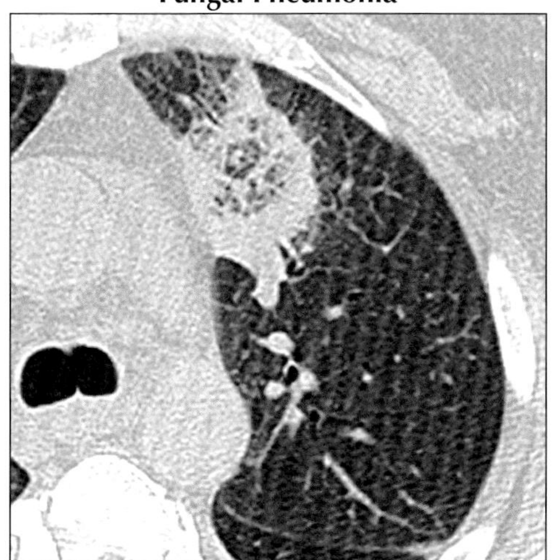

Fungal Pneumonia

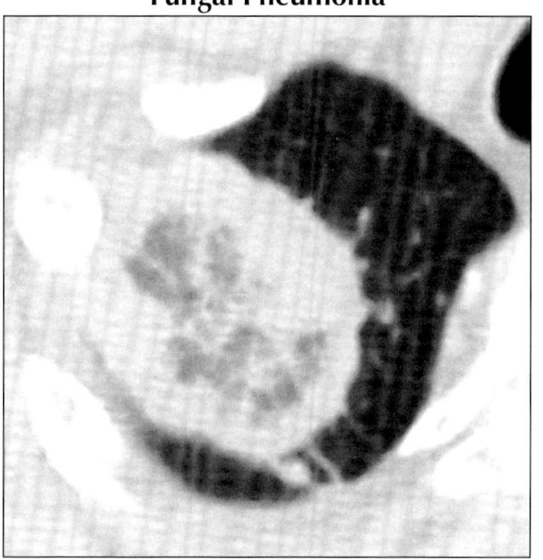

***(Left)** Axial NECT shows an irregular air-space opacity with a reverse halo configuration suggestive of an invasive fungal pneumonia in this neutropenic patient who presented with fever and chest pain. **(Right)** Axial NECT shows thick-walled consolidation in the right apex with a reverse halo configuration shown to represent aspergillosis. This lesion was followed to resolution given the imaging overlap with bronchogenic carcinoma.*

Bacterial Pneumonia

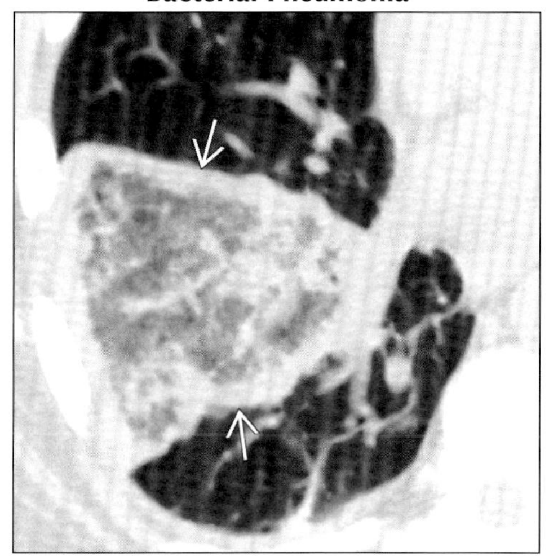

Bacterial Pneumonia

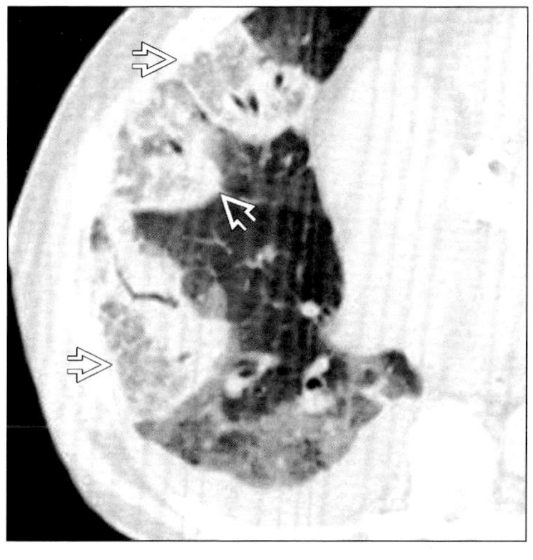

***(Left)** Axial NECT shows a large region of ground-glass opacity and peripheral rim of consolidation in the right lower lobe with superimposed interlobular and intralobular septal thickening ➔. The patient was not neutropenic and presented with fever and chills. **(Right)** Axial NECT shows multifocal regions of air-space opacity with a reverse halo configuration ➲ and patchy regions of ground-glass opacity. There is a small right pleural effusion.*

Pulmonary Infarct

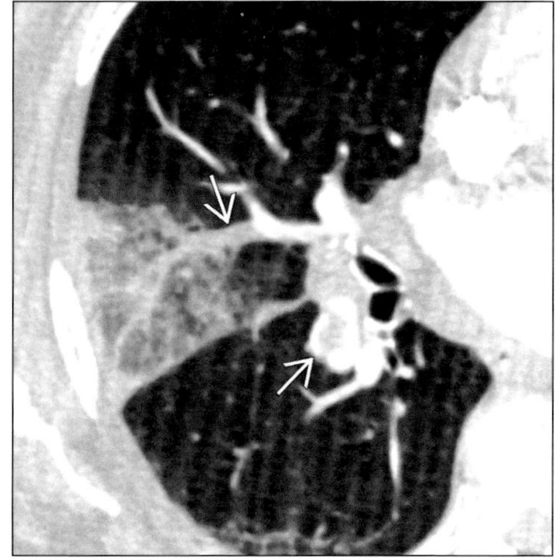

Tumor

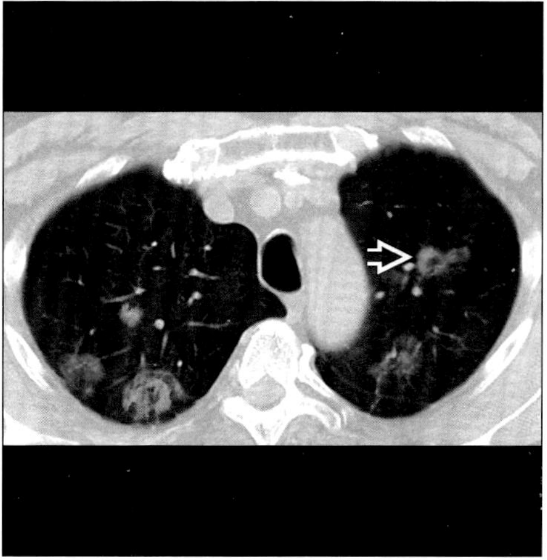

***(Left)** Axial CECT shows acute pulmonary emboli ➔ in the right lung. The peripheral focus of air-space opacity with partial reverse halo configuration is highly suggestive of pulmonary infarct in this setting. **(Right)** Axial NECT show multiple solid and ground-glass nodules, some of which have reverse halo configuration ➲. Tissue biopsy was diagnostic of melanoma metastases.*

SECTION 6
Interstitium

MILIARY PATTERN

DIFFERENTIAL DIAGNOSIS

Common

- Mycobacterial
- Metastases
- Viral Pneumonia
- Disseminated Fungal Disease

Less Common

- Sarcoidosis
- Silicosis/Coal Worker's Pneumoconiosis
- Talcosis
- Alveolar Microlithiasis
- Lung Ossification
- Bronchioloalveolar Cell Carcinoma

Rare but Important

- Intravesical Bacillus Calmette-Guérin (BCG) Immunotherapy

ESSENTIAL INFORMATION

Key Differential Diagnosis Issues

- Definition: Diffuse tiny lung nodules (< 5 mm in diameter)
  - Determine location of nodules with respect to secondary pulmonary lobule
    - Centrilobular or perilymphatic or random
  - Term "miliary" derived from Latin; related to millet seed, which it resembles
- Miliary pattern: Random pattern
  - Random distribution of nodules in secondary pulmonary lobule
  - Too numerous to count, < 5 mm in diameter
  - Pathophysiology: Random miliary pattern primarily due to hematogenous spread of disease
- Chest radiographs vs. HRCT
  - Chest radiograph may be normal even in biopsy-proven cases
    - Summation effect on radiograph: Superimposition of nodules otherwise below detection threshold allows detection
    - Sensitivity of chest radiographs in miliary tuberculosis: 60-70%
  - HRCT more sensitive than chest radiographs

Helpful Clues for Common Diagnoses

- **Mycobacterial**
  - Tuberculosis
    - Miliary spread may occur during primary or post-primary stages, usually with severe immunosuppression
    - Presentation in HIV depends on severity of immunosuppression: Miliary presentation usually occurs when CD4(+) < 200
    - Sputum often AFB negative; bronchoscopy with transbronchial biopsy or liver or bone marrow biopsy often necessary for diagnosis
    - Spectrum of illness: Asymptomatic to severe respiratory distress
  - Nontuberculous mycobacteria
    - Usually centrilobular nodules
    - Miliary pattern occasionally seen in immunocompromised hosts
    - May be associated with bronchiectasis
- **Metastases**
  - Most frequently seen with
    - Melanoma
    - Thyroid carcinoma
    - Choriocarcinoma
    - Renal cell carcinoma
  - Miliary metastases typically larger than those of tuberculosis
  - Tend to have more well-defined margins than miliary tuberculosis
  - Background ground-glass attenuation more common with miliary tuberculosis
  - Chronic miliary tuberculosis nodules usually more profuse in upper lung zones whereas metastases more common in lower lung zones
- **Viral Pneumonia**
  - Varicella (chickenpox)
    - Healed varicella pneumonia can present as miliary calcified nodules
  - Influenza
    - Miliary pattern rare but has been described; also seen in other viral infections, such as Cytomegalovirus
- **Disseminated Fungal Disease**
  - Usually occurs in those with impaired T-cell immunity, elderly, or debilitated
  - Pattern identical to miliary tuberculosis
  - Upper lung zone proclivity seen with blastomycosis; uncommon with other fungi
  - May progress to diffuse lung consolidation

- May complicate acute or chronic disease or be initial manifestation

Helpful Clues for Less Common Diagnoses

- **Sarcoidosis**
  - Usually nodules in a perilymphatic distribution, rarely miliary
  - Mid and upper zone predominance
  - May have symmetric hilar and mediastinal lymphadenopathy
- **Silicosis/Coal Worker's Pneumoconiosis**
  - Usually nodules in a perilymphatic distribution, rarely miliary
  - Occupational exposures essential
  - Tuberculosis can complicate both silicosis and coal worker's pneumoconiosis
  - May have symmetric hilar and mediastinal lymphadenopathy
- **Talcosis**
  - Talc: Common ingredient in oral medication ground-up with intent to inject intravenously
  - Initial miliary pattern may coalesce to progressive massive fibrosis, much like silicosis
  - Findings of pulmonary hypertension may be present
- **Alveolar Microlithiasis**
  - Calcification of nodules striking
  - Subpleural sparing results in "black pleura" sign
- **Lung Ossification**
  - Densely calcified, 1-5 mm nodules concentrated in middle and lower lungs
  - Associated with chronic severe mitral stenosis
  - Idiopathic form also exists, associated with pulmonary fibrosis
  - Tend to become confluent and may form osseous trabeculae (3-13%)
  - Tends not to be severe; miliary pattern uncommon
  - Typically patients are elderly and male; symptoms uncommon
- **Bronchioloalveolar Cell Carcinoma**
  - Predominant nodule distribution pattern is centrilobular
    - Reflects endobronchial spread of tumor
  - Nodules with random distribution occur less often
    - Reflects hematogenous spread of tumor
  - Nodules usually are ground-glass attenuation
  - Continued growth over weeks or months

Helpful Clues for Rare Diagnoses

- **Intravesical Bacillus Calmette-Guérin (BCG) Immunotherapy**
  - Intravesical instillation of attenuated *Mycobacterium bovis* for treatment of superficial transitional cell carcinoma of bladder
  - Indistinguishable from miliary tuberculosis except by history
  - Represents actual BCG bacteremia

Mycobacterial

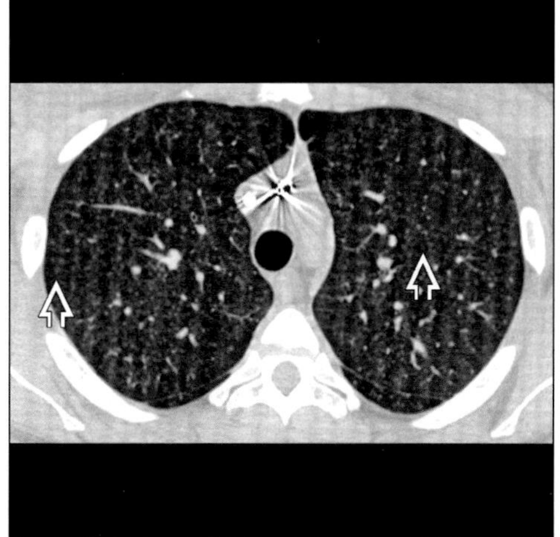

Axial HRCT shows the typical CT features of miliary tuberculosis. Pinpoint nodules ➔ are present in a random pattern of distribution.

Mycobacterial

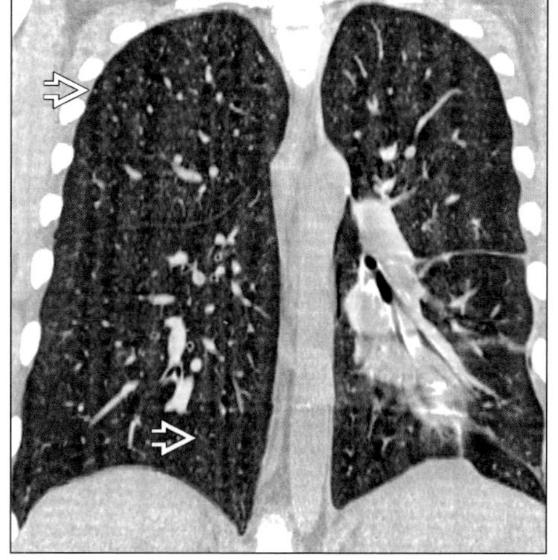

Coronal HRCT reconstruction in the same patient shows the uniform distribution of miliary nodules ➔ throughout the upper and lower lobes.

MILIARY PATTERN

*(**Left**) Coronal HRCT shows miliary nodules from thyroid metastases. Notice the large thyroid mass ⇨ causing deviation of the trachea to the left. Diffuse miliary nodules → demonstrate a random distribution. (**Right**) Axial HRCT shows miliary nodules from Cytomegalovirus pneumonia. There are diffuse miliary nodules ⇨ and patchy ground-glass opacities →. CMV pneumonia usually affects immunocompromised patients.*

Metastases

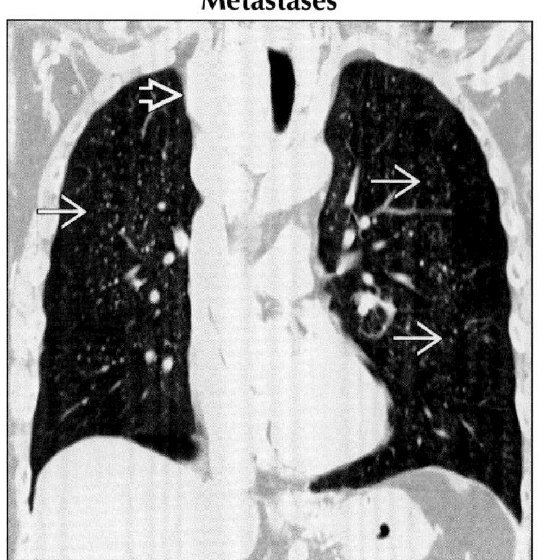

Viral Pneumonia

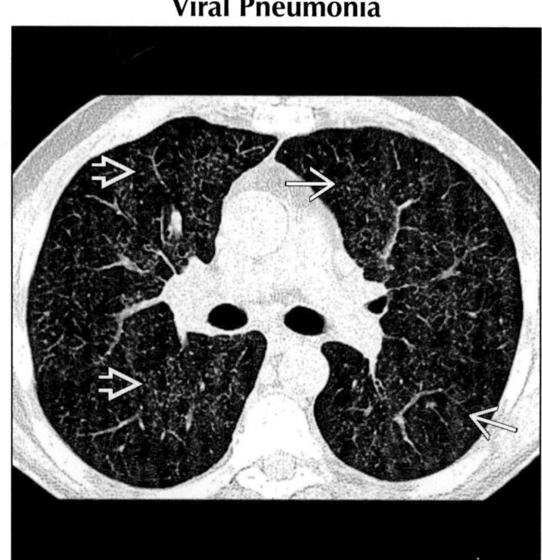

*(**Left**) Frontal radiograph coned down to the right lung shows variant radiographic features of blastomycosis with diffuse miliary nodules → and moderate pleural effusion ⇨. (**Right**) Axial HRCT in the same patient shows the miliary nodules (< 3 mm in size) →. Moderate-sized pleural effusions ⇨ are not frequently associated with blastomycosis. Other features of blastomycosis include osteolytic lesions.*

Disseminated Fungal Disease

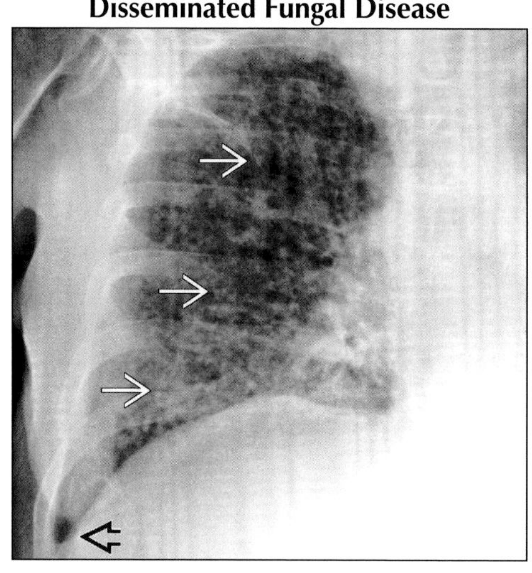

Disseminated Fungal Disease

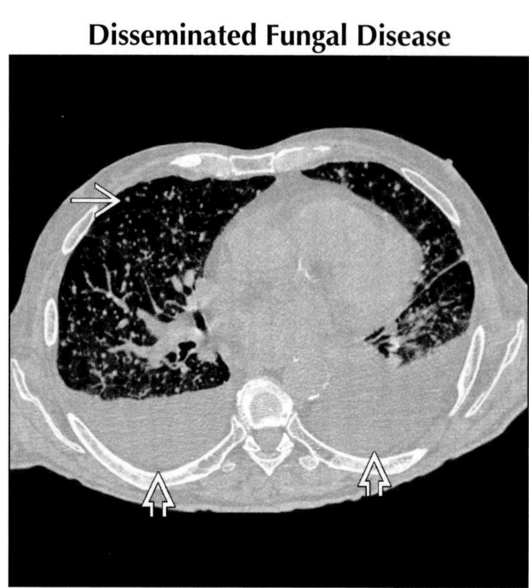

*(**Left**) Axial HRCT shows miliary nodules from histoplasmosis. The primary histoplasma pneumonia is in the left upper lobe →. Diffuse miliary nodules ⇨ are the result of hematogenous dissemination of histoplasmosis. (**Right**) Axial HRCT shows diffuse tiny nodules throughout the lungs. Some nodules are perilymphatic in location: Along the major fissures → and peripheral subpleural lung, locations commonly seen with sarcoidosis.*

Disseminated Fungal Disease

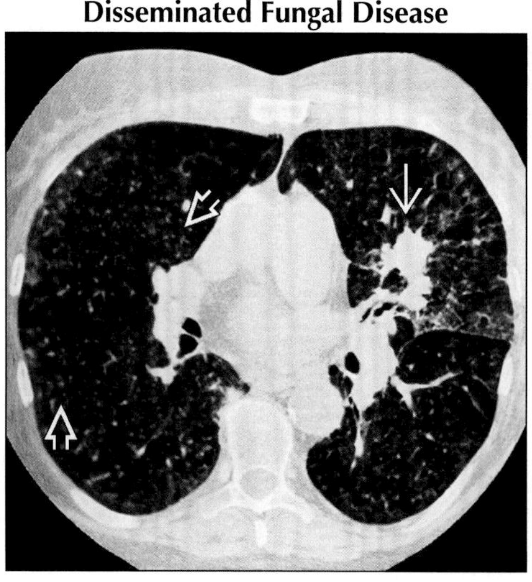

Sarcoidosis

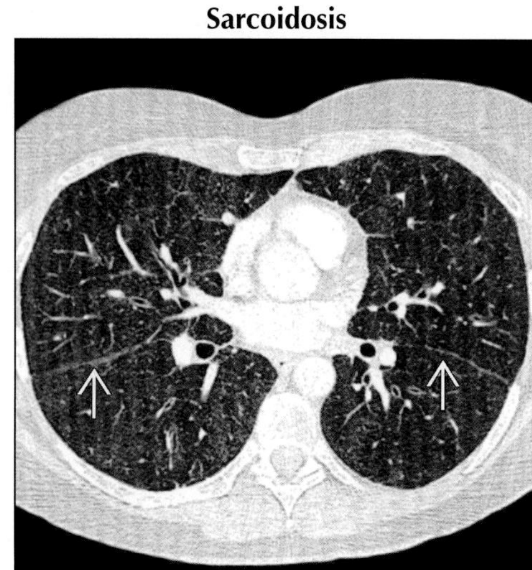

Silicosis/Coal Worker's Pneumoconiosis

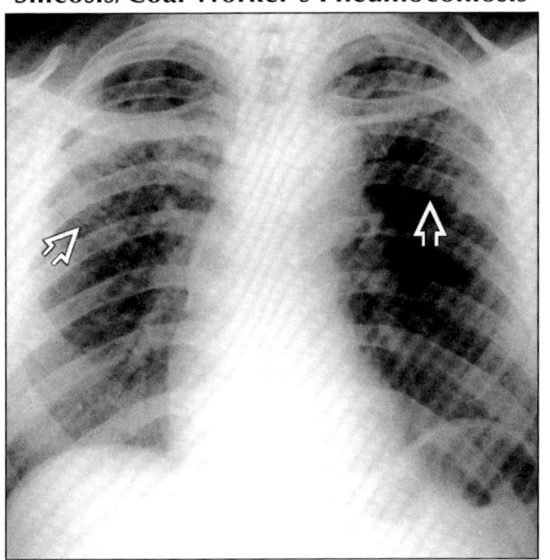

Talcosis

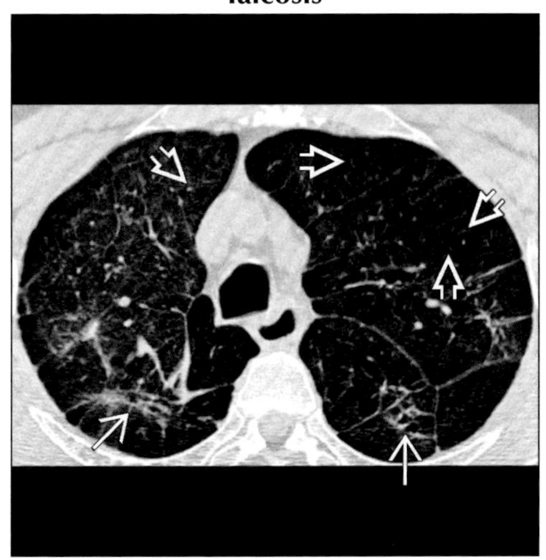

(Left) *Frontal radiograph shows miliary nodules ➡ in both lungs, predominating in the upper lobes in this patient with simple silicosis. Coalescence of the nodules over time results in development of progressive massive fibrosis.* ***(Right)*** *Axial HRCT shows developing fibrosis ➡ on a background of miliary nodules ➡ from talcosis resulting from intravenous drug abuse. Inhalational talcosis can also cause miliary nodules but is far less common.*

Alveolar Microlithiasis

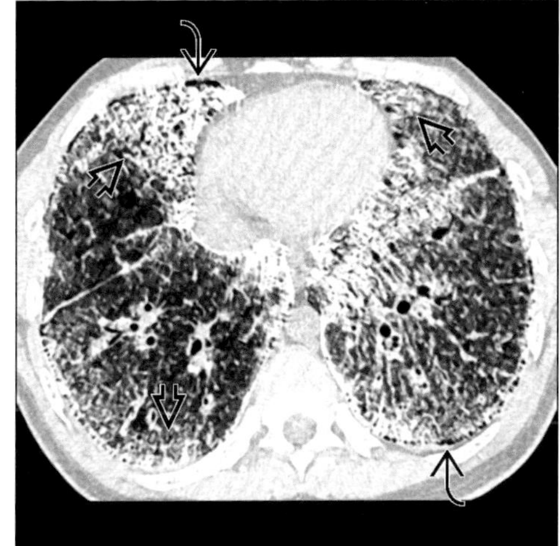

Lung Ossification

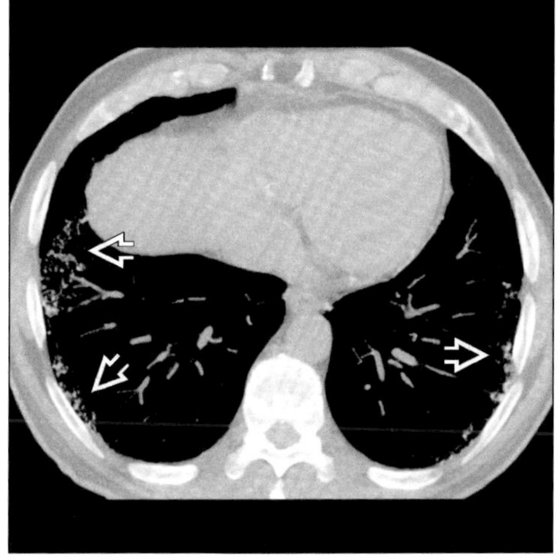

(Left) *Axial HRCT shows typical CT features of diffuse calcification due to alveolar microlithiasis. Confluent micronodular opacities ➡ are more extensive in the lower lobes and predominantly peripheral in distribution. Note the band-like sparing of the subpleural areas, "black pleural" sign ➡.* ***(Right)*** *Axial NECT at bone windows shows numerous peripheral miliary calcifications ➡ from lung ossification.*

Bronchioloalveolar Cell Carcinoma

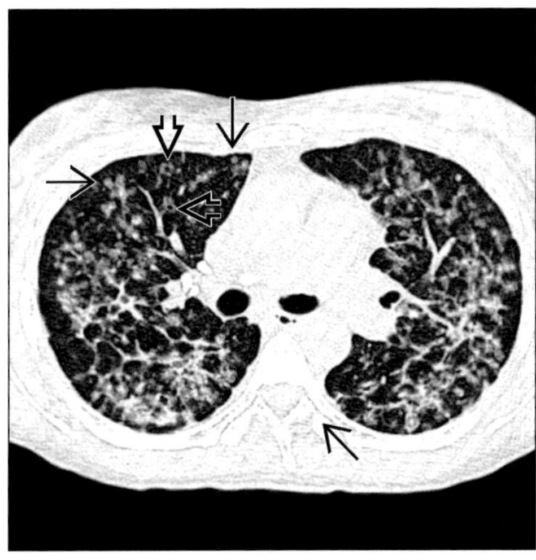

Intravesical Bacillus Calmette-Guérin (BCG) Immunotherapy

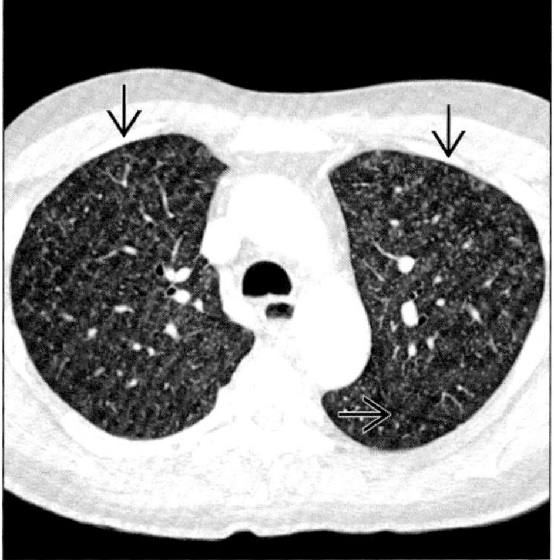

(Left) *Axial HRCT shows numerous small nodules ➡ throughout the lungs. Some of the nodules have central lucencies ➡ sometimes referred to as pseudocavitation, reflecting tumor growth around the airways.* ***(Right)*** *Axial HRCT shows innumerable tiny nodules ➡ in a patient treated with intravesicular BCG for transitional cell carcinoma of the bladder. Spread of BCG to the lungs is indistinguishable on CT from miliary tuberculosis.*

HONEYCOMBING

DIFFERENTIAL DIAGNOSIS

Common
- Usual Interstitial Pneumonia (UIP)
- Nonspecific Interstitial Pneumonia (NSIP)
- Chronic Hypersensitivity Pneumonitis

Less Common
- Sarcoidosis
- Asbestosis

Rare but Important
- Acute Interstitial Pneumonia

ESSENTIAL INFORMATION

Key Differential Diagnosis Issues
- Honeycombing represents end-stage lung fibrosis
  - As final common pathway, can be difficult to distinguish inciting cause
  - Honeycombing seen on CT (macroscopic) does not always correlate with microscopic honeycombing seen on histology
  - Poor prognostic indicator
- Characterized on imaging by
  - Clustered cysts with well-defined walls
  - 3-10 mm in diameter (up to 2.5 cm), similar size
  - Frequently form stacked rows in peripheral lung
  - Cystic spaces on occasion can become large
- Honeycombing always associated with other findings of lung fibrosis

Helpful Clues for Common Diagnoses
- **Usual Interstitial Pneumonia (UIP)**
  - Histologic pattern of interstitial fibrosis characterized by
    - Temporal and spatial heterogeneity
    - Patchy distribution
    - Subpleural and basal predominance
    - Fibroblastic foci
  - Most patients with histologic and CT pattern of UIP have idiopathic pulmonary fibrosis (IPF)
  - Other causes of UIP pattern
    - Collagen-vascular disease, especially rheumatoid arthritis
    - Drug toxicity
    - Asbestosis
    - Hypersensitivity pneumonitis
    - Familial fibrosis
    - Inflammatory bowel disease (rare)
  - Most common cause of honeycombing
  - Early honeycombing forms in subpleural lung
    - Basal predominance
    - Clusters and rows of honeycomb cysts
  - Other associated features of lung fibrosis
    - Reticulation
    - Traction bronchiectasis and bronchiolectasis
    - Architectural distortion
    - Ground-glass opacity less than extent of reticular abnormality
- **Nonspecific Interstitial Pneumonia (NSIP)**
  - Histological pattern of interstitial fibrosis characterized by
    - Spatial and temporal homogeneity
    - Basal predominant
    - Cellular, mixed, and fibrotic forms
  - Most patients have collagen vascular disease (especially scleroderma, mixed connective tissue disease, and polymyositis) or hypersensitivity pneumonitis
  - Other causes of NSIP pattern
    - Idiopathic (young women of east Asian ethnicity)
    - Drug toxicity
    - Familial fibrosis
    - Cigarette smoking (rare cause)
  - Honeycombing on CT is a late finding; less common with NSIP than UIP
  - Associated features
    - Basal predominant ground-glass opacity (most common)
    - Superimposed reticulation
    - Traction bronchiectasis and bronchiolectasis
    - Subpleural sparing (suggestive of diagnosis)
    - Peripheral and peribronchovascular distribution
    - Esophageal dilation (scleroderma and mixed connective tissue disease)
- **Chronic Hypersensitivity Pneumonitis**
  - Lung fibrosis resulting from chronic hypersensitivity reaction to organic antigen or low-molecular-weight inorganic compounds

- Mold and avian antigens most common causes
- Inorganic compounds include isocyanates (industrial paints)
  - Honeycombing infrequent
  - Associated features
    - Peripheral and peribronchial reticulation
    - Traction bronchiectasis and bronchiolectasis
    - Architectural distortion
    - Patchy ground-glass opacity
    - Lobular foci of air-trapping (very suggestive of diagnosis)
    - Poorly defined centrilobular nodules (very suggestive of diagnosis)
    - Extreme lung bases typically spared in contrast to idiopathic pulmonary fibrosis

Helpful Clues for Less Common Diagnoses

- **Sarcoidosis**
  - Honeycombing less common in sarcoidosis than with other end-stage lung diseases
  - Honeycomb cysts typically larger than those occurring with usual interstitial pneumonia
  - Subpleural and MID and UPPER lung zone distribution with basal sparing
  - Lymphadenopathy uncommon with end-stage sarcoidosis
- **Asbestosis**
  - Interstitial fibrosis from asbestos exposure
    - Histologically similar to UIP
  - Subpleural branching opacities (fibrosis centered on respiratory bronchioles where asbestos fibers deposited) earliest finding on CT
  - Honeycombing less common unless disease severe
  - Associated features
    - Parenchymal bands and subpleural curvilinear opacities
    - Calcified or noncalcified pleural plaques
    - Subpleural reticulation
    - Traction bronchiectasis and bronchiolectasis
    - Architectural distortion

Helpful Clues for Rare Diagnoses

- **Acute Interstitial Pneumonia**
  - Acute, rapidly evolving illness with respiratory failure requiring ventilatory support
    - 50% mortality rate
    - Idiopathic acute respiratory distress syndrome (ARDS)
    - Characterized histologically by diffuse alveolar damage
  - Predominant radiographic features
    - Consolidation (basal and posterior lungs)
    - Ground-glass opacity (superior and anterior lungs)
  - Honeycombing late finding in survivors
    - More common in anterior lung due to barotrauma (overinflating nondependent alveoli)

Usual Interstitial Pneumonia (UIP)

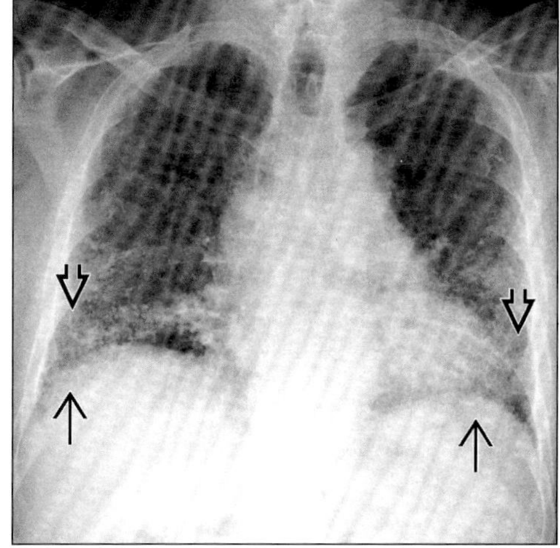

Frontal radiograph shows thin-walled honeycomb cysts in the lung bases ➔ with subpleural reticulation ➔. Honeycombing is only apparent on chest radiographs when it is advanced.

Usual Interstitial Pneumonia (UIP)

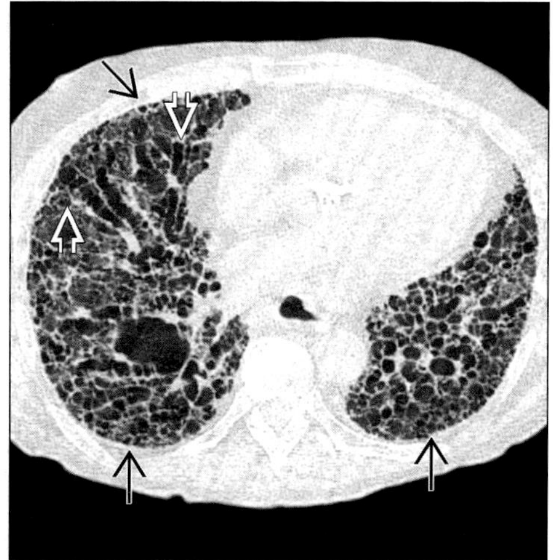

Axial HRCT shows diffuse honeycombing ➔ most pronounced posteriorly. Extensive traction bronchiectasis is present ➔ and can mimic honeycombing when seen on end.

HONEYCOMBING

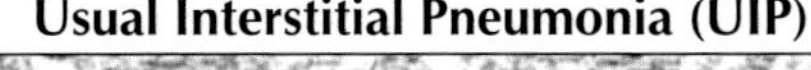

Usual Interstitial Pneumonia (UIP) | Usual Interstitial Pneumonia (UIP)

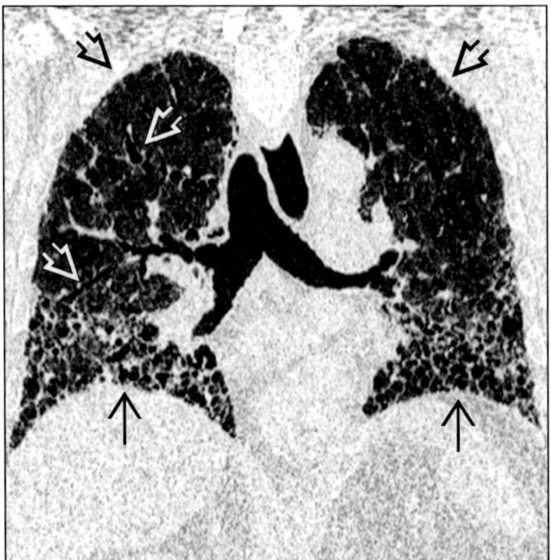

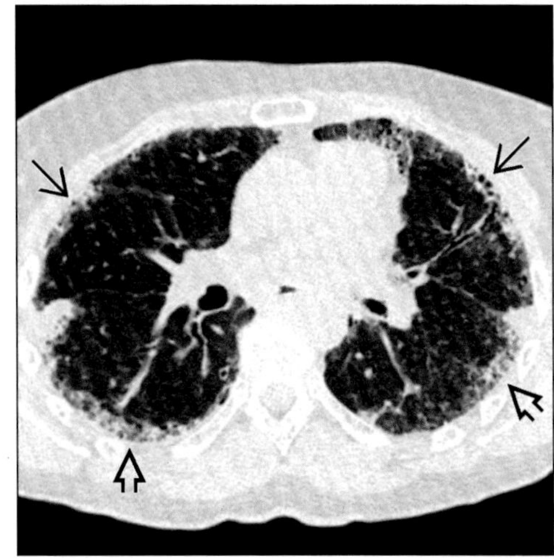

(Left) *Coronal CT reconstruction in a patient with idiopathic pulmonary fibrosis shows subpleural and basal predominant honeycombing →. Note low lung volumes, architectural distortion, traction bronchiectasis ➡, and subpleural reticulation ⇨.* ***(Right)*** *Axial HRCT in a patient with rheumatoid arthritis shows only mild subpleural honeycombing →. Note exquisitely subpleural distribution of reticulation ⇨ and architectural distortion.*

Nonspecific Interstitial Pneumonia (NSIP) | Nonspecific Interstitial Pneumonia (NSIP)

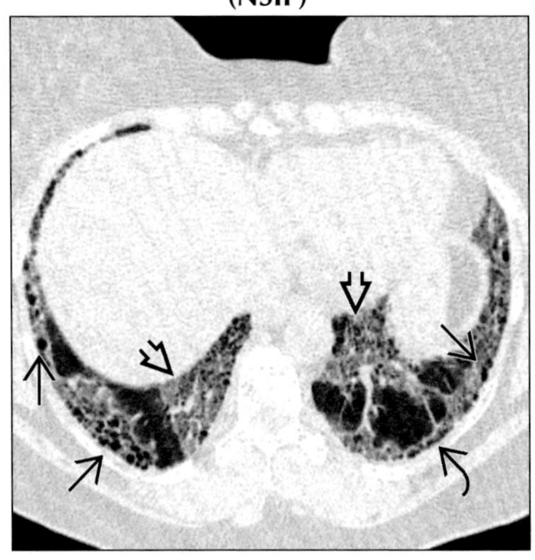

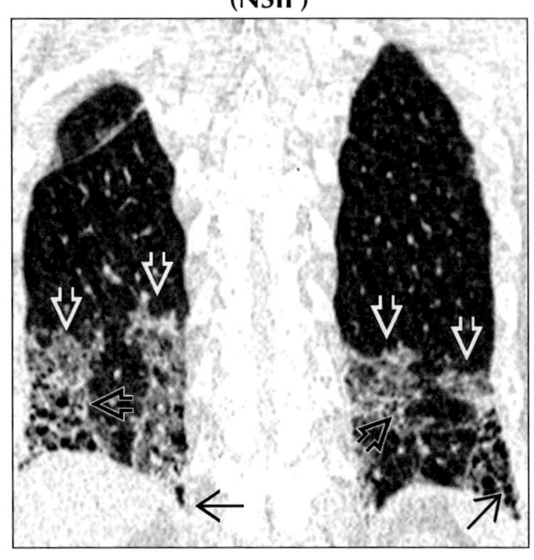

(Left) *Axial HRCT shows mild subpleural honeycombing → superimposed on ground-glass opacity ⇨ in this patient with scleroderma. Note focal subpleural sparing on the left ↷. Advanced fibrotic NSIP can be indistinguishable from UIP on HRCT.* ***(Right)*** *Coronal CT reconstruction shows patchy ground-glass opacity in the lung bases ➡ with superimposed architectural distortion and traction bronchiectasis ⇨. Honeycombing is mild →.*

Chronic Hypersensitivity Pneumonitis | Chronic Hypersensitivity Pneumonitis

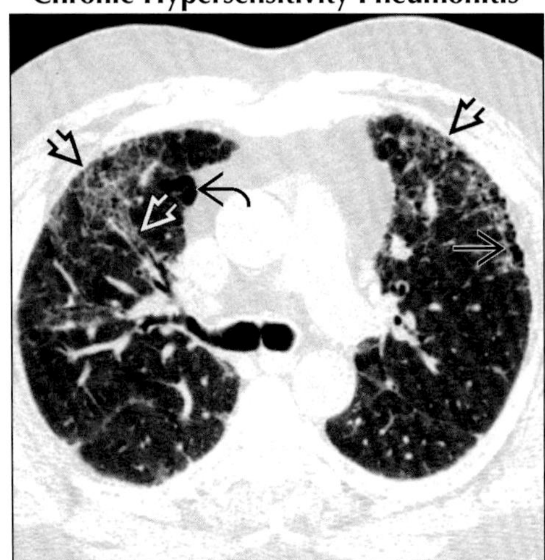

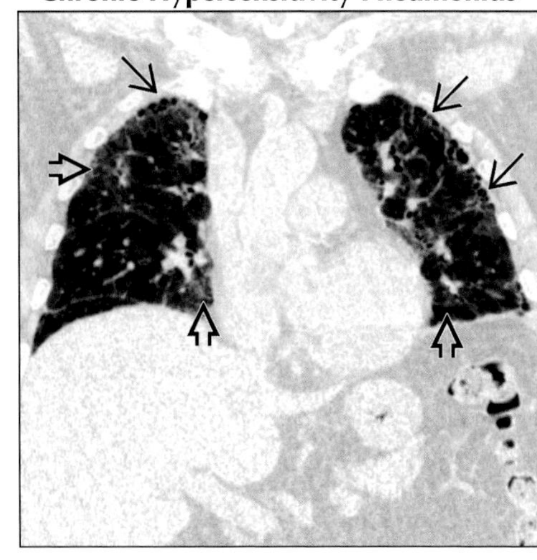

(Left) *Axial HRCT shows peripheral ⇨ and peribronchovascular ➡ reticulation and ground-glass opacity in the mid lungs with mild subpleural honeycombing in the left upper lobe →. Note the hyperinflated lobule in the right upper lobe ↷.* ***(Right)*** *Coronal CT reconstruction shows mild honeycombing in the mid and upper lungs → and patchy ground-glass opacity ⇨. Relative sparing of the bases is common in chronic hypersensitivity pneumonitis.*

HONEYCOMBING

Sarcoidosis

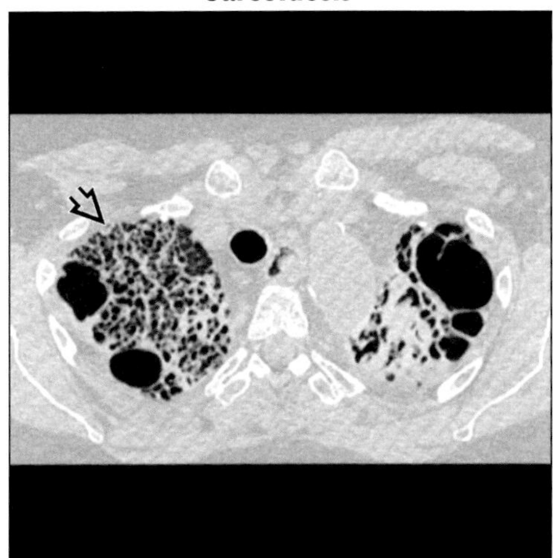

Sarcoidosis

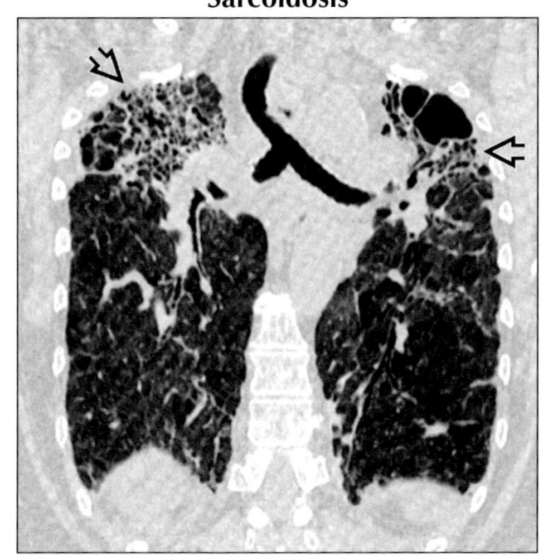

(Left) *Axial HRCT shows severe honeycombing and cystic spaces → primarily in the upper lung zones. Honeycombing is both subpleural and along the bronchovascular bundles.* ***(Right)*** *Coronal CT reconstruction shows severe fibrosis and honeycombing → in the upper lobes. No honeycombing is present at the bases. Note the upward traction of the hila.*

Asbestosis

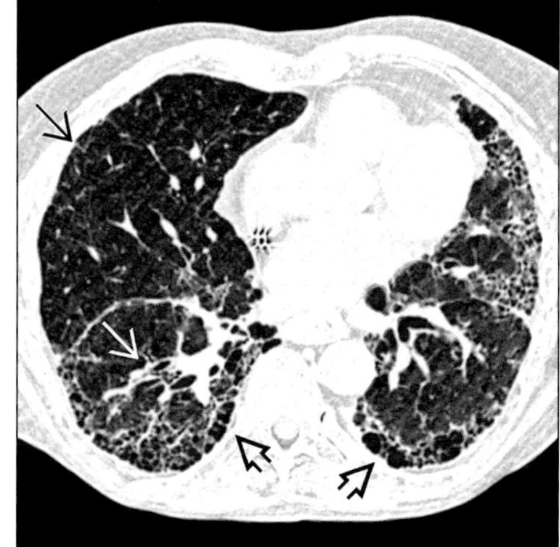

Asbestosis

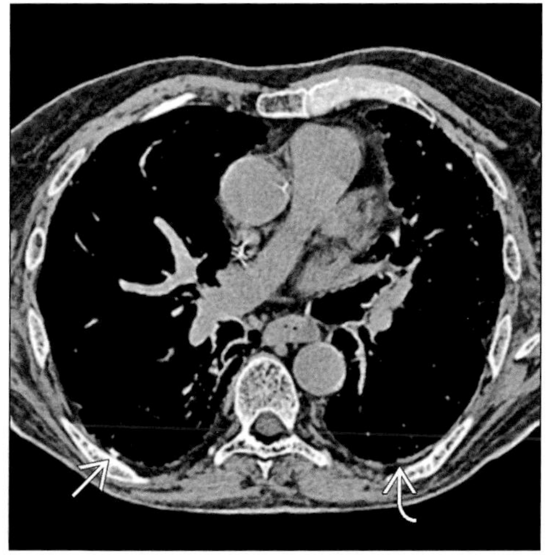

(Left) *Axial HRCT shows subpleural and basal predominant interstitial fibrosis characterized by honeycombing →, irregular interlobular septal thickening →, traction bronchiectasis →, and architectural distortion. Note bilateral lower lobe volume loss.* ***(Right)*** *Axial HRCT shows calcified → and noncalcified asbestos-related pleural plaques →. Pleural plaques are not a feature of idiopathic pulmonary fibrosis or other causes of UIP.*

Acute Interstitial Pneumonia

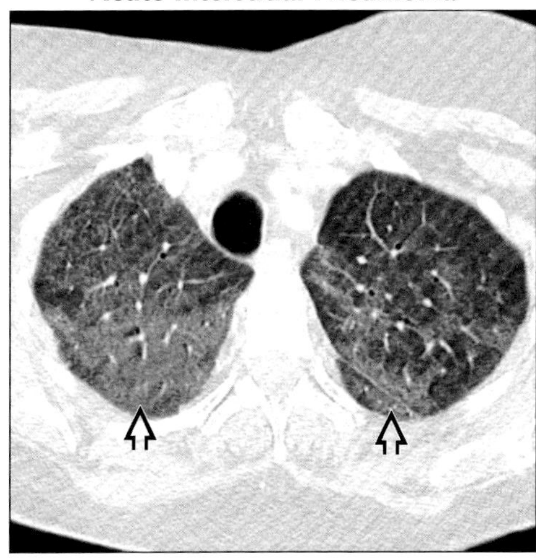

Acute Interstitial Pneumonia

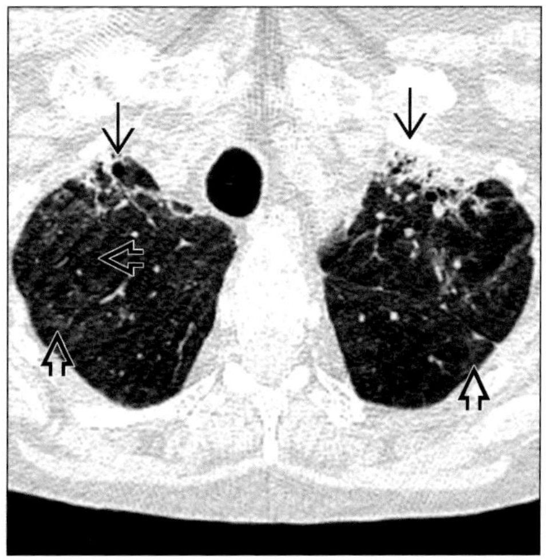

(Left) *Axial HRCT shows patchy ground-glass opacity in the upper lungs → in this patient with acute interstitial pneumonia. Consolidation may also occur in acute interstitial pneumonia, especially basally.* ***(Right)*** *Axial HRCT 3 months later shows development of peripheral fibrosis in the upper lobes anteriorly with minimal honeycombing →. Residual nodular foci of ground-glass opacity → remain in both lungs. Note relative sparing of the lungs posteriorly.*

RETICULAR PATTERN

DIFFERENTIAL DIAGNOSIS

Common

- Idiopathic Pulmonary Fibrosis (IPF)
- Pulmonary Edema
- Nonspecific Interstitial Pneumonitis (NSIP)
- Connective Tissue Diseases
  - Scleroderma
  - Rheumatoid Arthritis
- Sarcoidosis
- Asbestosis

Less Common

- Chronic Hypersensitivity Pneumonitis
- Drug-Induced Lung Disease
- Polymyositis/Dermatomyositis
- Lymphangitic Carcinomatosis

Rare but Important

- Diffuse Pulmonary Lymphangiomatosis

ESSENTIAL INFORMATION

Key Differential Diagnosis Issues

- Reticular pattern
  - Pattern produced by innumerable interlacing small linear opacities
    - Resembles fisherman's net; mesh-like
    - Fine, medium, or coarse reticulation may reflect disease progression
  - Connotation for pattern on chest radiographs similar; however, summation of cystic spaces may result in reticular pattern
  - HRCT specific components
    - Small, irregular linear opacities
    - Irregular interlobular septal thickening
    - Irregular intralobular linear opacities; interstitial thickening within secondary pulmonary lobule, usually fibrosis
    - Architectural distortion, traction bronchiectasis, and bronchiolectasis, due to fibrosis

Helpful Clues for Common Diagnoses

- **Idiopathic Pulmonary Fibrosis (IPF)**
  - Common interstitial lung disease of unknown etiology
  - Pathologically has usual interstitial pneumonia (UIP) pattern
  - Bilateral, symmetric, patchy reticular pattern; may involve all lobes but most severe in subpleural lung and lung bases
    - Traction bronchiectasis and bronchiolectasis; architectural distortion; irregular interfaces with pleural, vascular, and bronchial structures
  - Subpleural honeycombing often present (air-containing cysts measuring 2-25 mm)
- **Pulmonary Edema**
  - Smooth thickening of interlobular septa and bronchovascular bundles; gravity-dependent ground-glass opacities &/or consolidation
  - Associated cardiomegaly, pleural effusions
  - Rapidly evolves; may resolve quickly with diuretics
- **Nonspecific Interstitial Pneumonitis (NSIP)**
  - Most commonly in patients with connective tissue disease (scleroderma, rheumatoid arthritis) and drug-related lung disease
  - Histologic pattern of interstitial fibrosis and inflammation
  - Extent of ground-glass opacities > reticular opacities
  - Traction bronchiectasis usually out of proportion to severity of reticular opacities
  - Honeycombing uncommon
  - Distribution: Lower lung zones (60-90%), peripheral lung (50-70%); may be diffuse
    - Sparing of immediate subpleural lung in dorsal aspect of lower lobes (50%)
- **Scleroderma**
  - Pattern typically NSIP; UIP pattern less common
  - Dilated esophagus common
  - Consolidation may occur due to
    - Pneumonia, aspiration, organizing pneumonia, diffuse alveolar damage, diffuse pulmonary hemorrhage
- **Rheumatoid Arthritis**
  - Findings of NSIP (ground-glass opacities, fine reticulation), UIP pattern less common
  - Osseous erosions may be evident in humeral heads or sternoclavicular joints
- **Sarcoidosis**
  - Reticular pattern more common with end-stage fibrotic disease (stage IV)
  - Extensive reticulation, mainly involving perihilar regions of upper and middle lung zones; cystic changes may occur

- Architectural distortion, traction bronchiectasis, superior hilar retraction, compensatory overinflation of lower lobes
- Small perilymphatic nodules may be present in less involved lung
- Hilar and mediastinal adenopathy, common in early sarcoidosis; usually has resolved with extensive fibrosis

- **Asbestosis**
  - Irregular thickening of inter- and intralobular septa, subpleural curvilinear opacities, parenchymal bands
  - Predominantly involves peripheral and dorsal aspects of lower lung zones
  - Frequently associated pleural plaques (90%)
  - Occupational exposure important

Helpful Clues for Less Common Diagnoses

- **Chronic Hypersensitivity Pneumonitis**
  - Mid-lung predominance most common, especially in those with low-level continuous antigen exposure (bird breeders)
  - Upper lung zone predominance more common in those with intermittent exposure (farmers)
  - Fibrosis: Irregular linear opacities (40%), traction bronchiectasis (20%)
  - Often superimposed subacute findings
    - Poorly defined centrilobular opacities, ground-glass opacities, lobular areas of air-trapping
- **Drug-Induced Lung Disease**
  - Produces wide array of injury patterns, including reticular pattern
  - Reticular pattern may be due to UIP, NSIP, or pulmonary edema
- **Polymyositis/Dermatomyositis**
  - Symmetric basal reticular opacities, architectural distortion, irregular bronchovascular thickening; may progress to honeycombing
  - Early stages: Ground-glass opacities; bilateral, symmetric basal distribution
- **Lymphangitic Carcinomatosis**
  - Smooth &/or nodular thickening of interlobular septa, bronchovascular bundles, interlobar fissures, and subpleural interstitium
  - Distribution: Often spares lobe or whole lung
  - May have pleural effusions and mediastinal adenopathy
  - Usually known history of previous malignancy

Helpful Clues for Rare Diagnoses

- **Diffuse Pulmonary Lymphangiomatosis**
  - a.k.a. lymphangiectasis
  - Smooth, uniform thickening of interlobular septa and fissures
  - Marked, smooth thickening of bronchovascular bundles
  - Diffuse effacement of mediastinal fat and enlarged mediastinal lymph nodes key to recognition

Idiopathic Pulmonary Fibrosis (IPF)

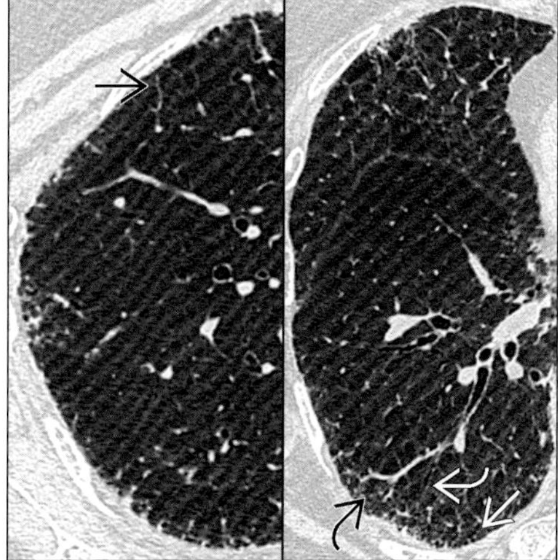

Axial HRCT of a patient with early IPF shows irregular thickened interlobular septa ➙, intralobular reticulation ➙, traction bronchiectasis ➙, and fine honeycombing ➙.

Idiopathic Pulmonary Fibrosis (IPF)

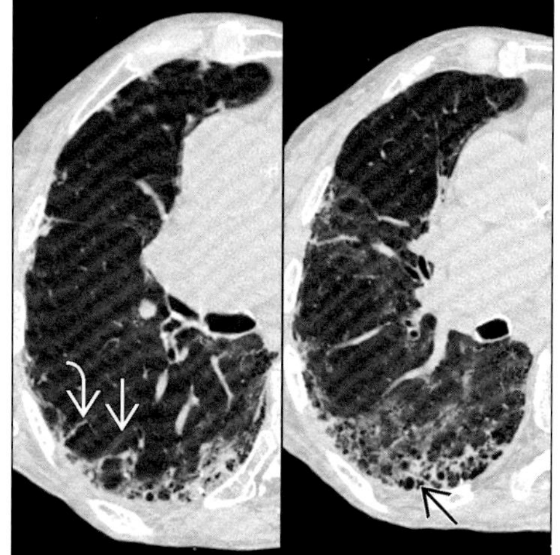

Axial HRCT of a patient with moderate IPF shows irregular interlobular septa ➙, traction bronchiectasis ➙, and subpleural honeycombing ➙ resulting in architectural distortion.

RETICULAR PATTERN

(Left) Frontal radiograph of the right lung shows coarse peripheral and basilar reticulation. HRCT shows extensive peripheral and basilar honeycombing and traction bronchiectasis ➔. (Right) Frontal radiograph coned to the right lung shows reticulation with blurring of the bronchovascular borders, septal (Kerley B) lines ➔, and thickening of the subpleural interstitium along the minor fissure ➔.

Idiopathic Pulmonary Fibrosis (IPF)

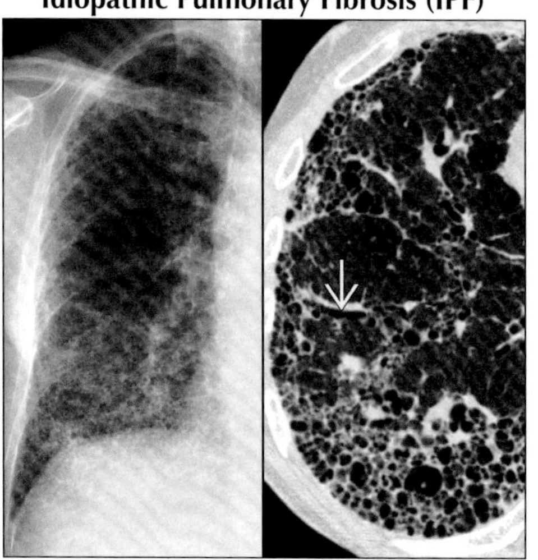

Pulmonary Edema

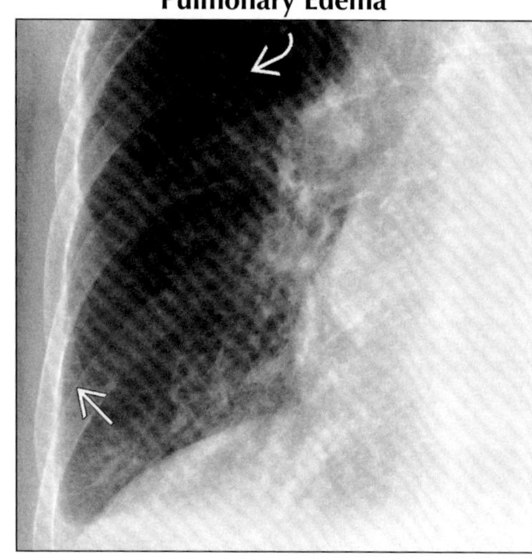

(Left) Axial HRCT shows a thickened interlobular septa ➔ outlining the secondary pulmonary lobules, centrilobular core structures ➔, and subpleural interstitium along the major fissure ➔. (Right) Frontal radiograph and HRCT of the right lung show predominant lower lung zone ground-glass opacities with fine reticulation. HRCT in particular shows traction bronchiectasis ➔.

Pulmonary Edema

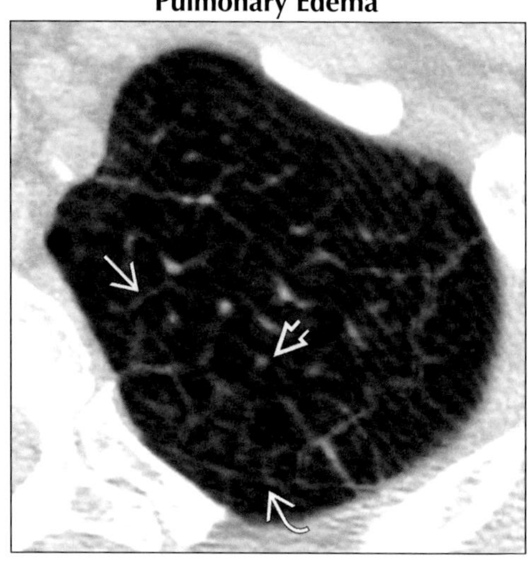

Nonspecific Interstitial Pneumonitis (NSIP)

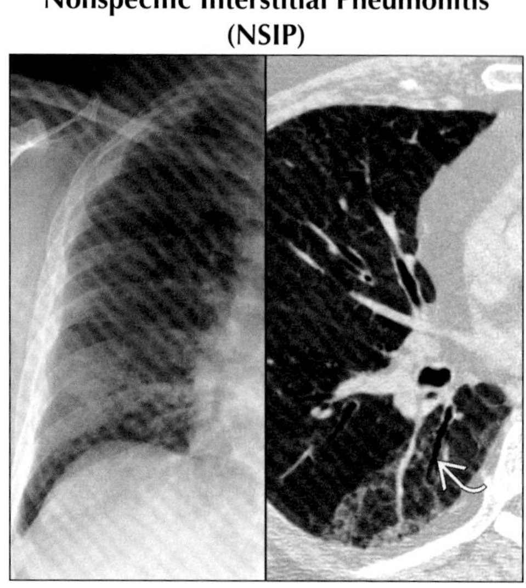

(Left) Axial HRCT shows a dilated esophagus ➔ and peripheral reticulation with irregular thickening of the interlobular septa ➔, intralobular reticulation ➔, and traction bronchiectasis ➔. Features consistent with NSIP. (Right) Axial CECT of a patient with rheumatoid arthritis shows peripheral subpleural interstitial thickening, architectural distortion, and early honeycombing ➔, most severe in the lung bases. Features consistent with UIP.

Scleroderma

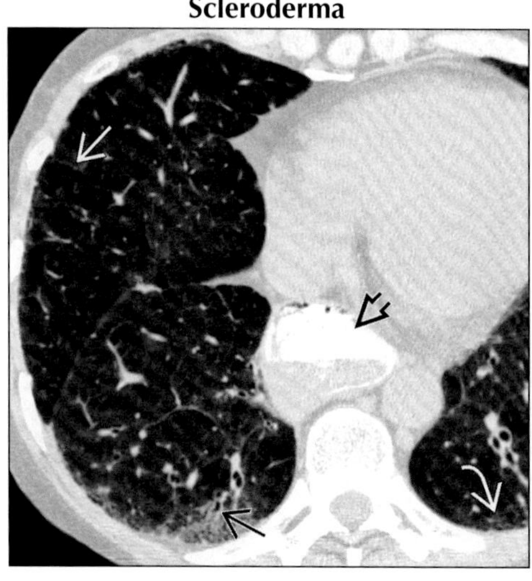

Rheumatoid Arthritis

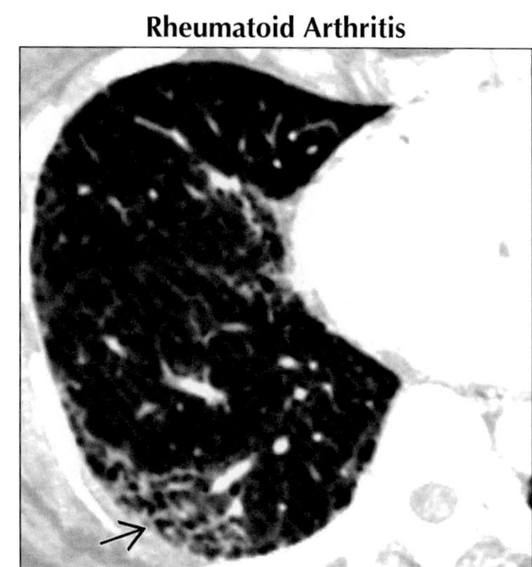

Asbestosis

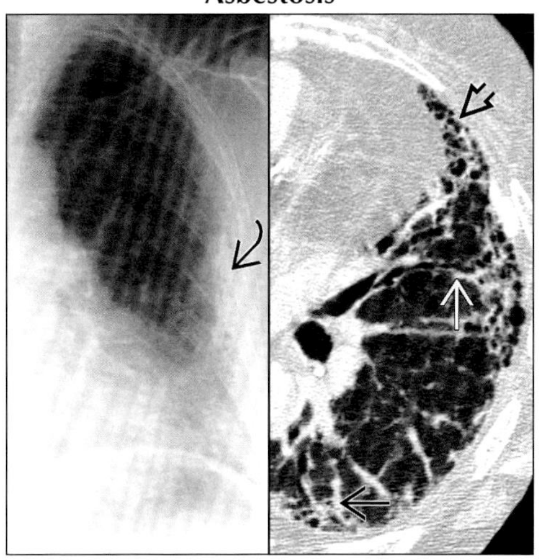

Chronic Hypersensitivity Pneumonitis

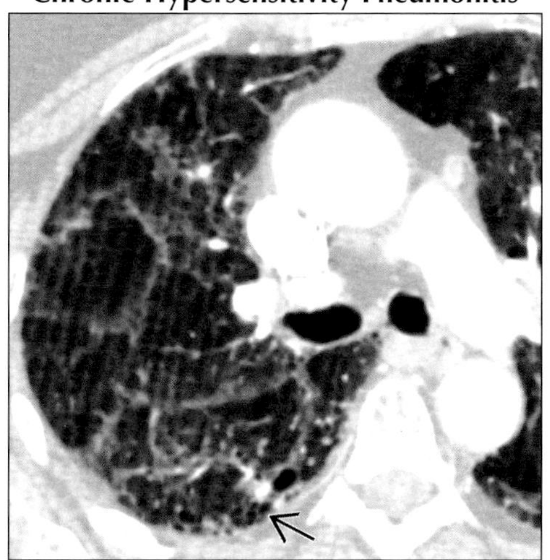

(Left) *Frontal radiograph of the left lung shows calcified pleural plaque ➔ and fine peripheral and basilar reticulation. HRCT shows peripheral reticulation, irregular thickening of interlobular septa ➔, traction bronchiectasis ➔, and honeycombing ➔.* ***(Right)*** *Axial HRCT shows a random distribution of coarse reticulation, architectural distortion, and fine honeycombing ➔. The findings were most prominent in the mid-lung zones.*

Drug-Induced Lung Disease

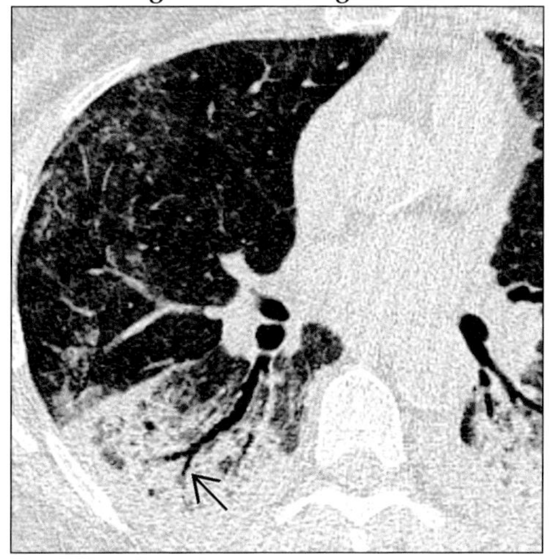

Lymphangitic Carcinomatosis

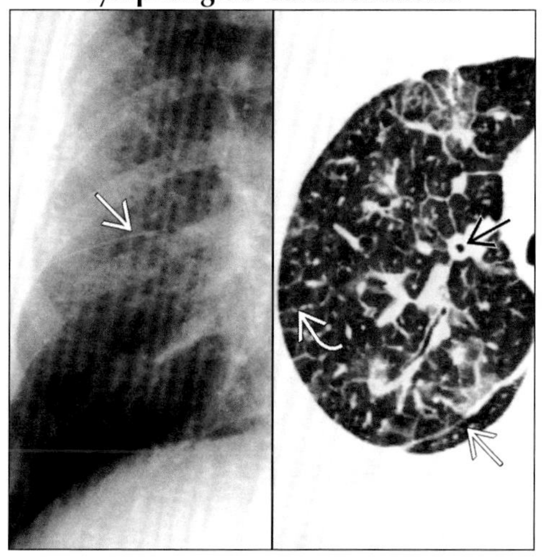

(Left) *Axial HRCT shows ground-glass opacity, mild reticulation, areas of consolidation, and traction bronchiectasis ➔ in the lower lungs of a patient with bleomycin toxicity.* ***(Right)*** *Frontal radiograph and HRCT show reticulation and thickening of the bronchovascular bundles ➔, interlobular septa ➔, and subpleural interstitium ➔.*

Diffuse Pulmonary Lymphangiomatosis

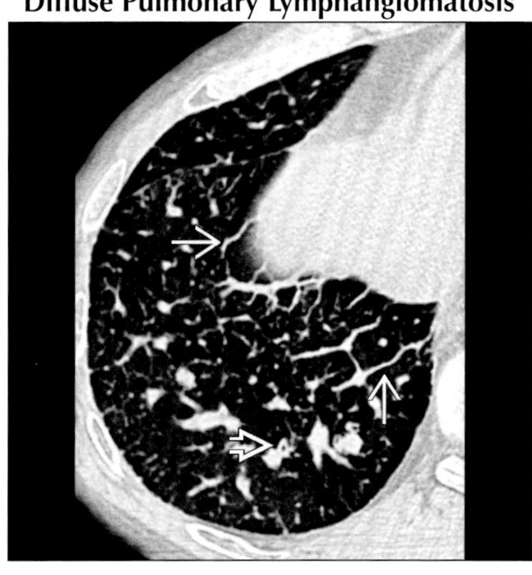

Diffuse Pulmonary Lymphangiomatosis

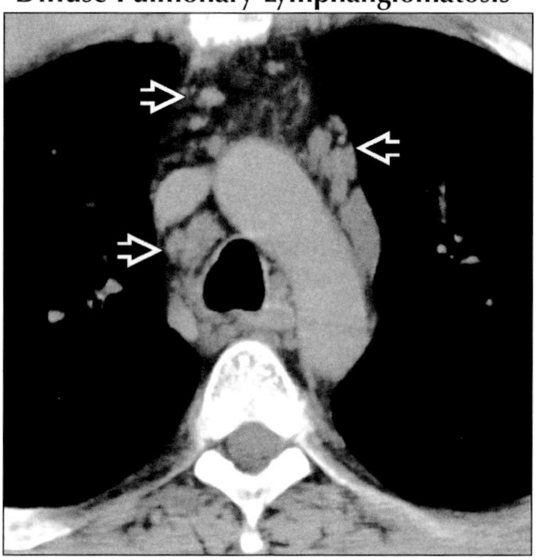

(Left) *Axial NECT shows diffuse smooth interlobular thickening ➔ and thickened bronchovascular bundles ➔. The mediastinum fat was effaced, and the mediastinal lymph nodes were enlarged (not shown).* ***(Right)*** *Axial NECT shows diffuse effacement of the mediastinal fat and multiple enlarged mediastinal lymph nodes ➔.*

GROUND-GLASS OPACITIES

DIFFERENTIAL DIAGNOSIS

Common

- Atypical Pneumonia
  - Pneumocystis Pneumonia
  - Viral Pneumonia
- Acute Airspace
  - Cardiogenic Pulmonary Edema
  - Noncardiac Pulmonary Edema
  - Diffuse Alveolar Hemorrhage (DAH)
  - Hypersensitivity Pneumonitis (HP)
  - Eosinophilic Pneumonia
- Chronic Infiltrative Lung Disease
  - Nonspecific Interstitial Pneumonitis
  - Smoking-Related Interstitial Lung Disease
    - Respiratory Bronchiolitis
    - Desquamative Interstitial Pneumonia (DIP)
  - Eosinophilic Pneumonia

Less Common

- Bronchioloalveolar Cell Carcinoma
- Atypical Adenomatous Hyperplasia (AAH)

Rare but Important

- Pulmonary Alveolar Proteinosis (PAP)
- Drug Reaction

ESSENTIAL INFORMATION

Key Differential Diagnosis Issues

- Definition of ground-glass opacity (GGO)
  - Hazy increased lung density with preservation of underlying vessels
- Recognition problems
  - Difficult if minimal or diffuse; pitfalls
    - Normally seen with exhalation
    - Volume averaging with thick collimation (> 5 mm)
    - Window settings too narrow or too wide
    - Normal in dependent lung from atelectasis
- Radiology-pathology correlation
  - Partial airspace filling by edema, hemorrhage, infection, or tumor
  - Interstitial thickening by inflammation, edema, or fibrosis
    - Presence of consolidation suggests that GGO represents alveolar filling
    - GGO with reticular opacities or traction bronchiectasis likely represents interstitial disease
  - Lepidic growth: Abnormal cells use alveolar septa and respiratory bronchioles as scaffolding to grow
    - Preserves lung architecture and often results in GGO

Helpful Clues for Common Diagnoses

- **Atypical Pneumonia**
  - Typically febrile immunocompromised patients, GGO should be considered opportunistic infection
- **Cardiogenic Pulmonary Edema**
  - GGO earliest parenchymal change, usually gravity-dependent distribution
  - Increased severity → septal thickening, consolidation, and pleural effusions
- **Noncardiac Pulmonary Edema**
  - Acute respiratory distress syndrome (ARDS)
  - GGO predominant abnormality, extent typically > 50% of lung
- **Diffuse Alveolar Hemorrhage (DAH)**
  - Lobular GGO often admixed with dense consolidation, gravity dependent
  - Hemorrhage may be associated with focal lesions, resulting in halos
    - Hemorrhagic metastases (e.g., renal cell carcinoma)
    - Invasive aspergillosis
    - Transbronchial biopsy site
- **Hypersensitivity Pneumonitis (HP)**
  - Typically diffuse; centrilobular ground-glass nodules 70%
  - Most specific pattern: Geographic GGO + normal lung + air-trapping (head cheese sign)
- **Eosinophilic Pneumonia**
  - Acute
    - Pattern identical to acute pulmonary edema
    - GGO (100%) admixed with septal thickening, consolidation, random distribution
    - Pleural effusions common (80%)
  - Chronic
    - Typical distribution: Peripheral and upper lobes
    - Consolidation > ground-glass opacities
    - Often migratory, waxing and waning over time
- **Nonspecific Interstitial Pneumonitis**
  - Idiopathic or associated with collagen vascular diseases

- GGO often basilar, follow bronchovascular pathways (fan- or wedge-shaped)
- Traction bronchiectasis often out of proportion to severity of reticular opacities

- **Smoking-Related Interstitial Lung Disease**
  - Spectrum of cigarette-related injuries from respiratory bronchiolitis to DIP
    - Generally dose related; more common with heavier cigarette smoking or use of unfiltered cigarettes
  - Respiratory bronchiolitis: Upper lobe centrilobular GGO
  - DIP: GGO in 100%, often diffuse, symmetric, and panlobular

Helpful Clues for Less Common Diagnoses

- **Bronchioloalveolar Cell Carcinoma**
  - GGO may be focal, typically lobulated, and sharply demarcated from surrounding lung
  - GGO may be combined with solid nodular tissue (part-solid nodule)
  - Most helpful characteristic is growth or presence of solid component within GGO
- **Atypical Adenomatous Hyperplasia (AAH)**
  - 3% of population; prevalence increases with age (7% over 60 years)
  - Importance unknown but may represent premalignant lesion
    - Prevalence of AAH in surgical specimens of patients with adenocarcinoma or bronchioloalveolar cell carcinoma (BAC) high (25%)
  - Imaging features that help differentiate between BAC and AAH
    - Air bronchograms; larger size associated with BAC
    - Sphericity associated with AAH

Helpful Clues for Rare Diagnoses

- **Pulmonary Alveolar Proteinosis (PAP)**
  - Typically admixed with interlobular reticular lines in crazy-paving pattern
- **Drug Reaction**
  - Histologic patterns include diffuse alveolar damage, hypersensitivity pneumonitis, eosinophilic lung disease, DAH
  - Best diagnostic clue: High index of clinical suspicion, diagnosis by exclusion

Alternative Differential Approaches

- If immunosuppression or bone marrow suppression is present
  - Consider infection, hemorrhage, edema, drug toxicity
- Acute presentation
  - Pneumonia
  - Edema (cardiogenic and noncardiogenic)
  - Hypersensitivity pneumonitis
  - DAH
- Multiple GGO nodules
  - Bronchioloalveolar cell carcinoma
  - AAH
- Multiple centrilobular ground-glass nodules
  - Hypersensitivity pneumonitis
  - Respiratory bronchiolitis

Pneumocystis Pneumonia

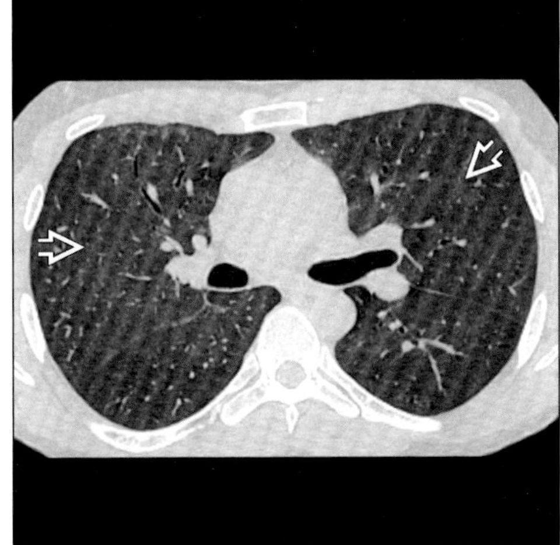

Axial HRCT in a patient with AIDS shows faint perihilar ground-glass opacities ⇨. This patient presented with fever and cough, but the chest radiograph was normal.

Viral Pneumonia

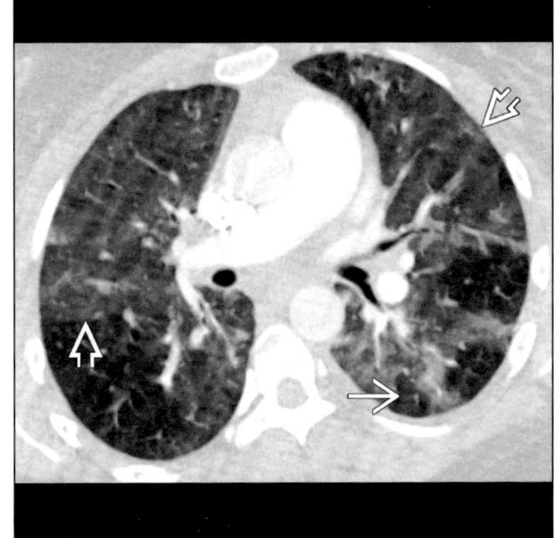

Axial CECT in a febrile immunocompromised patient shows diffuse ground-glass opacities ⇨ with lobular sparing or hyperinflation ➡.

GROUND-GLASS OPACITIES

(Left) *Axial CECT shows diffuse ground-glass opacities ➔, lobular sparing ➔, and bilateral pleural effusions ➔. The dorsal gradient in ground-glass opacities is consistent with pulmonary edema.* ***(Right)*** *Axial CECT shows ground-glass opacities ➔. The diagnosis in this patient was acute interstitial pneumonia, due to an idiopathic form of noncardiogenic pulmonary edema.*

Cardiogenic Pulmonary Edema

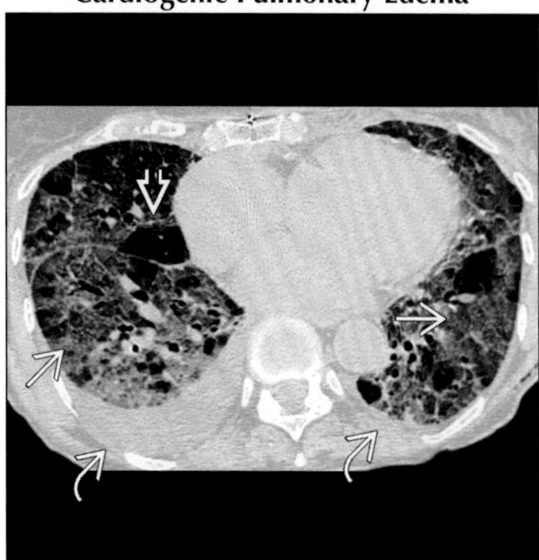

Noncardiac Pulmonary Edema

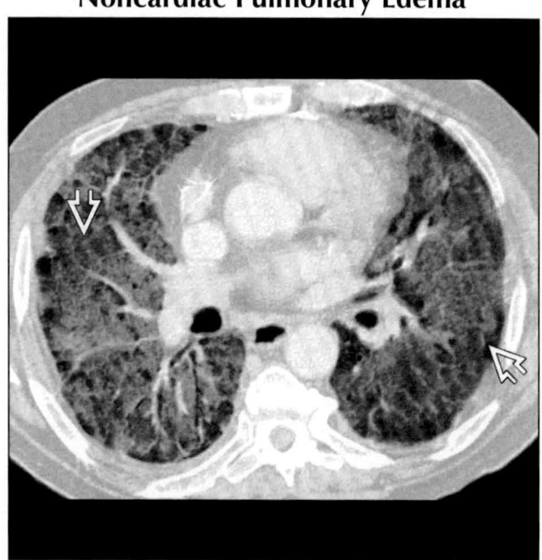

(Left) *Axial HRCT shows perihilar ground-glass opacities ➔ from diffuse alveolar hemorrhage.* ***(Right)*** *Axial CECT shows diffuse ground-glass opacities ➔ with lobular sparing ➔ in this example of subacute hypersensitivity. Expiratory scanning would be useful to look for air-trapping.*

Diffuse Alveolar Hemorrhage (DAH)

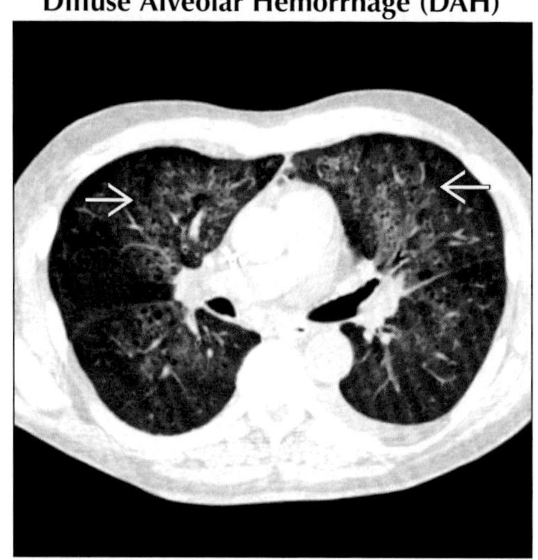

Hypersensitivity Pneumonitis (HP)

(Left) *Axial NECT shows ground-glass opacities ➔ admixed with reticular opacities. In nonspecific interstitial pneumonitis, ground-glass opacities often exceed reticular opacities, and traction bronchiectasis is out of proportion to the degree of reticular opacities.* ***(Right)*** *Axial NECT shows diffuse ground-glass opacities ➔ and a few small scattered cysts ➔ in this patient with desquamative interstitial pneumonia.*

Nonspecific Interstitial Pneumonitis

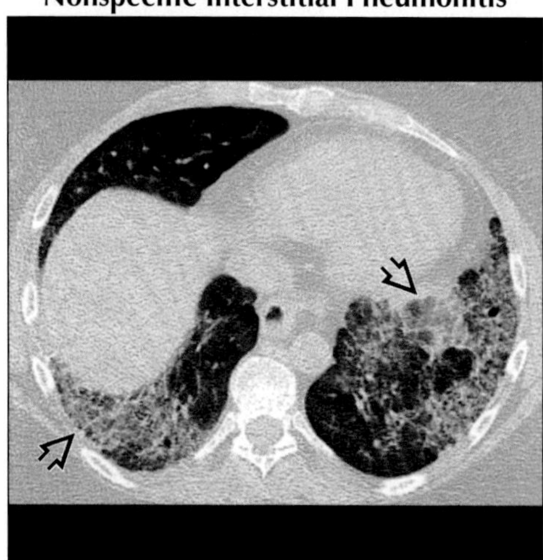

Desquamative Interstitial Pneumonia (DIP)

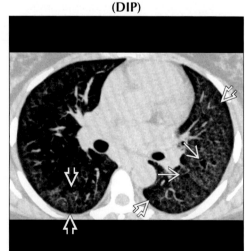

GROUND-GLASS OPACITIES

Desquamative Interstitial Pneumonia (DIP)

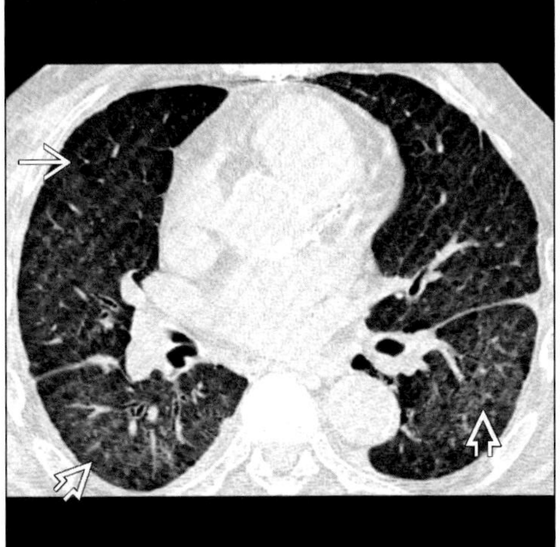

Eosinophilic Pneumonia

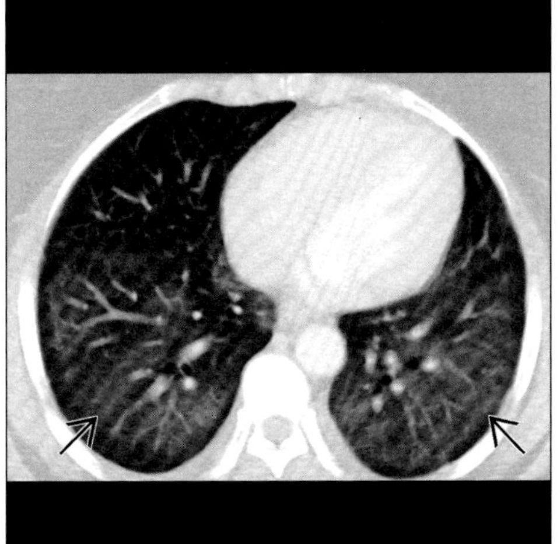

*(**Left**) Axial HRCT shows diffuse ground-glass opacities ➡ and scattered cysts ➡ in a patient with desquamative interstitial pneumonia. (**Right**) Axial CECT shows symmetric ground-glass opacities ➡ in the basilar lung. The subpleural lung is spared. The upper lobes were consolidated (not shown). Note the preservation of the bronchovascular structures, which defines the ground-glass pattern.*

Eosinophilic Pneumonia

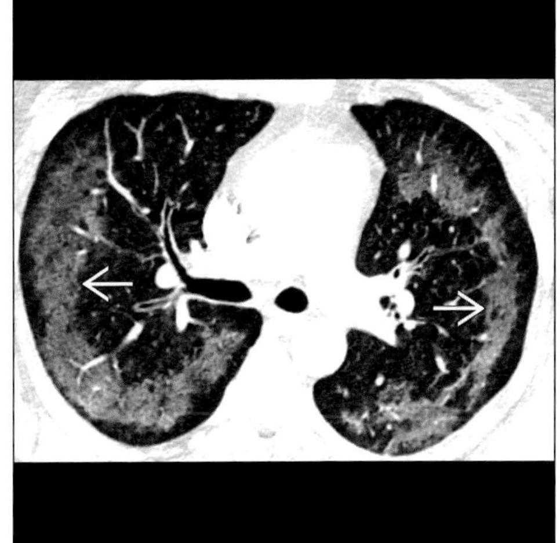

Bronchioloalveolar Cell Carcinoma

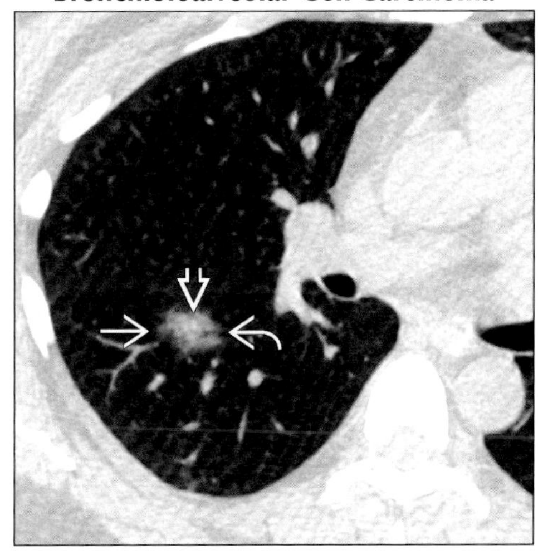

*(**Left**) Axial CECT shows peripheral bands of ground-glass opacities ➡ in the upper lobes from chronic eosinophilic pneumonia. (**Right**) Axial NECT shows a part-solid solitary pulmonary nodule with ground-glass ➡ and solid components ➡. An air-bronchogram ➡ is also noted.*

Bronchioloalveolar Cell Carcinoma

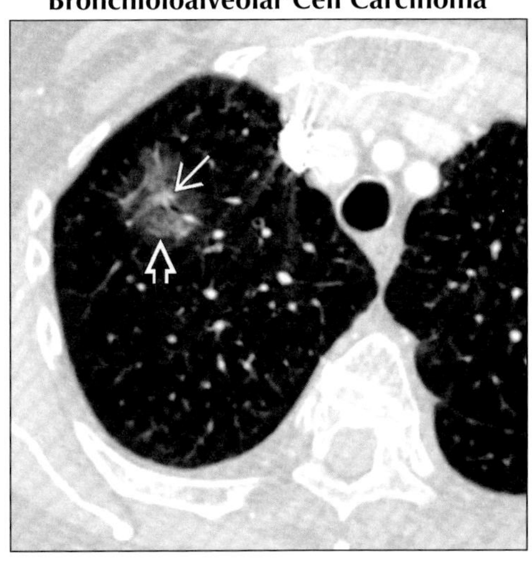

Pulmonary Alveolar Proteinosis (PAP)

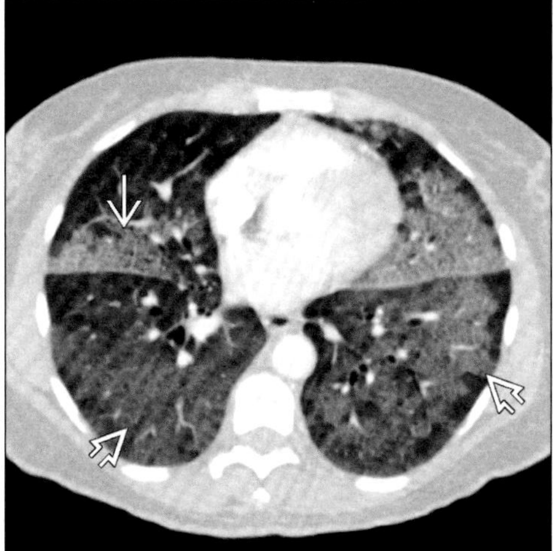

*(**Left**) Axial CECT shows focal ground-glass opacity ➡ and a small central solid nodule ➡ from bronchioloalveolar cell carcinoma. (**Right**) Axial HRCT shows central diffuse ground-glass opacities ➡ and crazy-paving pattern ➡ in the right middle lobe and lingula.*

CRAZY-PAVING PATTERN

DIFFERENTIAL DIAGNOSIS

Common
- Pulmonary Alveolar Proteinosis (PAP)
- Pneumocystis Pneumonia (PCP)
- Acute Interstitial Pneumonia (AIP)
- Diffuse Alveolar Damage (DAD)
- Edema

Less Common
- Diffuse Alveolar Hemorrhage
- Eosinophilic Pneumonia
- Cryptogenic Organizing Pneumonia (COP)

Rare but Important
- Bronchioloalveolar Cell Carcinoma (BAC)
- Lymphangitic Carcinomatosis
- Lipoid Pneumonia

ESSENTIAL INFORMATION

Key Differential Diagnosis Issues
- Crazy-paving definition: Combination of smooth interlobular septal thickening superimposed on areas of ground-glass attenuation
  - Resembles paths made of broken pieces of stone
  - Prevalence of pattern in those with diffuse lung disease (1%)
- Radiology-pathology correlation
  - Linear network due to thickening of interlobular septa
    - May also be due to preferential accumulation of material in periphery of airspaces
  - Ground-glass opacities result from partial alveolar filling
- Acute time course
  - Edema, PCP, hemorrhage, AIP, DAD
- Subacute or chronic time course
  - PAP, COP, hemorrhage, BAC, lymphangitic carcinomatosis, lipoid pneumonia, chronic eosinophilic pneumonia
- Focal crazy-paving pattern
  - Hemorrhage, BAC, lymphangitic carcinomatosis, lipoid pneumonia
- Topology
  - Upper lung zones predominant
    - Chronic eosinophilic pneumonia
    - Pneumocystis pneumonia
  - Basilar lung zones predominant
    - Edema
    - Cryptogenic organizing pneumonia
    - Lipoid pneumonia
- Extent of crazy-paving pattern
  - Greater number of segments involved, more likely PAP

Helpful Clues for Common Diagnoses
- **Pulmonary Alveolar Proteinosis (PAP)**
  - Classic disease with crazy-paving pattern, subsequently found in other diseases
  - Crazy-paving pattern often has sharply marginated geographic distribution
  - Widespread crazy-paving pattern not seen with other conditions
  - Symptoms usually less severe than radiographic abnormalities
    - Nonproductive cough, dyspnea (fever less common)
- **Pneumocystis Pneumonia (PCP)**
  - Typically perihilar or upper lung distribution
  - More severe in upper lung zones in patients on pentamidine aerosol prophylaxis
  - May have pneumatoceles, which typically develop in periphery of upper lobes
    - Curiously, pneumatoceles only seen in those with HIV infection
  - Cough, dyspnea, and fever
- **Acute Interstitial Pneumonia (AIP) and Diffuse Alveolar Damage (DAD)**
  - Cause severe respiratory failure requiring mechanical ventilation
  - AIP: Progressive respiratory disorder of unknown etiology with DAD on biopsy
  - ARDS: End result of multiple medical or surgical conditions with DAD on biopsy
  - AIP more often symmetrical than ARDS
  - Ground-glass opacities (and crazy-paving pattern) seen in all phases of DAD
    - Ground-glass opacities and consolidation are more common than crazy-paving pattern
- **Edema**
  - Crazy-paving pattern can be seen in both cardiogenic and noncardiogenic edema
  - Cardiogenic edema worse in gravity-dependent locations
  - Heart enlarged and pleural effusions common in cardiogenic edema
  - Resolves rapidly with treatment

Helpful Clues for Less Common Diagnoses

- **Diffuse Alveolar Hemorrhage**
  - Hemoptysis (80%) and anemia common
  - Acute onset with hemorrhage into alveolar spaces (results in consolidation or ground-glass opacities)
    - Blood removed from alveoli by macrophages (2-3 days)
    - Macrophages migrate into interstitium (septal thickening)
    - Macrophages removed by lymphatics (7-14 days)
    - Crazy-paving pattern may be seen when macrophages migrate into interstitium
  - Distribution typically perihilar or diffuse
- **Eosinophilic Pneumonia**
  - Peripheral eosinophilic lung consolidation more common in chronic (90%) than in acute pneumonia
  - Typically peripheral in lung
  - Consolidation and ground-glass opacities more common than crazy-paving pattern
- **Cryptogenic Organizing Pneumonia (COP)**
  - Reverse halo sign: Foci of ground-glass opacification surrounded by halo of consolidation
  - Opacities may be migratory, similar to eosinophilic pneumonia
  - Consolidation and ground-glass opacities more common than crazy-paving pattern

Helpful Clues for Rare Diagnoses

- **Bronchioloalveolar Cell Carcinoma (BAC)**
  - Mucinous well-differentiated adenocarcinoma
  - Lipidic growth results in ground-glass opacities, mixed ground-glass opacities & solid opacities, and solid nodules
  - Crazy-paving pattern uncommon
  - Interlobular septal thickening may be due to tumor infiltration or edema
- **Lymphangitic Carcinomatosis**
  - Often spares lobes or lungs (confined to 1 lung or lobe in 30%)
  - Interlobular septa often beaded or irregularly thickened, uncommon with other conditions
  - Associated findings more common, including pleural effusions, hilar and mediastinal lymphadenopathy
- **Lipoid Pneumonia**
  - Aspiration or inhalation of fatty or oily substances, animal or vegetable oils, oral laxatives, oil-based nose drops, and liquid paraffin
  - Chronic consolidation often has fat density (-30 to -150 Hounsfield units)
  - Distribution based on aspiration

Alternative Differential Approaches

- Prevalence of crazy-paving pattern in various diseases
  - Pulmonary alveolar proteinosis (100%)
  - Diffuse alveolar damage (66%)
  - Acute interstitial pneumonia (30%)
  - Hemorrhage, COP, eosinophilic pneumonia, edema (10-20%)

Pulmonary Alveolar Proteinosis (PAP)

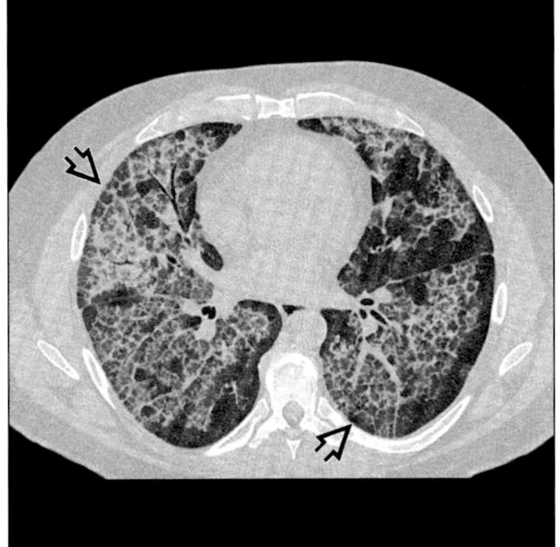

Axial HRCT shows crazy-paving pattern ➩ in alveolar proteinosis. Note the prominent and widespread distribution of this pattern.

Pulmonary Alveolar Proteinosis (PAP)

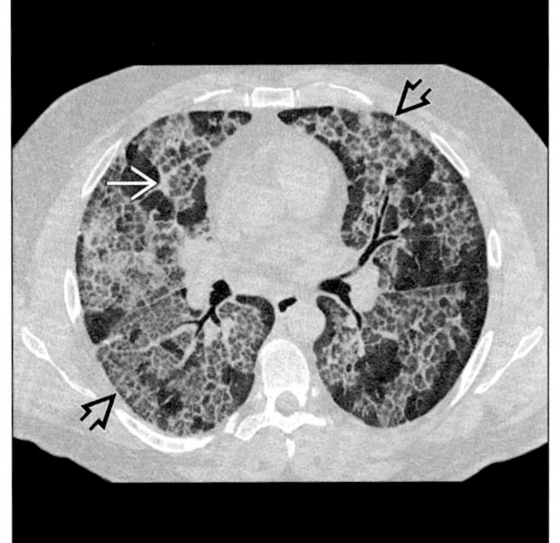

Axial HRCT shows crazy-paving pattern ➩ with a distinct geographic distribution. The more widespread the pattern of crazy-paving, the more likely the diagnosis of pulmonary alveolar proteinosis ➡.

CRAZY-PAVING PATTERN

(Left) Axial HRCT shows a geographic distribution of crazy-paving pattern ➡ in pulmonary alveolar proteinosis. Note the sharp demarcation from the surrounding normal lung. *(Right)* Coronal HRCT shows a widespread crazy-paving pattern ➡ in alveolar proteinosis. The more lung segment involved, the more likely the diagnosis is alveolar proteinosis.

Pulmonary Alveolar Proteinosis (PAP)

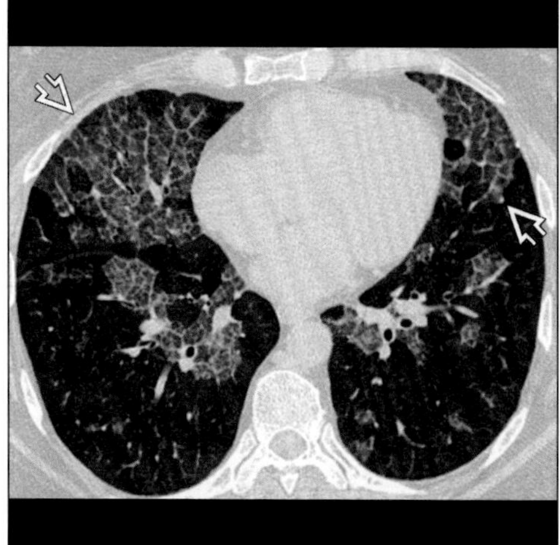

Pulmonary Alveolar Proteinosis (PAP)

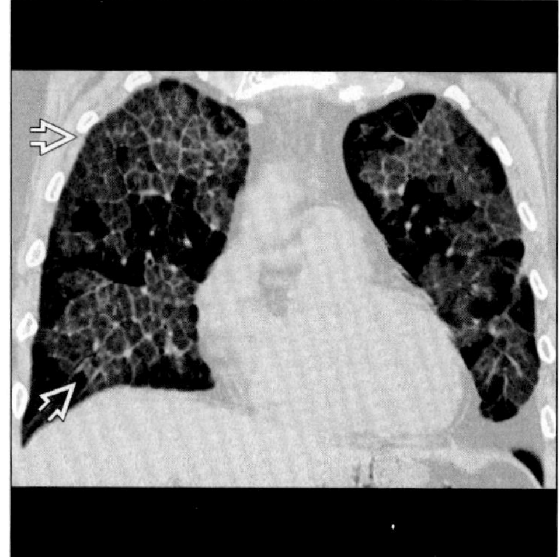

(Left) Axial NECT shows crazy-paving pattern ➡ and tiny pneumatoceles ➡ in a 31-year-old patient with AIDS. *(Right)* Axial CECT shows crazy-paving pattern ➡ from acute interstitial pneumonia. Distribution is also geographic, similar to alveolar proteinosis.

Pneumocystis Pneumonia (PCP)

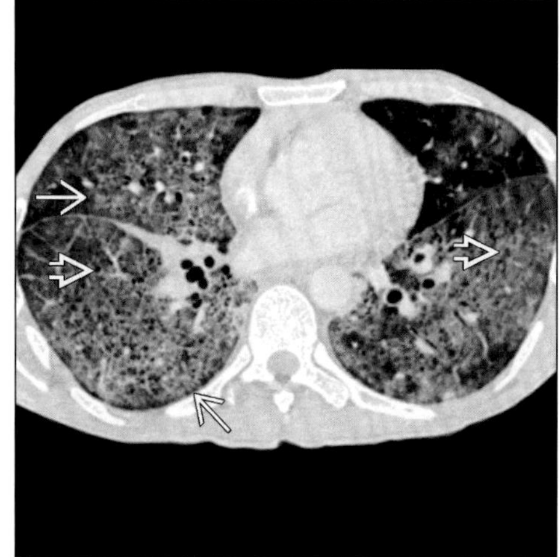

Acute Interstitial Pneumonia (AIP)

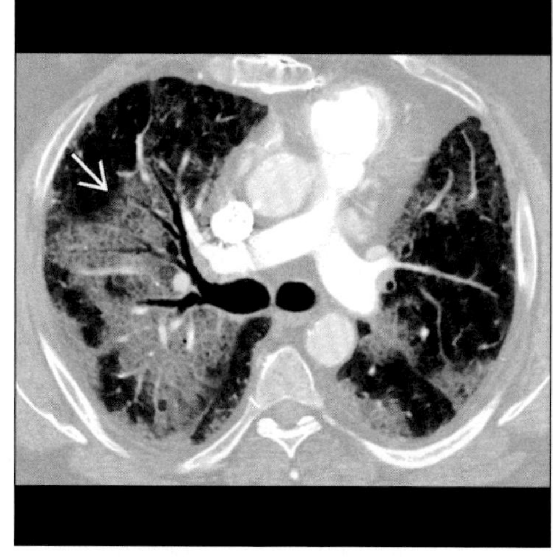

(Left) Axial CECT shows crazy-paving pattern ➡ in a patient with acute interstitial pneumonia. *(Right)* Axial CECT shows diffuse crazy-paving pattern ➡ from edema from crack abuse.

Acute Interstitial Pneumonia (AIP)

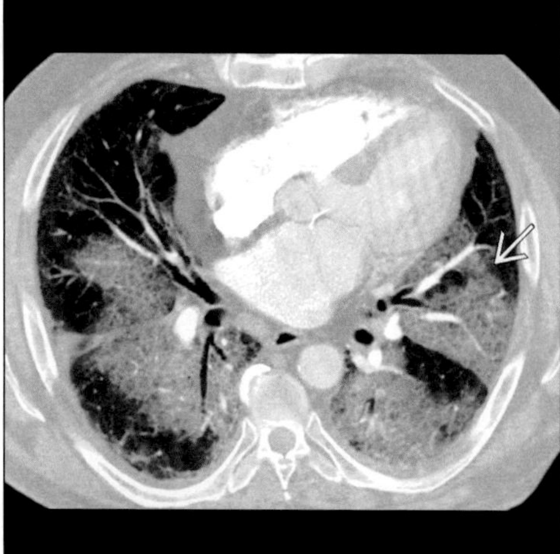

Edema

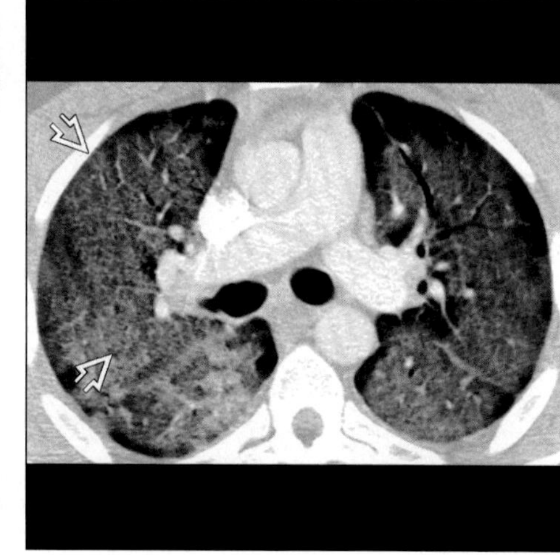

Diffuse Alveolar Hemorrhage

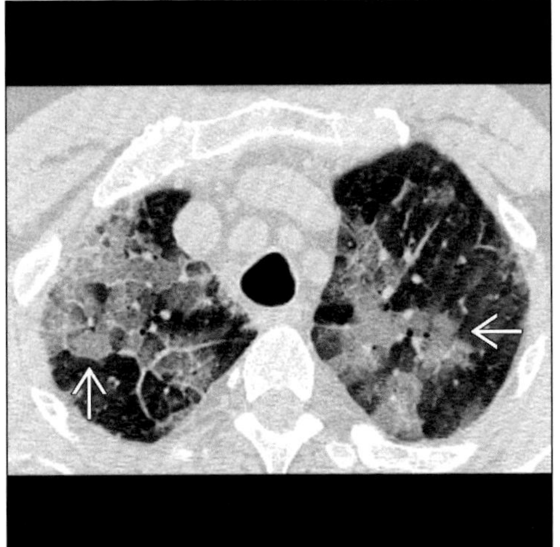

Eosinophilic Pneumonia

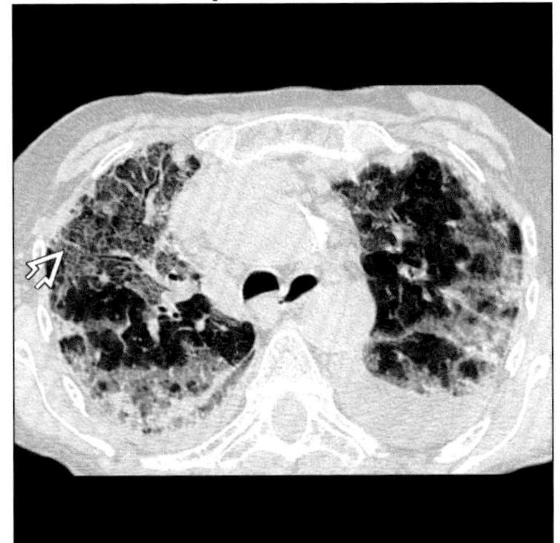

*(**Left**) Axial HRCT shows the typical features of crazy-paving pattern ➡ from diffuse alveolar hemorrhage. (**Right**) Axial HRCT shows crazy-paving pattern ➡ in chronic eosinophilic pneumonia. Note that the peripheral consolidation is more extensive than the crazy-paving pattern.*

Eosinophilic Pneumonia

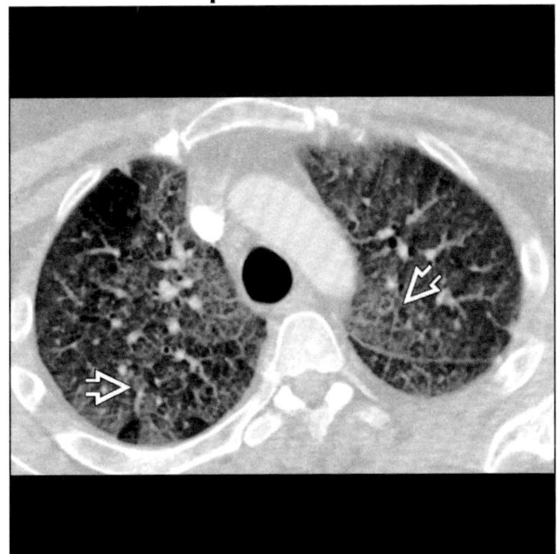

Cryptogenic Organizing Pneumonia (COP)

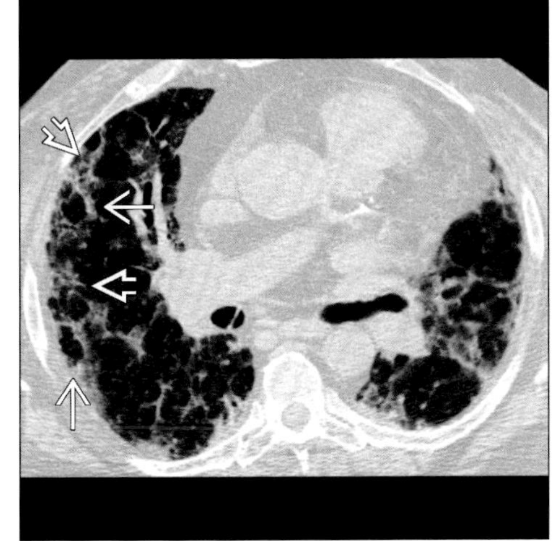

*(**Left**) Axial CECT shows a crazy-paving pattern in a patient with acute eosinophilic pneumonia. Ground-glass opacities ➡ represent the dominant finding. (**Right**) Axial HRCT shows small subpleural focal areas of crazy-paving pattern ➡ in cryptogenic organizing pneumonia. Perilobular distribution ➡ is also characteristic of COP.*

Bronchioloalveolar Cell Carcinoma (BAC)

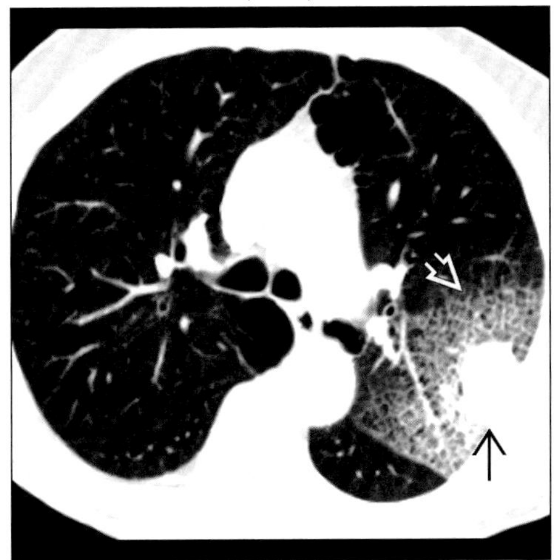

Lymphangitic Carcinomatosis

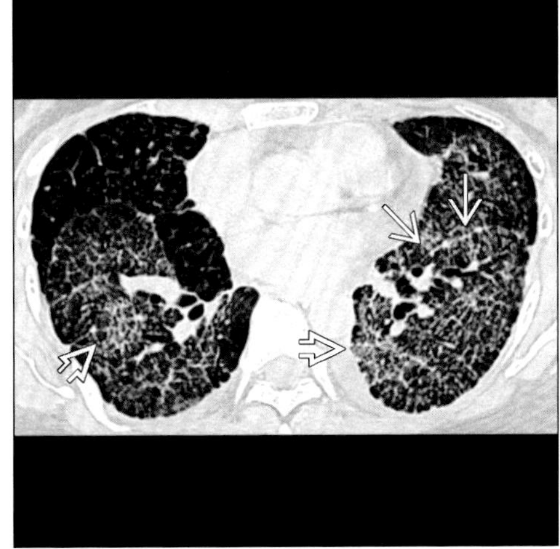

*(**Left**) Axial NECT shows a focal mass ➡ surrounded by crazy-paving pattern ➡ in a patient with bronchioloalveolar cell carcinoma. (**Right**) Axial HRCT shows widespread crazy-paving pattern ➡ in a patient with lymphangitic carcinomatosis. The beaded fissure ➡ is highly suspicious for lymphangitic tumor.*

RANDOM (MILIARY) DISTRIBUTION, CENTRILOBULAR NODULES

DIFFERENTIAL DIAGNOSIS

Common
- Metastases, Hematogenous
- Metastases, Miliary
- Infection, Miliary
  - Mycobacterial
  - Fungal
  - Viral

Less Common
- Infectious Bronchiolitis
- Sarcoidosis
- Hypersensitivity Pneumonitis

Rare but Important
- Talcosis, Intravenous
- Vasculitis
- Langerhans Cell Granulomatosis

ESSENTIAL INFORMATION

Key Differential Diagnosis Issues
- Random pattern
  - Nodules are diffuse and not clustered into rosettes (like grapes)
  - Feeding vessels to nodules helpful clue to random pattern
  - Blood flow to lung position is gravitationally dependent: Increased in bases in upright position, dorsal lung in supine position
  - Random pattern often more severe in lower lung zones and periphery
- Random vs. bronchovascular pattern
  - Bronchovascular centrilobular nodules clustered into rosettes
  - Bronchovascular pattern may have signs of small airways obstruction (mosaic attenuation, tree-in-bud opacities, bronchiectasis, air-trapping)
- Random vs. lymphatic pattern
  - Lymphatic centrilobular nodules clustered like grapes
  - Lymphatic nodules more profuse along pleura and fissures
  - Lymphatic nodules may be arranged in rays along blood vessels and airways
  - Lymphatic pattern often more severe in upper lung zones; random pattern often more severe in lower lung zones

Helpful Clues for Common Diagnoses
- **Metastases, Hematogenous**
  - Shape and margin characteristics
    - Round, sharply defined margins (40%), irregular shape, sharply defined (15%), round, ill-defined margins (15%), irregular shape, ill-defined margins (30%)
  - Variable size: Due to multiple episodes of primary tumor dissemination
  - Typically solid: Adenocarcinomas from gastrointestinal malignancies, lung, breast, melanoma, sarcoma
  - May be cavitary: Squamous cell carcinomas from primary head and neck, cervical, adenocarcinoma
  - May be calcified
    - Psammomatous calcification: Mucin-producing adenocarcinomas, such as from colon, ovary
    - Treated neoplasms: Thyroid, adenocarcinomas
    - Ossified metastases: Chondrosarcoma and osteosarcoma
  - May be surrounded by ground-glass halo
    - Vascular tumors with hemorrhage: Choriocarcinoma, angiosarcoma, renal cell carcinoma
- **Metastases, Miliary**
  - Tumors whose primary venous drainage is to lungs
    - Medullary thyroid carcinoma, renal cell carcinoma, head and neck tumors, ovarian or testicular tumors, melanoma
  - Nodules similar in size, too numerous to count
- **Infection, Miliary**
  - Nearly any organism, most commonly *Mycobacterium tuberculosis*, fungal, viral
  - Miliary tuberculosis
    - Disseminated disease in either primary or post-primary infection
    - Immunosuppressed patients most susceptible, especially those with impaired cellular immunity
    - **Chronic miliary tuberculosis:** Miliary nodules often **larger** in upper lung zones
  - Miliary histoplasmosis
    - Dissemination usually due to reactivation of latent disease

- In AIDS patients, dissemination usually when CD4 count is < 75 cells/mm^3, associated hilar and mediastinal lymphadenopathy
- Associated with adrenal insufficiency
- Miliary blastomycosis
  - Chronic miliary nodules: Often larger in upper lung zones
  - Disseminated disease may occur up to 3 years after primary infection
  - Extrathoracic involvement: Skin, bone, prostate, central nervous system
- Pneumonia, viral
  - Diffuse, often ill-defined nodules
  - Nodules may coalesce or have ground-glass halos

Helpful Clues for Less Common Diagnoses

- **Infectious Bronchiolitis**
  - Typical bronchovascular pattern
  - Fever, elevated white blood cell count
  - Typical pattern in tree-in-bud opacities
  - Patchy or diffuse
- **Sarcoidosis**
  - Typical lymphatic distribution
  - Nodules with heterogeneous distribution, cut swath through lung
  - May have symmetric hilar and mediastinal adenopathy
  - Nodules more profuse in upper lung zones
- **Hypersensitivity Pneumonitis**
  - Acute or subacute
  - Typical bronchovascular pattern
  - Centrilobular ground-glass nodules + lobular air-trapping
  - Environmental history important

Helpful Clues for Rare Diagnoses

- **Talcosis, Intravenous**
  - Found in illicit drug abuse
    - Talc common filler in oral medications, not meant to be injected intravenously
  - Nodules often pinpoint in size and may be of higher density
  - Nodules more profuse in mid and lower lung
    - In contrast, inhalational talcosis more common in upper lung zones
  - May result in progressive massive fibrosis
- **Vasculitis**
  - Centrilobular nodules from hemorrhage or hemosiderin deposits (often bronchovascular distribution with larger vessel involvement)
  - Often nodules follow episodes of hemorrhage (diffuse or patchy ground-glass opacities and consolidation)
  - Sedimentation rate usually elevated
- **Langerhans Cell Granulomatosis**
  - Typical bronchovascular pattern
  - Centrilobular nodules; with time nodules enlarge and cavitate
  - Eventually cavitated nodules form thin-walled cysts that aggregate into bizarre shapes
  - Usually seen in smokers

Metastases, Hematogenous

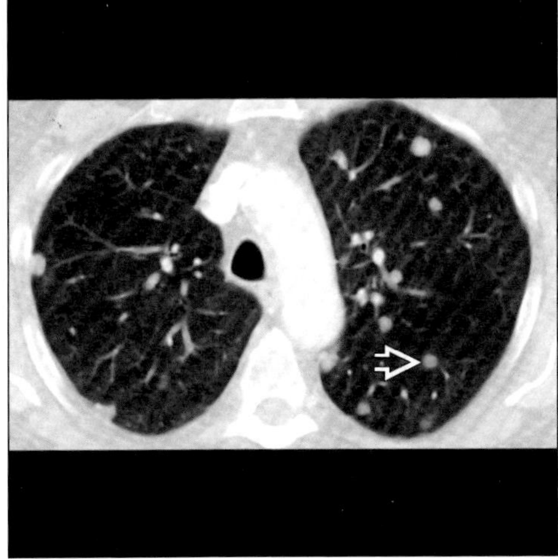

Axial CECT shows a random distribution of variably sized pulmonary nodules ➨. The nodules have smooth, sharply defined margins and are distributed primarily in the lung periphery.

Metastases, Hematogenous

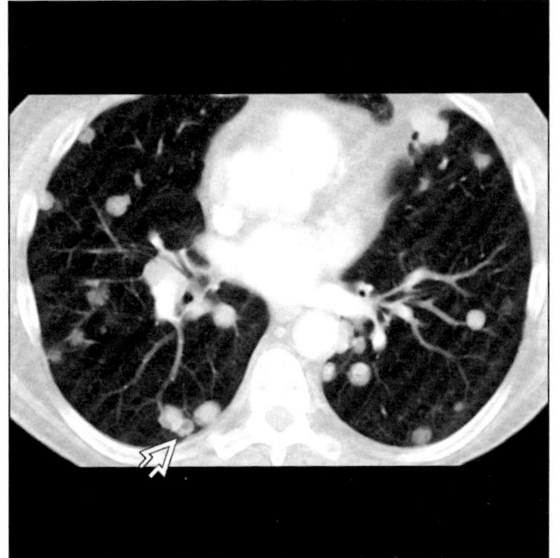

Axial CECT in the same patient shows increased profusion of nodules in the lower lungs. Note the nodule cavitation ➨ in this patient with head and neck squamous cell carcinoma.

RANDOM (MILIARY) DISTRIBUTION, CENTRILOBULAR NODULES

*(**Left**) Axial HRCT shows the typical features of hematogenous and lymphangitic involvement in a patient with lung cancer. Note the nodules ➔, septal thickening ➔, and ground-glass opacities ➔. (**Right**) Axial CECT shows typical features of variably sized, ill-defined nodules. Note the nodule with a ground-glass halo ➔, supplied by a feeding vessel ➔. The diagnosis was choriocarcinoma metastases.*

Metastases, Hematogenous

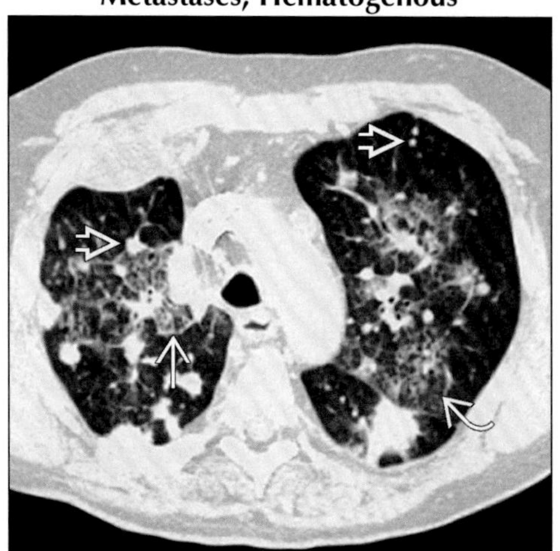

Metastases, Hematogenous

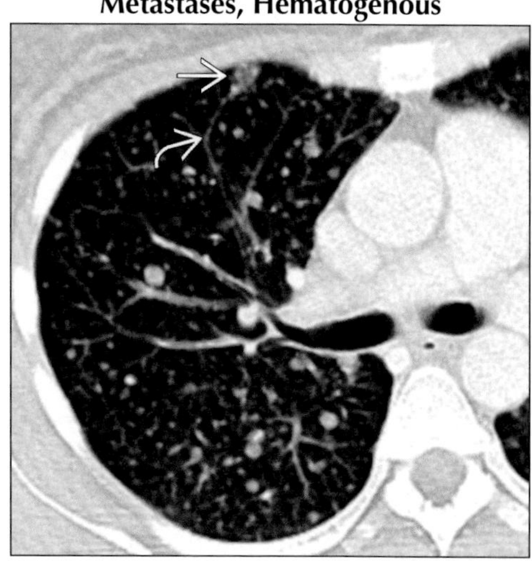

*(**Left**) Axial HRCT shows a random distribution of miliary nodules ➔ that represent treated metastases from thyroid cancer. Nodule calcification (not shown) is due to iodine-131 therapy. (**Right**) Axial HRCT shows innumerable miliary nodules ➔ from hematogenous dissemination of Mycobacterium tuberculosis. Note the absence of upper lobe cavitary disease.*

Metastases, Miliary

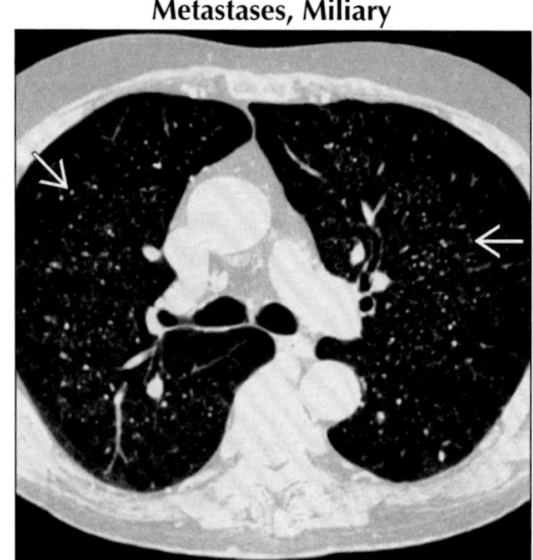

Mycobacterial

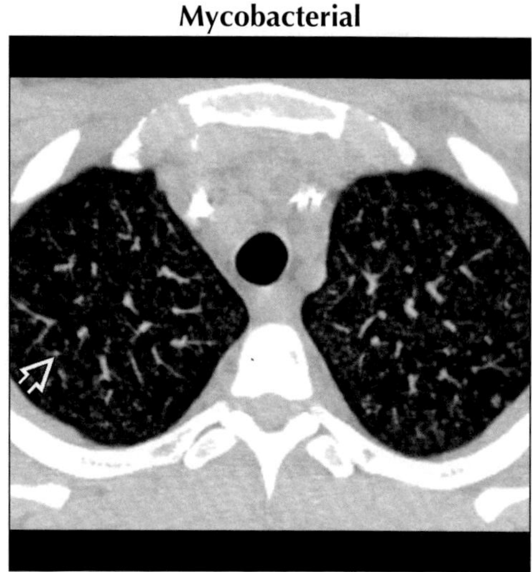

*(**Left**) Axial HRCT shows innumerable miliary nodules ➔ in both lungs due to the hematogenous spread of tuberculosis. The nodules show a random pattern of distribution. (**Right**) Axial CECT shows the typical CT features of diffuse, bilateral, random, small nodular opacities ➔. Hilar and mediastinal lymphadenopathy (not shown) was present in this patient with histoplasmosis.*

Mycobacterial

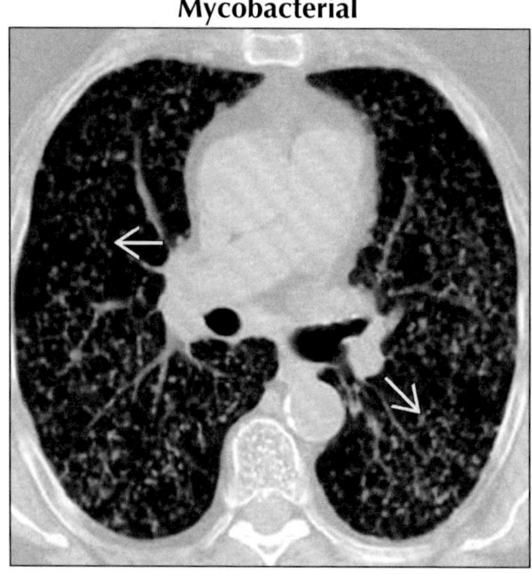

Fungal

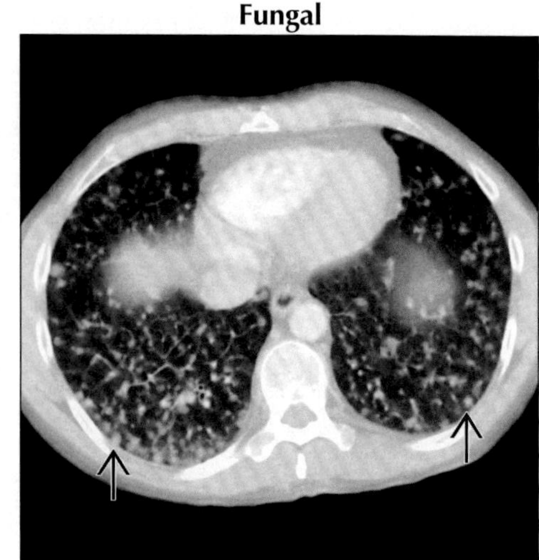

RANDOM (MILIARY) DISTRIBUTION, CENTRILOBULAR NODULES

Fungal

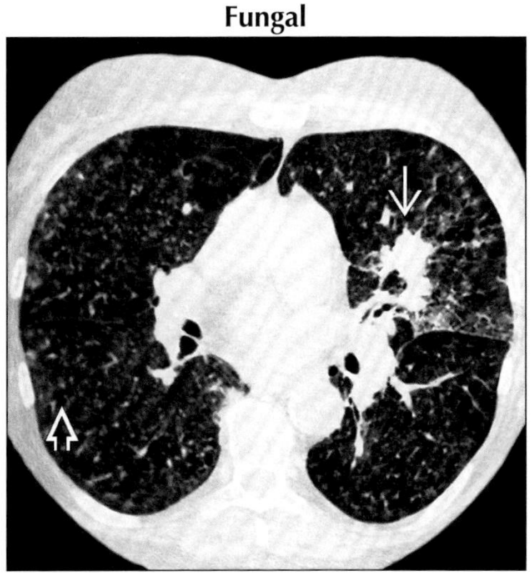

Fungal

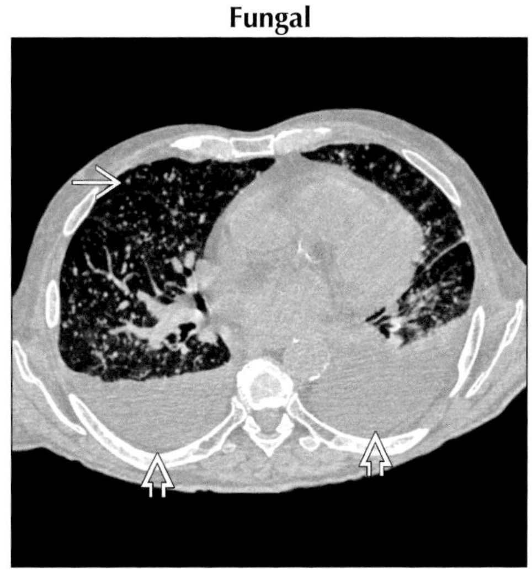

(Left) *Axial HRCT shows a mass-like opacity in the left upper lobe ➡ that represents histoplasma pneumonia. Left hilar lymphadenopathy is not shown. Note diffuse miliary nodules ⇨, the result of hematogenous dissemination of histoplasmosis.* ***(Right)*** *Axial HRCT shows variant features of blastomycosis with diffuse random miliary nodules ➡ indicating disseminated disease. Moderate effusions ⇨ are not frequently seen with blastomycosis.*

Fungal

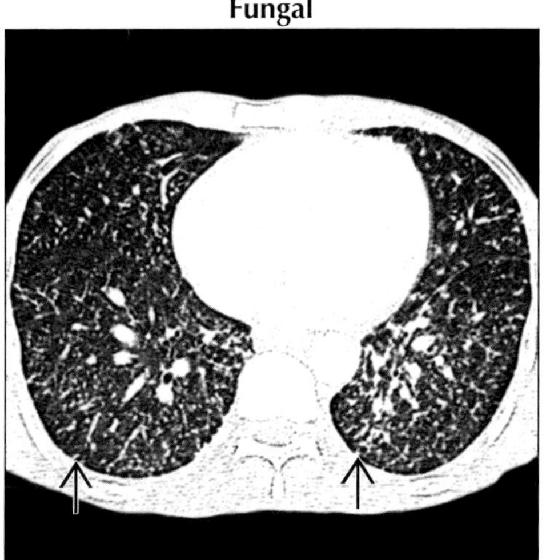

Viral

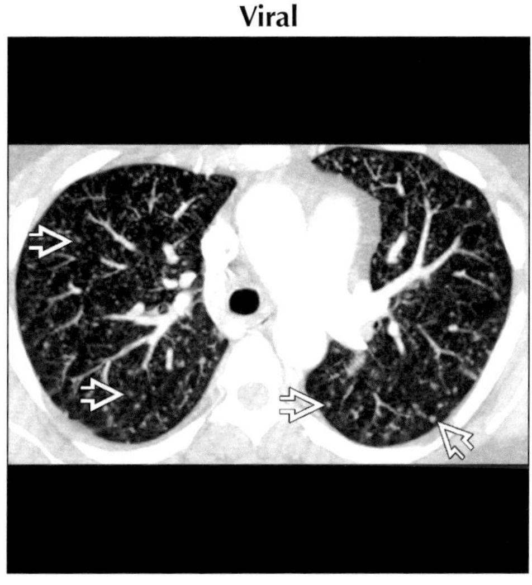

(Left) *Axial HRCT shows variant features of miliary disease from disseminated coccidioidomycosis in a patient with AIDS. The miliary nodules ➡ show random distribution.* ***(Right)*** *Tangential HRCT MIP shows a random distribution of miliary nodules ⇨. MIP images are often superior to standard axial images in demonstrating a miliary pattern.*

Talcosis, Intravenous

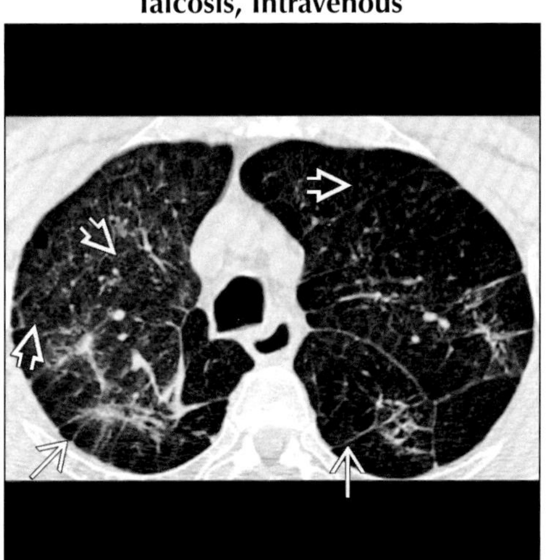

Vasculitis

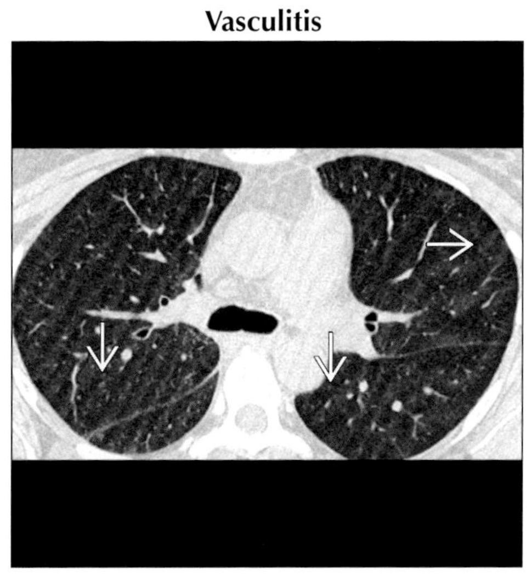

(Left) *Axial HRCT shows micronodules ⇨ and long linear lines ➡ with architectural distortion in this patient who was an IV drug abuser.* ***(Right)*** *Axial CECT shows faint diffuse micronodular and ground-glass nodules ➡ throughout both lungs. Histologic sections (not shown) revealed neutrophilic infiltrate within capillary endothelium and parenchymal hemorrhage.*

BRONCHOVASCULAR DISTRIBUTION, CENTRILOBULAR NODULES

DIFFERENTIAL DIAGNOSIS

Common

- Airways Disease
  - Infectious Bronchiolitis
  - Subacute Hypersensitivity Pneumonitis
  - Aspiration
  - Respiratory Bronchiolitis
  - Follicular Bronchiolitis
  - Laryngeal Papillomatosis
- Vascular Disease
  - Vasculitis
  - Metastatic Pulmonary Calcification

Less Common

- Lymphatic Pattern
  - Pulmonary Sarcoidosis
  - Silicosis/Coal Worker's Pneumoconiosis
  - Lymphocytic Interstitial Pneumonia

Rare but Important

- Intravascular Pulmonary Metastases

ESSENTIAL INFORMATION

Key Differential Diagnosis Issues

- Definition of bronchovascular pattern
  - Nodules (< 1 cm diameter) centered on small airways or blood vessels (centrilobular)
- Bronchovascular pattern may result in small airways obstruction
  - Mosaic attenuation, tree-in-bud opacities, air-trapping, bronchiectasis
  - Ground-glass nodules usually signify bronchovascular pattern
- Bronchovascular vs. lymphatic pattern
  - Lymphatic pattern may have subpleural and fissural nodules that comprise > 10% of total nodules
  - Lymphatic pattern may not involve peripheral lymphatics
    - Thus differential overlaps with bronchovascular pattern
  - Bronchovascular pattern may have signs of small airways obstruction
  - Ground-glass nodules usually signify bronchovascular pattern
- Bronchovascular vs. random pattern
  - Centrilobular nodules clustered like grapes
    - Hematogenous, usually randomly dispersed
  - Hematogenous nodules may have **feeding** vessels
  - Bronchovascular pattern may have signs of small airways obstruction
  - Ground-glass nodules usually signify bronchovascular pattern
  - For less profuse nodules, separation of centrilobular nodules from random difficult
    - Consider both in differential

Helpful Clues for Common Diagnoses

- **Infectious Bronchiolitis**
  - Classically described with mycobacterial disease (endobronchial spread) but nonspecific
    - Includes bacterial, fungal, and viral pneumonias
- **Subacute Hypersensitivity Pneumonitis**
  - Upper lobe centrilobular indistinct ground-glass nodules
  - Confluent lower lobe ground-glass nodules
  - Lobular air-trapping on exhalation CT
  - Rare in smokers
- **Aspiration**
  - Tree-in-bud opacities especially common in chronic aspiration of legumes
  - Primarily involves gravity-dependent lung regions
    - Posterior segments and superior segments of lower lobe in supine position
    - Basilar segments in upright position
- **Respiratory Bronchiolitis**
  - Upper lobe faint centrilobular ground-glass nodules
    - Profusion & severity of nodules usually much less than in hypersensitivity pneumonitis
  - May be precursor to centrilobular emphysema
  - Smoking-related lung disease, responds to smoking cessation
- **Follicular Bronchiolitis**
  - Lymphoid hyperplasia of bronchus-associated lymphoid tissue (BALT)
  - Associated with collagen vascular diseases (rheumatoid arthritis), AIDS, infections, hypersensitivity reaction

- Centrilobular nodules most common, usually associated with subpleural nodules and ground-glass opacities
- **Laryngeal Papillomatosis**
  - Usually associated with nodules within airways
  - Distribution often in gravity-dependent lung regions
  - Nodules may cavitate
- **Vasculitis**
  - Centrilobular nodules from hemosiderin-laden macrophages
  - Nodules follow episodes of hemorrhage (seen as consolidation and ground-glass opacities)
- **Metastatic Pulmonary Calcification**
  - Usually seen in conditions associated with hypercalcemia (especially renal failure)
  - Typically upper lobes
  - Nodules often clustered into rosettes (resembles mulberry)
    - Often have ground-glass density or high attenuation

Helpful Clues for Less Common Diagnoses

- **Lymphatic Pattern**
  - If disease does not involve peripheral lymphatics, lymphatic pattern may be indistinguishable from bronchovascular pattern
  - **Pulmonary Sarcoidosis**
    - Bronchovascular nodules
    - Nodularity more profuse in upper lung zones
    - Usually associated with subpleural fissural nodules
    - Noncaseating granulomas concentrated in lymphatics
    - May have symmetric hilar and mediastinal adenopathy
  - **Silicosis/Coal Worker's Pneumoconiosis**
    - Nodularity more profuse in upper and dorsal lung zones
    - Usually associated with subpleural fissural nodules
    - May have adenopathy (typically with "eggshell" calcification)
    - Nodules may aggregate into masses known as progressive massive fibrosis
  - **Lymphocytic Interstitial Pneumonia**
    - Associated with viral infections: HIV and Epstein-Barr virus
    - Also associated with Sjögren syndrome or dysproteinemias
    - Thin-walled cysts distinctive (80%)

Helpful Clues for Rare Diagnoses

- **Intravascular Pulmonary Metastases**
  - Tumor origin typically angiosarcoma, renal cell carcinoma, hepatoma

Alternative Differential Approaches

- Predominant distribution in upper lung zones
  - Respiratory bronchiolitis
  - Sarcoidosis
  - Silicosis/coal worker's pneumoconiosis
  - Metastatic pulmonary calcification

Infectious Bronchiolitis

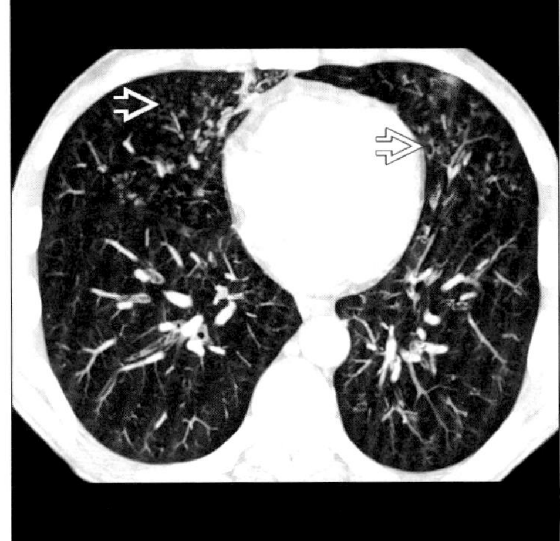

Axial HRCT shows branching tree-in-bud opacities ➔ in the middle lobe and lingula from Mycobacterium avium complex.

Infectious Bronchiolitis

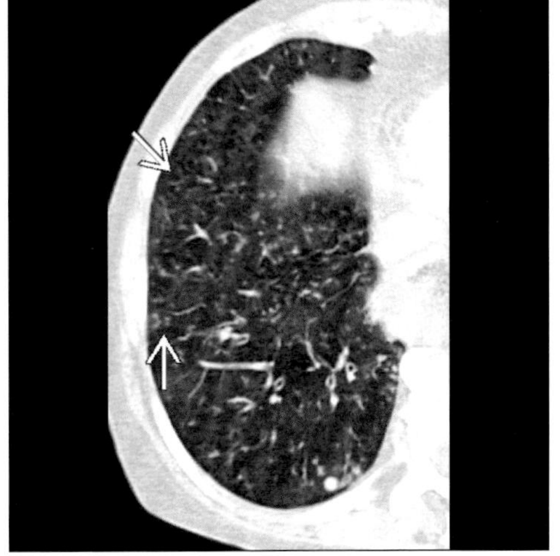

Axial CT shows diffuse tree-in-bud opacities ➔ in the lower lobe from infectious bronchiolitis.

BRONCHOVASCULAR DISTRIBUTION, CENTRILOBULAR NODULES

Subacute Hypersensitivity Pneumonitis

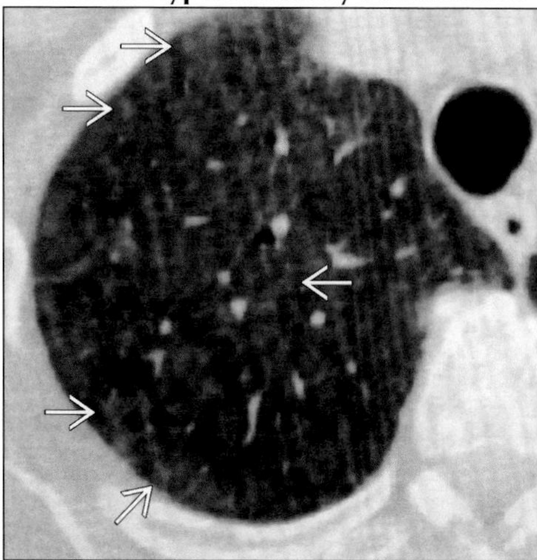

Subacute Hypersensitivity Pneumonitis

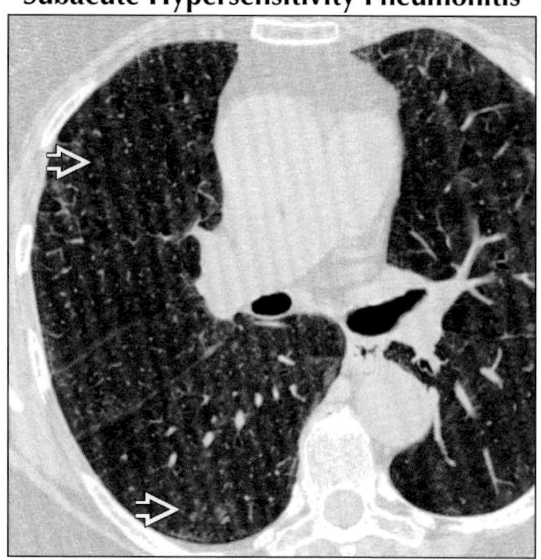

(Left) *Axial supine HRCT shows numerous ground-glass upper lobe centrilobular nodules ➔ that improved with steroids. The diagnosis was a hypersensitivity to a variety of molds in the patient's log home.* ***(Right)*** *Axial HRCT shows faint ground-glass centrilobular nodules ➔ and patchy ground-glass opacities diffusely throughout the lung in a patient with subacute hypersensitivity pneumonitis.*

Subacute Hypersensitivity Pneumonitis

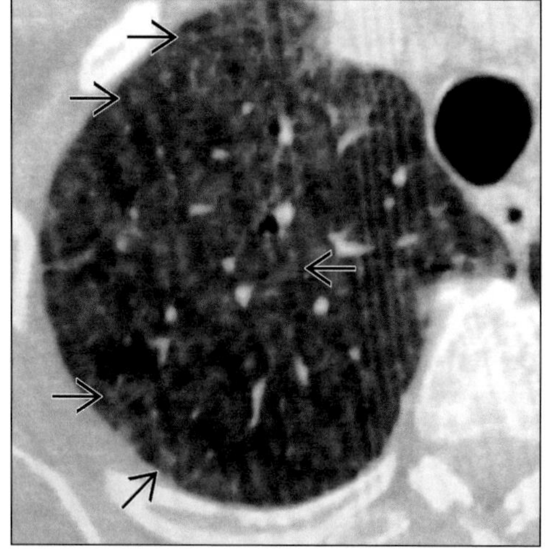

Aspiration

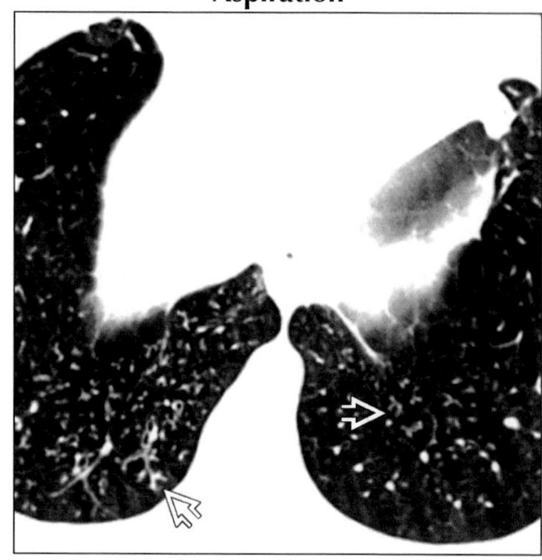

(Left) *Axial supine HRCT shows ground-glass centrilobular nodules ➔ from subacute hypersensitivity pneumonitis. This patient with chronic shortness of breath had repeated exposures to parakeets.* ***(Right)*** *Axial HRCT shows typical tree-in-bud opacities ➔ from chronic aspiration in the basilar segments of the lower lobes. This appearance can occur from any aspirated material but is also seen from endobronchial spread of infected material.*

Respiratory Bronchiolitis

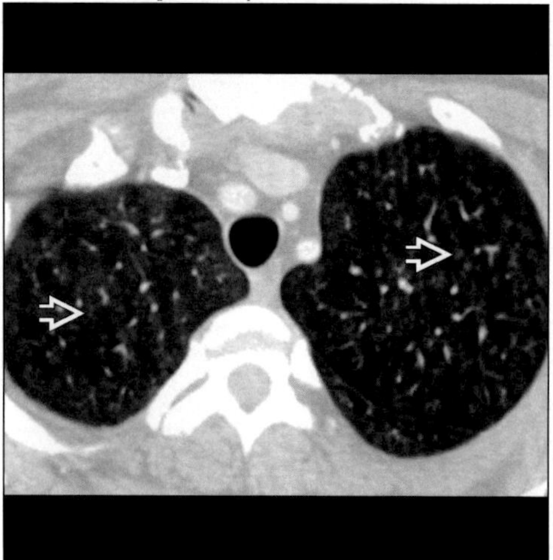

Follicular Bronchiolitis

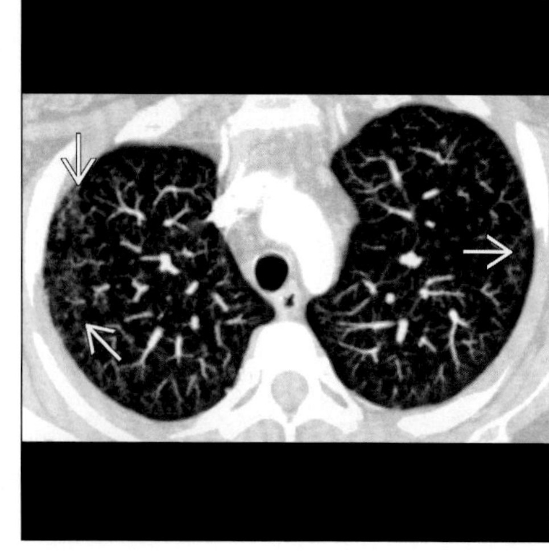

(Left) *Axial CECT shows faint centrilobular nodules ➔ from respiratory bronchiolitis. Note the difference in severity of the nodules when compared with hypersensitivity pneumonitis.* ***(Right)*** *Axial CECT MIP reconstruction shows a peripheral tree-in-bud pattern ➔ in a patient with rheumatoid arthritis.*

BRONCHOVASCULAR DISTRIBUTION, CENTRILOBULAR NODULES

Vasculitis

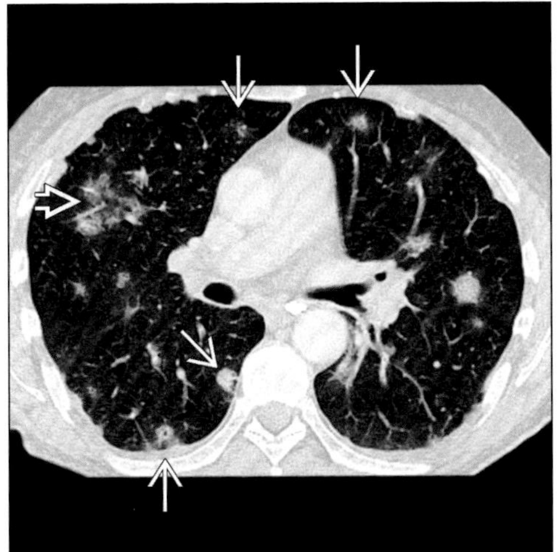

Metastatic Pulmonary Calcification

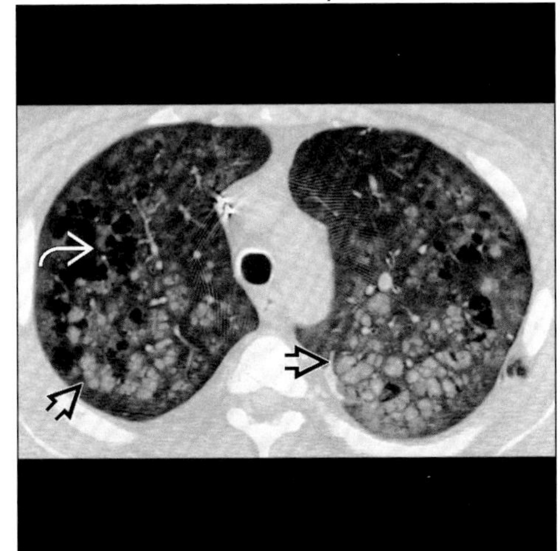

(Left) Axial CECT shows focal, variably sized ground-glass opacities ➡ and "target" lesions ➡ centered on pulmonary arterioles. (Right) Axial NECT shows emphysema ➡ and clustered rosettes of high-density centrilobular nodules ➡ in metastatic pulmonary calcification from chronic renal failure. The calcification pattern has also been described as resembling the mulberry.

Pulmonary Sarcoidosis

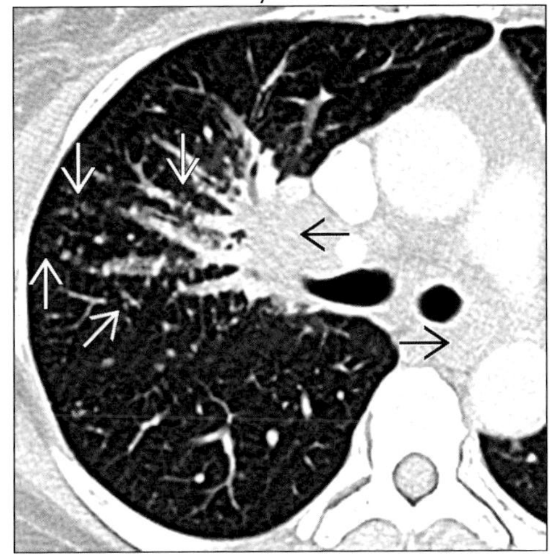

Silicosis/Coal Worker's Pneumoconiosis

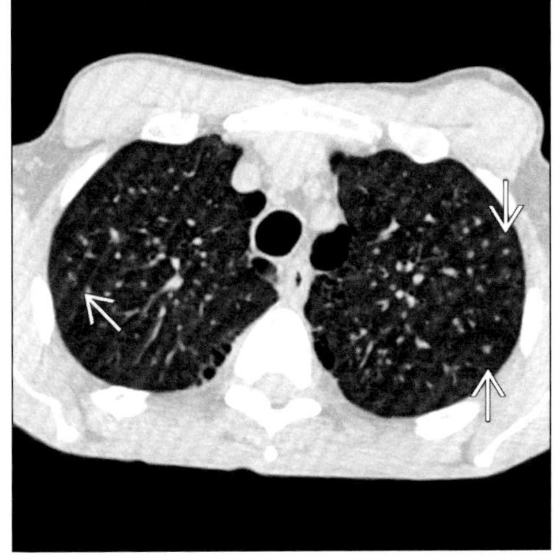

(Left) Axial NECT shows nodules ➡ in peribronchovascular distribution in a patient with sarcoidosis. Note the extensive mediastinal and hilar lymphadenopathy ➡. (Right) Axial HRCT shows centrilobular nodules ➡ in the upper lobes in a patient with mild occupational lung disease, silicosis. In more severe cases, the nodules can become confluent and lead to progressive massive fibrosis.

Lymphocytic Interstitial Pneumonia

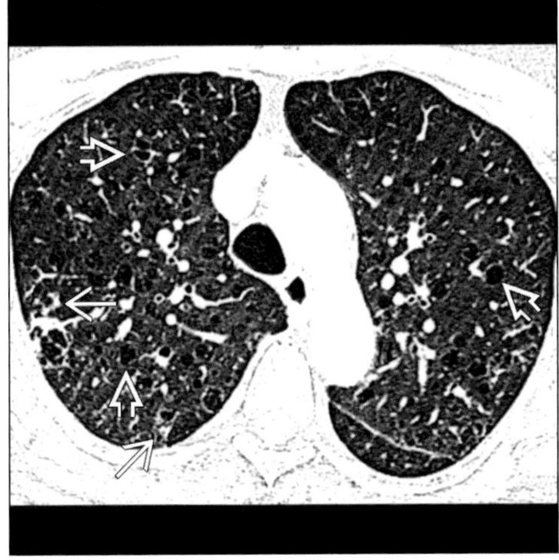

Intravascular Pulmonary Metastases

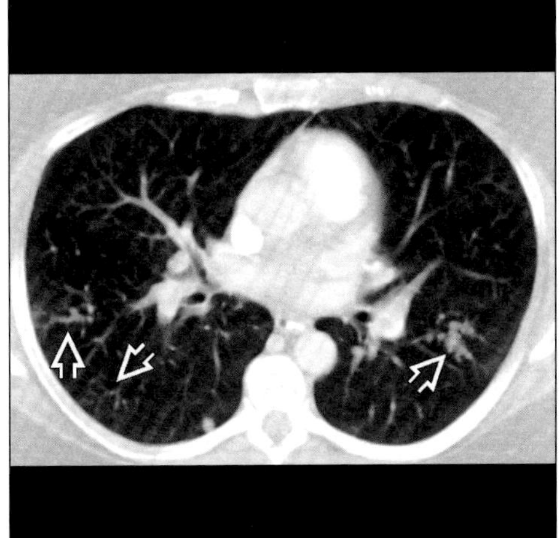

(Left) Axial HRCT shows multiple thin-walled cysts ➡ and nodules in a bronchocentric location ➡. This disease pattern can be seen with Sjögren syndrome. (Right) Axial CECT shows tree-in-bud opacities ➡ and beading along pulmonary arteries from intravascular metastases from chondrosarcoma. This beaded vessel appearance is characteristic but easily confused with airway or lymphatic distributed disease.

LYMPHATIC DISTRIBUTION, CENTRILOBULAR NODULES

DIFFERENTIAL DIAGNOSIS

Common
- Sarcoidosis, Pulmonary
- Silicosis/Coal Worker's Pneumoconiosis
- Lymphangitic Carcinomatosis

Less Common
- Lymphoma, Non-Hodgkin or Hodgkin
- Bronchiolitis, Follicular
- Amyloidosis
- Berylliosis

Rare but Important
- Lymphocytic Interstitial Pneumonia

ESSENTIAL INFORMATION

Key Differential Diagnosis Issues
- Definition of lymphatic pattern
  - Predominant abnormality is nodules (< 1 cm diameter) in pulmonary lymphatics
  - Often called "**perilymphatic**" (pathology, however, usually in lymphatics)
- Lymphatic compartments
  - **Axial**: Follows bronchi and arteries to level of terminal bronchioles in secondary pulmonary lobule
  - **Peripheral**: Follows veins, septa, and pleura
  - Alveoli and respiratory bronchioles devoid of lymphatics
  - **Same disease process may sometimes preferentially involve axial lymphatics, sometimes peripheral lymphatics**
- Pathophysiology of disease
  - Inhalational: Especially from **rounded** dust particles
  - Hematogenous less common, implies migration into adjacent lymphatics (lymphohematogenous dissemination)
- Lymphatic vs. hematogenous pattern
  - Lymphatic nodules
    - Clustered like grapes, unlike dispersion in random distribution pattern
    - May be focal and localized; random is usually diffuse
  - Lymphatic pattern
    - Nodules arranged in rays along bronchovascular pathways
    - Usually associated with subpleural and fissural nodules that comprise > 10% of total number of nodules
    - Often more severe in upper lung zones, random pattern often more severe in lower lung zones
    - Often associated with hilar and mediastinal adenopathy
- Lymphatic vs. bronchovascular pattern
  - Bronchovascular pattern nodules less common along fissure and subpleural lung (< 10% of total number of nodules)
    - Associated with small airways disease: Mosaic attenuation, air-trapping, tree-in-bud opacities
    - May be focal (from aspiration) or diffuse (from inhalation disorders)
  - Some diseases **start** as bronchovascular pattern (from acute-semiacute reaction from inhaled pathogen) and **evolve** into lymphatic pattern (as pathogen migrates to draining lymphatics)
  - Lymphatic pattern often associated with hilar and mediastinal adenopathy

Helpful Clues for Common Diagnoses
- **Sarcoidosis, Pulmonary**
  - Focal aggregation of nodules along bronchovascular bundles
  - Nodules may be clustered into large masses (called **alveolar sarcoid**)
    - **Galaxy sign**: Coalescent mass surrounded by its constituent smaller nodules
  - Nodules more profuse in upper lung zones
  - Symmetric hilar and mediastinal adenopathy common
    - Nodes may contain **chalky-smudgy or eggshell pattern** calcification
- **Silicosis/Coal Worker's Pneumoconiosis**
  - Work history of occupational exposure to silica particles or coal
  - Nodules more profuse in upper lung zones
  - Nodules tend to aggregate in **dorsal** aspect of lung; right lung usually more severely involved than left
  - Severity and time results in progressive massive fibrosis (PMF)
  - Hilar and mediastinal lymphadenopathy may show "**eggshell**" calcification (5%)
  - Inhalational **talcosis** and **siderosis** give identical findings (reflects lung's ability to chronically handle small rounded dusts)
- **Lymphangitic Carcinomatosis**
  - Seen primarily with adenocarcinomas

- Frequency of involvement: Axial lymphatics (75%), axial + peripheral (20%), peripheral (5%)
- Characteristically **spares** whole lobe or even whole lung
- Lung architecture **preserved**, unlike sarcoidosis and silicosis, which show architectural distortion
- Pleural effusion(s) common (unusual in sarcoidosis or silicosis)
- May have adenopathy

Helpful Clues for Less Common Diagnoses

- **Lymphoma, Non-Hodgkin or Hodgkin**
  - Pulmonary involvement in Hodgkin (40%) and non-Hodgkin (25%) disease
    - Primarily involves axial lymphatics
    - Pulmonary nodules, usually > 1 cm (often with air-bronchograms)
  - Associated with bulky lymphadenopathy, effusion(s) also common
- **Bronchiolitis, Follicular**
  - Synonym: Lymphoid hyperplasia of bronchus-associated lymphoid tissue (BALT)
  - Pathology: Similar to lymphocytic interstitial pneumonia (LIP)
    - Follicular bronchiolitis: Centered on airway lymphatics
  - Interlobular septal thickening, bronchiolectasis, thin-walled cysts
  - Associated with collagen vascular diseases (rheumatoid arthritis, Sjögren syndrome), AIDS, infections, hypersensitivity reaction
- **Amyloidosis**
  - Primary (associated with myeloma) and secondary (associated with chronic inflammatory disease)
  - Wide spectrum findings: Tracheobronchial thickening and nodularity, centrilobular nodules, septal thickening
  - Diffuse septal form more commonly has nodules in subpleural lung
  - Nodules may calcify
- **Berylliosis**
  - Gives identical findings, occupational history important
  - Beryllium lightweight metal with high melting point, used in wide variety of industries
  - Latent period after exposure of 1 month to 40 years
  - Incites hypersensitivity reaction with granulomas

Helpful Clues for Rare Diagnoses

- **Lymphocytic Interstitial Pneumonia**
  - Also associated with viral infection: HIV and Epstein-Barr virus, dysproteinemias, or Sjögren syndrome
  - Thin-walled cysts distinctive (80%)
  - Usually associated with nonspecific ground-glass opacities (100%)
  - Diffuse distribution

Sarcoidosis, Pulmonary

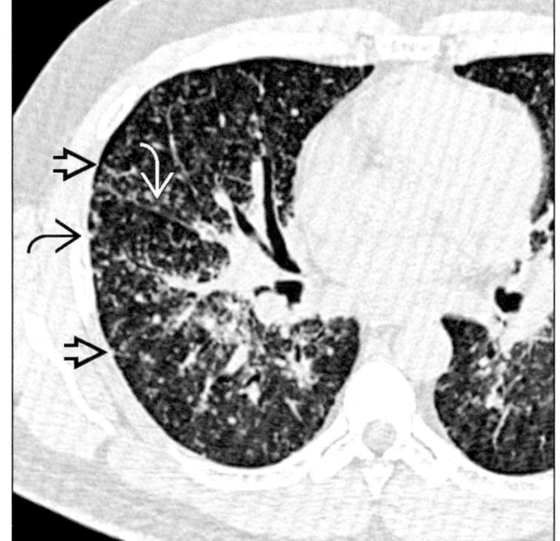

Axial HRCT shows typical perilymphatic distribution of subpleural, interlobular septal, and major fissure nodules.

Sarcoidosis, Pulmonary

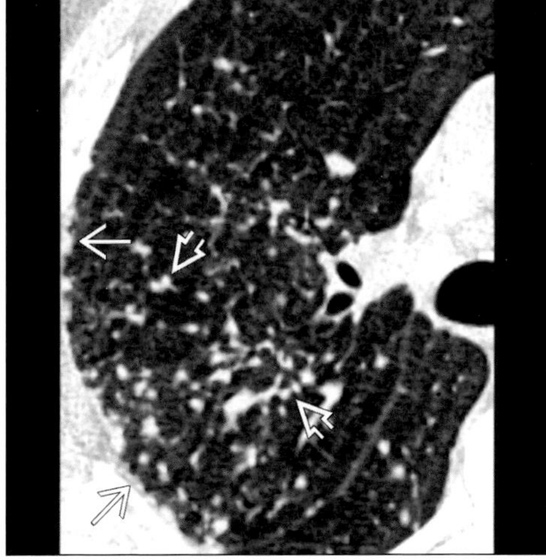

Axial HRCT shows perivascular & subpleural nodules from sarcoidosis.

LYMPHATIC DISTRIBUTION, CENTRILOBULAR NODULES

*(**Left**) Axial HRCT shows perilymphatic nodules at left major fissure ➡ and subpleural lung ↪. Note the nodular conglomeration at left major fissure and interlobular septa ⇨. (**Right**) Axial HRCT shows centrilobular nodules ➡ & subpleural nodules ⇨ in silicosis.*

Silicosis/Coal Worker's Pneumoconiosis

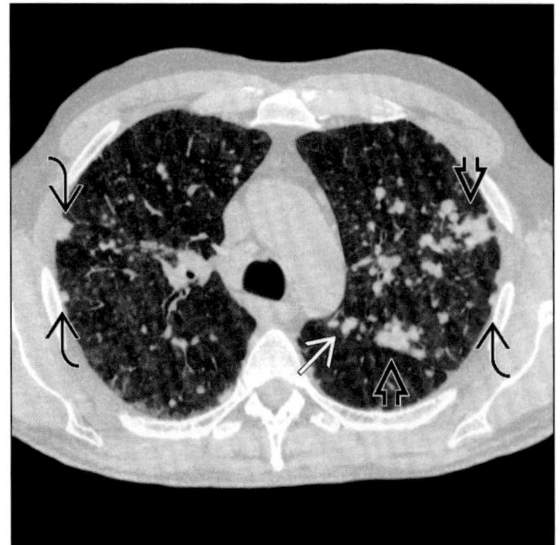

Silicosis/Coal Worker's Pneumoconiosis

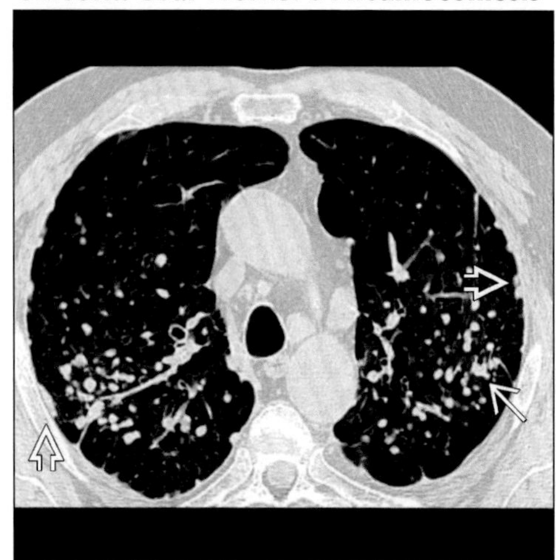

*(**Left**) Axial HRCT shows the typical features of diffuse, irregular, and beaded thickening of interlobular septa, producing polygonal structures ⇨ of variable size and thickening of central bronchovascular bundles ➡. (**Right**) Axial CECT shows the typical CT features of irregular septal thickening ⇨ and central bronchovascular wall thickening ➡. Note the perilymphatic pattern of tumor extension in this patient with breast cancer.*

Lymphangitic Carcinomatosis

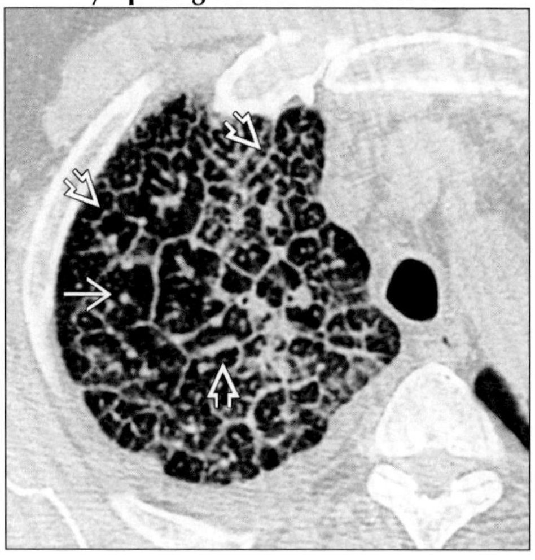

Lymphangitic Carcinomatosis

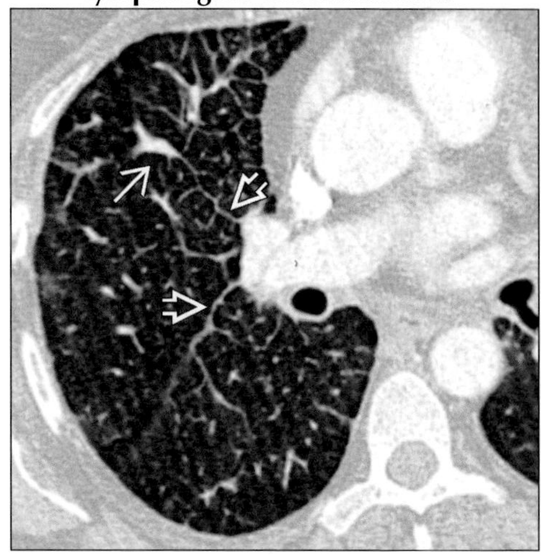

*(**Left**) Axial HRCT shows typical features of bronchocentric soft tissue and nodularity extending along the airways ➡ in this patient with subpleural and sub-fissural perilymphatic disease ⇨. (**Right**) Axial prone HRCT in the same patient shows interlobular septal and subpleural perilymphatic disease ⇨. Core biopsy showed pulmonary B-cell lymphoma.*

Lymphoma, Non-Hodgkin or Hodgkin

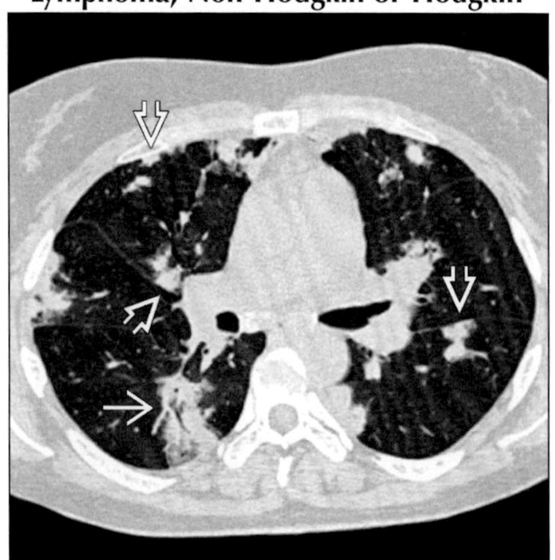

Lymphoma, Non-Hodgkin or Hodgkin

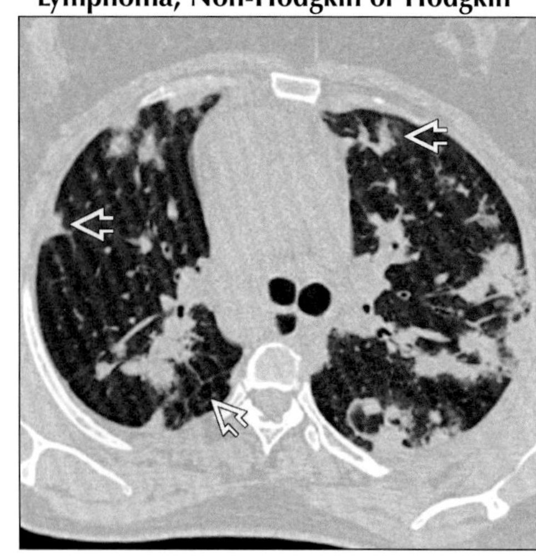

LYMPHATIC DISTRIBUTION, CENTRILOBULAR NODULES

Bronchiolitis, Follicular

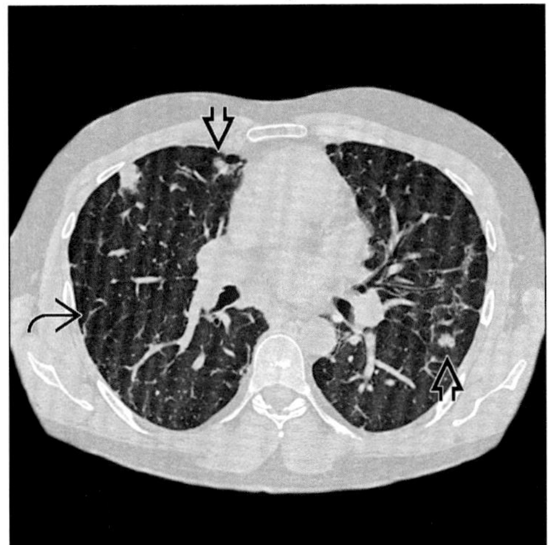

Bronchiolitis, Follicular

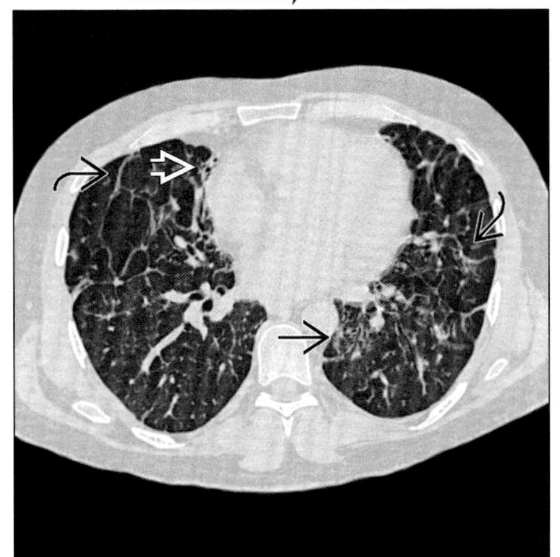

(Left) Axial HRCT image shows the typical findings of centrilobular nodules ⇨ and septal lines ↗. (Right) Axial HRCT in the same patient shows variant features of perilymphatic, irregular, interlobular, septal thickening ↗, ground-glass opacity →, and bronchiectasis ⇨.

Amyloidosis

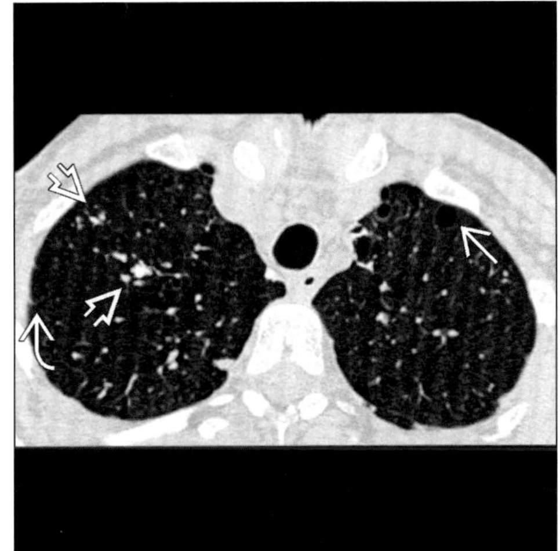

Berylliosis

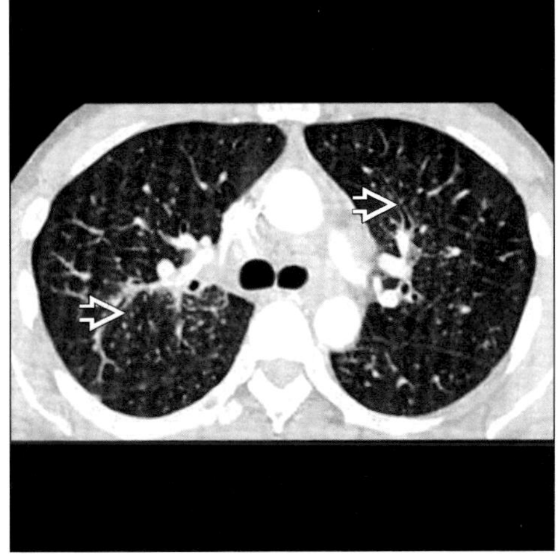

(Left) Axial HRCT shows nodular amyloidosis. Centrilobular nodules ⇨, cysts →, and tiny subpleural nodules ↗ are also present. (Right) Axial CECT shows nodular peribronchial thickening ⇨ extending from the hilum to the central part of the lung in this patient with berylliosis.

Lymphocytic Interstitial Pneumonia

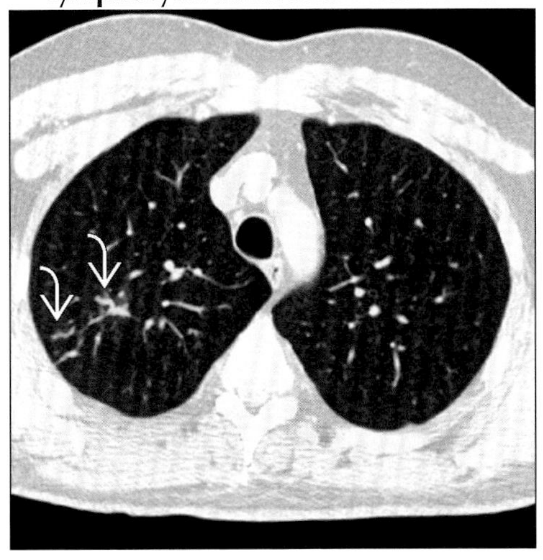

Lymphocytic Interstitial Pneumonia

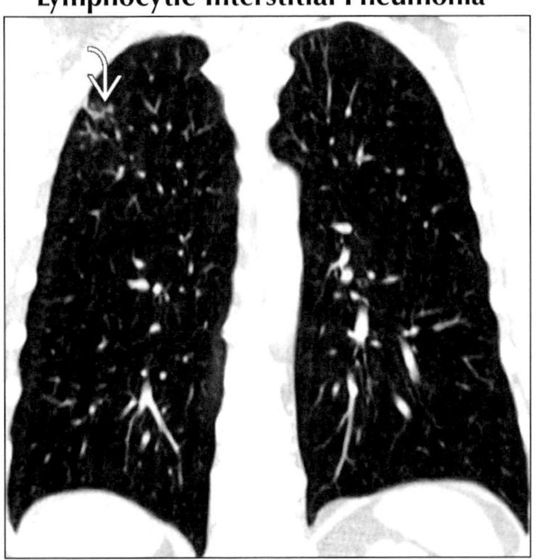

(Left) Axial HRCT shows right upper lobe interlobular septal thickening ↗ indicating perilymphatic involvement. (Right) Coronal NECT in the same patient shows nodularity at the septa ↗. Fine-needle aspiration biopsy showed lymphocytic interstitial pneumonia.

PERIBRONCHIAL INTERSTITIAL THICKENING

DIFFERENTIAL DIAGNOSIS

Common
- Acute and Chronic Bronchitis
- Asthma
- Aspiration
- Cardiogenic Pulmonary Edema
- Bronchiectasis
- Sarcoidosis
- Cystic Fibrosis

Less Common
- Allergic Bronchopulmonary Aspergillosis
- Langerhans Cell Histiocytosis
- Chronic Hypersensitivity Pneumonitis
- Cryptogenic Organizing Pneumonia
- Lymphoma
- Lymphangitic Carcinomatosis
- Lymphocytic Interstitial Pneumonia

Rare but Important
- Kaposi Sarcoma
- Laryngeal Papillomatosis
- Amyloidosis

ESSENTIAL INFORMATION

Key Differential Diagnosis Issues
- Normally 23 generations of airways from trachea to respiratory bronchiole
  - CT can visualize to 8 generation branches
- Airways parallel course of arteries, both enclosed in connective tissue sheath known as peribronchovascular or axial interstitium
  - Components include airway and arterial wall and central lymphatics
- Normally bronchi slightly smaller than artery (normal bronchoarterial ratio [B/A] = 0.65-0.70)
  - B/A > 1 seen in elderly (> 65 years old) or those living at high altitude (due to mild hypoxia that dilates bronchi and causes vasoconstriction)
  - B/A > 1.5 indicative of bronchiectasis

Helpful Clues for Common Diagnoses
- **Acute and Chronic Bronchitis**
  - Acute bronchitis usually secondary to viral upper respiratory infection; chronic bronchitis due to inhaled irritants (cigarette smoke and air pollution)
  - CT insensitive, nonspecific findings of smooth bronchial wall thickening, narrowed lumen, mucus-filled airway
- **Asthma**
  - Reactive airways disease
  - Heterogeneous distribution in lung
  - Affects mainly small and medium-sized bronchi
  - Degree of bronchial wall thickening correlates with severity of airflow obstruction
- **Aspiration**
  - Recurrent aspiration typically in elderly with neurologic disorders, dementia, or swallowing disorder
  - Gravity-dependent opacities
  - Consolidation and interstitial fibrosis centered on airways
- **Cardiogenic Pulmonary Edema**
  - Smooth bronchovascular bundle thickening due to peribronchovascular edema
  - Usually seen with associated findings: Septal thickening, cardiomegaly, pleural effusions
- **Bronchiectasis**
  - Integrity of bronchial wall dependent on normal immune system, normal structural integrity of airways (normal cartilage), and normal ciliary function
  - Bronchiectasis most commonly involves medium-sized bronchi of 4th-9th generations
  - Bronchi diameter larger than adjacent pulmonary artery: Cylindrical to saccular morphology
  - Focal or diffuse; when confined to 1 lobe, usually postinfectious or secondary to aspiration
  - Bronchial wall thickening may be absent even with dilatation
- **Sarcoidosis**
  - Perilymphatic nodules (granulomas) along axial interstitium
  - Often associated with septal and subpleural nodules
- **Cystic Fibrosis**
  - Bronchial wall thickening earliest finding, precedes development of bronchiectasis
  - Leads to diffuse bronchiectasis, usually more severe in upper lobes

Helpful Clues for Less Common Diagnoses

- **Allergic Bronchopulmonary Aspergillosis**
  - Hypersensitivity reaction to *Aspergillus fumigatus* in asthmatics or cystic fibrosis
  - Central bronchiectasis, usually more severe in upper lobes
- **Langerhans Cell Histiocytosis**
  - Strongly associated with smoking
  - Bronchocentric nodules evolving into cysts in upper and mid lung zones
- **Chronic Hypersensitivity Pneumonitis**
  - Chronic granulomatous lung disease caused by inhalation of organic or chemical antigens
  - Chronic disease leads to fibrosis, usually centered on airways
- **Cryptogenic Organizing Pneumonia**
  - Clinicopathological entity characterized by polypoid plugs of granulation tissue within airspaces
  - Most common pattern is multiple alveolar opacities (90%) centered on airways
  - Air-bronchograms common, often dilated
  - Other patterns: Multiple pulmonary nodules (may have air-bronchograms), solitary mass, perilobular pattern, reverse halo sign
- **Lymphoma**
  - May be either non-Hodgkin or Hodgkin
  - Multifocal masses centered on airways with air-bronchograms
  - Masses are usually nonobstructive
- **Lymphangitic Carcinomatosis**
  - Typically adenocarcinomas
  - Nodular or beaded thickening of bronchovascular bundles
  - Frequency of involvement: Axial (75%) > axial + peripheral (20%) > peripheral (5%)
- **Lymphocytic Interstitial Pneumonia**
  - Spectrum of lymphoproliferative disorder
  - Ground-glass opacities, centrilobular nodules, and thin-walled cysts
  - Findings centered on lymphatic pathways: Peribronchovascular, septa, and pleura

Helpful Clues for Rare Diagnoses

- **Kaposi Sarcoma**
  - AIDS-related neoplasm with propensity to involve skin, lymph nodes, GI tract, and lungs
  - Nodular perihilar thickening of bronchovascular bundles
- **Laryngeal Papillomatosis**
  - Due to human papilloma virus, < 1% seed lung
  - Multiple solid or cavitated nodules centered on airways
- **Amyloidosis**
  - Tracheobronchial most common form
  - Focal or diffuse thickening of airway wall with intraluminal nodules and submucosal foci of calcification

Acute and Chronic Bronchitis

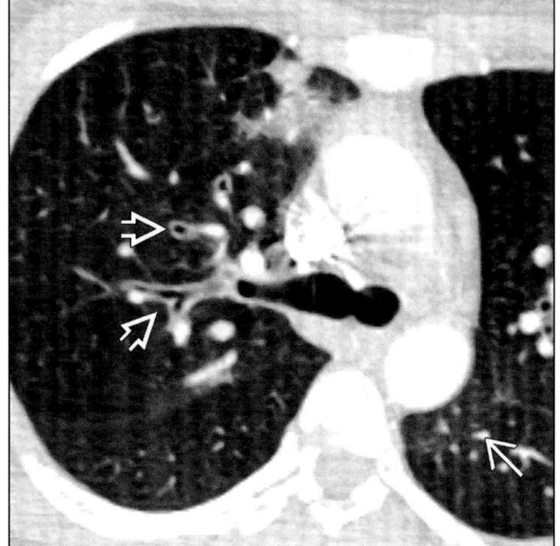

Axial CECT shows bronchial wall thickening ➡ and patchy ground-glass opacities ➡ from an acute viral pneumonia.

Acute and Chronic Bronchitis

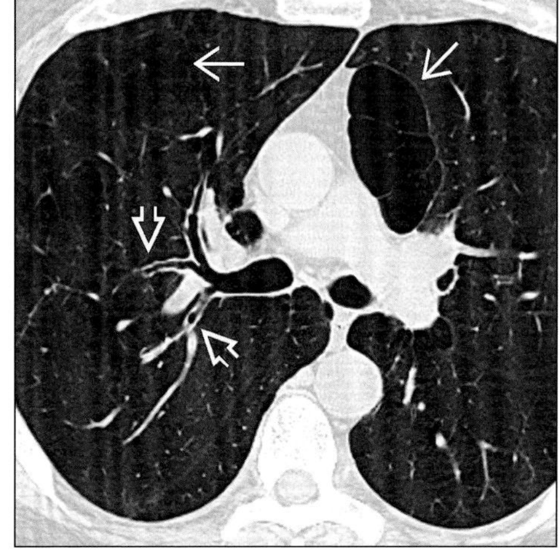

Axial HRCT shows diffuse bronchial wall thickening ➡ and focal areas of emphysema ➡ in this patient with smoking-related chronic bronchitis and emphysema.

PERIBRONCHIAL INTERSTITIAL THICKENING

(Left) *Axial NECT shows smooth thickening of the walls of the central bronchi → from chronic bronchitis. Note the areas of emphysema ⇨.* **(Right)** *Axial CECT shows diffuse bronchial wall thickening → and mucus plugging ⇨ of subsegmental airways. Note that the distal lung is normal. Patient had acute asthma and had a study to rule out pulmonary embolus.*

Acute and Chronic Bronchitis

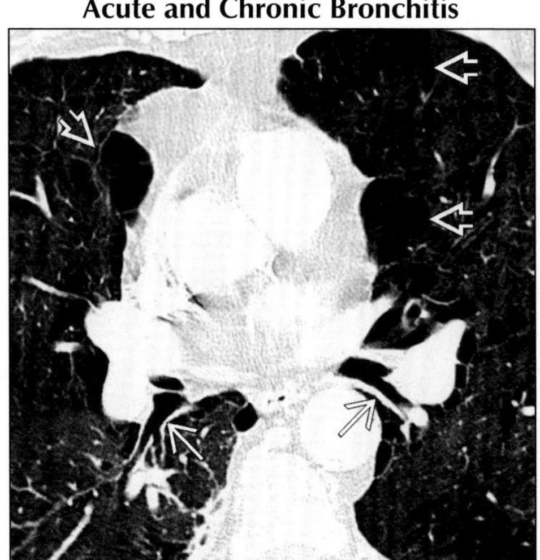

Asthma

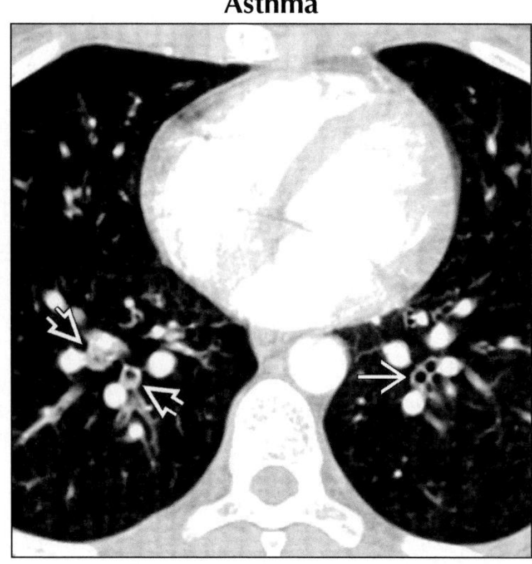

(Left) *Axial HRCT in a different patient shows bronchial wall thickening ⇨ and mucus plugs →. Asthma may not affect all of the airways. Imaging asthma is becoming more common as patients are suspected of having a pulmonary embolus in the emergency room.* **(Right)** *Axial CECT shows peribronchovascular thickening and consolidation ⇨ from aspiration. Aspiration tends to follow dependent segments depending on the position at time of aspiration.*

Asthma

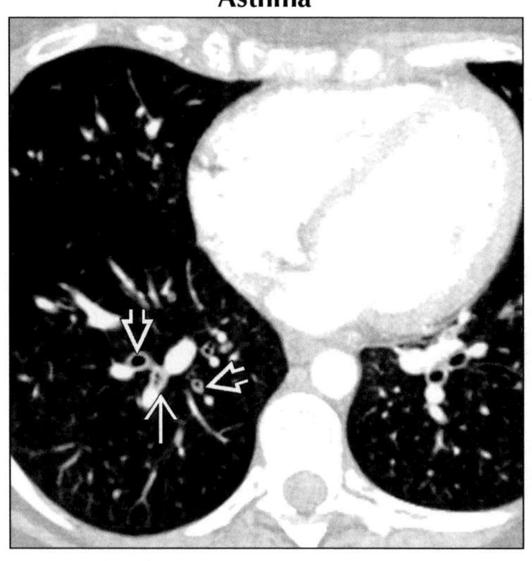

Aspiration

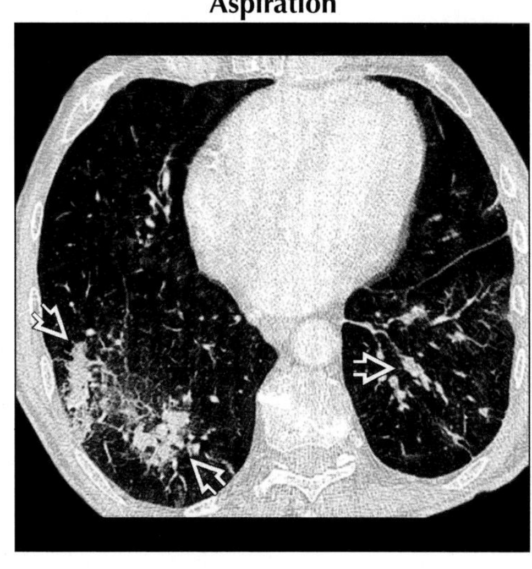

(Left) *Axial CECT shows smooth septal thickening ⇨, smooth bronchial wall thickening →, and bilateral pleural effusions ↷.* **(Right)** *Axial CECT shows subtle bronchiectasis ⇨ in the right upper lobe. Note that the airways are larger than the adjacent artery and fail to taper. Bronchial wall is not thickened.*

Cardiogenic Pulmonary Edema

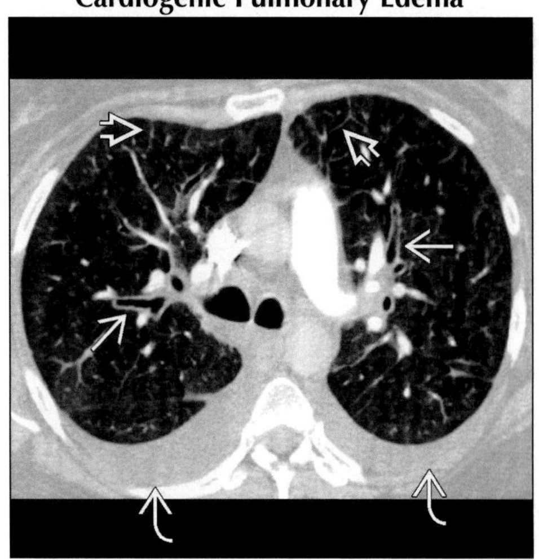

Bronchiectasis

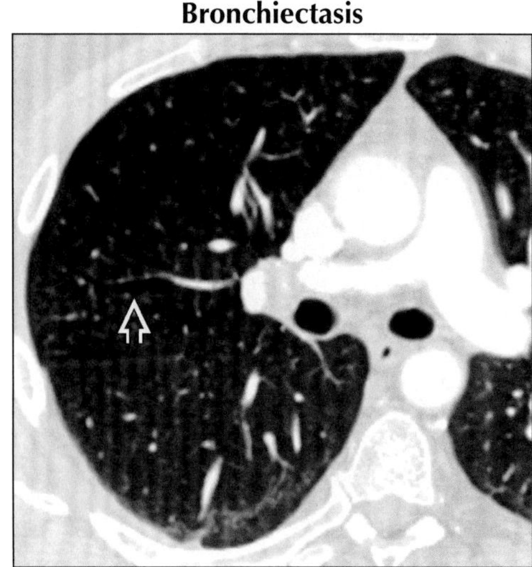

Bronchiectasis

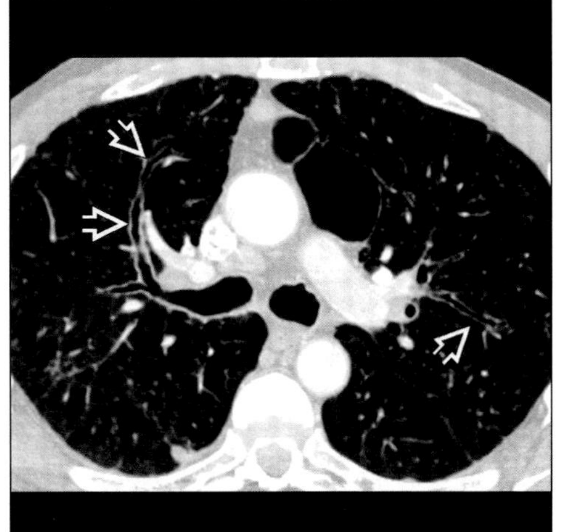

Bronchiectasis

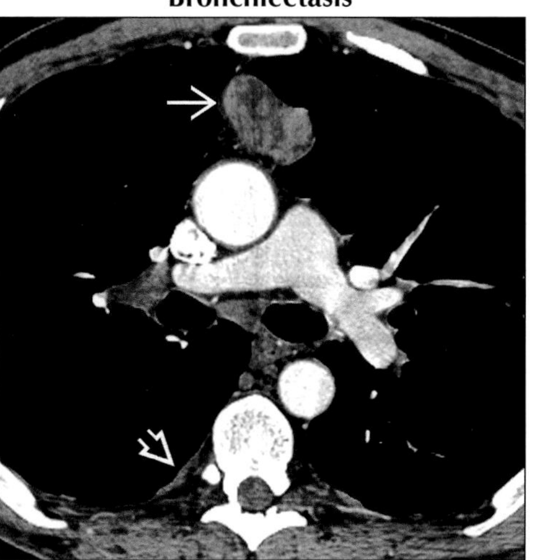

(Left) *Axial CECT shows bronchial wall thickening and mild bronchiectasis ➯.* ***(Right)*** *Axial CECT from the same patient shows a heterogeneous mass ➔ in the anterior mediastinum. Focal pleural thickening is from drop metastases ➯. Association of thymoma, immunodeficiency, and bronchiectasis is known as Good syndrome.*

Bronchiectasis

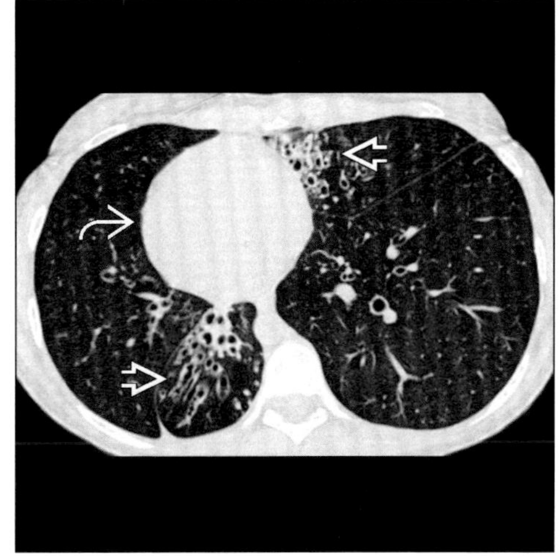

Sarcoidosis

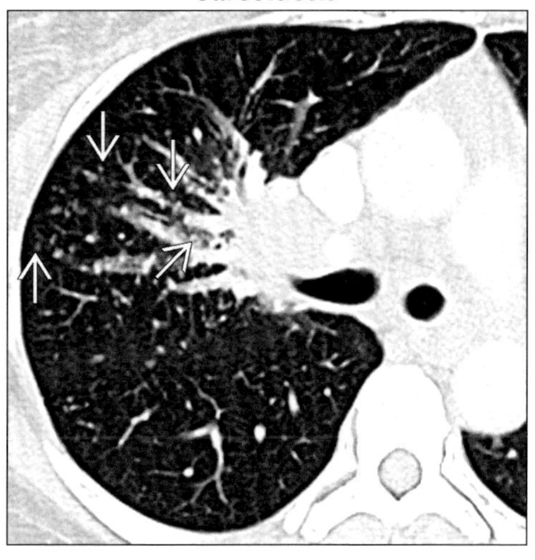

(Left) *Axial NECT shows bronchial wall thickening and bronchiectasis ➯. Patient had dextrocardia ➚ and situs inversus. Diagnosis is immotile cilia syndrome (Kartagener syndrome).* ***(Right)*** *Axial NECT shows multiple small nodules predominantly along the bronchovascular bundles ➔. Mediastinal and right hilar nodes are also enlarged.*

Sarcoidosis

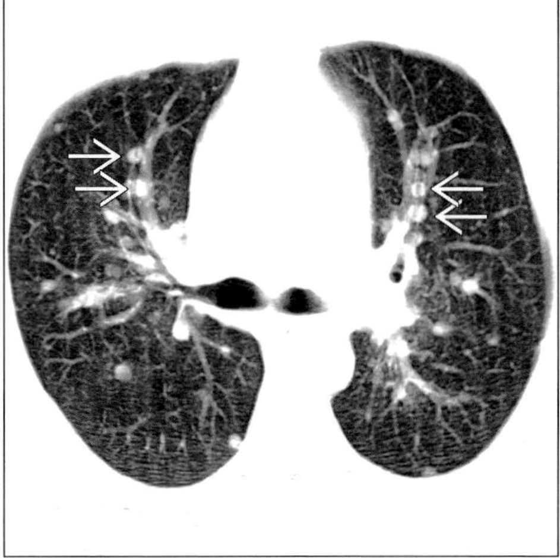

Sarcoidosis

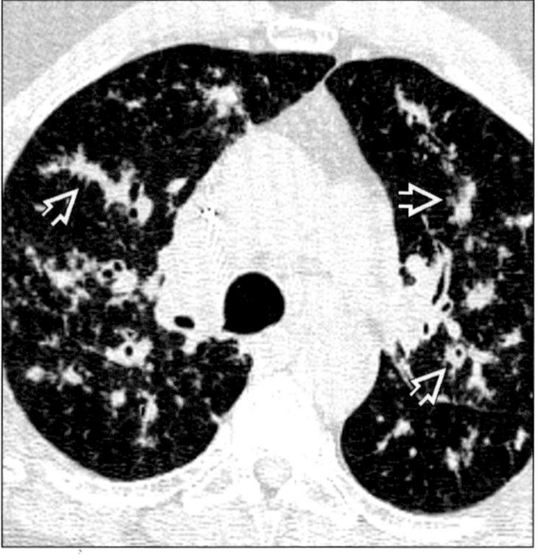

(Left) *Axial NECT MIP reconstruction show numerous discrete sharply marginated peribronchial nodules ➔.* ***(Right)*** *Axial NECT shows interstitial thickening and nodularity along bronchovascular pathways ➯.*

PERIBRONCHIAL INTERSTITIAL THICKENING

Cystic Fibrosis

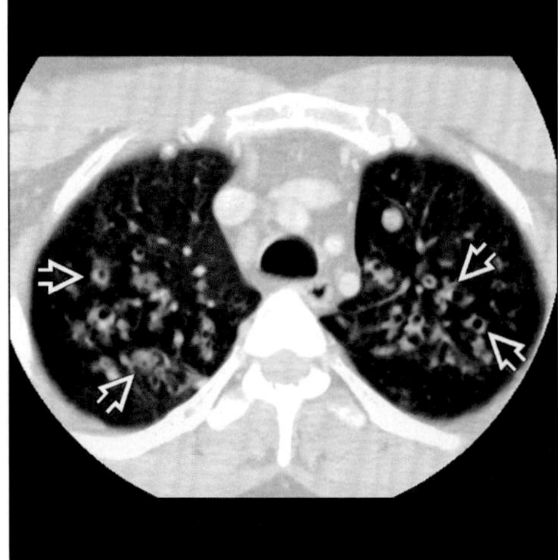

Allergic Bronchopulmonary Aspergillosis

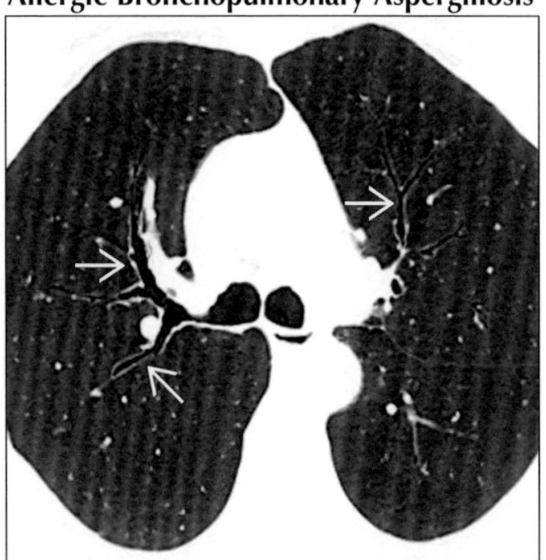

(Left) Axial CECT shows bronchial wall thickening and bronchiectasis ➲. Several of the airways are filled with mucus plugs. (Right) Axial HRCT MinIP reconstruction shows mild bronchiectasis ➲. Peripheral lung and airways were normal. Bronchial wall is minimally thickened. Typically allergic bronchopulmonary aspergillosis demonstrates central bronchiectasis.

Langerhans Cell Histiocytosis

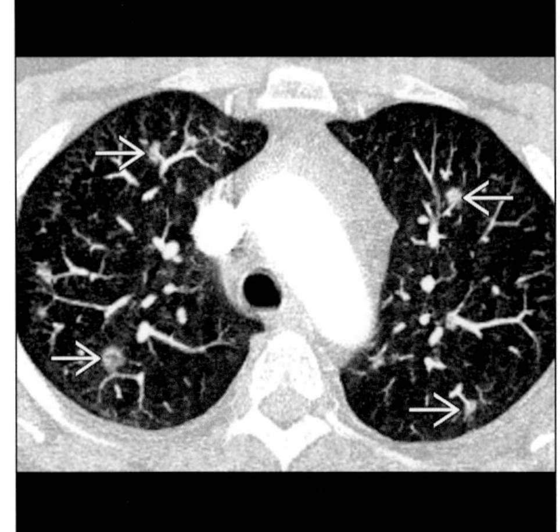

Chronic Hypersensitivity Pneumonitis

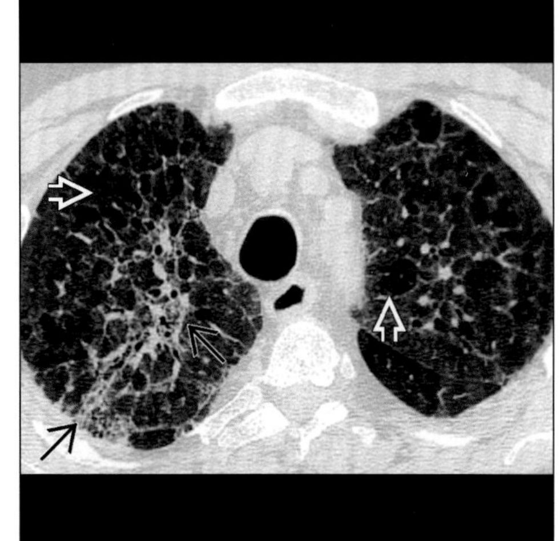

(Left) Axial CECT MIP reconstruction shows bronchocentric nodules ➲. Both nodules and cysts tend to be centered on airways. (Right) Axial HRCT shows bronchocentric fibrosis → and hyperinflated lobules ➲ from farmer's lung.

Cryptogenic Organizing Pneumonia

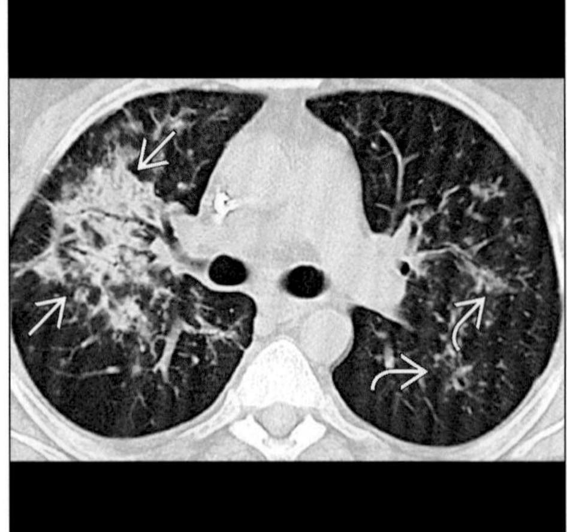

Cryptogenic Organizing Pneumonia

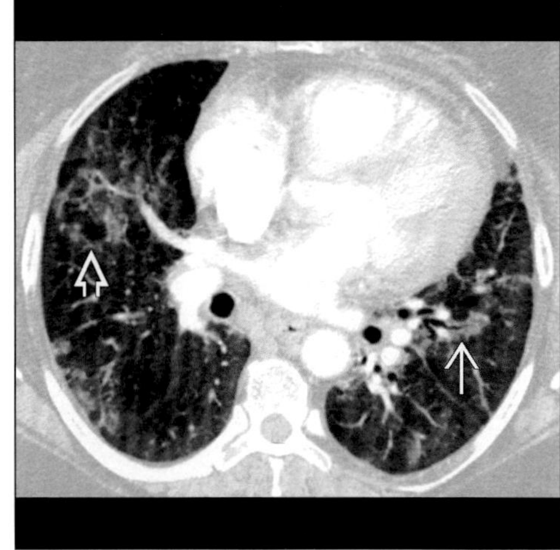

(Left) Axial HRCT shows focal consolidation in the right upper lobe ➲. Smaller areas are centered on airways within the left mid lung ➲. (Right) Axial CECT in a different patient shows peribronchial ground-glass opacities ➲ and reverse halo sign ➲.

PERIBRONCHIAL INTERSTITIAL THICKENING

Lymphoma

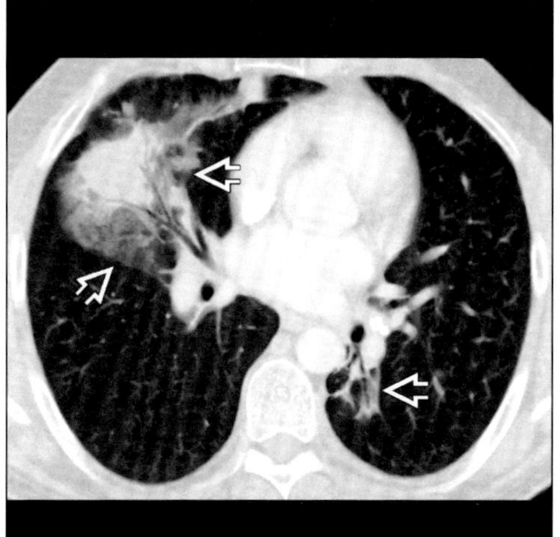

Lymphangitic Carcinomatosis

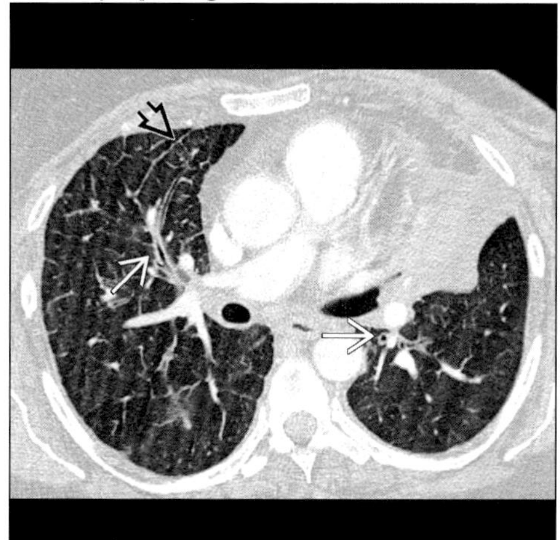

*(**Left**) Axial CECT shows peribronchial consolidation and ground-glass opacities ➡ in a patient with non-Hodgkin lymphoma. Atelectasis is uncommon even with airway involvement. (**Right**) Axial CECT shows diffuse bronchial wall thickening ➡ and mild septal thickening ➡ in a patient with breast carcinoma.*

Lymphocytic Interstitial Pneumonia

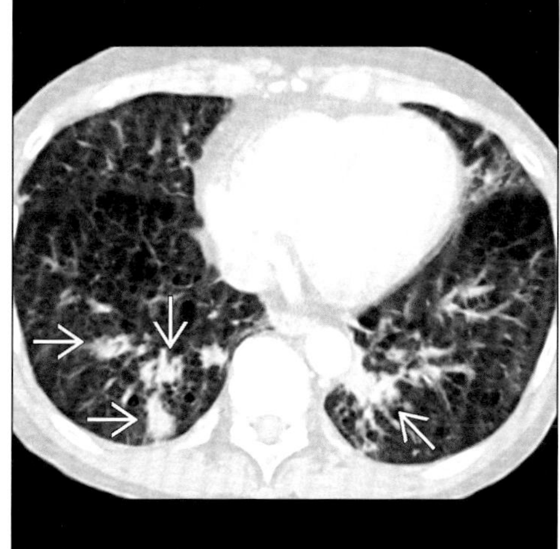

Kaposi Sarcoma

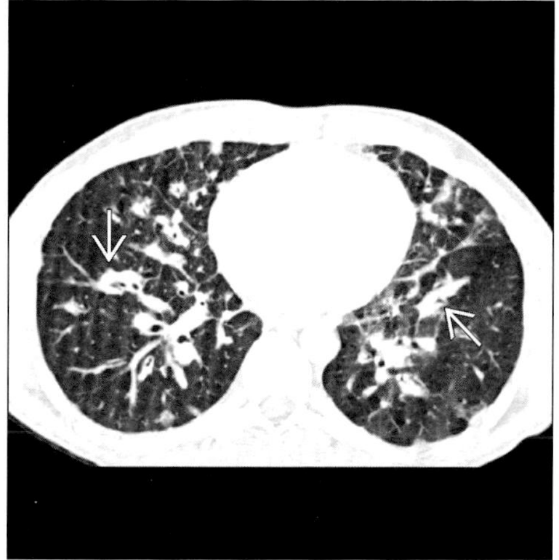

*(**Left**) Axial NECT shows marked bronchial wall thickening ➡ in the lower lobes. Other sections showed a few scattered cysts. (**Right**) Axial HRCT shows ill-defined nodular opacities located along the bronchovascular bundles ➡. Patient had skin lesions. Nodules tend to spread from hilum into the periphery of the lung.*

Laryngeal Papillomatosis

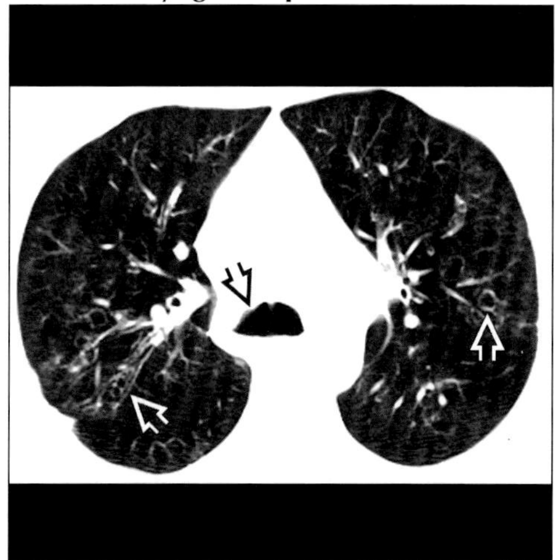

Amyloidosis

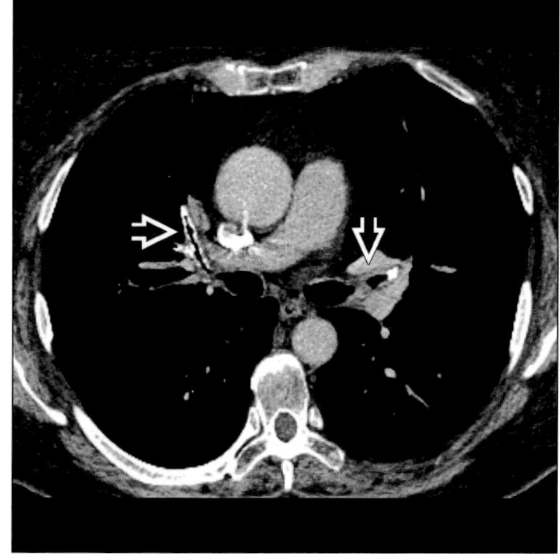

*(**Left**) Axial NECT shows bronchial wall thickening and peribronchial cysts ➡. Note nodularity along airway wall from intratracheal papillomas ➡. Nodules and cysts tend to be more common in the dependent lung. (**Right**) Axial CECT shows diffuse thickening and calcification of airway walls ➡. Tracheobronchial amyloid is the most common form of pulmonary amyloid.*

CYST(S)

DIFFERENTIAL DIAGNOSIS

Common

- Emphysema
- Pneumatoceles

Less Common

- Idiopathic Pulmonary Fibrosis
- Pulmonary Langerhans Cell Histiocytosis
- Lymphocytic Interstitial Pneumonia
- Hypersensitivity Pneumonitis
- Coccidioidomycosis

Rare but Important

- Lymphangioleiomyomatosis
- Cystic Adenomatoid Malformation
- Laryngeal Papillomatosis
- Birt-Hogg-Dubé Syndrome
- Desquamative Interstitial Pneumonia

ESSENTIAL INFORMATION

Key Differential Diagnosis Issues

- Definition of cysts
  - Round well-demarcated lung lesion with thin wall (< 2 mm)
  - Usually air-filled but may contain fluid
- Large emphysematous bullae can mimic cysts
  - Compress adjacent lung
- Distribution and morphology of cysts key to narrowing differential diagnosis

Helpful Clues for Common Diagnoses

- **Emphysema**
  - Permanent enlargement of air spaces distal to terminal bronchiole
    - Not true cysts
    - No perceptible wall
  - Centrilobular emphysema
    - Associated with cigarette smoking
    - Upper lung zone predominant
  - Panlobular emphysema
    - Most frequently from alpha-1 antitrypsin deficiency
    - Intravenous methylphenidate abuse
    - Basal lung zone predominant
  - Paraseptal
    - Subpleural and peribronchovascular
    - May be paracicatricial as in sarcoidosis, silicosis, and coal worker's pneumoconiosis
    - Spontaneous pneumothorax from rupture into pleural space
- **Pneumatoceles**
  - Transient thin-walled cysts in association with pneumonia
  - Commonly develop later during course of pneumonia
  - Up to 30% in *Pneumocystis pneumonia*, almost exclusively in patients with AIDS
  - Other causes
    - Hydrocarbon ingestion
    - Trauma (pulmonary laceration)

Helpful Clues for Less Common Diagnoses

- **Idiopathic Pulmonary Fibrosis**
  - Honeycomb cysts
    - Subpleural and basal predominant
    - Frequently occur in rows
    - Begins in subpleural lung and progresses centrally
  - Associated with reticulation, traction bronchiectasis, and architectural distortion
- **Pulmonary Langerhans Cell Histiocytosis**
  - > 95% of adult patients cigarette smokers
  - Polyclonal proliferation of CD1a(+) histiocytes (Langerhans cells) in lungs
  - Disseminated, monoclonal form in children
  - Cysts of varying shapes and sizes
    - Upper lung zone predominant
    - Larger cysts frequently have bizarre shapes
  - Associated findings
    - Small nodules ± central lucency progressing to cysts over time
    - Ground-glass opacity
  - Spontaneous pneumothorax in < 10%
- **Lymphocytic Interstitial Pneumonia**
  - Most commonly occurs in adults with Sjögren syndrome
  - Less commonly occurs in children with HIV and other immunodeficiency diseases
  - Cysts in about 80%
    - Usually < 20 in number, ranging from 2-30 mm in diameter
    - Basal predominance typical
  - Perilymphatic distribution of nodules (peribronchovascular, centrilobular, septal, and subpleural)
  - Associated patchy ground-glass opacity throughout lungs
- **Hypersensitivity Pneumonitis**

- Cysts few in number and occur in 10%
- Other findings
  - Poorly defined centrilobular nodules
  - Lobular air-trapping characteristic
  - Patchy or diffuse ground-glass opacity
- Higher incidence in nonsmokers
- Agricultural and avian antigens most common

- **Coccidioidomycosis**
  - Endemic fungal infection most common in arid regions of southwestern USA
  - Thin-walled cysts occasional in acute infection (5%) or later with evolution of pneumonia
  - Usually solitary (90%) and located in upper lobes

Helpful Clues for Rare Diagnoses

- **Lymphangioleiomyomatosis**
  - Occurs exclusively in women of child-bearing age or patients with tuberous sclerosis
  - Diffuse lung cysts
    - 2-20 mm with thin, smooth walls
    - May completely replace lung in advanced disease
  - Associated findings
    - Chylous pleural effusions
    - Renal angiomyolipomas
    - Lymphangiomas (mediastinal, retroperitoneal)
    - Pulmonary hyperinflation
  - Spontaneous and recurrent pneumothoraces may develop
- **Cystic Adenomatoid Malformation**
  - Congenital hamartomatous malformation of the lungs with cysts resembling bronchioles
  - Comprise approximately 25% of all congenital lung lesions
  - Focal multiloculated cystic lesion with cysts of varying sizes
  - May have fluid or solid components
- **Laryngeal Papillomatosis**
  - Infection with human papilloma virus
  - < 1% involve lower respiratory tract and lungs
  - Combination of solid and cystic nodules in lung
  - Airway nodules in trachea or other airways distinctive
  - Rare degeneration into squamous cell carcinoma
- **Birt-Hogg-Dubé Syndrome**
  - Autosomal dominant triad of fibrofolliculomas, renal cell carcinoma, and lung cysts
  - Cysts usually few in number, similar to lymphocytic interstitial pneumonia
- **Desquamative Interstitial Pneumonia**
  - Characterized by extensive ground-glass opacity with basal predominance
    - Superimposed reticulation
    - Cysts infrequent and few in number
  - Most patients heavy cigarette smokers
  - Occasionally associated with connective tissue disease or dust and fume inhalation

Emphysema

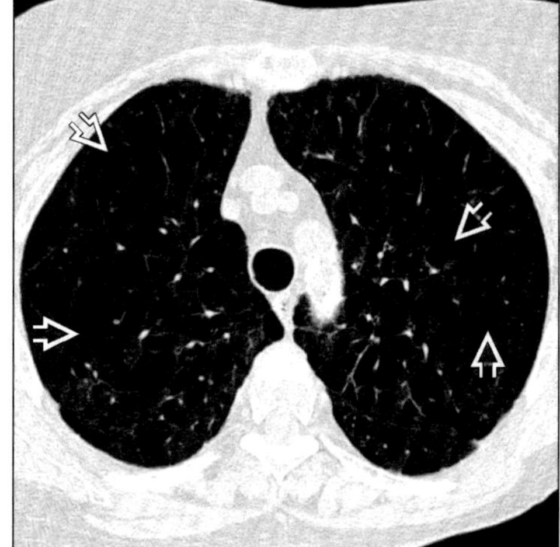

Axial HRCT shows numerous large cystic lesions ➡ in the lungs in this patient with smoking-related emphysema. Note the lack of perceptible walls, typical of centrilobular emphysema.

Pneumatoceles

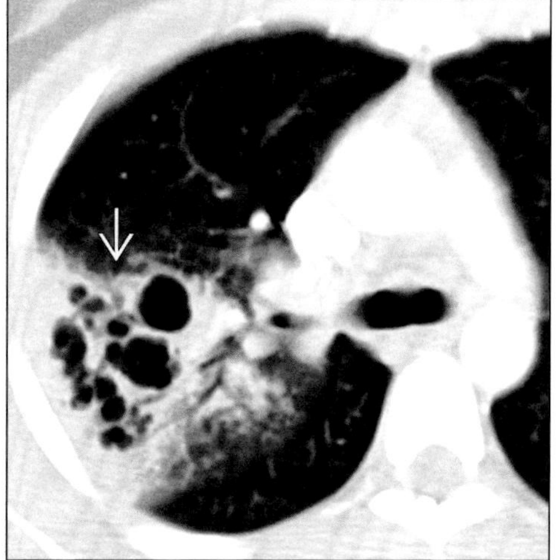

Axial CECT shows numerous variable-sized pneumatoceles ➡ in a patient with staphylococcal pneumonia. Pneumatoceles developed several days after the onset of pneumonia.

CYST(S)

(Left) Axial HRCT shows subpleural honeycomb cysts → in the left lower lobe. Other signs of interstitial fibrosis include subpleural reticulation → and traction bronchiectasis →. The honeycomb cysts of idiopathic pulmonary fibrosis initially develop in the subpleural lung and progress centrally. **(Right)** Axial HRCT shows multiple cysts of varying shapes (some bizarre) and sizes → in addition to scattered nodules →.

Idiopathic Pulmonary Fibrosis

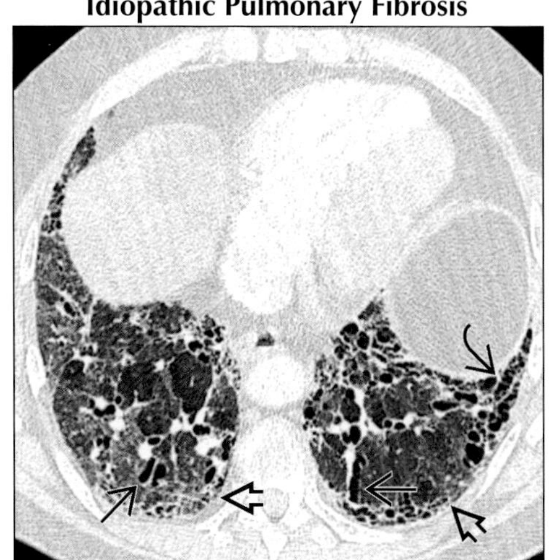

Pulmonary Langerhans Cell Histiocytosis

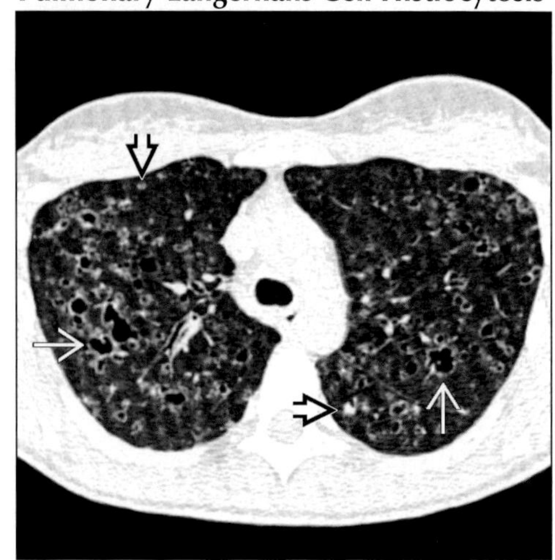

(Left) Coronal CT reconstruction shows an upper lobe predominance of cysts →, some with bizarre shapes, and nodules →. The combination of cysts and nodules with an upper lobe predominance is typical of Langerhans cell histiocytosis. **(Right)** Axial HRCT shows cysts → with scattered ground-glass attenuation nodules → in this patient with Sjögren syndrome. Cysts are typically fewer in number and larger than those of lymphangioleiomyomatosis.

Pulmonary Langerhans Cell Histiocytosis

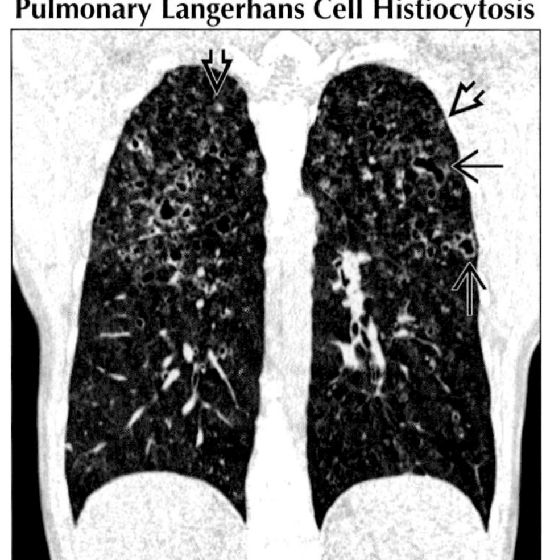

Lymphocytic Interstitial Pneumonia

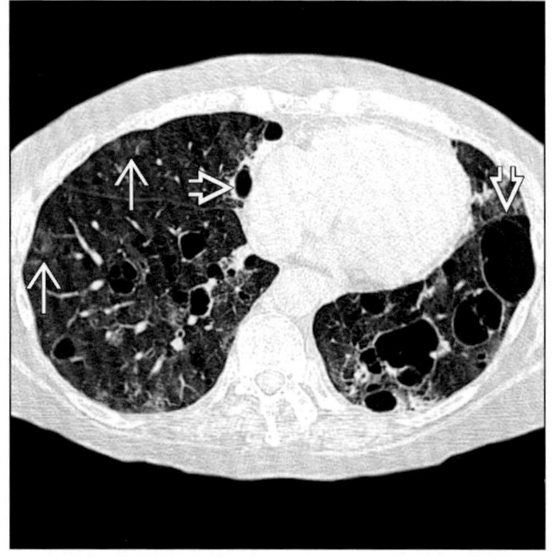

(Left) Axial HRCT shows a solitary cyst → in a patient with chronic hypersensitivity pneumonitis related to domestic mold exposure. Note the fairly extensive ground-glass opacity →. Reticulation → indicates lung fibrosis. Cysts in hypersensitivity pneumonitis are usually few in number. **(Right)** Axial HRCT shows a single thin-walled cyst → in the right lower lobe. Cysts may remain following resolution of acute infection.

Hypersensitivity Pneumonitis

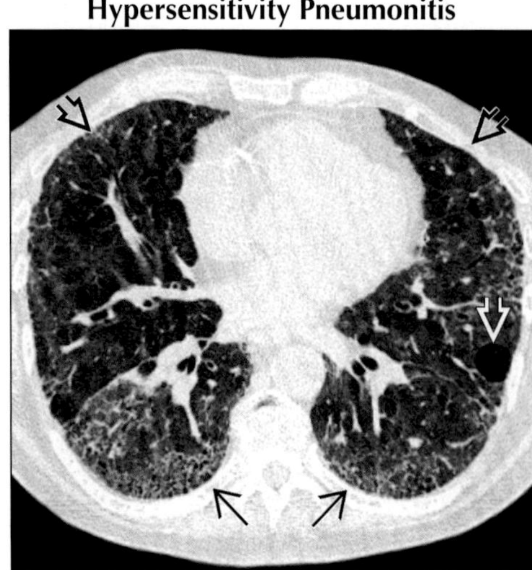

Coccidioidomycosis

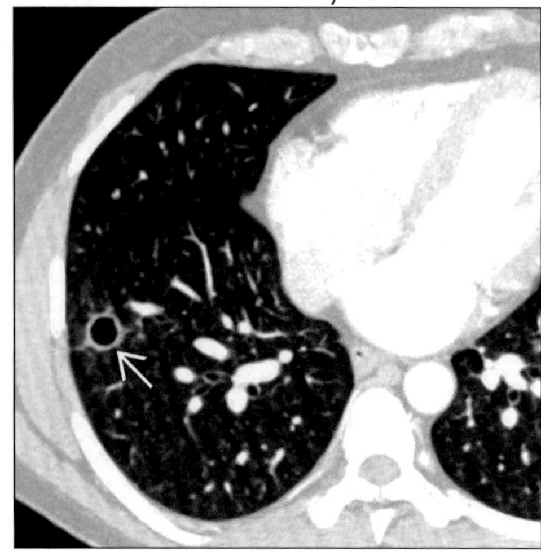

CYST(S)

Lymphangioleiomyomatosis

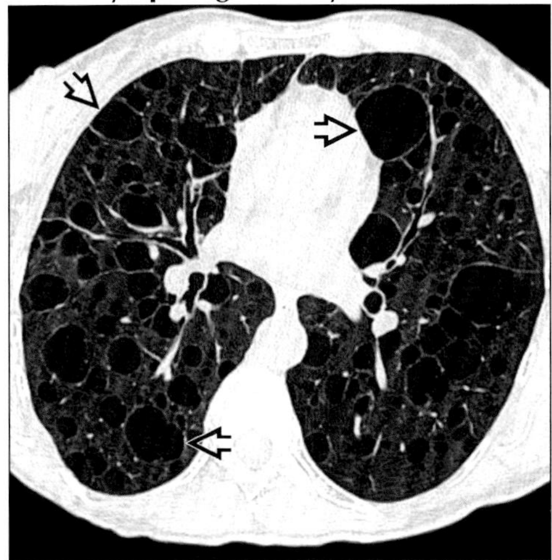

Lymphangioleiomyomatosis

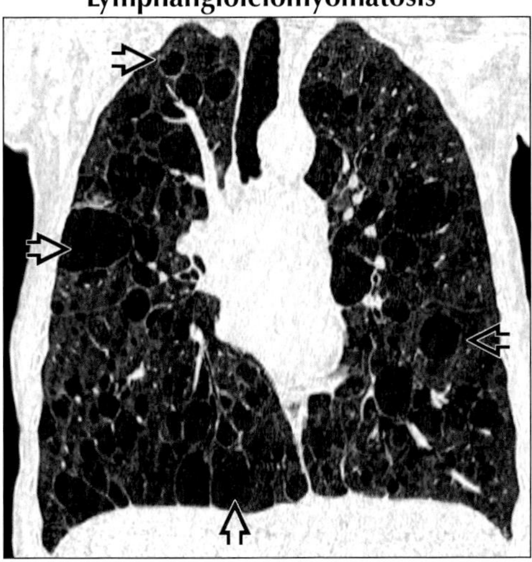

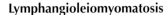

(Left) *Axial HRCT shows diffuse thin-walled cysts ➲ surrounded by normal lung. Cysts in lymphangioleiomyomatosis are usually distributed evenly throughout the lungs and have thin walls.* ***(Right)*** *Coronal CT reconstruction shows diffuse thin-walled cysts ➲ in both lungs. The diffuse nature of the cysts and uniform distribution are highly suggestive of lymphangioleiomyomatosis in a young woman or patient with tuberous sclerosis.*

Cystic Adenomatoid Malformation

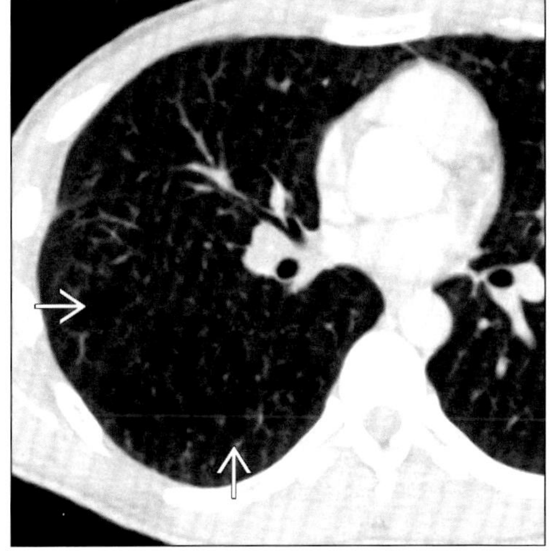

Laryngeal Papillomatosis

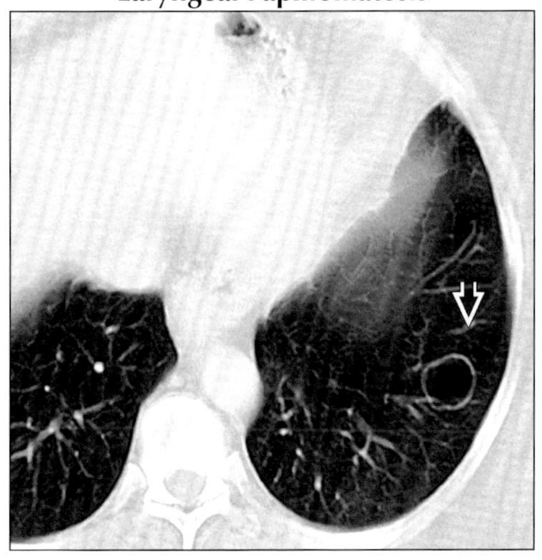

(Left) *Axial CECT shows multiple cysts with very thin walls ➡ in the right lower lobe. These cystic areas may represent abnormal airways, hence the term congenital pulmonary airway malformation is more commonly used.* ***(Right)*** *Axial NECT shows a thin-walled cyst ➡ in this patient with laryngeal papillomatosis. In patients with thin-walled cysts, closely examine the trachea and main bronchi for nodular wall thickening from papillomas.*

Birt-Hogg-Dubé Syndrome

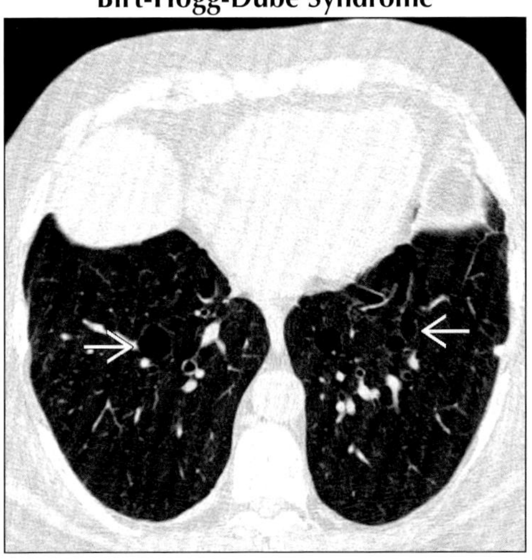

Desquamative Interstitial Pneumonia

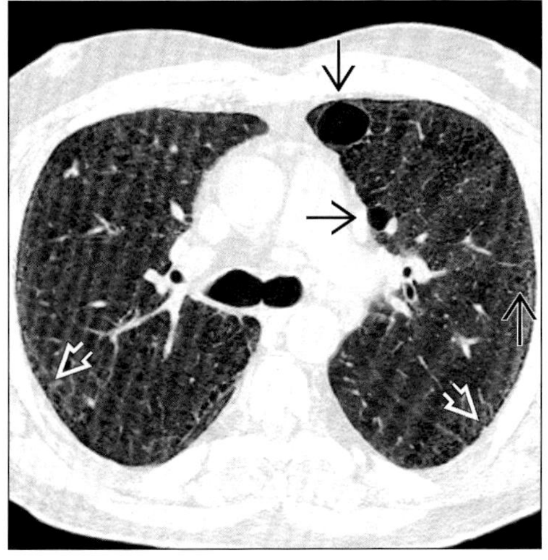

(Left) *Axial HRCT shows scattered thin-walled cysts in the lung bases of a patient with Birt-Hogg-Dubé ➡. The cysts generally have a basal and subpleural distribution. Associated features include renal neoplasms and facial fibrofolliculomas.* ***(Right)*** *Axial HRCT shows a few cysts → with thin walls and varying sizes on a background of diffuse ground-glass opacity. Note fine peripheral reticulation ➡, suggestive of mild fibrosis.*

INTERLOBULAR SEPTAL THICKENING

DIFFERENTIAL DIAGNOSIS

Common
- Cardiogenic Pulmonary Edema
- Lymphangitic Carcinomatosis
- Sarcoidosis
- Usual Interstitial Pneumonitis

Less Common
- Pulmonary Vein Stenosis
- Pulmonary Alveolar Proteinosis
- Venoocclusive Disease
- Alveolar Septal Amyloidosis

Rare but Important
- Erdheim Chester Disease
- Leukemic Infiltration
- Diffuse Pulmonary Lymphangiomatosis
- Acute Eosinophilic Pneumonia

ESSENTIAL INFORMATION

Key Differential Diagnosis Issues
- Most often due to pulmonary edema or lymphangitic carcinomatosis
- Smooth thickening
  - Cardiogenic pulmonary edema
  - Lymphangitic carcinomatosis
- Nodular or irregular thickening
  - Lymphangitic carcinomatosis or sarcoidosis

Helpful Clues for Common Diagnoses
- **Cardiogenic Pulmonary Edema**
  - Due to imbalances in Starling forces: Usually due to increased pulmonary venous pressure
    - Left-sided heart failure (myocardial infarct or ischemic cardiomyopathy)
    - Fluid overload or renal failure
    - Mitral valvular disease
  - Interlobular septal thickening; Kerley B and Kerley A lines on chest radiograph
  - Diffuse hazy, air-space opacities
    - Characteristically central predominant due to higher concentration of lymphatics in peripheral aspect of lungs
  - Cardiomegaly
  - Signs of coronary artery disease (coronary artery calcification, CABG, coronary artery stents, subendocardial fatty metaplasia)
- **Lymphangitic Carcinomatosis**
  - Most common with primary lung adenocarcinoma
    - Also breast, stomach, pancreas adenocarcinoma
  - Asymmetric nodular (beaded) or smooth interlobular septal thickening
  - Peribronchial and peribronchovascular thickening
  - Pleural effusion and hilar/mediastinal lymphadenopathy common
- **Sarcoidosis**
  - Upper and mid lung, small perilymphatic nodules (along interlobular septa, subpleural, peribronchovascular)
  - Subcentimeter centrilobular nodules
  - Air-trapping
  - Nodular interlobular septal thickening
  - Symmetric hilar and mediastinal lymphadenopathy; ± calcification
  - Perilymphatic nodules may coalesce into focal nodular consolidation or foci of ground-glass opacity
  - Low-density lesions in spleen and liver; hepatosplenomegaly, upper abdominal lymphadenopathy
- **Usual Interstitial Pneumonitis**
  - Interlobular and intralobular septal thickening predominate in peripheral and basilar aspects of lungs
  - Costophrenic angles most severely affected
  - Traction bronchiectasis, honeycombing, and architectural distortion
  - Mild mediastinal lymphadenopathy not uncommon

Helpful Clues for Less Common Diagnoses
- **Pulmonary Vein Stenosis**
  - Multiple etiologies
    - Extrinsic compression or invasion of pulmonary vein, thrombosis of pulmonary vein, post ablation stenosis
  - Asymmetric interlobular septal thickening, peribronchial thickening, and peribronchovascular thickening
  - In distribution of affected pulmonary vein
  - Ipsilateral pleural effusion
- **Pulmonary Alveolar Proteinosis**
  - Diffuse or patchy airspace opacities often with geographic distribution
  - Interlobular and intralobular septal thickening common
  - Most often idiopathic

- Much less often secondary to hematological malignancy, massive silica inhalation, drugs, infection, or congenital causes
- **Venoocclusive Disease**
  - Rare cause of pulmonary arterial hypertension
  - Pulmonary arterial dilation
  - Smooth or nodular interlobular septal thickening
  - Centrilobular ground-glass nodules
  - Pericardial and pleural effusions
- **Alveolar Septal Amyloidosis**
  - Respiratory involvement in amyloidosis common though respiratory symptoms uncommon
  - Alveolar septal subtype of amyloidosis least common
  - Interlobular and intralobular septal thickening with micronodules (often in subpleural distribution)
  - Affected areas may calcify; ossification less common

Helpful Clues for Rare Diagnoses

- **Erdheim Chester Disease**
  - Non-Langerhans cell histiocytosis primarily involving long bones; up to 1/3 have pulmonary involvement
  - Smooth interlobular septal thickening
  - Smooth pleural thickening or pleural effusions
  - Soft tissue encasement of aorta, great vessels, and kidneys
  - Bilateral symmetric osteosclerosis of metaphyses and diaphyses of long bone
- **Leukemic Infiltration**
  - History of leukemia
  - Asymmetric or symmetric interlobular septal thickening, may be nodular
  - Peribronchial and peribronchovascular thickening
  - Patchy, multifocal airspace opacities
  - Intrathoracic lymphadenopathy common
- **Diffuse Pulmonary Lymphangiomatosis**
  - Congenital proliferation and dilatation of lymphatics
  - Diffuse interlobular septal and peribronchial thickening
  - Extensive infiltration of mediastinal fat
  - Pleural or pericardial effusions
  - Mild mediastinal lymphadenopathy
- **Acute Eosinophilic Pneumonia**
  - Probable hypersensitivity reaction to inhaled agents; possible association with smoking
  - Imaging mimics pulmonary edema
    - Ground-glass opacities > consolidation
    - Interlobular septal thickening
    - Pleural effusions
  - Acute high fever, profound dyspnea, myalgia, pleuritic chest pain
  - Responds rapidly to corticosteroids

Cardiogenic Pulmonary Edema

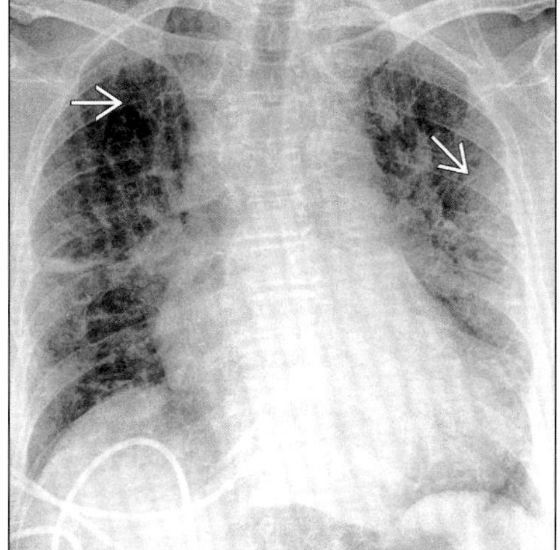

Frontal radiograph shows thickening of the pulmonary interstitium ➔ and cardiomegaly consistent with interstitial pulmonary edema from left-sided congestive heart failure.

Cardiogenic Pulmonary Edema

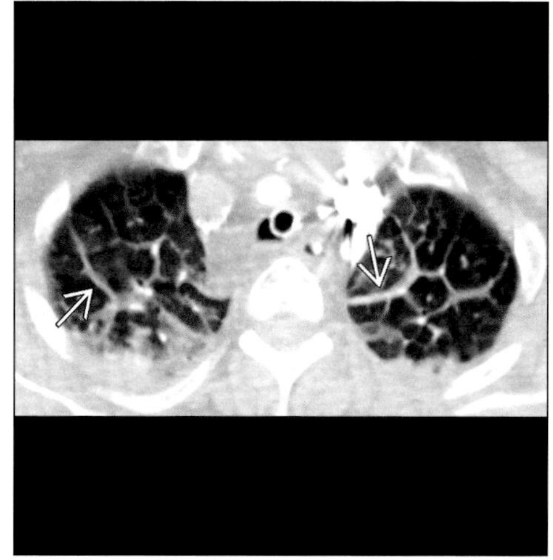

Axial CECT shows marked thickening of the interlobular septa ➔ and dependent pleural effusions.

INTERLOBULAR SEPTAL THICKENING

(Left) *Frontal radiograph shows diffuse pulmonary opacities most consistent with pulmonary edema in this patient with history of coronary artery disease.* **(Right)** *Axial NECT shows central pulmonary ground-glass opacities and superimposed interlobular septal thickening* ⇨ *highly suggestive of pulmonary edema in this patient with coronary artery disease. Large pleural effusions are also present.*

Cardiogenic Pulmonary Edema

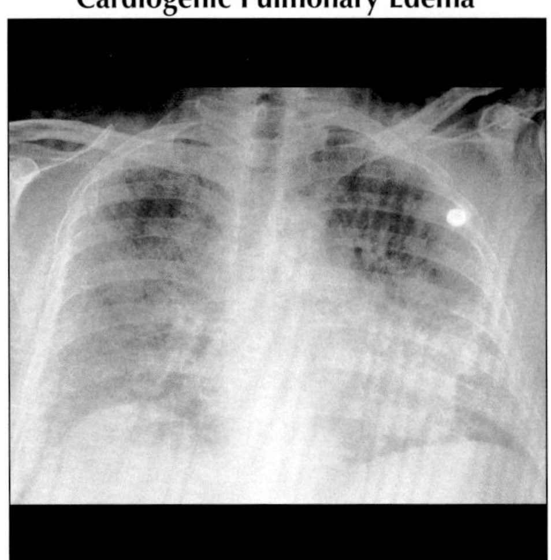

Cardiogenic Pulmonary Edema

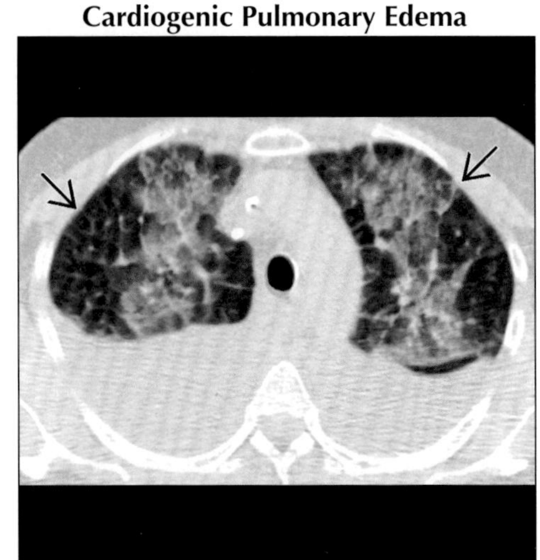

(Left) *Frontal radiograph (magnified) shows multiple pulmonary nodules in the right lower lung and multiple Kerley B lines* ➡ *in the right lung periphery. No Kerley B lines were present in the contralateral lung.* **(Right)** *Axial CECT shows multiple pulmonary nodules and patchy ground-glass opacity; superimposed interlobular septal thickening* ➡ *is highly suggestive of lymphangitic spread of tumor. There is a small right pleural effusion.*

Lymphangitic Carcinomatosis

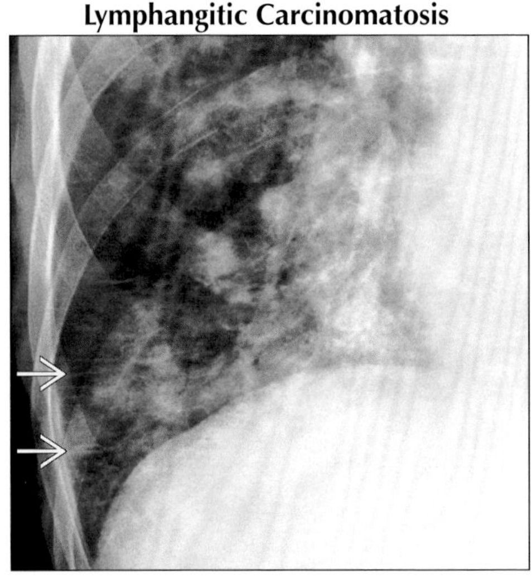

Lymphangitic Carcinomatosis

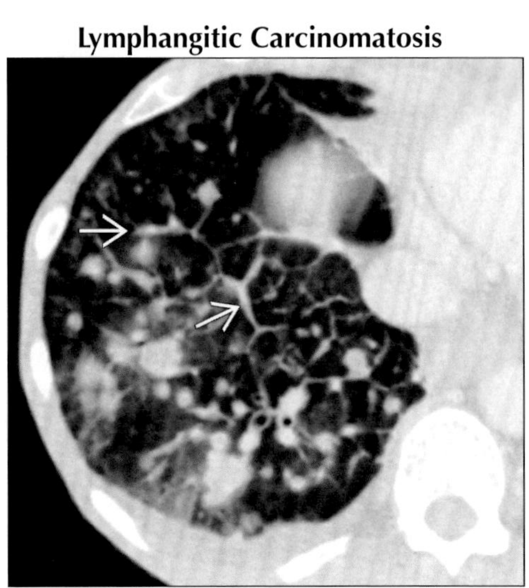

(Left) *Frontal radiograph shows a poorly marginated right upper lung malignancy. There is ipsilateral prominence of the interstitial markings consistent with lymphangitic carcinomatosis. The right heart border is obscured by the hazy opacity.* **(Right)** *Axial CECT shows a spiculated right upper lobe nodule with superimposed interlobular septal* ⇨ *and centrilobular* ➡ *thickening from a primary lung cancer with lymphangitic carcinomatosis.*

Lymphangitic Carcinomatosis

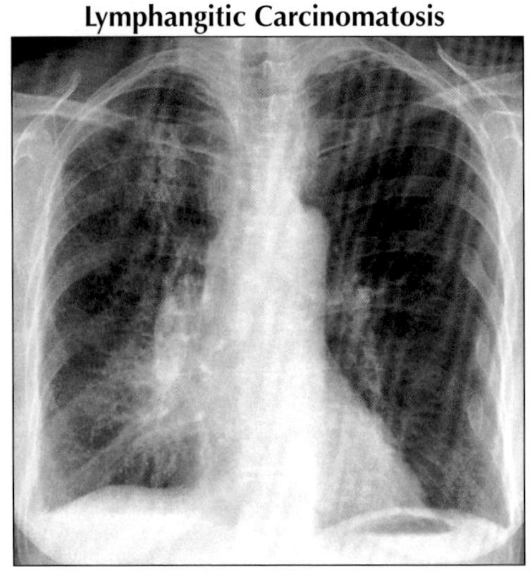

Lymphangitic Carcinomatosis

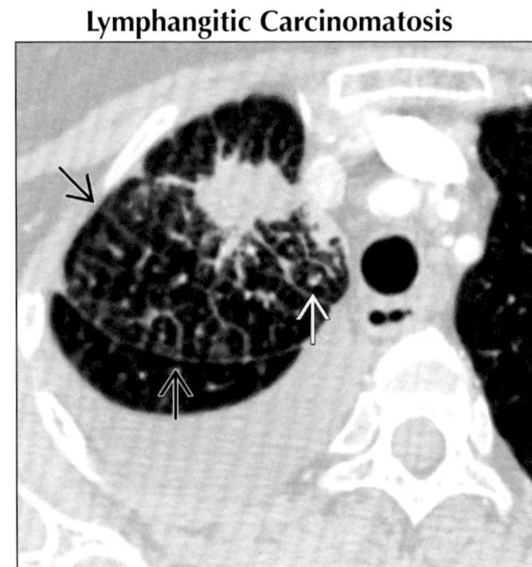

Lymphangitic Carcinomatosis

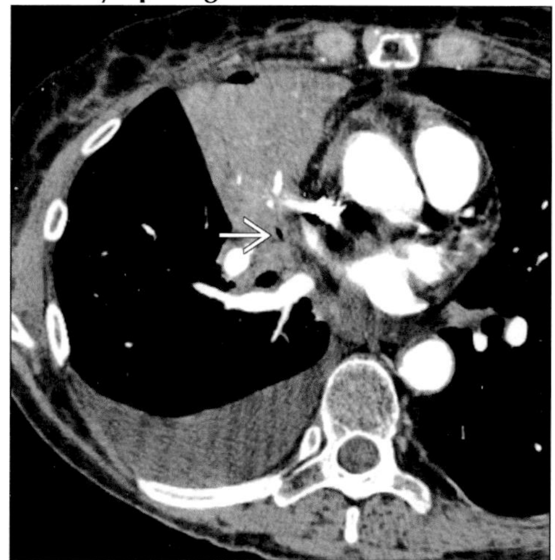

Sarcoidosis

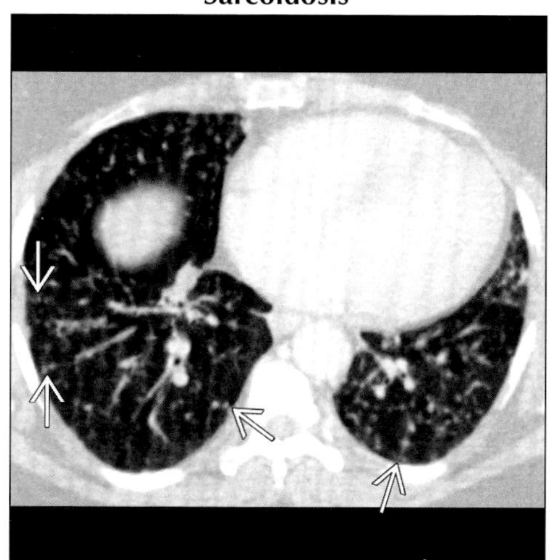

(Left) *Axial CECT in the same patient shows resorptive right middle lobe atelectasis from bronchial narrowing ➔ from right peribronchial lymphadenopathy. There is a moderate-sized right pleural effusion.* ***(Right)*** *Axial NECT shows nodular patchy interlobular septal thickening ➔ in this patient with sarcoidosis.*

Sarcoidosis

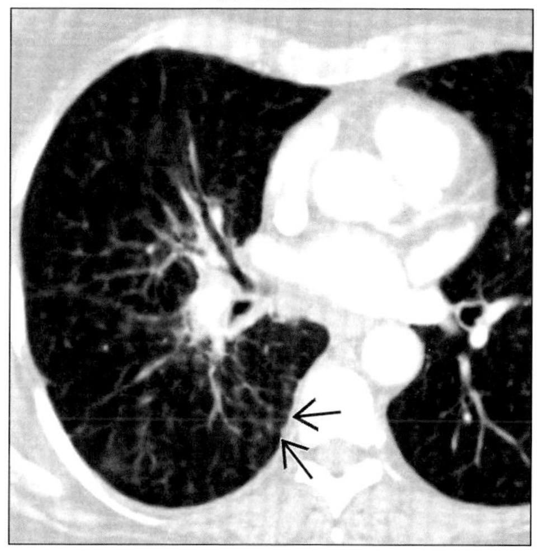

Usual Interstitial Pneumonitis

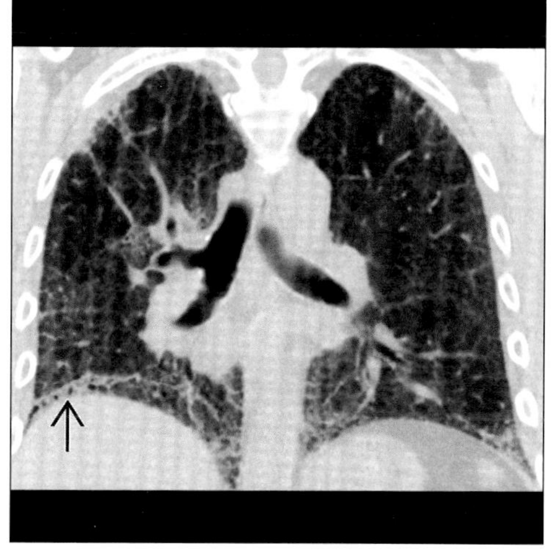

(Left) *Axial CECT shows irregular thickening of the right central bronchovasculature and ipsilateral nodular interlobular septal thickening ➔ representing sarcoidosis. The asymmetric involvement is atypical.* ***(Right)*** *Coronal NECT shows peripheral and basilar interlobular and intralobular septal thickening and patchy areas of hazy ground-glass opacity. There is mild, right basilar traction bronchiolectasis ➔.*

Pulmonary Vein Stenosis

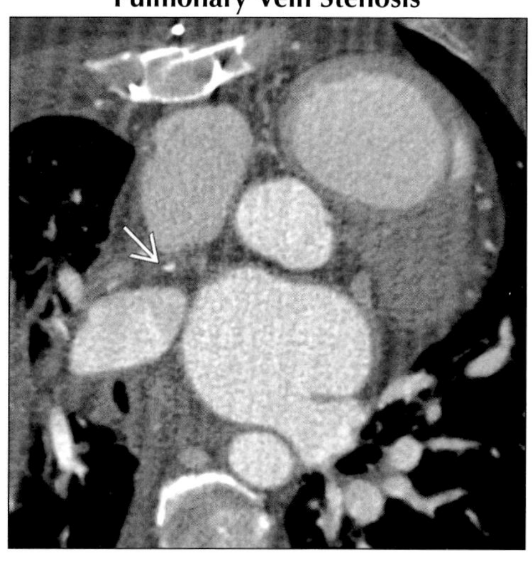

Pulmonary Vein Stenosis

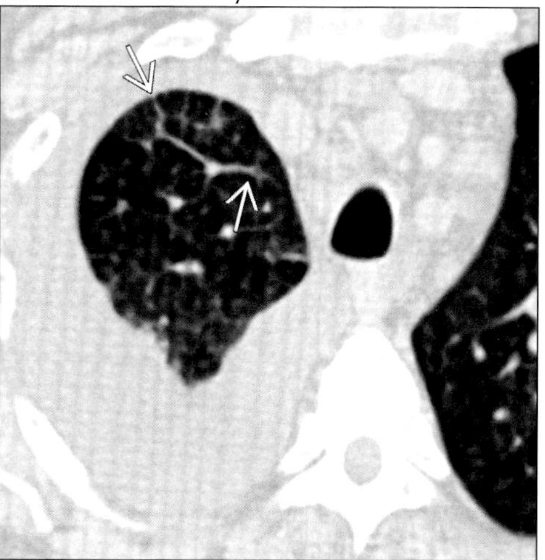

(Left) *Axial CECT shows chronic occlusion ➔ of the right superior pulmonary vein.* ***(Right)*** *Axial NECT from the same patient shows asymmetric right upper lobe interlobular septal thickening ➔ and a large right pleural effusion from abnormally high right-sided pulmonary venous pressure.*

INTERLOBULAR SEPTAL THICKENING

*(**Left**) Coronal NECT in a different patient shows bilateral ground-glass opacity with superimposed interlobular and intralobular septal thickening. There is asymmetric emphysema, worse in the right lung. (**Right**) Axial NECT shows patchy, geographic regions of ground-glass opacity with superimposed interlobular and intralobular septal thickening in a crazy-paving pattern. Pulmonary opacities decreased after high volume bronchoalveolar lavage.*

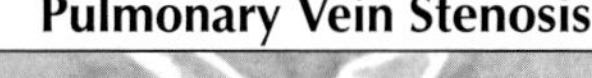

Pulmonary Vein Stenosis

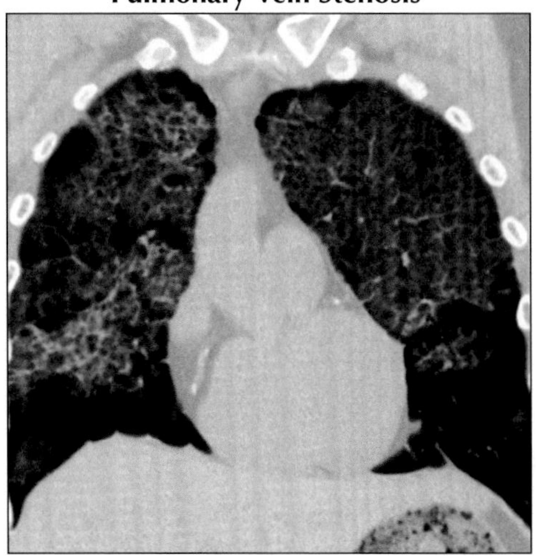

Pulmonary Alveolar Proteinosis

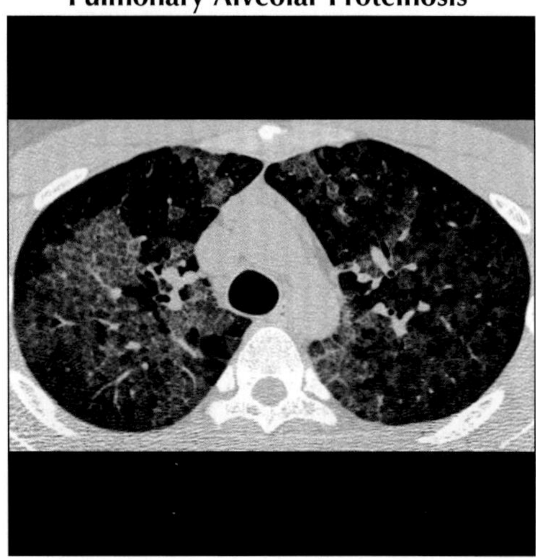

*(**Left**) Axial CECT shows an enlarged main pulmonary artery suggestive of pulmonary arterial hypertension and small bilateral pleural effusions. (**Right**) Axial CECT in the same patient shows subtle bilateral interlobular septal and mild peribronchial thickening consistent with pulmonary venoocclusive disease in this patient with pulmonary arterial hypertension and normal capillary wedge pressure.*

Venoocclusive Disease

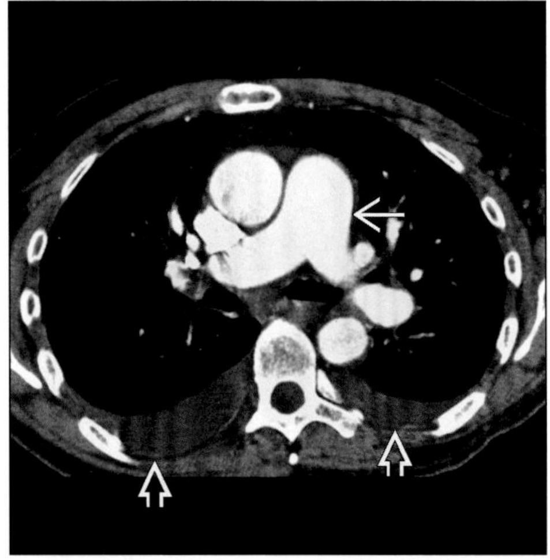

Venoocclusive Disease

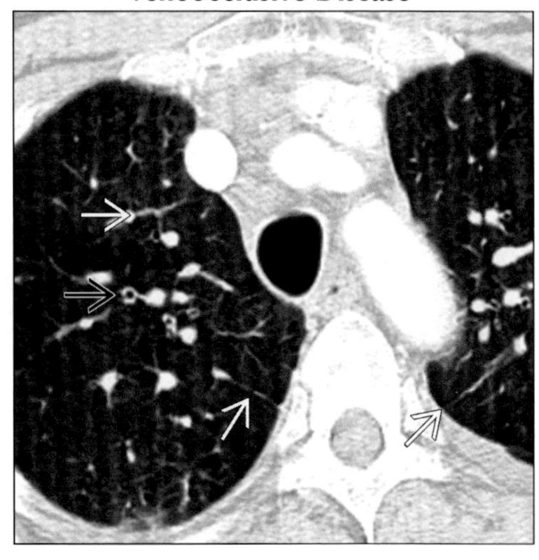

*(**Left**) Axial HRCT shows interlobular septal thickening and scattered nodules in this patient with history of alveolar septal amyloidosis, a rare form of pulmonary amyloidosis. (**Right**) Axial NECT shows bilateral interlobular septal thickening and patchy ground-glass opacities in this patient with Erdheim Chester disease.*

Alveolar Septal Amyloidosis

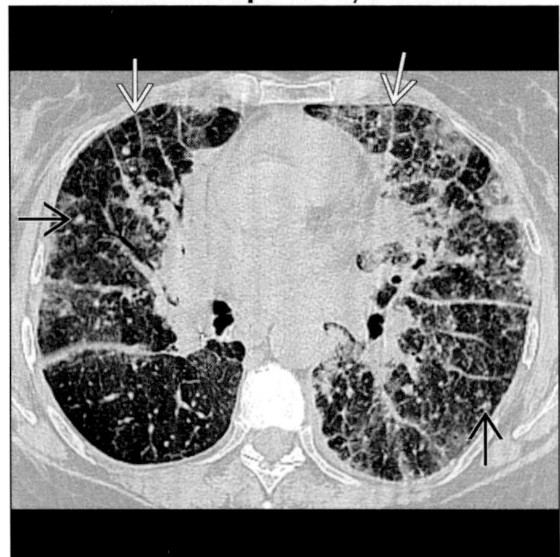

Erdheim Chester Disease

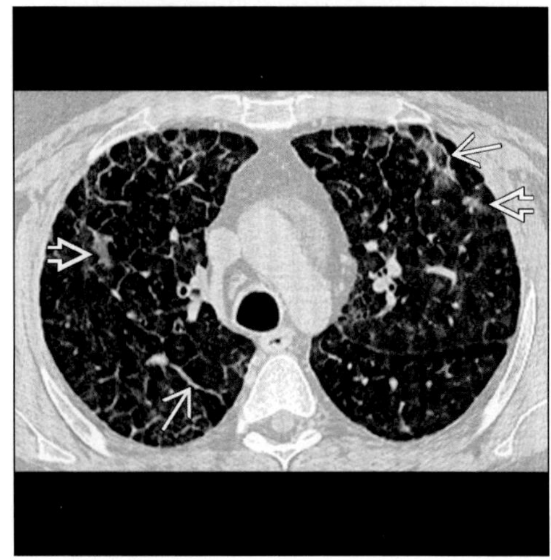

Erdheim Chester Disease

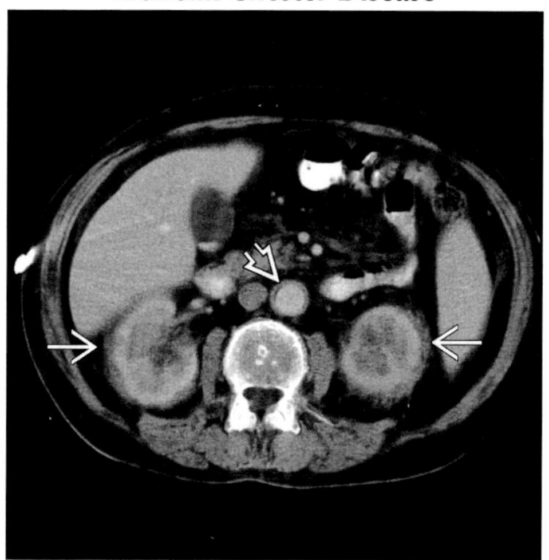

Leukemic Infiltration

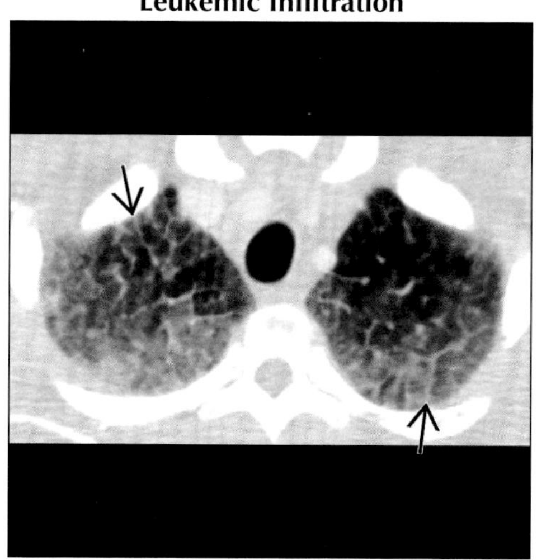

(Left) *Axial CECT in the same patient shows soft tissue attenuation surrounding the kidneys ➡ and aorta ➡, highly suggestive of Erdheim Chester disease given concomitant pulmonary interlobular septal thickening.* ***(Right)*** *Axial NECT shows symmetric upper lung ground-glass opacity and superimposed interlobular septal thickening → in this patient with leukemia.*

Leukemic Infiltration

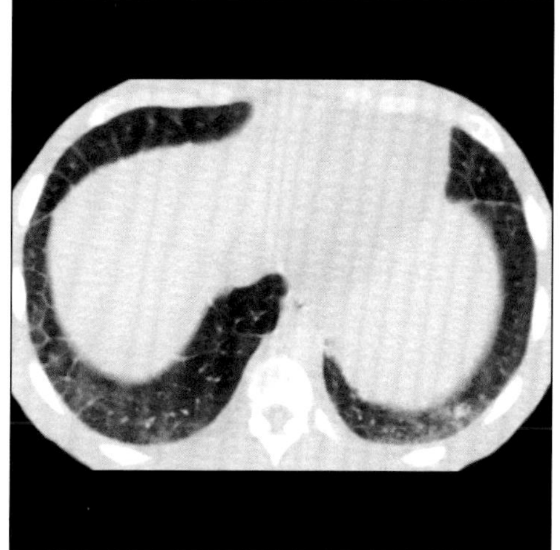

Diffuse Pulmonary Lymphangiomatosis

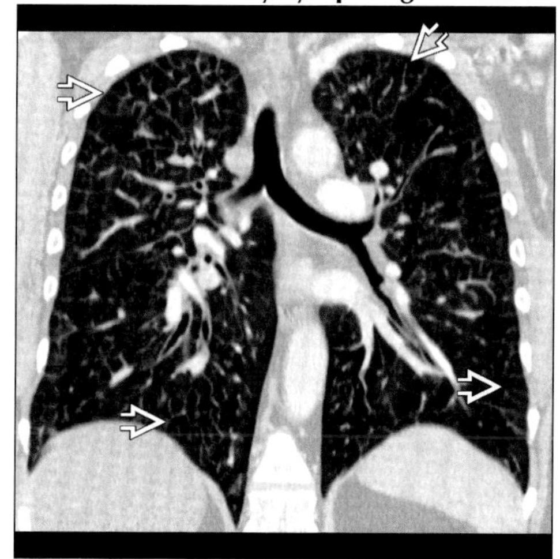

(Left) *Axial NECT in the same patient shows interlobular septal thickening bilaterally without pleural effusions most consistent with leukemic infiltration given the young age of the patient and the absence of cardiac history.* ***(Right)*** *Coronal CECT shows diffuse smooth interlobular septal thickening ➡ and peribronchial thickening in this patient with diffuse pulmonary lymphangiomatosis.*

Diffuse Pulmonary Lymphangiomatosis

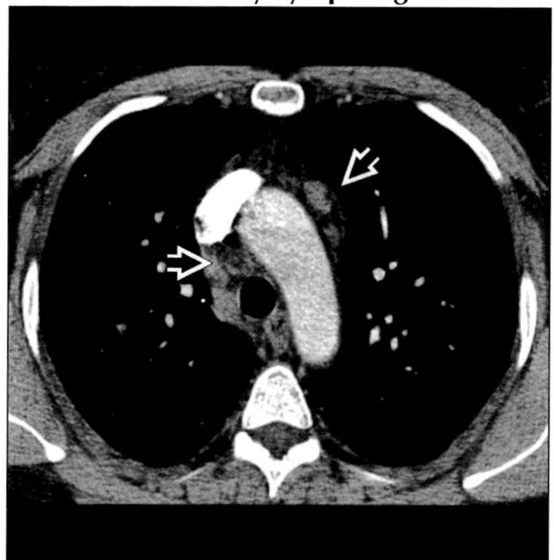

Acute Eosinophilic Pneumonia

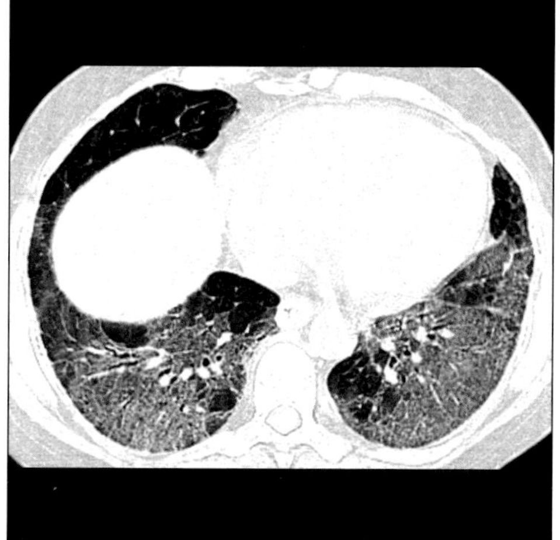

(Left) *Axial CECT in the same patient shows mildly enlarged prevascular and paratracheal lymph nodes ➡ in this patient with diffuse pulmonary lymphangiomatosis.* ***(Right)*** *Axial HRCT shows ground-glass opacity in the basilar aspects of the lungs with interlobular and intralobular septal thickening shown to represent acute eosinophilic pneumonia.*

UPPER LUNG ZONE DISEASE DISTRIBUTION

DIFFERENTIAL DIAGNOSIS

Common
- Post-Primary Tuberculosis
- Sarcoidosis
- Centrilobular Emphysema
- Bronchiolitis, Respiratory
- Langerhans Cell Histiocytosis

Less Common
- Silicosis/Coal Worker's Pneumoconiosis
- Chronic Hypersensitivity Pneumonitis
- Cystic Fibrosis
- Chronic Eosinophilic Pneumonia
- Allergic Bronchopulmonary Aspergillosis

Rare but Important
- Neurogenic Pulmonary Edema
- Smoke Inhalation
- Metastatic Pulmonary Calcification
- Ankylosing Spondylitis
- Chronic Lung Allograft Rejection

ESSENTIAL INFORMATION

Key Differential Diagnosis Issues
- Pneumonic: CHEST CASES
  - **C**ystic fibrosis, **H**istiocytosis X or **H**ypersensitivity pneumonitis, **E**mphysema, **S**arcoidosis, **T**uberculosis
  - **C**alcification-metastatic pulmonary, **A**BPA or **A**nkylosing spondylitis, **S**ilicosis, **E**osinophilic pneumonia, **S**moke inhalation
- Normal physiologic gradients in upright lung create zones or regions of lung that differ in terms of blood flow, ventilation, lymphatic function, stress, and concentration of inhaled gases
  - Consider lung as a map, with zones not defined by anatomy but by regional differences produced by physiology
  - End result of interaction between pathologic process with its environment
  - Soil and seed concept: Seeds (pathologic process) finds certain soils (physiologic regions) more conducive to growth
- Distribution of disease usually readily apparent from frontal radiograph
  - Caveats: Normally lung much thicker at base than at apex
    - Truly uniform distribution of pathology will be more apparent in lower lung zones due to summation across greater thickness of lower lobes
    - Uniform radiographic distribution may actually be more profuse in upper lung zones pathologically due to less summation across thinner upper lobes

Helpful Clues for Common Diagnoses
- **Post-Primary Tuberculosis**
  - Proclivity for apical posterior segments of upper lobes
  - Cavitary disease combined with consolidation and bronchial wall thickening
- **Sarcoidosis**
  - Chronic granulomatous process of unknown etiology
  - Peribronchial and perilymphatic nodules
  - Identical findings in **berylliosis**
- **Centrilobular Emphysema**
  - Sequelae of long-term smoking
  - Punched out holes in centrilobular distribution
- **Bronchiolitis, Respiratory**
  - Clustered "dirty" macrophages in and around respiratory bronchioles from cigarette smoking
  - Faint, ill-defined centrilobular nodules in upper lung zones
  - May be precursor of centrilobular emphysema
- **Langerhans Cell Histiocytosis**
  - Granulomas contain Langerhans cell (that processes antigen)
  - Seen almost exclusively in smokers
  - Probably allergic reaction to constituent of cigarette smoke
  - Centrilobular nodules that eventually evolve into bizarre-shaped cysts, paracicatricial emphysema

Helpful Clues for Less Common Diagnoses
- **Silicosis/Coal Worker's Pneumoconiosis**
  - Long-term exposure to occupational dusts
  - Simple (nodular interstitial thickening) may progress to progressive massive fibrosis (PMF)
  - Nodules follow lung lymphatics, tends to be more profuse in dorsal upper lung
- **Chronic Hypersensitivity Pneumonitis**

- History of inhaled organic antigen exposure
- Upper lung zone distribution, especially common in those with intermittent exposure (like farmer's lung)
  - Midlung predominance seen in many other antigen exposures that occur continuously (like bird breeder's lung)
- Centrilobular ground-glass nodules and hyperinflated lobules (head-cheese sign) evolves into peribronchial fibrosis

- **Cystic Fibrosis**
  - Autosomal recessive gene disorder that results in thick viscous secretions
  - Primary pathology occurs in airways
  - Bronchiectasis more severe in upper lobes, especially right upper lobe
- **Chronic Eosinophilic Pneumonia**
  - Predominant involvement in upper peripheral lung ("photographic negative" of pulmonary edema)
  - Ground-glass opacities and consolidation
    - Opacities resolve from periphery, leaving lines (inner edge) paralleling chest wall
  - Rapid response to corticosteroid therapy
- **Allergic Bronchopulmonary Aspergillosis**
  - Asthma history, abnormal hypersensitivity reaction to *Aspergillus* organisms
  - Central upper lobe bronchiectasis with peripheral sparing

Helpful Clues for Rare Diagnoses

- **Neurogenic Pulmonary Edema**
  - Any central nervous system (CNS) insult that acutely raises intracranial pressure
  - Edema is due to both hydrostatic and capillary leak
- **Smoke Inhalation**
  - Burning wood or plastic products create volatile compounds that produce chemical pneumonitis and edema within hours of exposure
  - High ventilation/perfusion ratio in upper lung zones concentrates inhaled gases
- **Metastatic Pulmonary Calcification**
  - Definition: Deposition of calcium in otherwise normal tissue in hypercalcemic states, such as renal failure
  - High pH in upper lung zones, calcium is less soluble in alkaline environment
    - Calcium also tends to deposit in gastric wall and renal medulla, regions with relative alkaline pH
  - High-attenuation centrilobular ground-glass nodules clustered into rosettes, resemble mulberries
- **Ankylosing Spondylitis**
  - Fibrocystic change in upper lobes
  - Seen in < 2% of patients with ankylosing spondylitis
- **Chronic Lung Allograft Rejection**
  - Seen 18-72 months (mean: 42 months) following transplantation
  - Starts as interstitial opacities in lung periphery, progressing to honeycombing

Post-Primary Tuberculosis

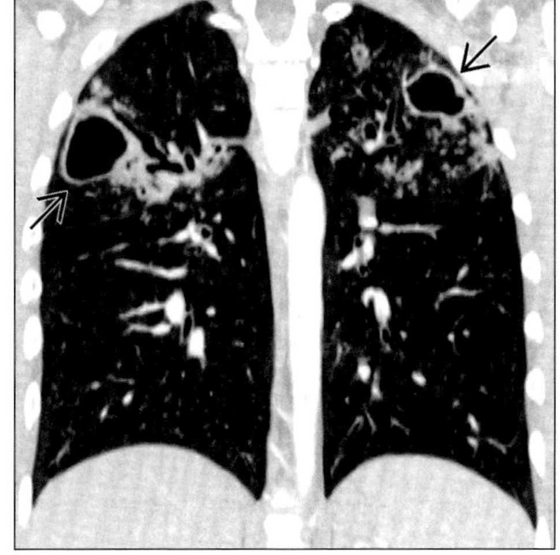

Coronal CECT reconstruction shows biapical cavities ➔ and adjacent nodules and consolidation. Bronchogenic spread to other areas of the lung is common.

Sarcoidosis

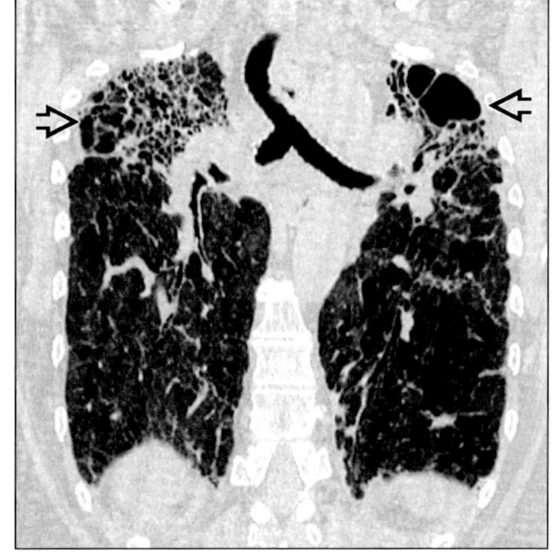

Coronal HRCT reconstruction shows severe traction bronchiectasis and fibrosis in the upper lobes with honeycombing ➪.

UPPER LUNG ZONE DISEASE DISTRIBUTION

*(**Left**) Coronal HRCT reconstruction shows upper lung zone distribution of low-attenuation holes ➔ from emphysema. Upper lobes contribute less to overall pulmonary function and so emphysema is often severe before patient has symptoms. (**Right**) Coronal HRCT reconstruction shows faint centrilobular nodules → in respiratory bronchiolitis. Respiratory bronchiolitis develops within months of onset of cigarette smoking.*

Centrilobular Emphysema

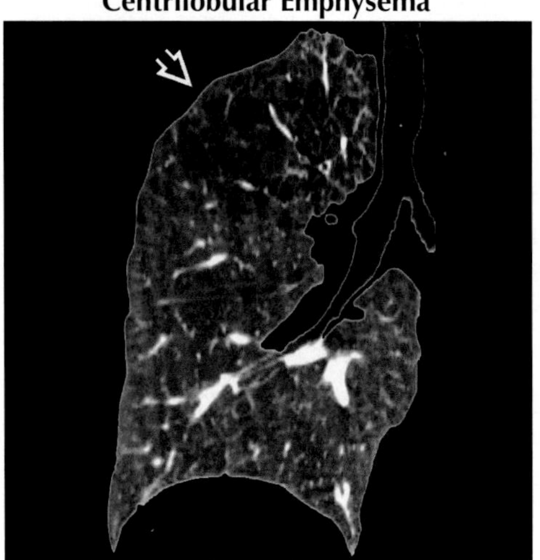

Bronchiolitis, Respiratory

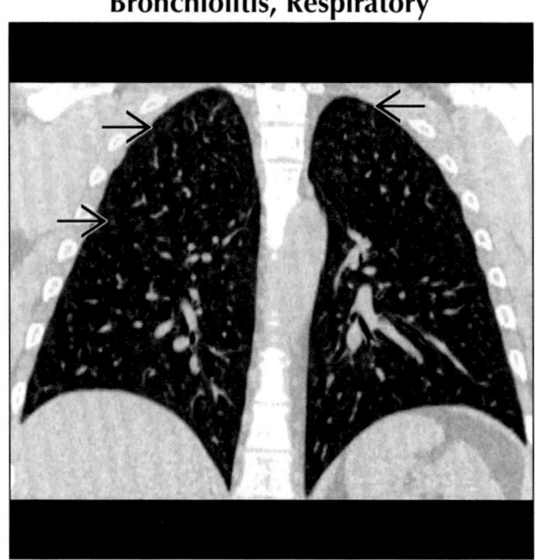

*(**Left**) Coronal NECT reconstruction shows nodules → and cysts ➔ predominantly in the upper lung. Note that the largest hole has a bizarre shape ➔. (**Right**) Coronal HRCT reconstruction shows progressive massive fibrosis ➔ with cavitation. PMF is surrounded by clustered nodules. Peripheral lung is emphysematous. Cavitation may be related to tuberculosis, which must be excluded.*

Langerhans Cell Histiocytosis

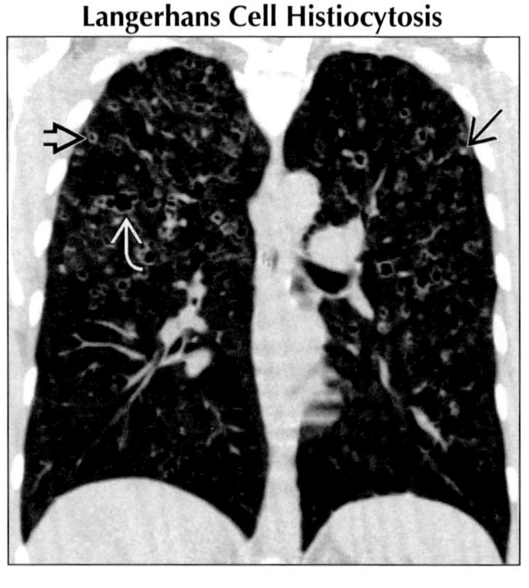

Silicosis/Coal Worker's Pneumoconiosis

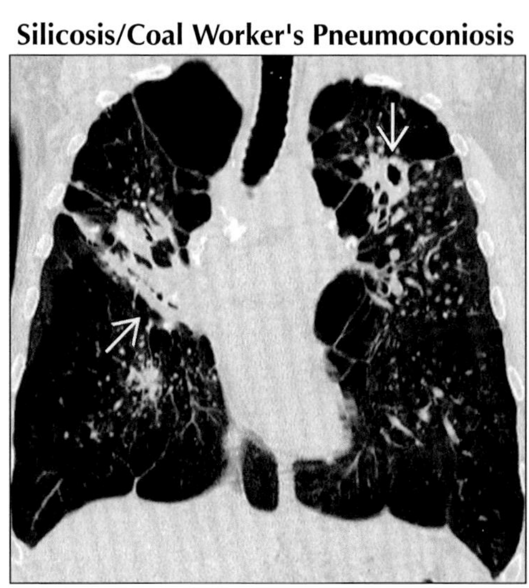

*(**Left**) Coronal HRCT reconstruction shows irregular interstitial thickening predominately in the upper and mid lung zones ➔. This patient had farmer's lung. (**Right**) Coronal HRCT reconstruction shows distribution of upper lobe bronchiectasis ➔. Note that the lungs are hyperinflated. Bronchiectasis is often more severe in the right upper lobe as compared to the left upper lobe.*

Chronic Hypersensitivity Pneumonitis

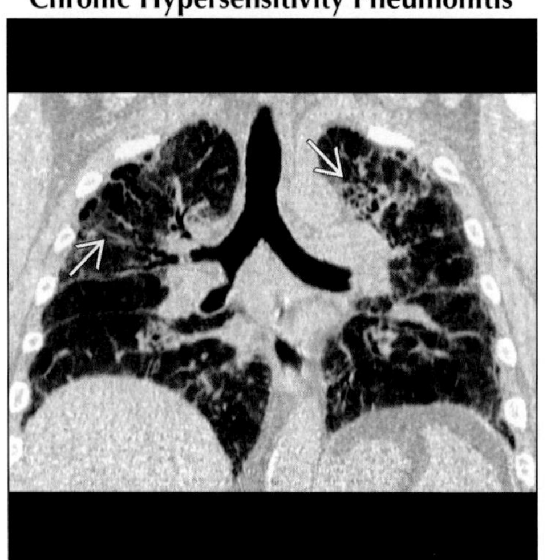

Cystic Fibrosis

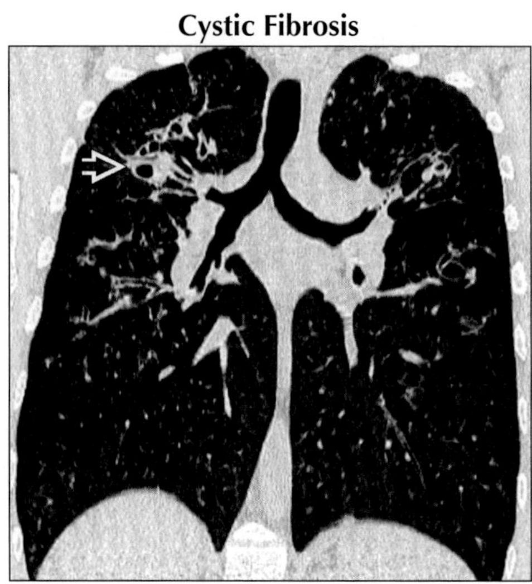

UPPER LUNG ZONE DISEASE DISTRIBUTION

Chronic Eosinophilic Pneumonia

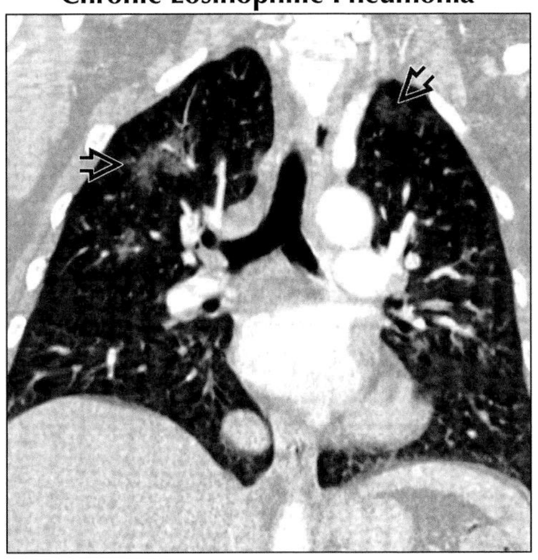

Allergic Bronchopulmonary Aspergillosis

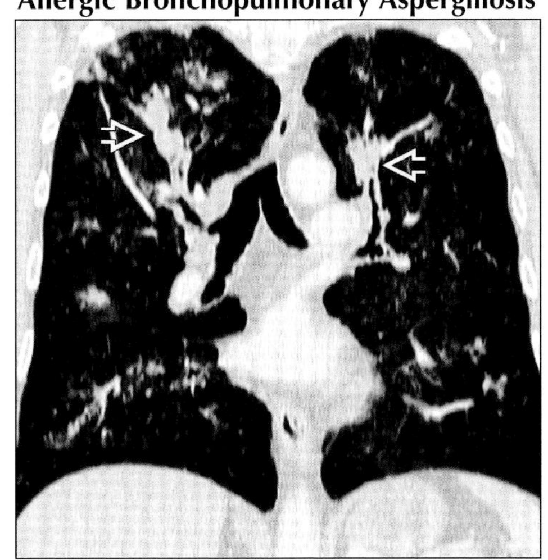

*(**Left**) Coronal CECT reconstruction shows multifocal ground-glass opacities ⇒. Patient had been previously diagnosed with eosinophilic pneumonia, which recurred when corticosteroids were decreased. (**Right**) Coronal HRCT reconstruction shows distribution of finger in glove opacities ⇒ that are most severe in the upper lobes.*

Neurogenic Pulmonary Edema

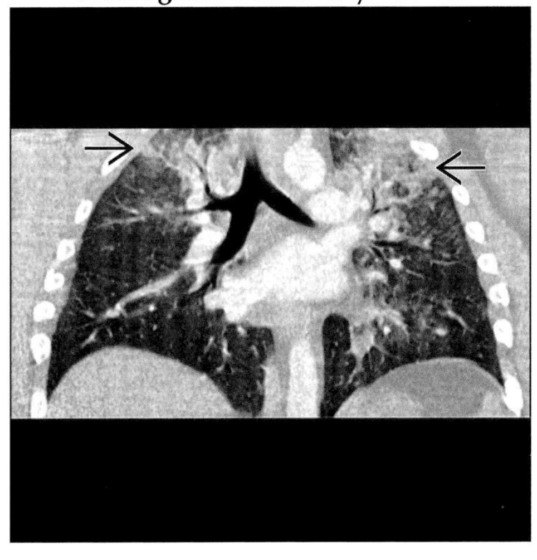

Smoke Inhalation

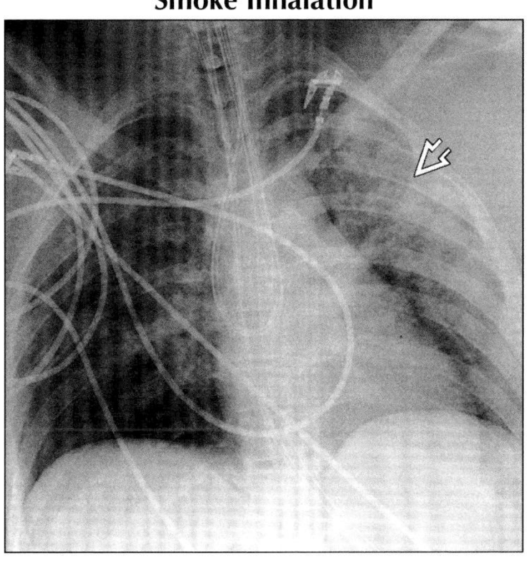

*(**Left**) Coronal CECT reconstruction shows ground-glass opacities and consolidation in both apices → from pulmonary edema. Patient had subarachnoid hemorrhage. (**Right**) Anteroposterior radiograph shows perihilar consolidation, slightly more severe in the upper lung zones ⇒. The soft tissues of the chest wall are thickened from edema from upper body burn.*

Metastatic Pulmonary Calcification

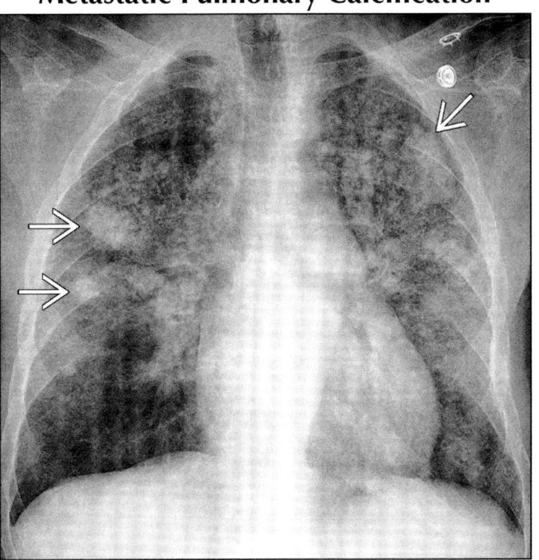

Ankylosing Spondylitis

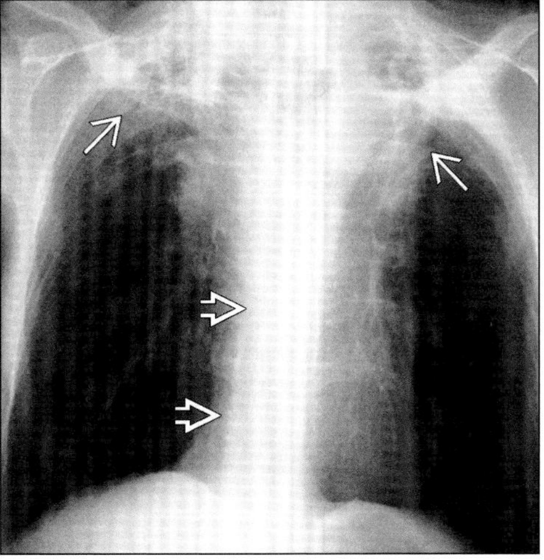

*(**Left**) Frontal radiograph shows diffuse nodular interstitial thickening primarily in the upper lung zones. Aggregated nodules are dense →, suggesting they are calcified. (**Right**) Frontal radiograph shows marked interstitial fibrosis and volume loss → in the upper lobes. Thoracic spine was ankylosed ⇒.*

BASILAR LUNG ZONE DISEASE DISTRIBUTION

DIFFERENTIAL DIAGNOSIS

Common
- Idiopathic Pulmonary Fibrosis
- Nonspecific Interstitial Pneumonitis
- Aspiration

Less Common
- Cryptogenic Organizing Pneumonia
- Asbestosis

Rare but Important
- Alpha-1 Antiprotease Deficiency
- Desquamative Interstitial Pneumonia
- Immotile Cilia Syndrome

ESSENTIAL INFORMATION

Key Differential Diagnosis Issues
- Tobacco abuse
  - Desquamative interstitial pneumonia (90% are smokers)
  - Alpha-1 antiprotease deficiency
- Occupational exposures
  - Asbestosis
  - Desquamative interstitial pneumonia (dusts, fumes)

Helpful Clues for Common Diagnoses
- **Idiopathic Pulmonary Fibrosis**
  - Characterized histologically by usual interstitial pneumonia (UIP)
    - Temporal and spatial heterogeneity
    - Fibroblastic foci
  - Radiographic findings
    - Honeycombing
    - Reticulation
    - Traction bronchiectasis and bronchiolectasis
    - Architectural distortion
  - Subpleural and basal predominant
- **Nonspecific Interstitial Pneumonitis**
  - Histological pattern of interstitial inflammation characterized by
    - Spatial and temporal heterogeneity
    - Cellular, mixed, and fibrotic forms
  - Most patients have collagen vascular disease (especially scleroderma, mixed connective tissue disease, and polymyositis)
  - Other causes of nonspecific interstitial pneumonitis (NSIP) pattern
    - Idiopathic (especially in young women of east Asian ethnicity)
    - Drug toxicity
    - Familial fibrosis
    - Hypersensitivity pneumonitis
    - Cigarette smoking (rare cause)
  - Radiographic findings
    - Basal predominant ground-glass opacity
    - Superimposed reticulation
    - Subpleural sparing (suggestive of diagnosis)
    - Traction bronchiectasis and bronchiolectasis (usually mild)
    - Esophageal dilation (scleroderma and mixed connective tissue disease)
- **Aspiration**
  - Ranges from innocuous intake of solids or liquids into airways to extensive lung injury
  - Common causes
    - Alcohol and drug abuse
    - Neuromuscular disease
    - Loss of consciousness
    - Disorders of esophagus and pharynx, reflux disease
  - Radiographic findings
    - Consolidation in dependent portions of lungs, often peribronchial
    - May lead to lung abscess formation (cavitation with fluid level)
    - Associated bronchial wall thickening, endobronchial debris, centrilobular nodules, and tree-in-bud opacities
    - Esophageal dilation or retained debris or liquid in esophagus suggestive

Helpful Clues for Less Common Diagnoses
- **Cryptogenic Organizing Pneumonia**
  - Histologic pattern defined by
    - Granulation tissue polyps in lumens of alveolar ducts and surrounding alveoli
  - Common causes of organizing pneumonia
    - Connective tissue disease
    - Drug reaction
    - Infection
    - Inhalational injury
  - Radiographic findings
    - Bilateral symmetric or asymmetric lung consolidation ± air bronchograms
    - Mid and basal lung zone predominance
    - Subpleural or peribronchial (60-80%) distribution

- Perilobular (60%) distribution
- Reverse halo or atoll sign (20%)
- Ground-glass opacity (more common in immunocompromised patients)

- **Asbestosis**
  - Interstitial fibrosis from asbestos exposure
    - Histological similar to UIP
  - Subpleural branching opacities (fibrosis centered on respiratory bronchioles where asbestos fibers deposited) earliest finding on CT
  - Honeycombing less common except in severe disease
  - Associated features
    - Parenchymal bands and subpleural curvilinear opacities
    - Calcified or noncalcified pleural plaques
    - Subpleural reticulation
    - Tractions bronchiectasis and bronchiolectasis
    - Architectural distortion

Helpful Clues for Rare Diagnoses

- **Alpha-1 Antiprotease Deficiency**
  - Accounts for < 1% of patients with chronic obstructive pulmonary disease (COPD)
  - Homozygous deficiency (PiZZ) increases risk of COPD 30x
  - Cigarette smoking major contributory factor
  - Manifests in lungs as panlobular (panacinar) emphysema
  - Radiographic findings
    - Hyperinflation
    - Ill-defined absence of normal lung, wispy "cotton candy" lung markings
    - Homogeneous appearance
    - Marked basal predominance
- **Desquamative Interstitial Pneumonia**
  - Histologic pattern of widespread accumulation of intraalveolar pigmented macrophages
  - Heavy smokers (90%)
  - Other causes of desquamative interstitial pneumonia-like reaction
    - Dust inhalation
    - Drug reaction
    - Connective tissue disease
  - Radiographic findings
    - Basal predominant ground-glass opacity (75%)
    - Subpleural distribution (50%)
    - Mild reticulation
- **Immotile Cilia Syndrome**
  - Autosomal recessive disorders of ciliary structure and function
  - Patients predisposed to sinusitis, recurrent respiratory tract infections, bronchiectasis, and infertility
  - Situs abnormalities occur in up to 50%
  - Radiographic findings
    - Situs inversus or heterotaxy
    - Bronchiectasis (50% lower lobe predominant)
    - Centrilobular nodules and tree-in-bud opacities

Idiopathic Pulmonary Fibrosis

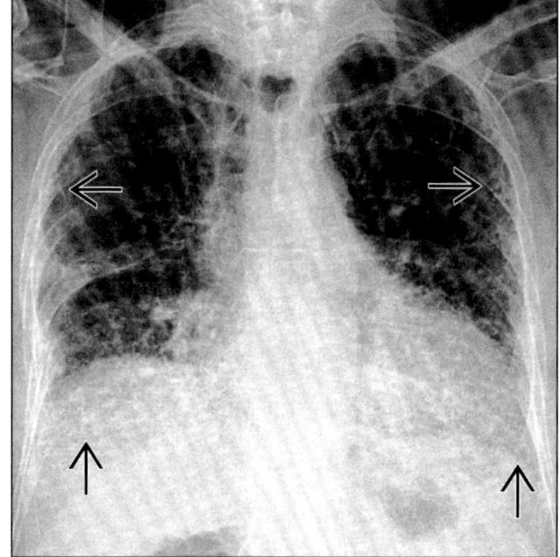

Frontal radiograph shows low lung volumes with subpleural and basal predominant reticulation ⇒ and architectural distortion. The distribution of fibrosis is highly suggestive of a UIP pattern.

Idiopathic Pulmonary Fibrosis

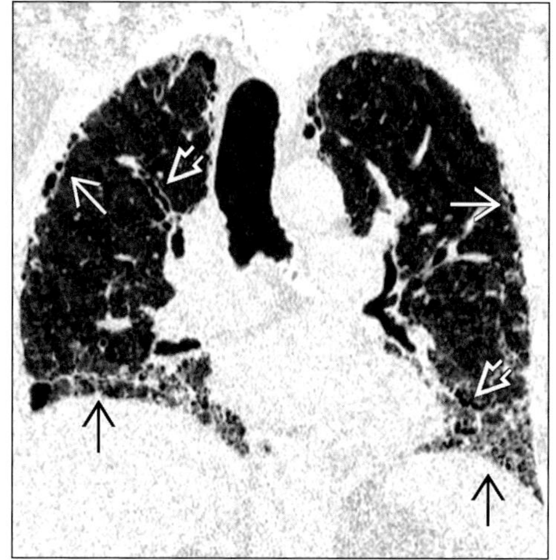

Coronal CT reconstruction shows subpleural honeycombing ➡ and reticulation ⇒ with a basal and subpleural predominance. Note traction bronchiectasis ➡.

BASILAR LUNG ZONE DISEASE DISTRIBUTION

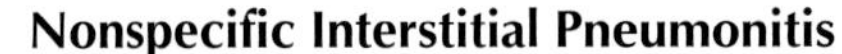

Nonspecific Interstitial Pneumonitis | **Nonspecific Interstitial Pneumonitis**

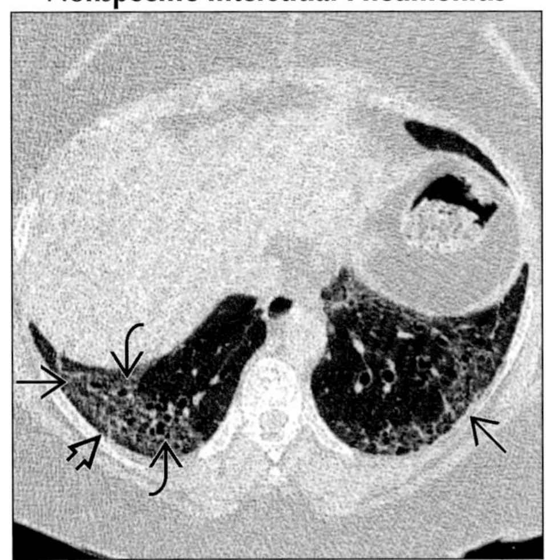

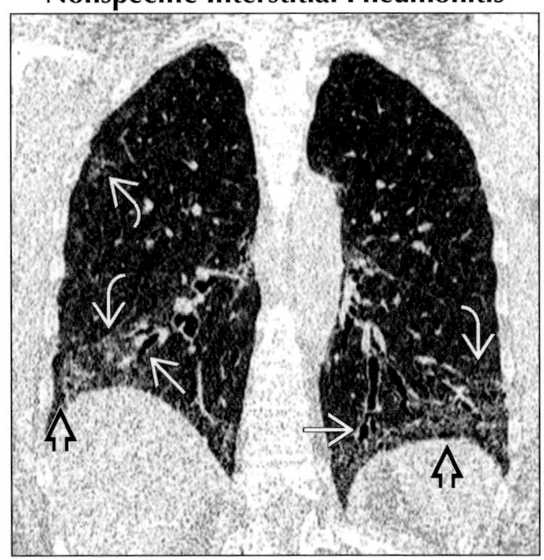

(Left) *Axial HRCT shows patchy ground-glass opacity in the lung bases in this patient with scleroderma. Note subpleural sparing on the right, a feature that strongly favors NSIP over UIP. Traction bronchiectasis is mild, and there is no honeycombing.* ***(Right)*** *Coronal CT reconstruction shows basal predominant ground-glass opacity with some subpleural sparing and mild traction bronchiectasis. Honeycombing is absent.*

Aspiration | **Aspiration**

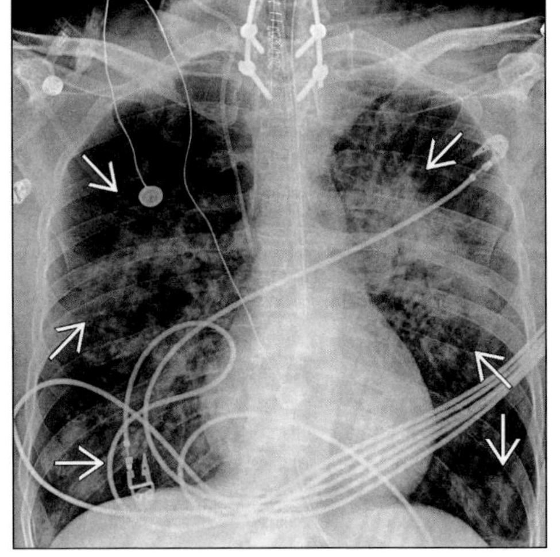

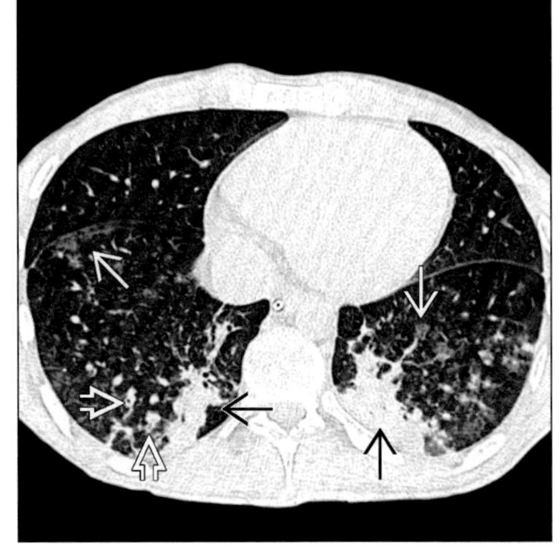

(Left) *Anteroposterior radiograph shows fluffy and nodular bilateral perihilar and bibasilar lung consolidation in this patient who aspirated following major trauma. The distribution of disease often depends on body position.* ***(Right)*** *Axial HRCT shows bilateral lower lobe dependent consolidation in a peribronchial distribution. Other features of aspiration present include peribronchial ground-glass opacity and bronchial wall thickening.*

Cryptogenic Organizing Pneumonia | **Cryptogenic Organizing Pneumonia**

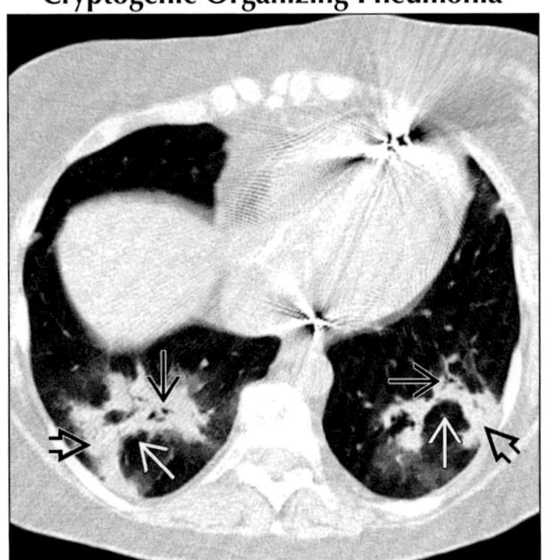

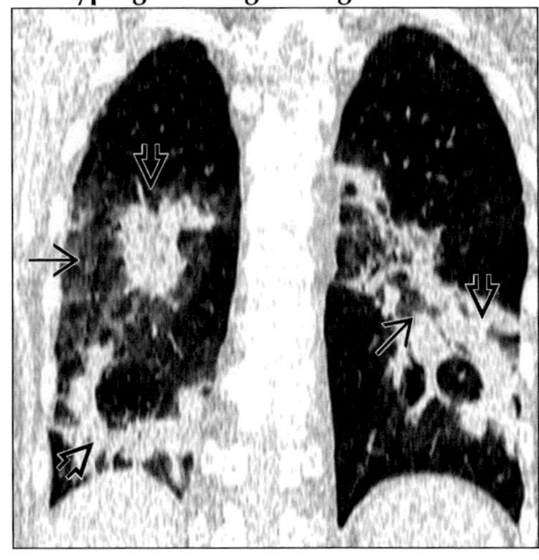

(Left) *Axial HRCT shows bilateral lower lobe peribronchial consolidation with air bronchograms. The curvilinear shape of the foci of consolidation surrounding secondary pulmonary lobules has been described as perilobular.* ***(Right)*** *Coronal CT reconstruction shows mid and basal lung zone predominant peripheral and peribronchial consolidation with some adjacent ground-glass opacity typical of organizing pneumonia.*

BASILAR LUNG ZONE DISEASE DISTRIBUTION

Asbestosis

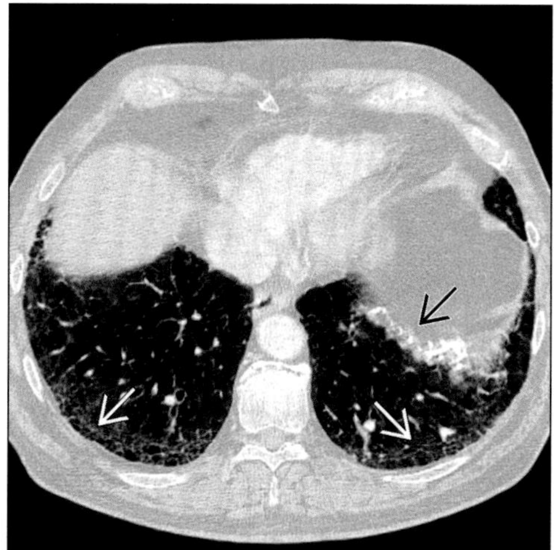

Alpha-1 Antiprotease Deficiency

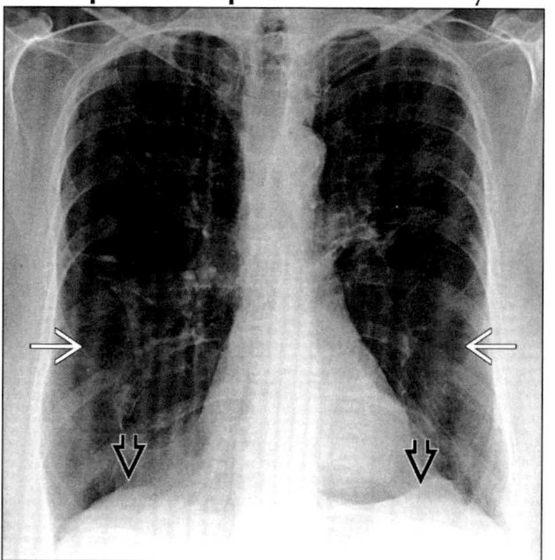

(Left) *Axial HRCT shows mild peripheral reticulation → and architectural distortion typical of asbestosis. The presence of pleural plaques →, calcified in this patient, is a biomarker of asbestos exposure. Asbestosis should not be diagnosed by CT alone in the absence of pleural plaques.* ***(Right)*** *Frontal radiograph shows hyperinflation, especially of the lower lobes, with flattening of the hemidiaphragms →. Marked basal hyperlucency → is present.*

Alpha-1 Antiprotease Deficiency

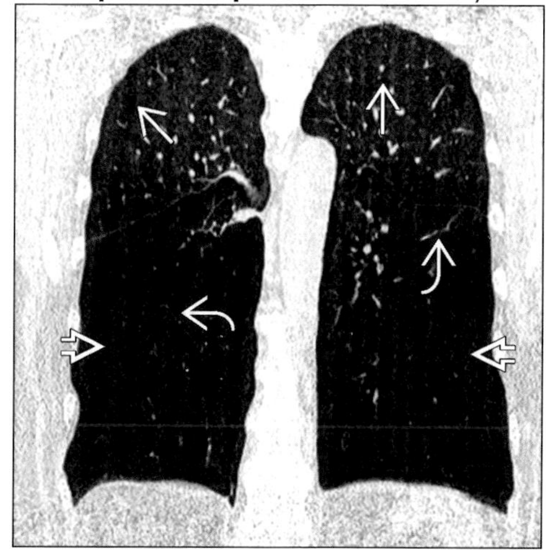

Desquamative Interstitial Pneumonia

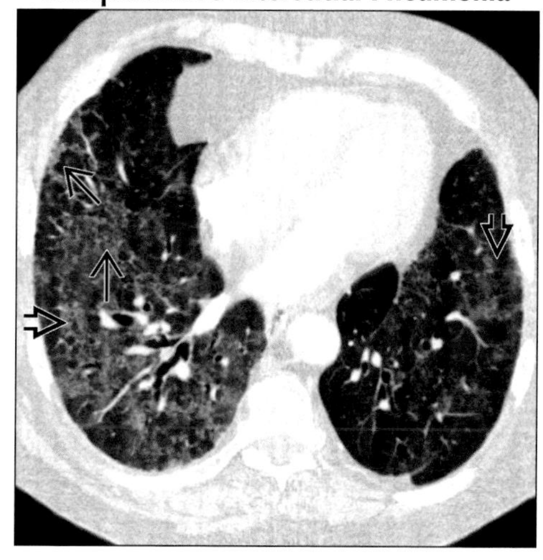

(Left) *Coronal CT reconstruction shows severe, diffuse panlobular emphysema in the lower lobes →, which are hyperinflated. Upper lobe emphysema → is very mild. The lower lobe vessels are very small →.* ***(Right)*** *Axial HRCT shows patchy ground-glass opacity in the lower lobes → in this heavy smoker. The reticular abnormality → is much milder than that typically seen in UIP or NSIP. Most patients with DIP are heavy smokers.*

Immotile Cilia Syndrome

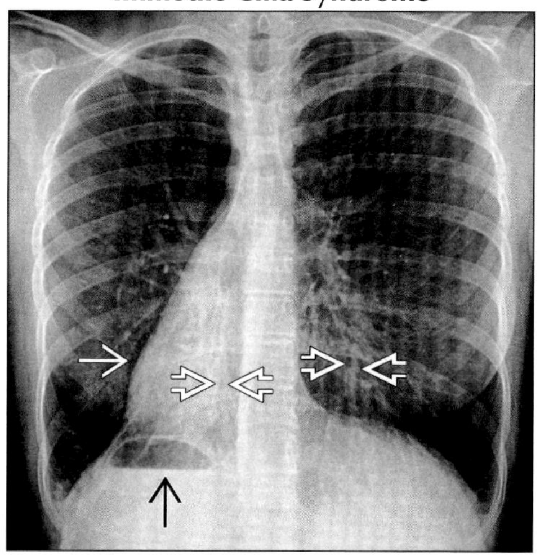

Immotile Cilia Syndrome

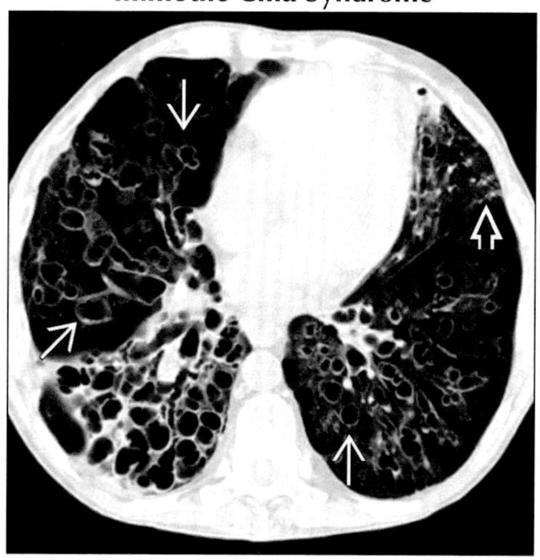

(Left) *Frontal radiograph shows dextrocardia → and the stomach on the right →, consistent with situs inversus totalis. Cylindrical bronchiectasis is in both lower lobes →. Situs inversus totalis, chronic sinusitis, and bronchiectasis comprise Kartagener syndrome.* ***(Right)*** *Axial NECT shows severe cystic bronchiectasis in both lungs →. Small nodules are in the lingula →. Recurrent infection is thought to lead to development of bronchiectasis.*

PERIPHERAL (SUBPLEURAL) LUNG DISEASE DISTRIBUTION

DIFFERENTIAL DIAGNOSIS

Common
- Pneumonia
- Lung Cancer
- Rounded Atelectasis
- Septic Emboli
- Pulmonary Contusions

Less Common
- Pulmonary Infarction
- Cryptogenic Organizing Pneumonia
- Chronic Eosinophilic Pneumonia
- Usual Interstitial Pneumonitis
- Desquamative Interstitial Pneumonia

Rare but Important
- Amyloidosis

ESSENTIAL INFORMATION

Key Differential Diagnosis Issues
- Acute vs. chronic
  - Acute abnormalities
    - Pneumonia
    - Septic emboli
    - Pulmonary infarctions (within 12-24 hours of embolic event); slow resolution
  - Chronic abnormalities
    - Lung cancer
    - Round atelectasis
    - Cryptogenic organizing pneumonia
    - Chronic eosinophilic pneumonia
    - Chronic interstitial lung diseases

Helpful Clues for Common Diagnoses
- **Pneumonia**
  - Airspace opacities: Ground-glass opacities to dense consolidation
  - Reactive lymphadenopathy; very large lymph nodes unusual
  - Parapneumonic pleural effusion or empyema
  - Correlation with sputum, WBC count, and clinical presentation paramount
- **Lung Cancer**
  - Suggestive findings include
    - Focal mass-like consolidation larger than 3 cm
    - Spiculated margins
    - Thick-walled or nodular cavitation
    - Large hilar &/or mediastinal lymphadenopathy (> 2 cm)
    - Concomitant emphysema and smoking history
- **Rounded Atelectasis**
  - Definitive diagnosis on CT requires 4 findings
    - Pleural abnormality: Pleural thickening, pleural effusion, or pleural plaque
    - Broad-based intimate attachment of mass-like consolidation to pleural abnormality
    - Volume loss
    - Comet tail (or hurricane) sign: Swirling of bronchovasculature into mass-like consolidation
- **Septic Emboli**
  - Patients with indwelling catheters or IV drug users at risk
  - Multiple peripheral/subpleural nodules and wedge-shaped consolidation with rapid cavitation
  - Feeding vessel sign: Vessel leads directly to peripheral nodule or wedge-shaped consolidation
  - Exudative pleural effusion, often loculated
- **Pulmonary Contusions**
  - Acute trauma clinical setting
  - Peripheral
  - Under point of blunt kinetic energy absorption
    - Often lateral portions of lung away from overlying musculature
  - Overlying rib fractures
    - Can occur without rib fractures in children and young adults
  - Appear at time of injury
  - Resolve in 3-5 days
  - Associated with other injuries but can be isolated
  - Associated with ballistic injuries

Helpful Clues for Less Common Diagnoses
- **Pulmonary Infarction**
  - Most often from pulmonary arterial embolism
  - Often in setting of superimposed cardiac dysfunction (cardiomyopathy, congestive heart failure)
    - Both pulmonary and bronchial arterial supply to lung reduced
  - Lower lung predominant, peripheral/subpleural, wedge-shaped consolidation

- Resolves over months (retains its original shape) rather than patchy resolution as in pneumonia

- **Cryptogenic Organizing Pneumonia**
  - Bilateral, basal-predominant, peripheral and peribronchovascular consolidation
  - Scattered areas of ground-glass opacities and nodules
  - Atoll sign (a.k.a. reversed halo sign): Central ground-glass opacity surrounded by rim of consolidation
  - Perilobular opacities: Ill-defined opacities outlining interlobular septa of secondary pulmonary lobule
- **Chronic Eosinophilic Pneumonia**
  - Peripheral, upper lung consolidation (so-called photographic negative of pulmonary edema)
  - Ground-glass opacities do not predominate
  - Waxing and waning disease course
  - Tendency to resolve centripetally (from outer to inner)
  - Residual band of linear opacities parallels chest wall late in evolution of disease
- **Usual Interstitial Pneumonitis**
  - Peripheral and basal predominant distribution; costophrenic angles most affected
  - Volume loss
  - Reticular opacities, linear opacities, architectural distortion
  - Traction bronchiectasis and honeycombing
  - Ground-glass opacities do not predominate
  - Mild mediastinal lymphadenopathy not uncommon
- **Desquamative Interstitial Pneumonia**
  - Slowly progressive dyspnea and cough in smoker
  - Basal and peripheral/subpleural ground-glass opacities; may be diffuse
  - Consolidation does not predominate
  - Scattered, thin-walled lung cysts
  - Basal reticular opacities common; honeycombing rare
  - Concomitant smoking-related disease, most commonly centrilobular emphysema

Helpful Clues for Rare Diagnoses

- **Amyloidosis**
  - Nodular parenchymal subtype
    - Nodules that slowly grow over time
    - Peripheral, sharply marginated
    - Cavitation highly uncommon
    - Calcification (osseous metaplasia) in up to half of cases
  - Diffuse alveolar septal subtype
    - Least common type of thoracic amyloidosis
    - Interlobular and intralobular septal thickening
    - Micronodules often in subpleural distribution
  - Mediastinal or hilar lymphadenopathy not uncommon; ± calcification
  - Amyloidosis rare cause of pulmonary infarcts

Pneumonia

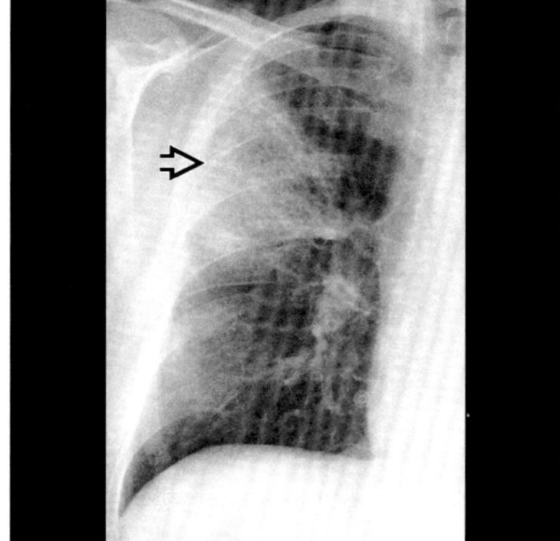

Frontal radiograph shows peripheral consolidation ➲ in the right upper lobe in a patient presenting with fever and chills. Consolidation resolved with antibiotics.

Lung Cancer

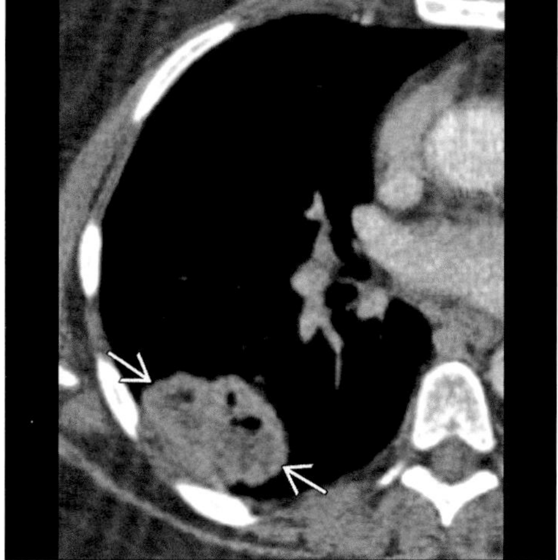

Axial CECT shows a necrotic and cavitary mass ➡ in the peripheral aspect of the right lower lobe.

PERIPHERAL (SUBPLEURAL) LUNG DISEASE DISTRIBUTION

*(**Left**) Axial NECT shows small peripheral adenocarcinoma in the left upper lobe ➙. Also note the fairly extensive paraseptal emphysema ➙. (**Right**) Axial NECT shows a rounded mass in the right lower lobe with broad-based attachment to calcified pleural thickening ➙; there is characteristic swirling of the bronchovasculature into the mass-like consolidation ➙ (the comet tail sign).*

Lung Cancer

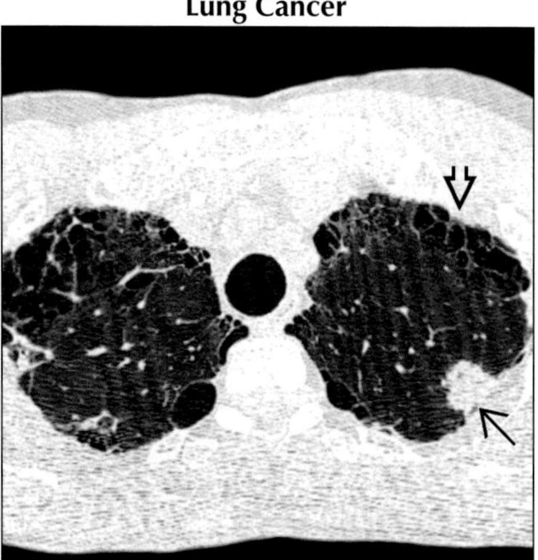

Rounded Atelectasis

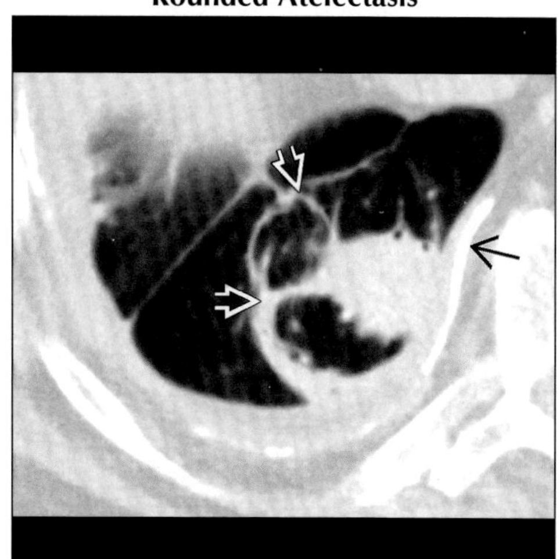

*(**Left**) Axial CECT shows multiple peripheral nodules in this patient with high fever and history of IV drug abuse. There is cavitation in a left upper lobe nodule ➙. (**Right**) Coronal CECT shows multiple lung nodules, some of which are cavitary ➙, highly suggestive of septic emboli in this patient with high fever and history of IV drug use.*

Septic Emboli

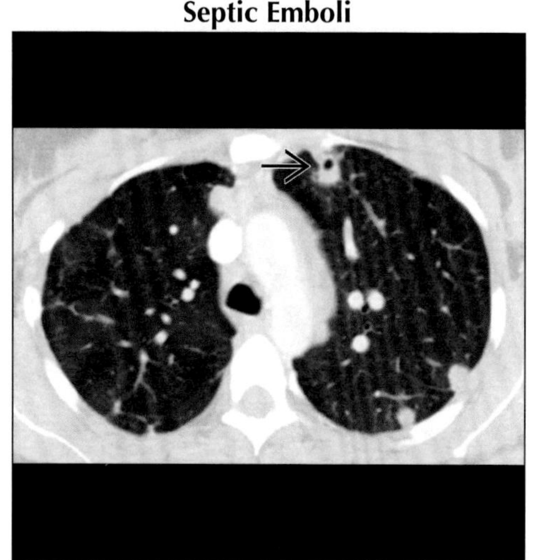

Septic Emboli

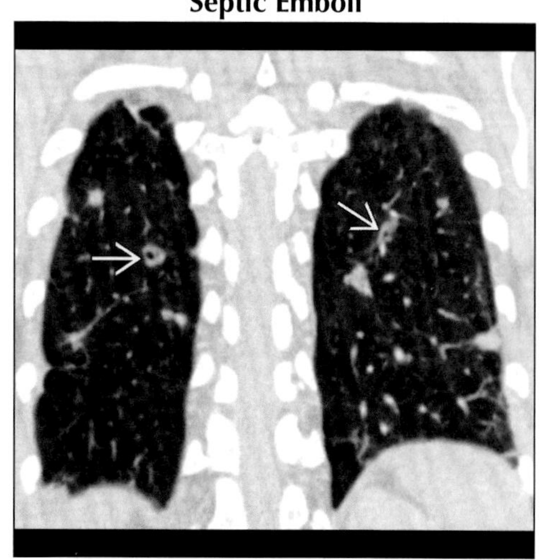

*(**Left**) Axial CECT shows peripheral wedge-shaped ground-glass opacity and consolidation in the right middle lobe; acute pulmonary emboli ➙ are present. (**Right**) Axial NECT shows peripheral and subpleural lung consolidation ➙ and ground-glass opacity ➙ in a patient with biopsy-proven organizing pneumonia.*

Pulmonary Infarction

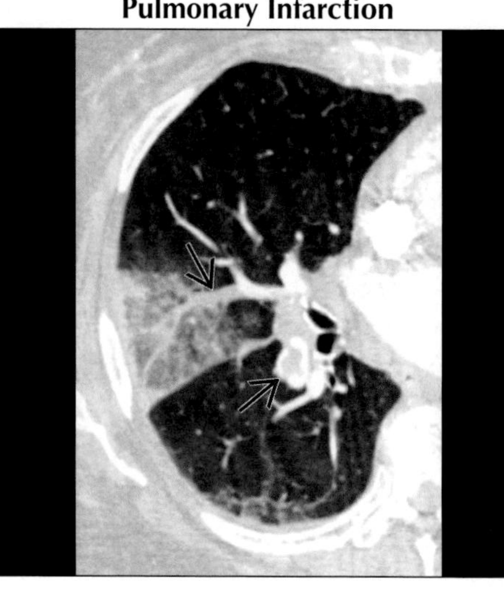

Cryptogenic Organizing Pneumonia

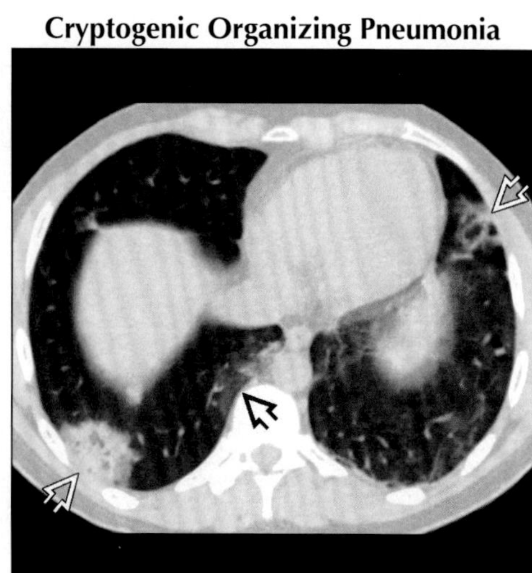

Cryptogenic Organizing Pneumonia

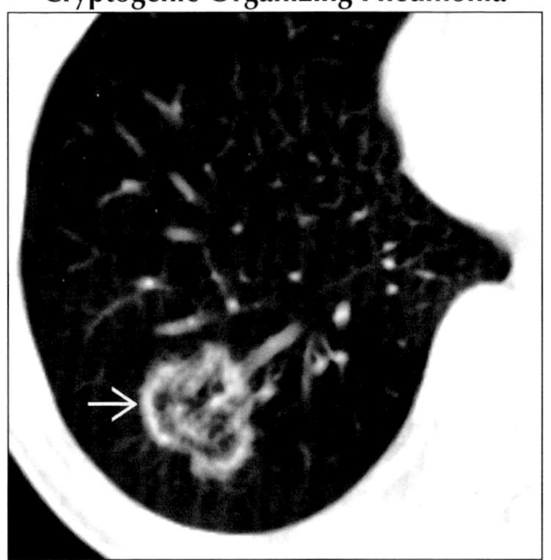

Chronic Eosinophilic Pneumonia

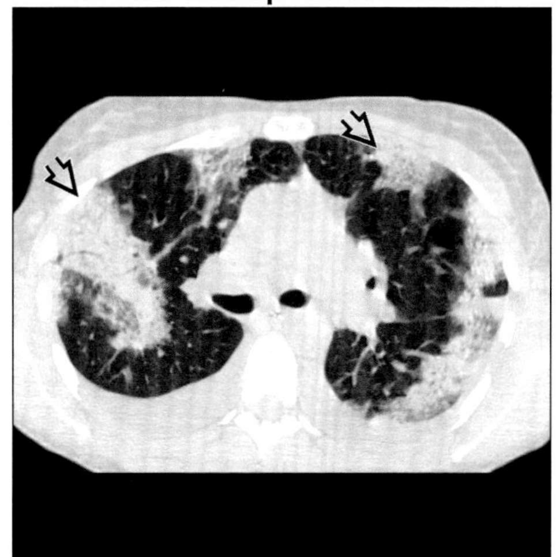

(Left) Axial NECT shows central ground-glass opacity with a peripheral rim of consolidation (atoll sign or reversed halo sign) in the right lower lobe ➔, typical of cryptogenic organizing pneumonia. *(Right)* Axial NECT shows peripheral consolidation ➔ and small pleural effusions.

Usual Interstitial Pneumonitis

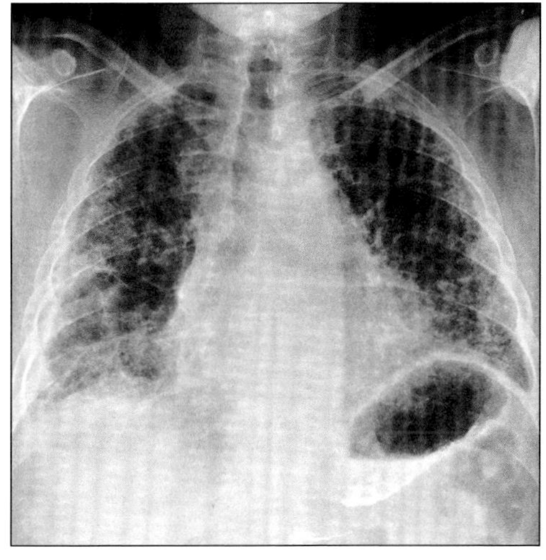

Usual Interstitial Pneumonitis

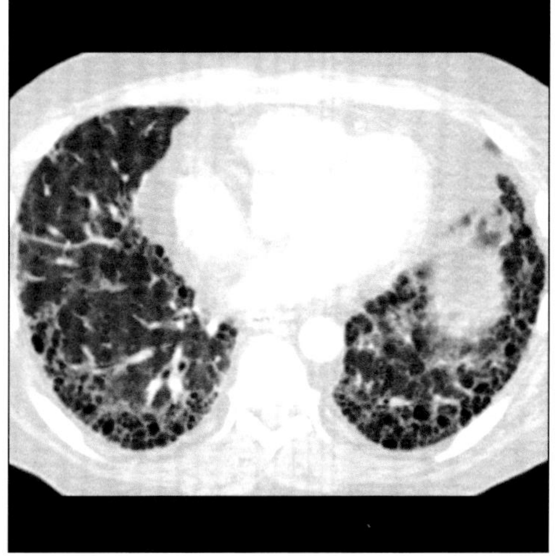

(Left) Frontal radiograph shows low lung volumes and peripheral and basilar predominant reticular opacities and cystic lucencies highly suggestive of interstitial lung fibrosis. *(Right)* Axial CECT shows peripheral predominant honeycombing with minimal patchy areas of ground-glass opacity highly suggestive of usual interstitial pneumonitis.

Desquamative Interstitial Pneumonia

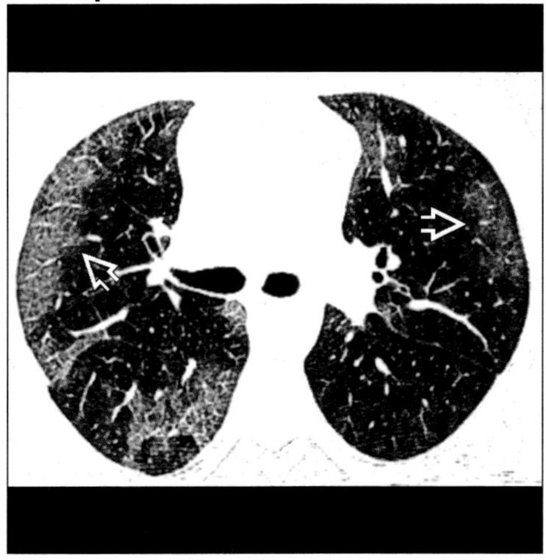

Amyloidosis

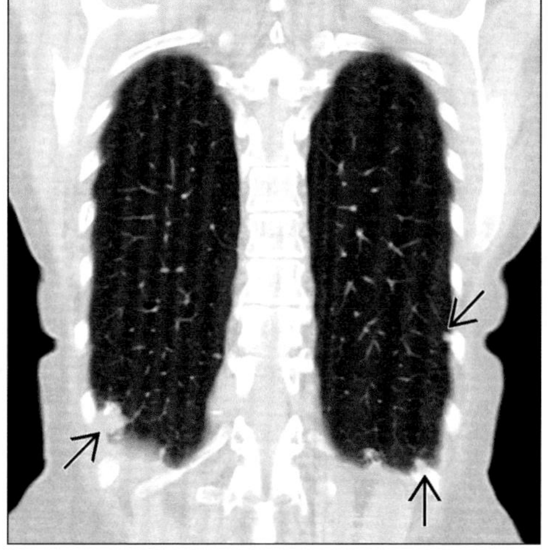

(Left) Axial HRCT shows patchy peripheral ground-glass opacities ➔ with superimposed areas of interlobular and intralobular septal thickening in this patient with history of smoking. *(Right)* Coronal NECT shows peripheral calcified and noncalcified pulmonary nodules ➔ consistent with nodular amyloidosis.

INTERSTITIAL PATTERN, HYPERINFLATION

DIFFERENTIAL DIAGNOSIS

Common
- Emphysema with Superimposed Process
- Asthma
- Viral or Atypical Pneumonia

Less Common
- Cystic Fibrosis (Mimic)
- Sarcoidosis

Rare but Important
- Lymphangiomyomatosis
- Pulmonary Langerhans Cell Histiocytosis

ESSENTIAL INFORMATION

Key Differential Diagnosis Issues
- Age, gender, and clinical presentation are key discriminators

Helpful Clues for Common Diagnoses
- **Emphysema with Superimposed Process**
  - Chronic bronchitis with bronchial wall thickening
  - Pulmonary edema
  - Pneumonia involving interstitium
  - Interstitial lung disease
    - Usual interstitial pneumonia
    - Desquamative interstitial pneumonia
    - Respiratory bronchiolitis
- **Asthma**
  - Normal radiograph is most common radiographic manifestation during acute attack
  - Radiographic findings slightly more common and more severe in children
    - Secondary to smaller diameter of bronchioles
  - Radiographs show
    - Hyperinflated lungs
    - Areas of atelectasis secondary to mucus plugging of small airways
    - Bronchial wall thickening
  - HRCT demonstrates
    - Bronchial wall thickening
    - Mosaic perfusion and air-trapping on expiratory images
    - Mucous plugging
    - May be complicated by allergic bronchopulmonary aspergillosis
- **Viral or Atypical Pneumonia**
  - Discriminators are age and symptoms of infection
  - Causes hyperinflation in small children secondary to
    - Poorly developed collateral ventilation
    - Small airway diameter that easily plugs with mucus
    - More abundant mucus production
  - Less frequent to see hyperinflation in adults
  - Interstitial abnormality secondary to
    - Inflammation of small airways
    - Peribronchial edema
  - Radiographic findings (more common in children)
    - Course markings radiating from hila into lungs (busy or dirty lungs)
    - Hyperinflation
    - Subsegmental atelectasis

Helpful Clues for Less Common Diagnoses
- **Cystic Fibrosis (Mimic)**
  - Common autosomal recessive disease
  - Causes recurrent infections in children
  - Early radiographic findings
    - Hyperinflation secondary to obstruction of small airways
    - Nodular or reticular opacities secondary to impaction of small airways
    - Tram-tracking indicating bronchial wall thickening or bronchiectasis
    - Upper lung predominant disease
  - Late radiographic findings
    - Pulmonary hypertension
    - Cystic bronchiectasis with more diffuse distribution
    - Mucoid impaction of larger airways
    - Atelectasis
  - HRCT findings
    - Bronchiectasis
    - Bronchial wall thickening
    - Tree-in-bud opacities secondary to mucoid impaction of small airways which ± indicate infection
    - Mucous plugging of larger airways
    - Mosaic perfusion and air-trapping on expiratory views indicates small airways involvement
- **Sarcoidosis**
  - Systemic granulomatous disease
  - May involve almost any organ
  - 90% have pulmonary involvement

- Radiographs demonstrate
  - Hilar and right paratracheal lymphadenopathy ± calcification
  - Well- or ill-defined nodules with upper lung predominance
  - Lungs may be hyperinflated secondary to small airways involvement by noncaseating granulomas
- HRCT findings
  - Upper lung predominance
  - Perilymphatic distribution of nodules (along fissures, subpleural lung, and bronchovascular bundles)
  - Uncommonly a random distribution of nodules
  - Nodular bronchial wall thickening
  - Small airways involvement demonstrated by mosaic perfusion or air-trapping

Helpful Clues for Rare Diagnoses

- **Lymphangiomyomatosis**
  - Exclusively women of childbearing age
  - May exacerbate during pregnancy
  - Identical disease can be seen in tuberous sclerosis
  - Radiographic findings
    - Normal or large lungs
    - Normal radiograph early
    - Fine or coarse reticular opacities with diffuse distribution
    - Pneumothorax (up to 80%)
    - Pleural effusions (chylous)
  - HRCT findings
    - Diffuse distribution of round cysts
    - Cysts start small and increase in size with disease progression
    - ± chylous pleural effusions (indistinguishable from simple pleural fluid)
    - ± pneumothorax
    - 10-15% have angiomyolipomas in kidneys
    - ± mediastinal or retroperitoneal lymphadenopathy
- **Pulmonary Langerhans Cell Histiocytosis**
  - 20-40-year-old male Caucasian cigarette smoker presenting with cough and dyspnea
  - Peribronchiolar proliferation of Langerhans cells
  - Radiographic findings
    - Nodular or reticulonodular opacities in upper 2/3 of lung
    - Preserved or increased lung volumes
    - Spares lung bases
    - 30% have pneumothoraces
  - HRCT findings
    - Centrilobular nodules ± central cavities
    - Cystic spaces ≤ 10 mm in diameter
    - Round or bizarrely shaped cysts
    - Spares costophrenic sulci
    - ± pneumothorax
    - Rare association with lytic bone lesions
    - Disease progresses from nodules to cavitating nodules to cysts
    - Cysts thought to represent enlarged airway lumina (paracicatricial emphysema)

Emphysema with Superimposed Process

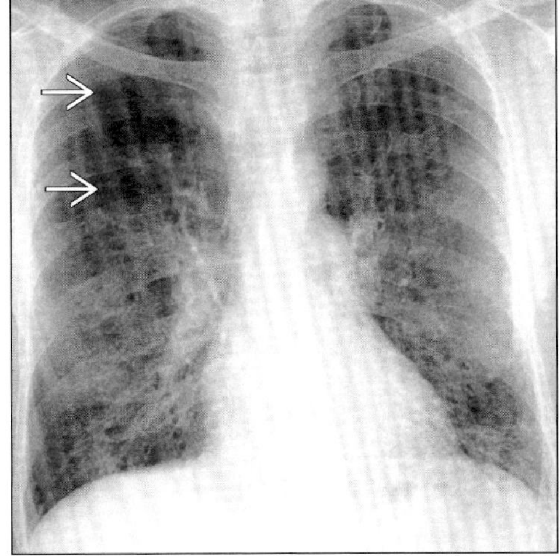

Frontal radiograph shows increased linear opacities bilaterally, representing bronchial wall thickening, and increased lucency in the right upper lung ➔, representing emphysema.

Emphysema with Superimposed Process

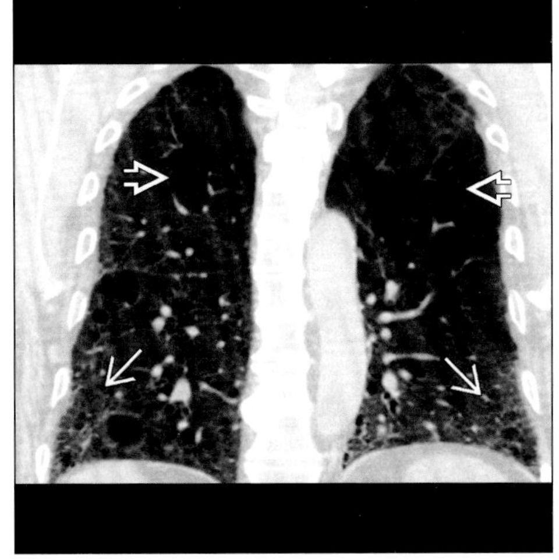

Coronal NECT shows subpleural and basal predominant reticular opacities and architectural distortion ➔ in this patient with usual interstitial pneumonia. Note emphysema in the upper lungs ➔.

INTERSTITIAL PATTERN, HYPERINFLATION

*(**Left**) Frontal radiograph shows hyperinflated lungs and distended central pulmonary arteries ➡, consistent with pulmonary arterial hypertension due to chronic hypoxia. Streaky opacities at the bases likely represent bronchial wall thickening ➡. (**Right**) Frontal radiograph shows emphysema complicated by DIP. Note slight increase in interstitial opacities in the lung bases ➡ from the chronic inflammation associated with smoking cigarettes.*

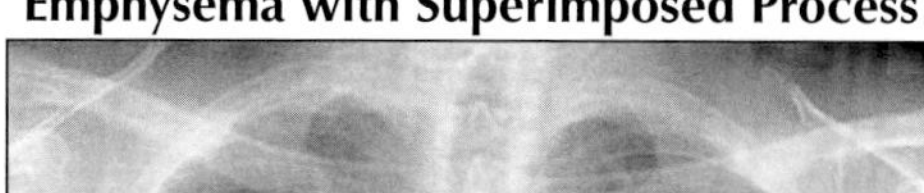

Emphysema with Superimposed Process

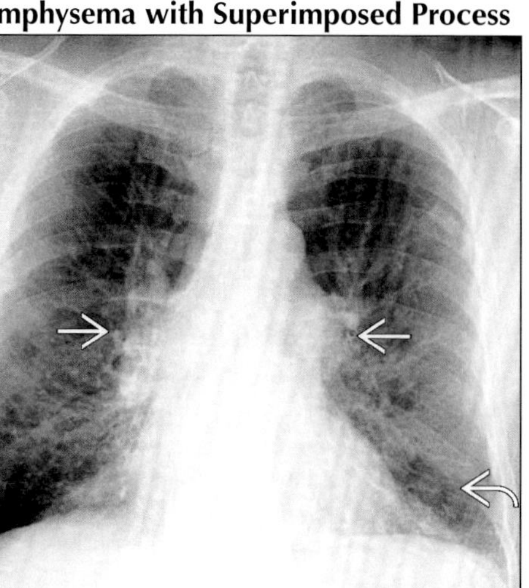

Emphysema with Superimposed Process

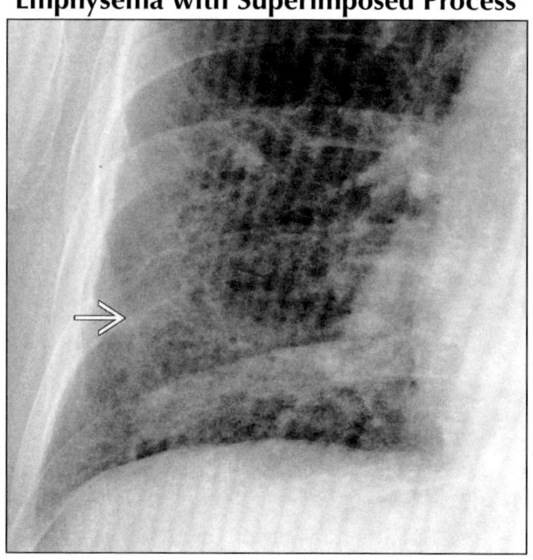

*(**Left**) Frontal radiograph shows subtle diffuse increased reticular pattern in an otherwise normal examination. (**Right**) Axial HRCT shows an expiratory image with multifocal areas of sharply marginated air-trapping ➡ explaining the hyperinflated lungs. Note the geographic distribution and vessel caliber difference between regions.*

Asthma

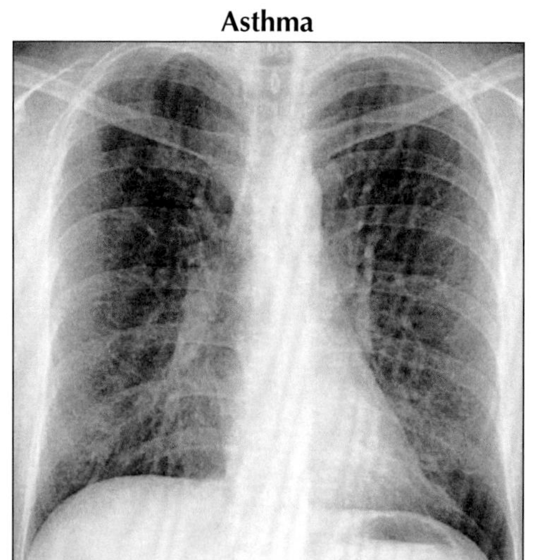

Asthma

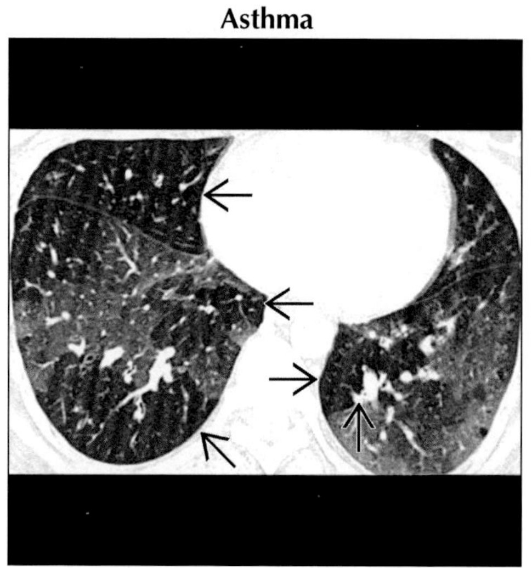

*(**Left**) Frontal radiograph shows lung hyperinflation. Note bronchial wall thickening ➡ in this patient with longstanding asthma. (**Right**) Frontal radiograph shows typical radiographic features of influenza A viral pneumonia. Note faint streaky opacities in the right lung ➡. Clinical history is key in diagnosing this patient.*

Asthma

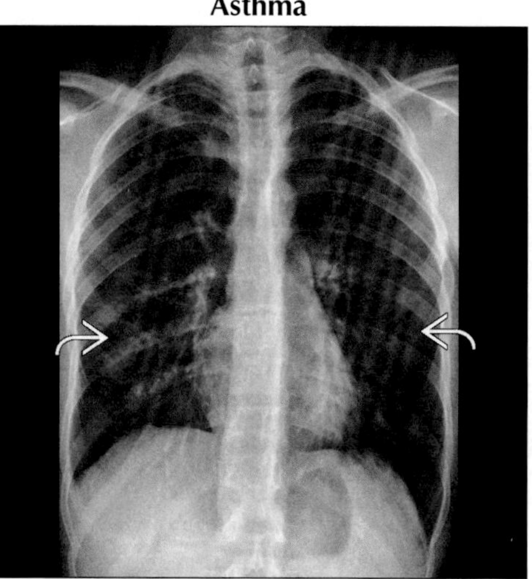

Viral or Atypical Pneumonia

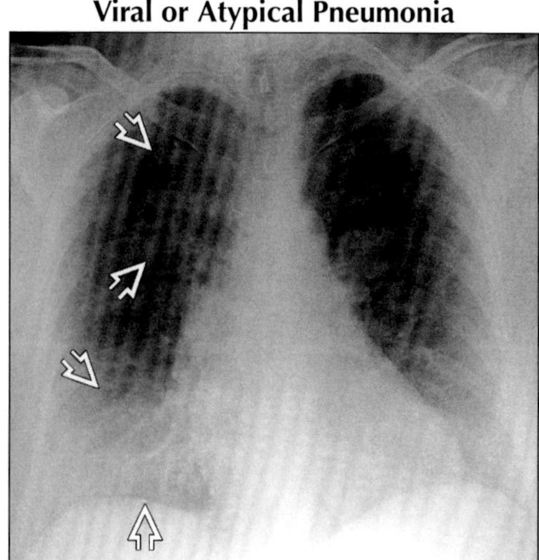

Viral or Atypical Pneumonia

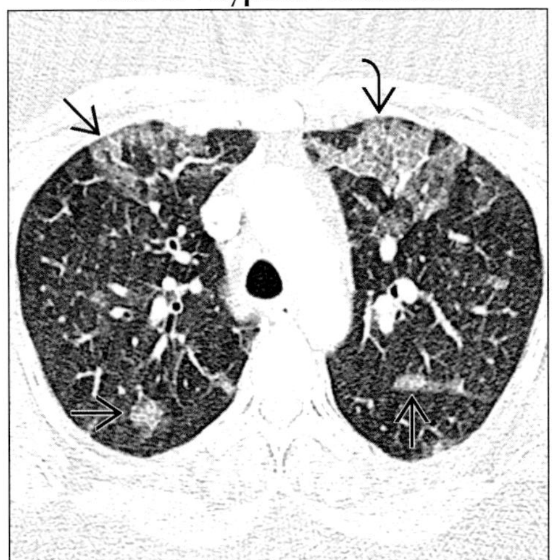

Cystic Fibrosis (Mimic)

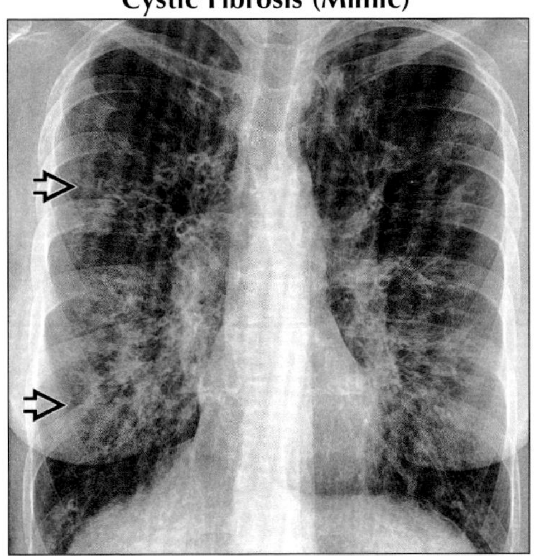

(Left) *Axial NECT shows bilateral ground-glass opacities in the lungs ➔ related to influenza A. Some thickening of the peripheral intralobular interstitium is also visible at some locations ➔.* ***(Right)*** *Frontal radiograph shows tram-tracking, rings, and small opacities ➔. Lungs are hyperinflated. Findings are largely the result of bronchiectasis with associated bronchial wall thickening.*

Cystic Fibrosis (Mimic)

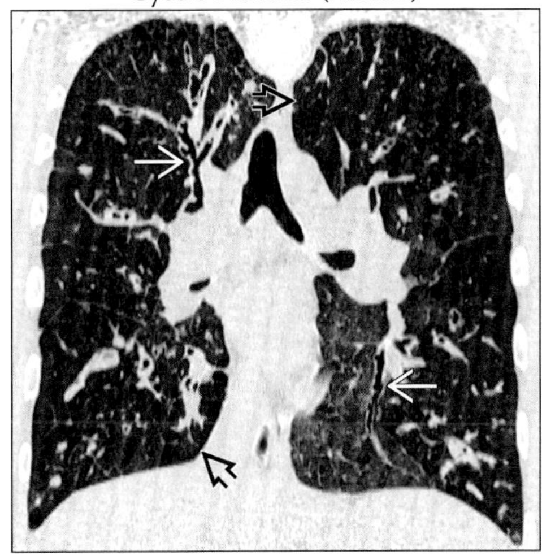

Cystic Fibrosis (Mimic)

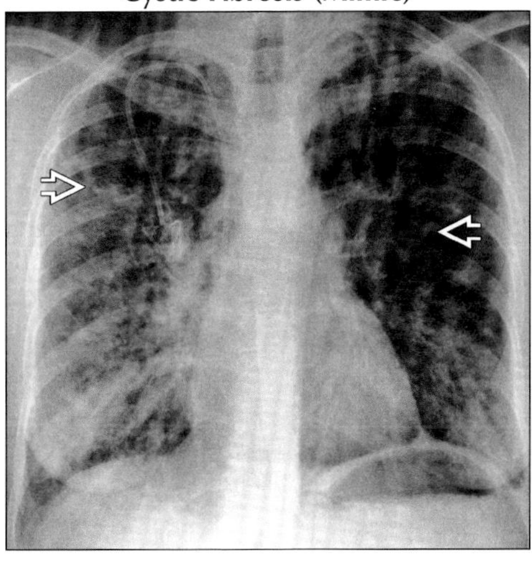

(Left) *Coronal HRCT shows multilobar, distorted, bronchiectatic airways ➔ and associated mosaic perfusion ➔ secondary to small airways obstruction with resultant decrease in perfusion to these areas.* ***(Right)*** *Frontal radiograph shows diffuse mucus plugging and bronchiectasis ➔. Note mildly hyperinflated lungs.*

Cystic Fibrosis (Mimic)

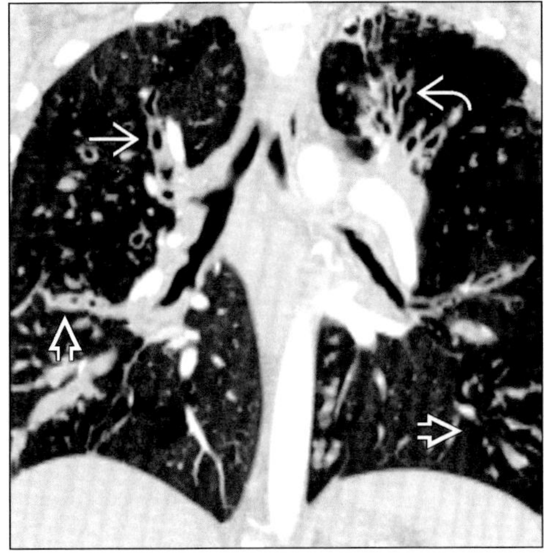

Sarcoidosis

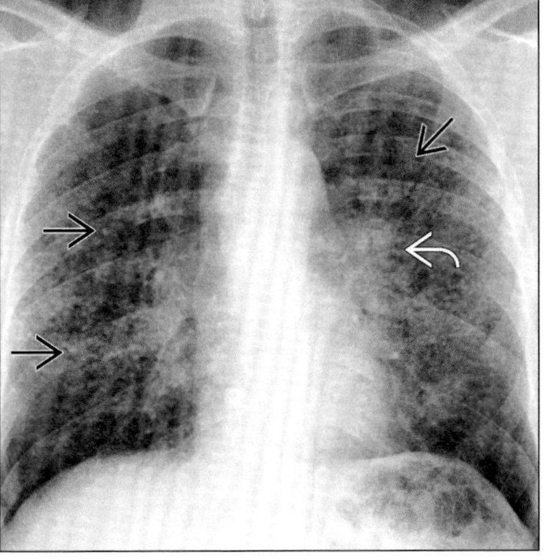

(Left) *Coronal CECT shows extensive diffuse bronchial wall thickening ➔, multilobar bronchiectasis ➔, and mucus plugging ➔. Patchy differential attenuation is secondary to small airways disease and mosaic perfusion.* ***(Right)*** *Frontal radiograph shows small nodular opacities ➔ in the mid lungs and slightly enlarged hili ➔ from lymphadenopathy. The lungs are mildly hyperinflated.*

INTERSTITIAL PATTERN, HYPERINFLATION

(Left) Axial HRCT shows typical subpleural nodules and peribronchovascular nodules ➡ extending from the hila. There is sparing of the anterior lung ➡ making this a perilymphatic pattern of nodules and not a random distribution. *(Right)* Frontal radiograph shows bilateral hilar and right paratracheal adenopathy ➡ and focal consolidation in the left upper lobe ➡ from nodules coalescing.

Sarcoidosis

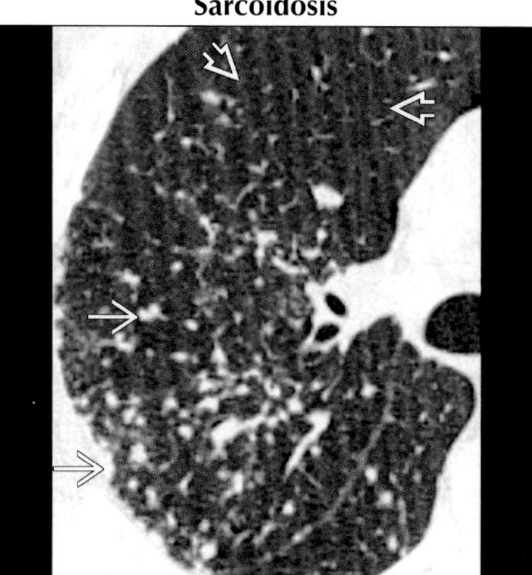

Sarcoidosis

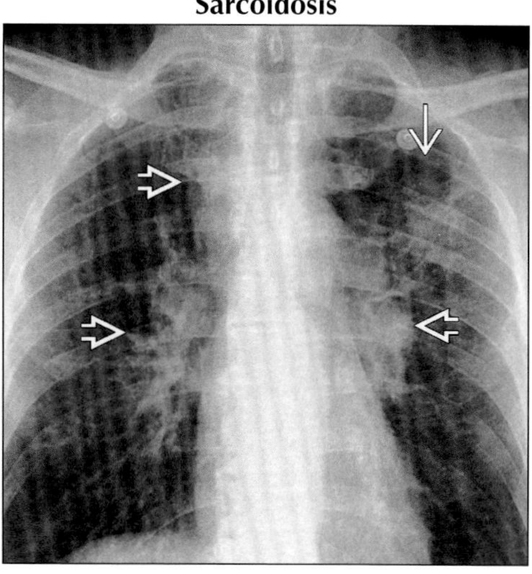

(Left) Frontal radiograph shows linear and faint nodular opacities scattered throughout the lungs, which are large lungs. *(Right)* Coronal NECT shows near-uniform distribution and appearance of innumerable thin-walled, round cysts ➡ throughout all lobes bilaterally. No lung nodules are present. Note large lung volumes.

Lymphangiomyomatosis

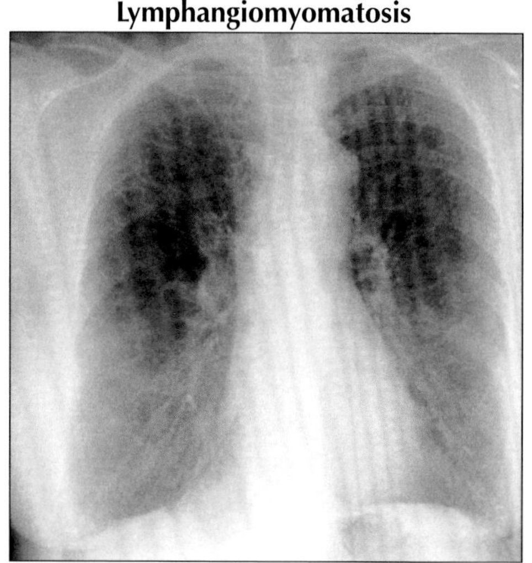

Lymphangiomyomatosis

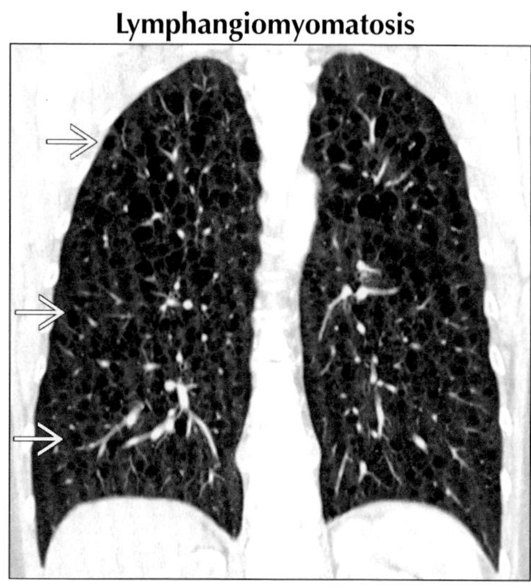

(Left) Axial HRCT demonstrates numerous thin-walled cysts ➡. Note well-defined wall, with no centrilobular core structure, helping to differentiate this appearance from centrilobular emphysema. *(Right)* Frontal radiograph shows extensive "interstitial thickening" ➡ as a result of the overlap of the underlying variable-sized lung cysts ➡.

Lymphangiomyomatosis

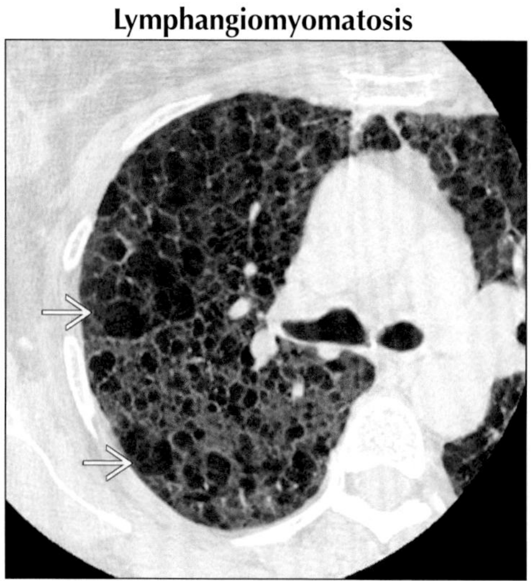

Lymphangiomyomatosis

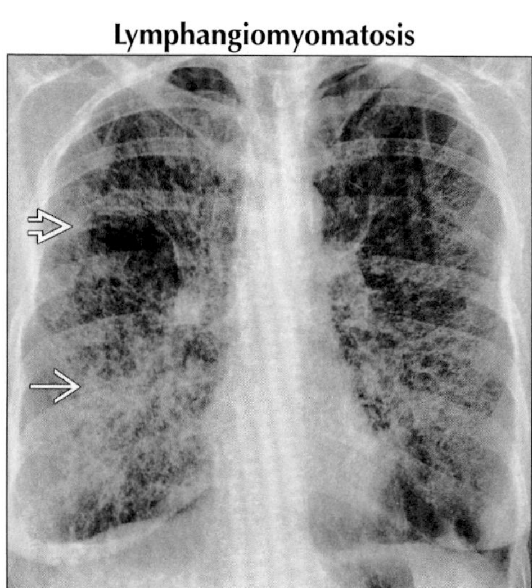

Lymphangiomyomatosis

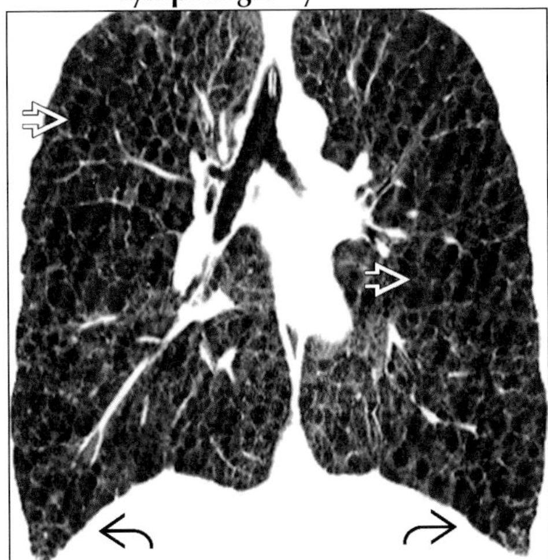

Pulmonary Langerhans Cell Histiocytosis

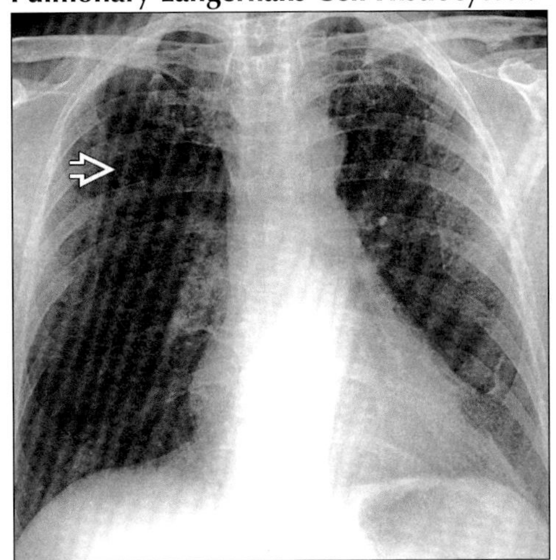

*(**Left**) Coronal HRCT shows diffuse distribution of cysts and marked hyperinflation with flattening of the diaphragms. (**Right**) Frontal radiograph shows subtle reticular opacities in both upper lobes. Note mild hyperinflation and sparing of the lower lungs.*

Pulmonary Langerhans Cell Histiocytosis

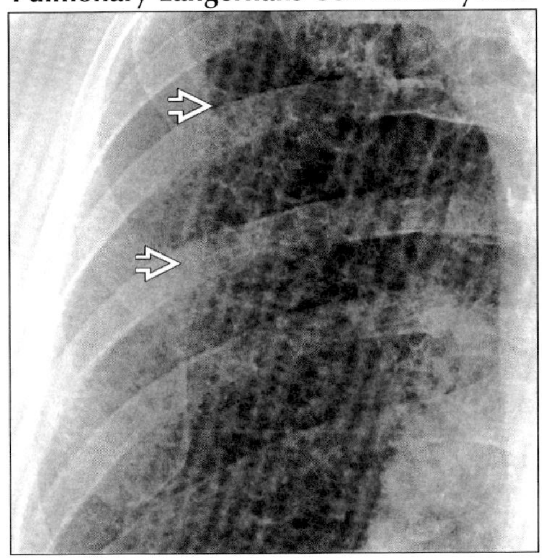

Pulmonary Langerhans Cell Histiocytosis

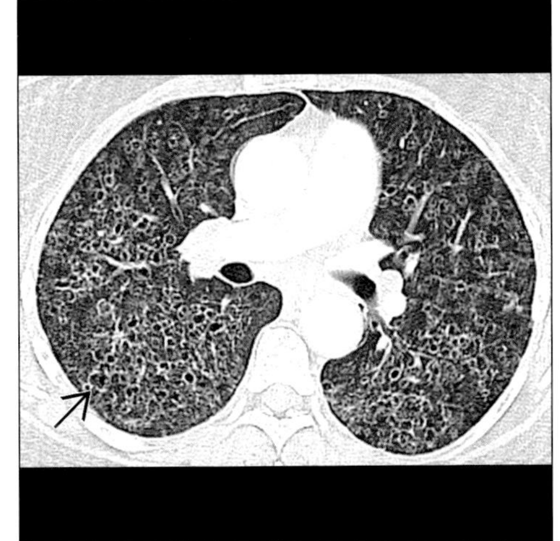

*(**Left**) Frontal radiograph shows a magnified view of the right upper lung with multiple irregular reticular opacities representing superimposition of the innumerable cyst walls. (**Right**) Axial HRCT shows a severe case with innumerable thick-walled, somewhat irregularly shaped cysts, more abundant in upper lobes. Some appear as cavitating nodules.*

Pulmonary Langerhans Cell Histiocytosis

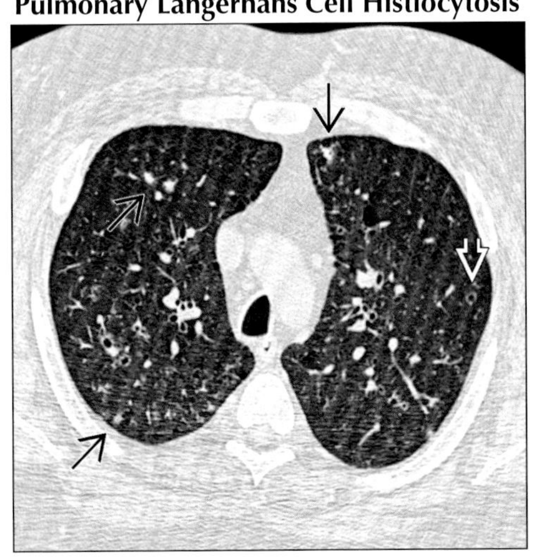

Pulmonary Langerhans Cell Histiocytosis

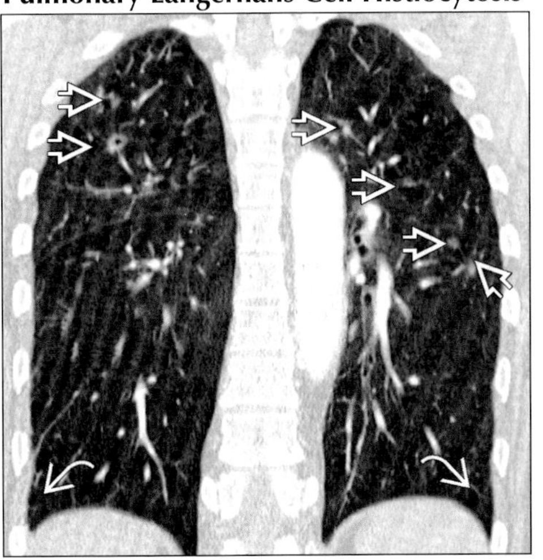

*(**Left**) Axial HRCT shows a milder case with multiple centrilobular nodules and cavities with variable shape and wall thickness. (**Right**) Coronal CECT shows upper lung distribution of nodules. Note hyperinflation and sparing of the costophrenic angles.*

INTERSTITIAL PATTERN, MEDIASTINAL-HILAR ADENOPATHY

DIFFERENTIAL DIAGNOSIS

Common
- Sarcoidosis
- Lymphangitic Carcinomatosis
- Cystic Fibrosis (Mimic)

Less Common
- Silicosis/Coal Worker's Pneumoconiosis
- Usual Interstitial Pneumonia

Rare but Important
- Berylliosis
- Lymphocytic Interstitial Pneumonia
- Diffuse Pulmonary Lymphangiomatosis
- Pulmonary Langerhans Cell Histiocytosis
- Lymphangioleiomyomatosis

ESSENTIAL INFORMATION

Key Differential Diagnosis Issues
- Age of patient
- Gender
- Race
- Presenting symptoms

Helpful Clues for Common Diagnoses
- **Sarcoidosis**
  - Systemic granulomatous disease of unknown etiology
  - Common demographics
    - Women
    - Child-bearing age
    - African-American race
  - Radiography
    - Symmetric hilar and mediastinal lymphadenopathy
    - Mid to upper lobe reticulonodular opacities in ≤ 50% of patients
  - HRCT
    - Bilateral hilar and mediastinal lymphadenopathy
    - Perilymphatic nodules involving fissures, subpleural lung, and bronchovascular bundles
    - Air-trapping secondary to granulomas obstructing small airways
- **Lymphangitic Carcinomatosis**
  - Tumor growth in pulmonary lymphatics
  - Common causes include metastases from
    - Breast carcinoma
    - Bronchogenic carcinoma
    - Pancreatic carcinoma
    - Gastric carcinoma
    - Thyroid carcinoma
    - Adenocarcinoma of unknown primary
  - Unilateral disease occurs most commonly with lung carcinoma
  - Radiography
    - Reticulonodular opacities (unilateral or bilateral)
    - Hilar &/or mediastinal lymphadenopathy
    - Pleural effusions
  - HRCT
    - Nodular or beaded interlobular septal thickening
    - Perilymphatic nodules
    - Hilar or mediastinal lymphadenopathy in 30-50% of patients
    - Pleural effusions
- **Cystic Fibrosis (Mimic)**
  - Autosomal recessive condition occurring primarily in Caucasians
    - Results in defective chloride transport across epithelial membranes
    - Causes variety of problems involving respiratory and gastrointestinal systems
  - Radiograph
    - Large lungs with bronchiectasis or bronchial wall thickening mimicking interstitial pattern
    - Small peribronchovascular nodular opacities secondary to impaction of small airways
  - Prominent hila indicate
    - Lymphadenopathy from recurrent infections
    - Enlarged pulmonary arteries from pulmonary hypertension
  - Early disease predominates in upper lobes
  - Uncontrollable hemoptysis may necessitate bronchial artery embolization

Helpful Clues for Less Common Diagnoses
- **Silicosis/Coal Worker's Pneumoconiosis**
  - Radiography
    - Well-circumscribed small nodules predominating in upper lungs
    - Small percentage of pulmonary nodules may calcify
    - Nodules may coalesce to form masses with upward retraction of hila; so-called "progressive massive fibrosis"
    - Hilar lymphadenopathy

- HRCT
  - Centrilobular and subpleural nodules
  - Posterior upper lung predominance
  - 40% of patients have hilar or mediastinal lymphadenopathy
  - 5% of lymph nodes show peripheral "egg shell" calcification
- **Usual Interstitial Pneumonia**
  - Basilar and subpleural predominant fibrosis with honeycombing
  - Mild mediastinal lymphadenopathy in majority of cases

Helpful Clues for Rare Diagnoses

- **Berylliosis**
  - Identical appearance to sarcoidosis
    - Perilymphatic nodules, lymphadenopathy, and noncaseating granulomas
    - Upper lung predominant disease
  - Key discriminator is occupational exposure to beryllium
    - Workers in nuclear power, ceramics, aerospace, and electronics
    - Occurs most commonly 10-15 years after exposure
  - Most common symptom is dyspnea
  - Positive beryllium lymphocyte proliferation test via blood or bronchoalveolar lavage
- **Lymphocytic Interstitial Pneumonia**
  - Strong association with Sjögren syndrome
  - AIDS defining in children
  - Diffuse distribution
  - Poorly defined centrilobular nodules
  - Diffuse or patchy ground-glass opacity
  - Isolated or diffuse cystic lung disease
  - ± mediastinal or hilar lymphadenopathy
- **Diffuse Pulmonary Lymphangiomatosis**
  - Congenital lymphatic disorder
  - Diffuse smooth interlobular septal thickening
  - Mild mediastinal lymphadenopathy
  - 50% have associated pleural effusions
- **Pulmonary Langerhans Cell Histiocytosis**
  - Young male smokers
  - Radiography
    - Normal or large lungs
    - Nodular opacities in upper 2/3 of lung
    - Interstitial pattern results from "moire effect" of superimposed cysts
    - Pneumothoraces in 30% of cases
  - HRCT
    - Bizarrely shaped cysts
    - Relative sparing of lung bases
    - Paracicatricial emphysema
    - Centrilobular nodules ± cavitation
- **Lymphangioleiomyomatosis**
  - Women of child-bearing age
  - Radiography and HRCT
    - Pleural effusions
    - Pneumothoraces
    - Uniformly distributed similar-sized cysts
    - Interstitial pattern results from "moire effect" of superimposed cysts
    - Mediastinal or retroperitoneal lymphadenopathy

Sarcoidosis

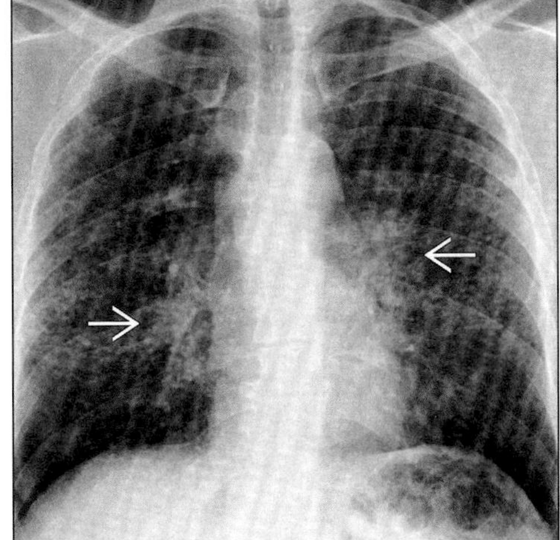

Frontal radiograph shows bilateral mid lung nodular opacities. Note the symmetric hilar enlargement from lymphadenopathy ➡.

Sarcoidosis

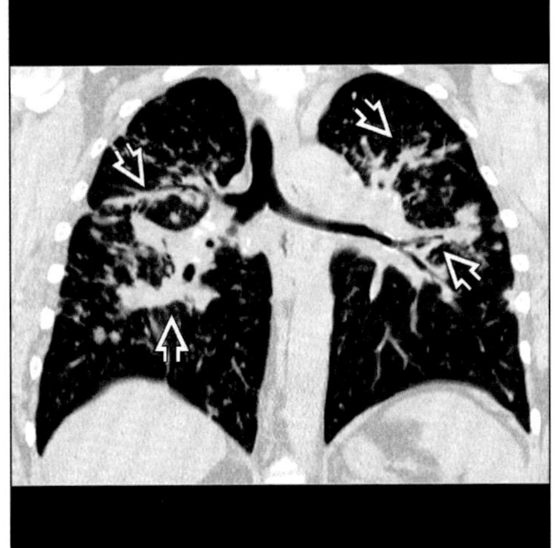

Coronal NECT shows marked nodular thickening along bronchovascular bundles ➡ indicating a perilymphatic distribution.

INTERSTITIAL PATTERN, MEDIASTINAL-HILAR ADENOPATHY

Sarcoidosis

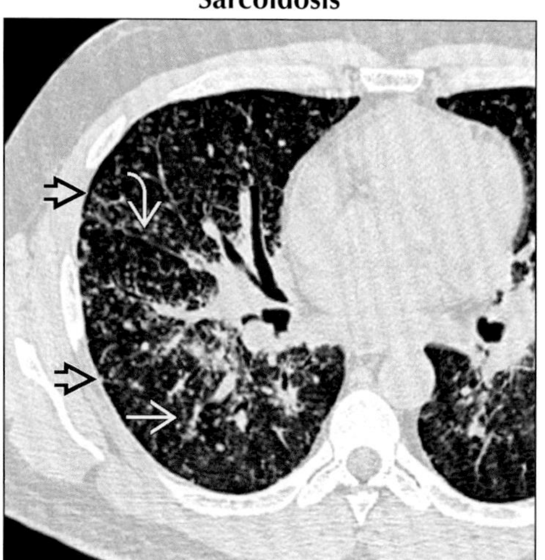

Sarcoidosis

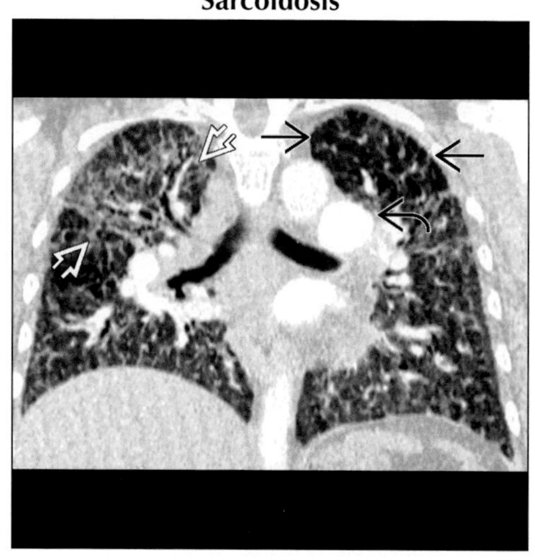

(Left) *Axial HRCT shows a perilymphatic distribution of nodules along interlobular septa ⇨, the major fissure ➢, and bronchovascular bundles ➡. **(Right)** Coronal CECT shows diffuse interstitial thickening most marked in the right upper lobe ➡. Enlarged pulmonary arteries are secondary to pulmonary hypertension ⇗. Lucency in the left upper lobe is secondary to mosaic perfusion from small airways involvement by sarcoid granulomas →.*

Lymphangitic Carcinomatosis

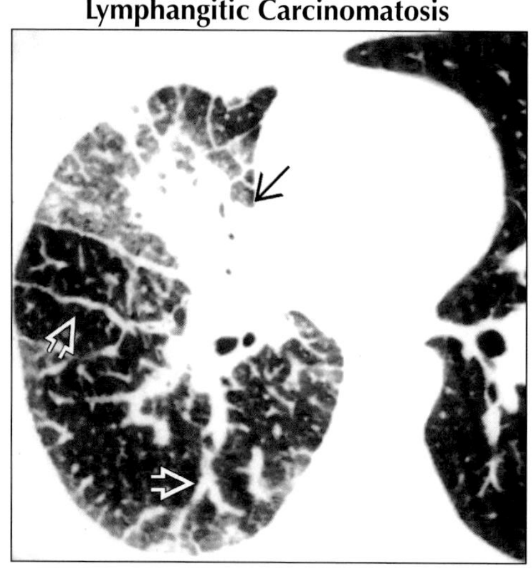

Lymphangitic Carcinomatosis

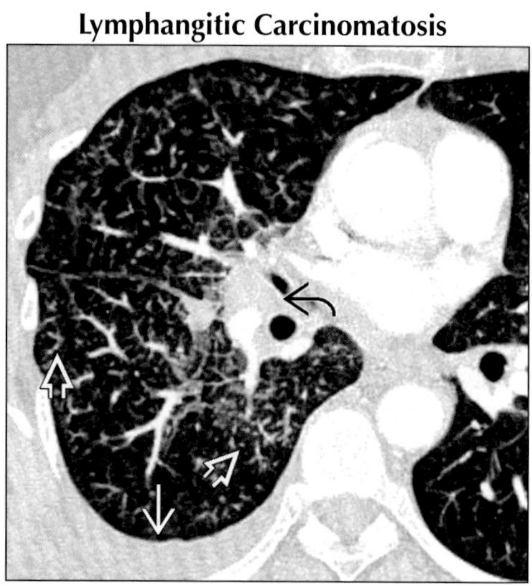

(Left) *Axial HRCT shows diffuse lobulated bronchovascular bundle thickening ➡ from adenocarcinoma of the lung →. Left lung is normal. **(Right)** Axial CECT shows interstitial thickening in the right lung ➡, including the bronchovascular bundles and interlobular septa. Note the right pleural effusion ➡ and right hilar lymphadenopathy ⇗ in this patient with bronchogenic carcinoma.*

Lymphangitic Carcinomatosis

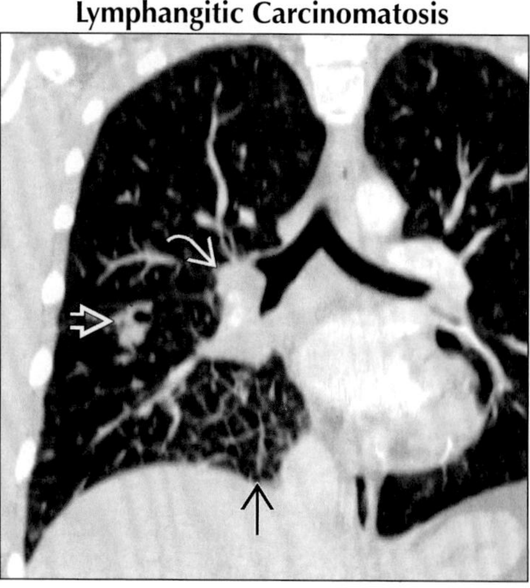

Cystic Fibrosis (Mimic)

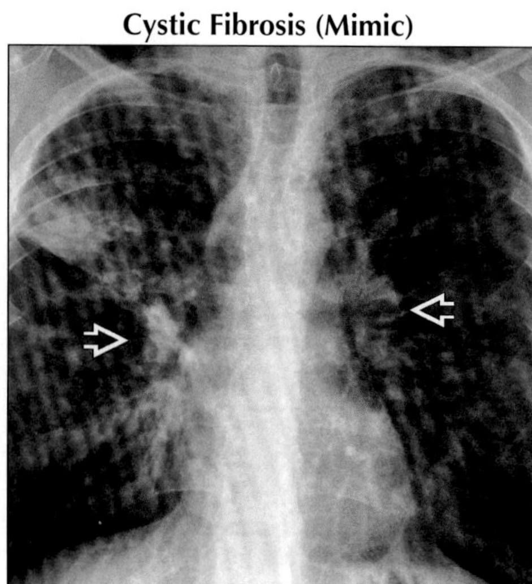

(Left) *Coronal CECT shows the primary cavitary squamous cell carcinoma ➡, lymphadenopathy ➡, and focal thickening of interlobular septa → in the right lower lobe. **(Right)** Frontal radiograph shows upper lobe predominant bronchiectasis and bronchial wall thickening, which mimics an interstitial abnormality. Note the bilateral hilar prominence ➡, likely lymphadenopathy from longstanding recurrent infections.*

Cystic Fibrosis (Mimic)

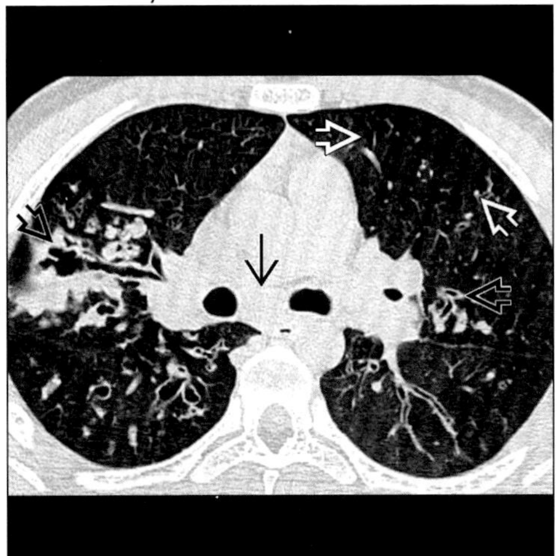

Silicosis/Coal Worker's Pneumoconiosis

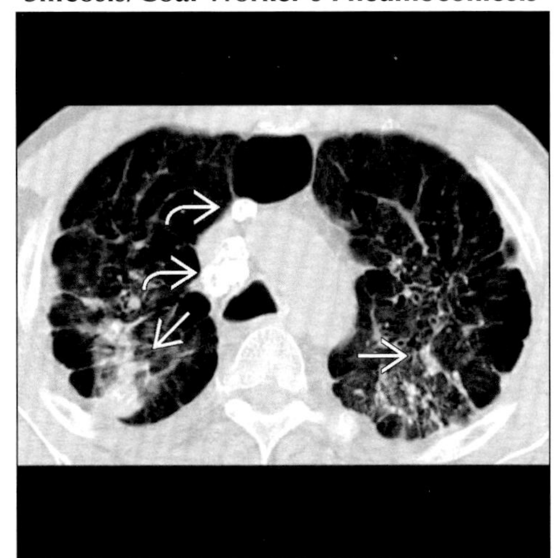

(Left) Axial NECT shows bilateral bronchiectasis and bronchial wall thickening ➩. Note the subcarinal lymph node enlargement → and mosaic perfusion ➩ reflecting small airways disease. *(Right)* Axial NECT shows parenchymal opacities from progressive massive fibrosis ➡. Note the calcification of mediastinal lymph nodes ➡ and subpleural nodules in this patient with silicosis.

Usual Interstitial Pneumonia

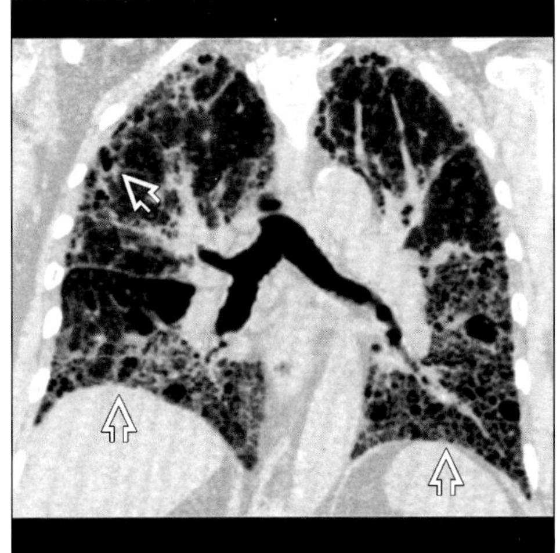

Usual Interstitial Pneumonia

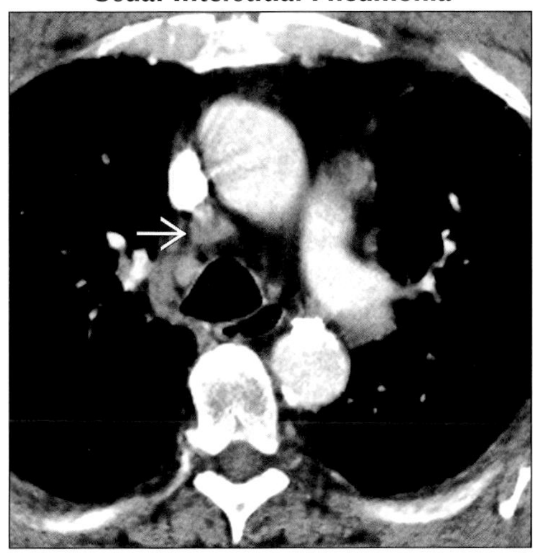

(Left) Coronal HRCT shows basilar predominant fibrosis with peripheral honeycombing ➡. Note the diffuse nature of disease, but still most severe in the lower lungs. Patchy areas of well preserved lung are common. *(Right)* Axial CECT shows mild enlargement of mediastinal lymph nodes ➡.

Berylliosis

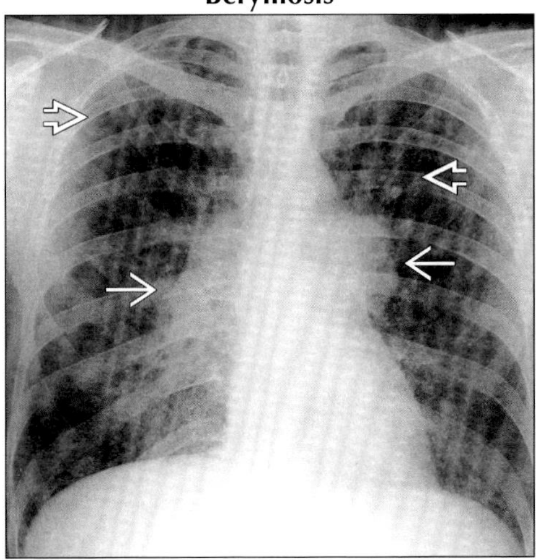

Berylliosis

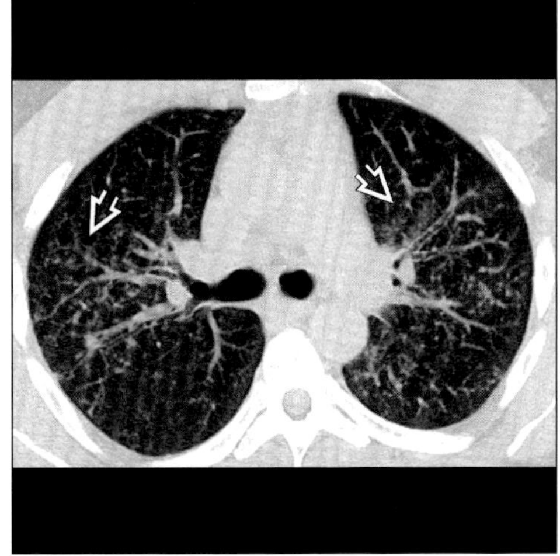

(Left) Frontal radiograph shows bilateral hilar lymphadenopathy ➡ and diffuse nodular interstitial thickening ➡ most predominant in the upper lungs. *(Right)* Axial MIP shows the relationship of nodules ➡ to the bronchovascular bundles indicating a perilymphatic distribution of nodules.

INTERSTITIAL PATTERN, MEDIASTINAL-HILAR ADENOPATHY

Lymphocytic Interstitial Pneumonia

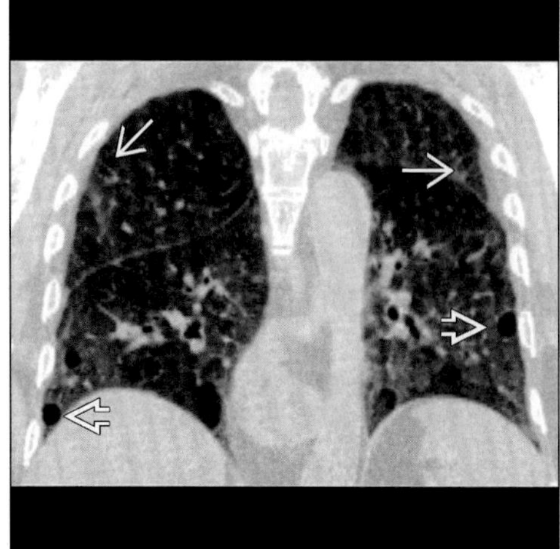

Lymphocytic Interstitial Pneumonia

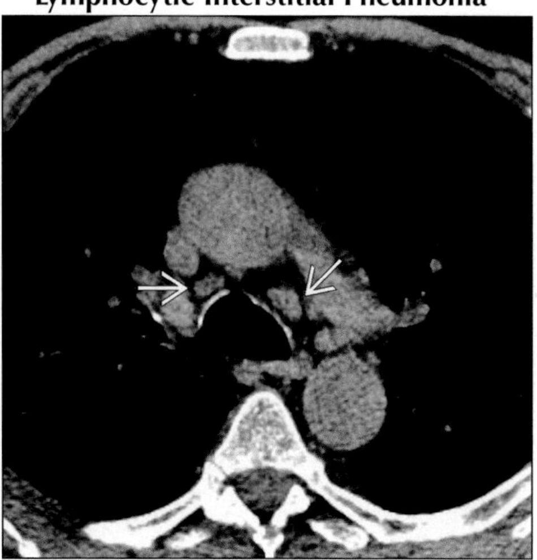

*(**Left**) Coronal NECT shows CT features of Dilantin toxicity causing lymphocytic interstitial pneumonia. Note the slight overall increase in lung density, septal thickening, and nodules of ground-glass opacity ➔. Scattered cysts ➔ are seen in the lower lungs. (**Right**) Axial NECT in the same patient shows mild enlargement of mediastinal lymph nodes ➔.*

Lymphocytic Interstitial Pneumonia

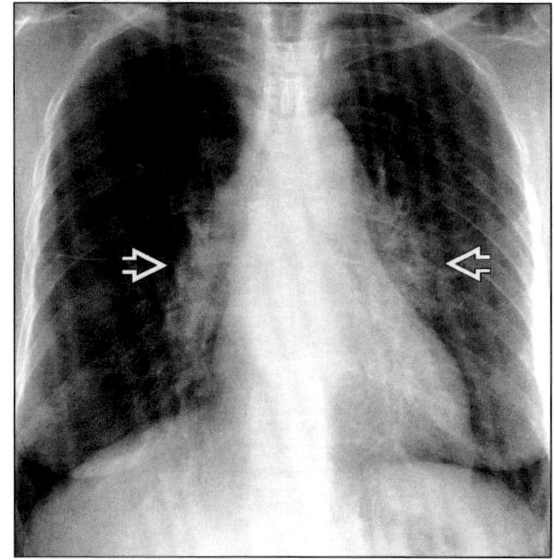

Lymphocytic Interstitial Pneumonia

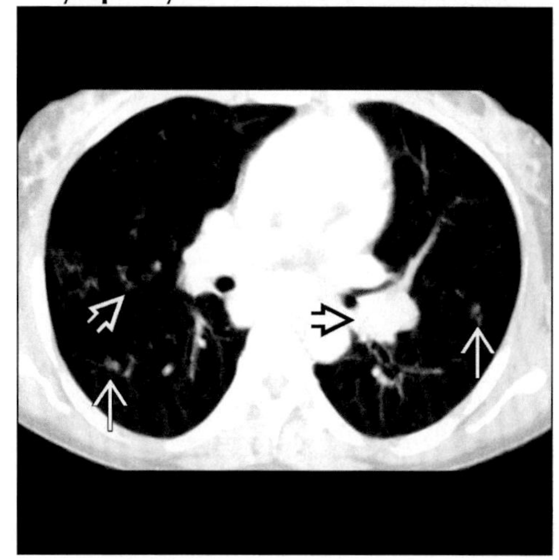

*(**Left**) Frontal radiograph shows bilateral hilar lymphadenopathy ➔. (**Right**) Axial CECT shows a thin-walled cyst ➔ and pulmonary nodules ➔. Left hilar prominence ➔ is secondary to lymphadenopathy and better seen on mediastinal windows.*

Diffuse Pulmonary Lymphangiomatosis

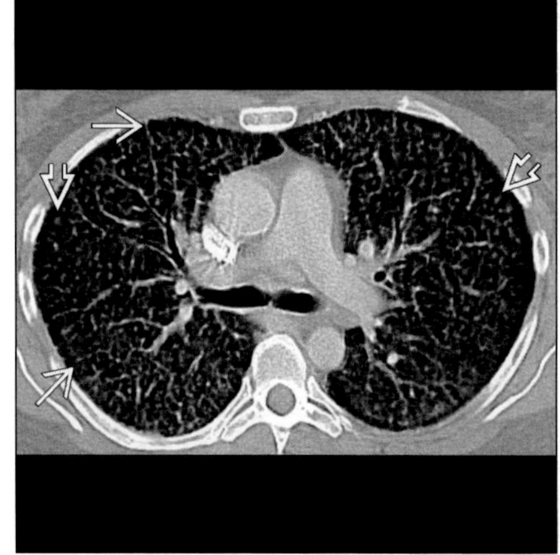

Diffuse Pulmonary Lymphangiomatosis

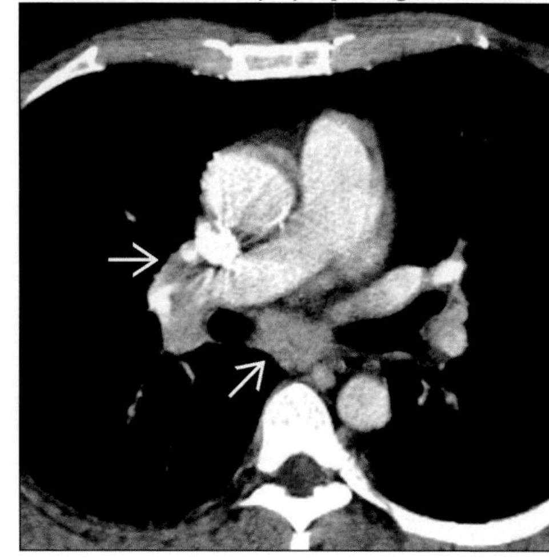

*(**Left**) Axial CECT shows centrilobular nodules ➔ and smooth interlobular septal thickening ➔. (**Right**) Axial CECT shows mediastinal lymph nodes and effacement of mediastinal fat ➔.*

Diffuse Pulmonary Lymphangiomatosis

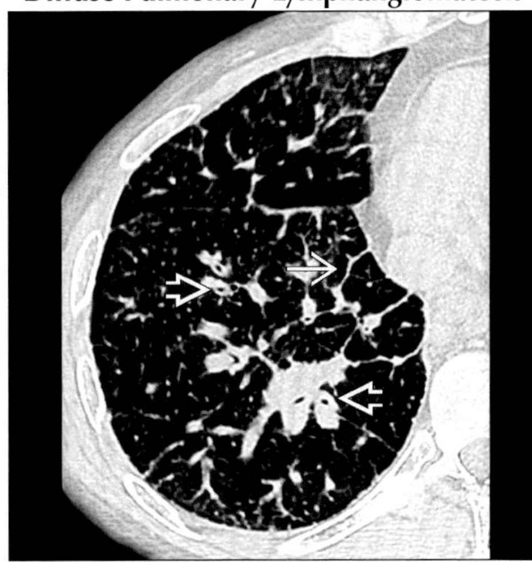

Diffuse Pulmonary Lymphangiomatosis

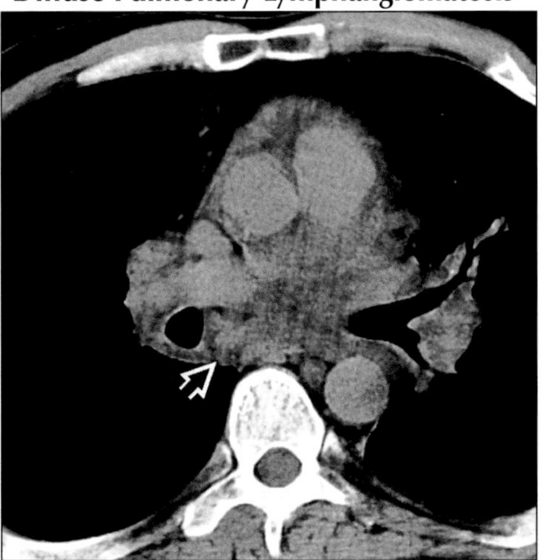

(Left) *Axial NECT shows diffuse smooth interlobular septal thickening* ➡ *and thickened bronchovascular bundles* ➡. ***(Right)*** *Axial NECT shows diffusely enlarged mediastinal and hilar lymph nodes* ➡, *without evidence of necrosis.*

Pulmonary Langerhans Cell Histiocytosis

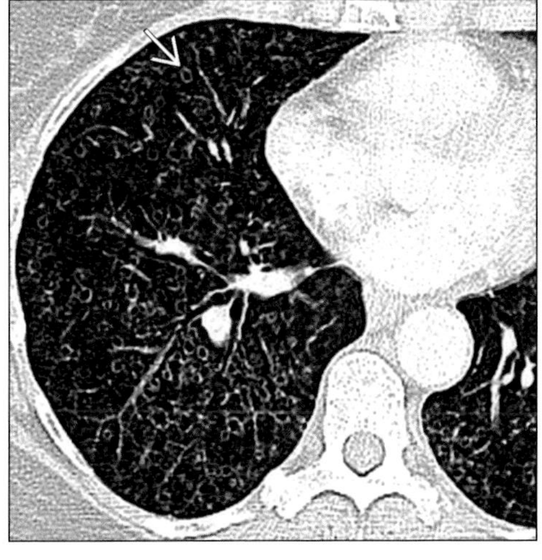

Pulmonary Langerhans Cell Histiocytosis

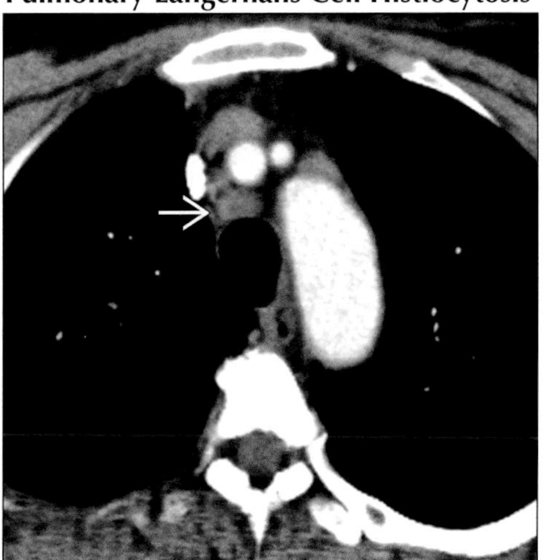

(Left) *Axial HRCT shows multiple cysts* ➡ *in the upper lobes in this young smoker. There was sparing of the costophrenic angles.* ***(Right)*** *Axial CECT in the same patient shows mildly enlarged lymph nodes* ➡.

Lymphangioleiomyomatosis

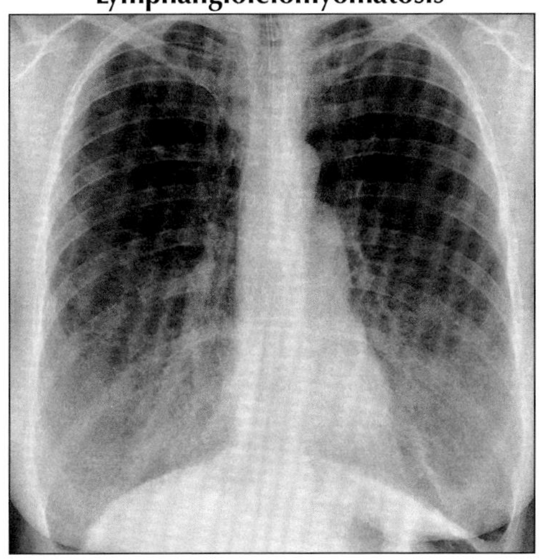

Lymphangioleiomyomatosis

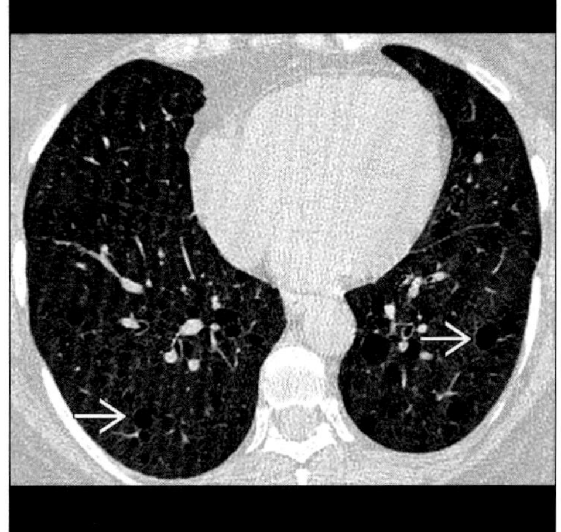

(Left) *Frontal radiograph shows marked hyperinflation of the lungs. Note the subtle reticular opacities best seen in the lower lungs corresponding to cysts on CT.* ***(Right)*** *Axial HRCT shows multiple uniformly distributed thin-walled cysts* ➡ *that vary slightly in size.*

INTERSTITIAL PATTERN, PLEURAL THICKENING AND EFFUSION

DIFFERENTIAL DIAGNOSIS

Common
- Pulmonary Edema

Less Common
- Lymphangitic Carcinomatosis
- Asbestosis
- Systemic Lupus Erythematosus
- Rheumatoid Arthritis

Rare but Important
- Lymphangiomyomatosis
- Diffuse Pulmonary Lymphangiomatosis
- Pulmonary Venoocclusive Disease
- Pulmonary Capillary Hemangiomatosis
- Erdheim Chester Disease

ESSENTIAL INFORMATION

Key Differential Diagnosis Issues
- Chronicity of process and response to diuretics helps guide differential

Helpful Clues for Common Diagnoses
- **Pulmonary Edema**
  - Caused by increased capillary hydrostatic pressure
  - New onset edema in outpatient without apparent cause may be secondary to myocardial infarction
  - Radiographic and CT findings
    - Cardiomegaly
    - Right ≥ left pleural effusions
    - Smooth interlobular septal thickening or Kerley B lines
    - Dependent lung distribution (posterior lung in supine patient and lower lung in upright patient)
    - ± lobular or centrilobular ground-glass opacity with fissural thickening
    - Spared lobules among affected lobules secondary to differing lobular perfusion
    - Crazy-paving; intralobular interstitial thickening superimposed on ground-glass opacity
    - Mild lymph node enlargement secondary to increased lymphatic drainage

Helpful Clues for Less Common Diagnoses
- **Lymphangitic Carcinomatosis**
  - Metastatic disease to lymphatics from
    - Breast, lung, stomach, colon, cervix, prostate, pancreas, and thyroid carcinoma among others
  - Smooth or nodular or "beaded" thickening of interlobular septa and peribronchovascular interstitium
  - Preserves underlying lung architecture
  - No change with diuretics
  - ± hilar/mediastinal lymphadenopathy
  - ± pleural effusions
  - Unilateral disease more common in lung carcinoma
  - Look for other sites of metastatic disease (liver or bone)
- **Asbestosis**
  - Prone imaging important in diagnosis
  - HRCT findings
    - Posterior and basal subpleural lung
    - Subpleural reticular or dot-like opacities indicates early fibrosis
    - Subpleural lines parallel pleural surface
    - Short or long parenchymal bands extend inward from abnormal pleural surfaces
    - Pleural plaques
    - Late fibrosis shows honeycombing and thickening of interlobular septa
- **Systemic Lupus Erythematosus**
  - Elevated antinuclear antibodies in young women
  - HRCT shows
    - Ground-glass and reticular opacities in a basal, posterior, and subpleural distribution
    - Traction bronchiectasis or bronchiolectasis
    - Pleural thickening or effusion seen in 50% of patients
    - ± anterior upper lobe involvement
    - Honeycombing is rare
  - Ground-glass opacity
    - Represents lupus pneumonitis, pneumonia, or hemorrhage
- **Rheumatoid Arthritis**
  - Subpleural basal predominant fibrosis in UIP, NSIP, or OP patterns
  - ± unilateral pleural effusion or pleural thickening
  - Bronchiectasis in 30% of patients secondary to chronic infection
  - Rheumatoid nodules in ≤ 5% of patients

- ± distal clavicular erosions or high-riding humeral head

Helpful Clues for Rare Diagnoses

- **Lymphangiomyomatosis**
  - Women of childbearing age
  - Large lungs with pleural effusions and associated pneumothoraces
  - Diffuse distribution of round lung cysts
  - ± renal angiomyolipomas
  - ± mediastinal and retroperitoneal lymphadenopathy
- **Diffuse Pulmonary Lymphangiomatosis**
  - Congenital lymphatic disorder with proliferation and dilatation of lymphatics
  - Findings confined to thorax
    - Smooth thickening of interlobular septa and bronchovascular bundles
    - ± pleural and pericardial effusions
    - Mediastinal lymphadenopathy with effacement of mediastinal fat
    - ± centrilobular nodules
- **Pulmonary Venoocclusive Disease**
  - Occlusion of small pulmonary veins and venules leading to pulmonary hypertension
  - Fatal pulmonary edema can follow standard vasodilator therapy
  - CT shows
    - Pulmonary arterial diameter ≥ 29 mm
    - ± pleural effusions
    - Smooth or nodular interlobular septal thickening
    - Diffuse, geographic, perihilar or centrilobular ground-glass opacity
- **Pulmonary Capillary Hemangiomatosis**
  - Proliferation of thin-walled capillaries leading to obstruction of pulmonary venules
  - Fatal pulmonary edema can follow standard vasodilator therapy
  - Overlap with imaging findings of venoocclusive disease
  - CT shows
    - Pulmonary arterial diameter ≥ 29 mm
    - Diffuse ill-defined centrilobular nodules of ground-glass opacity
    - ± pleural effusions
    - Sparse interlobular septal thickening
- **Erdheim Chester Disease**
  - Non-Langerhans cell histiocytosis
  - 1/3 have pulmonary involvement
    - Visceral pleural thickening with effusions
    - Smooth interlobular septal and fissural thickening
  - Extrapulmonary findings
    - Symmetric osteosclerosis of metadiaphysis of long bones
    - ± circumferential long segment aortic wall thickening
    - ± soft tissue encasement of kidneys
    - ± pericardial thickening
    - ± nodular thickening of dura
    - ± T2/FLAIR hyperintensity within brainstem

Pulmonary Edema

Axial HRCT shows a crazy-paving pattern, i.e., ground-glass opacities with intralobular interstitial thickening ➔. Note pleural effusion ⇨.

Pulmonary Edema

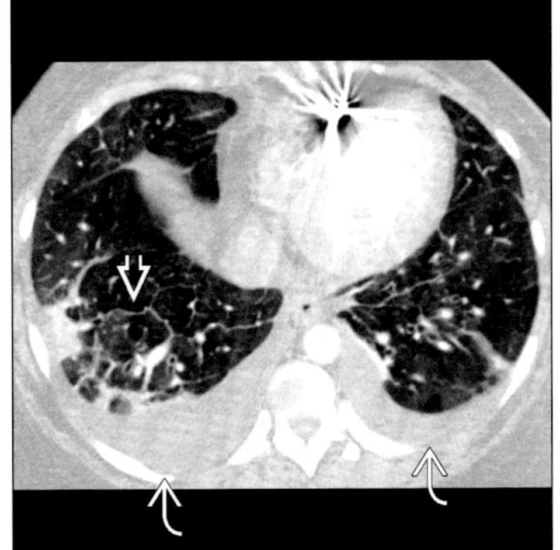

Axial CECT shows smooth septal thickening ⇨ and bilateral pleural effusions ➔.

INTERSTITIAL PATTERN, PLEURAL THICKENING AND EFFUSION

Pulmonary Edema

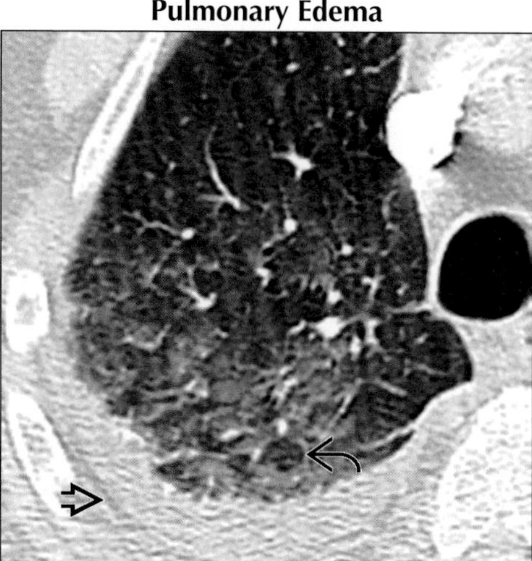

Lymphangitic Carcinomatosis

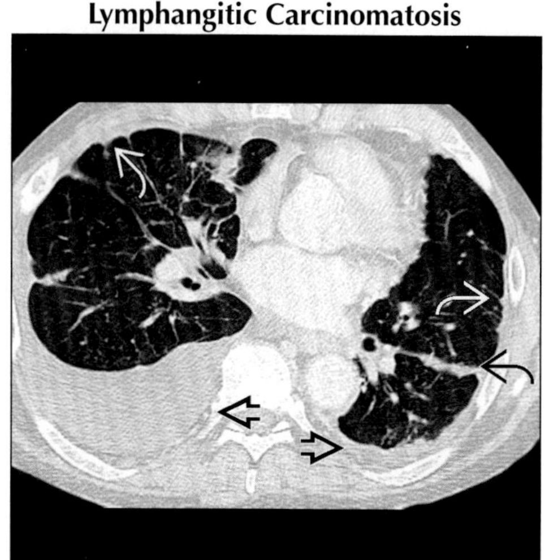

(Left) *Axial NECT shows dependent ground-glass opacity with right pleural effusion. Note characteristic, more normal-appearing lobules among lobules with ground-glass opacity. This is secondary to differing lobular perfusion.* ***(Right)*** *Axial CECT shows nodular thickening of the left major fissure. Note numerous subpleural nodules and bilateral right greater than left pleural effusions.*

Lymphangitic Carcinomatosis

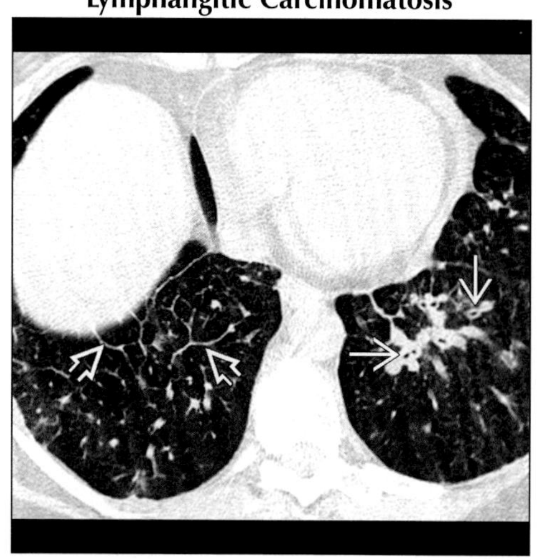

Asbestosis

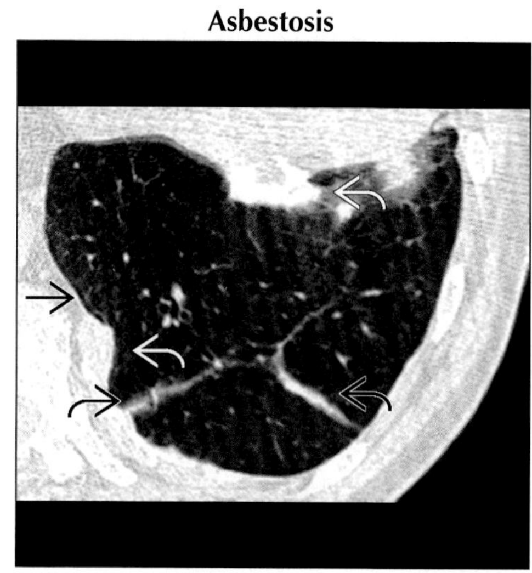

(Left) *Axial HRCT shows segmental bronchial wall thickening in the left lower lobe. Note relatively smooth thickening of interlobular septa in this patient with metastatic breast carcinoma.* ***(Right)*** *Axial HRCT prone image shows parenchymal bands, reticular opacities, and calcified pleural plaques as part of the fibrosis pattern associated with asbestosis.*

Asbestosis

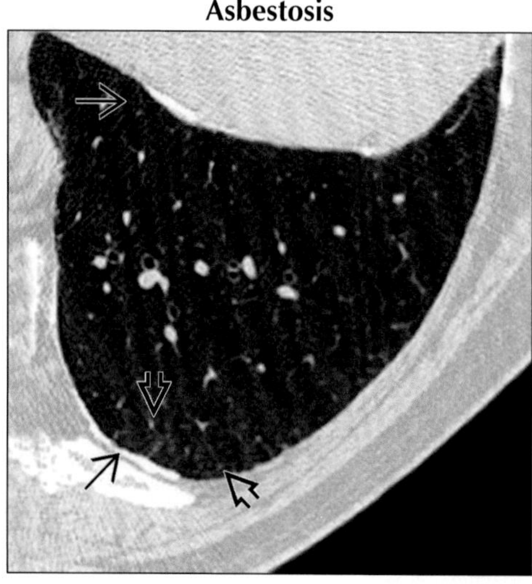

Systemic Lupus Erythematosus

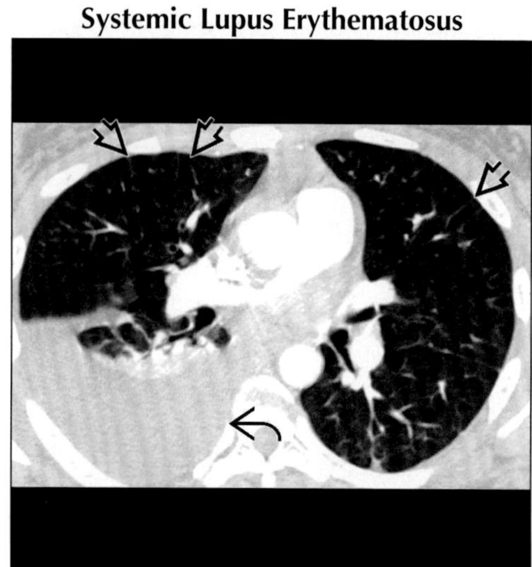

(Left) *Axial HRCT shows a prone image with subpleural reticular and dot-like opacities in the left lower lobe. Note calcified pleural plaques. This is the earliest manifestation of asbestosis.* ***(Right)*** *Axial CECT shows peripheral linear subpleural opacities and right pleural effusion.*

Rheumatoid Arthritis

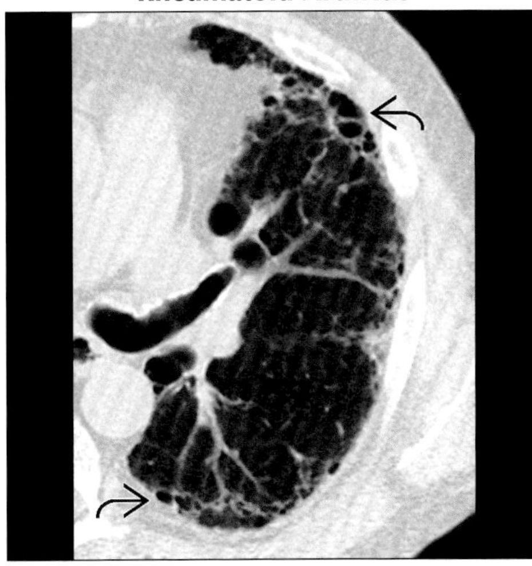

Lymphangiomyomatosis

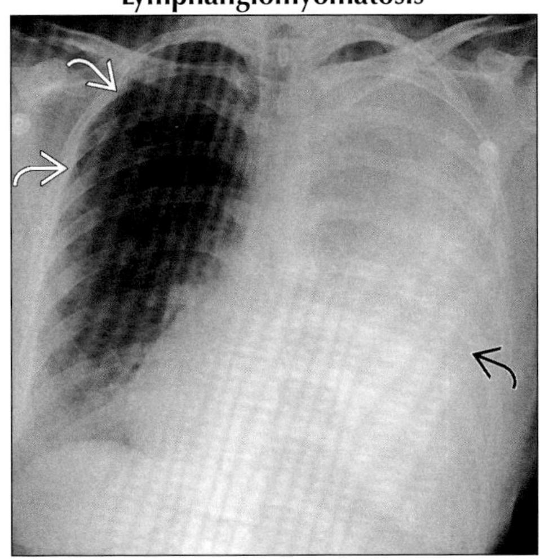

*(**Left**) Axial HRCT shows peripheral reticular opacities and honeycombing ➔ typical of usual interstitial pneumonia, a common manifestation of rheumatoid-associated interstitial lung disease. (**Right**) Frontal radiograph shows large left pleural effusion ➔ with contralateral mediastinal shift. Note right pneumothorax ➔. CT showed characteristic diffuse lung cysts. Pleural fluid was chylous in nature.*

Diffuse Pulmonary Lymphangiomatosis

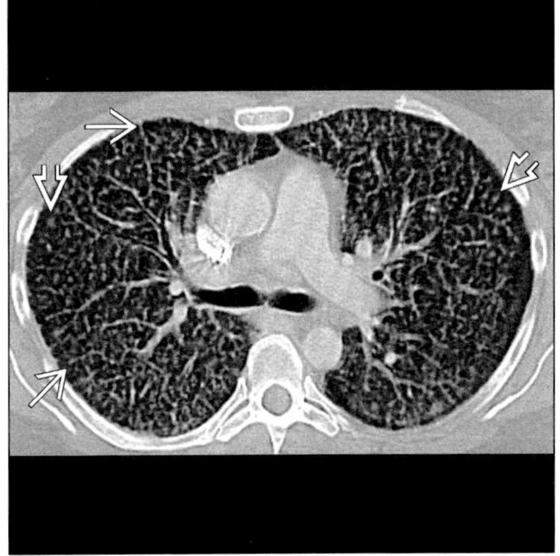

Pulmonary Venoocclusive Disease

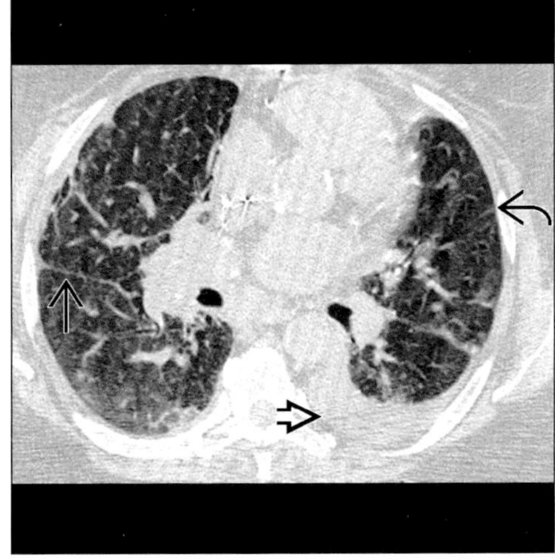

*(**Left**) Axial CECT shows centrilobular nodular thickening ➔ and smooth septal thickening ➔. Mediastinal windows showed effacement of mediastinal fat and lymphadenopathy (not shown). (**Right**) Axial NECT shows interlobular septal thickening ➔ and fissural thickening ➔. Note left pleural effusion ➔ and patchy ground-glass opacity. Dilatation of the pulmonary arteries and documented pulmonary hypertension were present.*

Pulmonary Capillary Hemangiomatosis

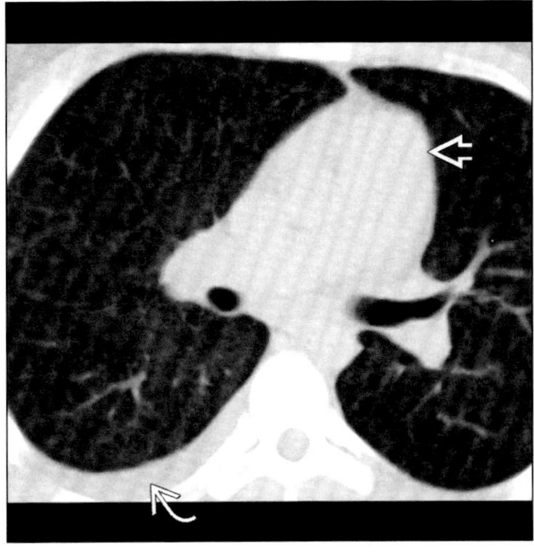

Erdheim Chester Disease

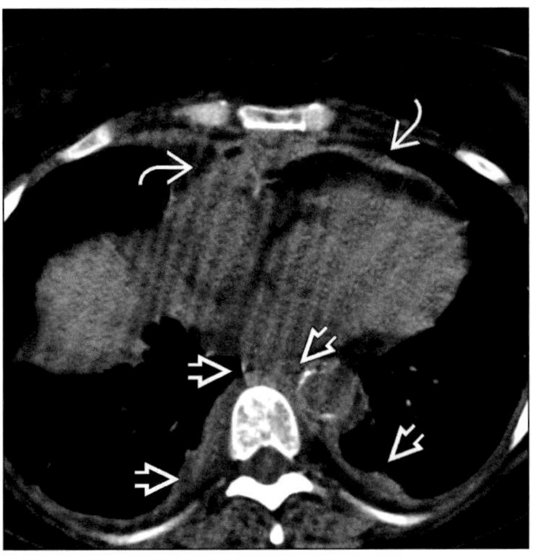

*(**Left**) Axial CECT shows small subtle centrilobular GGO nodules scattered throughout the lungs representing capillary proliferation. This can be confused with bronchiolitis. Main pulmonary artery ➔ is enlarged. Note small right pleural effusion ➔. (**Right**) Axial NECT shows relatively symmetric bilateral pleural thickening contiguous with mediastinum ➔ and pericardial thickening ➔. Smooth interlobular septal thickening was also present.*

CONGLOMERATE MASS (PROGRESSIVE MASSIVE FIBROSIS)

DIFFERENTIAL DIAGNOSIS

Common
- Sarcoidosis
- Radiation-Induced Lung Disease

Less Common
- Silicosis/Coal Worker's Pneumoconiosis
- Diffuse Alveolar Hemorrhage

Rare but Important
- Lipoid Pneumonia
- Pulmonary Talcosis

ESSENTIAL INFORMATION

Key Differential Diagnosis Issues
- Significant overlap of findings between sarcoidosis and silicosis and coal worker's pneumoconiosis
- Occupational and exposure history important
- Knowledge of treatment plan useful for recognizing radiation-induced lung fibrosis
  - Important for distinguishing radiation-induced lung disease from recurrent neoplasm

Helpful Clues for Common Diagnoses
- **Sarcoidosis**
  - Develops with progressive sarcoid-induced fibrosis
  - Conglomerate fibrosis difficult to distinguish from silicosis or coal worker's pneumoconiosis
    - Upper and mid lung zone predominant
    - Air bronchograms usually present
    - Associated traction bronchiectasis, architectural distortion, and volume loss
    - Punctate or coarse calcification frequently present
    - Perilymphatic nodules typically present bilaterally
  - Paracicatricial emphysema common peripheral to conglomerate mass
    - Increases with progressive fibrosis
  - Cavitation may occur from necrosis or infection
    - *Mycobacterium* species
  - Mediastinal and bilateral hilar lymphadenopathy often present
    - May be calcified (solid or "egg shell")
  - Honeycombing less common than with other end-stage lung diseases
    - Cysts usually larger
    - Basal sparing typical
- **Radiation-Induced Lung Disease**
  - Most commonly result of radiation for lung carcinoma
  - Less commonly for mediastinal lymphoma, esophageal carcinoma, or breast carcinoma
  - Radiation fibrosis
    - Typically occurs 6-12 months after completion of radiation therapy
    - Occurs within radiation field and can cross anatomic boundaries, such as pulmonary fissures
    - Straight lateral and medial margins with conventional therapy
    - May begin as small consolidative or ground-glass attenuation lung nodules
    - Nodules coalesce over time to form larger areas of fibrosis
    - Newer 3D radiation therapy techniques can result in lung abnormalities away from primary disease
    - Should stabilize within 2 years following therapy

Helpful Clues for Less Common Diagnoses
- **Silicosis/Coal Worker's Pneumoconiosis**
  - Exposure to coal dust or free silica
    - Coal miners
    - Quarry workers
    - Sand blasters
    - Foundry workers
    - Ceramics workers
    - Concrete cutters
  - Typically develops after 20 years of exposure
    - Can develop < 10 years with exposure to very high concentrations of dust
    - Progresses despite cessation of exposure
  - Silicosis and coal worker's pneumoconiosis indistinguishable radiographically
  - Large opacities > 1-2 cm
  - Begins in periphery of lung
    - Round or oval nodule or mass
    - Well-defined lateral margin paralleling chest wall
    - Posterior location on lateral radiograph or CT
    - Unilateral or asymmetric in early stages

- Becomes symmetric with progressive disease
- Difficult to distinguish from sarcoidosis
  - Develops in upper lobes
  - Air bronchograms less common than with sarcoidosis
  - Associated with bronchial distortion and upper lobe volume loss
  - Small perilymphatic nodules usually present
- Cavitation may occur from necrosis or infection, especially when > 5 cm
  - Predisposed to *Mycobacterium tuberculosis* infection
- Punctate calcifications common in conglomerate masses
- Mediastinal and hilar lymphadenopathy in up to 40%
  - Calcification in ~ 50% (diffuse, central, eccentric, and peripheral "egg shell")
- Paracicatricial emphysema common peripheral to conglomerate mass
- Increased risk of lung carcinoma independent of cigarette smoking
- Increased risk of developing connective tissue disease, especially systemic sclerosis

- **Diffuse Alveolar Hemorrhage**
  - Very rare cause of conglomerate mass
  - Occurs with recurrent alveolar hemorrhage
    - Subsequent hemosiderosis and fibrosis
  - Conglomerate mass with high attenuation

Helpful Clues for Rare Diagnoses

- **Lipoid Pneumonia**
  - Typically result of recurrent lipid aspiration
    - Most patients asymptomatic
    - Mineral oil ingestion most common
    - Occupational exposure to oil mist less frequent
  - Conglomerate mass with diffuse low attenuation
  - Usually gravitationally dependent (posterior lower lobes)
  - Cavitation uncommon
    - Usually from superinfection with nontuberculous mycobacteria
- **Pulmonary Talcosis**
  - Frequently results from chronic intravenous drug abuse
    - Granulomatous vasculitis from foreign body giant cell reaction to contaminants (talc) in drugs
    - Patients often initially asymptomatic
    - May progress to respiratory insufficiency and pulmonary hypertension
  - Early disease
    - Small nodules
    - Hyperinflation and emphysema (panlobular or panacinar)
  - Conglomerate masses develop with progressive disease
    - Similar to those of silicosis and coal worker's pneumoconiosis
    - May have diffuse or punctate calcification

Sarcoidosis

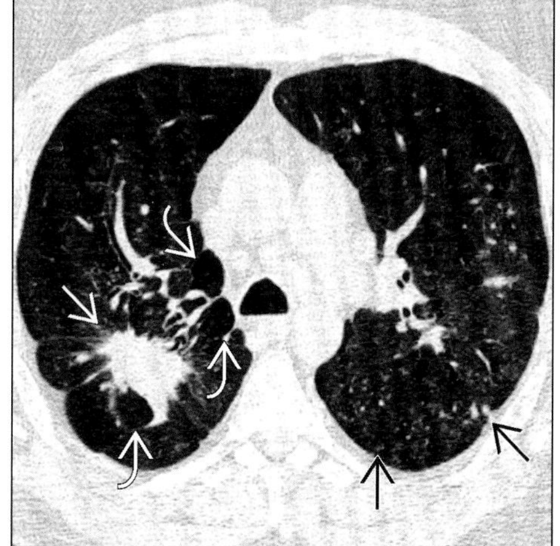

Axial HRCT shows a spiculated mass in the right lower lobe ➡. Note the nearby paracicatricial emphysema ➡. Scattered perilymphatic nodules typical of sarcoidosis are seen in the left lung ➡.

Sarcoidosis

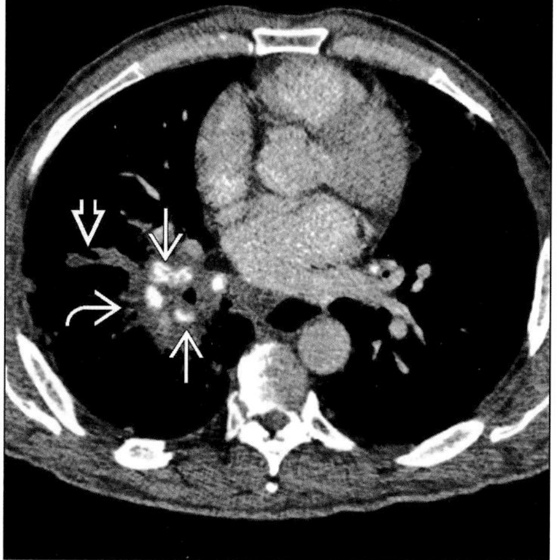

Axial NECT shows a right perihilar conglomerate mass ➡ containing large calcifications ➡. Note the dilated and impacted bronchus ➡ resulting from proximal stenosis.

CONGLOMERATE MASS (PROGRESSIVE MASSIVE FIBROSIS)

Sarcoidosis

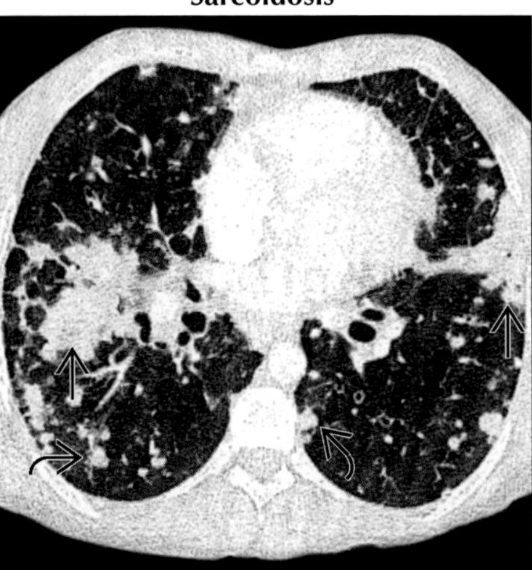

Sarcoidosis

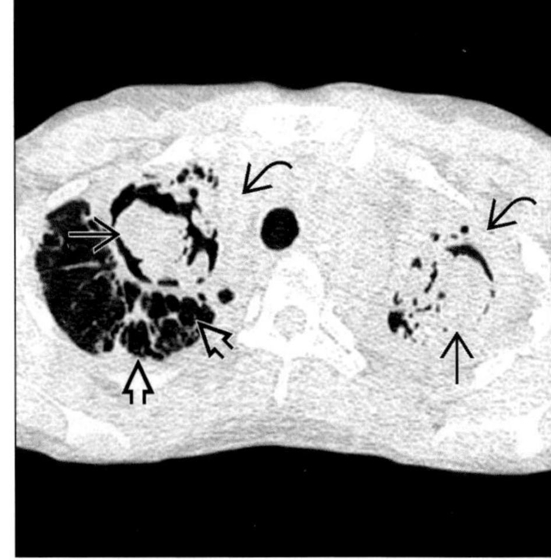

(Left) *Axial HRCT shows conglomerate masses ➔ in both lungs with numerous scattered nodules ➔. Note the relative symmetry typical of sarcoidosis.* ***(Right)*** *Axial HRCT shows large mycetomas ➔ in the upper lobes in this patient with severe fibrocavitary disease from sarcoidosis. Bilateral pleural thickening ➔ suggests chronicity of the inflammatory process. Note paracicatricial emphysema ➔ in the right upper lobe.*

Radiation-Induced Lung Disease

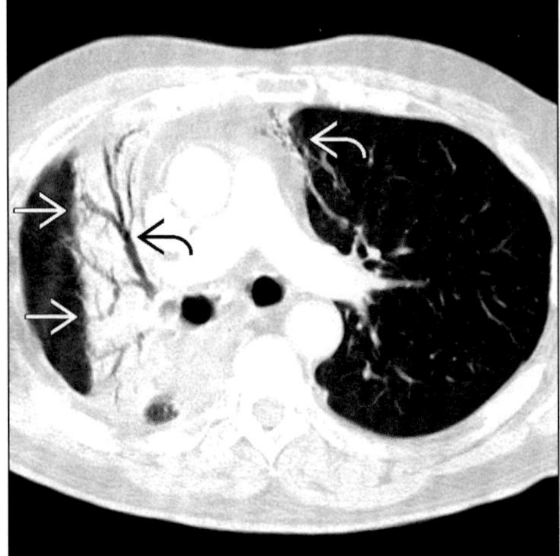

Radiation-Induced Lung Disease

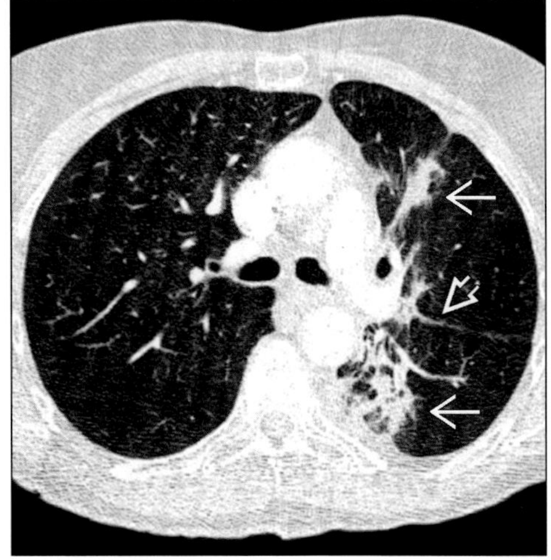

(Left) *Axial CECT shows consolidation in the right lung with straight margins ➔ in this patient treated for lung carcinoma. Note the dilated bronchi ➔. Mild radiation fibrosis ➔ is in the left lung.* ***(Right)*** *Axial HRCT shows nodular consolidation in the left lung in this patient treated with radiation therapy for lung carcinoma. Note relative linear lateral margin ➔ and crossing of the major fissure ➔, typical of radiation-induced fibrosis.*

Radiation-Induced Lung Disease

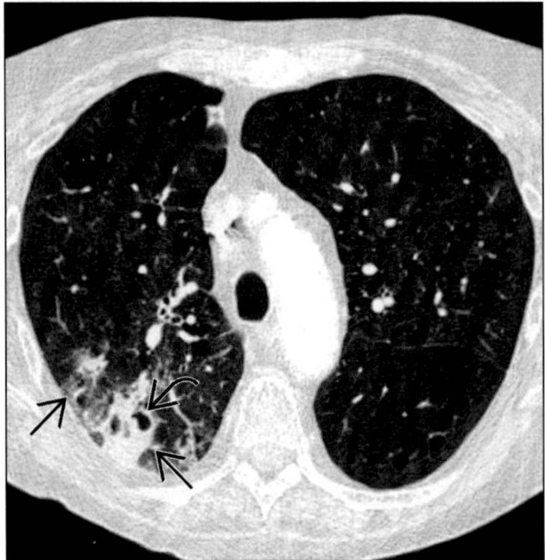

Silicosis/Coal Worker's Pneumoconiosis

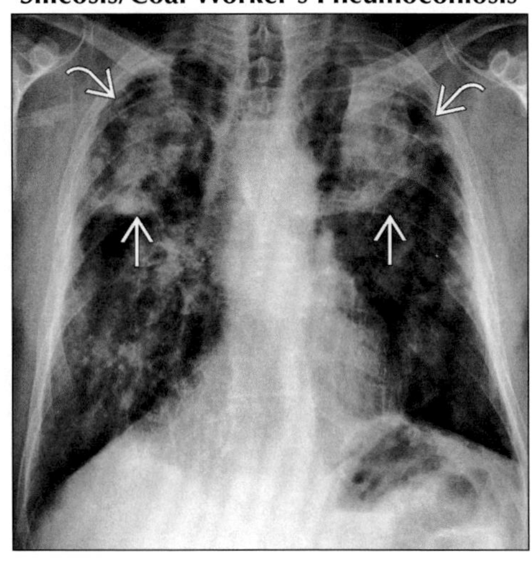

(Left) *Axial HRCT shows nodular consolidation in the right upper lobe ➔ with cavitation ➔ in this patient treated with stereotactic body radiotherapy (SBRT) for lung carcinoma. This can mimic acute infection.* ***(Right)*** *Frontal radiograph shows bilateral upper lobe masses ➔ in this foundry worker with complicated silicosis (progressive massive fibrosis). Note relative peripheral lucency from paracicatricial emphysema ➔.*

CONGLOMERATE MASS (PROGRESSIVE MASSIVE FIBROSIS)

Silicosis/Coal Worker's Pneumoconiosis

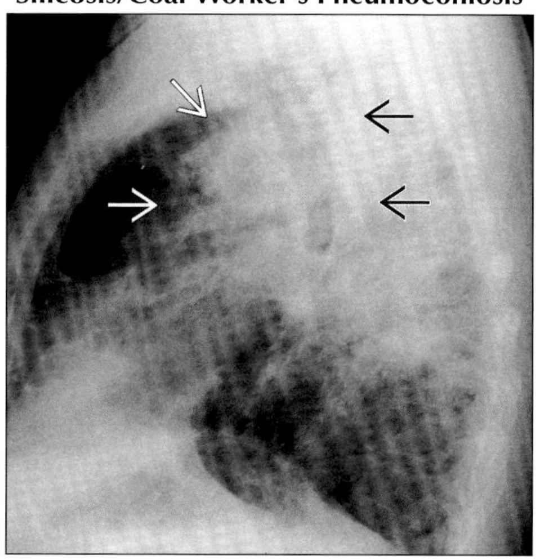

Silicosis/Coal Worker's Pneumoconiosis

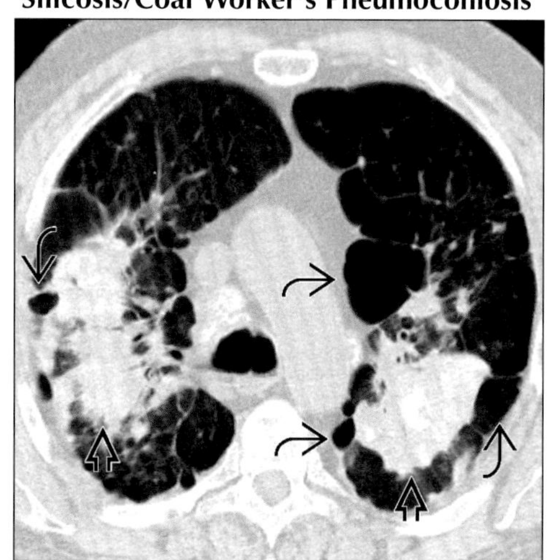

(Left) *Lateral radiograph shows typical upper lobe and posterior distribution of conglomerate masses* → *in this foundry worker with complicated silicosis. Note the smaller silicotic nodules anteriorly* ➡. ***(Right)*** *Axial NECT shows large, mass-like areas of consolidation* ⇨ *with adjacent paracicatricial emphysema* ↷ *in this foundry worker with complicated silicosis. Note how the lateral margins of the masses parallel the chest wall.*

Silicosis/Coal Worker's Pneumoconiosis

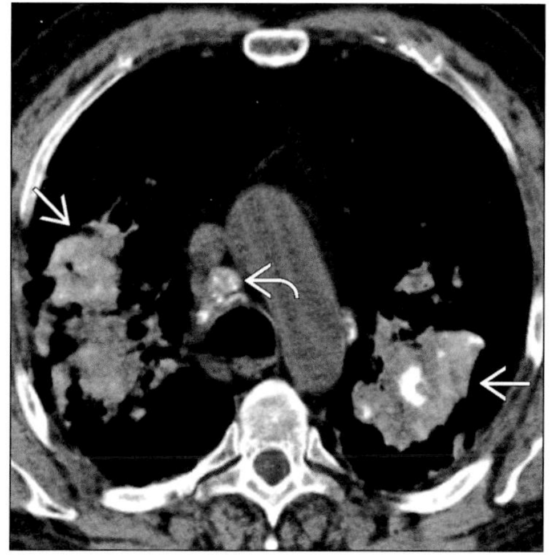

Diffuse Alveolar Hemorrhage

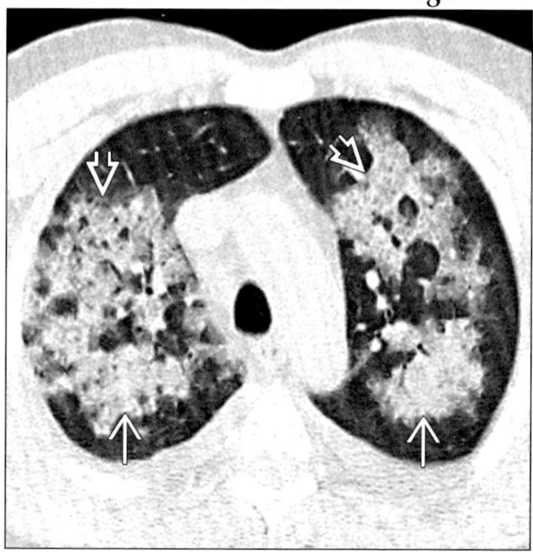

(Left) *Axial NECT shows large, mass-like areas of consolidation* ➡ *with varying degrees of calcification in this foundry worker with complicated silicosis. Calcified mediastinal lymph nodes are also present* ↶. ***(Right)*** *Axial HRCT shows patchy bilateral consolidation* ➡ *and ground-glass attenuation with superimposed septal thickening (crazy-paving)* ⇨ *in this patient with recurrent pulmonary hemorrhage.*

Lipoid Pneumonia

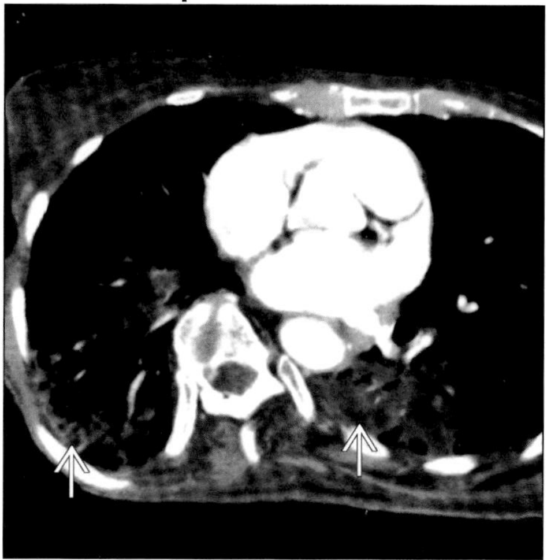

Pulmonary Talcosis

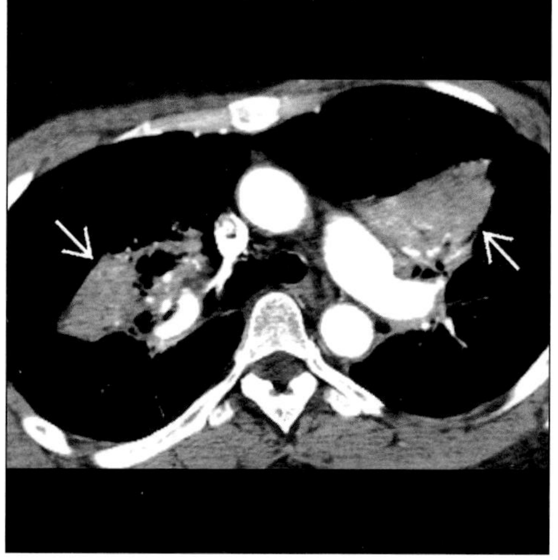

(Left) *Axial CECT shows bilateral gravitationally dependent consolidation* ➡ *in this patient with chronic mineral oil aspiration. Note the low attenuation characteristic of lipoid pneumonia.* ***(Right)*** *Axial CECT shows bilateral consolidative masses* ➡ *with high-attenuation foci in this intravenous drug abuser with talcosis. The presence of micronodules and panacinar or panlobular emphysema can be helpful in the diagnosis of talcosis.*

SECTION 7
Pulmonary Vasculature

PULMONARY ARTERIAL ENLARGEMENT

DIFFERENTIAL DIAGNOSIS

Common
- Pulmonary Arterial Hypertension (PAH)
- Pulmonic Valvular Stenosis (Post-Stenotic Dilatation)
- Atrial Septal Defect (ASD)

Less Common
- Takayasu Arteritis
- Pulmonary Artery Aneurysm

Rare but Important
- Mitral Stenosis or Regurgitation
- Pulmonary Venoocclusive Disease
- Pulmonary Capillary Hemangiomatosis

ESSENTIAL INFORMATION

Key Differential Diagnosis Issues
- Radiographic features of PAH
  - Disproportionate enlargement of central pulmonary arteries (PA)
  - Does not appear multilobular like hilar adenopathy
  - Right ventricular enlargement, especially with intracardiac shunt and right heart failure
- CT features of PAH
  - Increased main pulmonary artery (PA) measurement above 3 cm
  - Main PA to ascending thoracic aortic ratio of ≥ 1

Helpful Clues for Common Diagnoses
- **Pulmonary Arterial Hypertension (PAH)**
  - Enlargement of central PA and peripheral pruning
- **Pulmonic Valvular Stenosis (Post-Stenotic Dilatation)**
  - Disproportionate enlargement of main and left pulmonary arteries
  - Right ventricle enlargement
- **Atrial Septal Defect (ASD)**
  - Increased pulmonary vascular flow
  - Cardiomegaly: Enlarged right ventricle and right atrium

Helpful Clues for Less Common Diagnoses
- **Takayasu Arteritis**
  - Pulmonary artery wall thickening
  - Aneurysmal dilatation
- **Pulmonary Artery Aneurysm**
  - Focal dilatation in continuation with pulmonary artery

Helpful Clues for Rare Diagnoses
- **Mitral Stenosis or Regurgitation**
  - Cardiomegaly
  - Left atrial enlargement
- **Pulmonary Venoocclusive Disease**
  - Interlobular septal thickening
  - Ground-glass opacities but without centrilobular distribution
- **Pulmonary Capillary Hemangiomatosis**
  - Poorly defined ground-glass nodules in centrilobular or random distribution
  - Ground-glass represents capillary proliferation beyond resolution of imaging technique
  - No interlobular septal thickening

Pulmonary Arterial Hypertension (PAH)

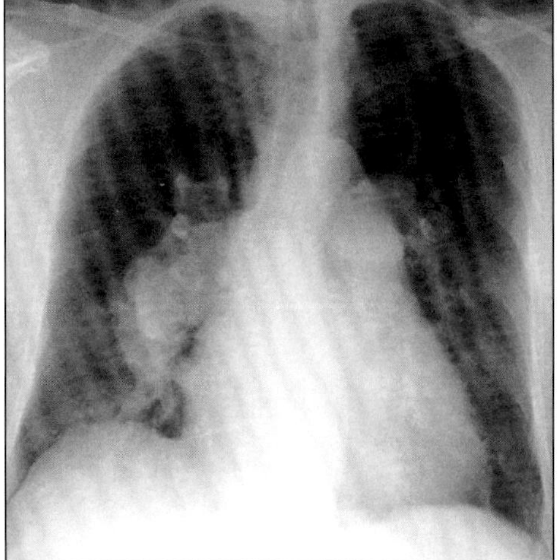

Frontal radiograph shows massively enlarged main and bilateral pulmonary arteries. Note rapid tapering and cardiomegaly. (Courtesy J.D. Godwin, MD.)

Pulmonic Valvular Stenosis (Post-Stenotic Dilatation)

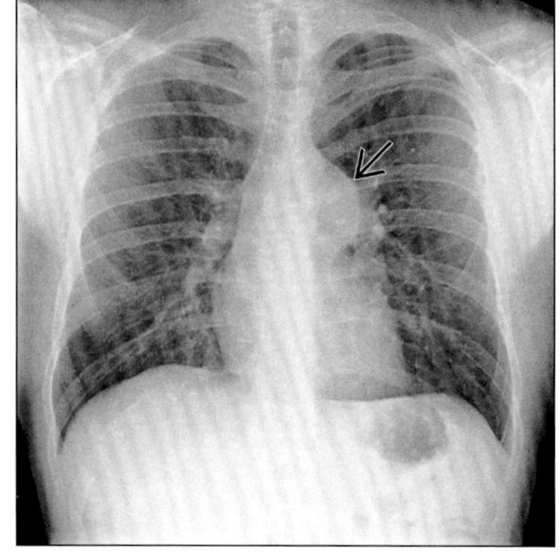

Frontal radiograph shows enlarged main and left pulmonary artery ⇒ with a right pulmonary artery of normal caliber. Heart size and peripheral pulmonary markings are normal.

PULMONARY ARTERIAL ENLARGEMENT

Atrial Septal Defect (ASD)

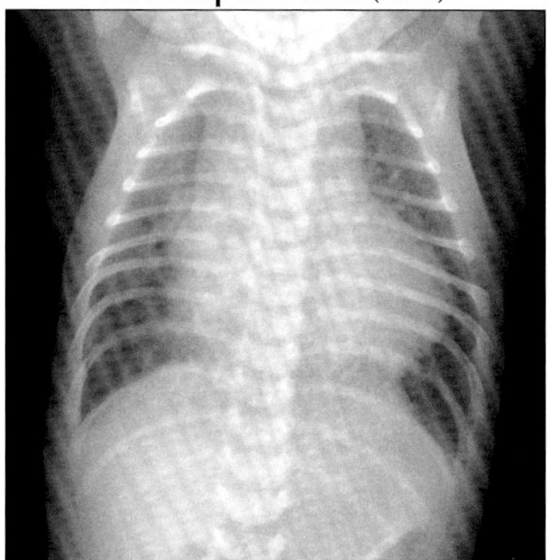

Takayasu Arteritis

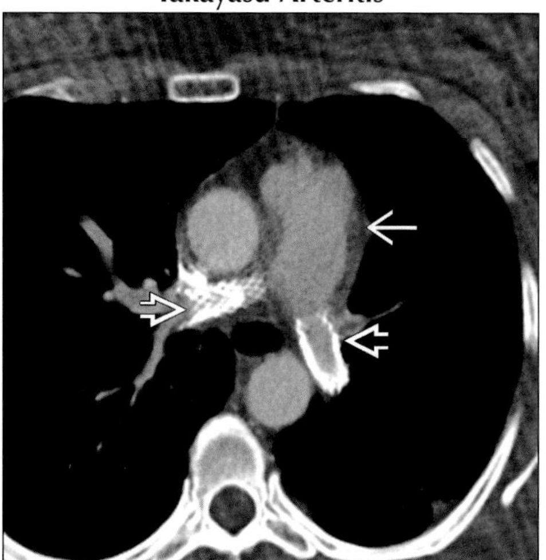

(Left) *Anteroposterior radiograph from an infant shows cardiomegaly and increased pulmonary vascular flow. Mediastinal widening is due to normal thymic tissue.* ***(Right)*** *Axial CECT shows dilation and mural (wall) thickening ➡ of the main pulmonary artery. Bilateral pulmonary artery stents were placed for vascular stenoses ➡.*

Pulmonary Artery Aneurysm

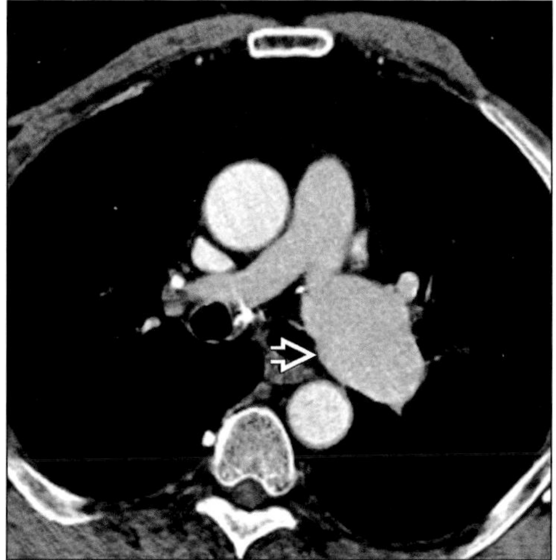

Mitral Stenosis or Regurgitation

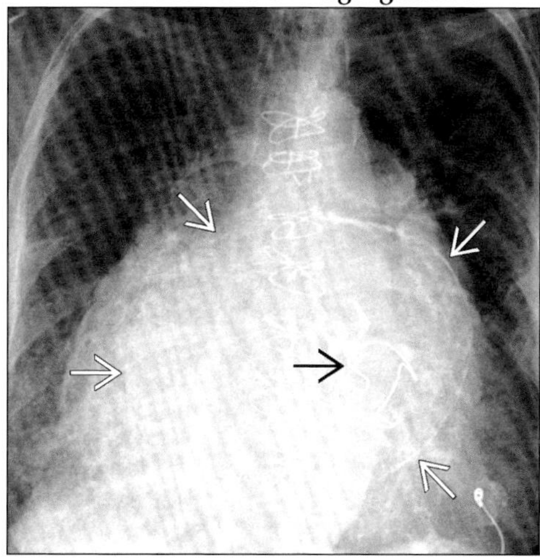

(Left) *Axial CECT shows a left pulmonary artery aneurysm ➡ in a patient with Hughes-Stovin syndrome, which is characterized by pulmonary artery and peripheral vein thrombosis and pulmonary artery aneurysms.* ***(Right)*** *Frontal radiograph shows cardiomegaly with an enlarged left atrium, outlined by a peripheral rim of calcification ➡. The mitral valve has been replaced →.*

Pulmonary Venoocclusive Disease

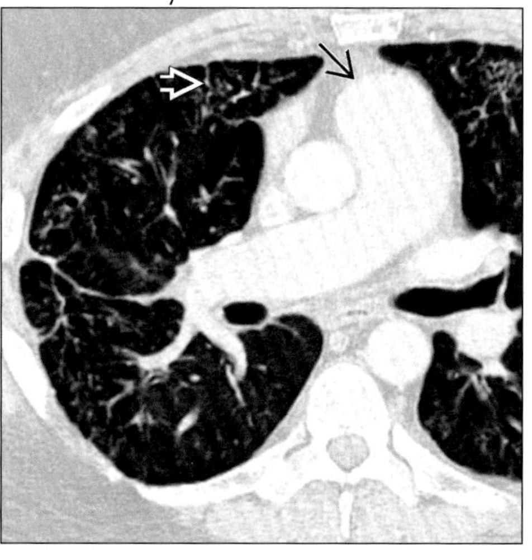

Pulmonary Capillary Hemangiomatosis

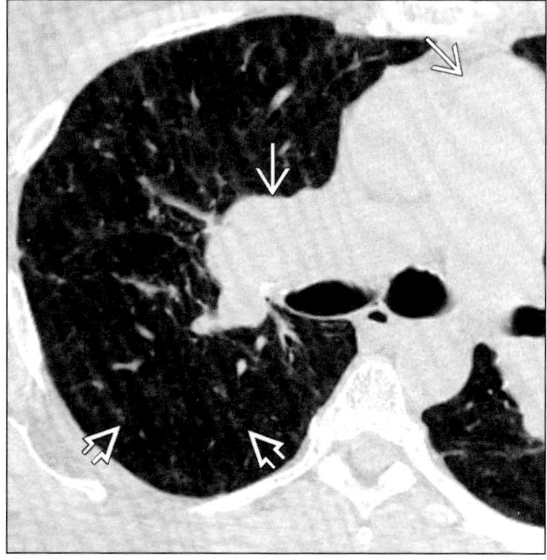

(Left) *Axial CECT shows septal thickening ➡ and enlarged central pulmonary arteries → indicative of pulmonary venoocclusive disease in a patient with pulmonary arterial hypertension. There are nonspecific patchy areas of ground-glass opacity.* ***(Right)*** *Axial NECT shows enlarged central pulmonary arteries ➡ and innumerable centrilobular ground-glass opacities ➡, indicating foci of capillary hemangiomatosis.*

FILLING DEFECT, PULMONARY ARTERY

DIFFERENTIAL DIAGNOSIS

Common
- Pulmonary Emboli

Less Common
- Tumor Embolism

Rare but Important
- Abnormal Tubes and Catheters
- Pulmonary Artery Sarcoma
- Air Embolism

ESSENTIAL INFORMATION

Key Differential Diagnosis Issues
- Bland thrombi, tumor thrombi, and pulmonary artery sarcoma can have similar imaging appearances

Helpful Clues for Common Diagnoses
- **Pulmonary Emboli**
  - Acute pulmonary thromboembolism
    - Complete or partial filling defect
    - Peripheral consolidation and ground-glass opacity from pulmonary hemorrhage or infarct
    - Residual thrombus in right heart
    - Right ventricular dilation from right heart strain (indicator of worse prognosis)
  - Chronic pulmonary thromboembolic disease
    - Eccentric clot contiguous with arterial wall
    - Uncommonly calcify
    - Webs and stenoses with post-stenotic dilation
    - Mosaic pattern of attenuation
    - Bronchial artery hypertrophy
  - Methylmethacrylate emboli
    - High-attenuation filling defect in pulmonary artery
    - Cement in spine from vertebroplasty

Helpful Clues for Less Common Diagnoses
- **Tumor Embolism**
  - Renal cell carcinoma, hepatocellular carcinoma, and carcinoma of breast, stomach, and prostate most common
  - Filling defect in central pulmonary arteries
  - Tumor thrombus in inferior vena cava suggestive

Helpful Clues for Rare Diagnoses
- **Abnormal Tubes and Catheters**
  - Retained or embolized catheter
- **Pulmonary Artery Sarcoma**
  - Vast majority arise in pulmonary valve or large pulmonary arteries
  - Large, lobulated, low-attenuation filling defect
  - Extension outside of vessel lumen
  - Enhancement on CT or MR or uptake on FDG PET/CT
- **Air Embolism**
  - Frequently iatrogenic
    - Intravenous line placement or utilization
    - Barotrauma from positive-pressure ventilation
  - Scuba diving

Pulmonary Emboli

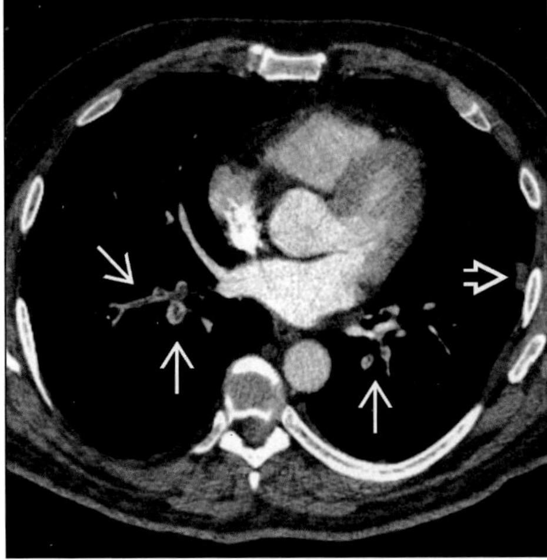

Axial CECT shows multiple acute pulmonary arterial filling defects ➡. Note dilation of the affected arteries. Focal atelectasis, hemorrhage, or infarct is present in the left lower lobe ⇨.

Pulmonary Emboli

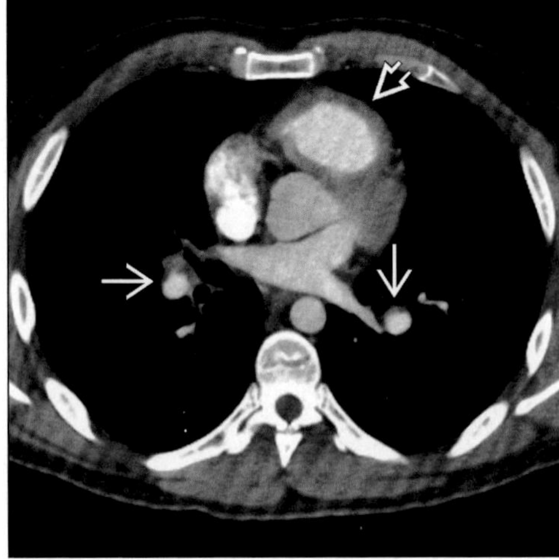

Axial CECT shows chronic eccentric pulmonary arterial filling defects ➡ and pulmonary arterial dilation. The right ventricular infundibulum is thickened from chronic pulmonary hypertension ⇨.

FILLING DEFECT, PULMONARY ARTERY

Pulmonary Emboli

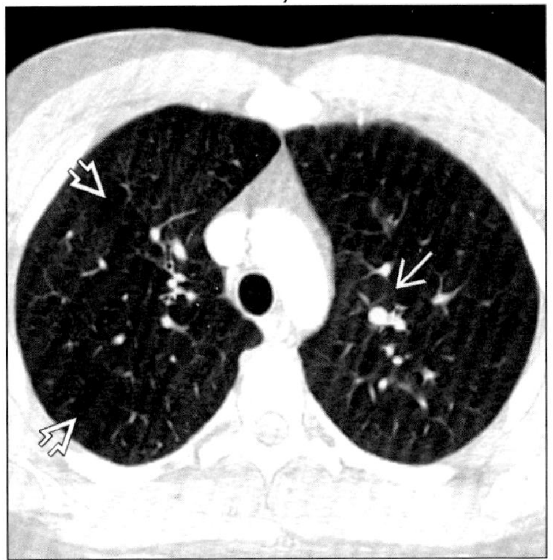

Tumor Embolism

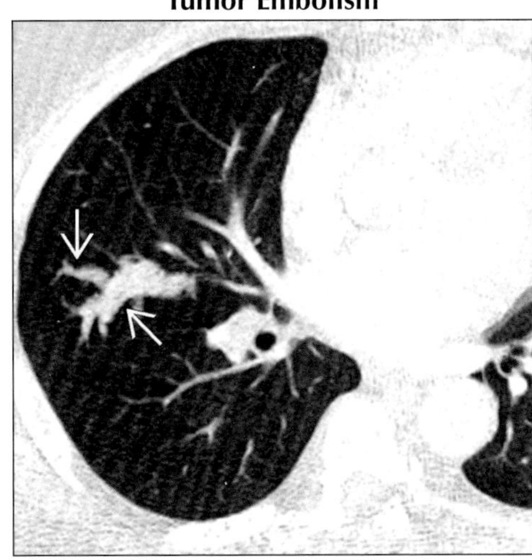

(Left) Axial HRCT shows heterogeneous or mosaic attenuation of the lungs in this patient with chronic pulmonary thromboembolic disease. Note the larger pulmonary vessels in areas of relative ground-glass opacity ➔ and relative paucity of vessels in areas of hypoperfusion ➪. (Right) Axial HRCT shows dilated right lower lobe pulmonary arteries ➔, which are filled with tumor, in this patient with metastatic renal cell carcinoma.

Abnormal Tubes and Catheters

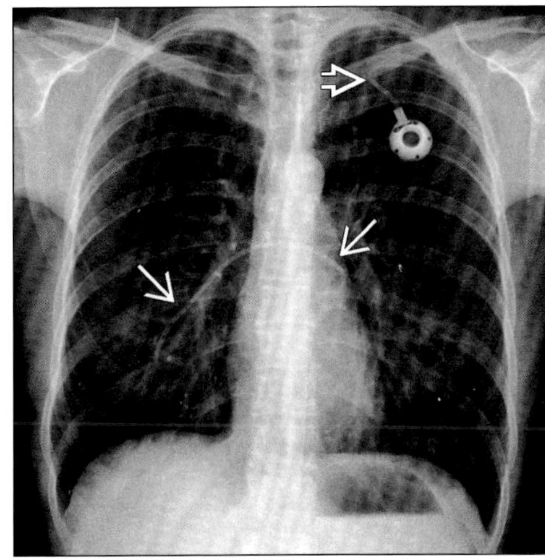

Pulmonary Artery Sarcoma

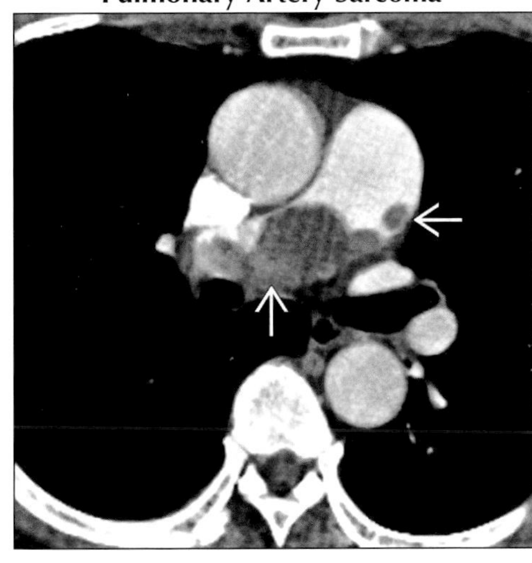

(Left) Frontal radiograph shows a large catheter fragment ➔, which has embolized into the central pulmonary arteries. Note the fracture site at the expected location of venous insertion of the tunneled catheter ➪. (Right) Axial CECT shows a large, nodular filling defect ➔ in the main pulmonary artery extending into the right main pulmonary artery in this patient with a primary pulmonary arterial pleomorphic sarcoma. Note mild pulmonary arterial dilation.

Pulmonary Artery Sarcoma

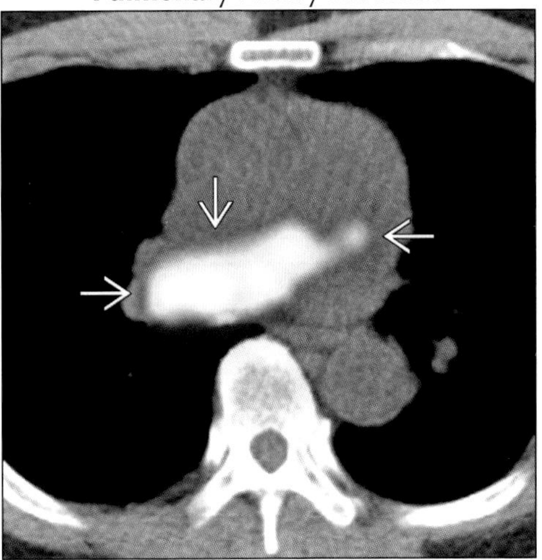

Air Embolism

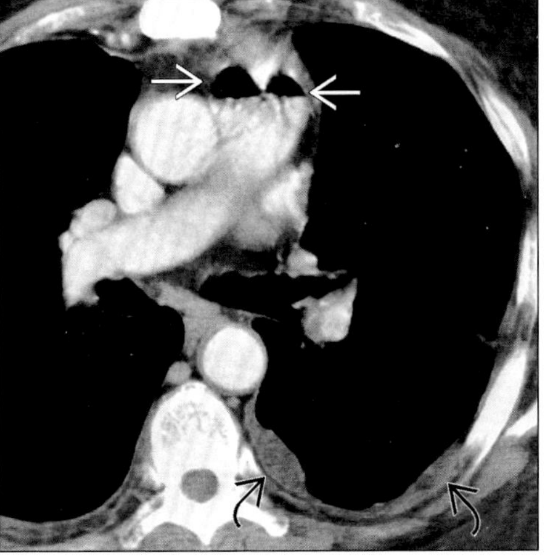

(Left) Axial PET shows marked heterogeneous FDG uptake ➔ in the main and right pulmonary artery in this patient with primary pulmonary arterial pleomorphic sarcoma. (Right) Axial CECT shows gas layering nondependently in the main pulmonary artery ➔. Left pleural metastases are present ➚.

SECTION 8
Mediastinum and Hilum

MEDIASTINAL SHIFT

DIFFERENTIAL DIAGNOSIS

Common
- Pleural Effusion
- Lobar Atelectasis
- Pneumothorax

Less Common
- Pneumonectomy
- Radiation Fibrosis
- Tuberculosis

Rare but Important
- Hemothorax
- Fibrothorax
- Malignancy
- Diaphragmatic Hernia
- Scimitar Syndrome

ESSENTIAL INFORMATION

Key Differential Diagnosis Issues
- Direction of shift
- Acuity of problem

Helpful Clues for Common Diagnoses
- **Pleural Effusion**
  - Contralateral mediastinal shift
  - Opaque hemithorax
  - Pleural nodularity or thickening raises suspicion of malignancy
  - Causes of large unilateral fluid collections include
    - Infection, primary or metastatic malignancy, chyle, blood
  - Smoothly thickened and enhancing parietal pleura indicates exudative effusion
  - Chylous effusions are indistinguishable from transudative effusions
    - Secondary to obstruction by tumor, iatrogenic from surgery or trauma
- **Lobar Atelectasis**
  - Ipsilateral mediastinal shift
  - Lobar collapse patterns
    - Obstructing neoplasm is more likely in outpatients
    - Mucus plug is more likely in inpatients
- **Pneumothorax**
  - Convex pleural line paralleling chest wall
  - No vascular markings lateral to pleural line
  - Tension pneumothorax is clinical diagnosis with symptoms/signs including
    - Chest pain, hypoxia, circulatory collapse
    - Physical examination findings of pneumothorax
  - Suggestive/concerning radiographic findings of tension pneumothorax
    - Contralateral mediastinal shift
    - Flattening of diaphragm
    - Widening of rib interspaces
    - Complete collapse of lung

Helpful Clues for Less Common Diagnoses
- **Pneumonectomy**
  - Small hemithorax with ipsilateral thoracotomy
  - Ipsilateral mediastinal shift
  - Opaque hemithorax secondary to fluid in pneumonectomy space
- **Radiation Fibrosis**
  - Important threshold doses
    - Seldom visible ≤ 30 Gy
    - Nearly always visible ≥ 40 Gy
  - Incidence increases with 2nd course of therapy
  - Occurs 6-12 months after radiotherapy
  - No further progression 2 years after radiotherapy
  - Radiographic and CT findings
    - Ipsilateral mediastinal shift
    - Traction bronchiectasis, pleural thickening, and volume loss
    - Fibrosis does not obey lobar or segmental boundaries
    - Sharp and straight demarcation corresponding to radiation portals
- **Tuberculosis**
  - Ipsilateral mediastinal volume loss with extensive post-primary tuberculosis
  - Activity difficult to determine without comparison radiographs
  - Common locations include
    - Upper lobes or superior segments of lower lobes
  - Radiographic or CT findings
    - Fibrosis
    - Traction bronchiectasis
    - Cavities
    - Adjacent emphysema
  - CT findings of active disease
    - Tree-in-bud opacities indicating endobronchial spread of infection
    - Cavitation
    - Consolidation
    - Rim-enhancing lymphadenopathy

Helpful Clues for Rare Diagnoses

- **Hemothorax**
  - Most common cause is penetrating or blunt trauma
  - Less common associations include
    - Aortic dissection, rupture of aneurysm, or coagulopathy
  - Contralateral mediastinal shift
  - CT demonstrates high-density fluid (≥ 30 HU)
  - May see fluid-fluid level representing hematocrit effect
  - Organization may lead to fibrothorax
- **Fibrothorax**
  - Marked unilateral pleural thickening ± calcification
  - Ipsilateral mediastinal shift
  - Causes include resolved
    - Hemothorax
    - Empyema
    - Tuberculosis effusion
- **Malignancy**
  - Contralateral mediastinal shift often caused by tumors metastatic to mediastinum or lung
  - Causes include
    - Primary or metastatic germ cell tumors
    - Thymoma or thymic carcinoma
    - Mesothelioma
    - Endobronchial or extrabronchial mass causing lung collapse
    - Pleural metastases with large pleural effusions
- **Diaphragmatic Hernia**
  - Diaphragmatic rupture with herniation of viscera into thorax
    - Secondary to high-energy blunt or penetrating trauma
    - Associated injuries can be many, including pneumo-/hemothorax, rib fractures, and pulmonary contusion
  - Bochdalek hernia
    - Bochdalek hernias are located "back and to the left"
    - Majority are small, contain fat, and are incidental
    - If containing bowel or kidney, may cause contralateral mediastinal shift
    - Large congenital hernias will usually be diagnosed prenatally by fetal ultrasound or MR
  - Morgagni hernia
    - Anterior and right-sided in location
    - Most contain omentum with small vessels
    - Most common viscera to herniate is colon
- **Scimitar Syndrome**
  - Right lung hypoplasia with ipsilateral mediastinal shift
  - Anomalous pulmonary venous return of a portion or all of affected lung
    - Vein parallels right heart border
  - Decreased size of right pulmonary artery
  - Systemic to pulmonary collaterals to portions of right lung
  - Associated congenital heart disease in 25%

Pleural Effusion

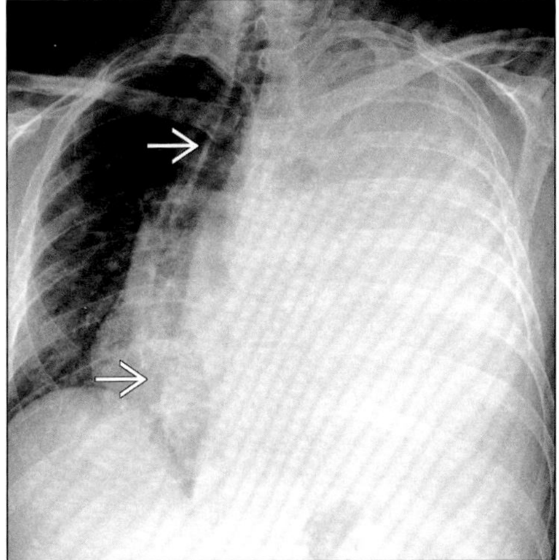

Frontal radiograph shows typical radiographic features of chylous effusion from thoracic duct obstruction. Note the left hemithorax opacification with rightward mediastinal shift ➡.

Pleural Effusion

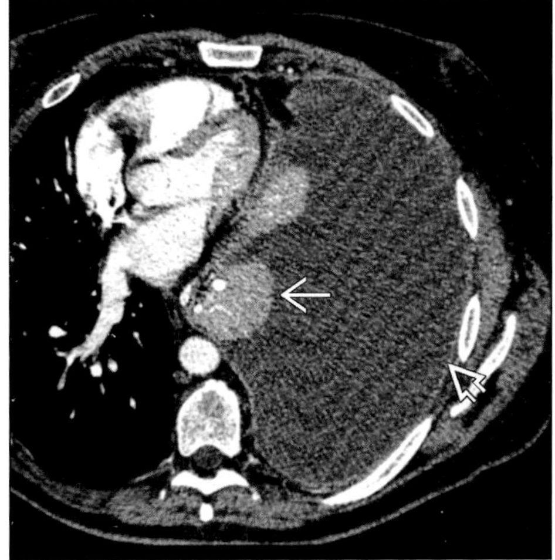

Axial CECT shows large pleural effusion. Pleura uniformly enhances ➡ indicating an exudative effusion. The left lung is completely atelectatic ➡.

MEDIASTINAL SHIFT

(Left) Frontal radiograph shows typical radiographic features of pleural effusion from mesothelioma. Note the complete opacification of the left hemithorax ➡ with mediastinal shift to the right ➡. Stomach bubble is displaced inferiorly and medially ➡. *(Right)* Coronal CECT shows inversion of the left hemidiaphragm ➡ and rightward mediastinal shift.

Pleural Effusion

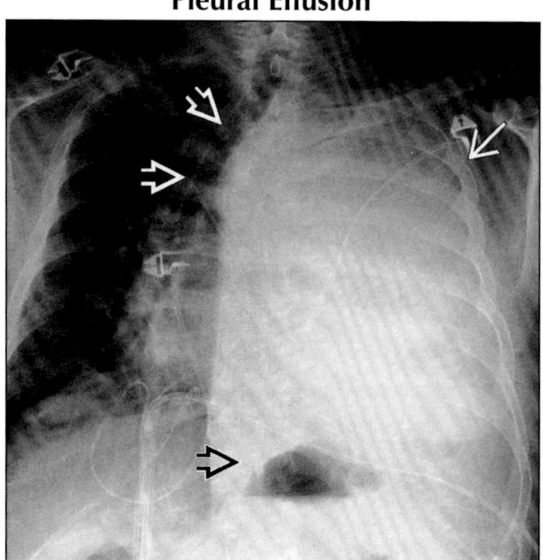

Pleural Effusion

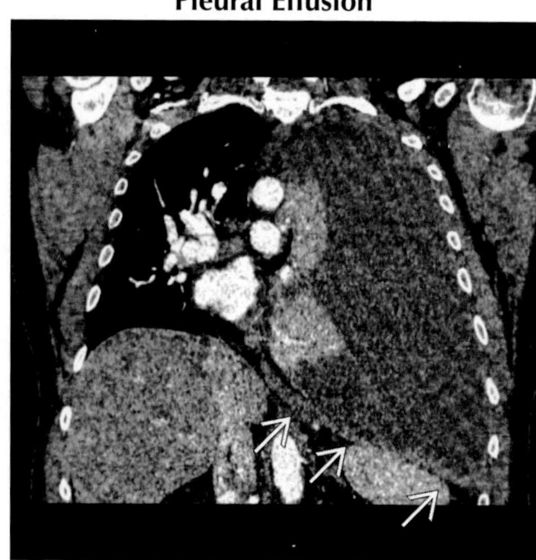

(Left) Axial CECT shows features of chylous effusion from thoracic duct obstruction. Note the large effusion ➡, contralateral mediastinal shift, and paraspinal adenopathy ➡. *(Right)* Axial CECT shows typical features of pleural effusion from malignant mesothelioma. There is a large pleural effusion ➡ and pleural thickening ➡. Note the rightward mediastinal shift ➡.

Pleural Effusion

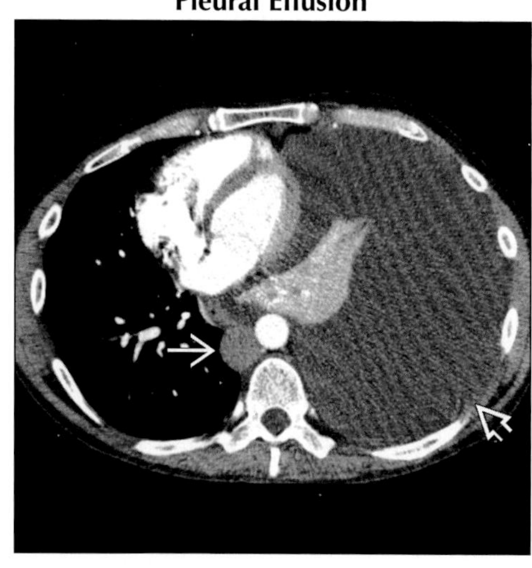

Pleural Effusion

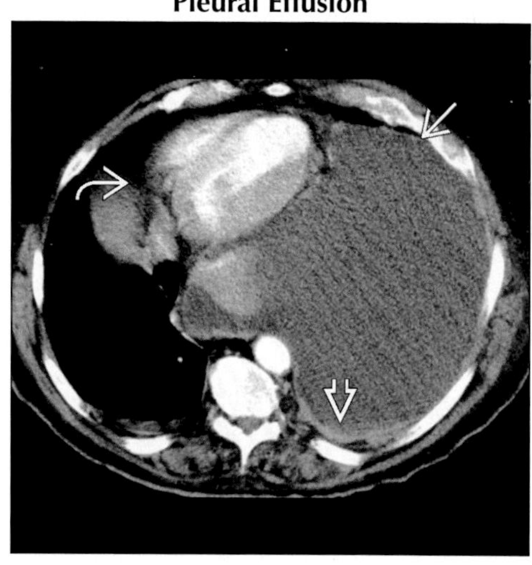

(Left) Anteroposterior radiograph shows right middle lobe and right lower lobe collapse ➡. The right hemithorax is small, and the trachea is shifted to the right. *(Right)* Frontal radiograph shows a triangular opacity behind the heart ➡ in this patient with left lower lobe collapse secondary to an obstructing bronchogenic carcinoma. Note the leftward mediastinal shift ➡ and compensatory hyperinflation of the left upper lung ➡.

Lobar Atelectasis

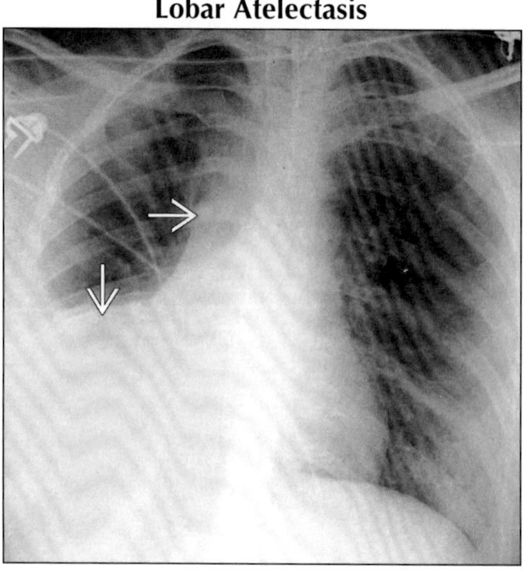

Lobar Atelectasis

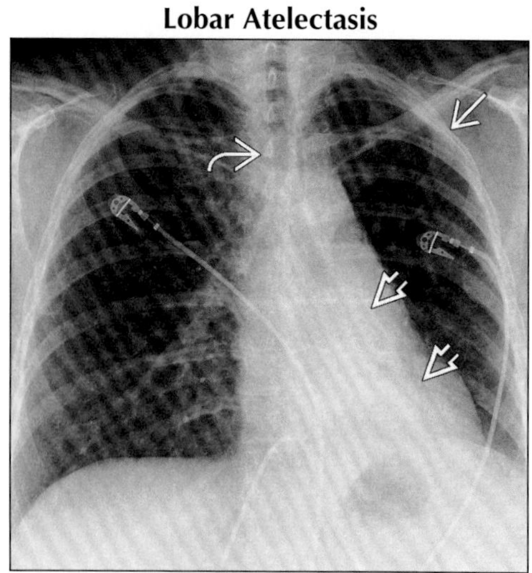

MEDIASTINAL SHIFT

Lobar Atelectasis

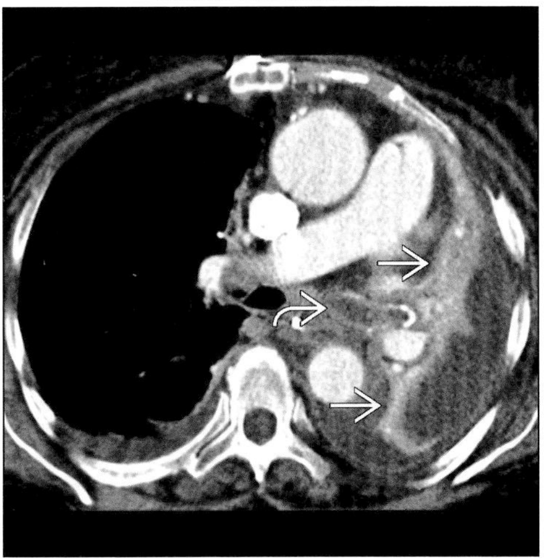

Lobar Atelectasis

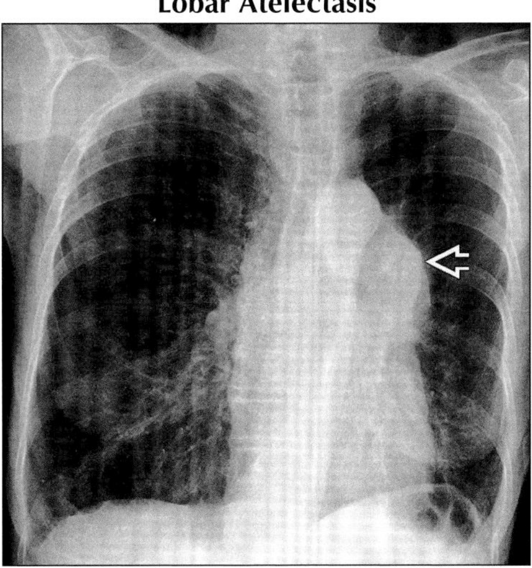

(Left) *Axial CECT shows typical features of left lung collapse secondary to mucus. Note the complete atelectasis of the left lung ➔, small pleural effusion, and obstructed left main bronchus ➔.* ***(Right)*** *Frontal radiograph shows typical features of LUL collapse from bronchogenic carcinoma. Note the mass over the left hilum ➔. The left hemithorax is small, the mediastinum is shifted to the left, and the left lung is more lucent, reflecting air-trapping.*

Pneumothorax

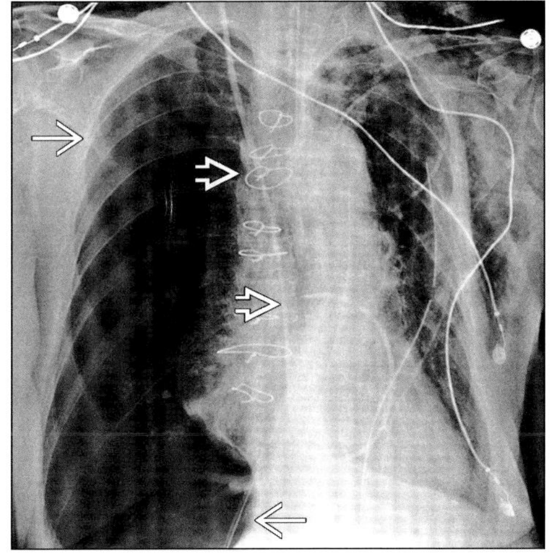

Pneumothorax

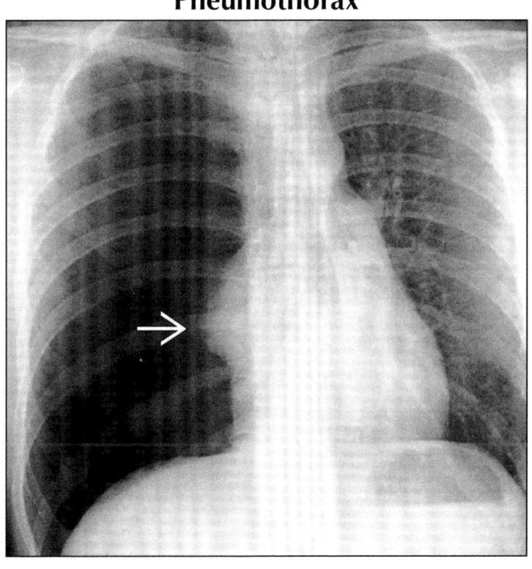

(Left) *AP radiograph shows a large pneumothorax ➔. The mediastinum is shifted to the left as marked by the Swan-Ganz catheter ➔. The hemidiaphragm is inverted and extends beyond the bottom of the radiograph.* ***(Right)*** *Frontal radiograph shows lucent right hemithorax and collapsed right lung ➔. Note the contralateral mediastinal shift, depression of the right hemidiaphragm, and widening of right rib interspaces, all concerning for tension physiology.*

Pneumonectomy

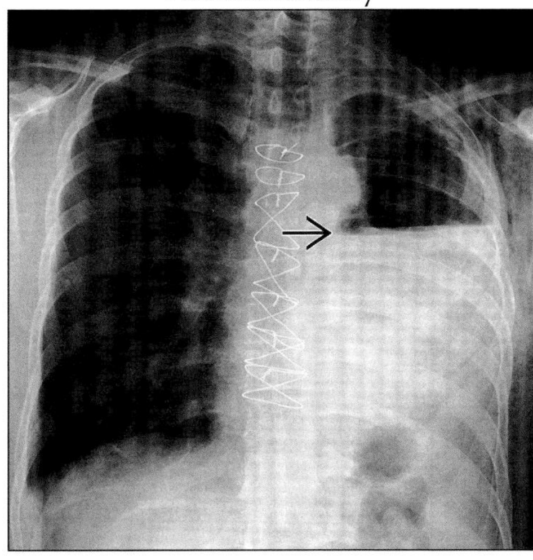

Pneumonectomy

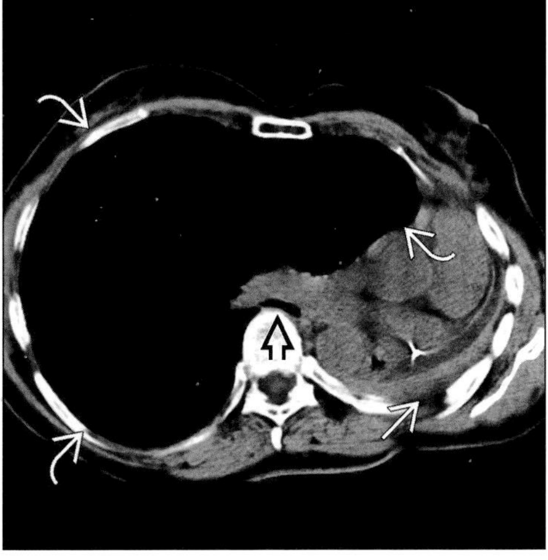

(Left) *Frontal radiograph shows an air-fluid level in the recent postoperative pneumonectomy space ➔ and mild ipsilateral mediastinal shift.* ***(Right)*** *Axial NECT shows typical features of left pneumonectomy syndrome following pneumonectomy. Note the pneumonectomy space ➔, marked hyperinflated right lung ➔, and narrowing of the airway as it crosses the spine ➔.*

MEDIASTINAL SHIFT

(Left) Frontal radiograph shows volume loss ➡ and reticular opacities in this patient with lung cancer treated primarily with radiation. Note the rightward tracheal deviation ⇨. *(Right)* Coronal CECT shows appearance of lung carcinoma at 36 months post radiation ⇨. Note the ipsilateral shift of the trachea ➡ and mediastinum.

Radiation Fibrosis

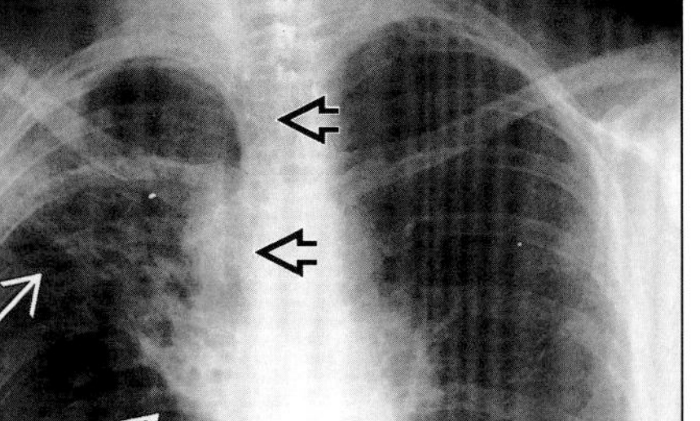

Radiation Fibrosis

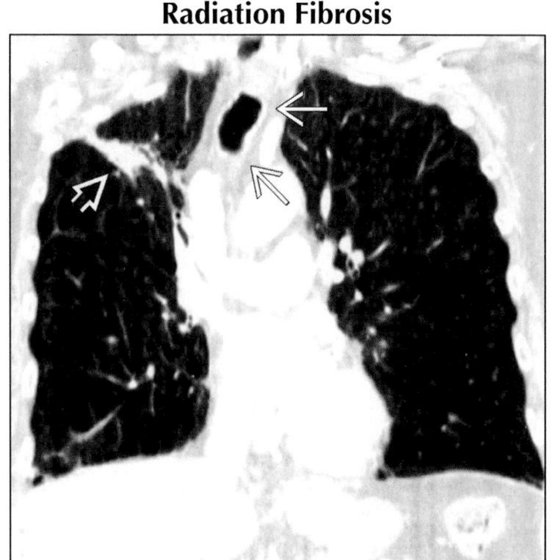

(Left) Coronal HRCT shows focal stenosis ➡ of the right main stem bronchus from tuberculosis infection. Note the rightward mediastinal shift of the trachea and elevation of the right hemidiaphragm ⇨. *(Right)* Coronal CECT shows basilar bronchiectasis ↪ and small right hemithorax with ipsilateral mediastinal shift in this "autopneumonectomy" patient following tuberculosis infection.

Tuberculosis

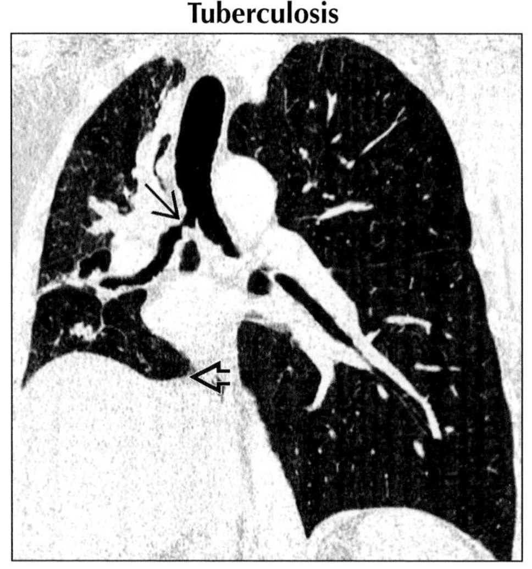

Tuberculosis

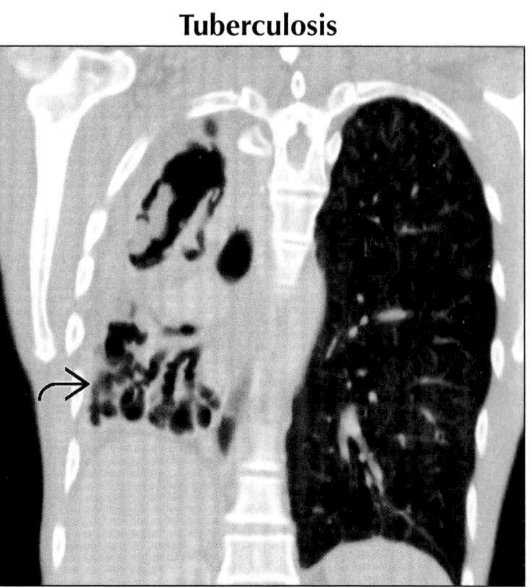

(Left) Anteroposterior radiograph shows radiographic features of hemothorax from rib trauma. Note the large left hemothorax ➡. There is rightward mediastinal shift. *(Right)* Axial CECT shows large pleural effusion ↪ and displaced extrapleural fat ⇨ from large extrapleural hematoma ➡. Note the rightward mediastinal shift. The rib fracture that caused the bleed was visualized on a lower section.

Hemothorax

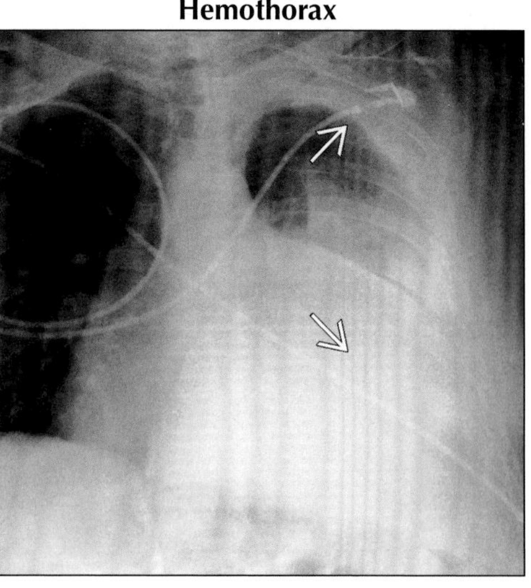

Hemothorax

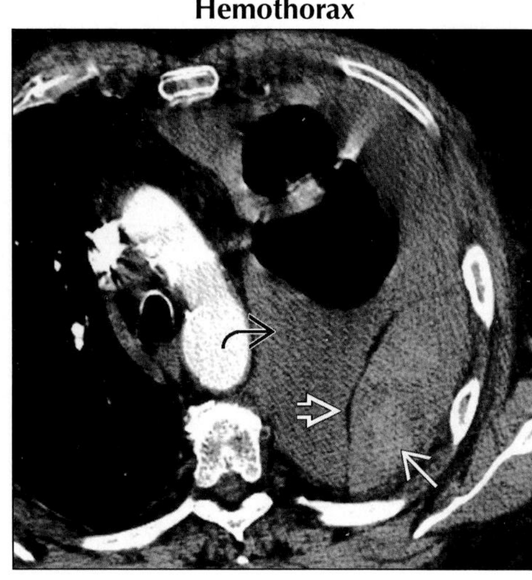

MEDIASTINAL SHIFT

Fibrothorax

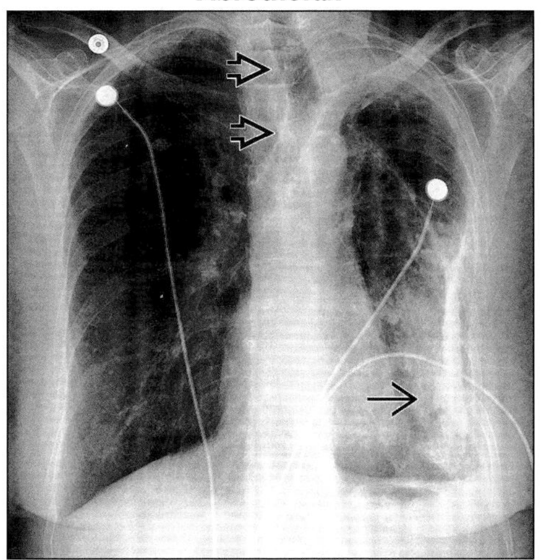

Fibrothorax

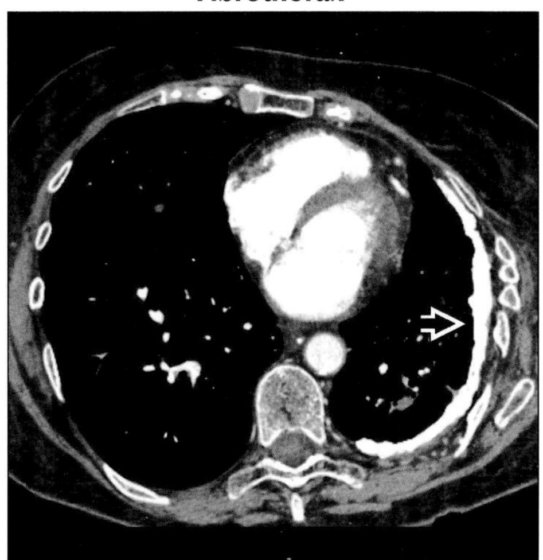

*(**Left**) Frontal radiograph shows small left hemithorax and diffuse calcified pleura* → *. The trachea is deviated leftward* ⇨ *. (**Right**) Axial CECT shows thick calcified pleural thickening* ➡ *with volume loss in the left hemithorax. Note the ipsilateral mediastinal shift in this patient with fibrothorax secondary to old tuberculosis empyema.*

Malignancy

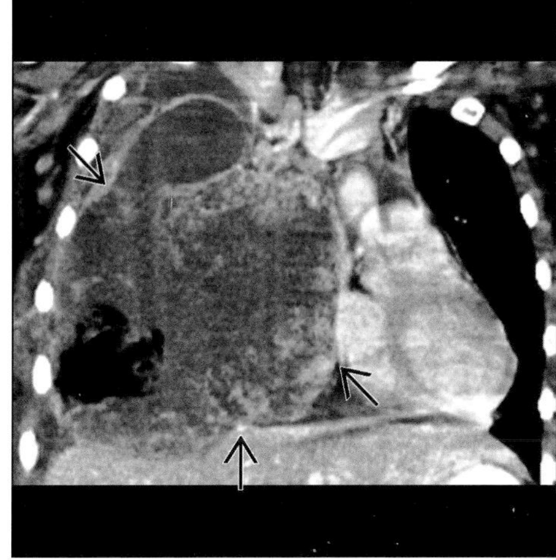

Malignancy

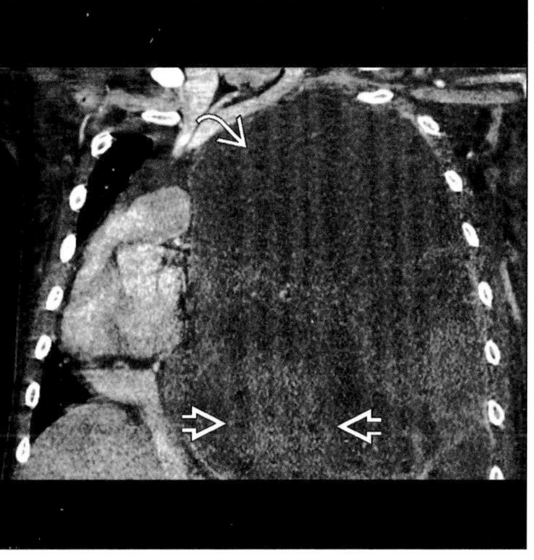

*(**Left**) Coronal CECT shows a large mass* → *causing contralateral mediastinal shift. This proved to be a yolk sac tumor. (**Right**) Coronal CECT shows a large heterogeneously enhancing mass with cystic* ↷ *and solid portions* ➡ *. Note the contralateral mediastinal shift in this patient with metastatic synovial cell sarcoma.*

Diaphragmatic Hernia

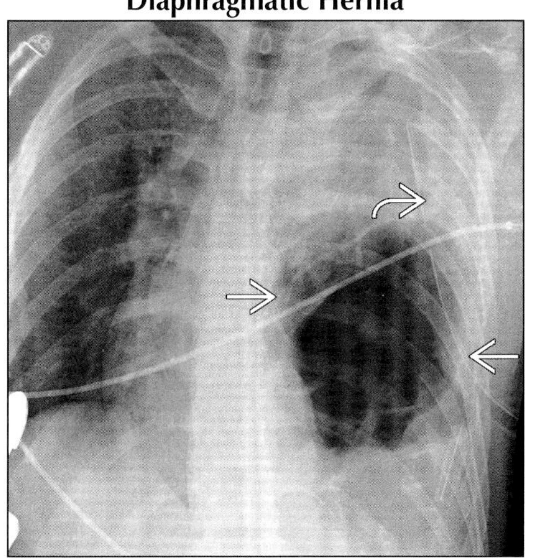

Scimitar Syndrome

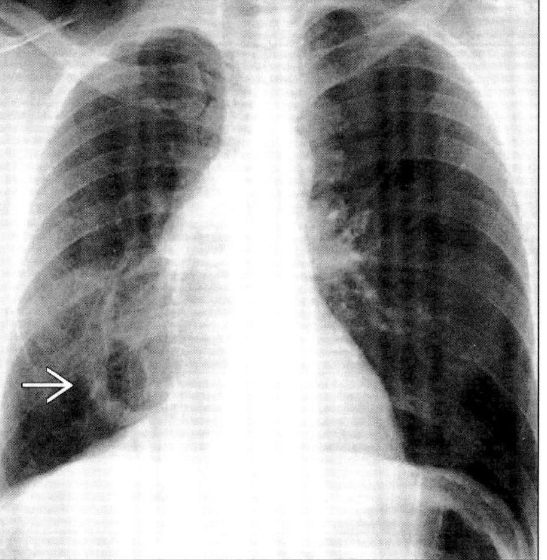

*(**Left**) Anteroposterior radiograph shows typical features of intrathoracic bowel in acute diaphragmatic tear. Note the intrathoracic bowel* ➡ *with mediastinal shift to the right. Left pleural effusion suggests strangulation* ↷ *. (**Right**) Frontal radiograph shows volume loss in the right lung as well as vertical vein extending inferiorly* ➡ *to the inferior vena cava.*

PNEUMOMEDIASTINUM

DIFFERENTIAL DIAGNOSIS

Common

- True Pneumomediastinum
  - Alveolar Rupture
  - Tracheobronchial Injury
  - Esophageal Injury
  - Iatrogenic Injury
  - Extension from Neck or Abdomen
  - Mediastinitis (Rare)
- Medial Pneumothorax (Mimic)
- Mach Band (Mimic)

Less Common

- Pneumopericardium
- Skin Fold (Mimic)
- Paratracheal Air Cyst (Mimic)

ESSENTIAL INFORMATION

Key Differential Diagnosis Issues

- CT generally diagnostic in differentiating pneumomediastinum from its mimics

Helpful Clues for Common Diagnoses

- **True Pneumomediastinum**
  - Alveolar rupture due to asthma, coughing, Valsalva maneuver, volutrauma, alveolar lung disease, or interstitial lung disease
  - Iatrogenic injury due to chest tube placement or tracheostomy
  - Ectopic gas in mediastinum; often clinically evident
  - Lucency along heart border that often extends into neck; lucent regions around mediastinal structures
  - Continuous diaphragm sign: Gas outlines inferior aspect of heart (also in pneumopericardium)
- **Medial Pneumothorax (Mimic)**
  - Pneumothorax in other portions of pleural space
  - If not loculated, will rapidly shift with change in position
- **Mach Band (Mimic)**
  - Lacks distinct pleural line of pneumomediastinum
  - Artifact no longer apparent when excluding dense heart from field of vision

Helpful Clues for Less Common Diagnoses

- **Pneumopericardium**
  - Does not extend above level of hila; continuous diaphragm sign
  - Rapidly shifts with change in position
- **Skin Fold (Mimic)**
  - Lacks distinct pleural line of pneumomediastinum; may see indistinct black line (gas in skin fold)
  - Often nonanatomic orientation; disappears on repeat studies
- **Paratracheal Air Cyst (Mimic)**
  - Small gas-filled foci at thoracic inlet along right posterolateral aspect of trachea
  - Connection to trachea rarely seen

True Pneumomediastinum

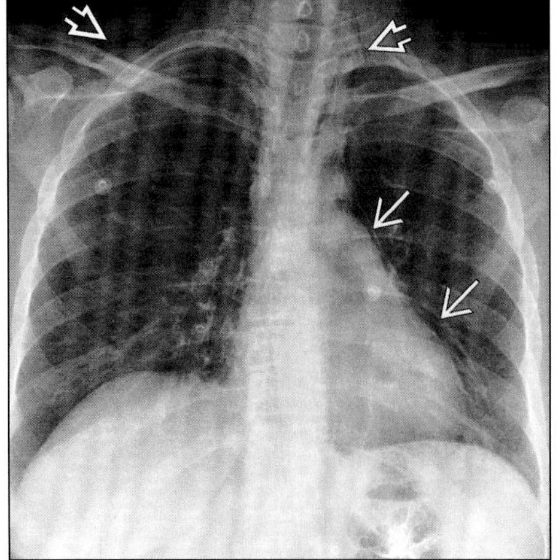

Frontal radiograph shows lucent regions along the left aspect of the mediastinum ➔ extending into the neck and shoulders ⇨, highly suggestive of pneumomediastinum.

True Pneumomediastinum

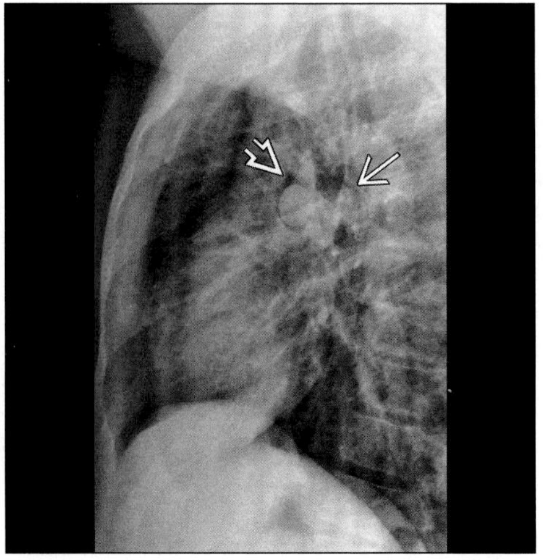

Lateral radiograph shows lucent regions within the mediastinum highly suggestive of pneumomediastinum. Gas outlines the right ⇨ and left ➔ pulmonary arteries.

Tracheobronchial Injury

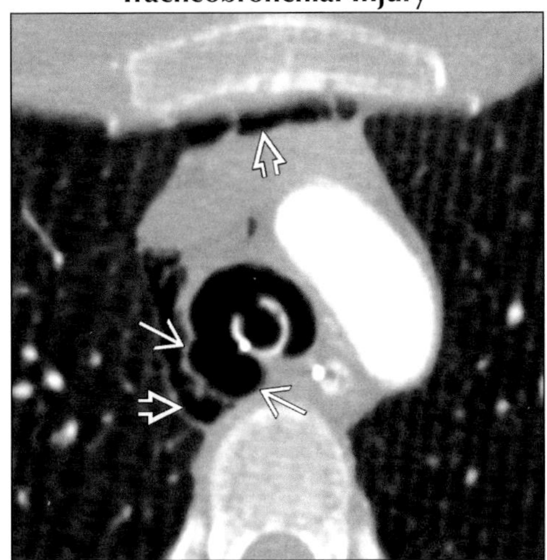

Esophageal Injury

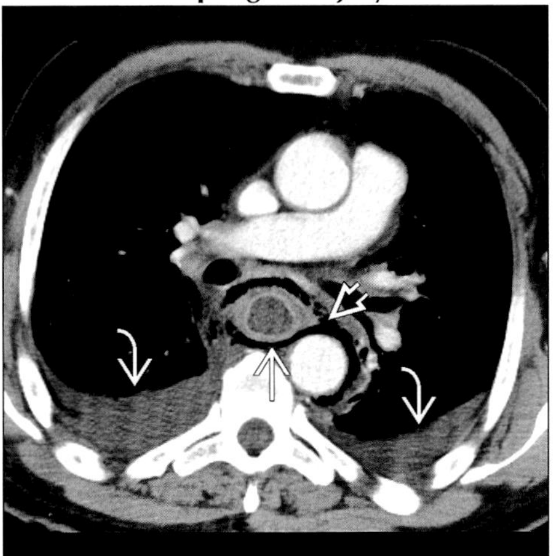

(Left) *Axial CECT shows focal outpouching ➡ along the right posterolateral aspect of the trachea highly suggestive of tracheal injury; there is associated pneumomediastinum ➡.* ***(Right)*** *Axial CECT shows a dilated, thick-walled esophagus ➡. Periesophageal pneumomediastinum ➡ and pleural effusions ➡ are consistent with Boerhaave syndrome (esophageal perforation).*

Medial Pneumothorax (Mimic)

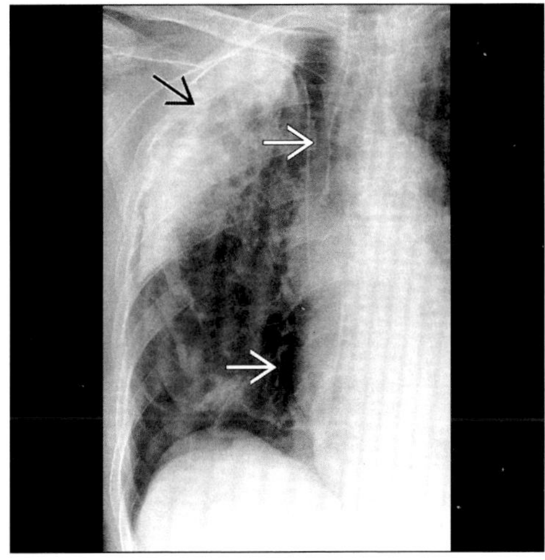

Mach Band (Mimic)

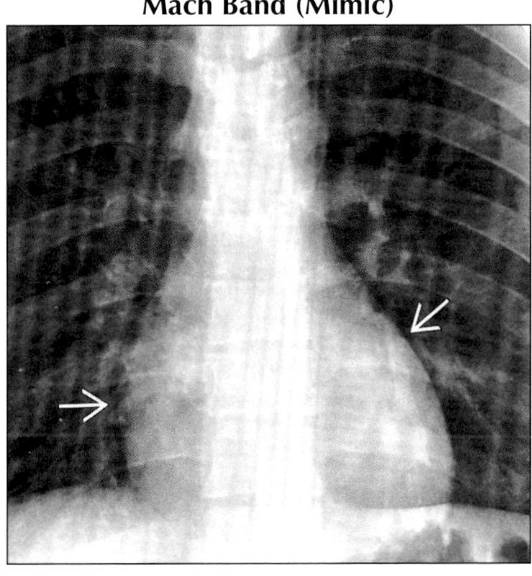

(Left) *Frontal radiograph shows lucent areas with elevation of the medial pleura ➡ along the right aspect of the mediastinum. Pneumothorax (caused by right upper lobe cavitary pneumonia ➡) is present in the right lateral pleural space, suggesting that medial lucent regions are likely pleural in location.* ***(Right)*** *Frontal radiograph shows lucent regions ➡ around the heart without visualization of distinct pleural lines, most consistent with mach bands.*

Pneumopericardium

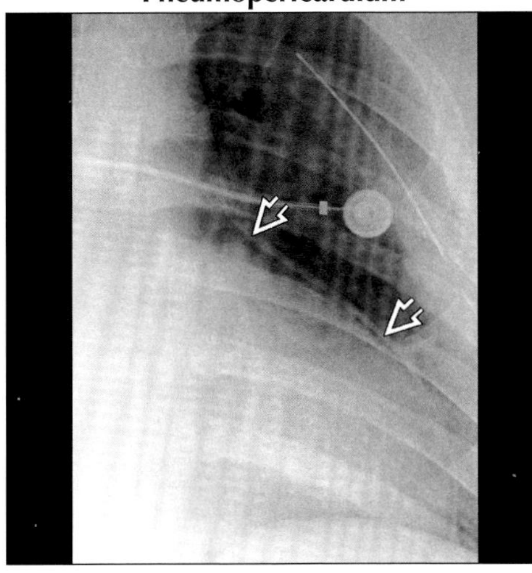

Paratracheal Air Cyst (Mimic)

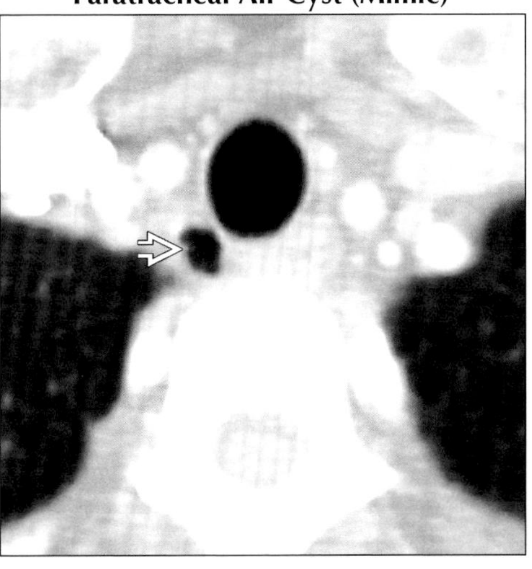

(Left) *Frontal radiograph shows a thin, lucent band that elevates the pericardium and pleura ➡ away from the left heart border. The lucent band terminates at the hilar level. The density of the heart is also lower than normal.* ***(Right)*** *Axial CECT shows a multiloculated air cyst ➡ along the right posterolateral aspect of the trachea at the level of the thoracic inlet. A connection to the trachea is often not apparent on CT, as in this case.*

ANTERIOR COMPARTMENT MASS

DIFFERENTIAL DIAGNOSIS

Common

- Lymphoma
- Germ Cell Tumor
  - Teratoma
  - Seminoma
- Thyroid Mass
- Thymoma
- Thymic Hyperplasia
- Lipomatosis
- Metastasis

Less Common

- Thymic Mass
  - Thymic Carcinoma
  - Thymic Carcinoid
  - Thymic Cyst
- Parathyroid Mass

Rare but Important

- Thymolipoma
- Lymphangioma
- Nonseminomatous Germ Cell Tumor

ESSENTIAL INFORMATION

Key Differential Diagnosis Issues

- Anatomy of anterior compartment
  - Radiologic description is based upon radiographic landmarks as defined by Fraser and Pare; note this differs from surgical description
  - Anterior border is sternum, and posterior border is anterior margin of vertebral column
- Normal contents: Thymus, ascending aorta, great vessels, part of main pulmonary artery, heart, pericardium, lymph nodes, adipose tissue
- CT is invaluable for determining site of origin and tissue characterization

Helpful Clues for Common Diagnoses

- **Lymphoma**
  - Hodgkin disease (HD) more common than non-Hodgkin lymphoma (NHL) within anterior compartment
  - Enlarged lymph nodes or nodal mass, usually displaying homogeneous soft tissue attenuation
  - Necrosis is occasionally present, usually detected after contrast administration
  - HD commonly involves several contiguous nodal groups in thorax
  - Involvement of single nodal group is more common with NHL
- **Germ Cell Tumor**
  - Most common age is 2nd-4th decades
  - More than 80% are benign
  - **Teratoma**
    - Most common benign germ cell tumor, though can be malignant
    - Display cystic areas, soft tissue, fat, and calcification
    - Fat-fluid level is diagnostic but usually not present
  - **Seminoma**
    - Most common malignant germ cell tumor and usually in males
    - Large homogeneous mass, which can have small focal areas of decreased attenuation
- **Thyroid Mass**
  - Caused by inferior extension of thyroid lesion
  - Direct connection to thyroid is usually evident on CT
  - High attenuation on noncontrast CT is due to iodine content
  - Differentiation of goiter and tumor may not be possible
- **Thymoma**
  - Most common in 6th decade
  - Associated with myasthenia gravis
  - Round or lobulated and usually homogeneous
  - Possible areas of necrosis, hemorrhage, calcification, and cyst formation
  - Does not conform to normal thymic contour and may be unilateral
  - Classified as invasive or noninvasive based upon invasion of adjacent structures (including vessels, heart, and pericardium); determination not always possible with CT
  - Pleural spread often produces multiple pleural implants
- **Thymic Hyperplasia**
  - Associated with recovery from chemotherapy or burn (thymic rebound) in children and young adults
  - Associated with Grave disease, myasthenia gravis, red cell aplasia, and other conditions in adults

- Thymic rebound often visible on chest radiograph; correlate with clinical history
- Enlarged thymus with normal homogeneous attenuation on CT

• **Lipomatosis**
- Excessive unencapsulated fat in mediastinum associated with Cushing syndrome, steroids, obesity
- Smooth, symmetric mediastinal widening on chest radiograph
- Homogeneous increased amount of mediastinal fat with smooth margins on CT

• **Metastasis**
- Lung and breast primaries are common
- May involve thymus or mediastinal lymph nodes
- Appearance is nonspecific

Helpful Clues for Less Common Diagnoses

• **Thymic Carcinoma**
- Large mass that can have areas of necrosis
- Similar to thymoma in appearance, but distant metastases are far more common than with thymoma
- Metastases often involve lungs, skeleton, liver, and brain

• **Thymic Carcinoid**
- Commonly secretes ACTH, which results in Cushing syndrome
- Appears similar to thymoma on imaging, though typically more aggressive

• **Thymic Cyst**
- Care should be taken not to confuse with cystic neoplasm
- Nonenhancing, thin-walled, water density, no soft tissue component

• **Parathyroid Mass**
- Normal glands are not visible on CT
- Ectopic glands often found in thymic bed
- Cannot distinguish adenoma, hyperplasia, and carcinoma on CT

Helpful Clues for Rare Diagnoses

• **Thymolipoma**
- Most common age is 1st-4th decades
- Usually asymptomatic and large at time of detection
- May appear to drape over heart on chest radiograph
- Primarily fat density on CT with strands of soft tissue attenuation

• **Lymphangioma**
- Usually congenital and often presents in childhood
- Well circumscribed with homogeneous water attenuation
- May wrap around mediastinal structures, such as great vessels

• **Nonseminomatous Germ Cell Tumor**
- Aggressive neoplasms with poor prognoses
- Infiltrative and heterogeneous with areas of hemorrhage and necrosis

Lymphoma

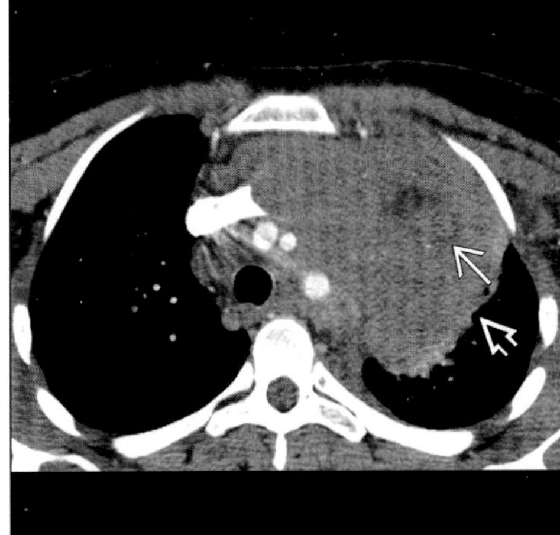

Axial CECT shows a large primarily homogeneous mass in the anterior and middle mediastinum ➡ in this 25-year-old man. There is some internal nodularity ➡. Biopsy revealed Hodgkin lymphoma.

Lymphoma

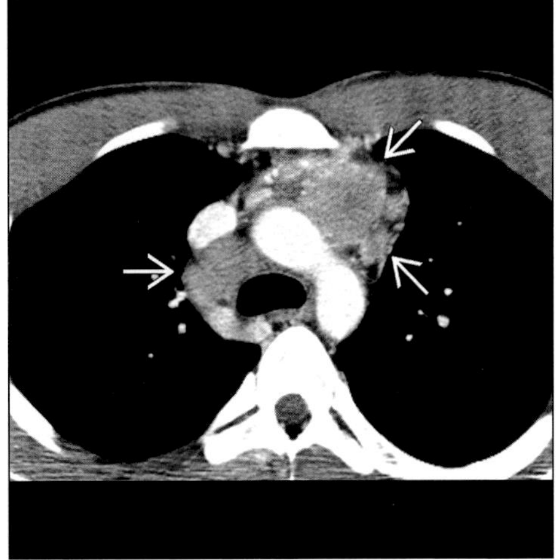

Axial CECT shows numerous nodular mediastinal masses in this 28-year-old man ➡. Involvement of multiple contiguous nodal groups is typical of Hodgkin lymphoma.

ANTERIOR COMPARTMENT MASS

*(**Left**) Axial CECT shows a large nodular mass in the anterior mediastinum ➡ with numerous areas of internal necrosis ➡. Note invasion of the superior vena cava ➡. Biopsy revealed non-Hodgkin lymphoma. (**Right**) Axial CECT shows a homogeneous anterior mediastinal mass in the prevascular space ➡. This lesion was radiographically occult and is biopsy-proven non-Hodgkin lymphoma.*

Lymphoma

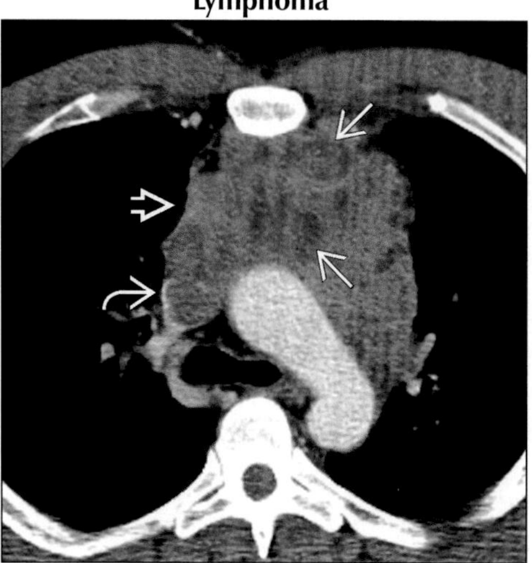

Lymphoma

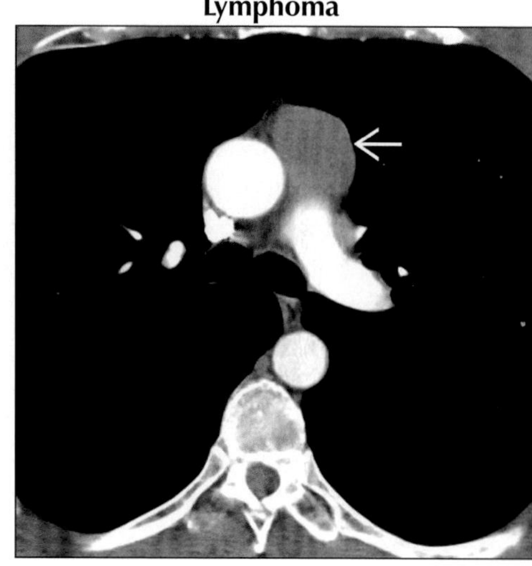

*(**Left**) Frontal radiograph shows an anterior mediastinal mass ➡ in this young adult. Notice the sharp lateral margin and indistinct medial margin. Also note absence of hilar distortion. These findings are suggestive of a mediastinal location. (**Right**) Axial CECT in the same patient shows a heterogeneous anterior mediastinal mass. Note the presence of fat within this lesion ➡, which is highly suggestive of the diagnosis of mediastinal teratoma.*

Teratoma

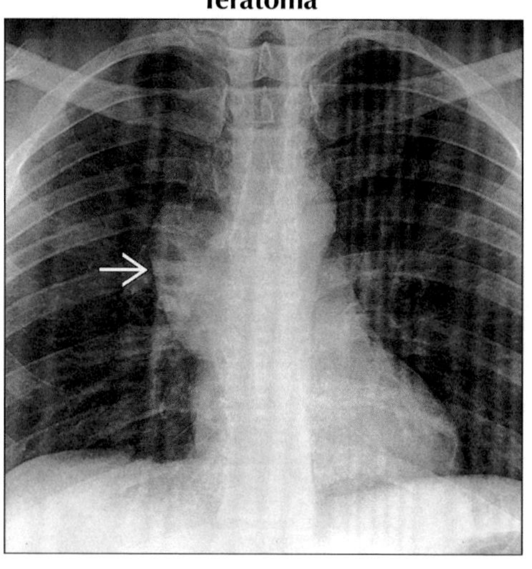

Teratoma

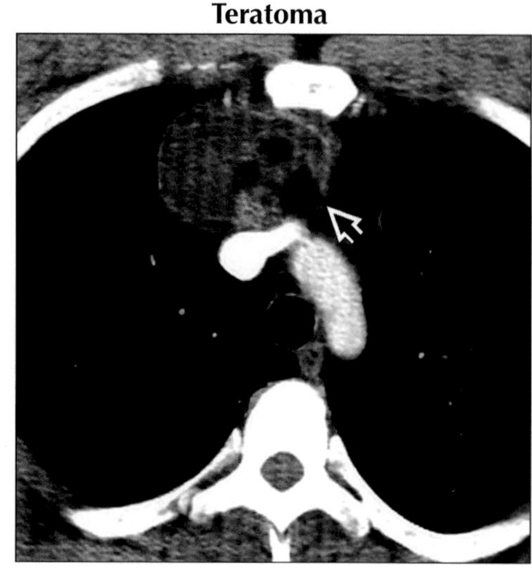

*(**Left**) Axial CECT shows a large homogeneous mass in the anterior mediastinum ➡. There is obstruction of the SVC with formation of venous collateral vessels ➡. This lesion is a biopsy-proven seminoma. (**Right**) Coronal CECT in the same patient again shows the large anterior mediastinal mass ➡ with invasion of the left brachiocephalic vein. Notice extension of thrombus within the left brachiocephalic vein ➡.*

Seminoma

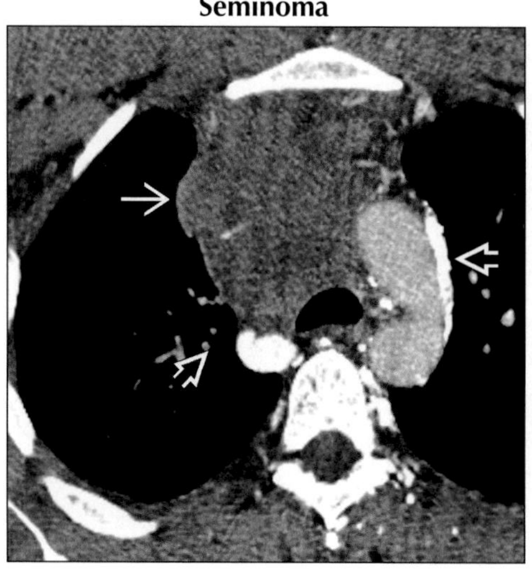

Seminoma

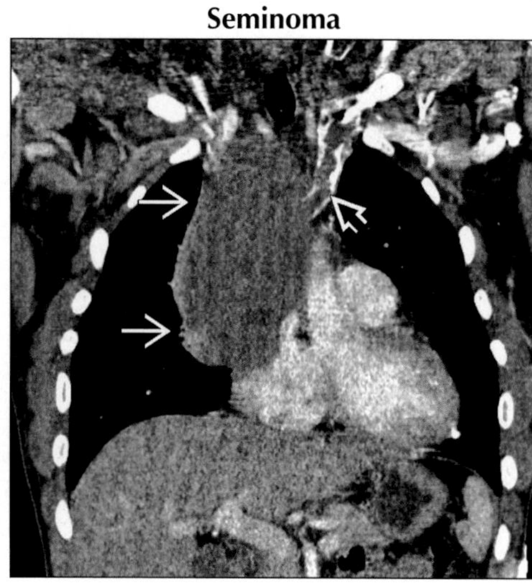

Thyroid Mass

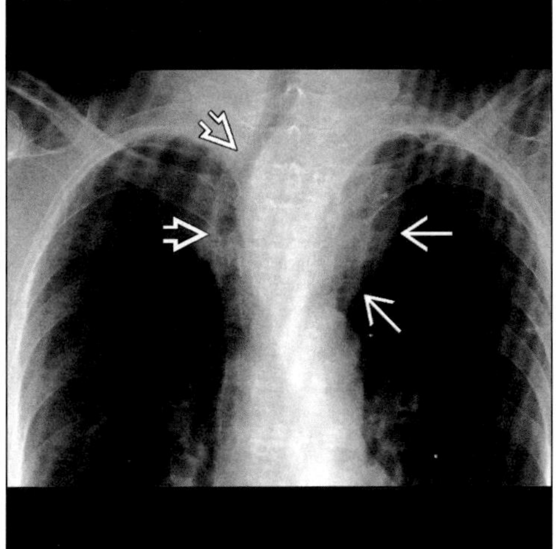

Thyroid Mass

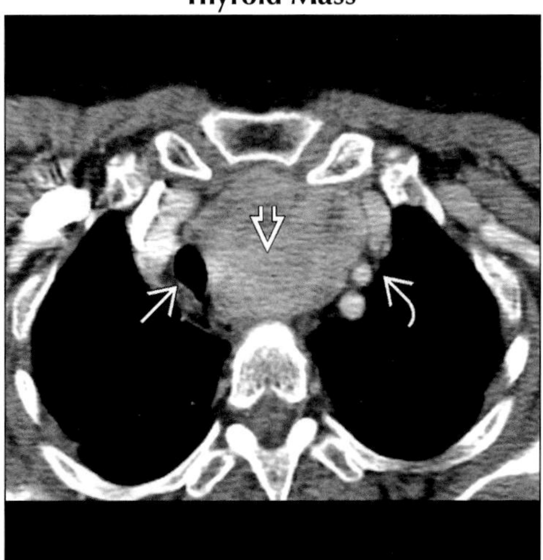

(Left) *Radiograph shows a large mediastinal mass ➡ displacing the trachea to the right ➡. This is a common appearance of goiter, though radiography is not specific.* ***(Right)*** *Axial CECT confirms the findings seen on radiograph. There is a large mediastinal mass ➡ with displacement of the trachea ➡ and great vessels ➡ and no evidence of invasion. Other images showed communication with the thyroid in this patient with a large substernal goiter.*

Thyroid Mass

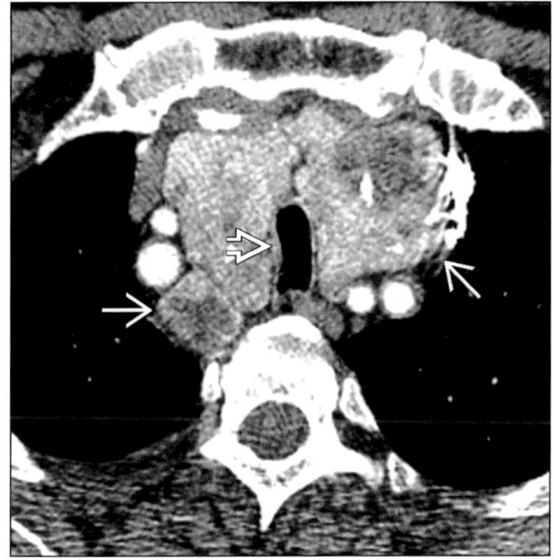

Thymoma

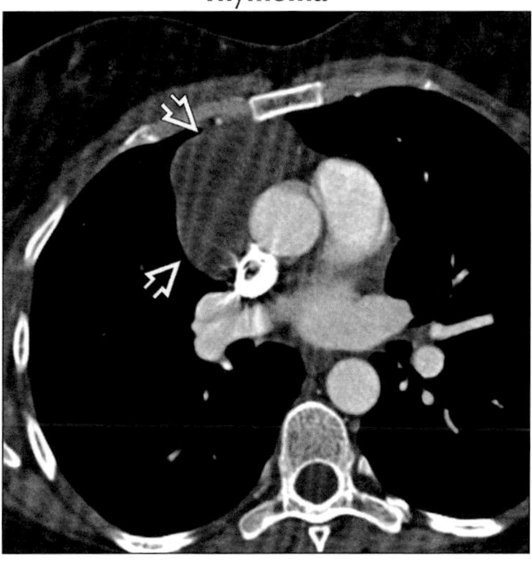

(Left) *Axial CECT shows an enlarged substernal thyroid ➡ with numerous nodules. Notice compression of the trachea ➡. Also notice the increased attenuation of the lesion due to internal iodine content.* ***(Right)*** *Axial CECT shows a homogeneous well-defined mass in the anterior mediastinum ➡ in a 45-year-old woman. This represents a thymoma, with no CT evidence of invasion of adjacent structures.*

Thymoma

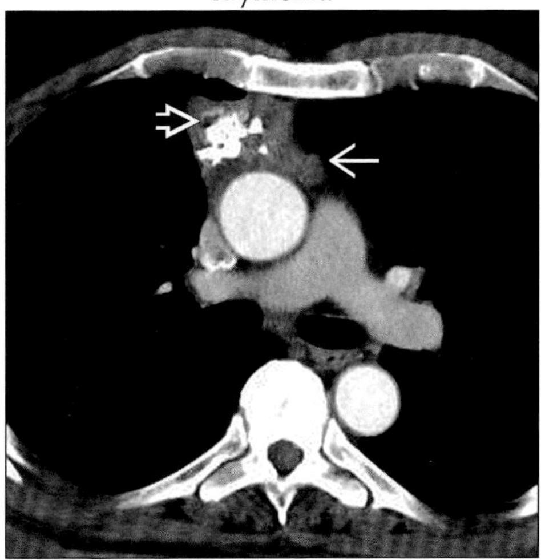

Thymoma

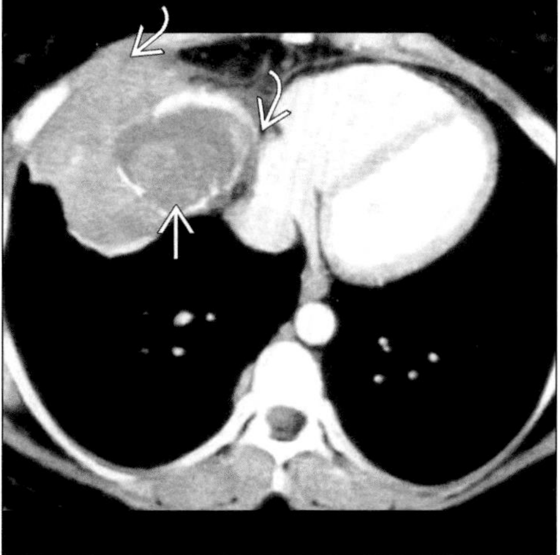

(Left) *Axial CECT shows an anterior mediastinal mass ➡ with coarse internal calcifications ➡. Calcifications are occasionally present within a thymoma and can be coarse, punctate, or peripheral.* ***(Right)*** *Axial CECT shows an anterior mediastinal mass with rim calcifications ➡. The mass infiltrates the adjacent heart and chest wall ➡. This lesion represents an invasive thymoma.*

ANTERIOR COMPARTMENT MASS

Thymoma

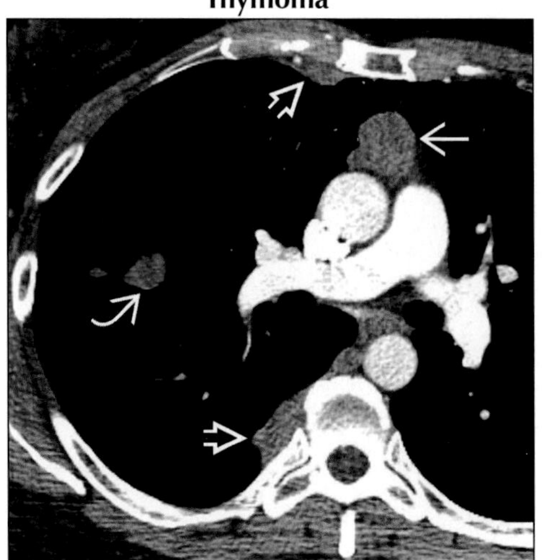

Thymic Hyperplasia

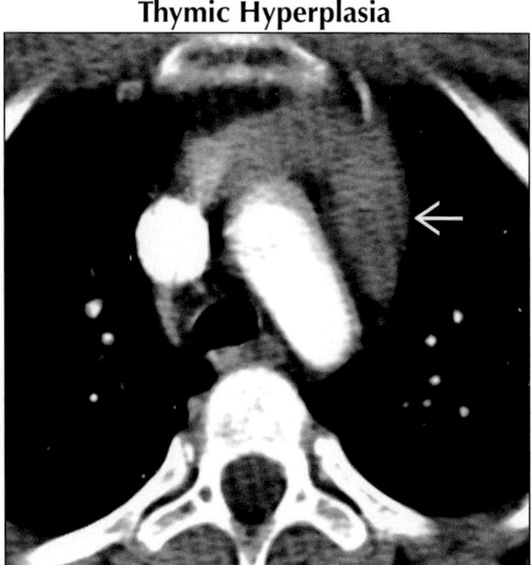

(Left) *Axial CECT shows a round anterior mediastinal mass ➡. There are several pleural masses ⇨, including masses within the major fissure ➦. This is a typical appearance of invasive thymoma with drop pleural metastases.* ***(Right)*** *Axial CECT shows an enlarged thymus ➡ in a 17-year-old patient who underwent chemotherapy. Given the appropriate history, this is consistent with thymic hyperplasia.*

Thymic Hyperplasia

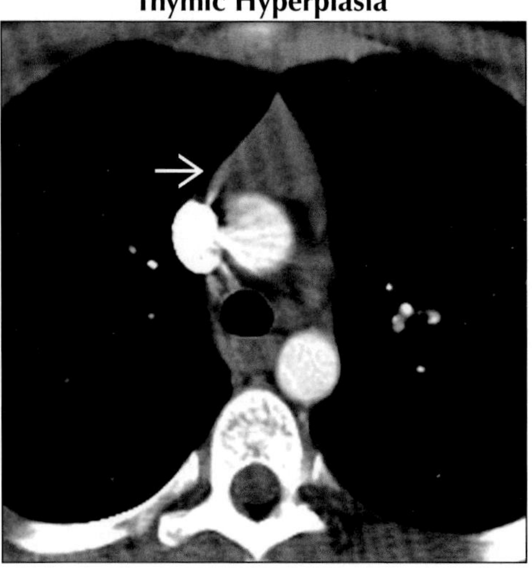

Thymic Hyperplasia

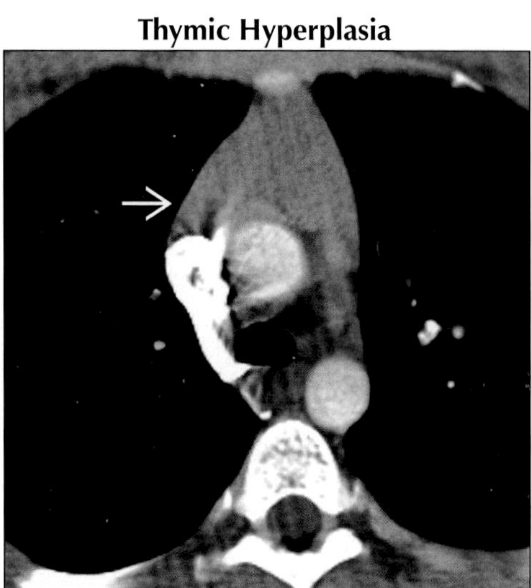

(Left) *Axial CECT shows a typical appearance of the normal thymus gland ➡ in a 13-year-old boy.* ***(Right)*** *Axial CECT obtained 3 months after treatment for lymphoma demonstrates enlargement of the thymus ➡, consistent with thymic hyperplasia (thymic rebound). Notice that the thymus remains homogeneous in attenuation and maintains its normal bilobed appearance.*

Lipomatosis

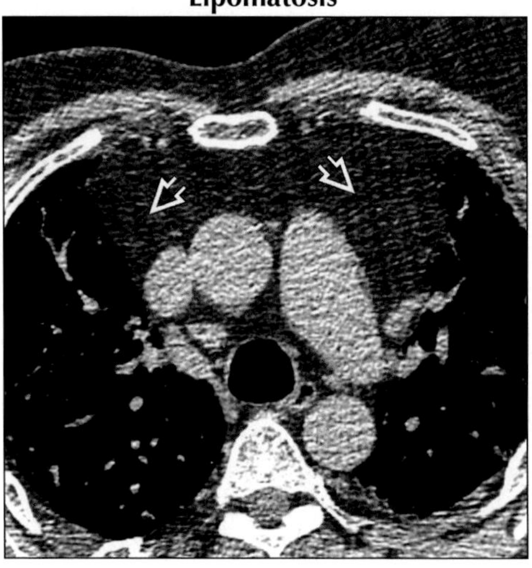

Metastasis

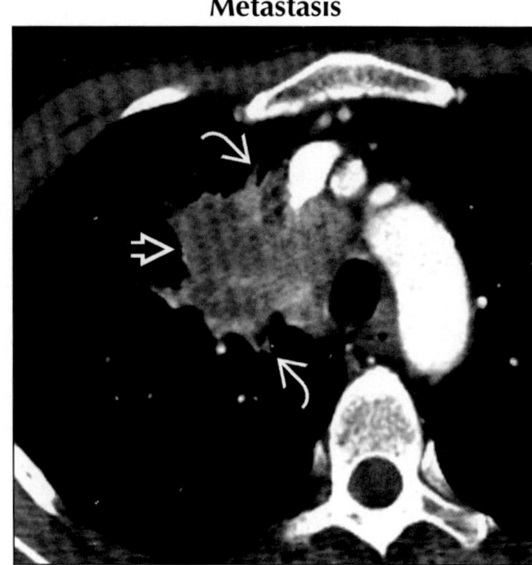

(Left) *Axial HRCT shows symmetric expansion of the mediastinal fat ⇨ without associated mass effect in this patient on steroid therapy for pulmonary fibrosis. This is typical of mediastinal lipomatosis.* ***(Right)*** *Axial CECT shows a large heterogeneous lesion involving the anterior and middle mediastinum, with extension into the adjacent right lung ⇨. Notice the spiculated margins ➦. This is a metastatic lesion from squamous cell lung carcinoma.*

ANTERIOR COMPARTMENT MASS

Thymic Carcinoma

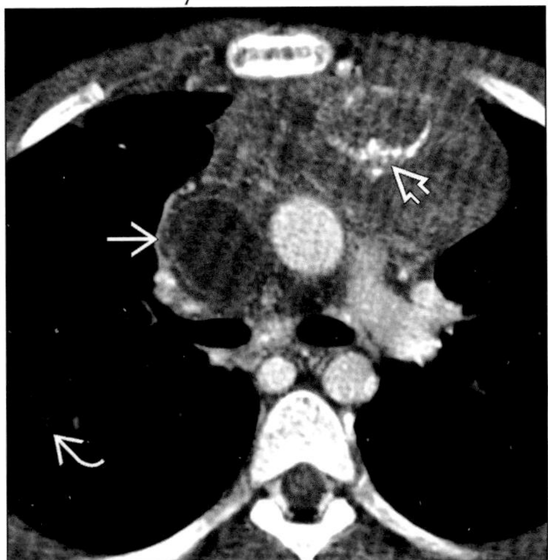

Thymic Carcinoid

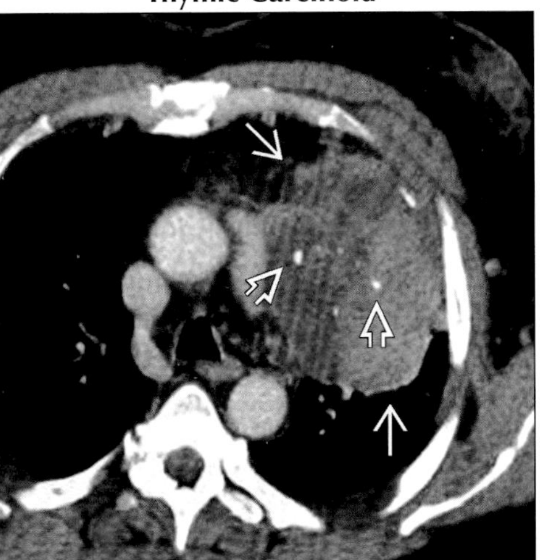

*(**Left**) Axial CECT shows a large heterogeneous mass with several cystic areas and ring-like calcifications in an elderly male patient. Although findings are suggestive of a malignant thymic tumor, the metastatic nodule in the right lung is more suggestive of thymic carcinoma. (**Right**) Axial CECT shows a large heterogeneous mediastinal mass with several focal calcifications. In a patient with elevated ACTH, this is consistent with thymic carcinoid.*

Thymic Cyst

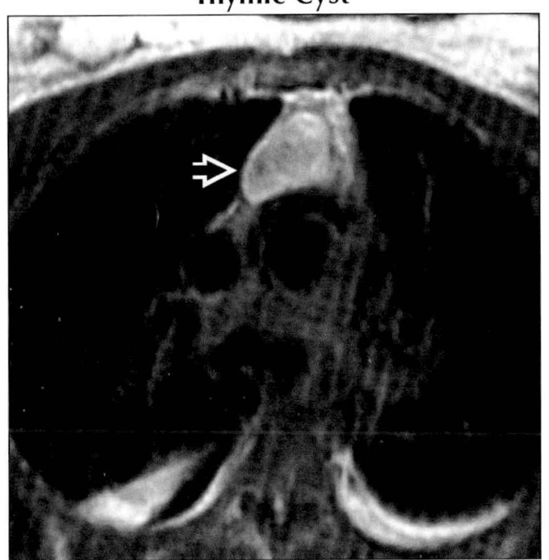

Thymolipoma

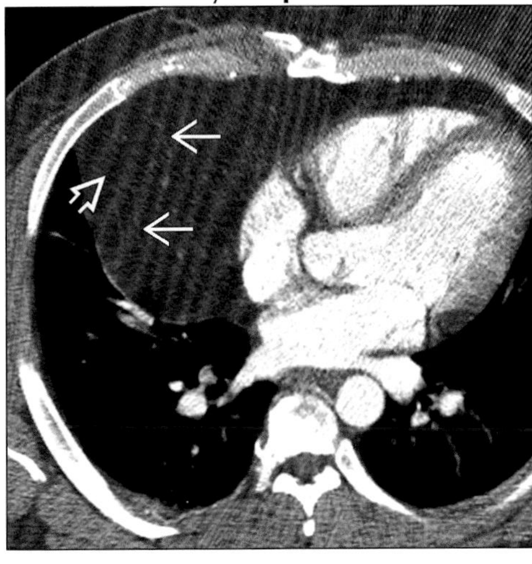

*(**Left**) Axial T2WI FS MR shows a well-defined hyperintense lesion in the anterior mediastinum. The high signal is suggestive of a cystic lesion. There is no soft tissue component in this pathologically proven thymic cyst. (**Right**) Axial CECT shows a large low-attenuation lesion draping over the right side of the heart. Notice the diffuse fat density with several streaks of interspersed soft tissue. This lesion was asymptomatic.*

Lymphangioma

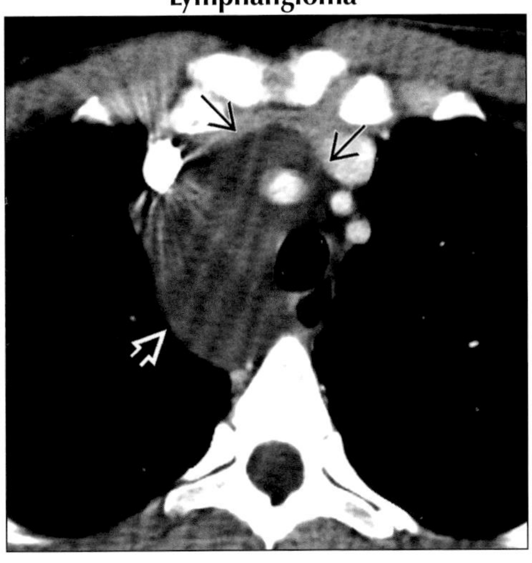

Nonseminomatous Germ Cell Tumor

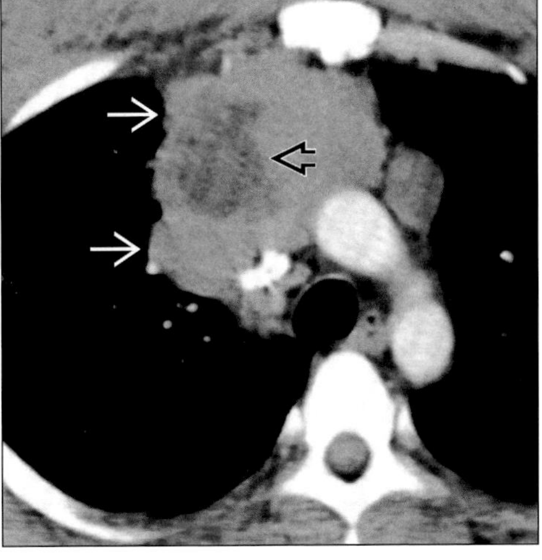

*(**Left**) Axial CECT shows a well-defined low-attenuation mediastinal mass. There are no solid or enhancing areas. Notice that the mass insinuates around the vessels without displacing them. This is typical of a lymphangioma. (**Right**) Axial CECT shows an anterior mediastinal mass with irregular margins and areas of decreased attenuation caused by internal necrosis. Findings are typical of an aggressive nonseminomatous germ cell tumor.*

MIDDLE COMPARTMENT MASS

DIFFERENTIAL DIAGNOSIS

Common
- Lymphadenopathy
  - Infection
  - Sarcoidosis
  - Lymphoma
  - Lung Carcinoma and Extrathoracic Metastases
- Foregut Duplication Cysts
- Hiatal Hernia

Less Common
- Aortic Aneurysm
- Lipomatosis
- Mediastinal Goiter

Rare but Important
- Esophageal Masses
- Mediastinitis
- Mediastinal Hemorrhage
- Tracheal Neoplasms

ESSENTIAL INFORMATION

Key Differential Diagnosis Issues
- Anatomic boundaries of middle mediastinum on lateral radiograph
  - Anterior boundary
    - Line drawn along anterior tracheal wall and posterior heart border
  - Posterior boundary
    - Line drawn 1 cm behind anterior margin of vertebral bodies
  - Contents include trachea, superior vena cava, mid aortic arch, lymph nodes, and esophagus
- Middle mediastinal mass deviates these normal radiographic lines and measurements
  - Right paratracheal stripe ≤ 4 mm
  - Concave interface in aortopulmonary window
  - Reverse S contour of azygoesophageal recess
  - Posterior tracheal stripe ≤ 6 mm on lateral radiograph
- Components to consider in differential diagnosis
  - Density of lesion (fat, calcium, soft tissue, fluid)
  - Number of lesions
  - Clinical history

Helpful Clues for Common Diagnoses
- **Lymphadenopathy**
  - Right paratracheal stripe thickening usually indicates lymphadenopathy
  - Subcarinal lymphadenopathy
    - Convexity in superior azygoesophageal recess
  - Calcified nodes
    - Dense calcification usually from prior granulomatous infection
    - Rim calcification, "eggshell" appearance with sarcoidosis, silicosis, and treated lymphoma
  - Necrotic or low-density nodes
    - Tuberculosis and histoplasmosis
    - Lymphoma, thymoma, metastases, and lung carcinoma
  - Enhancing lymphadenopathy
    - Vascular metastases (renal, thyroid, and melanoma)
    - Tuberculosis
    - Castleman disease
- **Foregut Duplication Cysts**
  - Round and well circumscribed
  - Highly variable Hounsfield units depending on fluid content
  - Bronchogenic cysts commonly subcarinal in location
    - Less commonly peripheral, hilar
  - Esophageal duplication cyst location
    - Paraesophageal or within esophageal wall
- **Hiatal Hernia**
  - Convexity of lower azygoesophageal recess
  - Easily diagnosed on CT by protrusion of stomach through esophageal hiatus

Helpful Clues for Less Common Diagnoses
- **Aortic Aneurysm**
  - Definitions
    - Dilated ≥ 4 cm
    - Aneurysmal ≥ 5 cm
    - High risk of rupture ≥ 6 cm
    - Saccular are focal outpouchings and are associated with trauma or infection
    - Fusiform is circumferential
    - Annuloaortic ectasia is a dilated aortic root and associated with Marfan syndrome
  - CT or MR are diagnostic
- **Lipomatosis**
  - Causes include

- Obesity, long-term steroid therapy, Cushing disease
  - Radiographs show smooth mediastinal widening without compression of trachea
  - CT shows homogeneous fat causing bulging of mediastinal contours
- **Mediastinal Goiter**
  - Radiographs reveal upper mediastinal mass with deviation of trachea
  - CT demonstrates connection to thyroid
    - Coronal images very helpful
  - Enhance avidly with contrast and are high in density on pre-contrast exams

Helpful Clues for Rare Diagnoses

- **Esophageal Masses**
  - Varices are secondary to portal hypertension
    - Abnormal convexity of lower azygoesophageal recess or paravertebral widening
    - CT with contrast is diagnostic and easily differentiates from hiatal hernia or tumor
- **Mediastinitis**
  - Associated with sternotomy, esophageal perforation, or spread of infection
  - Radiographs show widened mediastinum
  - CT findings include
    - Diffuse fat stranding replacing normal mediastinal fat
    - Pneumomediastinum
    - Fluid collections
  - Difficult to differentiate normal postoperative appearance from mediastinitis
    - Resolution of expected fluid collections occurs within 2-3 weeks after surgery
- **Mediastinal Hemorrhage**
  - Causes include
    - Acute aortic injury or venous bleeding secondary to severe blunt or penetrating trauma
    - Aneurysm or dissection rupture
  - Radiographs show nonspecific mediastinal widening
  - High-attenuation (blood density) fluid within mediastinum
  - Hematoma not adjacent to aorta is secondary to venous bleeding
  - Retrosternal hematoma in anterior compartment
- **Tracheal Neoplasms**
  - Usually secondary to primary squamous cell carcinoma or adenoid cystic carcinoma
  - Uncommonly single or multiple metastases from
    - Melanoma, breast carcinoma, colon carcinoma, or adjacent tumor extension
  - CT features include
    - Polypoid, sessile, or circumferential lesion
    - Adenoid cystic carcinoma usually originates from posterolateral wall
    - Important to define extraluminal extent of disease for surgical planning

Infection

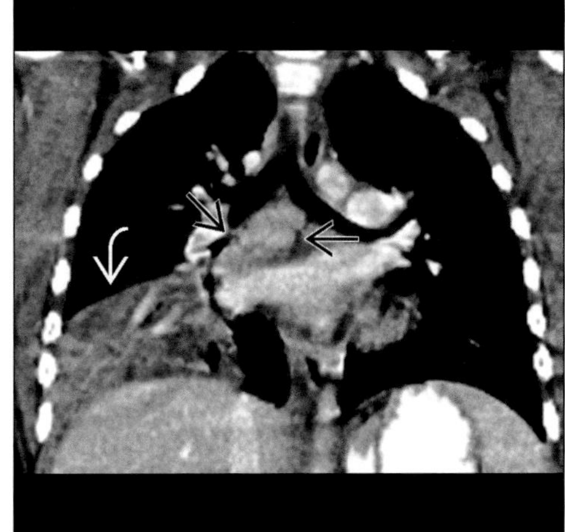

Coronal CECT shows subcarinal lymphadenopathy ➔ and right lower lung consolidation ➔ in this patient with bacterial pneumonia.

Infection

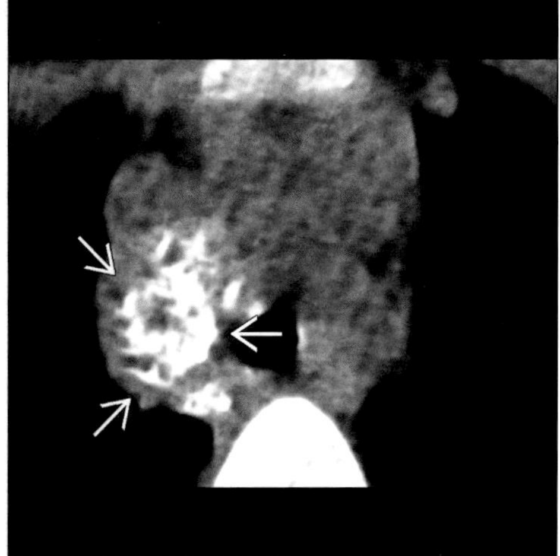

Axial NECT shows multiple calcified lymph nodes within the right paratracheal space ➔ in this patient with prior histoplasmosis infection.

MIDDLE COMPARTMENT MASS

Sarcoidosis

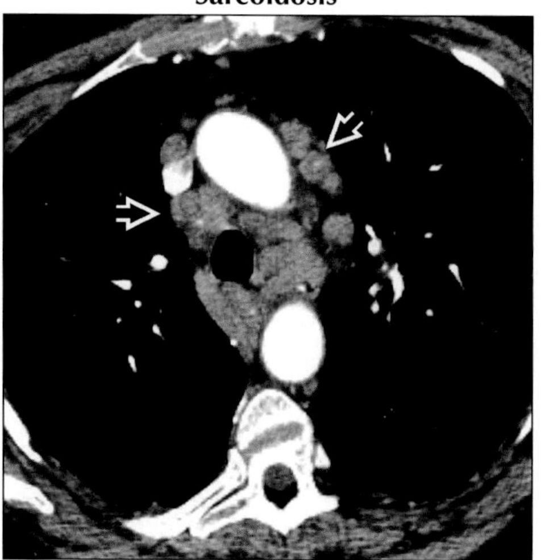

Sarcoidosis

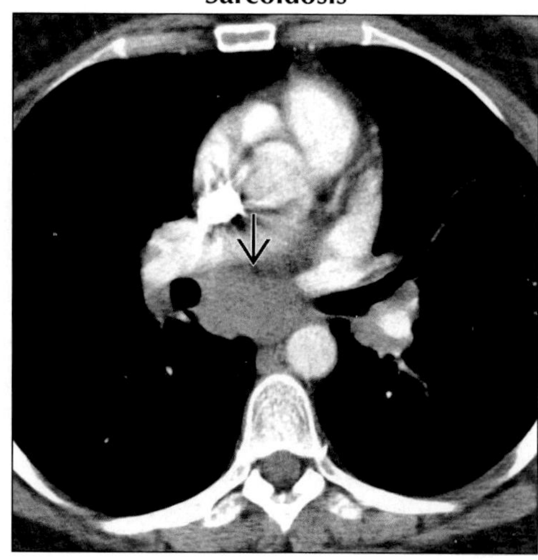

(Left) Axial CECT shows features of adenopathy in sarcoidosis. There is diffuse mediastinal adenopathy in the prevascular and paratracheal spaces. Lower sections revealed bilateral symmetric hilar lymphadenopathy. *(Right)* Axial CECT shows subcarinal lymphadenopathy in this asymptomatic patient. The symmetry of lymphadenopathy and age of the patient are important differential considerations to make the correct diagnosis.

Sarcoidosis

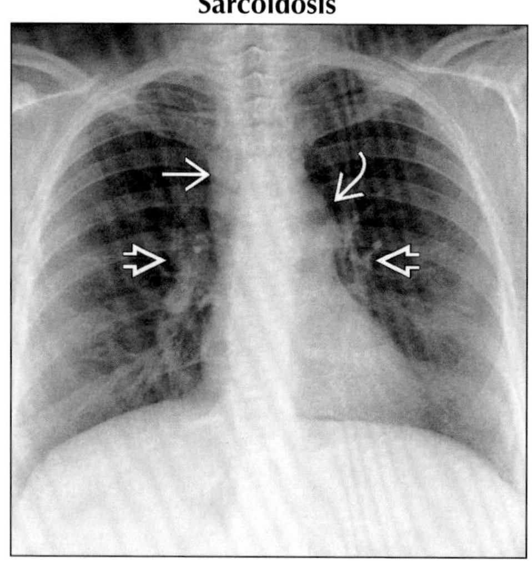

Sarcoidosis

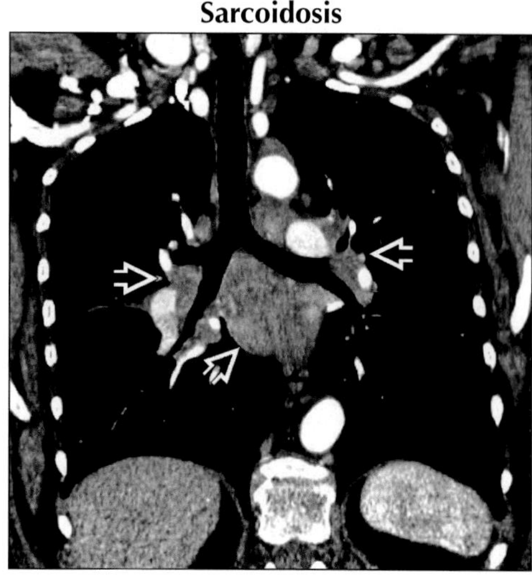

(Left) Frontal radiograph shows enlarged bilateral hilar, right paratracheal, and left aortopulmonary lymph nodes. This is a common finding in sarcoidosis. Presence of right paratracheal and bilateral hilar lymphadenopathy constitutes Garland triad. *(Right)* Coronal CECT shows typical CT features of lymphadenopathy in sarcoidosis. Note the diffuse hilar and mediastinal adenopathy.

Lymphoma

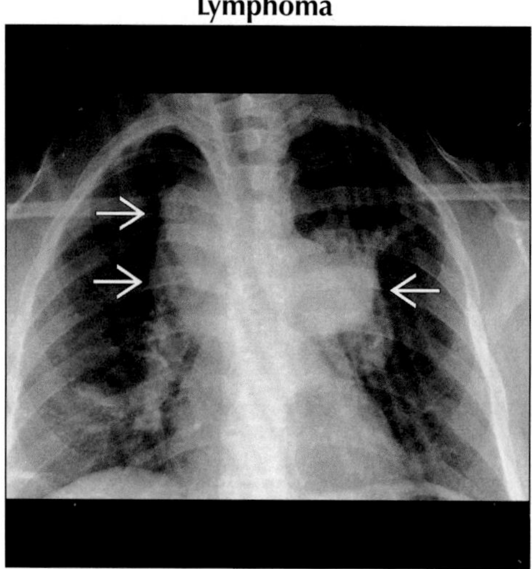

Lymphoma

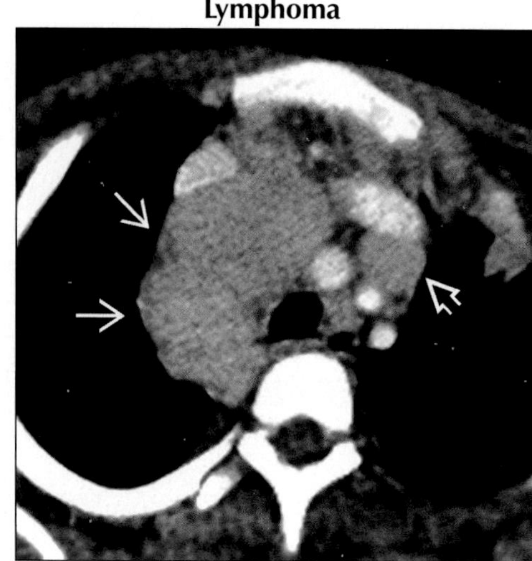

(Left) Frontal radiograph shows lobulated bilateral hilar and right paratracheal stripe thickening in this patient with Hodgkin lymphoma. This patient presented with "B symptoms" consisting of fever, night sweats, and weight loss. *(Right)* Axial CECT shows a homogeneous mass in the mediastinum crossing mediastinal compartments. Note the more solitary prevascular lymph node in this patient with Hodgkin lymphoma.

Lung Carcinoma and Extrathoracic Metastases

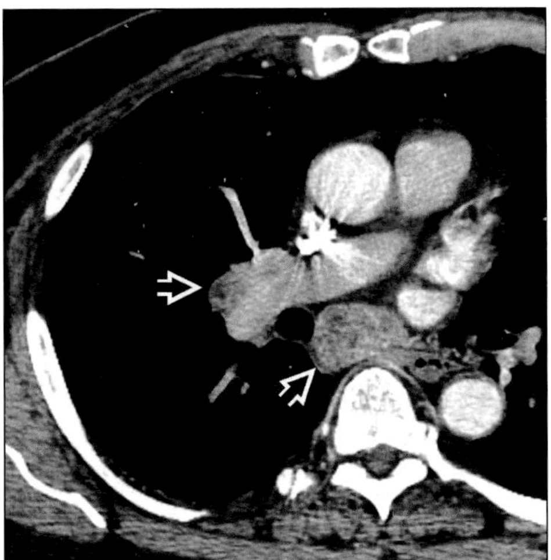

Lung Carcinoma and Extrathoracic Metastases

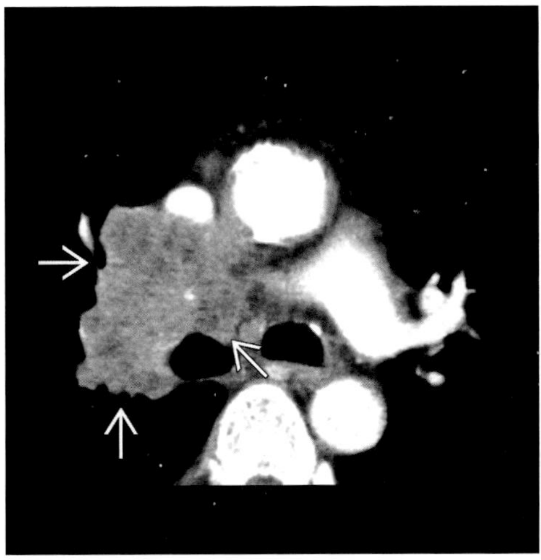

(Left) *Axial CECT shows typical CT features of metastases from renal cell carcinoma causing middle mediastinal widening with variable enhancing hilar and mediastinal adenopathy ⇨. Enhancing lymphadenopathy can be seen in metastatic disease, Castleman disease, and tuberculosis infection.* ***(Right)*** *Axial CECT shows middle mediastinal lymphadenopathy → in this patient with small cell lung carcinoma.*

Lung Carcinoma and Extrathoracic Metastases

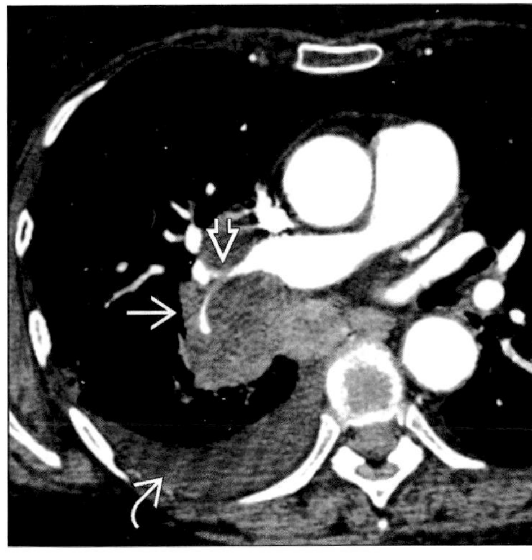

Foregut Duplication Cysts

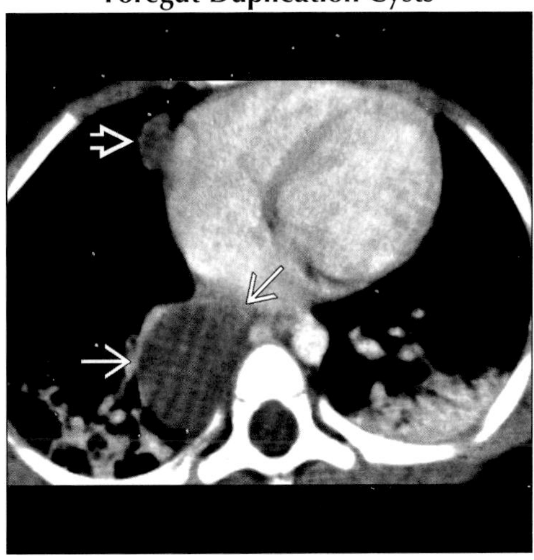

(Left) *Axial CECT shows typical features of a middle mediastinal mass from small cell carcinoma. Note the bulky mediastinal mass → and narrowing of the right pulmonary artery ⇨, as well as a small right pleural effusion ↗.* ***(Right)*** *Axial CECT shows a well-circumscribed mass within the subcarinal space →. No enhancement was noted on this post-contrast examination. Incidentally found was what proved to be a pericardial cyst adjacent to the heart ⇨.*

Hiatal Hernia

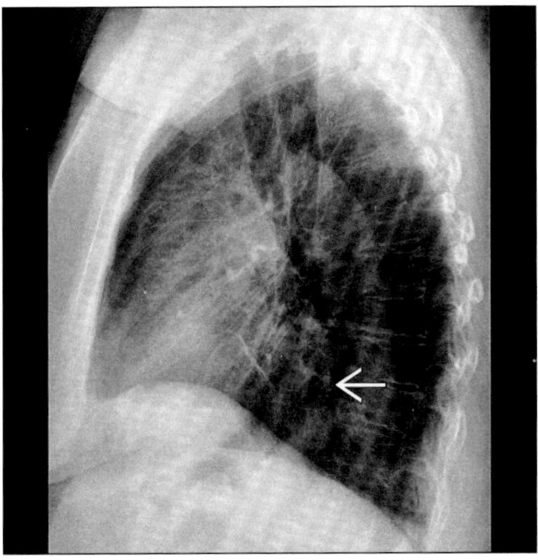

Hiatal Hernia

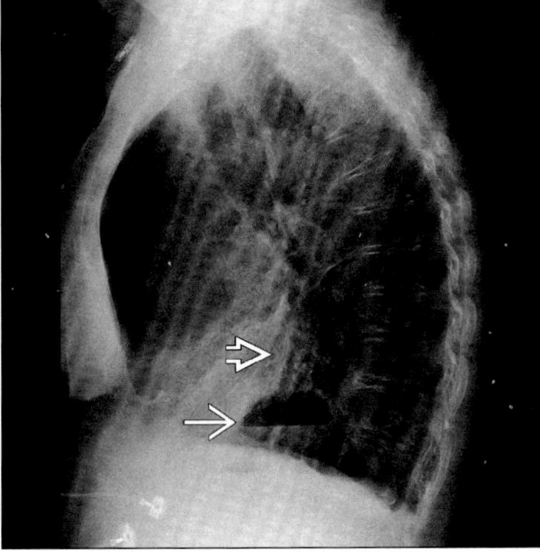

(Left) *Lateral radiograph shows typical radiographic features of a retrocardiac mass due to a hiatal hernia →. This was confirmed by reviewing previous cross-sectional imaging.* ***(Right)*** *Lateral radiograph shows a hiatal hernia with characteristic air-fluid level → and bronchiectasis ⇨. Situs inversus was noted on the PA chest radiograph in this patient with Kartagener syndrome.*

MIDDLE COMPARTMENT MASS

*(**Left**) Frontal radiograph shows typical radiographic features of a ruptured aortic aneurysm. There is marked mediastinal widening centered over the aortic arch ➔. Note the large left pleural effusion ➲. The patient was acutely hypotensive secondary to blood loss. (**Right**) Axial CECT shows a large, partially thrombosed aortic aneurysm off the aortic arch at the left apex ➲. Note the left pleural effusion ➔.*

Aortic Aneurysm

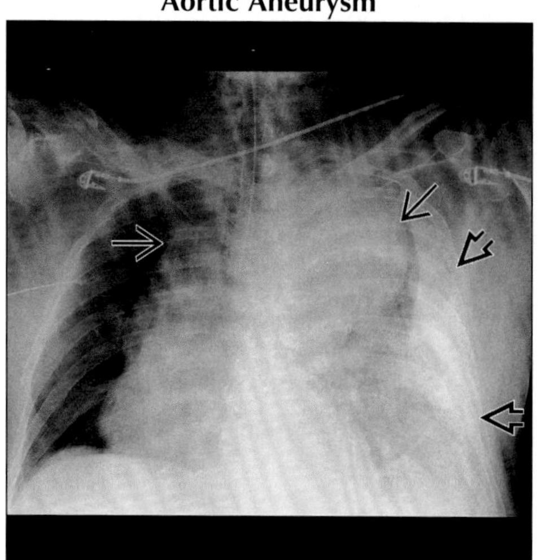

Aortic Aneurysm

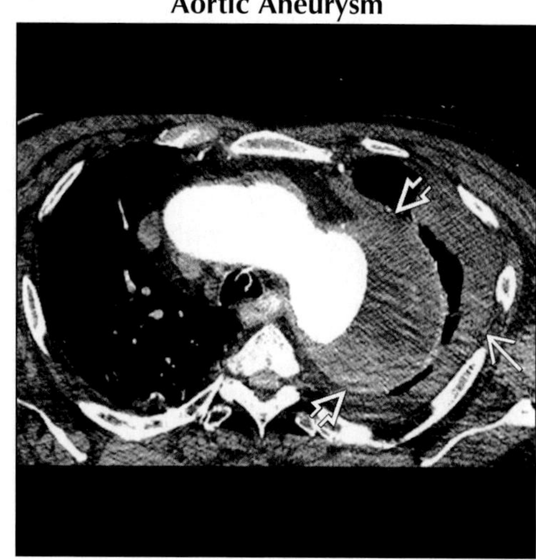

*(**Left**) Anteroposterior radiograph shows typical radiographic features of mediastinal lipomatosis with diffuse mediastinal widening ➔. Long-term stability by comparison to prior radiographs and CT would be helpful to make this diagnosis. Note absence of tracheal compression, an important differential consideration. (**Right**) Axial CECT shows typical CT features of mediastinal lipomatosis with diffuse smooth mediastinal widening from fat ➔.*

Lipomatosis

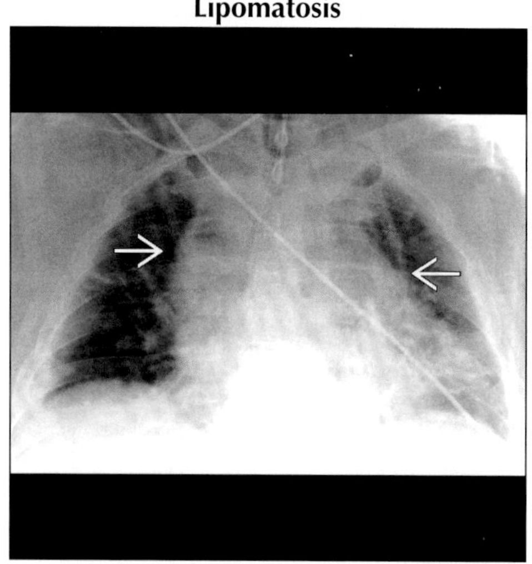

Lipomatosis

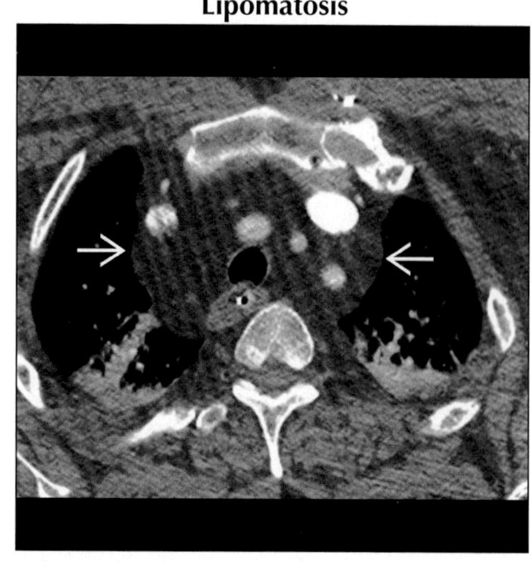

*(**Left**) Axial CECT demonstrates typical CT features of mediastinal mass due to goiter with an enlarged substernal thyroid ➔ with numerous nodules. Extension to the thyroid was shown on higher sections. (**Right**) Axial CECT shows a patient with multiple dilated varices ➔ secondary to chronic liver disease. There is lateral displacement of the azygoesophageal recess ➲. (Courtesy C. Rohrmann, MD.)*

Mediastinal Goiter

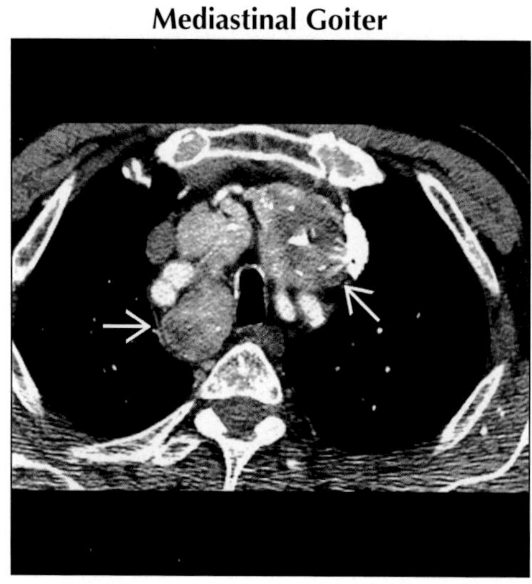

Esophageal Masses

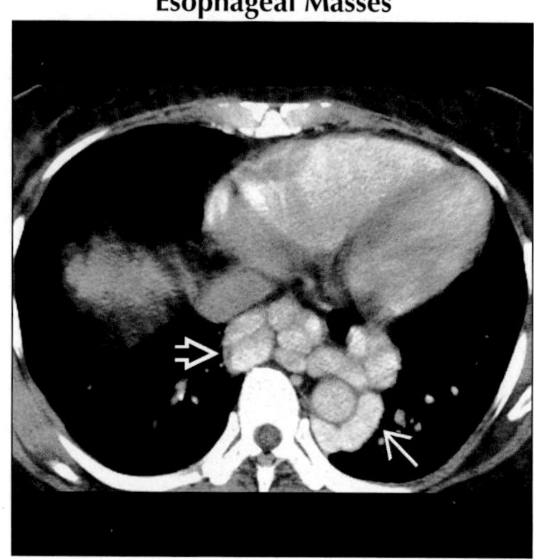

Esophageal Masses

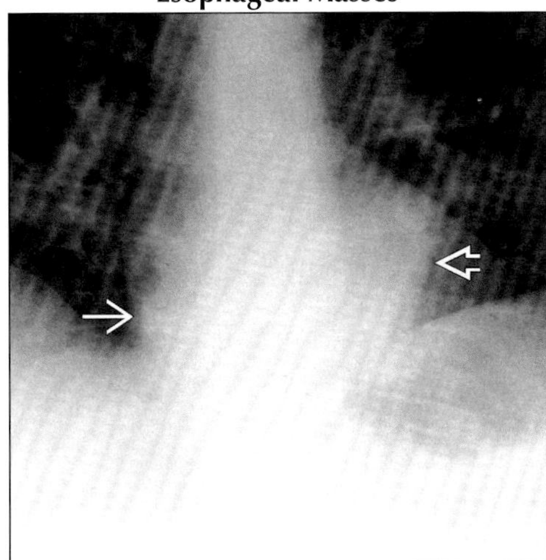

Esophageal Masses

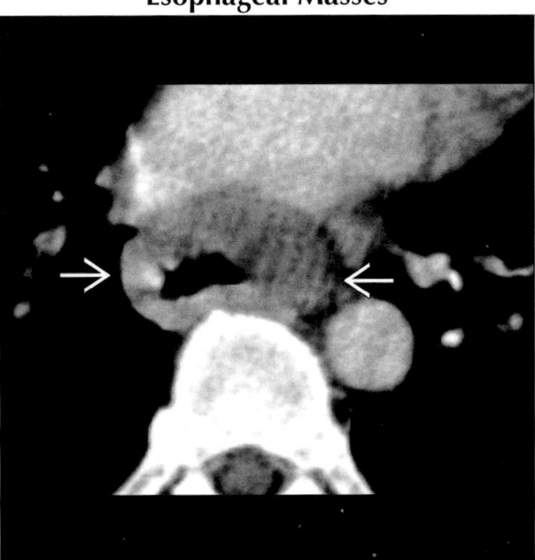

(Left) Frontal radiograph shows typical radiographic features of mediastinal mass from esophageal varices with an inferior retrocardiac mass. Note rightward bulging of the azygoesophageal recess ➡ and leftward displacement of the left paravertebral stripe ➡. *(Right)* Axial CECT shows diffuse esophageal widening ➡ in this patient with diffuse esophageal leiomyomatosis. (Courtesy C. Rohrmann, MD.)

Mediastinitis

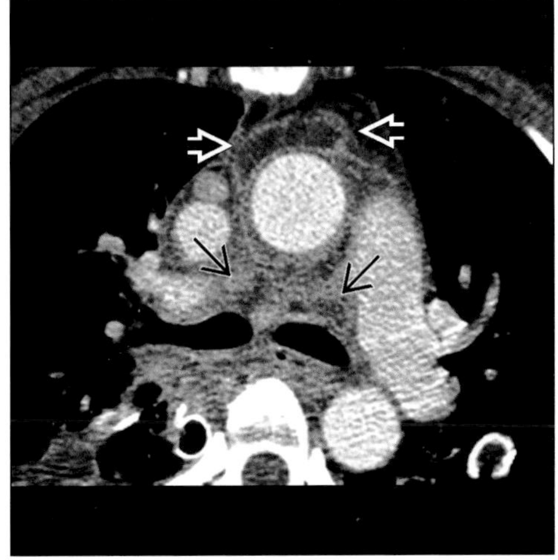

Tracheal Neoplasms

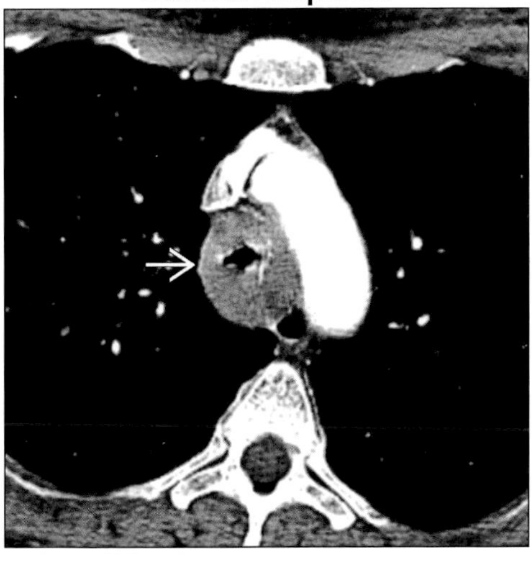

(Left) Axial CECT shows thickening and abnormal fluid collections within the anterior mediastinum ➡ and middle mediastinum ➡ in this patient with mediastinitis secondary to a spreading pharyngeal infection. Presence of infectious symptoms is an important factor in diagnosing this condition. *(Right)* Axial CECT shows diffuse circumferential tracheal wall thickening from adenoid cystic carcinoma ➡.

Tracheal Neoplasms

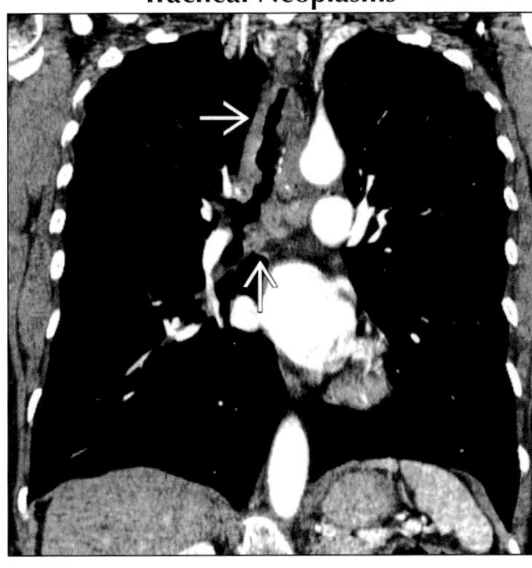

Tracheal Neoplasms

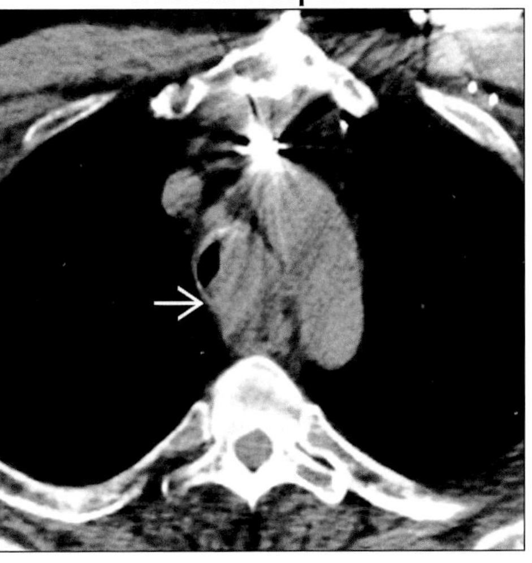

(Left) Coronal CECT shows the extent of the tumor spreading along the trachea ➡ in this patient with adenoid cystic carcinoma. There was no sparing of the noncartilaginous posterior wall. Adenoid cystic carcinoma is the 2nd most common primary tumor to affect the trachea. *(Right)* Axial NECT shows typical CT features of tracheal metastasis from renal cell carcinoma. Note the irregular-shaped lesion ➡ nearly completely occluding the tracheal lumen.

POSTERIOR COMPARTMENT MASS

DIFFERENTIAL DIAGNOSIS

Common
- Nerve Sheath Tumor
- Sympathetic Ganglion Tumor
- Lymphoma
- Hiatal Hernia
- Esophageal Tumor

Less Common
- Metastasis
- Foregut Duplication Cyst
- Extramedullary Hematopoiesis
- Aortic Aneurysm
- Esophageal Varices
- Spine Mass

Rare but Important
- Hemangioma
- Lymphangioma
- Meningocele

ESSENTIAL INFORMATION

Key Differential Diagnosis Issues
- Anatomy of posterior compartment
  - Description is based upon radiographic landmarks
    - Anterior border: Line 1 cm behind anterior margin of thoracic vertebrae
    - Posterior border: Chest wall
- Normal contents: Vertebral bodies, descending aorta, azygos vein, esophagus, lymph nodes, adipose tissue
- Cervicothoracic sign: Mediastinal mass outlined by lung on frontal radiograph above level of clavicle; indicates posterior location
- CT and MR are invaluable for determining site of origin and tissue characterization

Helpful Clues for Common Diagnoses
- **Nerve Sheath Tumor**
  - More common in adults
  - Schwannoma, neurofibroma, plexiform neurofibroma
  - Smooth, round or oval, often less dense than muscle
  - Enlargement of adjacent neural foramina with occasional extension into spinal canal
  - Often have internal foci of decreased attenuation due to lipid or cyst formation
  - Increased signal on T2 MR images and heterogeneous enhancement
- **Sympathetic Ganglion Tumor**
  - More common in children and young adults
  - Ganglioneuroma
    - Benign neoplasm of ganglion cells and Schwann cells
    - Most common in 2nd and 3rd decades
    - Calcification in 20%
    - May have whorled appearance on MR
  - Ganglioneuroblastoma
    - Intermediate histology between ganglioneuroma and neuroblastoma
    - Most common in older children
    - Imaging resembles neuroblastoma
  - Neuroblastoma
    - Malignant neoplasm associated with systemic symptoms
    - Most common in children less than 5 years old
    - Curvilinear and speckled calcification in 40%
    - May invade adjacent structures
- **Lymphoma**
  - Non-Hodgkin lymphoma is more common than Hodgkin disease in posterior compartment
  - Enlarged lymph nodes or nodal mass, often displaying homogeneous soft tissue attenuation
  - Necrosis is occasionally present, usually detected after contrast administration
- **Hiatal Hernia**
  - Superior herniation of stomach through esophageal hiatus
  - May see air-fluid level on upright radiograph
- **Esophageal Tumor**
  - Carcinoma
    - Thickening of esophageal wall that is often eccentric
    - Luminal narrowing
    - Invasion of adjacent tissues
  - Mesenchymal tumor
    - Most common histology is leiomyoma
    - Often asymptomatic
    - Margins are smooth

Helpful Clues for Less Common Diagnoses
- **Metastasis**
  - Often involves lymph nodes

- Involvement of posterior compartment lymph nodes is suggestive of primary malignancy within abdomen
- **Foregut Duplication Cyst**
  - Esophageal duplication cyst, bronchogenic cyst, neurenteric cyst
  - Round or oval with smooth borders
  - Thin wall with no enhancement; wall calcification is uncommon
  - Cyst contents may be proteinaceous, with increased attenuation and increased signal on T1 MR images
  - Neurenteric cysts are associated with adjacent vertebral anomalies
- **Extramedullary Hematopoiesis**
  - Associated with thalassemia, sickle cell anemia, and spherocytosis
  - Multiple bilateral paraspinal masses
  - Sharp borders with homogeneous attenuation
  - May be associated with skeletal abnormalities
- **Aortic Aneurysm**
  - May involve aortic arch or descending aorta
  - True aneurysm: Most commonly due to atherosclerotic disease
  - False aneurysm: Most commonly due to trauma
- **Esophageal Varices**
  - Result of liver disease with chronic portal hypertension
  - Vascular serpiginous masses within middle and posterior mediastinum
  - Connect with azygos system to bypass portal drainage
- **Spine Mass**
  - Neoplasms: Myeloma, metastasis, primary bone tumor
  - Infection: Spondylitis, paraspinous abscess
  - Look for disc space and vertebral body destruction
  - If mass is present, determine if it appears to arise from bone or soft tissues

Helpful Clues for Rare Diagnoses

- **Hemangioma**
  - Soft tissue mass
  - Clue to diagnosis is internal phlebolith
  - Appearance similar to soft tissue hemangiomas elsewhere in body
- **Lymphangioma**
  - Benign hyperplasia of lymphatic vessels
  - Low-density mass that insinuates between adjacent structures
- **Meningocele**
  - Herniation of meninges beyond spinal canal
  - Associated with neurofibromatosis and traumatic nerve root avulsion
  - Direct communication with subarachnoid space around spinal cord
  - Associated with adjacent vertebral anomalies in neurofibromatosis

Nerve Sheath Tumor

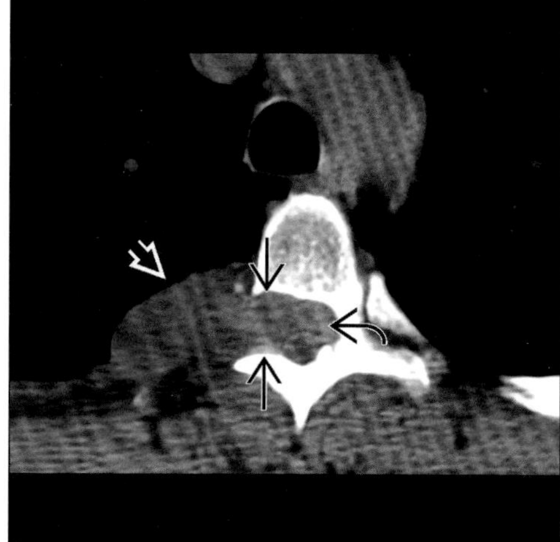

Axial NECT shows a soft tissue mass within the posterior mediastinum ➡ that has expanded the right neural foramen → and extends into the central canal ↪.

Nerve Sheath Tumor

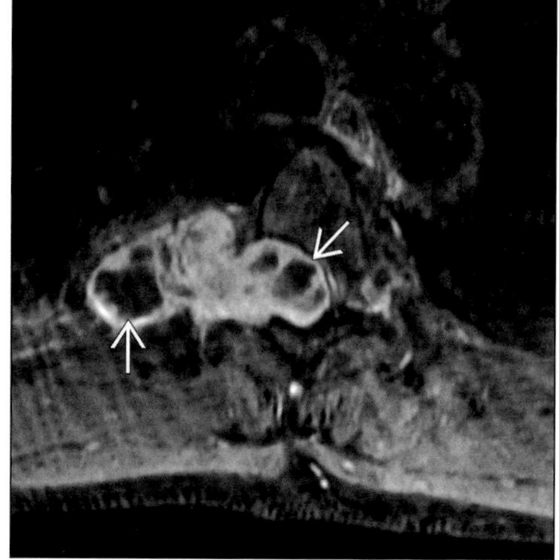

Axial T1WI C+ FS MR in the same patient shows intense enhancement of the mass with several nonenhancing areas ➡. These areas represent cystic regions, a common finding with schwannomas.

POSTERIOR COMPARTMENT MASS

Nerve Sheath Tumor

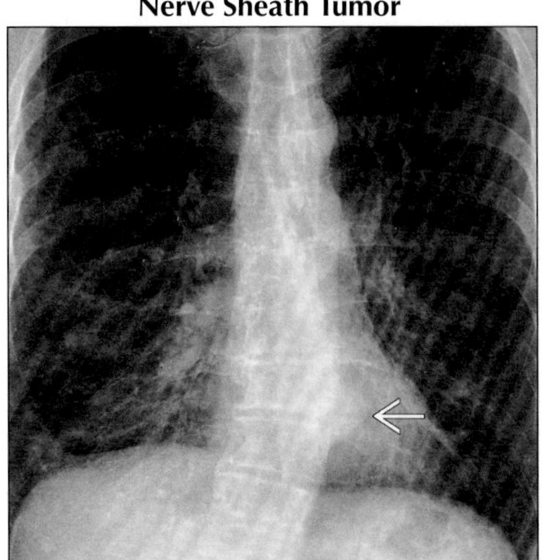

Nerve Sheath Tumor

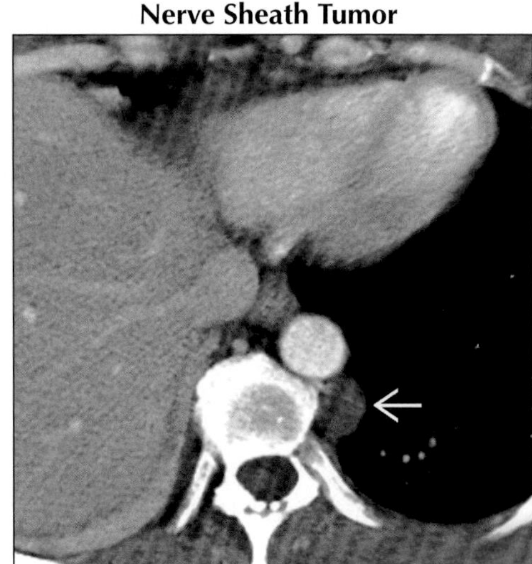

(Left) *Frontal radiograph shows mild levoscoliosis and a well-demarcated mediastinal soft tissue mass ➔. Note it does not silhouette with the descending thoracic aorta.* ***(Right)*** *Axial CECT in the same patient reveals a round homogeneous mass in the posterior mediastinum ➔. This patient has a history of neurofibromatosis, and this mass is consistent with a neurofibroma.*

Nerve Sheath Tumor

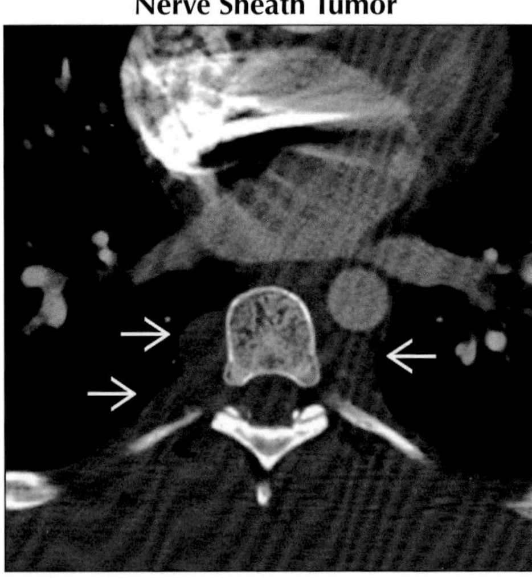

Sympathetic Ganglion Tumor

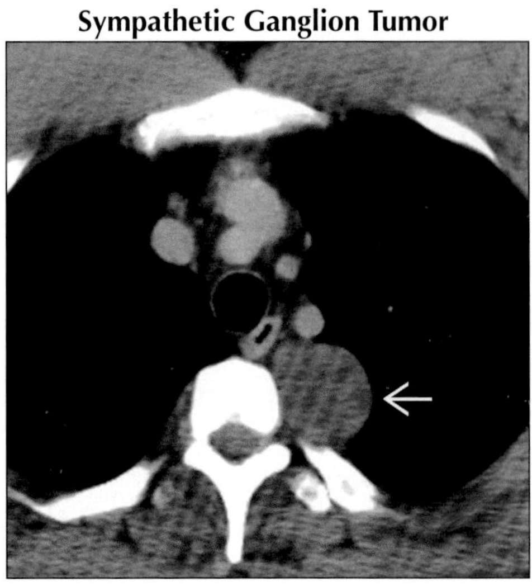

(Left) *Axial NECT shows several round and oval nonenhancing soft tissue masses bilaterally within the posterior mediastinum ➔. This is a typical appearance of multiple neurofibromas in a patient with neurofibromatosis.* ***(Right)*** *Axial CECT from a 28-year-old man shows a nonenhancing lobulated posterior mediastinal mass ➔. This was proven to represent a ganglioneuroma. Notice the lack of invasion into adjacent structures.*

Sympathetic Ganglion Tumor

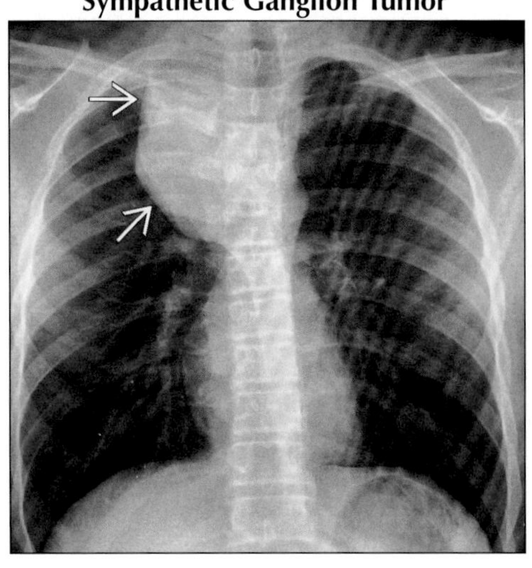

Sympathetic Ganglion Tumor

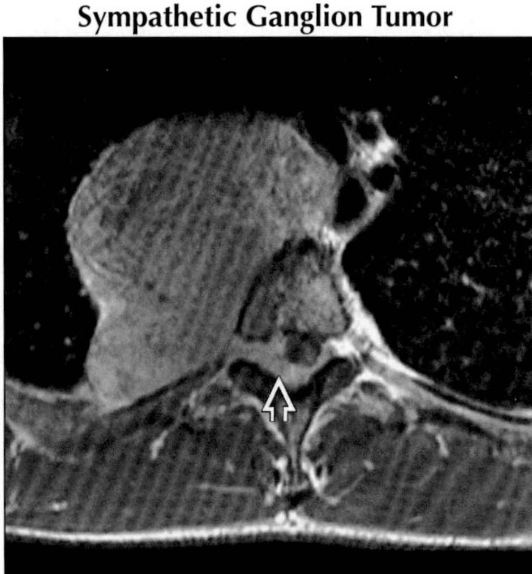

(Left) *Frontal radiograph shows a large paraspinous mass with sharp lateral margins ➔. There is mild mass effect upon the trachea with deviation to the left. Notice the presence of the cervicothoracic sign.* ***(Right)*** *Axial T1WI C+ FS MR in the same patient shows a large posterior and middle mediastinal mass with extension into the spinal canal through a neural foramen ➔. In this young child this lesion was a neuroblastoma.*

Sympathetic Ganglion Tumor

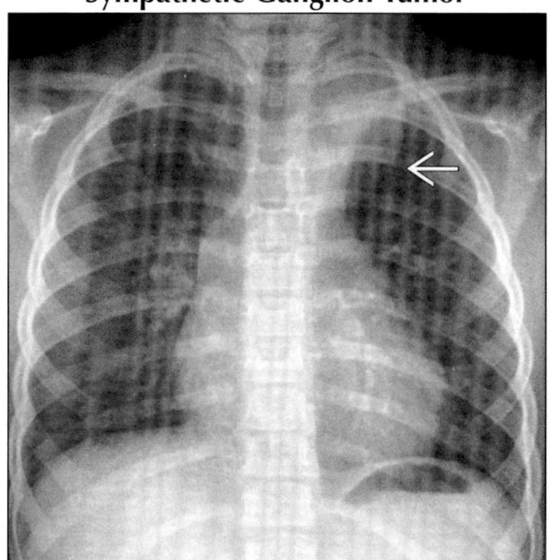

Sympathetic Ganglion Tumor

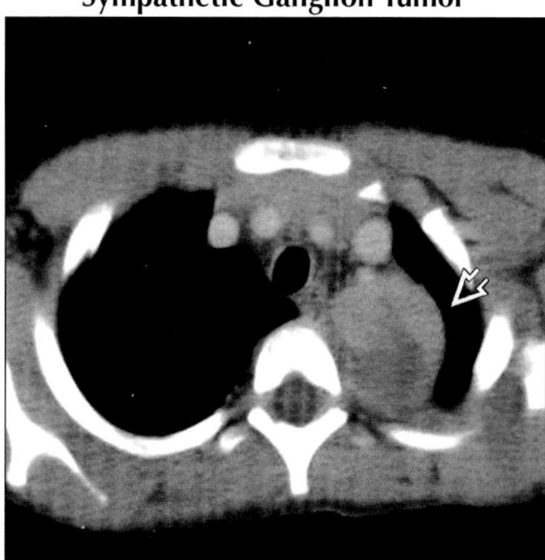

*(**Left**) Frontal radiograph shows a well-defined posterior mediastinal mass ➔. Notice the presence of the cervicothoracic sign with extension of the mass superior to the level of the clavicle, indicating a posterior location. (**Right**) Axial CECT in the same patient shows a heterogeneous mass in the posterior mediastinum ➔. This is a typical appearance of neuroblastoma in a young child.*

Sympathetic Ganglion Tumor

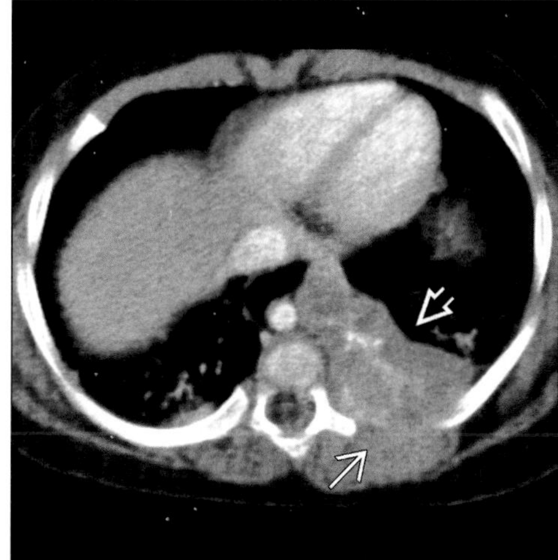

Lymphoma

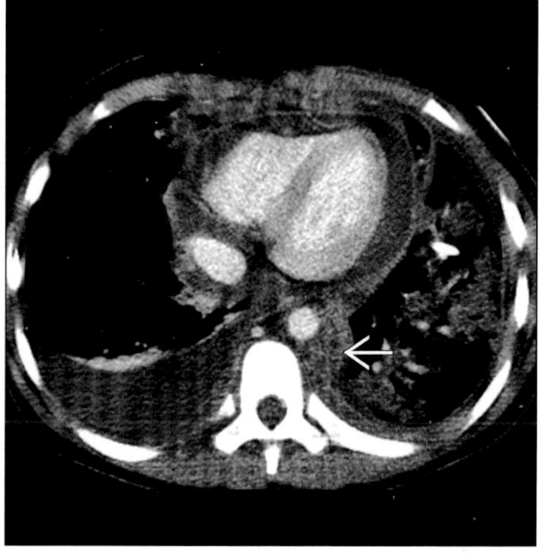

*(**Left**) Axial CECT shows a large mass in the left posterior mediastinum ➔. There is invasion of the adjacent chest wall ➔. Notice the internal calcifications. In a young child, this is highly suggestive of neuroblastoma. (**Right**) Axial CECT shows a soft tissue mass in the posterior mediastinum ➔ representing lymphoma. Several other lymph nodes were also involved. Notice the pericardial and right pleural effusions.*

Esophageal Tumor

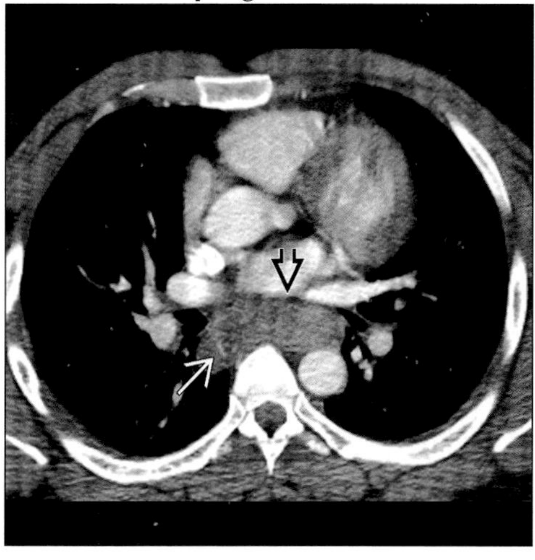

Esophageal Tumor

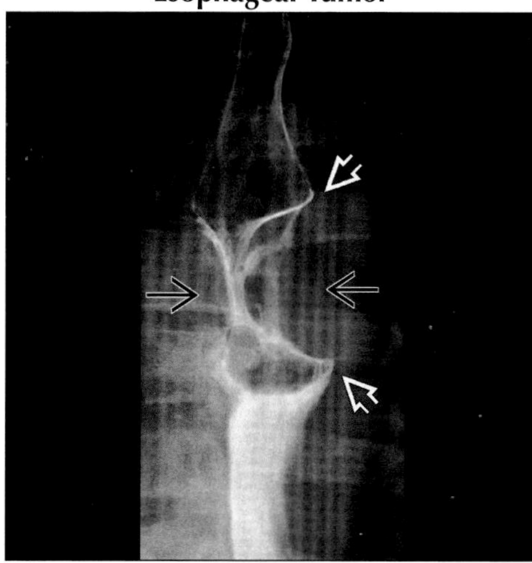

*(**Left**) Axial CECT shows an oblong, homogeneous, nonenhancing soft tissue mass in the expected location of the esophagus ➔. Small foci of hyperattenuation represent contrast or calcification ➔. (**Right**) Esophagram in the same patient shows a smooth circumferential esophageal "apple core" lesion ➔ forming obtuse angles with the esophageal lumen ➔, consistent with a submucosal lesion. Endoscopic biopsy revealed a benign leiomyoma.*

POSTERIOR COMPARTMENT MASS

Metastasis

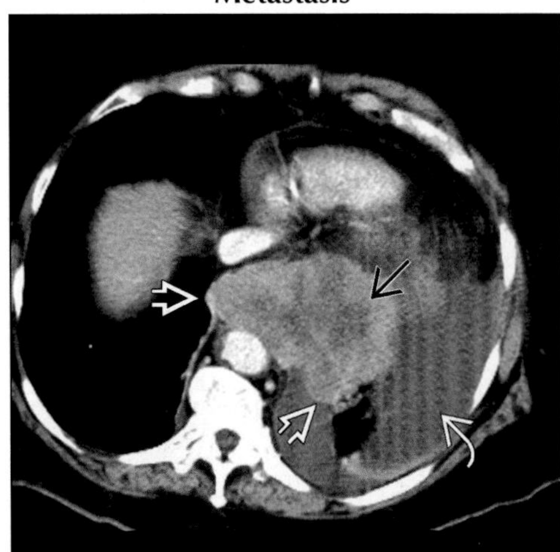

Foregut Duplication Cyst

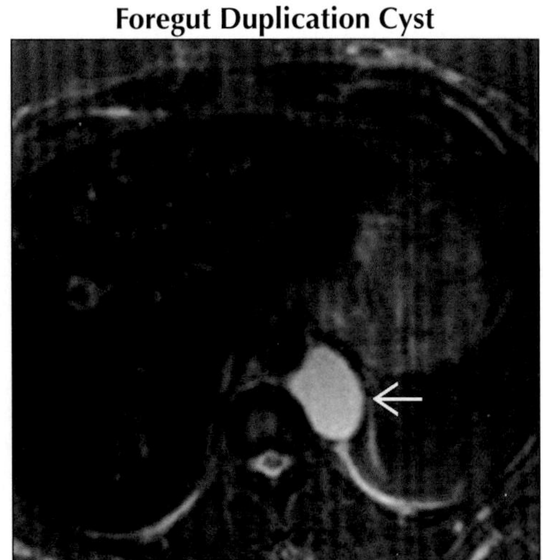

(Left) *Axial CECT shows a large mass invading the middle compartment, posterior compartment, and lung ➡. Central hypoattenuation represents necrosis ➡. Biopsy revealed small cell lung cancer. Also note left pleural effusion ➡.* ***(Right)*** *Axial T2WI FS MR shows a homogeneous smooth lesion with diffusely increased T2 signal ➡ adjacent to the esophagus. This was stable over several years and is consistent with a foregut duplication cyst.*

Extramedullary Hematopoiesis

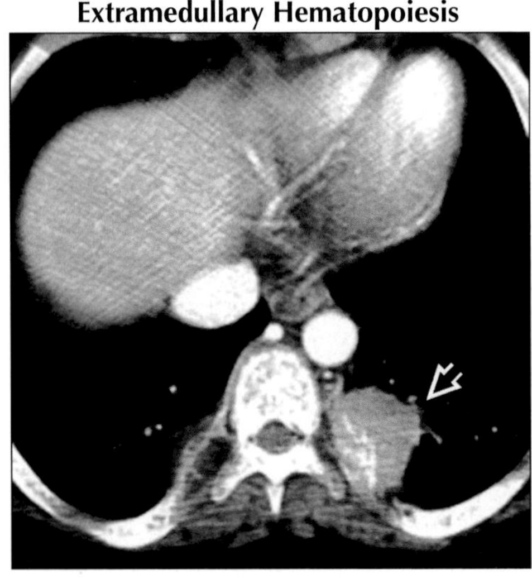

Extramedullary Hematopoiesis

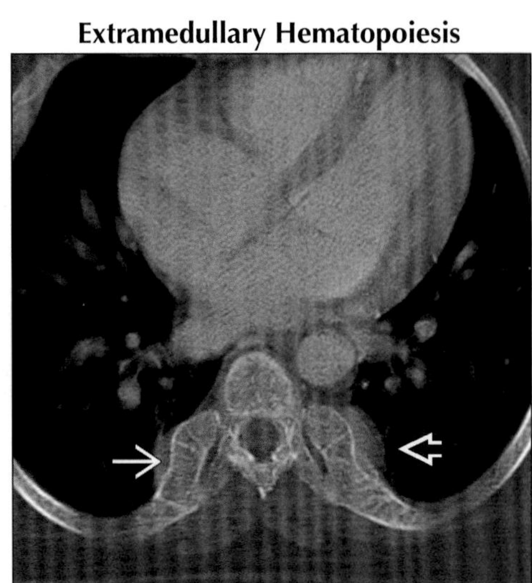

(Left) *Axial CECT shows a round, enhancing soft tissue mass to the left of the spine in the posterior mediastinum ➡. There was no association with any neural foramina.* ***(Right)*** *At a higher level, notice the bony expansion of the posterior ribs ➡ with small adjacent soft tissue masses ➡. Numerous masses were present along the thoracic spine. These findings are typical of extramedullary hematopoiesis in this patient with thalassemia.*

Aortic Aneurysm

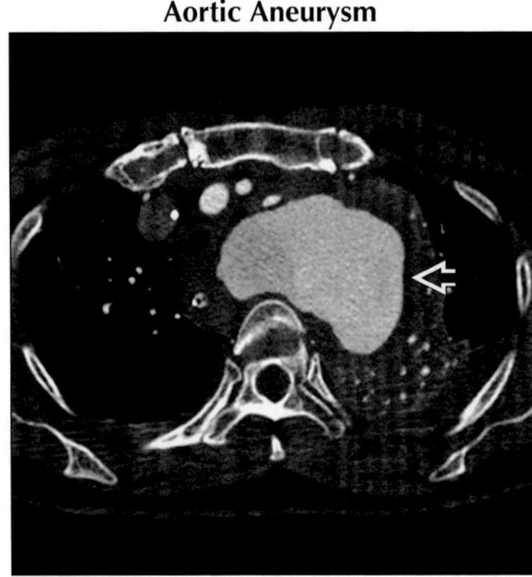

Esophageal Varices

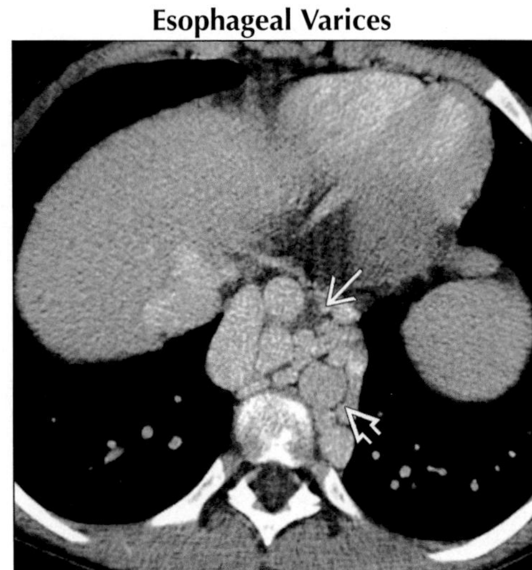

(Left) *Axial CTA shows a large pseudoaneurysm arising from the aortic arch ➡ as a complication of prior trauma. This will present as a large mediastinal mass on radiography and may be difficult to diagnose without CT.* ***(Right)*** *Axial CECT obtained during the venous phase of contrast administration shows numerous large varices around the esophagus ➡ and aorta ➡ caused by longstanding cirrhosis and portal hypertension.*

Spine Mass

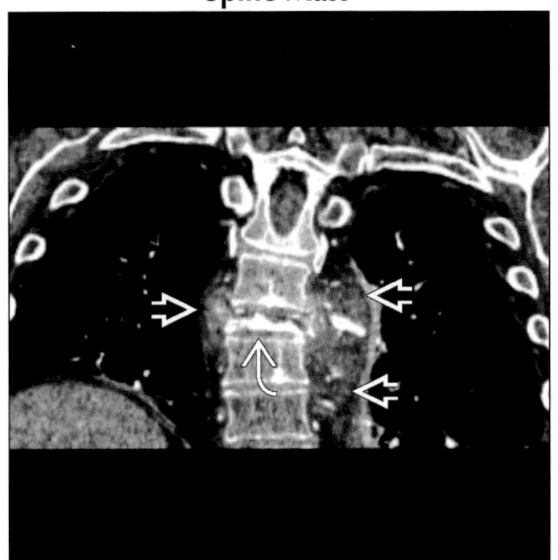

Spine Mass

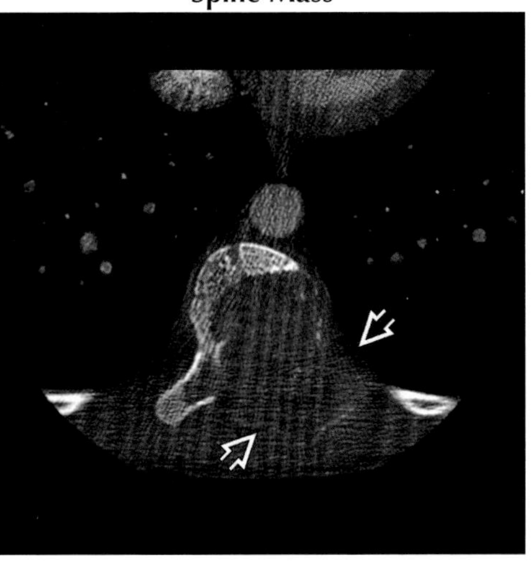

*(**Left**) Coronal CECT shows a large paraspinal abscess involving both sides of the spine ➔. There is near complete collapse of the adjacent vertebral body ➔ caused by osteomyelitis. (**Right**) Axial CECT shows an expansile lesion centered within the thoracic vertebra and involving the posterior elements ➔. Fluid-fluid levels were present on MR. Pathology revealed an aneurysmal bone cyst.*

Hemangioma

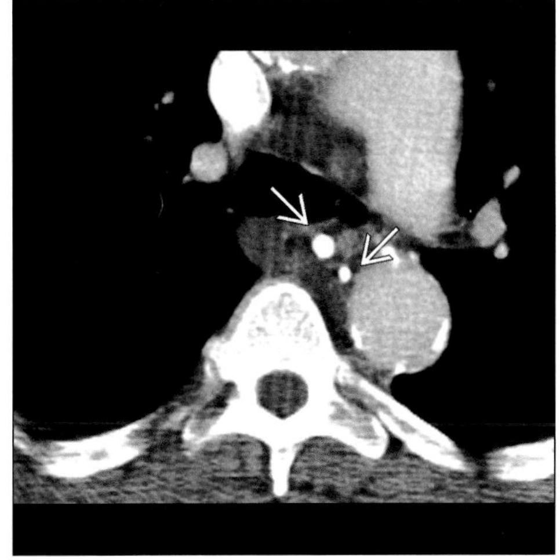

Lymphangioma

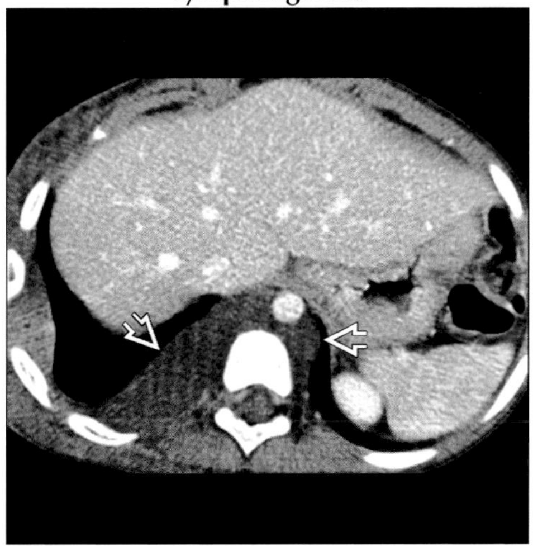

*(**Left**) Axial CECT shows a soft tissue mass adjacent to the esophagus. Notice the well-defined round calcifications within the mass, consistent with phleboliths ➔. This is highly suggestive of a hemangioma. (**Right**) Axial CECT shows a low-density mass in the posterior mediastinum that crosses midline ➔. Notice that the attenuation is near that of water. In a child, this is suggestive of a lymphangioma.*

Meningocele

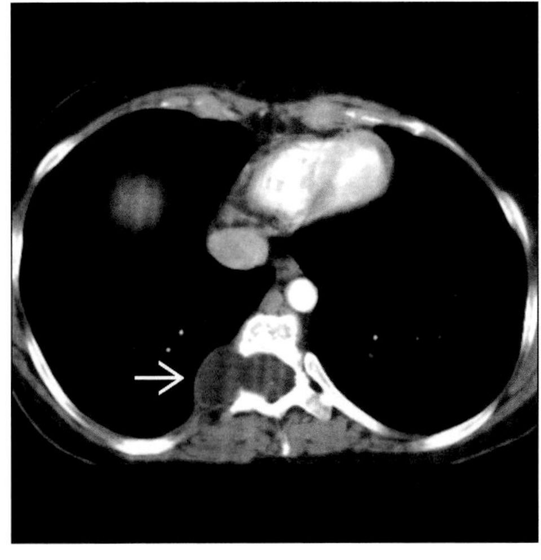

Meningocele

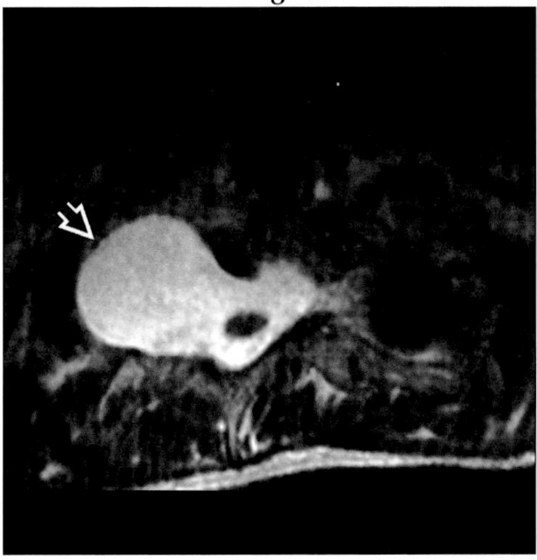

*(**Left**) Axial CECT shows a typical lateral meningocele ➔ in a patient with neurofibromatosis. Notice the low density, consistent with CSF and expansion of the neural foramen. (**Right**) Axial T2WI MR shows a large lateral meningocele arising from the right neural foramen of an upper thoracic vertebra ➔. Notice the contiguity with the central canal and homogeneous increased T2 signal, consistent with CSF.*

HIGH-ATTENUATION MASS, MEDIASTINUM OR HILUM

DIFFERENTIAL DIAGNOSIS

Common

- Calcified Lymphadenopathy
  - Histoplasmosis
  - Tuberculosis
  - Pneumocystis Pneumonia
  - Mediastinal Fibrosis
- Goiter
- Aneurysm
- Hematoma

Less Common

- Silicosis/Coal Worker's Pneumoconiosis
- Neoplastic
  - Treated Hodgkin Lymphoma
  - Thymoma
  - Teratoma
  - Neuroblastoma
  - Castleman Disease
  - Metastases
- Sarcoidosis

Rare but Important

- Amyloidosis
- Foregut Cyst
- Hemangiomas
- Gossypiboma
- Aluminum Pneumoconiosis
- Perflubron Ventilation

ESSENTIAL INFORMATION

Key Differential Diagnosis Issues

- Mnemonic: **EGGSHELL CA$^+$**
  - **E**nvironmental dusts (silica, coal, aluminum)
  - **G**oiter
  - **G**ossypiboma
  - **S**arcoidosis
  - **H**emangioma
  - **E**cchymosis (hematoma)
  - **L**ymphoma (treated Hodgkin)
  - **L**ymph nodes (histoplasmosis, tuberculosis, PCP)
  - **C**ancer (thymoma, teratoma, neuroblastoma, metastases, or Castleman)
  - **A**neurysm

Helpful Clues for Common Diagnoses

- **Calcified Lymphadenopathy**
  - **Histoplasmosis**
    - Calcification of granuloma and nodes age and time dependent
    - Calcification within months in children, years in adults
    - Either central nidus or diffuse calcification pattern
    - Nodes follow drainage pattern of lung granuloma
    - Splenic calcification common
    - Multiple small pulmonary calcifications in histoplasmosis; fewer, larger pulmonary calcifications in tuberculosis
  - **Tuberculosis**
    - Nodal calcification often diffuse
    - Seen in 50%
  - **Mediastinal Fibrosis**
    - Focal mediastinal mass > 5 cm diameter, most common paratracheal
    - Central calcification in mass (90%), also seen in peripheral granuloma
    - Eventually obstructs superior vena cava, airways, & pulmonary veins, in that order
- **Goiter**
  - Calcification: Coarse, punctate, or rings
- **Aneurysm**
  - Curvilinear calcification
  - Due to atherosclerosis, trauma, fungal infection, cystic medial necrosis, vasculitis
- **Hematoma**
  - Acute hematoma due to trauma, catheter insertion, surgery, clotting disorder, aneurysms, tumor
    - Consider ectopic parathyroid adenoma, which may spontaneously hemorrhage
  - 90% of clots have ↑ attenuation over 1st 72 hours

Helpful Clues for Less Common Diagnoses

- **Silicosis/Coal Worker's Pneumoconiosis**
  - Eggshell calcification in 3-6%
  - Associated with interstitial lung disease
- **Neoplastic**
  - **Treated Hodgkin Lymphoma**
    - Following radiation therapy, ~ 20% of nodal masses will calcify
    - 2 types: Eggshell or multiple discrete deposits (mulberry type)
    - Extremely rare (case reports) of calcification prior to treatment
  - **Thymoma**

  - 1/3 have calcification: Thin linear in capsule, scattered punctate calcification less commonly seen
  - Also seen in invasive thymomas
- ○ **Teratoma**
  - a.k.a. dermoid cyst
  - Teratomas: 70% of germ cell tumors
  - Fat: 75%, fluid: 90%, calcification: 40%
  - Calcification may have tooth shape
- ○ **Neuroblastoma**
  - Calcification (80%): Cloud-like, stippled, ring-shaped, solid
- ○ **Castleman Disease**
  - Calcification (5-10%): Discrete, coarse, or tree-like, rarely visible on radiographs
- ○ **Metastases**
  - Usually seen in those with known disease
  - Osteosarcoma, mucinous colon or ovarian, papillary thyroid carcinoma most common tumors

- **Sarcoidosis**
  - 50% have calcification, 40% within 1 year of diagnosis
  - Calcification typically central: Smudgy or putty-like, may be eggshell but uncommon

Helpful Clues for Rare Diagnoses

- **Amyloidosis**
  - Adenopathy, isolated or associated with interstitial lung disease (50%)
  - Usually multiple lymph node groups, may be massive
  - Calcification stippled, diffuse, or eggshell
  - Systemic disease common, typically Waldenström macroglobulinemia
- **Foregut Cyst**
  - Bronchogenic cysts most common (50%)
  - Calcification either in fluid (milk of calcium: 3%), less common curvilinear in wall
- **Hemangiomas**
  - Phleboliths: 10-40% (fat 40%)
    - Central area of decreased attenuation pathognomonic for phlebolith (in 7%)
    - More common: Multiple punctate round calcifications (30%)
- **Gossypiboma**
  - Retained surgical sponge or swab
  - Spongiform low-density mass with gas bubbles
  - Sponges in USA contain radiopaque markers, often 1 or 2 linear wires
  - Calcification also deposited along network architecture of surgical sponge ("calcified reticulate rind")
- **Aluminum Pneumoconiosis**
  - Nodes with diffuse homogeneous increased attenuation (from aluminum)
- **Perflubron Ventilation**
  - Used in severe respiratory failure
  - Contains bromine atoms, which makes agent radiopaque
  - May accumulate and remain long term in lymph nodes and efface mediastinal fat

Histoplasmosis

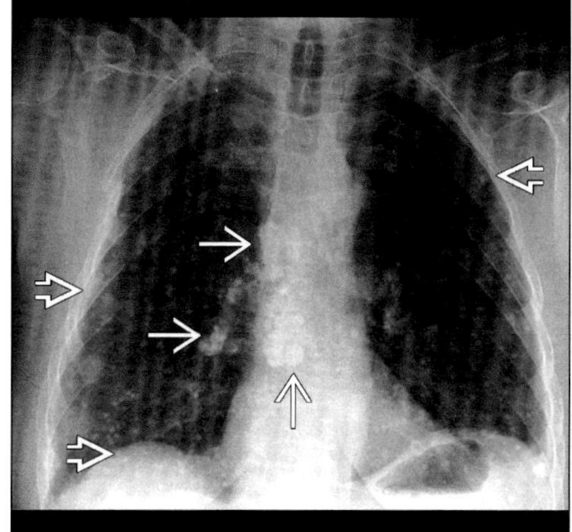

Frontal radiograph shows multiple small, peripheral, discrete, calcified granulomas ➾ and multiple enlarged, calcified hilar and mediastinal lymph nodes ➔ from histoplasmosis.

Pneumocystis Pneumonia

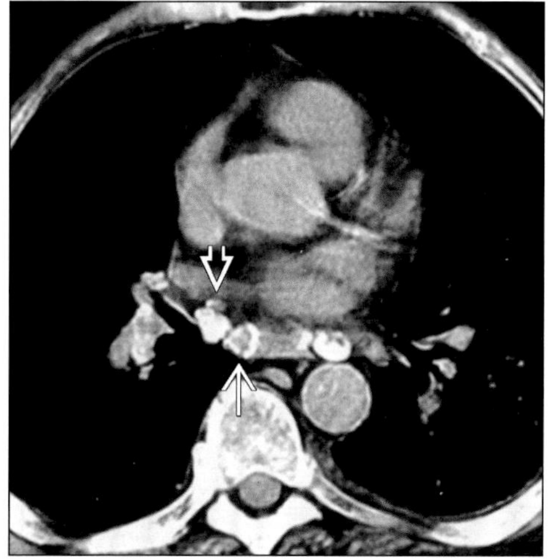

Axial CECT shows multiple calcified hilar and mediastinal lymph nodes in a patient with previous pneumocystitis pneumonia. Nodes are either diffusely calcified ➾ or show eggshell calcification ➔.

HIGH-ATTENUATION MASS, MEDIASTINUM OR HILUM

Mediastinal Fibrosis

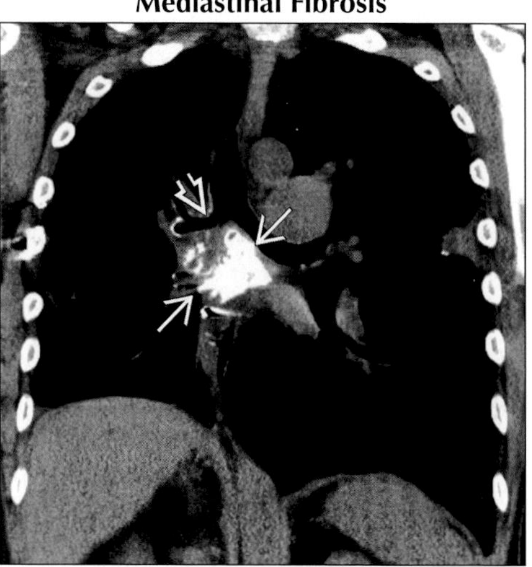

Goiter

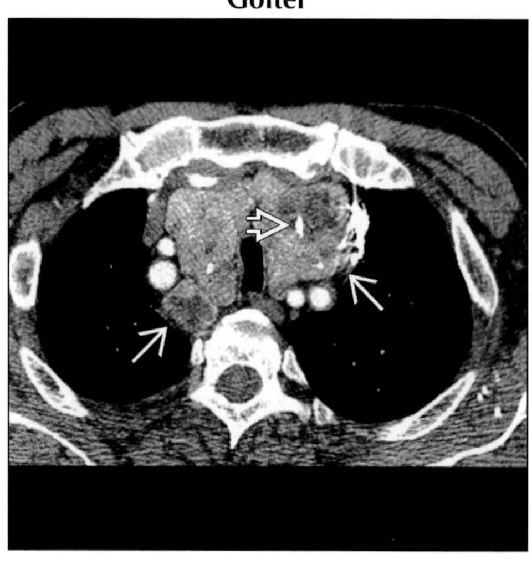

(Left) *Coronal NECT reconstruction shows a large subcarinal calcified mediastinal mass ➡ narrowing the right main bronchus ⇨. Subcarinal location is the 2nd most common location. Typically fibrosis in this area obstructs airways or pulmonary veins.* ***(Right)*** *Axial CECT shows a large superior mediastinal mass ➡ compressing the trachea. Goiter is high density from iodine and foci of calcification ⇨.*

Aneurysm

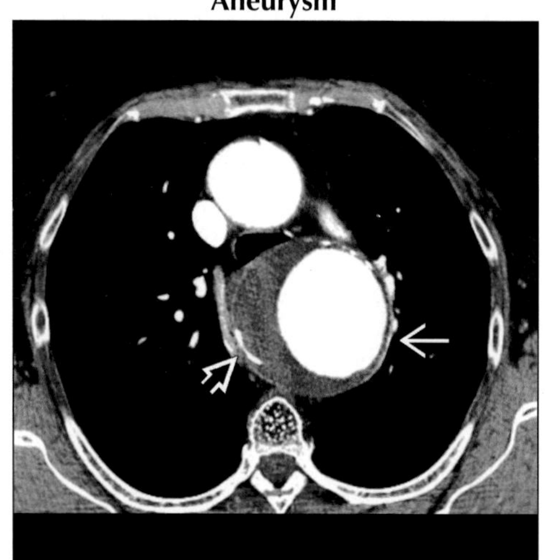

Hematoma

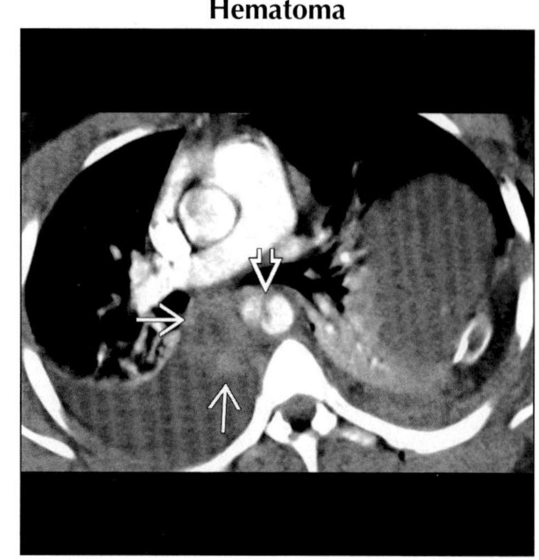

(Left) *Axial CECT shows an atherosclerotic aneurysm ➡ involving the proximal descending aorta. Aneurysm contains eggshell curvilinear calcification ⇨. Eggshell calcification may be seen with silicosis, sarcoid, aneurysms, foregut cysts, and treated Hodgkin lymphoma.* ***(Right)*** *Axial CECT shows high-density mediastinal hematoma ➡ and aortic laceration ⇨ from blunt chest trauma.*

Silicosis/Coal Worker's Pneumoconiosis

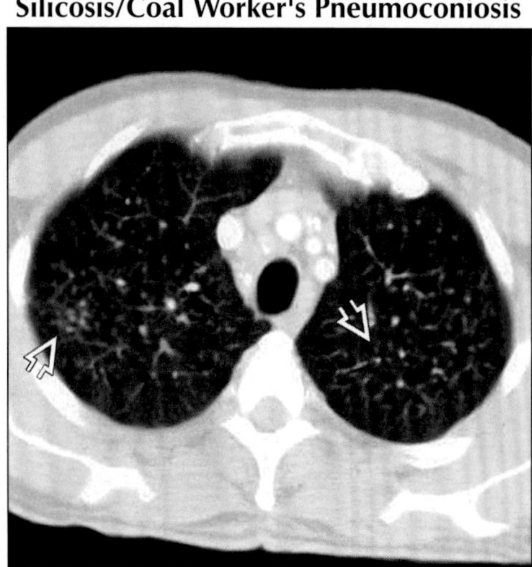

Silicosis/Coal Worker's Pneumoconiosis

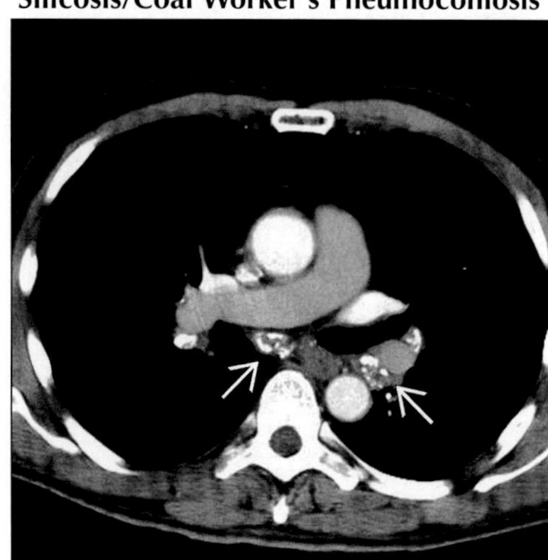

(Left) *Axial CECT shows numerous centrilobular nodules ⇨ in the upper lobes.* ***(Right)*** *Axial CECT in the same patient shows multiple enlarged hilar and mediastinal lymph nodes containing eggshell calcification ➡. Although classic in silicosis, such calcifications can also be seen with sarcoidosis, aneurysms, foregut cysts, treated Hodgkin disease, and fungal infections.*

Treated Hodgkin Lymphoma

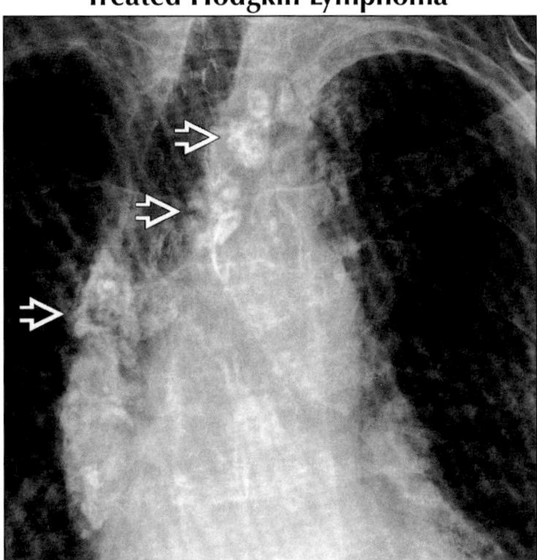

Teratoma

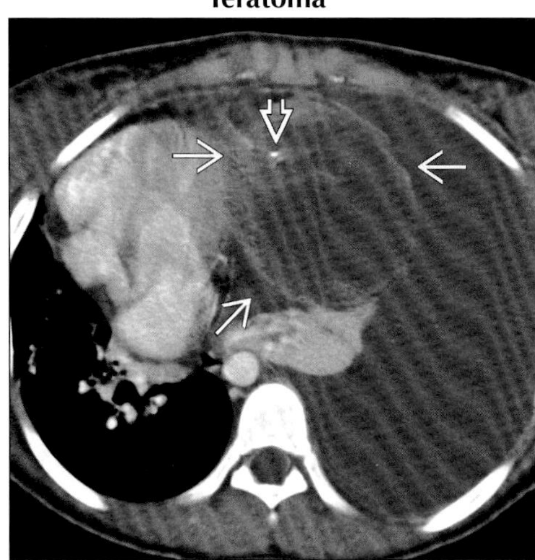

(Left) *Frontal radiograph shows mulberry-type calcifications ➡ within the lymph nodes. Patient had been treated 4 years previously with radiation therapy for Hodgkin disease.* ***(Right)*** *Axial CECT shows a large cystic anterior mediastinal mass ➡ with single punctate calcification ➡ and large left pleural effusion with shift of the heart into the right chest. Resected specimen showed mature teratoma with rupture into the pleural space.*

Thymoma

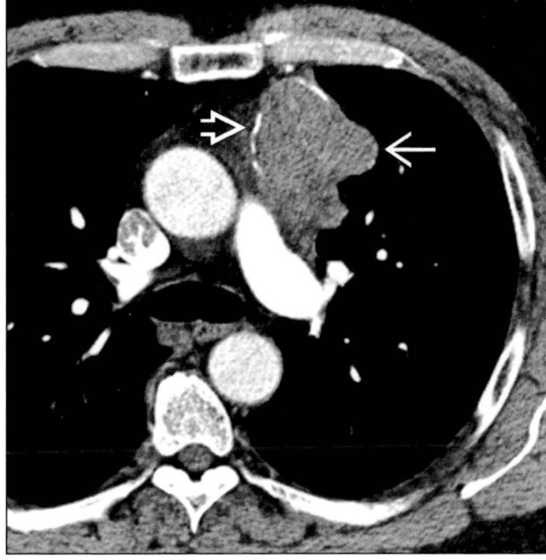

Thymoma

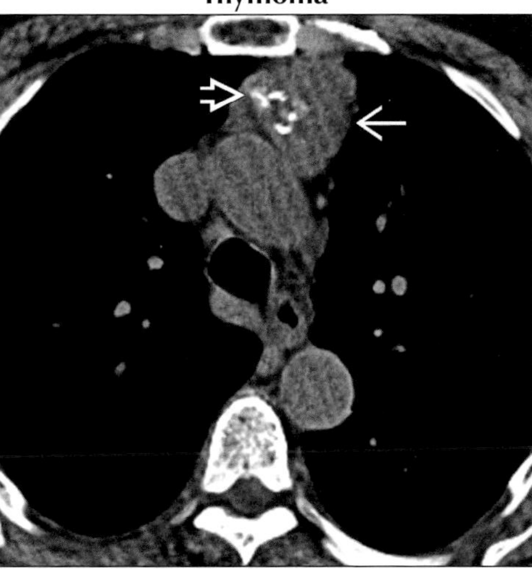

(Left) *Axial CECT shows lobulated anterior mediastinal mass ➡ with foci of eggshell calcification ➡. Calcification does not infer benign tumors. Indeed, this was an invasive thymoma with pleural drop metastases (not shown).* ***(Right)*** *Axial NECT shows a lobulated anterior mediastinal mass ➡ from thymoma. The mass contains foci of coarse calcification ➡. Removal showed benign thymoma.*

Castleman Disease

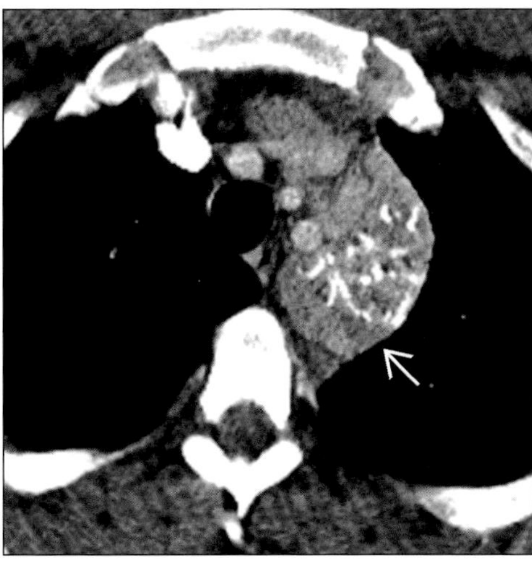

Metastases

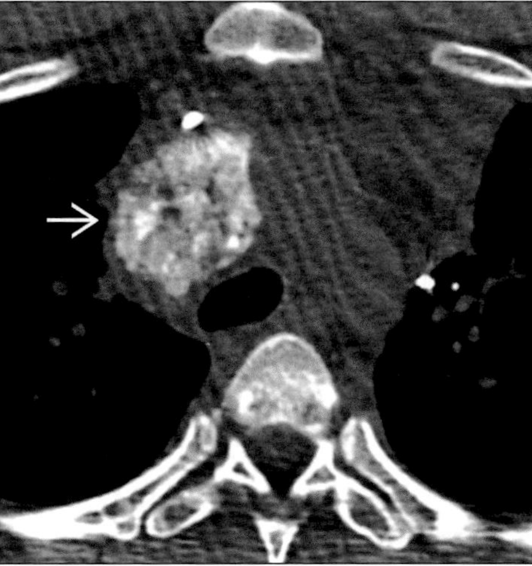

(Left) *Axial CECT shows solitary left-sided superior mediastinal mass ➡ containing flecks of calcification. Mass demonstrates faint contrast enhancement compared to muscle. Biopsy proved Castleman disease.* ***(Right)*** *Axial CECT shows a large right paratracheal mass with coarse calcification ➡ in this patient with metastases from osteosarcoma. Extrathoracic tumors that metastasize to the mediastinum include GU, H&N, breast, and melanoma malignancies.*

HIGH-ATTENUATION MASS, MEDIASTINUM OR HILUM

Sarcoidosis

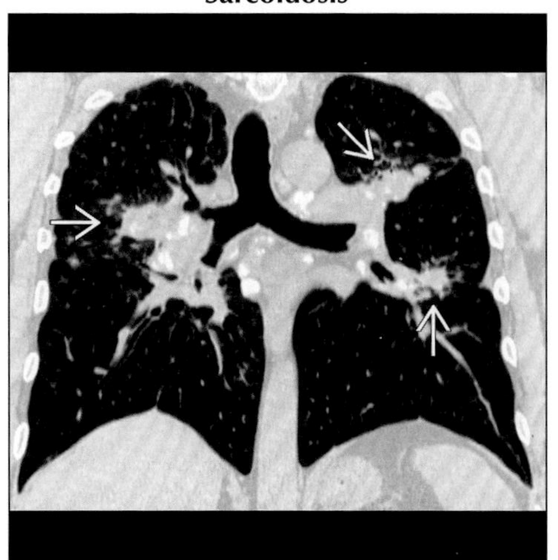

Sarcoidosis

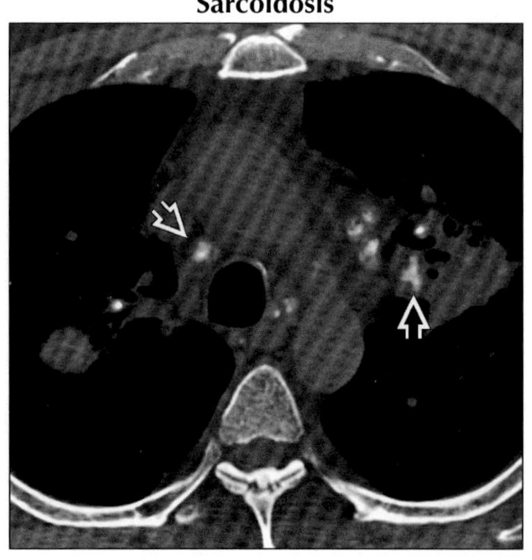

(Left) *Coronal NECT reconstruction shows typical peribronchovascular fibrosis ➔ in the mid-upper lung from sarcoidosis.* ***(Right)*** *Axial NECT shows chalky central lymph node ➔ calcification from sarcoidosis. Nodes tend to be multiple (mean = 20 nodes) and are bilateral and symmetrical in distribution.*

Sarcoidosis

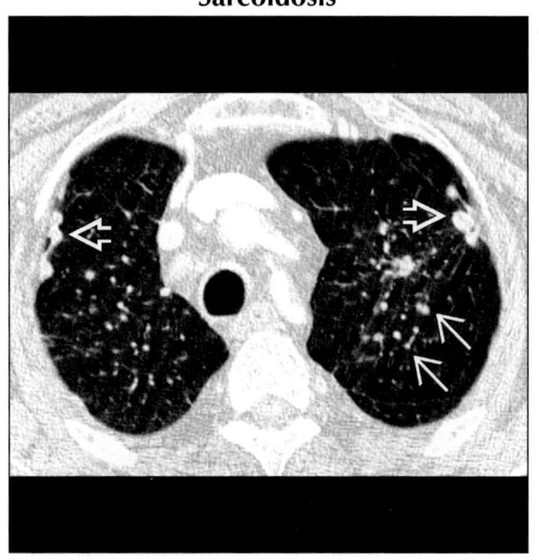

Sarcoidosis

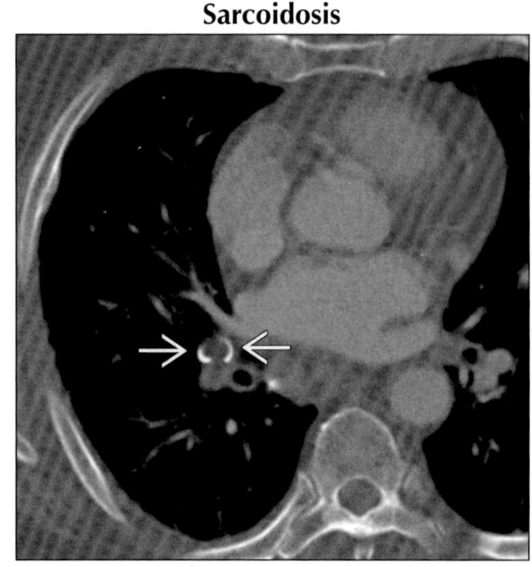

(Left) *Axial CECT shows subpleural nodules ➔ and interstitial nodules ➔.* ***(Right)*** *Axial CECT shows hilar lymph nodes with typical eggshell calcifications ➔. Eggshell calcification is not specific for silicosis and can be seen with other lung diseases.*

Amyloidosis

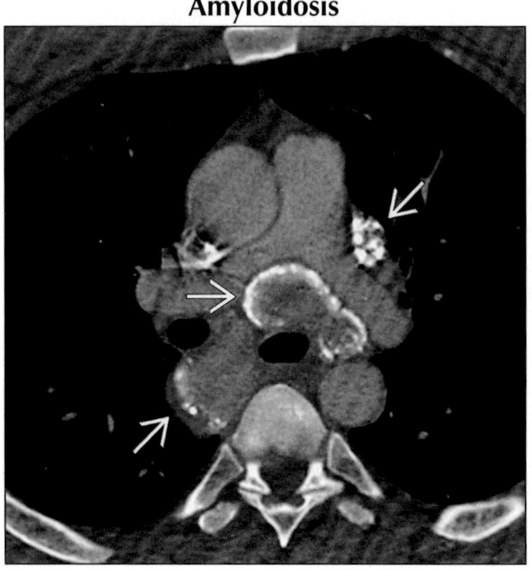

Amyloidosis

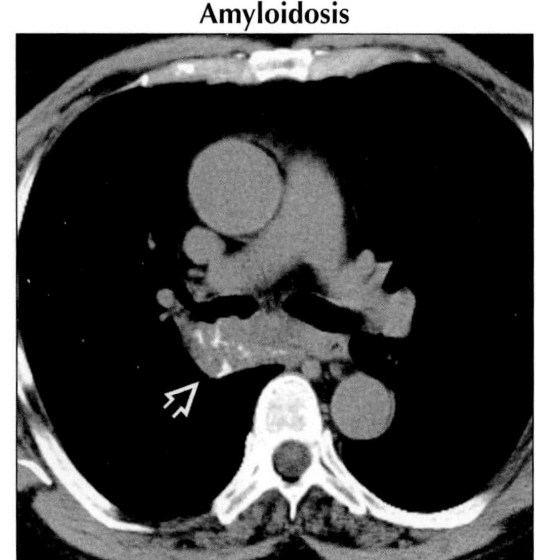

(Left) *Axial CECT shows multiple enlarged mediastinal lymph nodes that have eggshell calcification ➔. Lungs and airways were normal.* ***(Right)*** *Axial NECT shows a large subcarinal mass ➔ extending into the right main stem bronchus. The mass contains eccentric linear calcifications. Nodal amyloidosis is the least common form of pulmonary amyloidosis.*

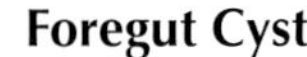

Foregut Cyst

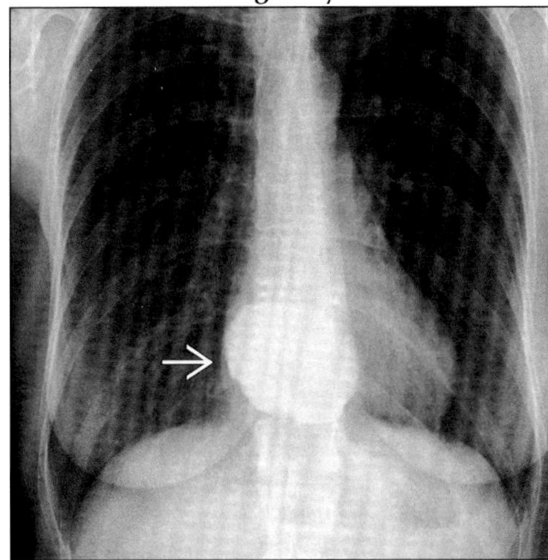

Foregut Cyst

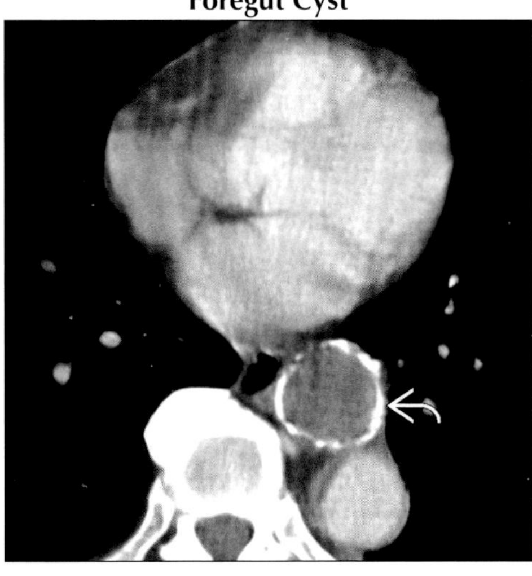

*(**Left**) Frontal radiograph shows an oval, sharply defined, calcified retrocardiac mass →. Bronchogenic cyst is filled with milk of calcium. Cysts may contain a small amount of milk of calcium and exhibit a fluid-fluid level. (**Right**) Axial CECT shows a periesophageal cyst with eggshell calcification →. This cyst is either a bronchogenic or esophageal duplication cyst. Given its location adjacent to the aorta, an aneurysm was excluded on serial sections.*

Hemangiomas

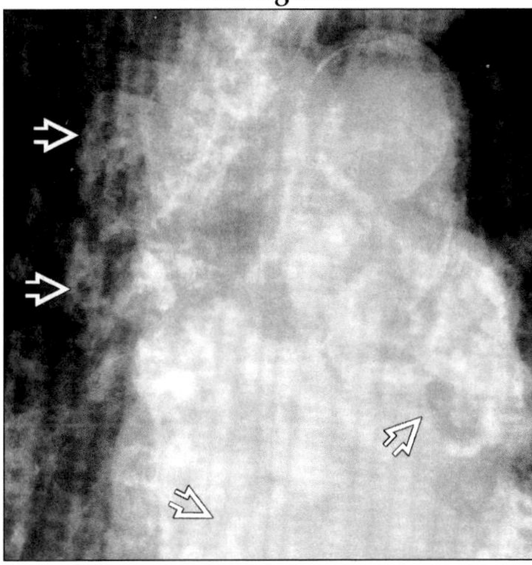

Gossypiboma

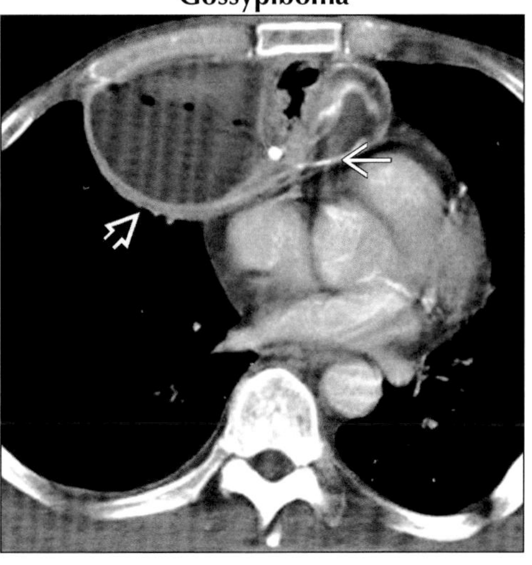

*(**Left**) Frontal radiograph magnified at the carina shows multifocal phleboliths throughout the mediastinum → from a hemangioma. (**Right**) Axial CECT shows mediastinal abscess → from gossypiboma → following median sternotomy. Curvilinear radiopaque markers are usually noted in the mass. As in this case, mass contains air, fluid, and an enhancing thick-walled rind.*

Aluminum Pneumoconiosis

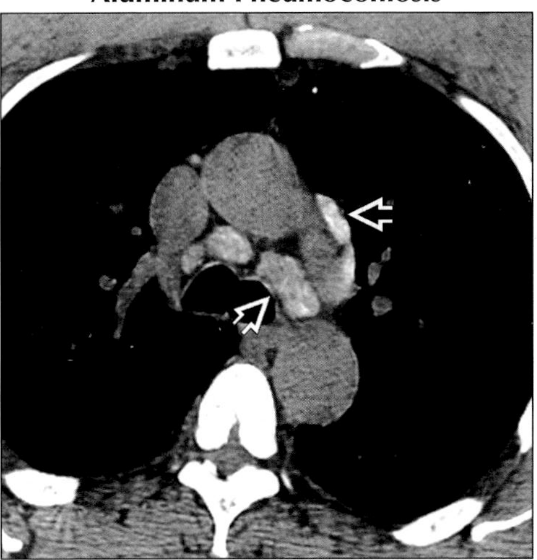

Perflubron Ventilation

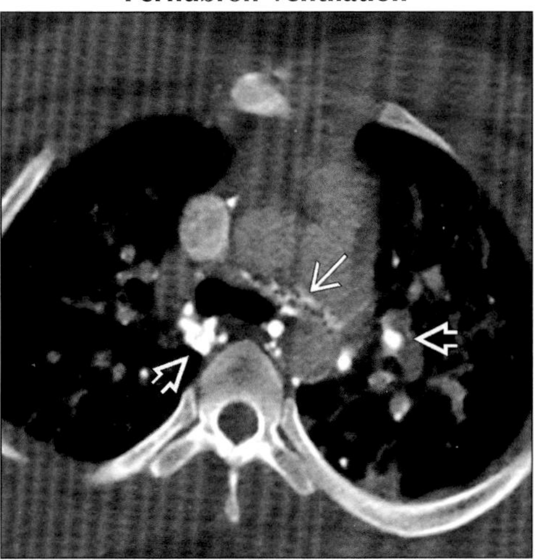

*(**Left**) Axial NECT shows multiple high-attenuation mediastinal lymph nodes →. Patient was an aluminum welder for 40 years. More cephalad lymph nodes will contain less aluminum and will be less dense. (**Right**) Axial CECT shows residual perflubron in lymph nodes → and free in mediastinal fat → a few years after liquid ventilation for acute respiratory distress syndrome. Residual lymphangiographic contrast material could give a similar appearance.*

LOW-ATTENUATION MASS, MEDIASTINUM OR HILUM

DIFFERENTIAL DIAGNOSIS

Common
- Diaphragmatic Hernia
- Lipomatosis
- Lipoma

Less Common
- Low-Attenuation Lymph Nodes
  - Mediastinal Metastases
  - Infection: Fungal & Tuberculosis
- Nerve Sheath Tumors
- Mediastinal Abscess
- Thymolipoma
- Teratoma (Dermoid Cyst)
- Mediastinal Cyst
- Liposarcoma
- Lymphangioma
- Hemangioma
- Thymic Cyst

Rare but Important
- Mediastinal Pseudocyst
- Lateral Meningocele
- Epipericardial Fat Pad Necrosis
- Extramedullary Hematopoiesis
- Whipple Disease (Intestinal Lipodystrophy)

ESSENTIAL INFORMATION

Key Differential Diagnosis Issues
- Fat (-70 to -130 HU) vs. fluid (0-30 HU)
- Mnemonic for fat-containing lesions: **LITHE** (yes, this is an oxymoron)
  - **L**ipomatosis, **l**ipoma, **l**iposarcoma
  - **I**ntestinal lipodystrophy
  - **T**hymolipoma, **t**eratoma (mature)
  - **H**ernias, **h**emangioma
  - **E**xtramedullary hematopoiesis, **e**pipericardial fat pad necrosis
- Mnemonic for water density lesions: **FLUIDS**
  - **F**oregut duplication cysts, **l**ymphangioma, pse**u**docyst, **i**nfection (nodes and abscess), **d**esmoid, **s**pine (meningocele)
- Enlarged normal lymph nodes often have central fat or fatty hilum

Helpful Clues for Common Diagnoses
- **Diaphragmatic Hernia**
  - Includes hiatal hernia, Bochdalek, Morgagni, and traumatic hernias
  - Contents typically include fat and bowel
- **Lipomatosis**
  - Location: Upper mediastinum, costophrenic angles, paraspinal
  - Unencapsulated fat
  - Associated with generalized obesity, Cushing disease, corticosteroid therapy
- **Lipoma**
  - Location: Typically anterior mediastinum
  - Encapsulated, may be pedunculated
  - Well-marginated, fat only
    - Any soft tissue component, consider liposarcoma or thymolipoma

Helpful Clues for Less Common Diagnoses
- **Low-Attenuation Lymph Nodes**
  - **Mediastinal Metastases**
    - Metastases may be low attenuation from necrosis or cystic degeneration
    - Typical tumors include bronchogenic carcinoma, testicular, ovarian, and treated lymphoma
  - **Infection: Fungal & Tuberculosis**
    - Enlarged nodes with rim enhancement and low-attenuation centers
    - Indicates active disease
- **Nerve Sheath Tumors**
  - Neurofibroma or schwannoma
  - Frequent low attenuation (15-20 HU) due to lipid content or cystic degeneration
- **Mediastinal Abscess**
  - Descending cervical mediastinitis usually from odontogenic or cervicofacial infection, esophageal perforation, or trauma
  - Caudal spread aided by gravity and negative intrapleural pressure
  - Irregularly shaped fluid collections, may contain air
- **Thymolipoma**
  - Anterior mediastinal mass, conforms to shape of adjacent structures
  - Typically large; mean length: 18 cm
  - Tumor contains mixture of fat (at least 50%) and soft tissue
    - Soft tissue seen as linear strands or whorls, uncommonly rounded nodules
- **Teratoma (Dermoid Cyst)**
  - Anterior mediastinal mass
  - Fat in 75%, fluid in 90%
  - Mixture of fat, soft tissue, fluid, and calcification (50%)
  - Cystic component often predominant (multilocular), 15% cystic only

- **Mediastinal Cyst**
  - Includes foregut duplication cysts, pericardial cysts
  - Cysts are thin walled, unilocular
  - Fluid attenuation variable: Water, hemorrhage, infection, milk of calcium
  - Bronchogenic cysts usually subcarinal; esophageal duplication cysts periesophageal; neurenteric cysts associated with adjacent vertebral body cleft
- **Liposarcoma**
  - Location: Typically posterior mediastinum
  - Inhomogeneous with large areas of soft tissue density
- **Lymphangioma**
  - Multilocular, well-defined, water density mass; may be septated
  - Location: Superior mediastinum adjacent to right lateral tracheal wall
  - Soft in composition, no mass effect
  - Intrathoracic lymphangiomas + cystic bone lesions = Gorham disease
- **Hemangioma**
  - Location: Superior mediastinum
  - Fat in 40%, phleboliths in 10-40%
- **Thymic Cyst**
  - Congenital cysts most common, usually unilocular
  - Acquired cysts usually multilocular
    - Occurs in patients after radiation therapy for Hodgkin disease, in association with thymic tumors, and after thoracotomy

Helpful Clues for Rare Diagnoses

- **Mediastinal Pseudocyst**
  - Pancreatic pseudocyst extending through esophageal or aortic hiatus
  - Location: Posterior inferior mediastinum
  - Fluid collection, thin or thick walled
  - Usually connects to pancreatic pseudocysts
- **Lateral Meningocele**
  - Associated with neurofibromatosis
  - May be multiple and bilateral
  - Typically enlarges neural foramen
- **Epipericardial Fat Pad Necrosis**
  - Patients usually present with acute pleuritic chest pain
  - Imaging and pathologic features similar to those of fat necrosis in epiploic appendagitis
- **Extramedullary Hematopoiesis**
  - Typically in patients with congenital hereditary anemias, especially thalassemia
  - Posterior mediastinal masses usually caudal to 6th thoracic vertebra
  - May contain fat, especially larger lesions
  - Centered on vertebral body with prominent trabeculae from marrow expansion
- **Whipple Disease (Intestinal Lipodystrophy)**
  - Infection caused by *Tropheryma whippelii*
  - Migratory polyarthritis followed by intestinal malabsorption
  - Low-density nodes from foamy lipid-containing macrophages

Diaphragmatic Hernia

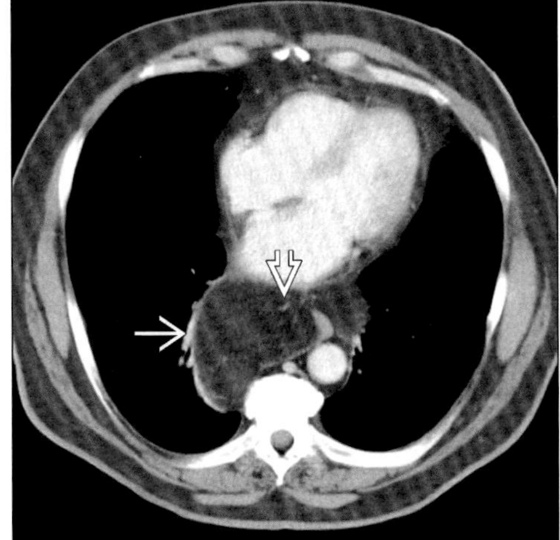

Axial CECT shows a hiatal hernia of peritoneal fat tissue through esophageal hiatus ➔. Note the sparse linear vessels ➔ typical for herniated abdominal fat.

Diaphragmatic Hernia

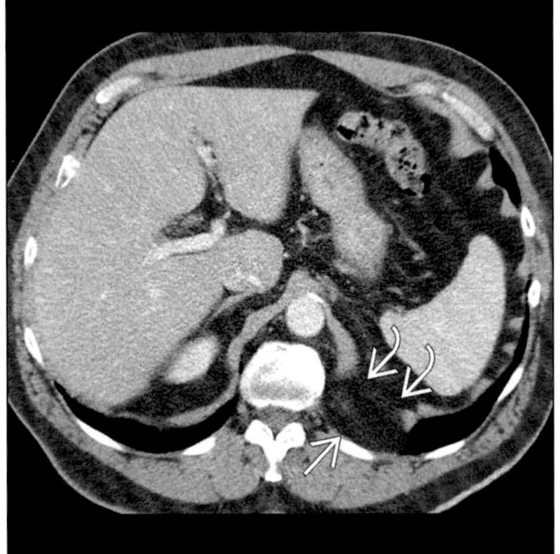

Axial CECT shows Bochdalek hernia containing retroperitoneal fat ➔. Note the localized discontinuity of the medial left hemidiaphragm ➔.

LOW-ATTENUATION MASS, MEDIASTINUM OR HILUM

Diaphragmatic Hernia

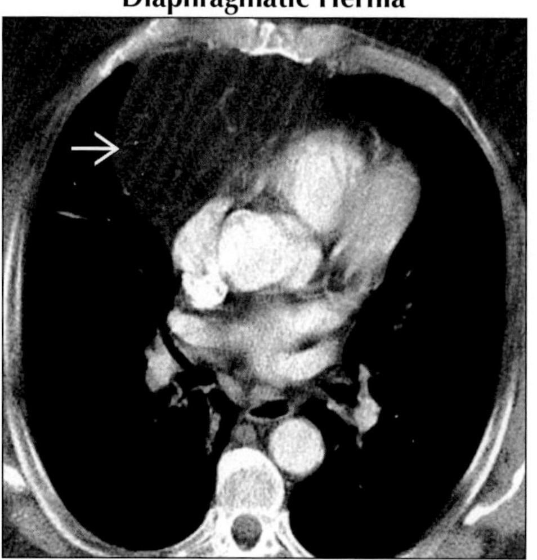

Diaphragmatic Hernia

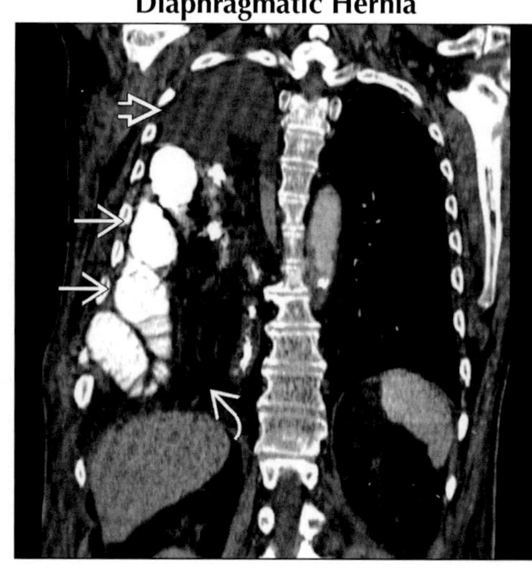

(Left) *Axial CECT shows herniation of peritoneal fat ➔ through Morgagni hiatus. Morgagni hernias are typically right-sided; the left side is blocked by the heart.* ***(Right)*** *Coronal CECT shows large right pleural effusion ➔, small bowel loops ➔, and peritoneal fat ➔ from traumatic diaphragmatic tear. Right-sided tears are less common than tears of the left hemidiaphragm. Coronal reconstructions are often useful for diaphragmatic hernias.*

Lipomatosis

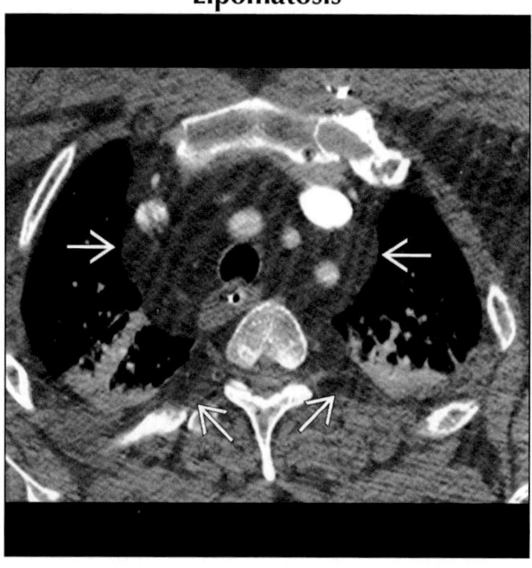

Lipoma

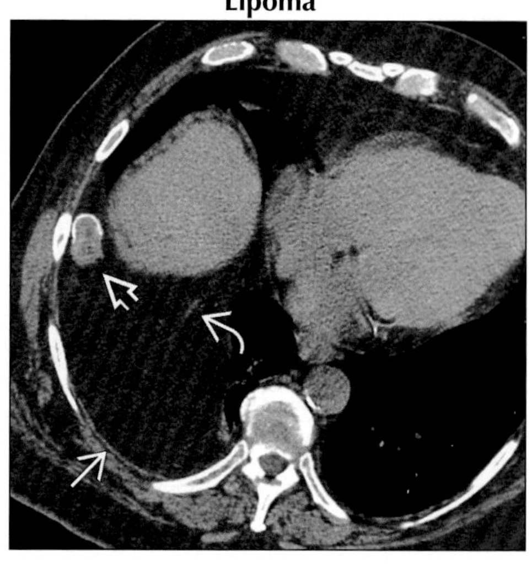

(Left) *Axial CECT shows diffuse mediastinal and paraspinal widening from fat ➔. Most commonly the largest quantity of fat is in the anterosuperior mediastinum.* ***(Right)*** *Axial NECT shows large lipoma ➔, old fat necrosis ➔, and vascular pedicle ➔. Lipoma was pedunculated from the anterior mediastinum. Note the lack of any soft tissue. Old fat necrosis is probably secondary to previous ischemia related to intermittent twisting of the pedicle.*

Mediastinal Metastases

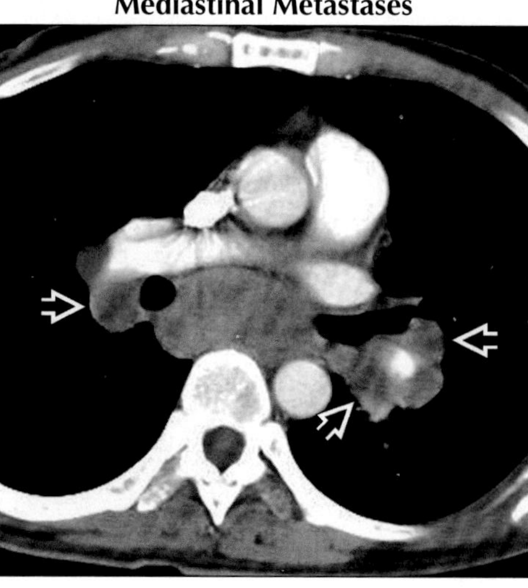

Infection: Fungal & Tuberculosis

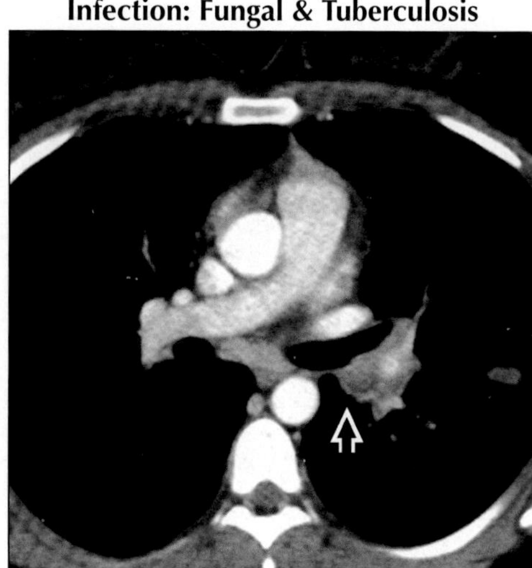

(Left) *Axial CECT shows numerous low-density nodes ➔ in the mediastinum. This patient had testicular metastases.* ***(Right)*** *Axial CECT shows left hilar lymphadenopathy ➔ with central low attenuation from necrosis in this immunocompromised patient with histoplasmosis. Infection by other fungi and tuberculosis would give identical findings. Generally this appearance is associated with active disease.*

Infection: Fungal & Tuberculosis

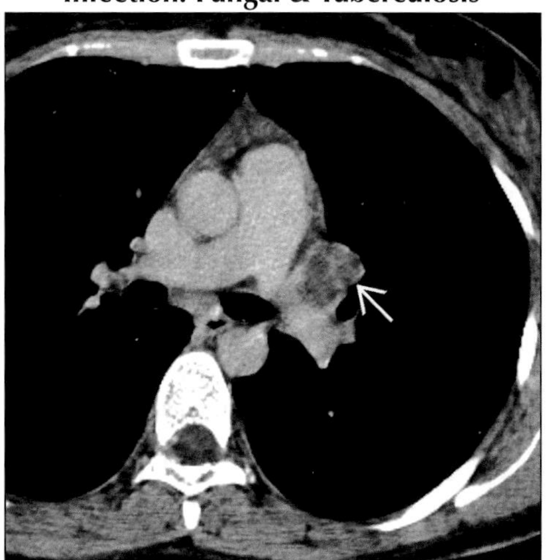

Nerve Sheath Tumors

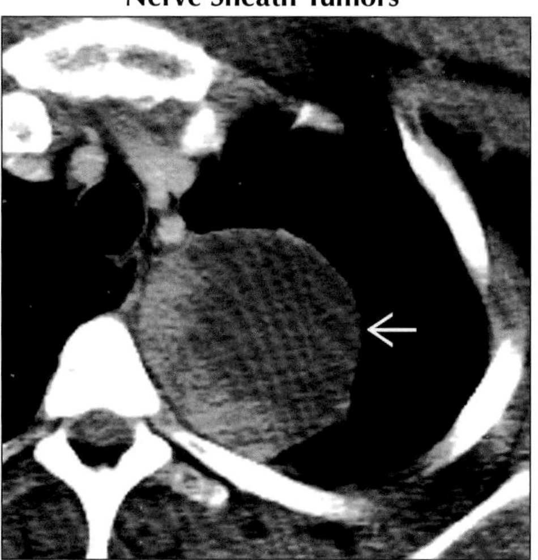

(Left) Axial CECT delayed imaging following IV contrast administration shows residual rim of contrast enhancement in the lymph nodes with low-attenuation centers ➡ from tuberculosis. (Right) Axial CECT shows a heterogeneous mass with large area of low attenuation ➡ representing a neurofibroma. The low attenuation is probably secondary to cystic degeneration.

Mediastinal Abscess

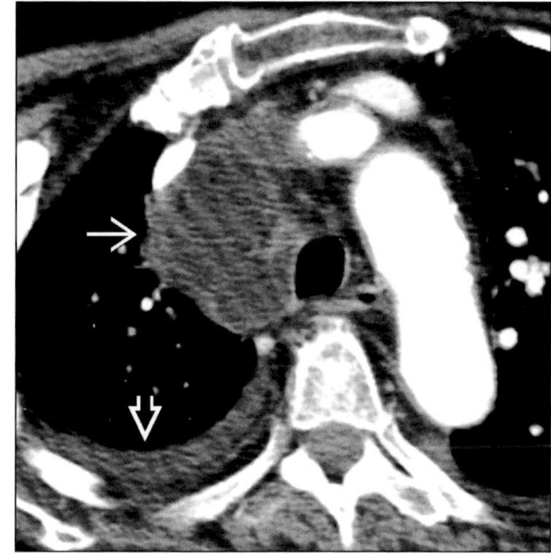

Thymolipoma

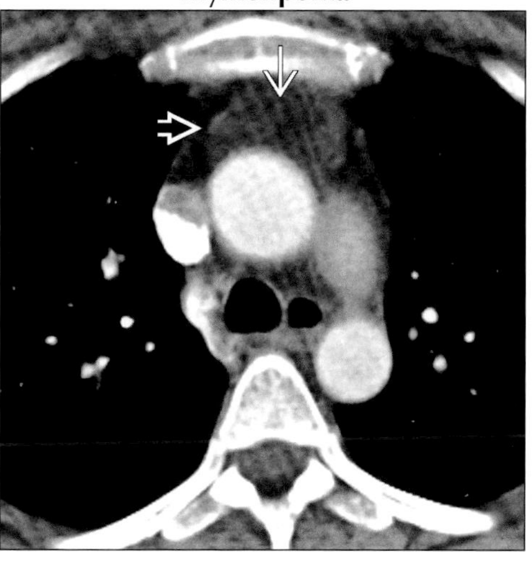

(Left) Axial CECT shows a thin-walled, fluid-filled mass ➡ that extended from the thoracic inlet to the right paratracheal space. Note the small right pleural effusion ⇨. Patient had retropharyngeal abscess. (Right) Axial CECT shows a predominant fatty anterior mediastinal mass ⇨. Residual thymic tissue is seen as thin linear strands ➡.

Teratoma (Dermoid Cyst)

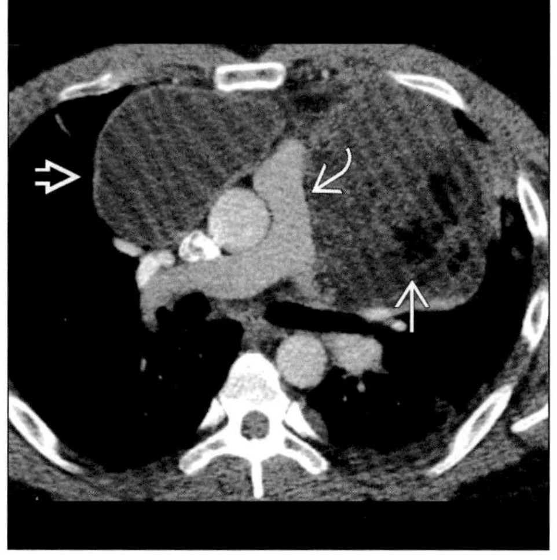

Mediastinal Cyst

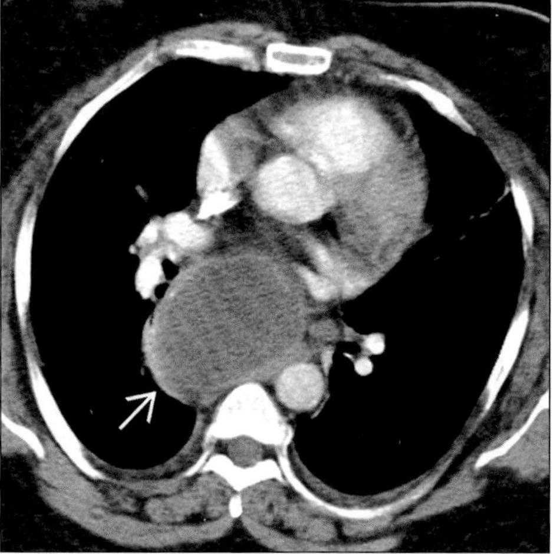

(Left) Axial CECT shows large heterogeneous anterior mediastinal mass ⇨, which compresses the main pulmonary artery ↪. Mass contains fat ➡ and fluid. A fat-fluid level is seen in 10% of dermoids and is pathognomonic. In this patient, biopsy showed embryonal cell germ cell tumor. (Right) Axial CECT shows a large, low-density, oval, subcarinal mass ➡ from bronchogenic cyst.

LOW-ATTENUATION MASS, MEDIASTINUM OR HILUM

Mediastinal Cyst

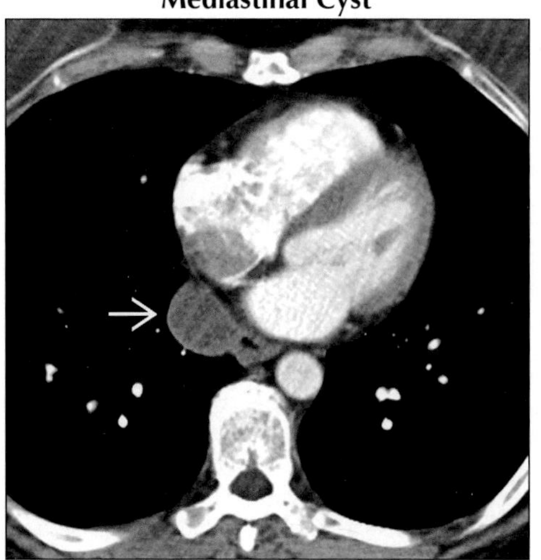

Liposarcoma

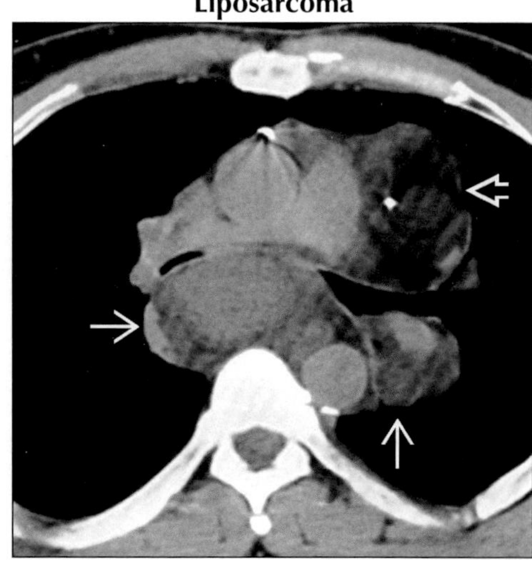

*(**Left**) Axial CECT shows a thin-walled, homogeneous, water density periesophageal cyst ➔ from an esophageal duplication cyst. (**Right**) Axial NECT shows complex soft tissue ➔ and fatty ➪ mass from liposarcoma. Typically, soft tissue component is more prominent than fat. However, soft tissue component may be minimal. One should include liposarcoma in differential of any fatty mass with a nodular soft tissue component.*

Lymphangioma

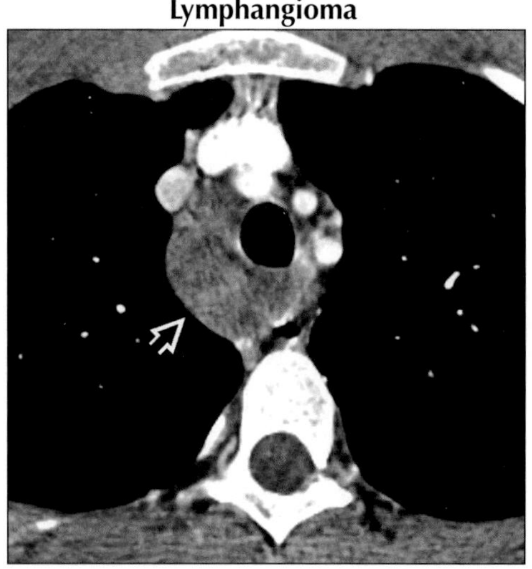

Lymphangioma

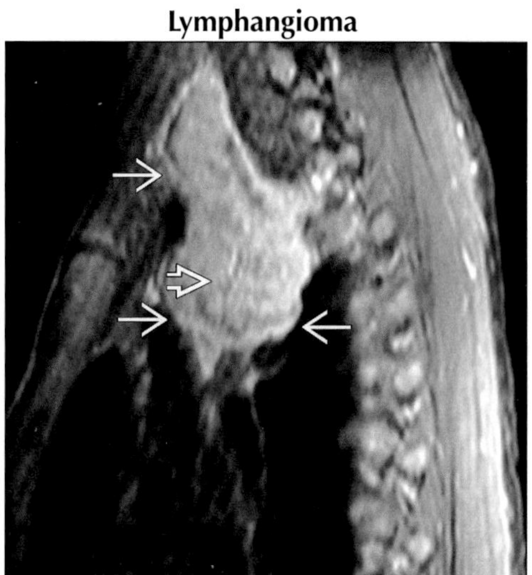

*(**Left**) Axial CECT shows a thin-walled, water density right paratracheal mass ➪. Notice that even though the mass is fairly large, there is no mass effect. (**Right**) Sagittal T1WI C+ FS MR in the same patient shows diffuse enhancement ➔ of the mass with extension into the neck. There is no mass effect on surrounding structures. Note the thin septa ➪.*

Hemangioma

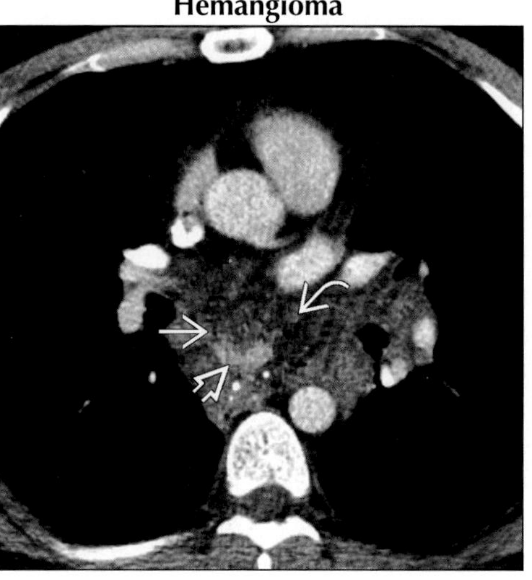

Thymic Cyst

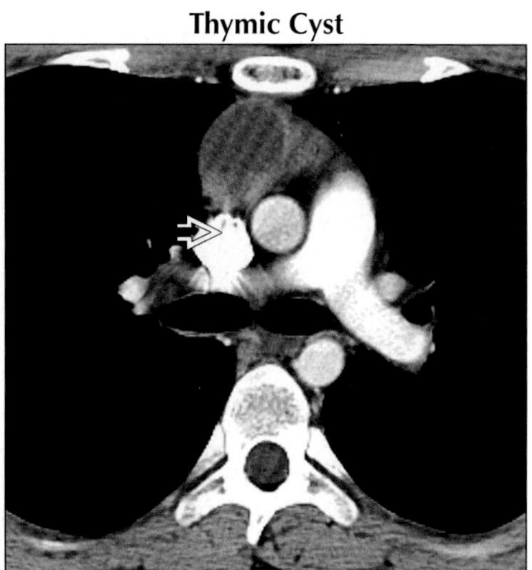

*(**Left**) Axial CECT shows a heterogeneous mass that contains multiple flecks of calcification ➪ and mild central contrast enhancement ➔ and fat ↗. In hemangiomas phleboliths are nearly as common as fat. (**Right**) Axial CECT shows a sharply defined cyst ➪ in the anterior mediastinum. Cyst contains a fluid level. This cyst is probably congenital, as the patient had no history of radiation therapy, no thymic tumor, and no history of thoracic surgery.*

Mediastinal Pseudocyst

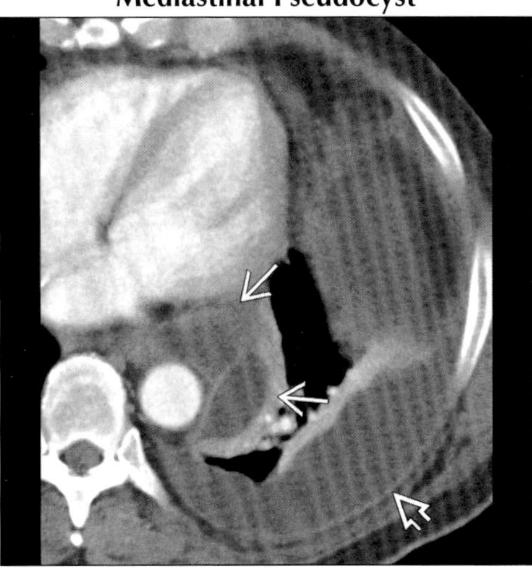

Mediastinal Pseudocyst

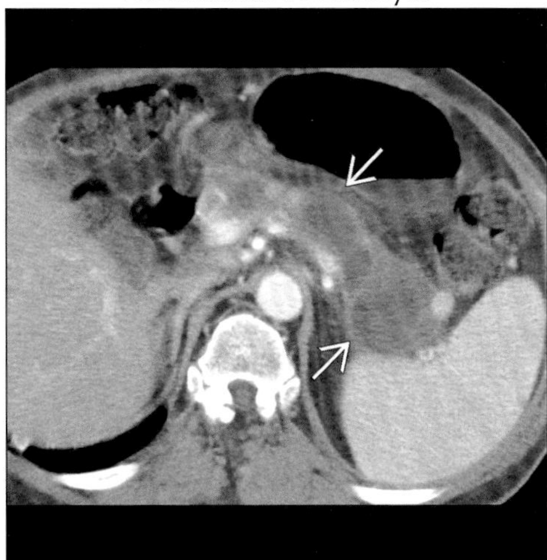

(Left) Axial CECT shows fluid density cysts surrounding the aorta ➡ and a moderate-sized left pleural effusion ➡. (Right) Axial CECT more inferiorly in the same patient shows that the periaortic cysts were continuous with pancreatic pseudocysts ➡ that had extended up through the aortic hiatus. Left pleural effusions are common in patients with inflammatory disease of the pancreas.

Lateral Meningocele

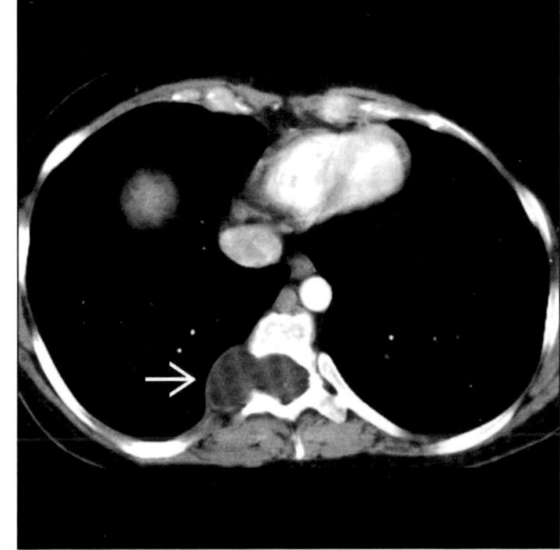

Epipericardial Fat Pad Necrosis

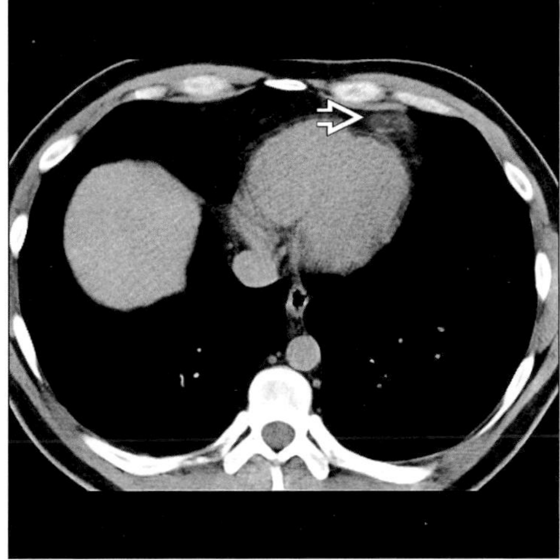

(Left) Axial CECT shows a thin-walled, water density lateral meningocele ➡. Neural foramen is widened. Patients with lateral meningocele commonly show scoliosis and present with neurofibromatosis. (Right) Axial NECT shows swirling high-density material in pericardial fat pad ➡ from epipericardial fat necrosis. Typically, the soft tissue density change will resolve over 2-3 weeks.

Extramedullary Hematopoiesis

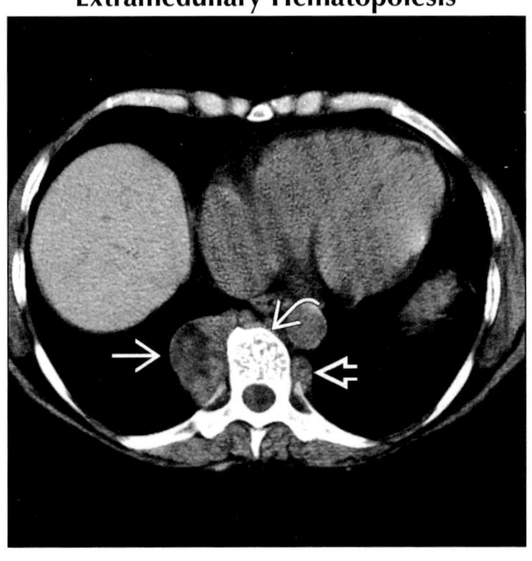

Whipple Disease (Intestinal Lipodystrophy)

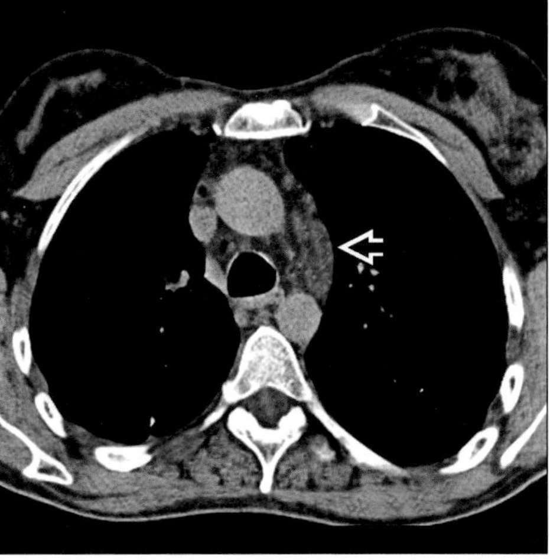

(Left) Axial NECT shows bilateral paraspinal masses. The larger mass ➡ contains fat. Vertebral body has prominent trabeculae ➡. Smaller lesions of extramedullary hematopoiesis ➡ tend to be homogeneous. (Right) Axial NECT shows mediastinal nodes and stranding ➡ in this patient with Whipple disease. 50% of patients with Whipple disease will have disseminated lymphadenopathy.

CONTRAST-ENHANCING MASS, MEDIASTINUM OR HILUM

DIFFERENTIAL DIAGNOSIS

Common
- Aneurysm
- Goiter

Less Common
- Varices
- Tuberculosis
- Castleman Disease
- Parathyroid Adenoma
- Acute Mediastinitis
- Kaposi Sarcoma
- Hemangioma
- Metastases
- Thymic Carcinoid

Rare but Important
- Paraganglioma
- Extramedullary Hematopoiesis
- Bacillary Angiomatosis
- Kimura Disease

ESSENTIAL INFORMATION

Key Differential Diagnosis Issues
- Mnemonic: **ATTACK PAIN**
  - **A**neurysm, **T**hyroid (goiter), **T**uberculosis, **A**ngiofollicular hyperplasia (Castleman), **C**arcinoid (thymic), **K**aposi sarcoma
  - **P**arathyroid Adenoma, **I**nfection (mediastinitis), **N**euroendocrine (paraganglioma)

Helpful Clues for Common Diagnoses
- **Aneurysm**
  - Due to atherosclerosis, trauma, mycotic infection, cystic medial necrosis, vasculitis
  - Wall may have curvilinear calcification
  - Consider perforation in patients with left pleural effusion
  - Any mediastinal mass should be considered as possible aneurysm
- **Goiter**
  - Develop in 5% worldwide
    - Up to 20% descend into mediastinum
  - NECT: High attenuation due to natural iodine; 70-120 HU
    - May also have calcifications (coarse, punctate, or rings)
    - Anterior to trachea (75%), usually left side predominant
    - Posterior to trachea (25%), usually right side predominant

Helpful Clues for Less Common Diagnoses
- **Varices**
  - From portal hypertension, flow through left gastric vein to esophageal venous plexus
  - Dilated serpiginous veins in azygoesophageal recess, may be unopacified on arterial phase imaging
  - CT findings include cirrhotic contour liver and splenomegaly
- **Tuberculosis**
  - Enlarged rim-enhanced lymph nodes
    - Low-attenuation center represents caseous necrosis
  - Indicates active disease, typically primary disease
- **Castleman Disease**
  - Angiofollicular lymph node hyperplasia
  - Histology: Hyaline vascular (90%), plasma cell (10%)
    - Localized: Hyaline vascular (90%) and asymptomatic
    - Multicentric: Plasma cell (80%) and often symptomatic
    - 70% occurs in thorax
    - Avid, uniform contrast enhancement is characteristic, especially in hyaline vascular type
- **Parathyroid Adenoma**
  - 10% ectopic (50% in anterior mediastinum usually near thymus)
    - Less common in paraesophageal region or aortopulmonary window
  - Benign tumor that results in hyperparathyroidism
  - Tumors usually < 3 cm diameter
  - 25% demonstrate mild enhancement
- **Acute Mediastinitis**
  - Most associated with median sternotomy or esophageal perforation
    - Less commonly descend from retropharyngeal infection
  - CT findings include effacement of normal mediastinal fat, fluid collections, extraluminal gas
- **Kaposi Sarcoma**
  - Imaging appearance overlaps with multicentric Castleman disease
    - Both associated with herpes virus-8

    - Kaposi and Castleman may be concurrently present in HIV patients
- **Hemangioma**
  - < 1% of mediastinal masses
  - Most common in superior or anterior mediastinum
    - Phleboliths (10-40%)
    - Intralesional fat also common (40%)
  - Heterogeneous contrast enhancement: 4 patterns
    - Central (60%), peripheral (10%), central and peripheral (20%), nonspecific (10%)
- **Metastases**
  - Vascular tumors: Renal cell carcinoma, papillary thyroid, small cell carcinoma, melanoma
  - Metastases to mediastinum from extrathoracic tumors uncommon
    - Genitourinary tumors: Renal cell, transitional cell, prostate, uterine, ovarian, testicular
    - Head & neck tumors: Squamous cell, thyroid
    - Breast
    - Melanoma
- **Thymic Carcinoid**
  - Large size is common, averaging 10-12 cm
  - May have metastases to lung, brain, lymph nodes, and pleura
    - Osseous metastasis often osteoblastic
  - 1/3 have paraneoplastic syndrome, usually Cushing syndrome
    - Curiously, carcinoid syndrome has not been reported
  - 20% associated with type 1 MEN syndrome

Helpful Clues for Rare Diagnoses

- **Paraganglioma**
  - Most are asymptomatic
  - Enhancement often intense
  - Most located in posterior mediastinum
    - Aortopulmonary recess, subcarinal or pericardiac region well-described locations
- **Extramedullary Hematopoiesis**
  - Posterior mediastinal masses usually caudal to 6th thoracic vertebra
  - May contain fat
  - Centered on vertebral body
  - Ribs usually demonstrate marrow expansion
- **Bacillary Angiomatosis**
  - Caused by *Bartonella henselae* or *B. quintana*
    - Transmitted by cats, fleas, and lice
  - Affects skin, lung, bone, brain, liver, spleen
    - Present with skin lesions that mimic Kaposi sarcoma
    - Lung nodules usually < 1.5 cm diameter
    - Nodes have intense contrast enhancement
  - Almost exclusively disease of AIDS
- **Kimura Disease**
  - Rare chronic inflammatory disease of unknown etiology primarily affecting young Asian males
  - Subcutaneous masses in head and neck + regional lymphadenopathy
  - Nodes moderately enhance with contrast

Aneurysm

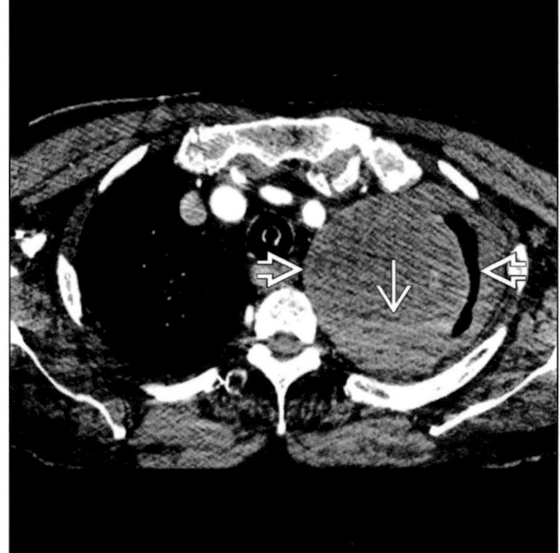

Axial CECT shows a large mass ➡ in the left upper lung. The mass contains a fluid-fluid level ➡.

Aneurysm

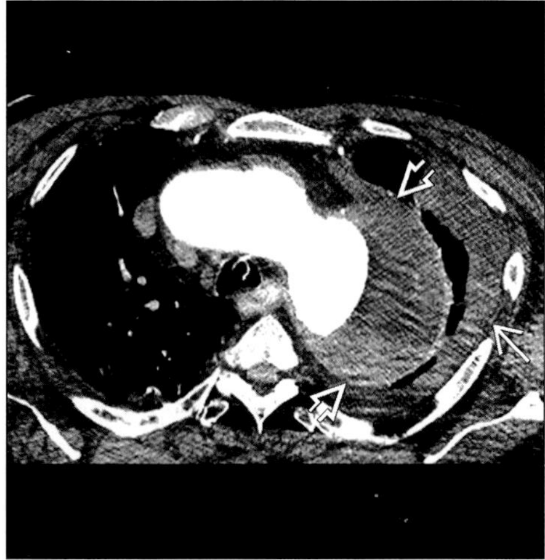

Axial CECT more inferiorly shows that the mass is a partially thrombosed aortic aneurysm ➡. The left pleural effusion ➡ is due to rupture.

CONTRAST-ENHANCING MASS, MEDIASTINUM OR HILUM

(Left) *Axial CECT shows a large, contrast-enhancing, superior mediastinal mass ➔ that compresses the trachea. Goiters may contain nodules and foci of calcification.* ***(Right)*** *Axial CECT shows contrast-enhancing varices ➔ surrounding the distal esophagus, anterior to the aorta. This patient had portal hypertension from cirrhosis. The esophageal wall is also slightly thickened ➲ from esophageal varices.*

Goiter

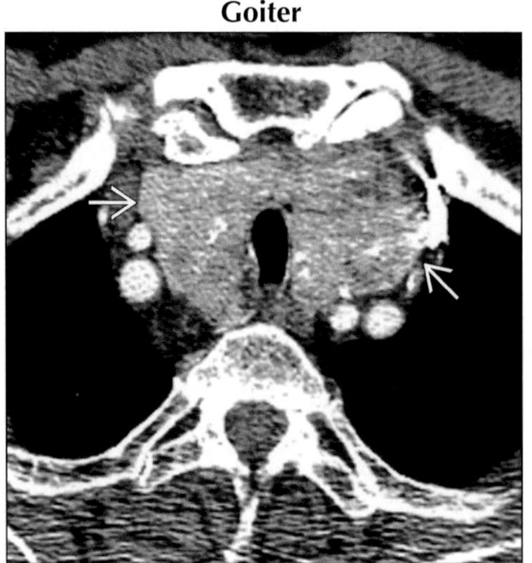

Varices

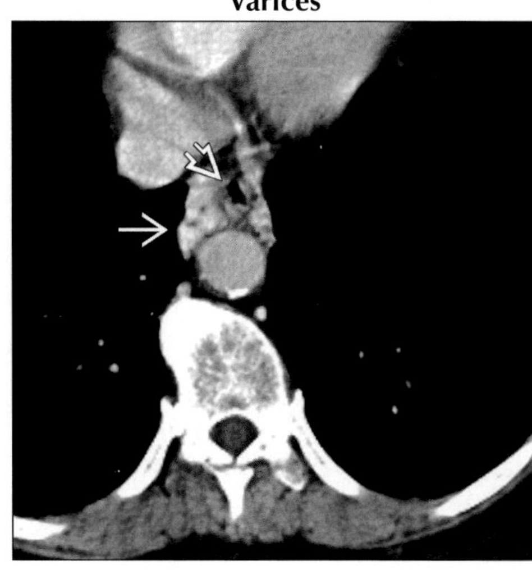

(Left) *Axial CECT shows enlarged mediastinal lymph nodes ➔ along the aortic arch.* ***(Right)*** *Axial CECT delayed image shows rim enhancement ➔ of the enlarged nodes. Rim enhancement is seen in up to 80% of patients with tuberculous lymphadenopathy. The outer wall is irregular in thickness. The most commonly involved nodes are the right paratracheal and tracheobronchial lymph nodes.*

Tuberculosis

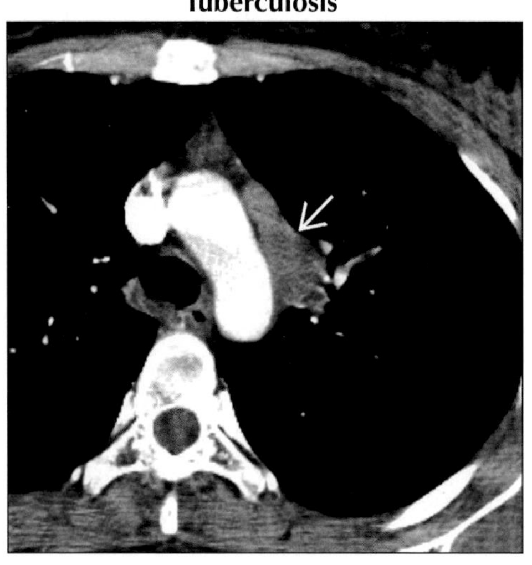

Tuberculosis

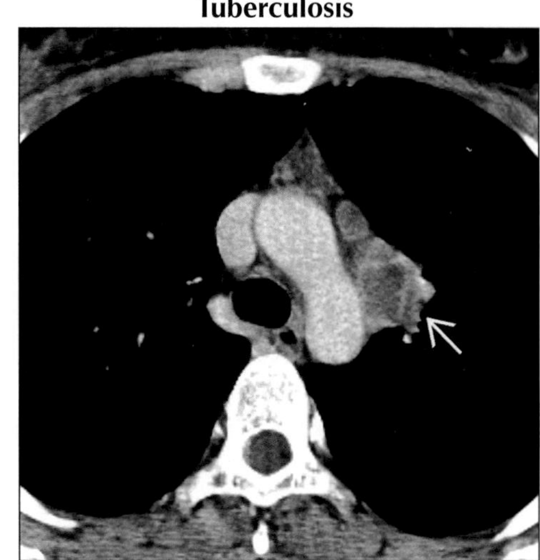

(Left) *Axial CECT shows an enhancing subcarinal mass ➔. Castleman disease may have calcification (5-10%), which is characteristically coarse or branch-like. Lung disease (interstitial thickening) is uncommon. Tumors larger than 5 cm may have heterogeneous contrast enhancement.* ***(Right)*** *Axial CECT shows a contrast-enhancing mass ➔ in tracheoesophageal groove. Parathyroid adenomas are often subtle, requiring careful examination of typical locations.*

Castleman Disease

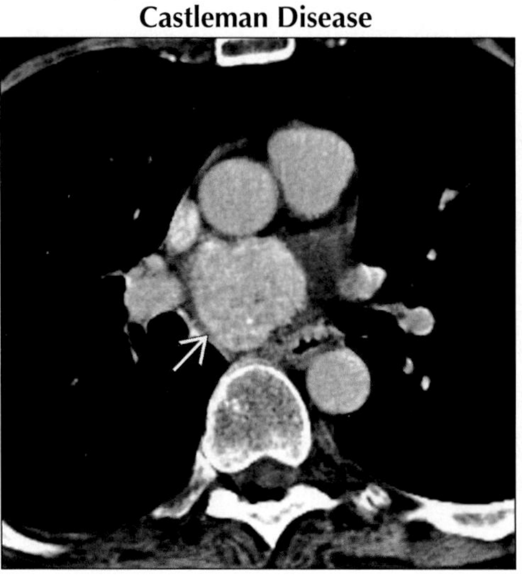

Parathyroid Adenoma

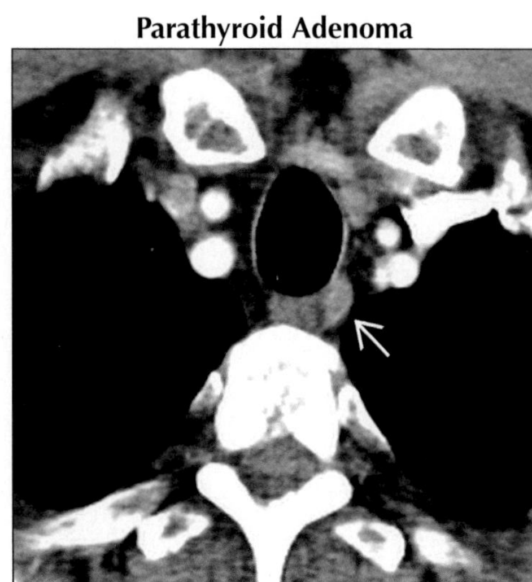

Acute Mediastinitis

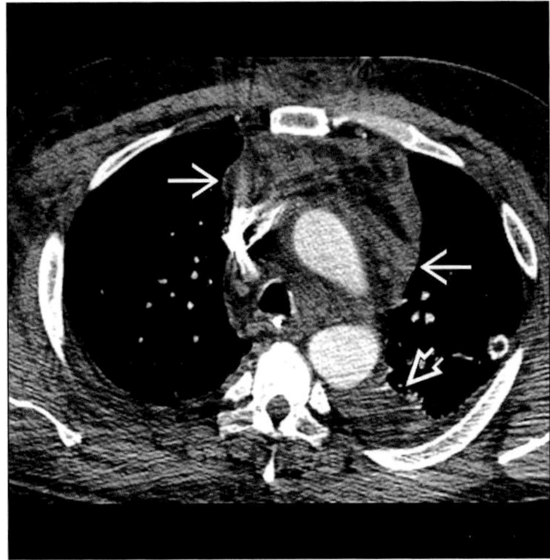

Kaposi Sarcoma

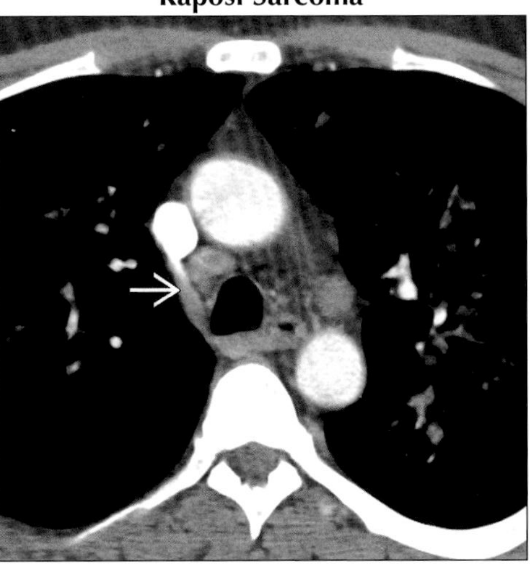

(Left) *Axial CECT shows diffuse infiltration of anterior mediastinal fat ➡ with slight contrast enhancement. Note the small left pleural effusion ⇨. Mediastinitis due to extension from head & neck infection.* ***(Right)*** *Axial CECT shows contrast-enhancing mediastinal lymph node ➡. Patient had diffuse peribronchial nodularity on lung windows (not shown). Differential includes bacillary angiomatosis; however, those nodes usually demonstrate more intense contrast enhancement.*

Hemangioma

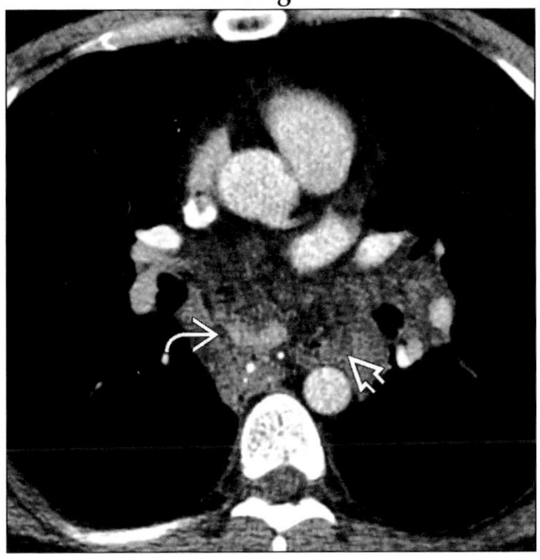

Metastases

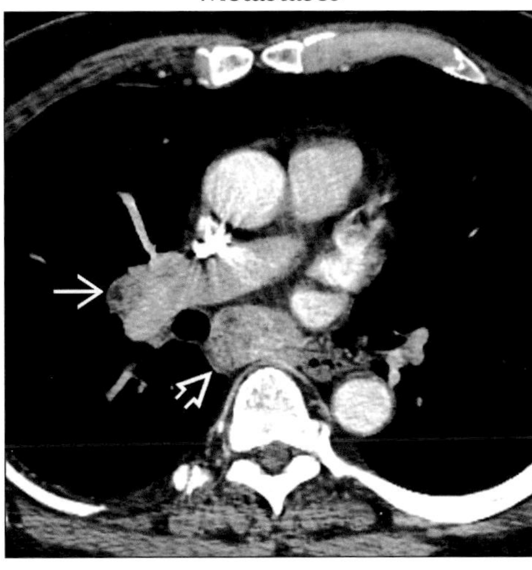

(Left) *Axial CECT shows a large subcarinal mass ⇨ that contains faint central contrast enhancement ↪. The mass also contains multiple small flecks of calcification. The mass infiltrated the entire middle mediastinum without obstructing adjacent veins or airways.* ***(Right)*** *Axial CECT shows an enlarged, heterogeneous, contrast-enhancing subcarinal mass ⇨ and right hilar mass ➡ in a patient with renal cell carcinoma metastasis.*

Thymic Carcinoid

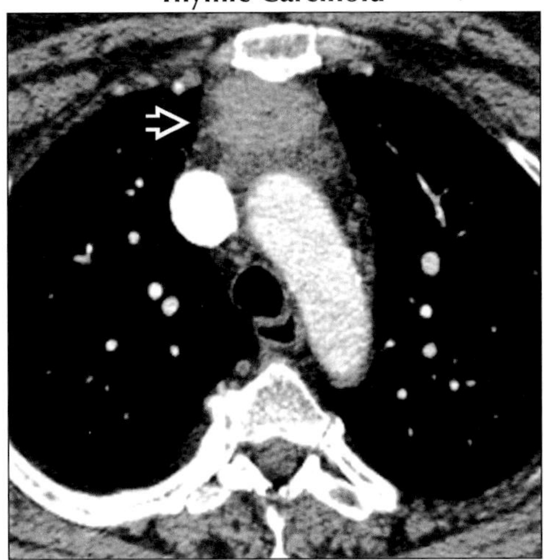

Paraganglioma

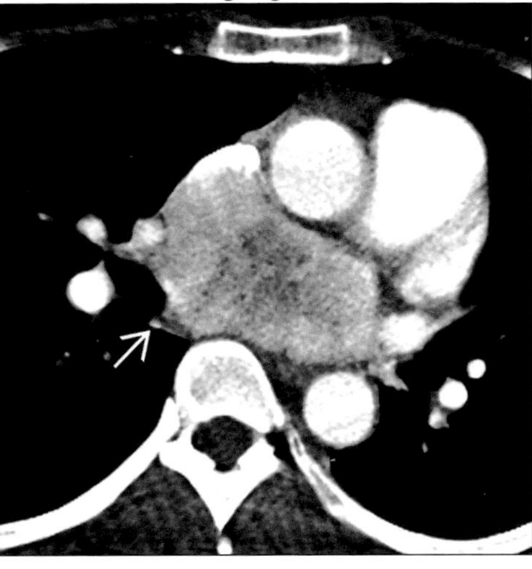

(Left) *Axial CECT shows a contrast-enhancing, anterior mediastinal mass ⇨ with irregular margins. The differential includes thymic carcinoma.* ***(Right)*** *Axial CECT shows a large, heterogeneous, contrast-enhancing subcarinal mediastinal mass ➡. Patient had severe hypertension. Smaller tumors usually demonstrate more homogeneous contrast enhancement. Enhancement may be intense.*

UNILATERAL MEDIASTINAL MASS

DIFFERENTIAL DIAGNOSIS

Common
- Thyroid Goiter
- Thymoma
- Teratoma
- Lymphoma
- Pericardial Cyst
- Bronchogenic Cyst
- Neurogenic Tumors
- Pleuropericardial Fat Pad
- Aortic Aneurysm

Less Common
- Thymic Carcinoma
- Thymic Cyst
- Lymphangioma
- Malignant Germ Cell Tumors
- Esophageal Duplication Cyst

Rare but Important
- Parathyroid Adenoma
- Thymolipoma
- Hemangioma
- Meningocele
- Thoracic Duct Cyst
- Gastroenteric (Neurenteric) Cyst

ESSENTIAL INFORMATION

Key Differential Diagnosis Issues
- Chest radiograph is of limited value in differential diagnosis of mediastinal masses
- Combination of location of mass, demographics, and imaging (CT, MR) may allow confident diagnosis
- Clinical history is key in diagnosing lymphoma, extramedullary hematopoiesis, thymoma (myasthenia gravis), thymic carcinoid (hormone syndrome, e.g., Cushing or MEN)

Helpful Clues for Common Diagnoses
- **Thyroid Goiter**
  - Most commonly in women
  - Right-sided mediastinal mass with contralateral tracheal displacement
  - High attenuation value (> 100 HU) on NECT
- **Thymoma**
  - Well-defined, round or ovoid, anterior mediastinal mass
  - Variable size
  - Homogeneous or heterogeneous
  - Areas of hemorrhage, necrosis, or cyst formation (CT, MR)
  - Punctate, linear, or ring-like calcification (CT)
  - May result in pleural dissemination ("drop metastases")
- **Teratoma**
  - In anterior mediastinum (> 80%)
  - Adipose tissue component is common (> 80%)
  - Heterogeneous appearance on CT and MR
  - CT and MR useful to identify small foci of fat
- **Lymphoma**
  - Non-Hodgkin lymphoma
    - Most frequent lymphoma (> 75%)
    - Large B-cell lymphoma: Young adults (20s and 30s), female predominance
  - Hodgkin lymphoma (nodular sclerosis)
    - Bulky anterior mass (40%)
    - Young adults (20s and 30s)
- **Pericardial Cyst**
  - Usually in cardiophrenic angle
- **Bronchogenic Cyst**
  - Variable origin: Paratracheal, carinal, hilar, paraesophageal, and extramediastinal
  - CT: 50% have high attenuation value (> 130 HU); wall calcification in 10%; rarely, milk of calcium in cyst fluid
- **Neurogenic Tumors**
  - Neurofibroma
    - Paravertebral region or along nerve
    - Low attenuation value (20-25 HU) on NECT
  - Neurilemoma (schwannoma)
    - Paravertebral region or along nerve
    - Adjacent bone changes may be present (50%)
  - Ganglioneuroma
    - Predominantly in infants and children; 60% in patients < 20 years old
    - Low attenuation value on NECT
  - Ganglioneuroblastoma
    - Rare after age 10; oval lesions oriented in vertical axis (sympathetic chain)
    - Variable appearance: Homogeneous solid to cystic masses
  - Paraganglioma
    - Near base of heart and great vessels (adjacent to pericardium)

- Usually bilateral; may be asymmetrical
- **Aortic Aneurysm**
  - Consider aneurysm of any mass contiguous with any part of aorta

Helpful Clues for Less Common Diagnoses

- **Thymic Carcinoma**
  - Most common histologic subtypes: Squamous cell carcinoma and neuroendocrine carcinoma
  - CT and MR: Irregular contour, necrotic or cystic component, heterogeneous contrast enhancement, great vessel invasion
  - Higher maximal standardized uptake values and homogeneous FDG uptake than thymoma
- **Thymic Cyst**
  - Congenital
    - Unilocular; homogeneous water density (0-20 HU) on NECT
    - Wall imperceptible on CT
  - Acquired
    - Multilocular; higher attenuation than water
    - Evident cyst wall on CT
- **Lymphangioma**
  - Usually found in neck or axilla; anterior mediastinum (10%); unilocular or multilocular (30%)
  - May insinuate around normal structures
- **Esophageal Duplication Cyst**
  - Sharply marginated masses in middle or posterior mediastinum
  - CT: Round or tubular water attenuation masses near or within (intramural) esophageal wall

Helpful Clues for Rare Diagnoses

- **Parathyroid Adenoma**
  - Most are very small; appearance similar to that of a lymph node
  - Optimal assessment by Tc-99m sestamibi combined with SPECT
- **Thymolipoma**
  - Entirely asymptomatic
  - May mimic cardiomegaly
  - Positional changes in shape (soft consistency)
- **Hemangioma**
  - Most are asymptomatic
  - Phleboliths visible (10%)
  - Heterogeneous appearance in both NECT and CECT
- **Meningocele**
  - Classic location: Between thoracic inlet and diaphragm
  - Continuity between CSF in thecal sac and meningocele typical
- **Thoracic Duct Cyst**
  - Small round or oval cystic mass in posterior mediastinum
- **Gastroenteric (Neurenteric) Cyst**
  - Diagnosis: Childhood
  - Round or lobulated mass; homogeneously dense
  - Neurenteric: When it is associated with spinal column anomalies (symptomatic)

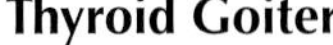

Thyroid Goiter

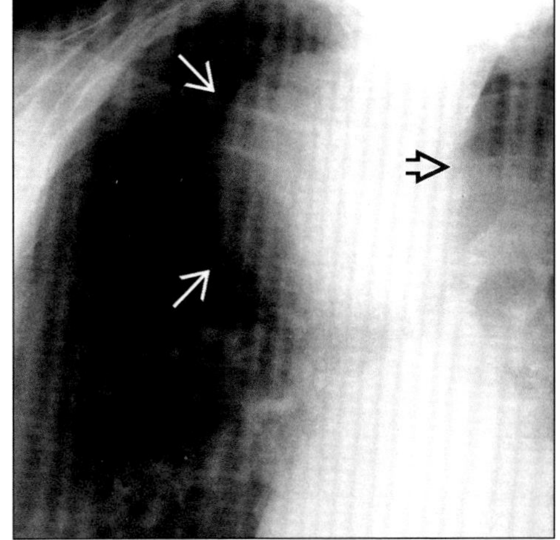

Frontal radiograph shows a large mass in the superior mediastinum ➔ displacing the trachea laterally ➲.

Thyroid Goiter

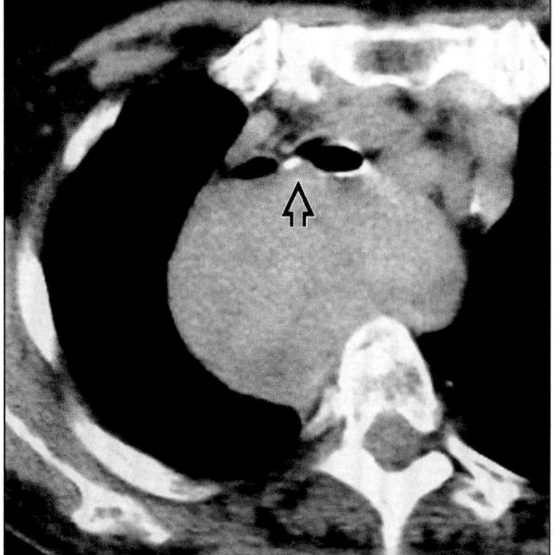

Axial NECT shows a large, homogeneous, middle mediastinal mass displacing the bronchi anteriorly with resulting airway compression ➲.

UNILATERAL MEDIASTINAL MASS

*(**Left**) Sagittal CECT shows a homogeneous anterior solid mediastinal mass ➔ located in the mid-retrosternal region. CT also shows the close relationship of the mass to the aortic arch without associated obliteration of the fat planes ➔. (**Right**) Axial CECT shows heterogeneous thymoma with cyst degeneration and punctate calcifications. Note multiple nodular areas of pleural thickening characteristic of disseminated pleural metastases ("drop metastases") ➔.*

Thymoma

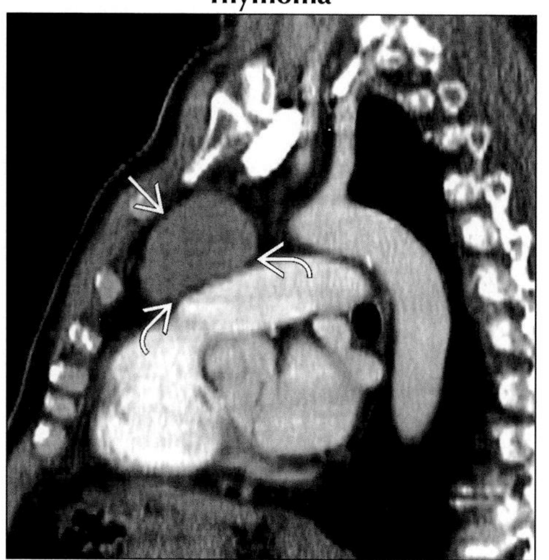

Thymoma

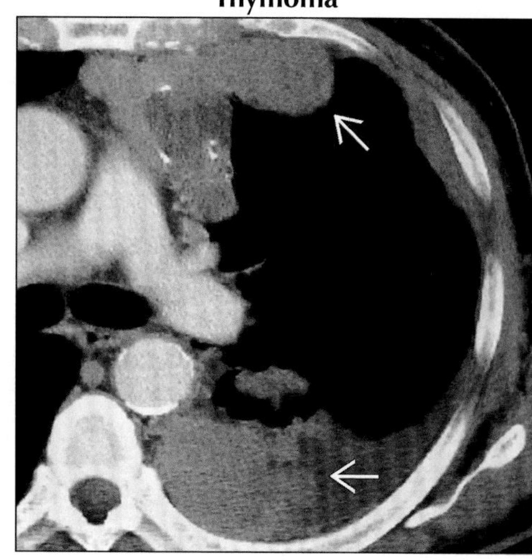

*(**Left**) Sagittal CECT shows a large, hypodense, predominantly cystic mass ➔ involving the anterior mediastinum. Note a solid focal intracystic lesion ➔. Pathology demonstrated a thymoma with an important cystic component. (**Right**) Axial NECT shows large, well-defined, heterogeneous anterior mediastinal mass. Note different tissue components: Soft tissue ➔, calcium ➔, and fat ➔. These findings are characteristic of mature teratoma.*

Thymoma

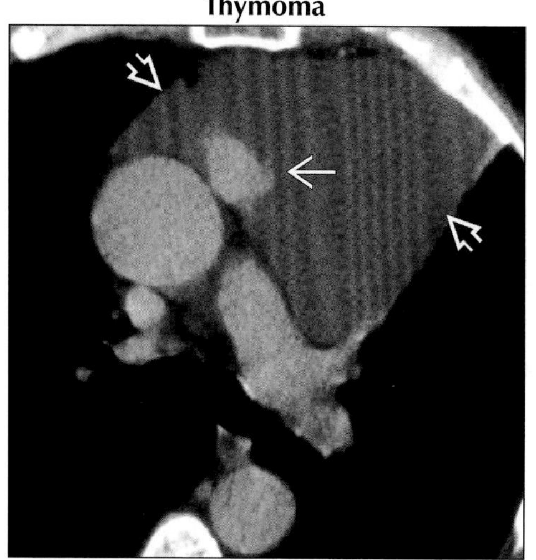

Teratoma

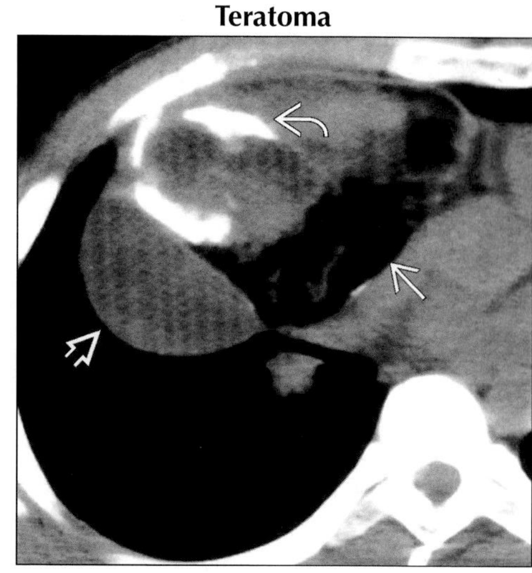

*(**Left**) Axial CECT shows a large, heterogeneous, polylobulated mass situated in the anterior mediastinum. Note that the lesion is composed of different soft tissue densities, including fat ➔ and calcium ➔. Histologically, a mature teratoma was diagnosed. (**Right**) Axial CECT shows a large right paratracheal mass with slightly heterogeneous enhancement. Biopsy confirmed large B-cell lymphoma.*

Teratoma

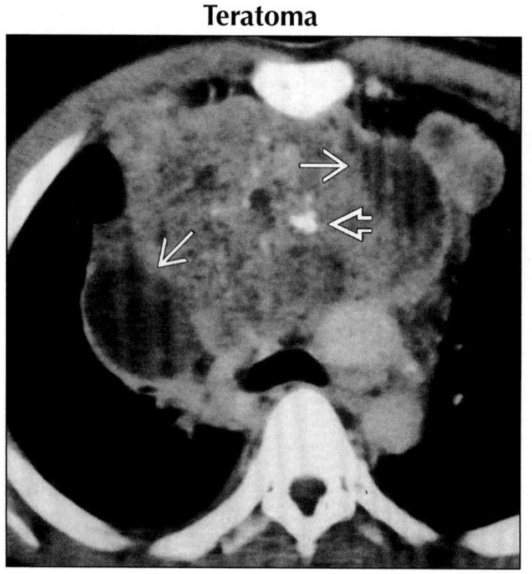

Lymphoma

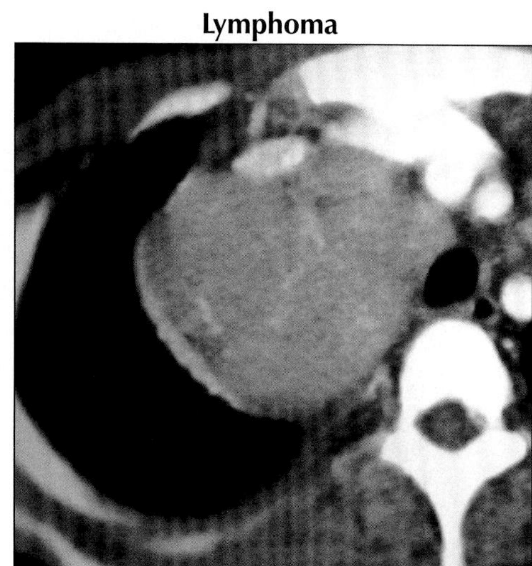

Pericardial Cyst

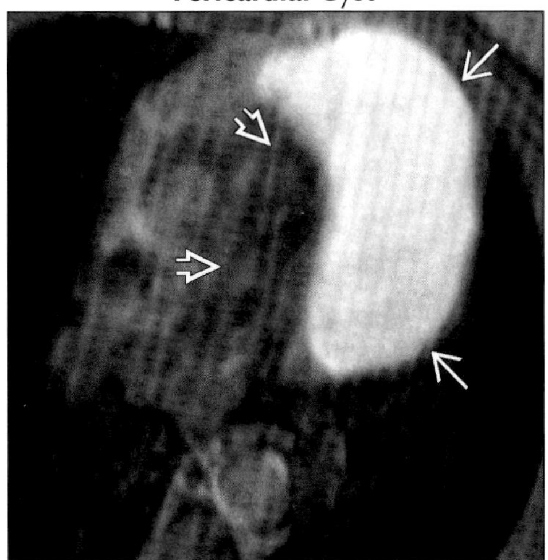

Bronchogenic Cyst

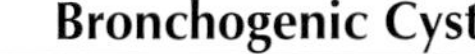

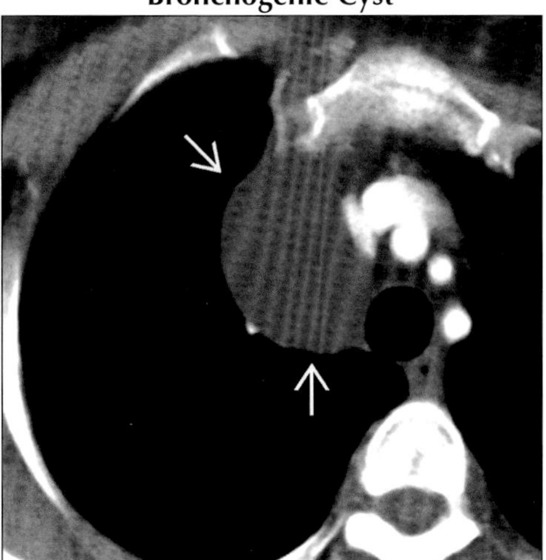

(Left) *Axial T2WI FS MR in a 45-year-old man shows a smoothly marginated large mediastinal mass. The mass has homogeneous increased signal intensity without septations ➔, characteristic of a cystic nature. Note the close relationship of the mass to the main pulmonary artery ➔.* ***(Right)*** *Axial CECT shows a right paratracheal homogeneous fluid-filled mass with an imperceptible wall ➔.*

Neurogenic Tumors

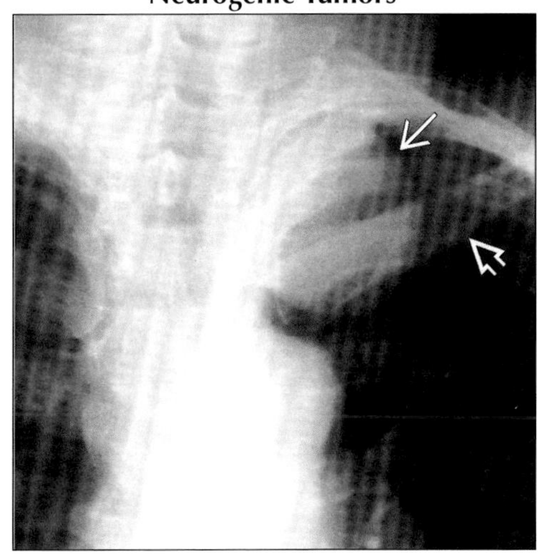

Neurogenic Tumors

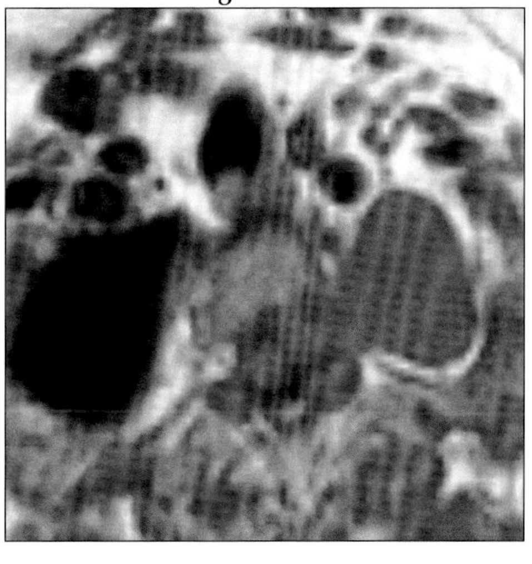

(Left) *Frontal radiograph shows a large well-circumscribed mass ➔ situated in the left superior paramediastinal area. Note that the lesion is clearly visible above the clavicle ➔, confirming an intrathoracic and posterior location. Ganglioneuroma was confirmed at histology.* ***(Right)*** *Axial T1WI MR shows a homogeneous, sharply marginated mass showing dumbbell extension into the spinal canal. This was confirmed as schwannoma at surgery.*

Pleuropericardial Fat Pad

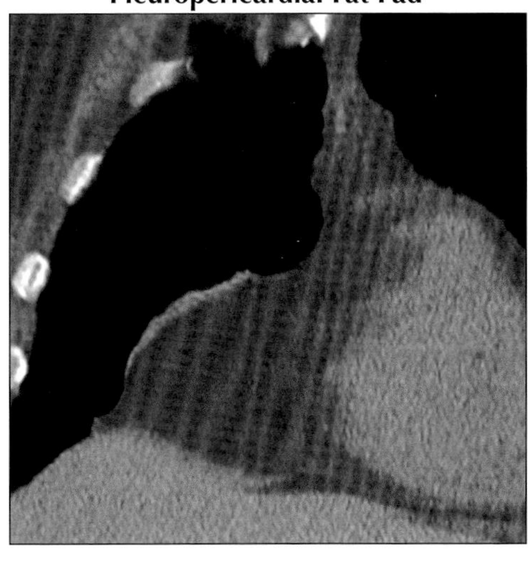

Aortic Aneurysm

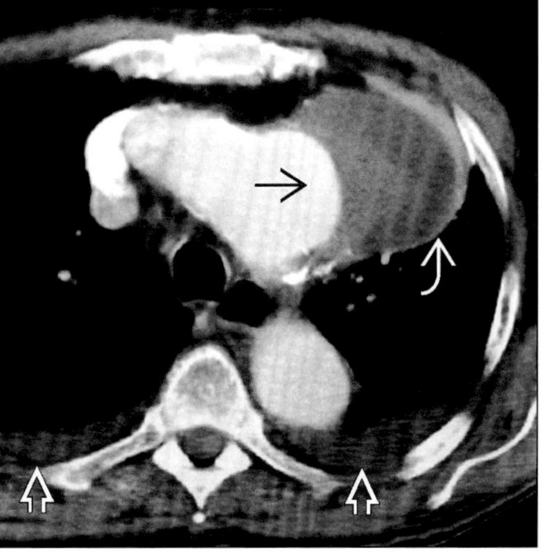

(Left) *Coronal NECT shows abundant homogeneous mediastinal fat at the right cardiophrenic angle without mass effect on cardiac chambers. Absence of vessels is characteristic of excessive fat accumulation, thus excluding intrathoracic omental fat extension (Morgagni hernia).* ***(Right)*** *Axial CECT shows a large aneurysm of the aortic arch → with extensive mural thrombus ➔. Note bilateral small pleural effusion ➔.*

(Left) *Axial CECT shows a large, heterogeneous, necrotic mass. Biopsy demonstrated a thymic carcinoma.* ***(Right)*** *Axial CECT shows a large, well-circumscribed, anterior mediastinal mass with homogeneous water density. The mass compresses and displaces mediastinal vascular structures.*

Thymic Carcinoma

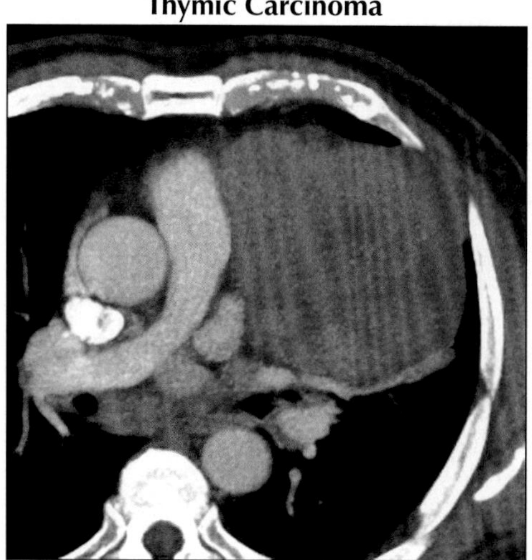

Thymic Cyst

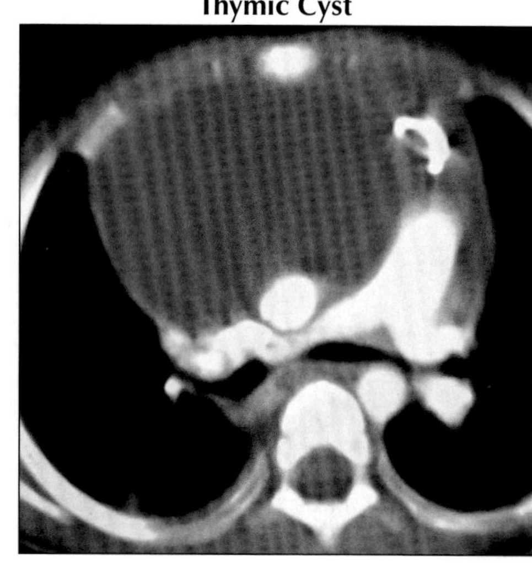

(Left) *Axial T2WI FS MR shows a homogeneous, hyperintense, sharply marginated anterior mediastinal mass. A thymic cyst was proven histologically.* ***(Right)*** *Axial T2WI FS MR shows a homogeneous, hyperintense mediastinal mass. Note the infiltrative component of the tumor → without distortion of adjacent vascular structures. This finding is commonly associated with mediastinal lymphangioma.*

Thymic Cyst

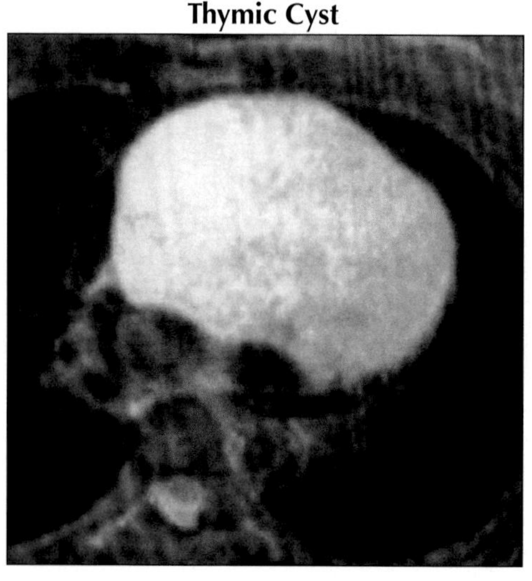

Lymphangioma

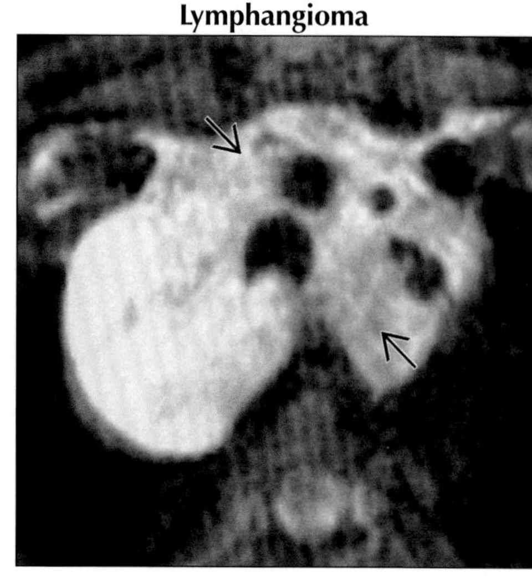

(Left) *Axial CECT shows a homogeneous subcarinal oval cystic mass → adjacent to the esophageal wall ↪.* ***(Right)*** *Axial CECT shows a large well-defined low-density mass → with rim calcification ↪ adjacent to the esophagus ⇒. Calcification is not a common feature associated with esophageal duplication cyst.*

Esophageal Duplication Cyst

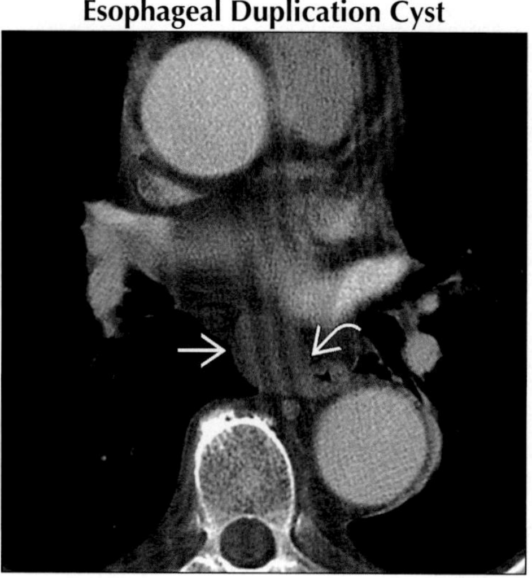

Esophageal Duplication Cyst

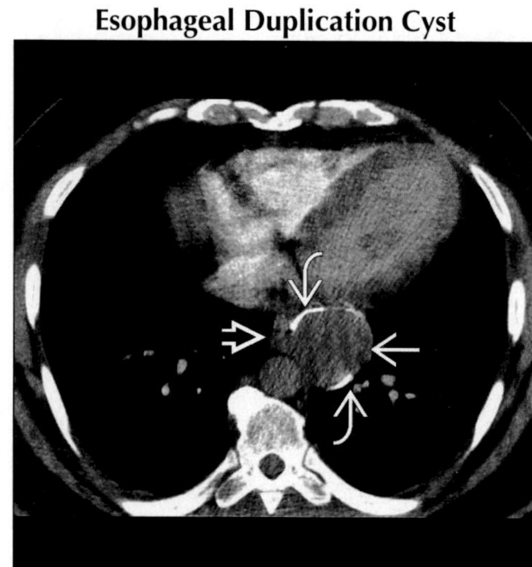

Thymolipoma

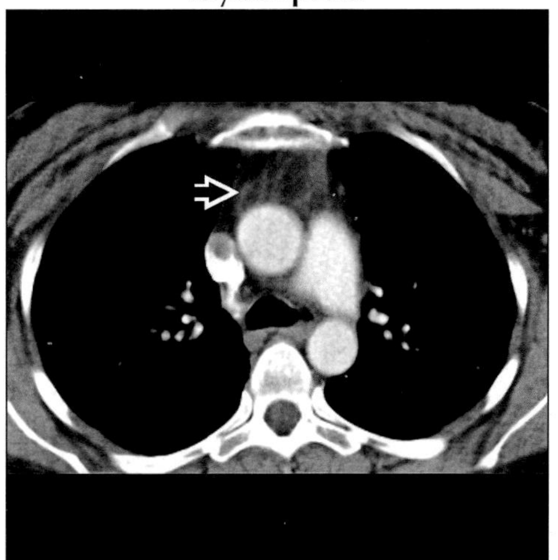

Hemangioma

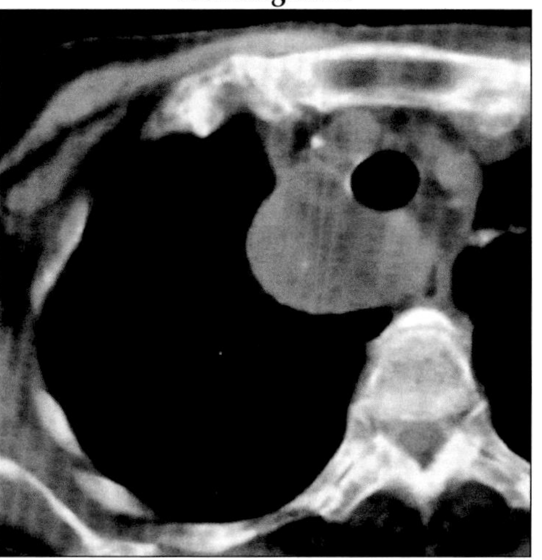

(Left) *Axial CECT shows typical CT features of a predominant fatty anterior mediastinal mass* ➡. ***(Right)*** *Axial NECT shows a well-circumscribed, heterogeneous anterior mediastinal mass. Note punctate calcification (phlebolith) within the mass.*

Hemangioma

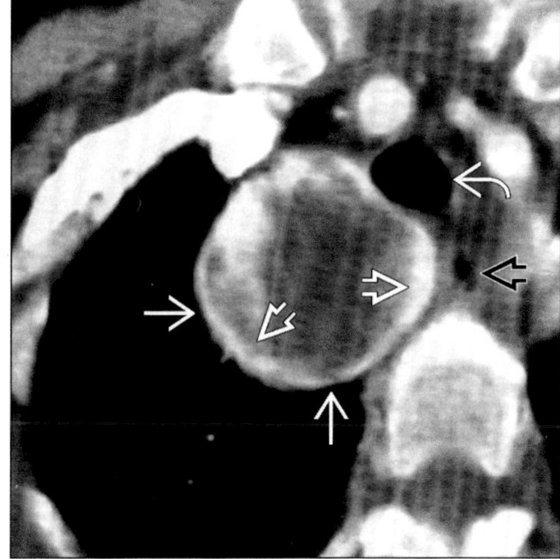

Meningocele

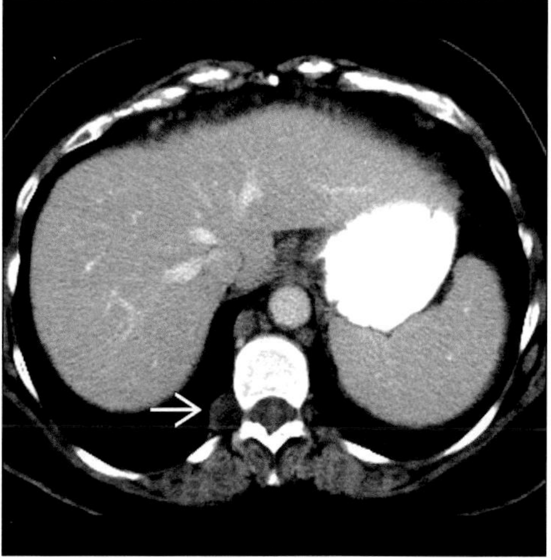

(Left) *Axial CECT shows a well-circumscribed, heterogeneous anterior mediastinal mass* ➡. *The mass lies lateral to the trachea* ↗ *and esophagus* ➡. *After intravenous administration of contrast, the mass shows a peripheral rim enhancement* ➡. ***(Right)*** *Axial CECT shows a well-defined paraspinal tumor* ➡. *The mass has characteristic fluid attenuation features of a small lateral meningocele.*

Meningocele

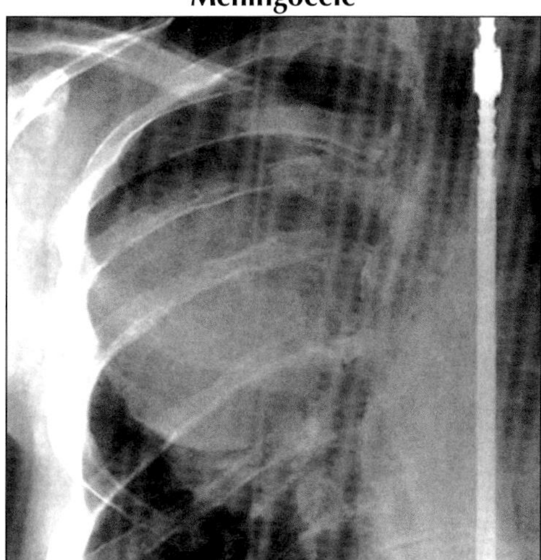

Meningocele

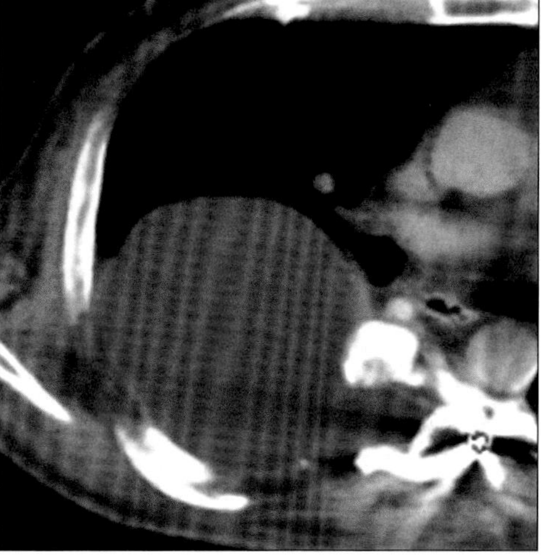

(Left) *Frontal radiograph shows a large rounded mass associated with intercostal space widening and multiple rib erosions. The patient had neurofibromatosis.* ***(Right)*** *Axial CECT shows a large, well-marginated, water attenuation mass arising from spinal canal. Note marked widening of neural foramen. The patient had neurofibromatosis. (Courtesy J. Vilar, MD.)*

BILATERAL MEDIASTINAL MASS

DIFFERENTIAL DIAGNOSIS

Common
- Mediastinal Lipomatosis
- Normal and Hyperplastic Thymus
- Thyroid Goiter
- Lymphoma
- Germ Cell Tumors

Less Common
- Lymphangioma
- Extramedullary Hematopoiesis

Rare but Important
- Liposarcoma

ESSENTIAL INFORMATION

Key Differential Diagnosis Issues
- Most common cause of diffuse mediastinal widening is mediastinal lipomatosis

Helpful Clues for Common Diagnoses
- **Mediastinal Lipomatosis**
  - Large amounts of normal fat; smooth symmetrical mediastinal widening without mass effect
  - Associated with Cushing syndrome, steroid treatment, and obesity
- **Normal and Hyperplastic Thymus**
  - Normal: Generalized thymic enlargement (< 5 years old)
  - Hyperplasia: Immunologic rebound phenomenon
- **Thyroid Goiter**
  - Most common cause of tracheal deviation; anterosuperior or posterosuperior mediastinal mass
- **Lymphoma**
  - Non-Hodgkin lymphoma: Bulky, bilaterally asymmetrical, mediastinal-hilar adenopathy
  - Hodgkin lymphoma: Due to nodal aggregation; rounded or bulky soft tissue masses; prevascular and paratracheal nodes
- **Germ Cell Tumors**
  - Teratoma: Multiple tissue densities
  - Nonseminomatous GCT: Large, irregular-shaped anterior mediastinal mass; pleural effusions and pulmonary metastasis common

Helpful Clues for Less Common Diagnoses
- **Lymphangioma**
  - Unilocular or multilocular (30%); may insinuate around normal structures
  - Low signal intensity on T1WI; high signal intensity on T2WI
- **Extramedullary Hematopoiesis**
  - Compensatory phenomenon due to inadequate production or excessive destruction of blood cells, e.g., sickle cell disease
  - Paravertebral masses: Single or multiple; unilateral or bilateral

Helpful Clues for Rare Diagnoses
- **Liposarcoma**
  - Rare malignant mediastinal tumor

Mediastinal Lipomatosis

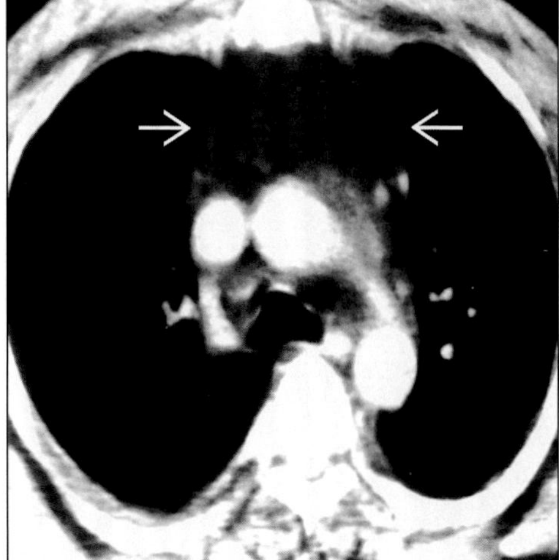

Axial CECT shows abundant homogeneous mediastinal fat that displaces the anterior junction line laterally ➡ without mass effect on adjacent vascular structures.

Thyroid Goiter

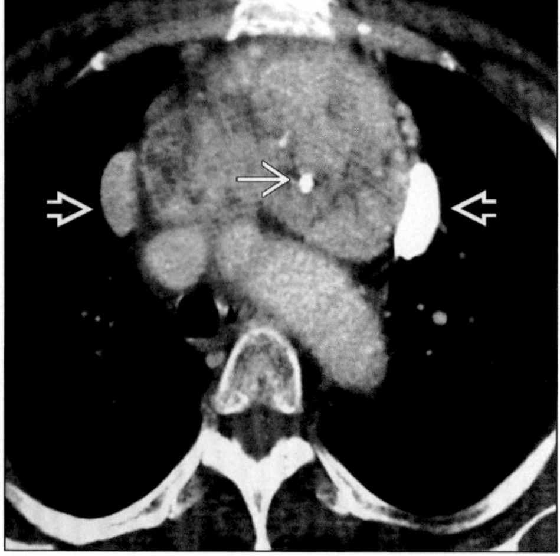

Axial CECT shows a sharply demarcated heterogeneous mediastinal mass that extended from the thyroid bed. The mass contains punctate calcification ➡ and displaces adjacent vascular structures ⇨.

Lymphoma

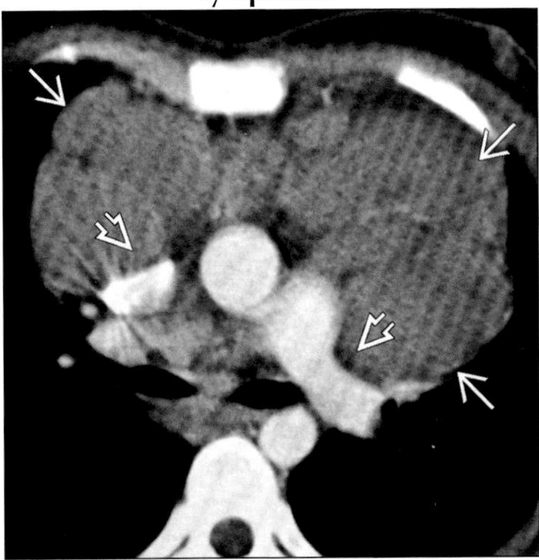

Germ Cell Tumors

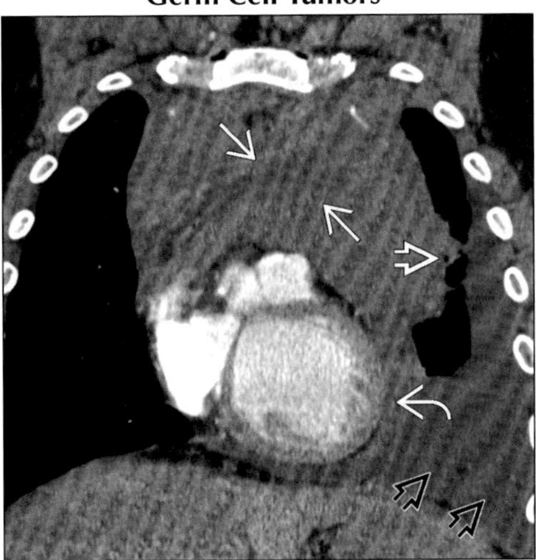

*(**Left**) Axial CECT shows nonenhancing anterior mediastinal lymphadenopathies ➔. Vascular structures are posteriorly displaced ➔. The diagnosis was non-Hodgkin lymphoma. (**Right**) Coronal CECT shows a large anterior mediastinal mass with inhomogeneous attenuation ➔ and poorly defined left margins ➔. Notice the left pleural effusion ➔ and pericardial involvement ➔ in this patient with malignant nonseminomatous germ cell tumor.*

Lymphangioma

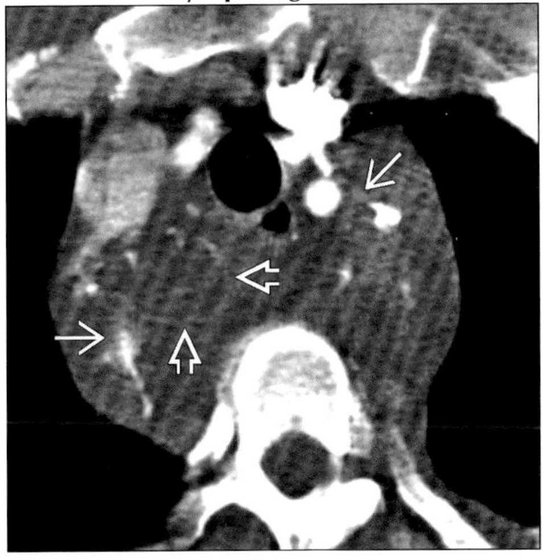

Liposarcoma

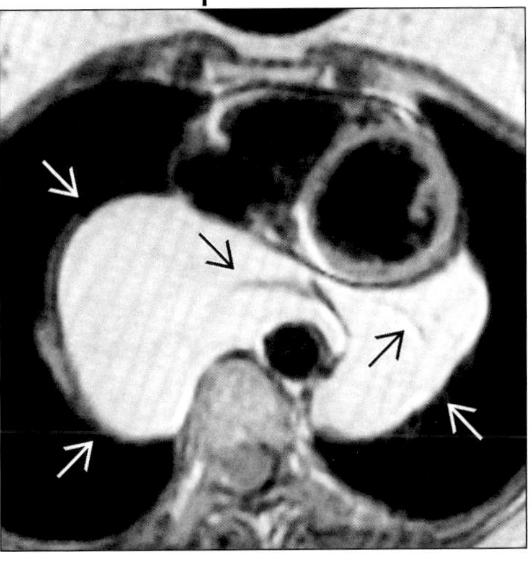

*(**Left**) Axial CECT shows an extremely large, low-attenuation, cystic-appearing mass infiltrating and displacing mediastinal vessels ➔. The mass contains few soft tissue septations ➔. (**Right**) Axial T1WI MR shows a liposarcoma, appearing as a dumbbell-shaped, high signal retrocardiac mass ➔. The mass contains fine septations ➔.*

Extramedullary Hematopoiesis

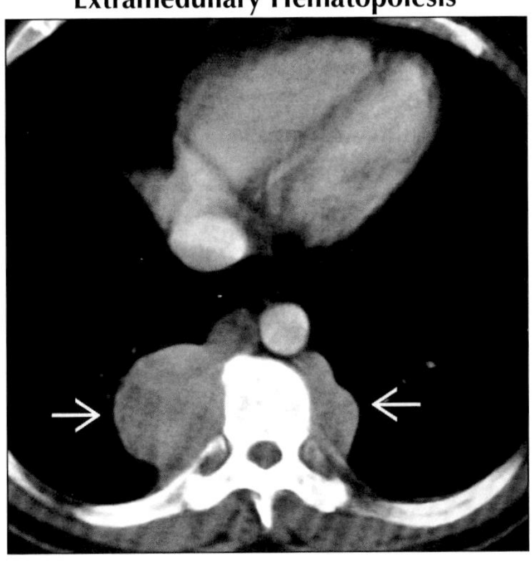

Extramedullary Hematopoiesis

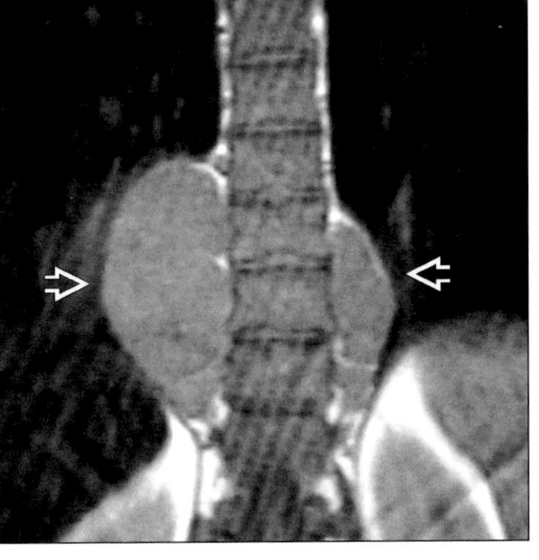

*(**Left**) Axial CECT from a patient with sickle cell disease shows bilateral lower thoracic paraspinal masses with mild variable contrast enhancement ➔. No bony erosions are seen, and the neural foramina were normal. (**Right**) Coronal T1WI MR in the same patient shows bilateral paraspinal hypointense lobulated masses ➔.*

AIR-CONTAINING MEDIASTINAL MASS

DIFFERENTIAL DIAGNOSIS

Common
- Hiatal Hernia
- Esophageal Diverticulum
- Zenker Diverticulum

Less Common
- Achalasia
- Esophageal Perforation
- Mediastinal Abscess

Rare but Important
- Bronchogenic Cyst
- Loculated Pneumomediastinum

ESSENTIAL INFORMATION

Key Differential Diagnosis Issues
- Location of air is key
  - Retrocardiac mass with air or air-fluid level is characteristic of esophageal hiatus hernia
  - Superior mediastinal air-fluid level often Zenker diverticulum
  - Bronchogenic cyst usually subcarinal

Helpful Clues for Common Diagnoses
- **Hiatal Hernia**
  - ± air-fluid level
- **Esophageal Diverticulum**
  - Air-fluid level in mid-esophagus (traction) or in epiphrenic region (pulsion)
- **Zenker Diverticulum**
  - Air-fluid level in superior mediastinum (pharyngoesophageal junction)
  - Complications: Aspiration pneumonia and bronchiolitis

Helpful Clues for Less Common Diagnoses
- **Achalasia**
  - Esophageal dilatation with air-fluid level
- **Esophageal Perforation**
  - Penetrating trauma (90%): Iatrogenic following endoscopic procedures, postsurgical and ingested foreign bodies (e.g., bones)
  - Spontaneous: Boerhaave syndrome (esophageal rupture after emesis)
  - Radiographic findings: Pneumomediastinum and subcutaneous emphysema in soft tissues of neck
  - NECT: Gas collections centered around esophagus (90%)
- **Mediastinal Abscess**
  - Usually secondary to erosion from esophageal carcinoma
  - Following cardiac or esophageal surgery

Helpful Clues for Rare Diagnoses
- **Bronchogenic Cyst**
  - Spontaneous cyst ruptures into airways, esophagus, pleural cavity, and pericardial cavity
    - Radiograph & CT: Large subcarinal cyst with air-fluid level (rupture)
- **Loculated Pneumomediastinum**
  - In neonates, air in mediastinum often loculates locally; tends not to dissect widely as in adults

Hiatal Hernia

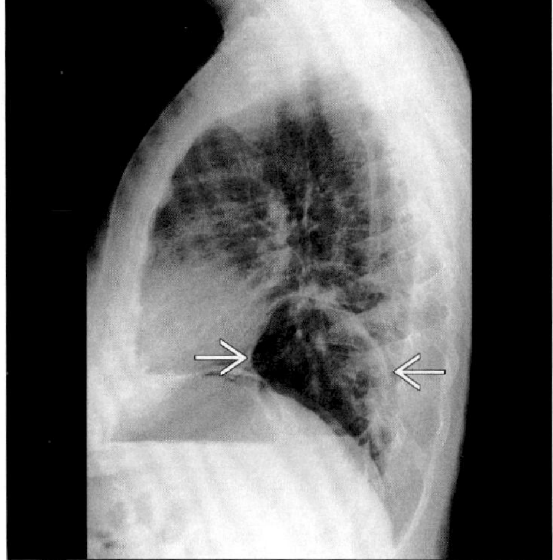

Lateral radiograph shows an abnormal, thin-walled, air-filled mass ➡ in the retrocardiac space, representing the stomach herniating through a diaphragmatic defect.

Esophageal Diverticulum

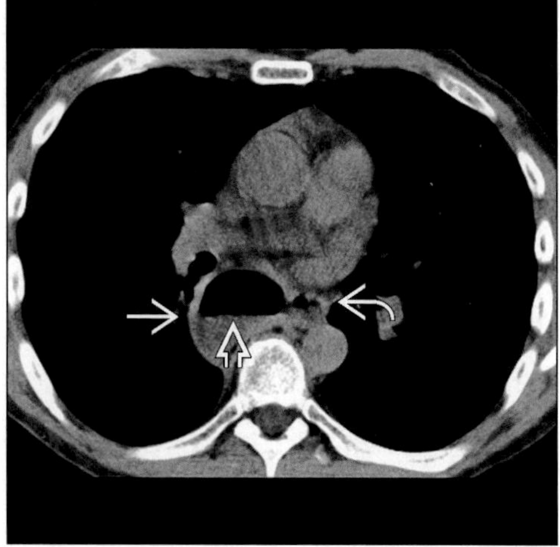

Axial NECT shows esophageal diverticulum ➡ with a visible air-fluid level ⇨. Adjacent esophagus is also seen ↪. This is consistent with a pulsion esophageal diverticulum.

Zenker Diverticulum

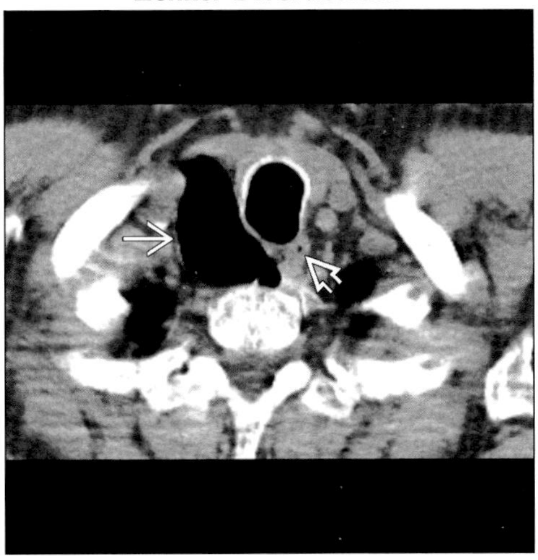

Achalasia

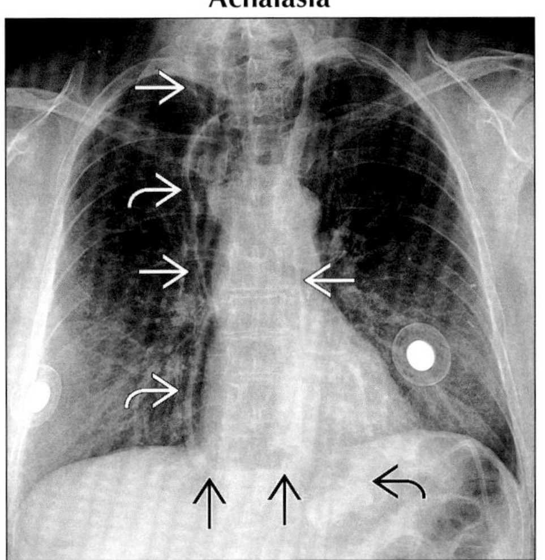

*(**Left**) Axial NECT shows thin-walled, air-filled right paratracheal mass ➔ adjacent to esophagus ➔, which is displaced to the left. (**Right**) Frontal radiograph shows a thin-walled, air-filled esophageal dilatation ➔. Dilated aperistaltic esophagus is projected to the right side of the mediastinum ➔. An air-fluid level is also visible ➔, and an absent gastric air bubble is confirmed ➔.*

Achalasia

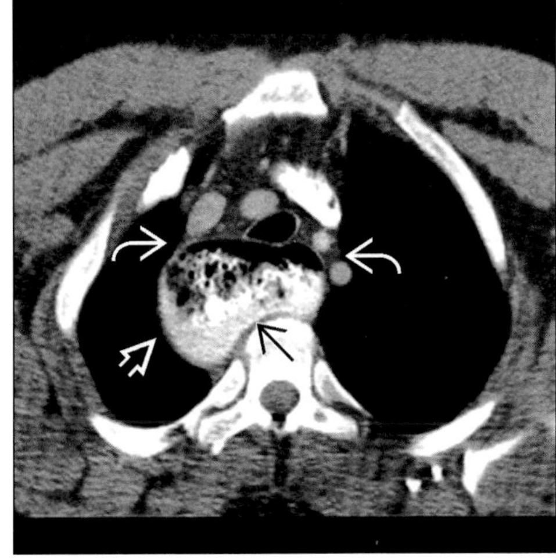

Esophageal Perforation

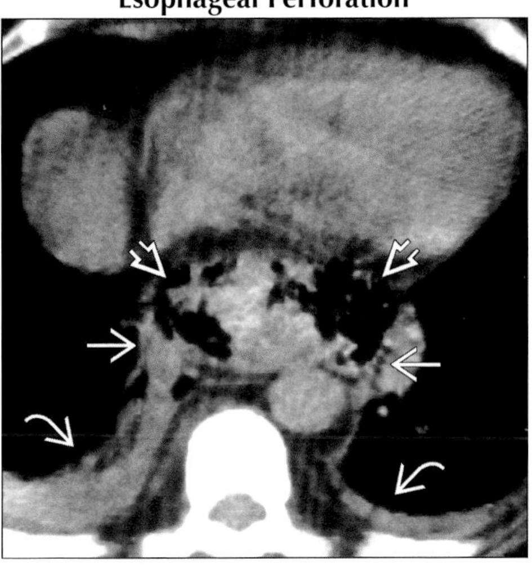

*(**Left**) Axial CECT shows dilated esophagus ➔ containing debris. Mediastinal widening is present ➔, and the dilated esophagus projects to the right side of the mediastinum ➔. (**Right**) Axial NECT in a 58-year-old man with burning substernal pain shows periesophageal soft tissue infiltration ➔, extraluminal gas ➔, and bilateral pleural effusion ➔. The diagnosis was mediastinal abscess due to perforation of the esophagus (Boerhaave syndrome).*

Mediastinal Abscess

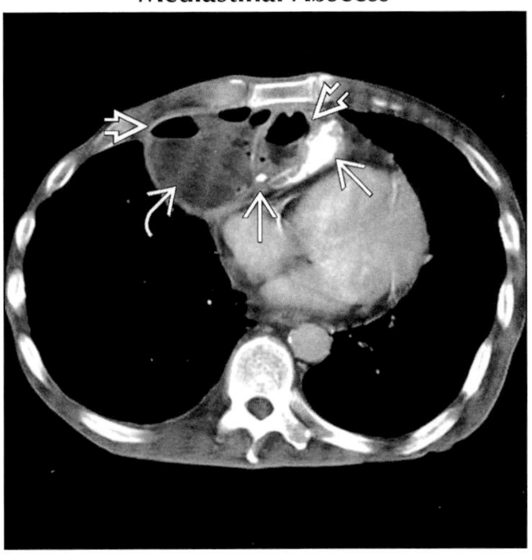

Loculated Pneumomediastinum

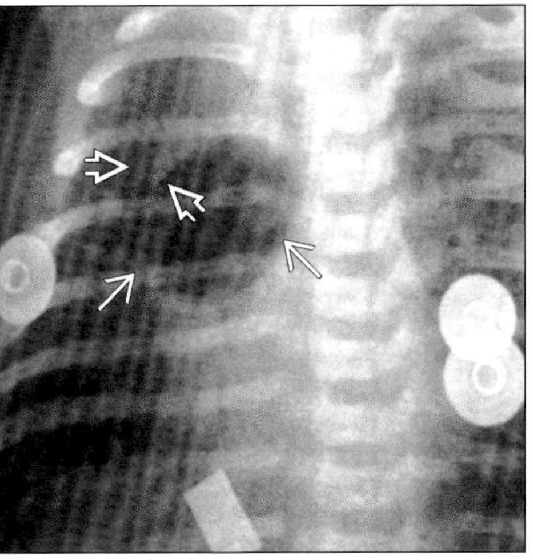

*(**Left**) Axial CECT shows a large heterogeneous mass containing high- ➔ and low-attenuation ➔ areas. Note multiple air-fluid levels ➔. The diagnosis was mediastinal abscess from gossypiboma. (Courtesy C. White, MD.) (**Right**) Frontal radiograph shows a rounded area of lucency, representing loculated air within mediastinum ➔. Air is located over the thymic area. If there is sufficient air, the thymus can become elevated to produce thymic sail sign ➔.*

CYSTIC MEDIASTINAL MASS

DIFFERENTIAL DIAGNOSIS

Common

- Bronchogenic Cyst
- Thyroid Goiter
- Pericardial Cyst

Less Common

- Necrotic Lymph Nodes
- Necrotic or Cystic Neoplasms

Rare but Important

- Other Foregut Duplication Cysts
- Lymphangioma
- Pseudocyst from Pancreatitis
- Mediastinal Abscess
- Lateral Meningocele
- Thymic Cyst

ESSENTIAL INFORMATION

Key Differential Diagnosis Issues

- Key diagnostic feature is location and clinical presentation
- 10% of mediastinal masses in adults and children are cysts
- Most mediastinal cysts are congenital in origin

Helpful Clues for Common Diagnoses

- **Bronchogenic Cyst**
  - Most common foregut duplication cyst
  - Occur in middle or posterior mediastinum
  - Paratracheal or subcarinal in location
  - Round and smooth in contour
  - Wall typically thin or imperceptible
  - Water to soft tissue density
  - Radiograph shows
    - Smooth and sharply marginated round mass
    - May displace bronchi or trachea
    - Rarely cause collapse of a lobe secondary to mass effect on bronchi
  - Distinguish from soft tissue neoplasm by
    - Lack of enhancement
    - Characterization by MR
  - May abruptly increase in size secondary to hemorrhage or infection
  - MR shows
    - High T1 signal secondary to proteinaceous content
    - High T2 signal in nearly all cases
- **Thyroid Goiter**
  - 10% of mediastinal masses
  - Radiograph shows
    - Leftward tracheal deviation
    - Mass in superior mediastinum
  - Noncontrast CT shows
    - High-attenuation cystic or heterogeneous lesion
    - Connection to thyroid on sequential images
    - Coronal images are key to demonstrate connection
  - Factors that suggest thyroid malignancy
    - Lymphadenopathy or metastases
    - Invasion of adjacent structures
- **Pericardial Cyst**
  - Smooth and well marginated
  - Most contact diaphragm
  - Majority right-sided and asymptomatic
  - Low Hounsfield units by CT
  - Single layer of mesothelial cells

Helpful Clues for Less Common Diagnoses

- **Necrotic Lymph Nodes**
  - Rim-enhancing lymph node with central low density indicating necrosis
  - Infectious causes include tuberculosis and histoplasmosis
  - Malignant causes include lymphoma or lung cancer
  - Extrathoracic malignancies, such as head and neck carcinoma, seminoma, or gastric carcinoma
- **Necrotic or Cystic Neoplasms**
  - Germ cell tumors (teratoma, seminomas, and nonseminomatous tumors)
    - Teratomas are anterior mediastinal, well defined, cystic in appearance, ± fat and calcification
    - Seminomas are anterior mediastinal, homogeneous in density, ± low-attenuation areas, in younger men
    - Nonseminomas are anterior mediastinal, heterogeneous with areas of necrosis or cystic areas
  - Large thymomas or thymic carcinomas
    - Anterior mediastinal mass
    - May have cystic or necrotic centers
    - So-called "drop metastases" to pleura may be seen
    - Thymic carcinoma invades great vessels and mediastinal structures in 40%

- Thymic carcinoma may demonstrate hematogenous metastases

Helpful Clues for Rare Diagnoses

- **Other Foregut Duplication Cysts**
  - Esophageal duplication cyst
    - Similar appearance to bronchogenic cyst
    - Occur within esophageal wall or contact esophagus
    - Lined by gastrointestinal mucosa
  - Neurenteric cyst
    - Posterior mediastinal mass
    - Connection to meninges through a vertebral defect
    - Vertebral anomalies include scoliosis or hemivertebrae
    - Identical appearance to other duplication cysts
    - Composed of neural and gastrointestinal components
- **Lymphangioma**
  - Most common in childhood; extend down from neck
  - Commonly localized to mediastinum in adults
  - Unilocular or multilocular ± thin septations
  - May drape over structures and can grow to large size
  - MR demonstrates heterogeneously increased T2 signal
- **Pseudocyst from Pancreatitis**
  - Located in lower mediastinum with access via esophageal or aortic hiatus
  - Clinical history of pancreatitis ± lesion tracking from abdomen
- **Mediastinal Abscess**
  - Recent history of median sternotomy, esophageal perforation, or head and neck infection
  - Typical rim-enhancing lesion with central low density
  - May demonstrate air bubbles with communication to adjacent infection
  - Difficult to differentiate from postoperative hematoma/seroma
    - May require needle aspiration
    - Postoperative hematoma/seroma should resolve after 2-3 weeks
- **Lateral Meningocele**
  - Strong association with neurofibromatosis type 1 or connective tissue disorders
  - Posterior mediastinal cystic mass with extension into spinal canal
  - Associated scoliosis and interpediculate widening
  - MR or myelogram are diagnostic by showing connection to spinal canal
- **Thymic Cyst**
  - Usually incidental; may be unilocular or multilocular
  - Thin walls
  - Congenital or acquired secondary to radiotherapy after Hodgkin disease
  - Fluid density
  - Occasionally may contain fat or hemorrhage

Bronchogenic Cyst

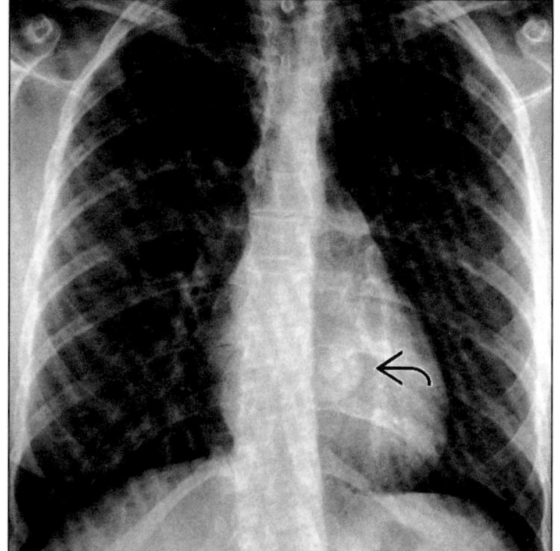

Frontal radiograph shows a round retrocardiac opacity obscuring a portion of the descending aorta ➙. Differential considerations would include lymphadenopathy.

Bronchogenic Cyst

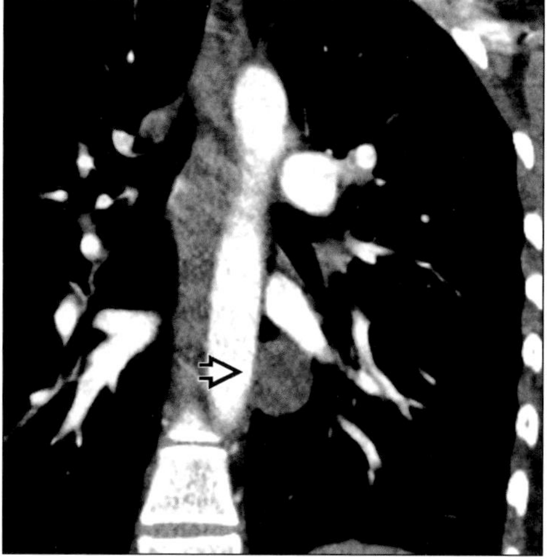

Coronal CECT shows a round lesion of fluid attenuation abutting the descending aorta ➙. The most common location for this lesion is in the subcarinal space.

CYSTIC MEDIASTINAL MASS

(Left) Esophagram shows external mass effect on the anterior esophagus ➔. The underlying mucosa is intact indicating this is an external process. Cross-sectional imaging would need to be performed for further characterization. (Right) Coronal CECT shows a well-circumscribed, low-attenuation mass ➔ causing compression of the left mainstem bronchus (not shown) with complete collapse of the left lung ➔. Note the reduced volume of left hemithorax.

Bronchogenic Cyst

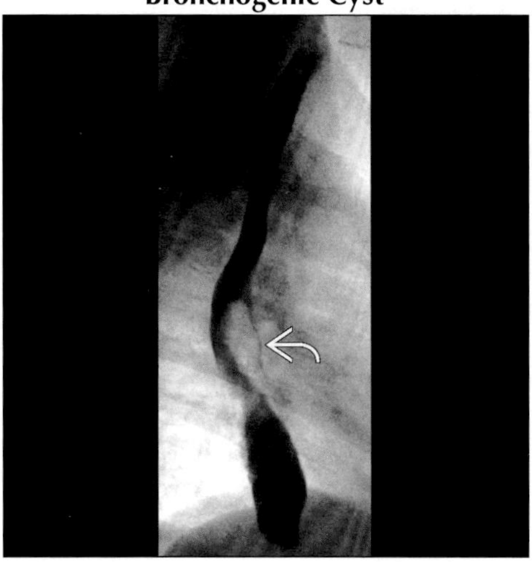

Bronchogenic Cyst

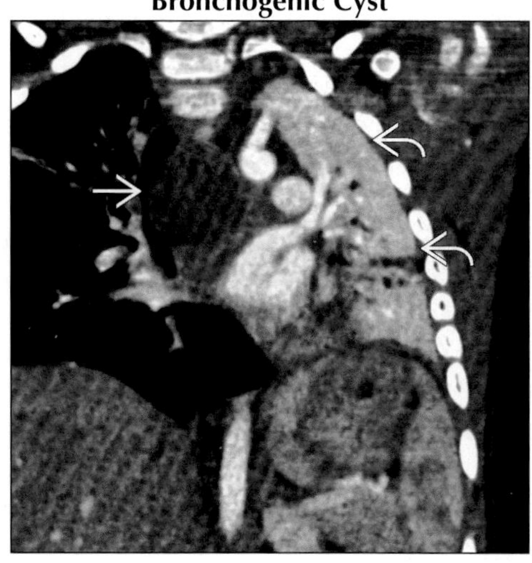

(Left) Frontal radiograph shows a large right paratracheal mass ➔. The trachea is deviated to the left ➔ and partially compressed. This is the most common appearance of an intrathoracic thyroid goiter. (Right) Axial NECT shows an enlarged, somewhat necrotic/cystic-appearing thyroid goiter ➔ descending into the right paratracheal space. Deviation of the trachea ➔ and esophagus ➔ are noted.

Thyroid Goiter

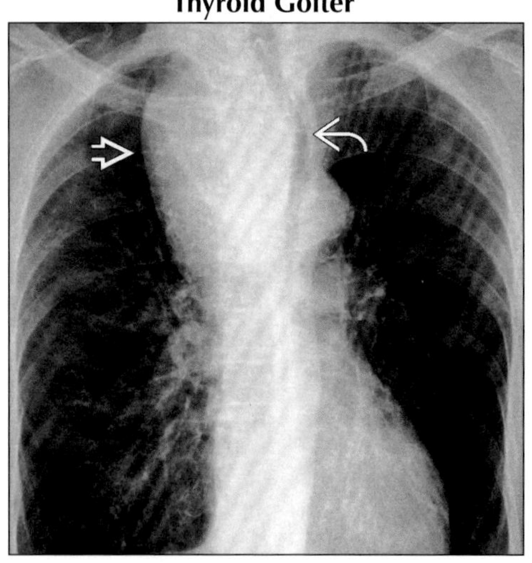

Thyroid Goiter

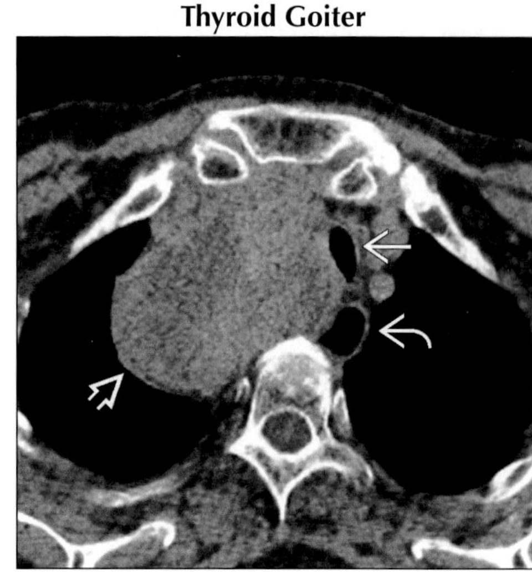

(Left) Frontal radiograph shows an oval mass ➔ in the cardiophrenic angle. Differential considerations would also include lymphadenopathy, a hernia, and a prominent pericardial fat pad. (Right) Axial CECT shows a well-circumscribed oval mass of fluid attenuation in the cardiophrenic angle ➔. No enhancement was noted on this post-contrast examination, an important differential point in making this diagnosis.

Pericardial Cyst

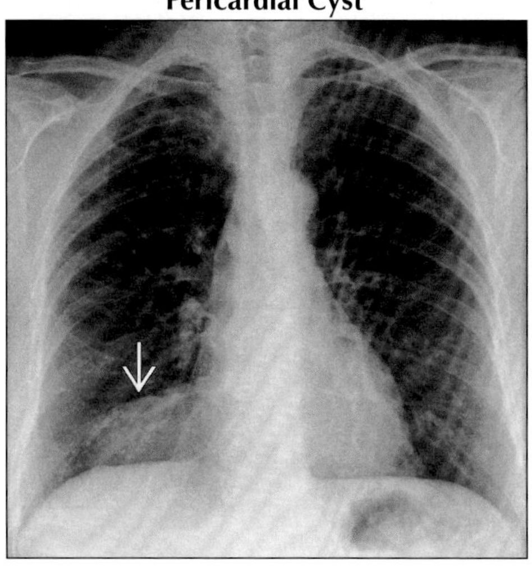

Pericardial Cyst

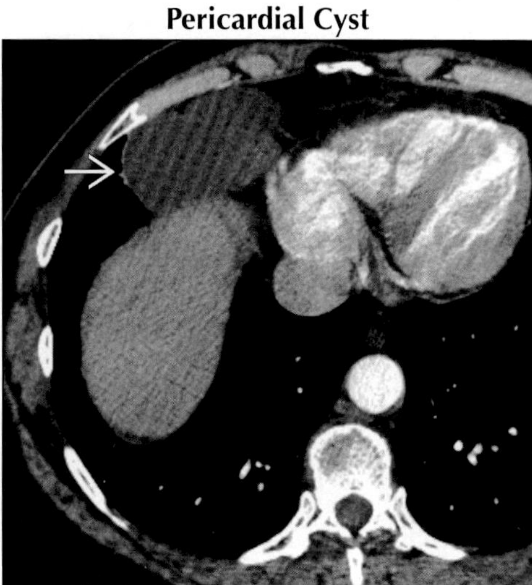

Necrotic Lymph Nodes

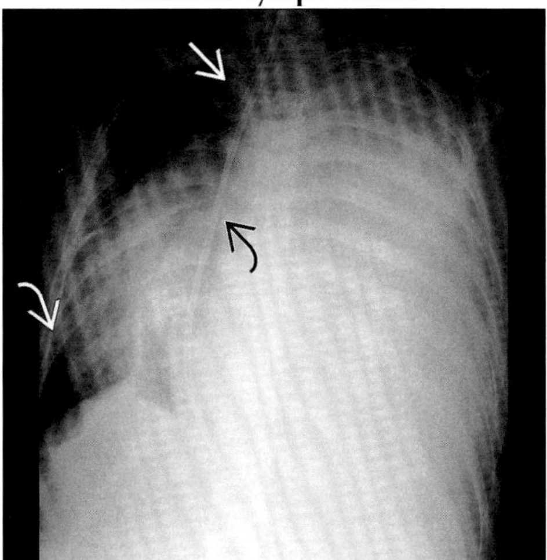

Necrotic Lymph Nodes

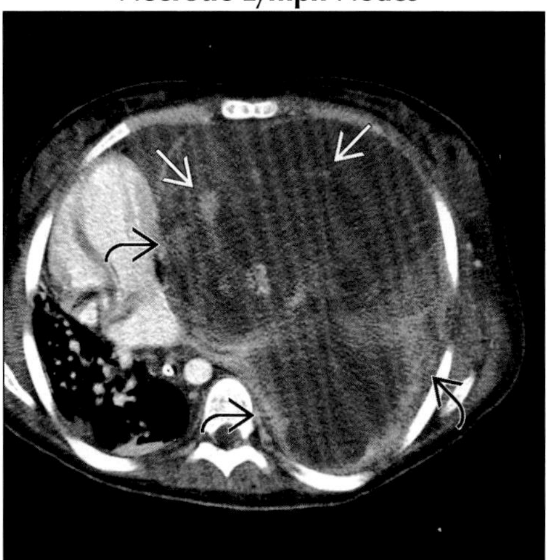

(Left) *Frontal radiograph shows left hemithorax opacification with rightward mediastinal shift. Note displacement of the heart, endotracheal tube, and enteric tube.* ***(Right)*** *Axial CECT shows a large heterogeneous mass with cystic and enhancing vascular components. There is extensive rightward mediastinal shift and complete left lung collapse in this patient with metastatic synovial cell sarcoma.*

Necrotic Lymph Nodes

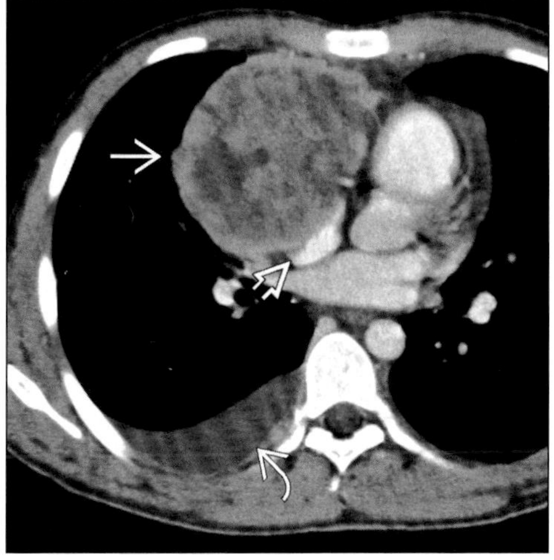

Necrotic Lymph Nodes

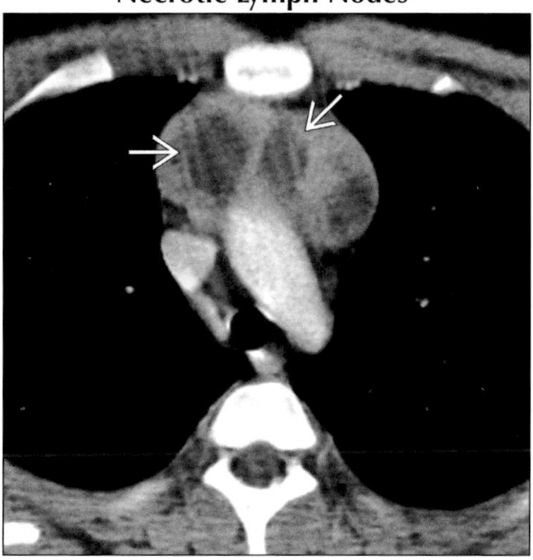

(Left) *Axial CECT shows a heterogeneously mixed cystic and solid mass in the anterior mediastinum. Note the compression of the right atrium and right-sided pleural effusion in this patient with lymphoblastic lymphoma.* ***(Right)*** *Axial CECT shows an anterior mediastinal mass with multiple low-density central areas in this patient with Hodgkin lymphoma involving the thymus.*

Necrotic Lymph Nodes

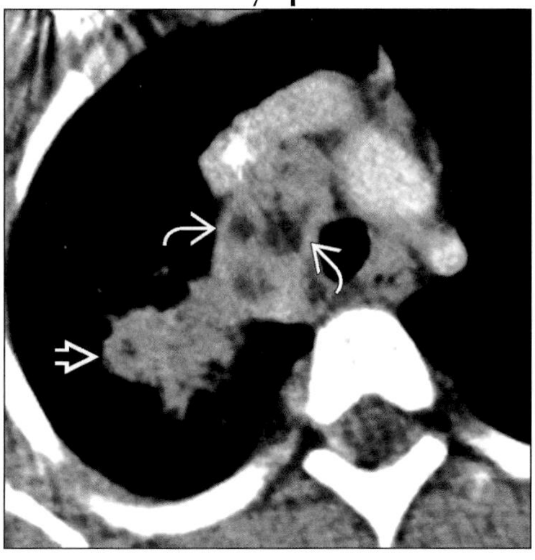

Necrotic or Cystic Neoplasms

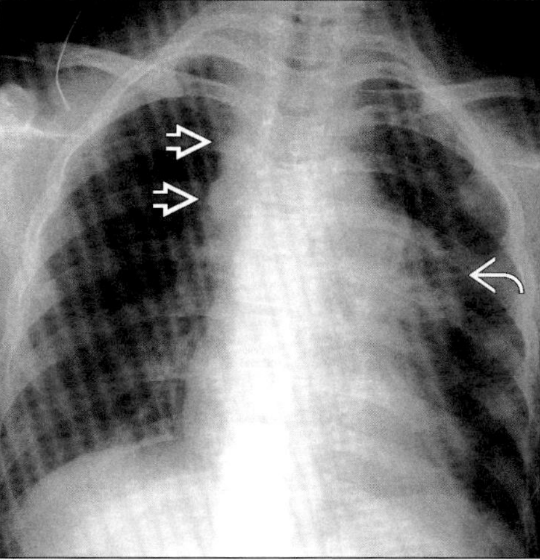

(Left) *Axial CECT shows right upper lobe lobulated consolidation. There are multiple coalescent lymph nodes in the right paratracheal area with low-density centers in this patient with tuberculosis.* ***(Right)*** *Frontal radiograph shows lobulated widening of the right paratracheal stripe. In addition, note a large left mediastinal mass.*

CYSTIC MEDIASTINAL MASS

*(**Left**) Axial CECT shows a heterogeneous anterior mediastinal cystic, calcified →, and solid lesion →. There is thrombosis and expansion of the superior vena cava secondary to tumor invasion →. Note the hematogenous lung metastasis → in this patient with thymic carcinoma. (**Right**) Frontal radiograph shows a large right-sided mass with leftward displacement of the heart and mediastinum. Note large right pleural effusion → in this yolk sac tumor.*

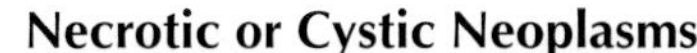

Necrotic or Cystic Neoplasms

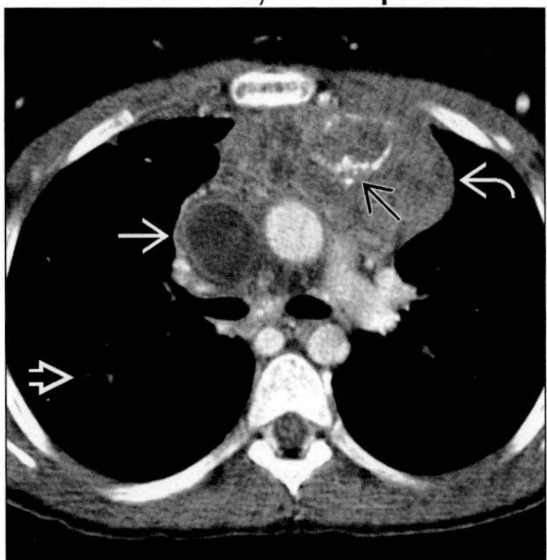

Necrotic or Cystic Neoplasms

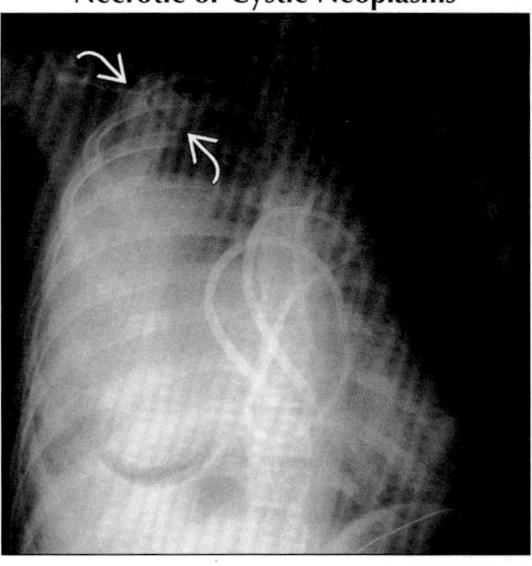

*(**Left**) Axial CECT shows a large predominantly cystic lesion → in the mediastinum with leftward mass effect on the right atrium and heart → in this patient with yolk sac tumor. (**Right**) Axial CECT shows an esophagus → and fluid-filled paraesophageal mass → in this esophageal duplication cyst. Connection to the esophagus is an important point in suggesting this diagnosis. Bronchogenic cyst could have a similar appearance.*

Necrotic or Cystic Neoplasms

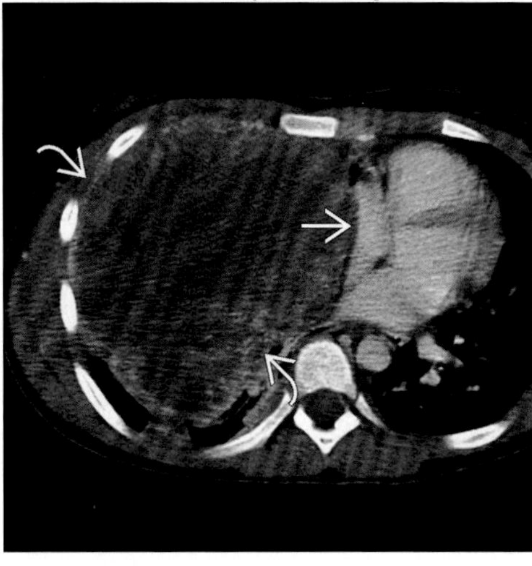

Other Foregut Duplication Cysts

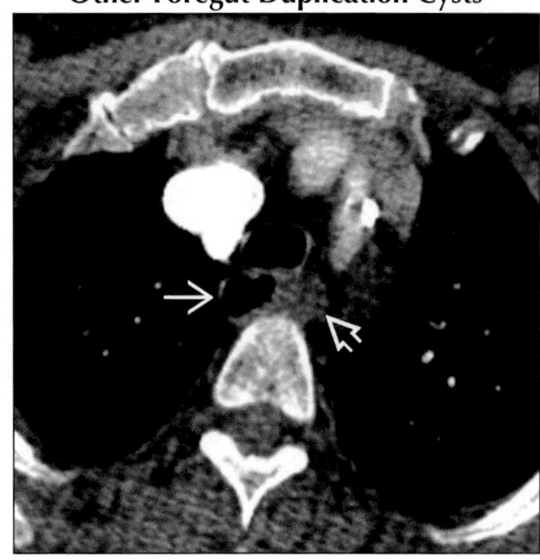

*(**Left**) Axial CECT shows a multiloculated cystic lesion located adjacent to the heart with no superior connection to the neck. The thick septations → are explained by superinfection. (**Right**) Axial STIR MR in the same patient reveals a predominantly cystic lesion adjacent to the heart with thick septations →. Note the extension along the lateral left chest wall →.*

Lymphangioma

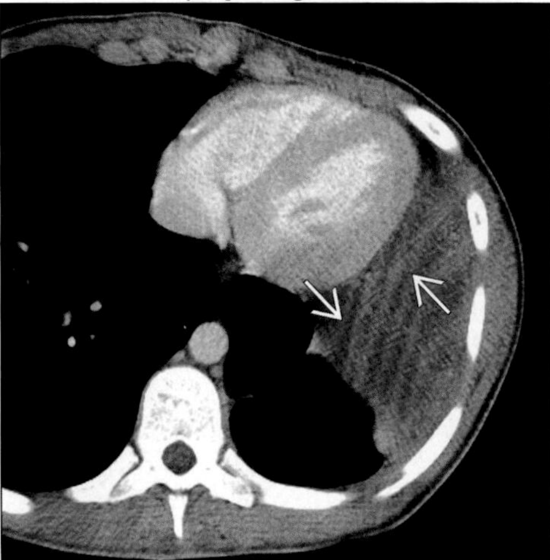

Lymphangioma

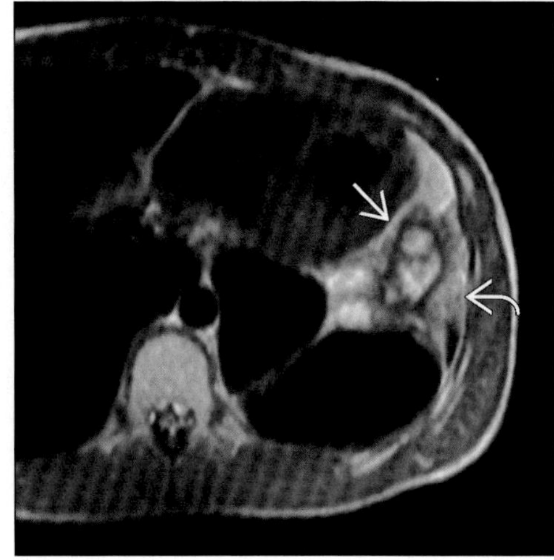

Pseudocyst from Pancreatitis

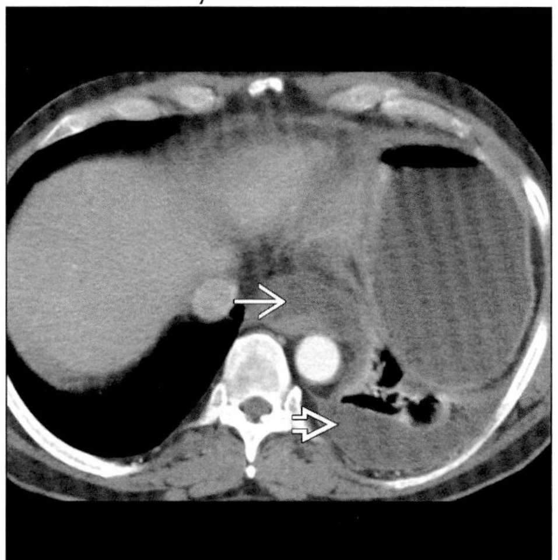

Pseudocyst from Pancreatitis

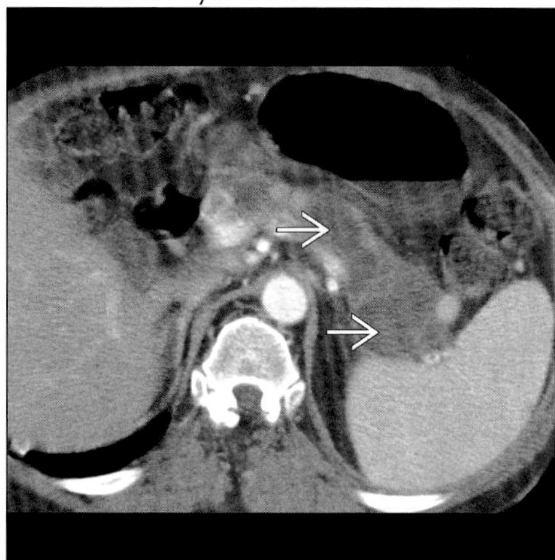

(Left) *Axial CECT demonstrates fluid-density cysts surrounding the aorta ➡. Note left pleural effusion ⇨. Lower sections revealed a peripancreatic cyst, and the patient had a remote history of severe pancreatitis. The pseudocyst resolved on follow-up imaging.* ***(Right)*** *Axial CECT shows pseudocysts within the pancreas ➡, which on sequential images communicated with the mediastinal fluid collections.*

Mediastinal Abscess

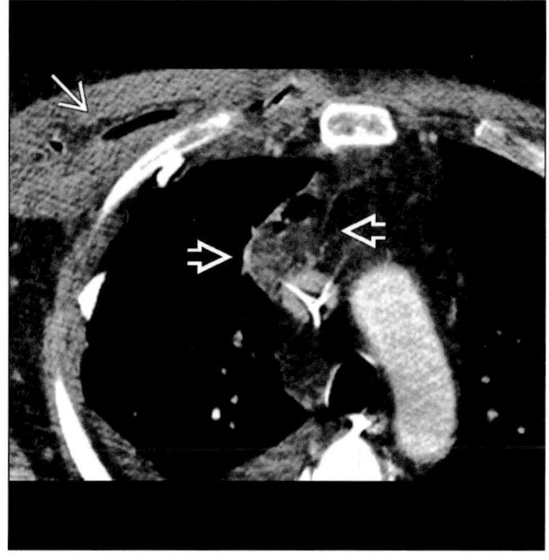

Lateral Meningocele

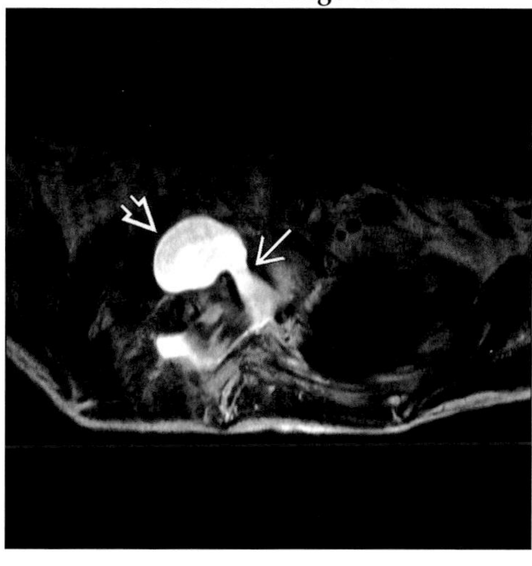

(Left) *Axial CECT shows enhancing air- and fluid-containing abscess within the anterior mediastinum ⇨. Note the abscess from source infection within the right pectoralis major muscle ➡.* ***(Right)*** *Axial T2WI FS MR shows a cystic lesion ⇨ extending out of the spinal canal ➡ into the posterior mediastinum. Note the associated thoracic scoliosis in this patient with neurofibromatosis type 1.*

Thymic Cyst

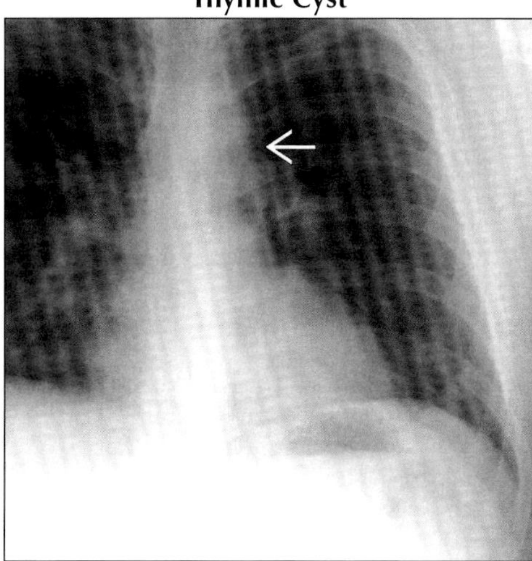

Thymic Cyst

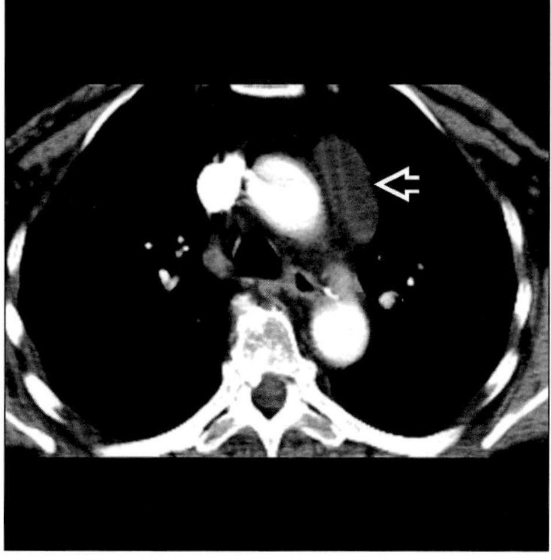

(Left) *Frontal radiograph shows abnormal contour along the left side of the mediastinum ➡ in this patient with a thymic cyst.* ***(Right)*** *Axial CECT shows sharply defined, elliptical, thin-walled cyst in the anterior mediastinum and prevascular space ⇨, probably arising from the thymus.*

UNILATERAL HILAR MASS

DIFFERENTIAL DIAGNOSIS

Common
- Bronchogenic Carcinoma
- Lymphadenopathy Associated with Infections

Less Common
- Lymphadenopathy Secondary to Metastatic Disease
- Lymphoma

Rare but Important
- Sarcoidosis
- Pulmonary Artery Enlargement
- Bronchogenic Cyst
- Carcinoid
- Castleman Disease

ESSENTIAL INFORMATION

Key Differential Diagnosis Issues
- Infection and malignancy dominate differentials in category
- Key features of clinical history help determine diagnosis
  - Signs and symptoms of infection
  - Presence of known malignancy
- Clues to distinguish hilar mass from lymphadenopathy
  - Nodes are well defined and smooth and occur in nodal stations
  - Masses may have infiltrating edges

Helpful Clues for Common Diagnoses
- **Bronchogenic Carcinoma**
  - Small cell lung carcinoma
    - Mediastinal mass involving 1 hilum
    - Typically large at diagnosis
    - May cause lobar or complete lung collapse
    - Ill-defined borders on CT and radiographs
    - Frequently metastatic at presentation
  - Squamous cell carcinoma
    - Most common tumor to cavitate
    - Often central in location
  - Adenocarcinoma
    - Spiculated lung nodule or mass
    - Ipsilateral hilar lymphadenopathy
  - Important to note contralateral mediastinal/hilar or supraclavicular lymphadenopathy
    - Could indicate N3 disease, which is unresectable
  - Abnormal lymph nodes
    - ≥ 1.2 cm short axis diameter for subcarinal lymph nodes
    - ≥ 1 cm short axis diameter for all other nodal groups
- **Lymphadenopathy Associated with Infections**
  - Signs/symptoms of infection
  - Seen with
    - Primary tuberculosis, endemic fungi, mononucleosis, severe bacterial pneumonia
  - TB: Nodes show central necrosis
  - Ipsilateral lung consolidation
  - Travel history important for endemic fungi

Helpful Clues for Less Common Diagnoses
- **Lymphadenopathy Secondary to Metastatic Disease**
  - History of extrathoracic malignancy
  - Common primary tumors
    - Head and neck malignancies, breast carcinoma, melanoma, and genitourinary malignancies
  - Lymph nodes are typically sharply marginated and round
  - Enhancing lymph nodes
    - Renal cell carcinoma, thyroid carcinoma, or melanoma
  - Necrotic lymph nodes
    - Breast carcinoma, testicular carcinoma, or renal cell carcinoma
  - Calcified lymph nodes
    - Treated metastases, thyroid carcinoma, mucinous adenocarcinoma
- **Lymphoma**
  - Bulky asymmetric mediastinal/hilar lymphadenopathy
  - Displaces but rarely constricts mediastinal structures
  - B symptoms
    - Night sweats, fever, and weight loss
  - Hodgkin lymphoma
    - Prevascular, paratracheal, and aorticopulmonary nodal involvement in nearly all cases
    - 25-35% have concomitant hilar nodal disease
    - Nodes may calcify after radiotherapy

- Spreads via contiguous lymph node groups
- Lung disease in 10% of patients
- Peak incidence in 3rd and 8th decades of life
- Ann Arbor system stages disease
  - Non-Hodgkin lymphoma (NHL)
    - Thoracic involvement in 50% of cases
    - Most patients with thoracic disease have anterior mediastinal disease
    - Hilar adenopathy in 10-20% of patients with thoracic involvement
    - Binodal peak incidence in 5th-8th decades of life
    - Spreads via noncontiguous lymph node groups
    - Multifocal disease at presentation is observed frequently
  - Extrathoracic lymphadenopathy seen more commonly with NHL

Helpful Clues for Rare Diagnoses

- **Sarcoidosis**
  - Unilateral hilar enlargement seen in minority of cases
  - Perilymphatic distribution of lung nodules
    - Nodules along fissures, pleural surfaces, and bronchovascular bundles
    - Predilection for upper lungs
  - Child-bearing females
- **Pulmonary Artery Enlargement**
  - CECT diagnostic
  - Causes include
    - Pulmonary valve stenosis
    - Pulmonary artery aneurysm
    - Intravascular tumor
    - Proximal interruption of pulmonary artery
  - Pulmonary artery aneurysm secondary to
    - Trauma from pulmonary arterial catheter
    - Mycotic aneurysm
    - Collagen vascular diseases
  - Main and left pulmonary artery enlargement
    - Pulmonic valve stenosis
    - Absent pulmonary valve
- **Bronchogenic Cyst**
  - Well-defined spherical mass
  - Highly variable internal HU secondary to varying protein content
  - Presence of air usually indicates infection
  - May displace or compress mediastinal structures
  - Wall is thin or not seen
  - No internal contrast enhancement
  - Abrupt increase in size secondary to hemorrhage or infection
- **Carcinoid**
  - Malignant tumor arising from central bronchi
    - Can cause lobar or segmental lung collapse
  - ± contrast enhancement
  - Chunky calcification common in hilum
- **Castleman Disease**
  - Solitary smooth or lobulated hilar mass
  - ± multifocal lymphadenopathy
  - Avid contrast enhancement

Bronchogenic Carcinoma

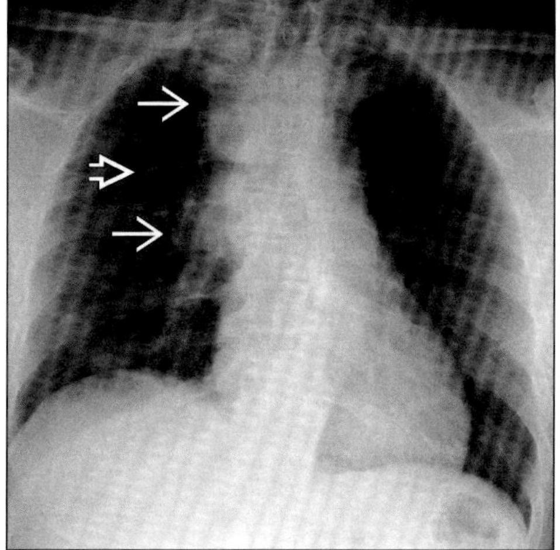

Anteroposterior radiograph shows a right lung nodule ⇨. Note mediastinal and right hilar lymphadenopathy → in this patient with small cell lung carcinoma.

Bronchogenic Carcinoma

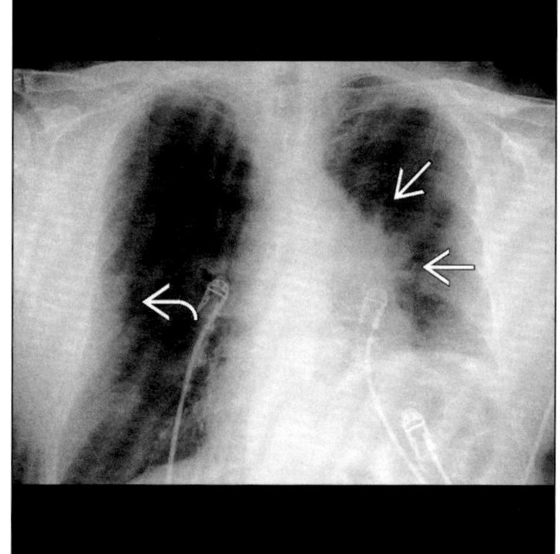

Frontal radiograph shows a left hilar mass with infiltrating margins →. Expansile right-sided rib metastasis ↩ makes this stage IV disease.

UNILATERAL HILAR MASS

*(**Left**) Frontal radiograph shows right hilar ➡ adenopathy. Note rightward bulge of the superior azygoesophageal recess ➡ suggesting subcarinal lymphadenopathy. (**Right**) Axial CECT shows extensive, centrally necrotic-appearing subcarinal → and right hilar ➡ lymph nodes associated with M. tuberculosis infection. Necrotic lymph nodes can be seen in fungal infections, lymphoma, lung carcinoma, and metastatic disease.*

Lymphadenopathy Associated with Infections

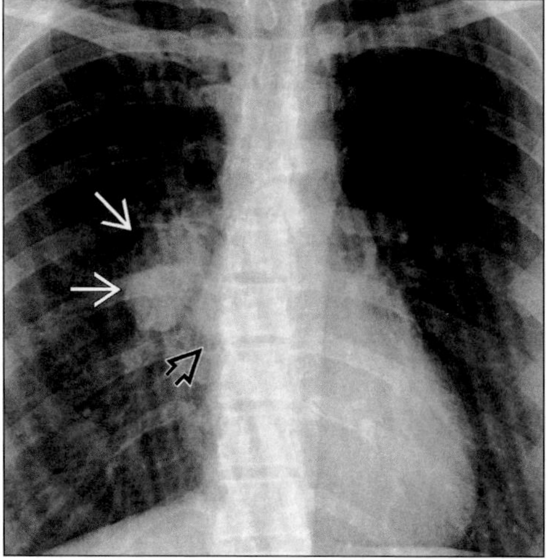

Lymphadenopathy Associated with Infections

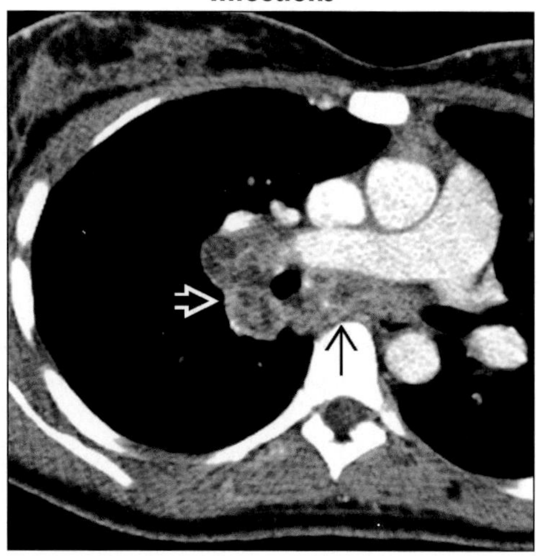

*(**Left**) Axial CECT shows right lower lobe consolidation ➡ and right hilar lymph node enlargement ➡ with associated narrowing of the lower lobe bronchus in a patient with bacterial pneumonia. This proved noncancerous on long-term follow-up despite bronchial narrowing. (**Right**) Axial CECT shows a necrotic left hilar lymph node metastasis ➡ in this patient with renal cell carcinoma. Presence of a known primary was important to make this diagnosis.*

Lymphadenopathy Associated with Infections

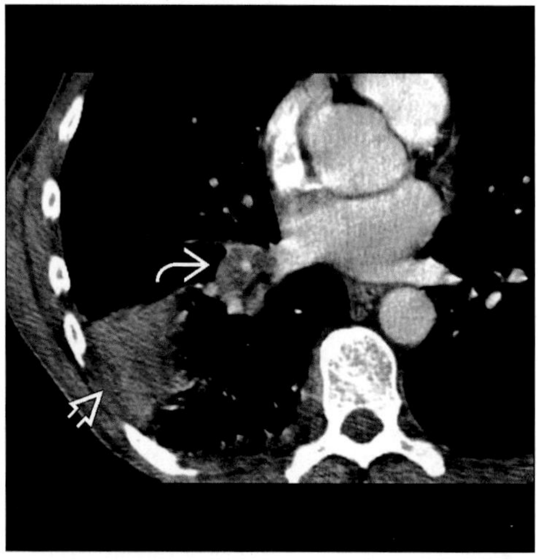

Lymphadenopathy Secondary to Metastatic Disease

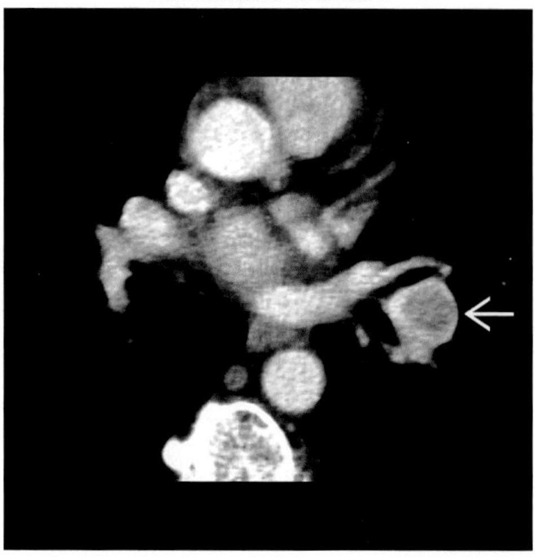

*(**Left**) Frontal radiograph shows a lobulated middle mediastinum mass ➡. Note right hilar nodal enlargement ➡ as well. (**Right**) Axial CECT shows a rounded soft tissue mass, representing enlarged subcarinal lymphadenopathy ➡. Note right hilar lymph node enlargement ➡. Prevascular nodal disease was noted on superior images. Isolated hilar lymphadenopathy without disease more superiorly is rarely related to lymphoma.*

Lymphoma

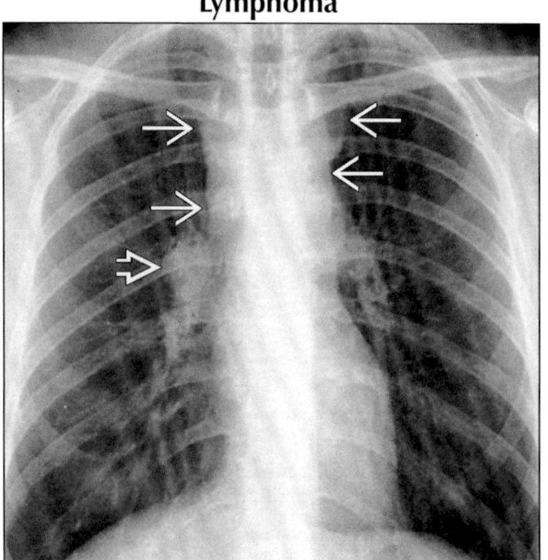

Lymphoma

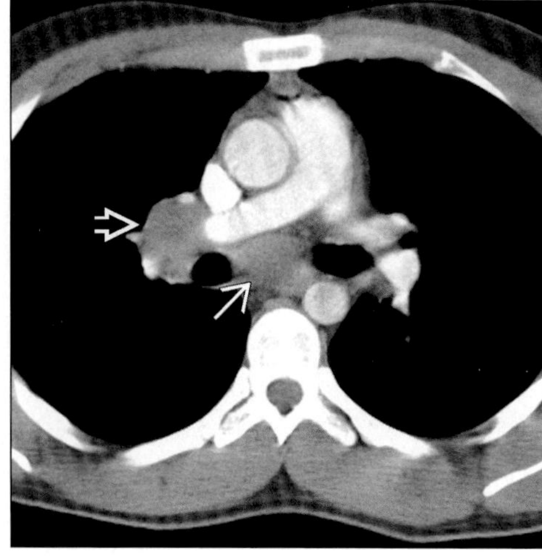

Sarcoidosis

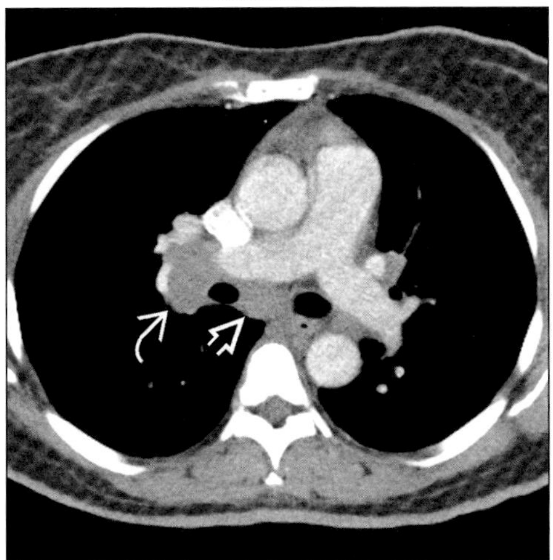

Pulmonary Artery Enlargement

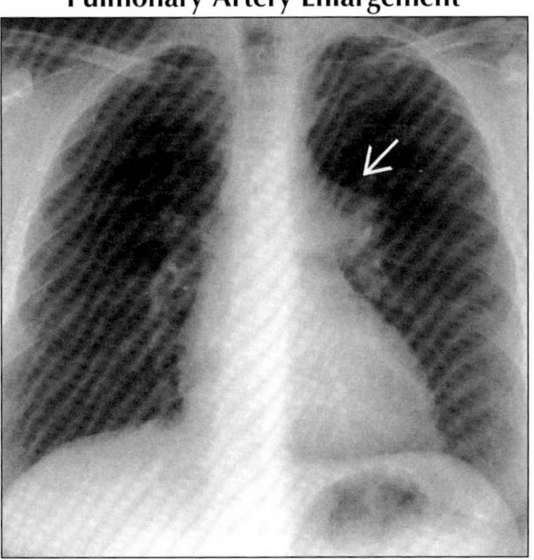

(Left) *Axial CECT shows asymmetric right hilar and subcarinal lymph node enlargement. Lung windows revealed perilymphatic lung nodules typical of sarcoidosis.* ***(Right)*** *Frontal radiograph shows smooth enlargement of the main and left pulmonary arteries. Pulmonary valve stenosis or an absent pulmonic valve should be considered as a potential cause in this setting. In this patient, the etiology was unknown.*

Pulmonary Artery Enlargement

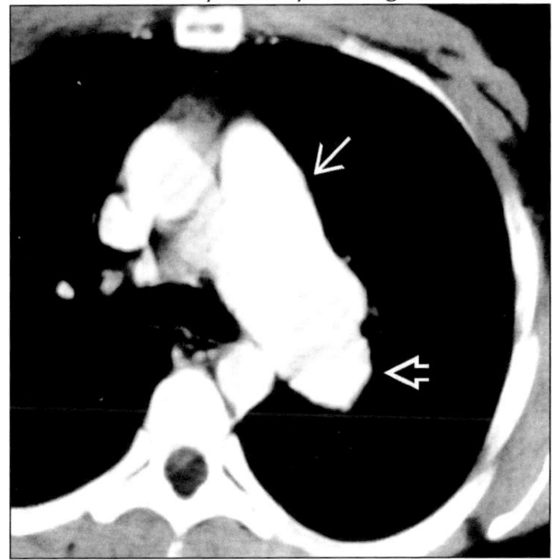

Bronchogenic Cyst

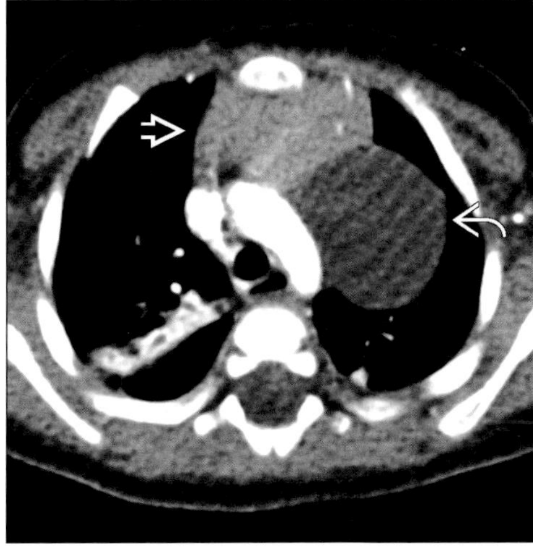

(Left) *Axial CECT shows dilated main and left pulmonary artery.* ***(Right)*** *Axial CECT shows a large round cystic lesion adjacent to the aorta in the region of the superior left hilum. This proved to be a bronchogenic cyst at resection. Note prominent normal thymus in this toddler. No enhancement of the lesion was identified when compared to the noncontrast CT examination.*

Carcinoid

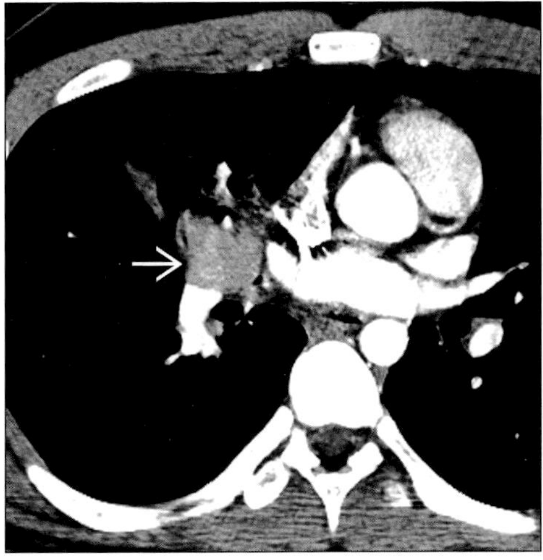

Castleman Disease

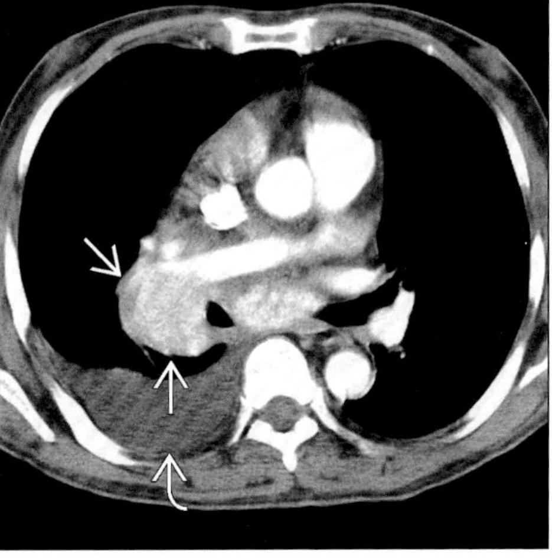

(Left) *Axial CECT shows a contrast-enhancing mass from carcinoid tumor causing right middle lobe collapse. In this case, there were no typical large central calcifications.* ***(Right)*** *Axial CECT shows enlarged, avidly enhancing right hilar lymph nodes typical of Castleman disease, plasma cell variant. Note incidental right pleural effusion. Vascular metastases could have a similar appearance.*

BILATERAL HILAR MASS

DIFFERENTIAL DIAGNOSIS

Common
- Sarcoidosis
- Pulmonary Arterial Enlargement

Less Common
- Lymphadenopathy Associated with Infections
- Lymphoma

Rare but Important
- Silicosis/Coal Worker's Pneumoconiosis
- Berylliosis
- Lymphadenopathy Secondary to Metastatic Disease
- Angioimmunoblastic Lymphadenopathy
- Amyloidosis

ESSENTIAL INFORMATION

Key Differential Diagnosis Issues
- Bilateral hilar mass usually secondary to pulmonary artery or hilar lymph node enlargement
  - Lobulated contour in lymph node enlargement
  - Smooth contour in pulmonary arterial enlargement

Helpful Clues for Common Diagnoses
- **Sarcoidosis**
  - Systemic disease of unknown etiology
  - Common in African-American females of childbearing age
  - Most patients present with thoracic lymph node enlargement
  - 50% have associated lung disease
  - Hilar lymph node enlargement in ≥ 80%
    - Lobulated and symmetric
    - ± calcification
  - 1, 2, 3 sign (Garland triad)
    - Right paratracheal (1), right hilar (2), and left hilar (3) nodal enlargement
  - CT findings
    - Symmetric hilar and mediastinal nodal disease
    - 25-50% of nodes show calcification
    - Eggshell calcification
    - Lung nodules (noncaseating granulomas) along fissures, subpleural lung, and bronchovascular bundles
    - Upper lung predominant
- **Pulmonary Arterial Enlargement**
  - CT angiogram diagnostic
  - Etiologies include
    - Pulmonary arterial hypertension, primary and secondary causes
    - Left-to-right shunts
    - Idiopathic with no associated pulmonary hypertension
  - Most common cause is pulmonary arterial hypertension
  - Radiographic and CT findings
    - Dilatation of central pulmonary arteries with pruning and tapering of distal vessels
    - Main pulmonary artery ≥ 29 mm
    - Main pulmonary artery ≥ size of ascending aorta
    - Calcification of pulmonary arterial wall seen with irreversible longstanding disease
    - ± mosaic perfusion due to associated small vessel disease
  - Examples of left-to-right shunts
    - Atrial septal defect
    - Ventricular septal defect
    - Partial anomalous pulmonary venous return
    - Patent ductus arteriosus
  - Eisenmenger syndrome
    - Reversal of left-to-right shunt caused by elevated pulmonary arterial pressure exceeding systemic pressure

Helpful Clues for Less Common Diagnoses
- **Lymphadenopathy Associated with Infections**
  - Most commonly seen with *Histoplasma* or *Coccidioides* infections
  - Primary *M. tuberculosis* usually unilateral disease
  - ± miliary lung nodules
  - ± lung consolidation
  - Low-attenuation lymph nodes common with endemic fungi
  - Elevated blood titers helpful in diagnosis
- **Lymphoma**
  - Hodgkin disease
    - Nearly all patients have superior mediastinal nodal involvement
    - 25-35% have hilar disease
    - Calcification occurs post radiotherapy
    - 20% of nodes appear necrotic

- 10% of patients have lung involvement
- Non-Hodgkin lymphoma
  - Hilar nodal disease less common than in Hodgkin disease

Helpful Clues for Rare Diagnoses

- **Silicosis/Coal Worker's Pneumoconiosis**
  - Hilar and mediastinal nodal enlargement in 30-40%
  - Eggshell calcification of lymph nodes in 5%
  - Upper lobe predominant centrilobular or perilymphatic lung nodules
  - ± calcification of lung nodules
  - Progressive massive fibrosis
    - Upper lobe conglomeration of nodules into large masses with volume loss and upward hilar retraction
    - Cavitation may indicate *Tuberculosis* superinfection
- **Berylliosis**
  - Occupational lung disease
  - Ceramic industry, aerospace industry, nuclear power production
  - Identical radiographic appearance to sarcoidosis
    - Symmetric hilar and mediastinal lymphadenopathy
    - ± lymph node calcification
    - Small nodules along fissures, subpleural lung, and bronchovascular bundles (perilymphatic distribution)
  - Positive BAL or serum beryllium lymphocyte proliferation test
  - Symptoms
    - Dyspnea most common
    - ± cough, chest pain, and fatigue
- **Lymphadenopathy Secondary to Metastatic Disease**
  - Unilateral hilar metastases are more common
  - Lymph nodes usually round and well defined
  - ± central low density
  - Most common cause is bronchogenic carcinoma
    - Presence of contralateral hilar lymph node metastases indicates N3 disease (unresectable)
- **Angioimmunoblastic Lymphadenopathy**
  - Erroneously called a systemic disease associated with immunodeficiency
  - Now accepted as peripheral T-cell lymphoma (non-Hodgkin lymphoma)
  - Mediastinal and hilar nodal enlargement ± lung disease
  - Pleural effusions in 40%
- **Amyloidosis**
  - Hilar enlargement secondary to
    - Thickening of central airways from amyloid deposition
    - Lymph node enlargement
  - Perilymphatic lung nodules
  - ± calcification in nodules and lymph nodes
  - Cardiac involvement leads to restrictive cardiomyopathy

Sarcoidosis

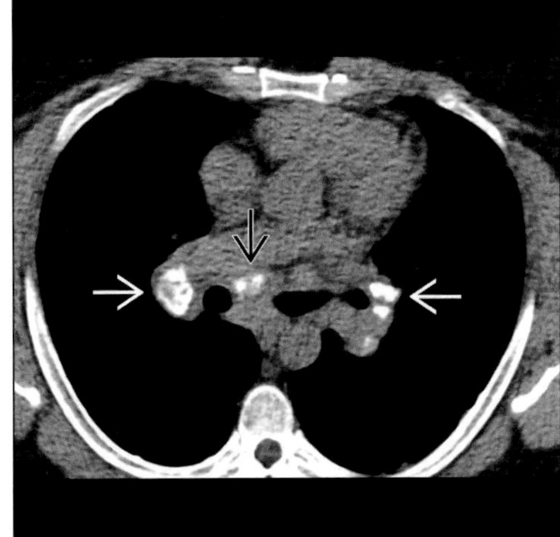

Axial NECT shows symmetric calcified hilar ➡ and subcarinal ➡ lymph nodes.

Sarcoidosis

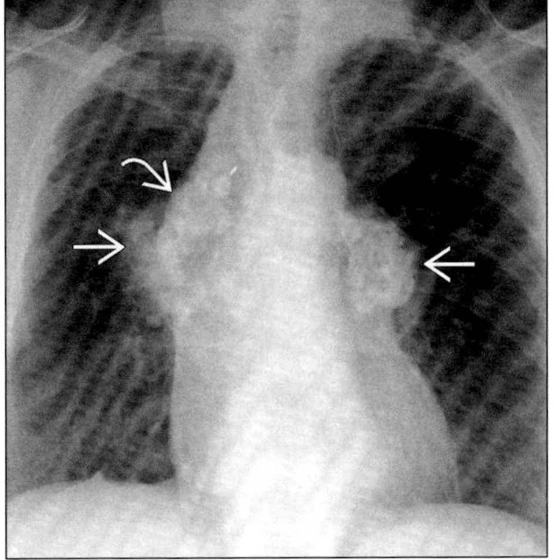

Frontal radiograph shows enlarged hili ➡ and right paratracheal lymph nodes ➡ with eggshell calcification.

BILATERAL HILAR MASS

(Left) Axial NECT shows typical mildly calcified symmetric hilar ➔ and subcarinal ➔ lymph nodes. Characteristic perilymphatic lung nodules are shown in the next image. *(Right)* Coronal NECT shows typical perilymphatic nodules in sarcoidosis. Note beading along the major fissure ➔, the subpleural nodules ➔, and the airway nodules ➔.

Sarcoidosis

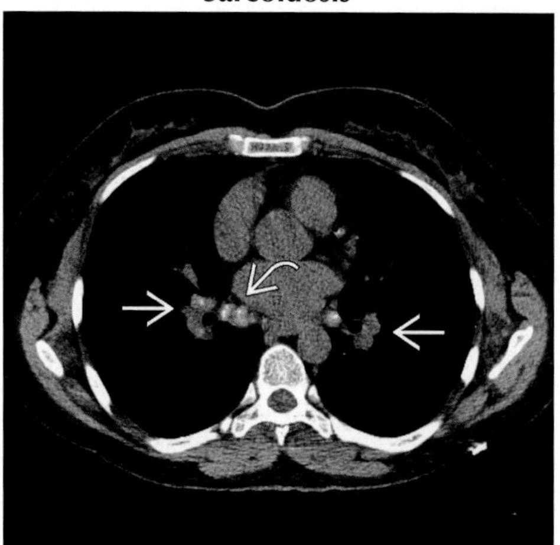

Sarcoidosis

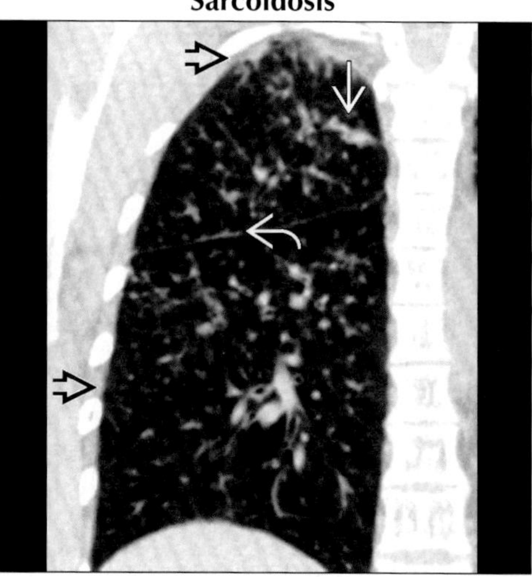

(Left) Lateral radiograph shows enlarged bilateral hilar nodes ➔. The presence of opacity in this location on the lateral view, called the inferior hilar window, usually indicates hilar lymphadenopathy. *(Right)* Frontal radiograph shows enlargement of central pulmonary arteries ➔ and main pulmonary artery ➔ with distal pruning.

Sarcoidosis

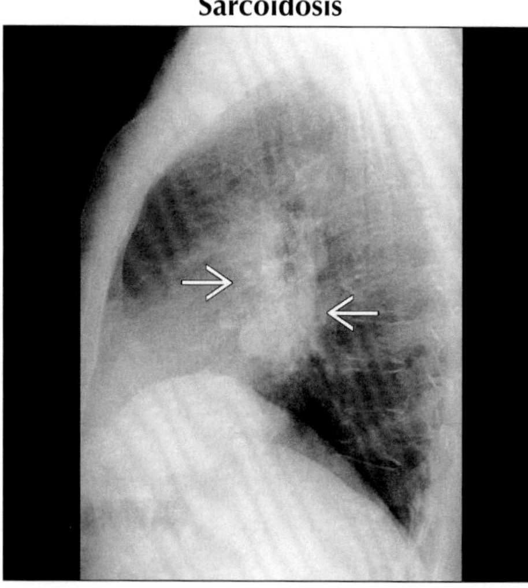

Pulmonary Arterial Enlargement

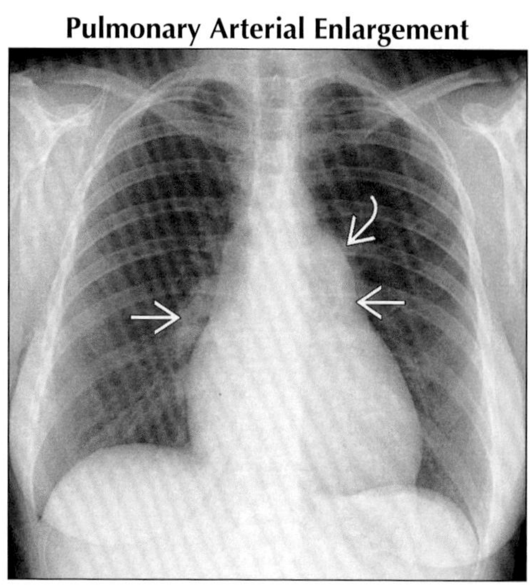

(Left) Axial CECT shows marked enlargement of the central pulmonary arteries ➔. Note the thrombosed dissection in right pulmonary artery ➔. *(Right)* Coronal CECT shows enlarged main pulmonary artery ➔ and associated mosaic perfusion with more lucent areas of abnormal lung ➔ and normal lung ➔. This patient had primary pulmonary hypertension.

Pulmonary Arterial Enlargement

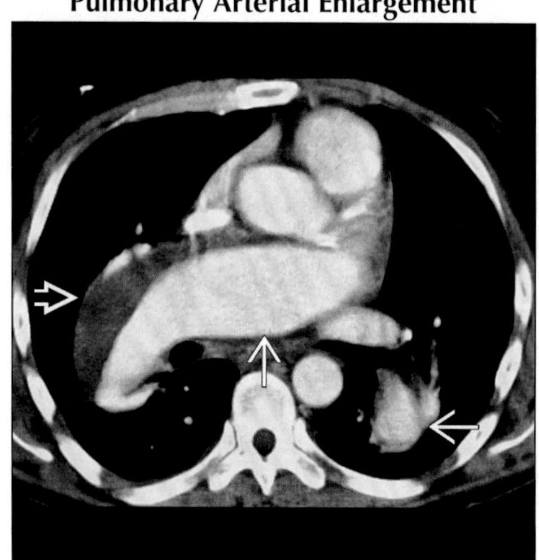

Pulmonary Arterial Enlargement

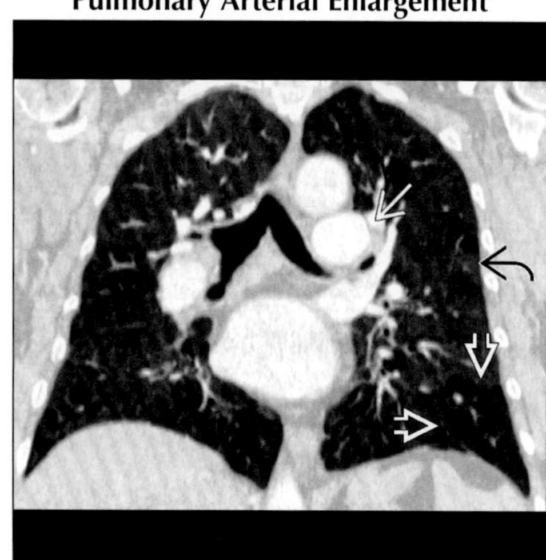

Lymphadenopathy Associated with Infections

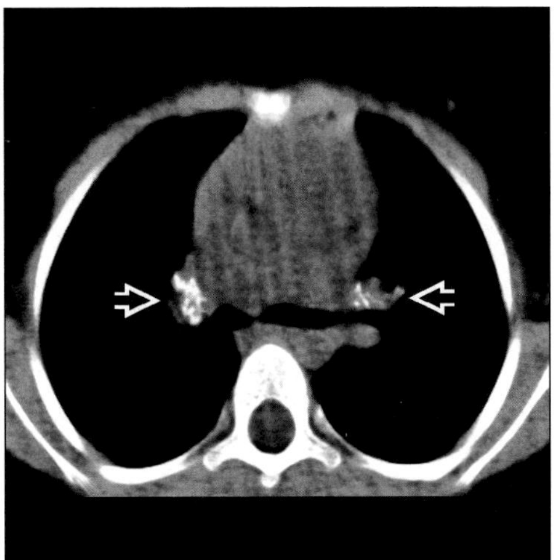

Lymphadenopathy Associated with Infections

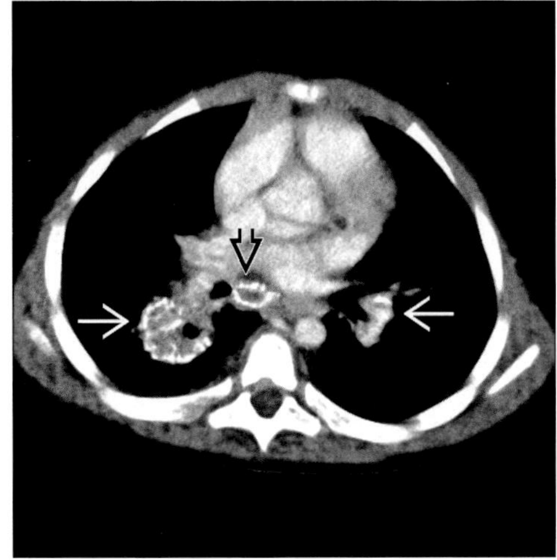

*(**Left**) Axial NECT shows bilateral calcified hilar lymph nodes ➡ in this patient with proven histoplasmosis 2 years prior. (**Right**) Axial CECT shows calcified hilar lymph nodes ➡, right more than left. Note calcified subcarinal lymph nodes ⇨. A psoas abscess and epidural abscess (not shown) were also discovered in this patient with symptoms of infection. This was secondary to tuberculosis.*

Lymphadenopathy Associated with Infections

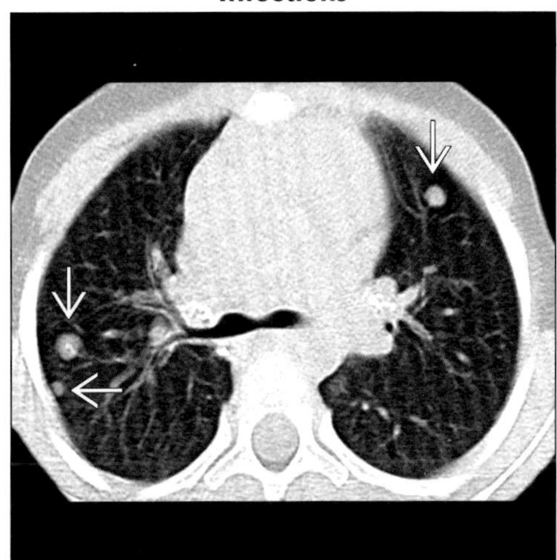

Lymphoma

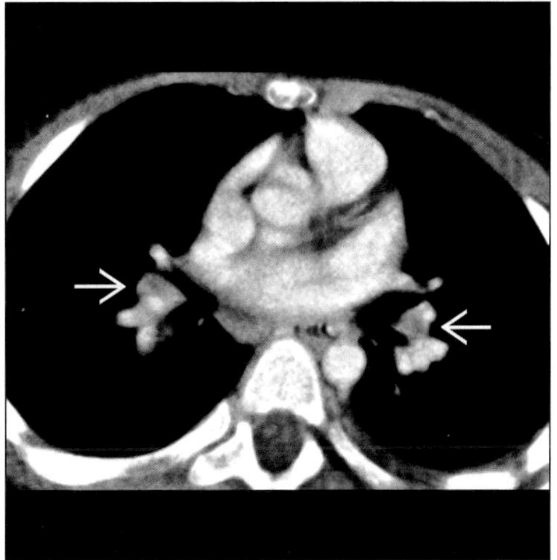

*(**Left**) Axial NECT shows bilateral round pulmonary nodules ➡. This proved to be histoplasmosis. (**Right**) Axial CECT shows mildly enlarged bilateral hilar lymph nodes ➡ in this patient with non-Hodgkin lymphoma (subtype lymphoblastic lymphoma). Involvement was also seen in the anterior mediastinum and inguinal lymph node regions.*

Lymphoma

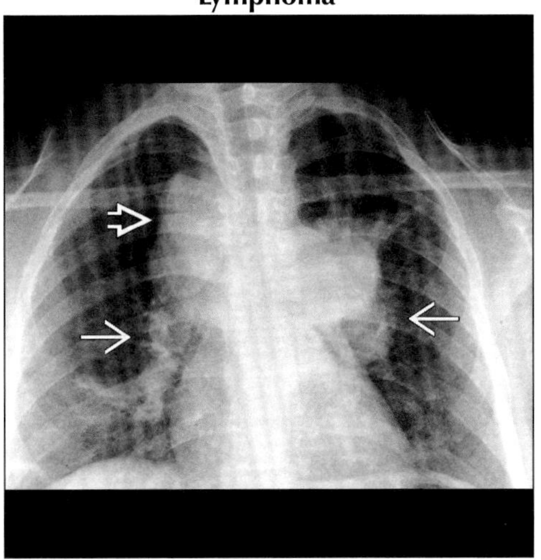

Silicosis/Coal Worker's Pneumoconiosis

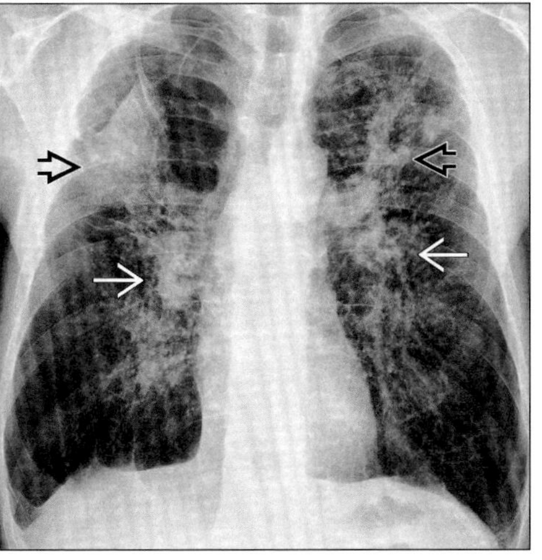

*(**Left**) Frontal radiograph shows asymmetric bilateral hilar lymph node enlargement ➡. Upper mediastinal nodal enlargement ➡ is seen characteristically in patients with Hodgkin lymphoma. (**Right**) Frontal radiograph shows large upper lobe opacities ⇨ with upward retraction of the hila typical of progressive massive fibrosis. Note bilateral hilar lymph node enlargement ➡. Innumerable small nodules represent silicotic lung nodules.*

BILATERAL HILAR MASS

(Left) Axial CECT shows left hilar lymph nodes containing eggshell calcification ➡. Right hilar lymph nodes reveal solid calcification ⇨. Centrilobular nodules were present on lung windows. *(Right)* Coronal NECT shows volume loss and progressive massive fibrosis ➡ in upper lobes. Note characteristic upward retraction of the hila and associated perilesional emphysema. Calcified hilar lymphadenopathy was better demonstrated on mediastinal windows.

Silicosis/Coal Worker's Pneumoconiosis

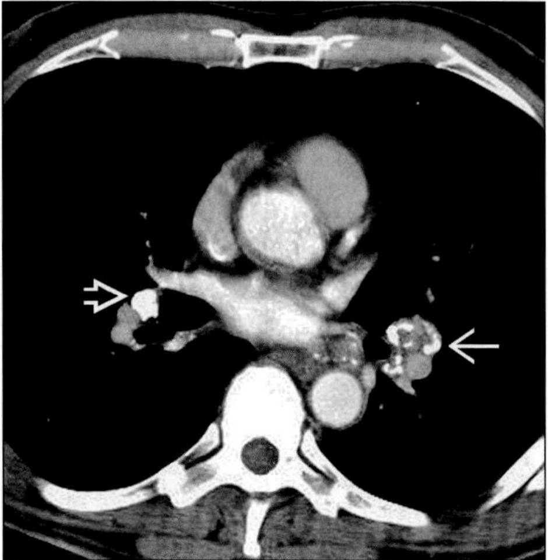

Silicosis/Coal Worker's Pneumoconiosis

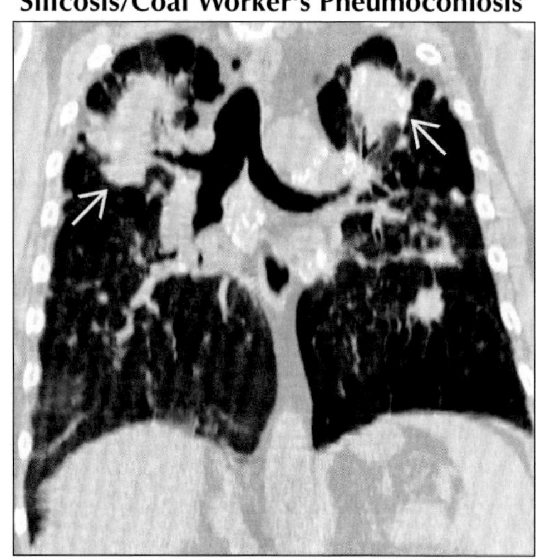

(Left) Frontal radiograph shows bilateral hilar adenopathy ➡ and diffuse nodular interstitial thickening ⇨, more profuse in the upper lung zones. This appearance is identical to that of sarcoidosis. *(Right)* Axial NECT shows typical nodules along the bronchovascular bundles ⇨ in a perilymphatic distribution.

Berylliosis

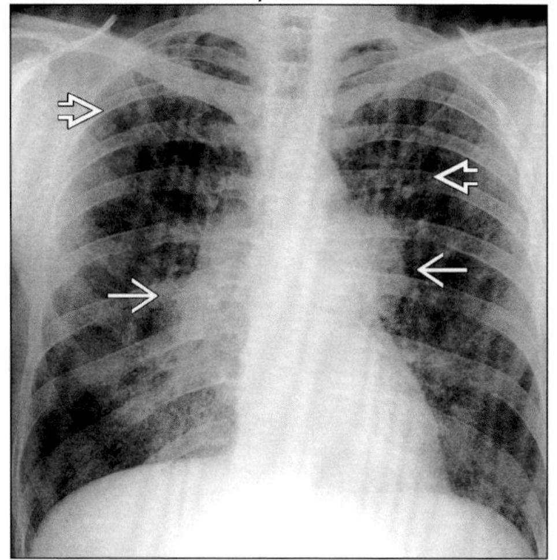

Berylliosis

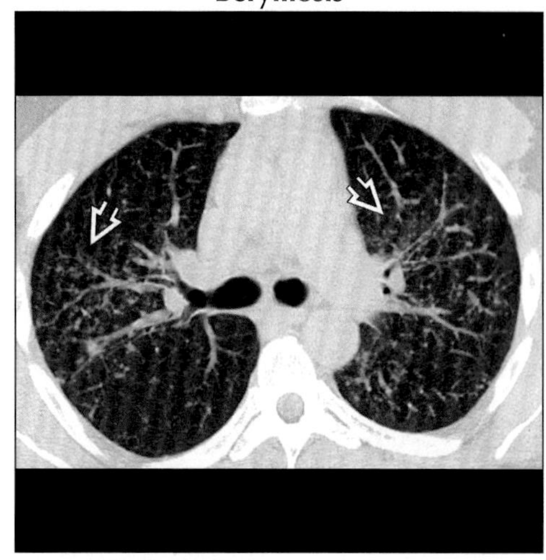

(Left) Frontal radiograph shows bilateral hilar adenopathy ➡ and diffuse nodular interstitial thickening ⇨. Blunting of the left costophrenic angle ↗ may represent pleural effusion. *(Right)* Frontal radiograph shows bilateral hilar and right paratracheal adenopathy ➡ in this patient with testicular metastases. Mediastinal metastases often mimic the pattern of adenopathy seen in sarcoidosis.

Berylliosis

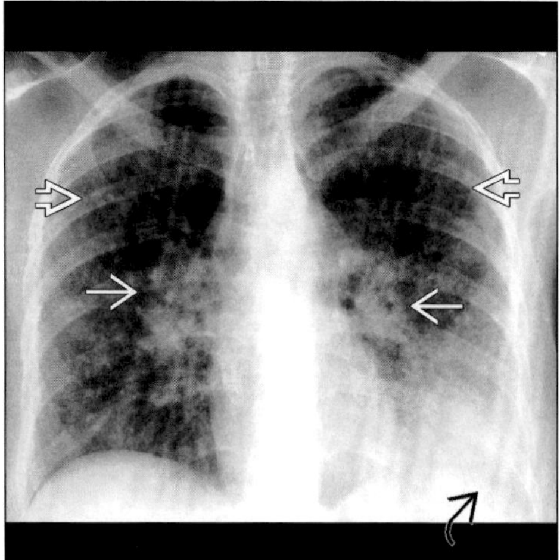

Lymphadenopathy Secondary to Metastatic Disease

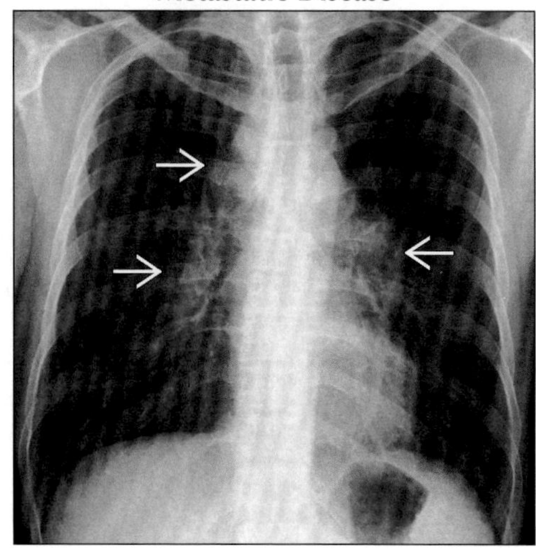

Lymphadenopathy Secondary to Metastatic Disease

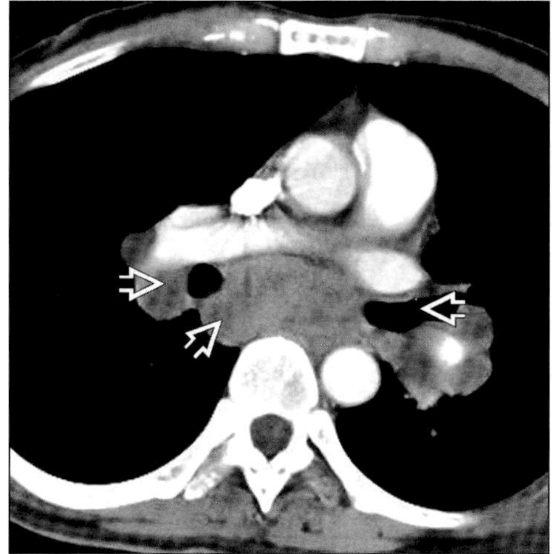

Lymphadenopathy Secondary to Metastatic Disease

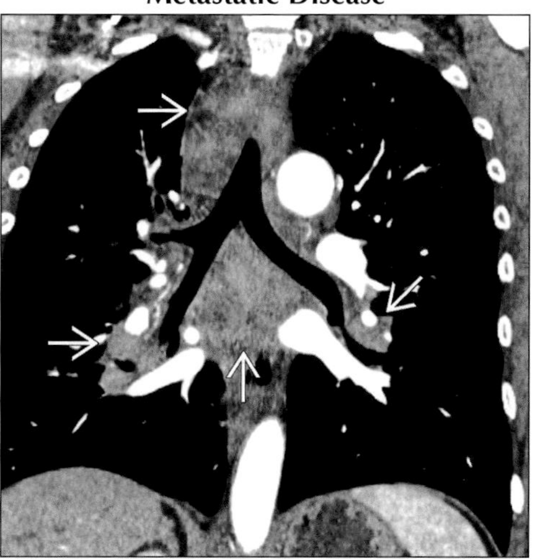

(Left) *Axial CECT shows numerous low-density nodes ➪ in the mediastinum in this patient with testicular metastases. Mediastinal metastases often mimic the pattern of adenopathy seen in sarcoidosis.* ***(Right)*** *Coronal CECT shows diffuse mediastinal adenopathy ➔ in this patient with small cell lung carcinoma.*

Angioimmunoblastic Lymphadenopathy

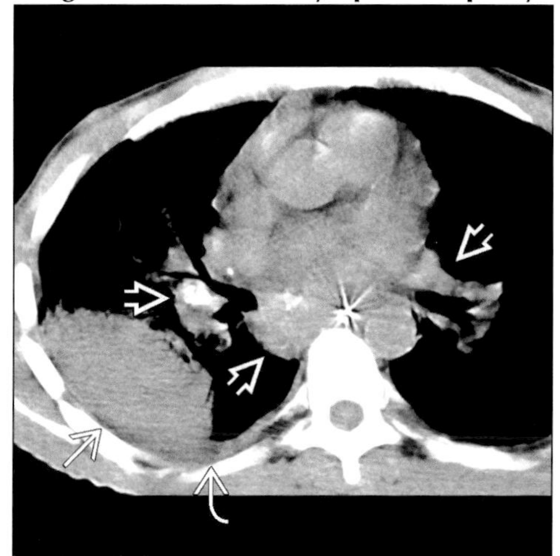

Amyloidosis

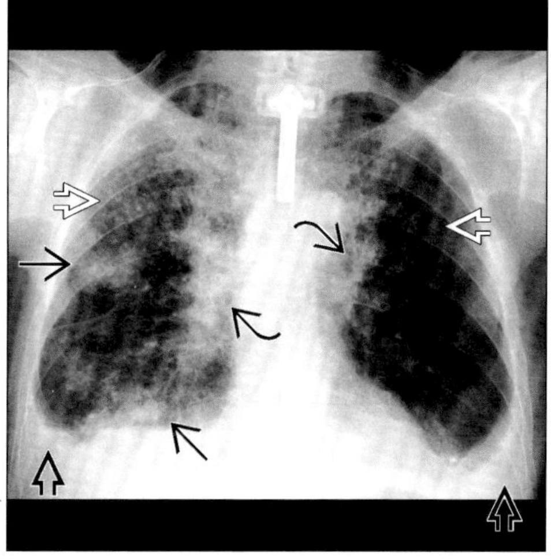

(Left) *Axial NECT shows mass ➔, pleural effusion ➚, and lymphadenopathy ➪. Biopsy was required for diagnosis.* ***(Right)*** *Frontal radiograph shows multiple pulmonary nodules ➪ and masses ➔, as well as small bilateral pleural effusions or pleural thickening ⇨. Note tracheostomy tube for amyloid involvement of airway. Indistinct hila ➚ probably represent peribronchial involvement.*

Amyloidosis

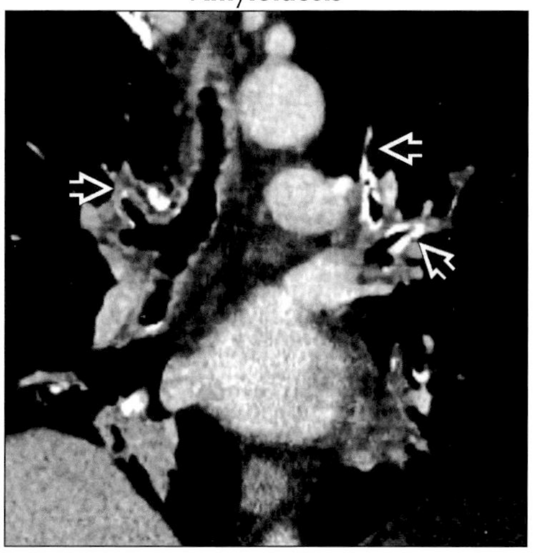

Amyloidosis

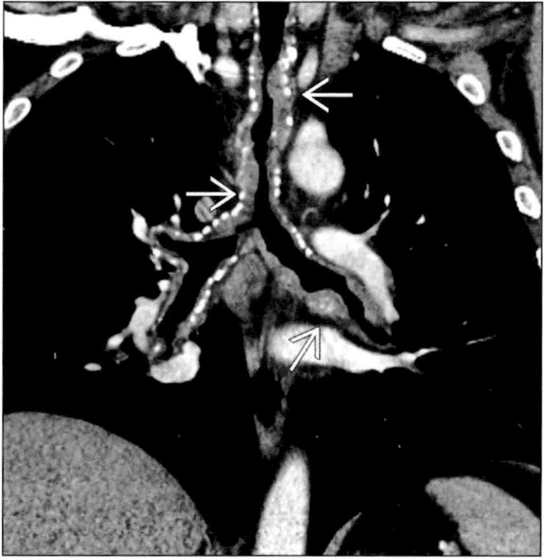

(Left) *Coronal CECT shows thickening and calcification of airway walls ➪.* ***(Right)*** *Coronal CECT shows diffuse tracheal wall thickening and calcification extending into the lobar and segmental bronchi ➔ in this patient with tracheobronchial amyloidosis.*

EGGSHELL CALCIFICATION, HILUM

DIFFERENTIAL DIAGNOSIS

Common
- Silicosis

Less Common
- Sarcoidosis
- Treated Lymphoma

Rare but Important
- Fungal Infection
- Scleroderma
- Amyloidosis

ESSENTIAL INFORMATION

Key Differential Diagnosis Issues
- Eggshell calcification usually relates specifically to lymph nodes
- Peripheral nodal calcifications < 2 mm in thickness
- May be continuous or broken ring of calcification
- May or may not be associated with internal calcifications
- Etiology of this calcification pattern is unknown
- Should be distinguished from calcified aneurysm or pulmonary artery

Helpful Clues for Common Diagnoses
- **Silicosis**
  - Due to chronic inhalation of silica dust
  - Usually requires at least 10 years of exposure
  - Disease will continue to progress despite discontinuation of exposure
  - Eggshell calcifications also occur with coal worker's pneumoconiosis (CWP)
  - CWP often coexists with silicosis, and differentiation is not possible with imaging
  - Mining occupations: Heavy metals and rock
  - Silica is ingested by macrophages, which break down and damage lung parenchyma
  - Multiple centrilobular and subpleural nodules
  - Nodules may be calcified
  - Progressive massive fibrosis
    - Coalescence of silicotic nodules
    - Results in mass > 1 cm in size
    - More common in upper lobes
    - May become necrotic and cavitate
    - Rarely occurs in pure CWP
  - Areas of emphysema often surround nodules
  - Disease predominates in upper and posterior lungs
  - Silicosis predisposes to tuberculosis infection
  - Acute silicoproteinosis: Due to acute exposure of a large amount of silica dust; imaging appearance resembles pulmonary alveolar proteinosis
  - Caplan syndrome: CWP with associated rheumatoid arthritis; may see large necrobiotic nodules

Helpful Clues for Less Common Diagnoses
- **Sarcoidosis**
  - Systemic disease of unknown etiology
  - Pulmonary disease predominates in most patients
  - Usually presents as restrictive lung disease
  - Commonly involves hilar, right paratracheal, and aortopulmonary window lymph nodes
  - Eggshell calcification is uncommon manifestation
  - Numerous lung nodules in perilymphatic distribution
  - Nodules may become calcified
  - Chronic disease may result in patchy upper lobe fibrosis with honeycombing
  - Radiographic stages
    - Stage 0: Normal appearance
    - Stage 1: Hilar &/or mediastinal lymphadenopathy without visible lung disease
    - Stage 2: Hilar &/or mediastinal lymphadenopathy with visible lung disease
    - Stage 3: Lung disease without lymphadenopathy
    - Stage 4: Chronic lung fibrosis
  - Associated with systemic disease
    - Cardiac: Conduction anomalies, myocardial infiltration
    - Ophthalmologic: Uveitis, retinitis
    - Neurologic: Basal meningitis, myelopathy, uveoparotid fever
    - Dermatologic: Alopecia, erythema nodosum

- Endocrine: Hypercalcemia, hyperprolactinemia

- **Treated Lymphoma**
  - Lymphoma may involve any lymph node within chest
  - Untreated nodes rarely calcify
  - Treatment with radiation &/or chemotherapy may result in calcification
  - Calcification occurs in 2-8% of cases post treatment
  - Rarely induces eggshell pattern
  - Post-treatment calcification may suggest better prognosis, especially with Hodgkin disease

Helpful Clues for Rare Diagnoses

- **Fungal Infection**
  - Endemic fungi live in soil
  - Organisms are geographically distributed
    - *Histoplasma capsulatum*: Midwestern and eastern USA
    - *Coccidioides immitis*: Southwestern USA and northern Mexico
    - *Blastomyces dermatitidis*: Midwestern and eastern USA
  - Imaging findings
    - Histoplasmosis: Multifocal consolidation, lymphadenopathy, scattered calcified and noncalcified nodules
    - Coccidioidomycosis: Consolidation, lymphadenopathy, nodules with cavitation, calcification uncommon
    - Blastomycosis: Consolidation, miliary disease, ARDS
  - Eggshell calcification is most common with histoplasmosis but rare overall
- **Scleroderma**
  - Most patients have interstitial fibrosis in UIP or NSIP pattern
  - Lower lungs and subpleural regions usually affected
  - Look for esophageal dilation, which is commonly present
  - Eggshell calcifications have been reported but are rare
- **Amyloidosis**
  - Caused by abnormal protein deposition
  - Amyloid L: Light chain disease usually associated with plasma cell disorders
  - Amyloid A: Secondary form caused by chronic inflammatory diseases and certain neoplasms
  - Radiologic presentations
    - Diffuse amyloidosis: Multiple lung nodules, patchy consolidation, parenchymal calcification, lymphadenopathy
    - Tracheobronchial amyloidosis: Mural airway infiltration, calcification common
    - Nodular amyloidosis: Single or several large nodule(s) and mass(es), calcification common
  - Eggshell calcification can occur in nodes or parenchymal nodules

Silicosis

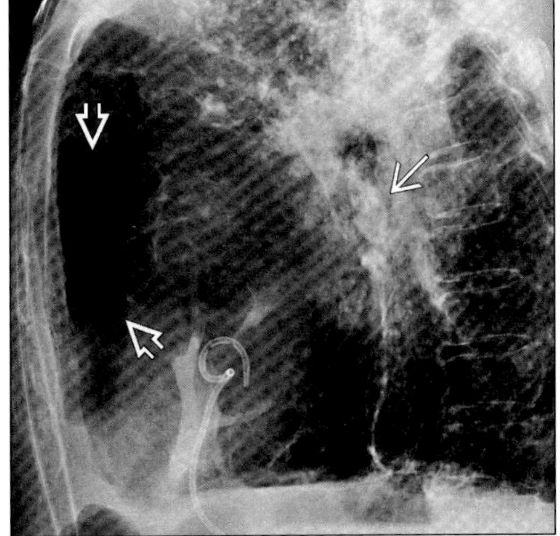

Lateral radiograph shows numerous calcified lymph nodes, many with an eggshell pattern ➔. Also notice the chronic lung opacities and emphysematous changes in the retrosternal space ➔.

Silicosis

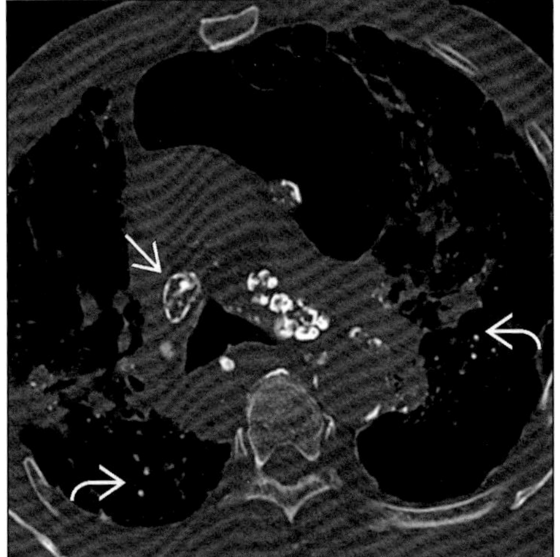

Axial NECT shows eggshell calcifications within the mediastinal lymph nodes ➔, calcified and noncalcified lung nodules ➔, scattered lung opacities, and emphysematous changes.

EGGSHELL CALCIFICATION, HILUM

Silicosis

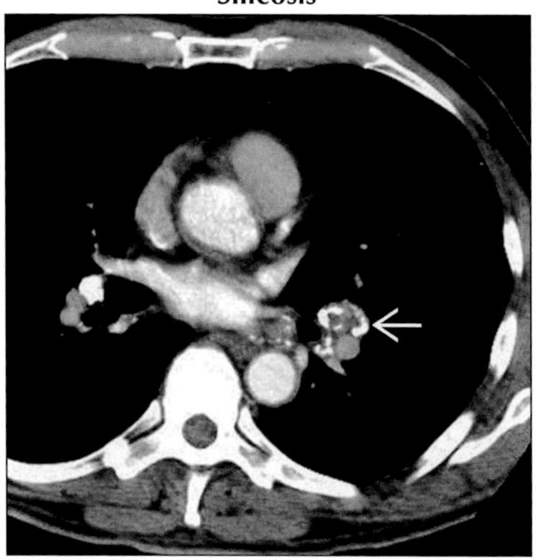

Silicosis

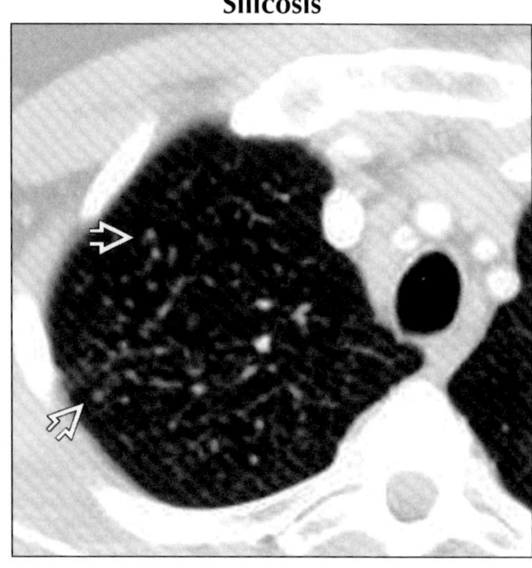

(Left) *Axial CECT shows eggshell calcification of the hilar lymph nodes ➔.* ***(Right)*** *Axial CECT in the same patient shows scattered centrilobular nodules ➔, many of which were calcified. The combination of eggshell calcifications and scattered lung nodules measuring 1-10 mm in size is suggestive of silicosis. The diagnosis requires a history of chronic exposure, usually for at least 10-20 years.*

Silicosis

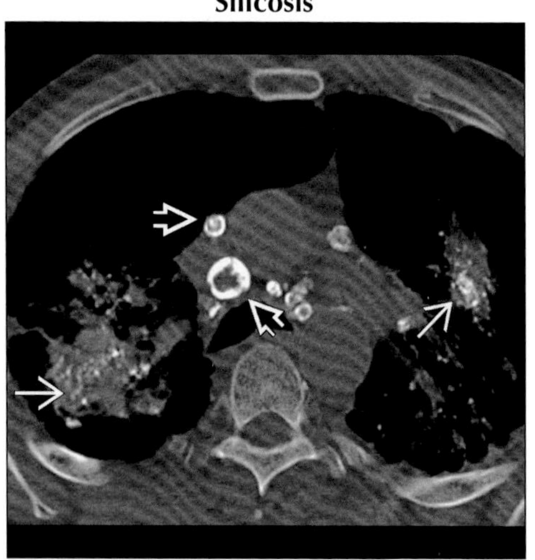

Sarcoidosis

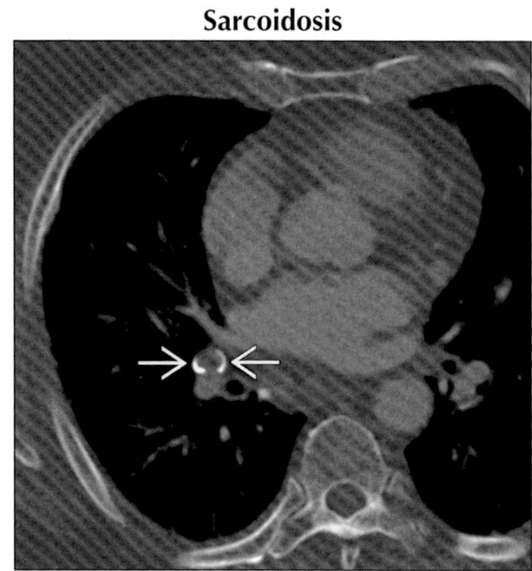

(Left) *Axial NECT shows typical CT features of progressive massive fibrosis in silicosis. There are parenchymal opacities with punctate calcification from progressive massive fibrosis ➔. Eggshell calcifications are present within mediastinal lymph nodes ➔.* ***(Right)*** *Axial CECT shows eggshell calcification of a right hilar lymph node ➔ in this patient with sarcoidosis. Look for characteristic lung findings to support the diagnosis.*

Sarcoidosis

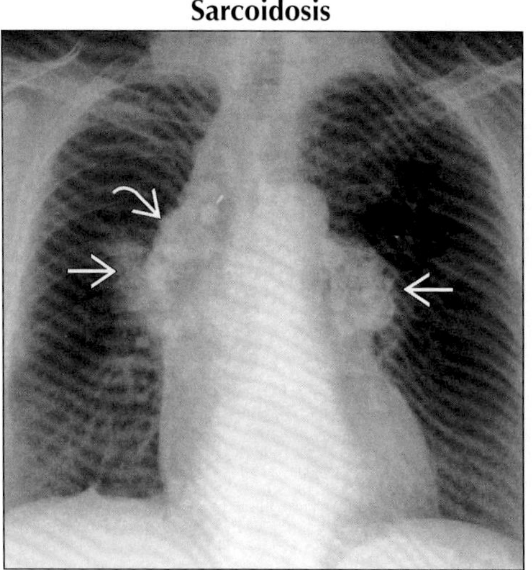

Sarcoidosis

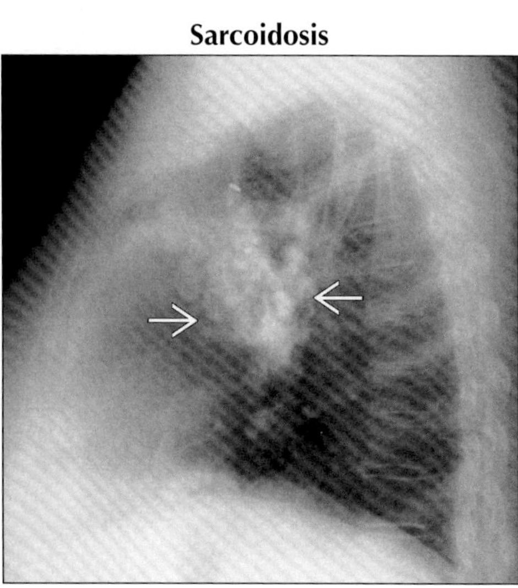

(Left) *Frontal radiograph shows bilateral hilar enlargement ➔ and right paratracheal lymph nodes ➔ with eggshell calcification.* ***(Right)*** *Lateral radiograph redemonstrates bilateral hilar enlargement with eggshell calcifications ➔. This characteristic pattern is typical of sarcoidosis.*

Sarcoidosis

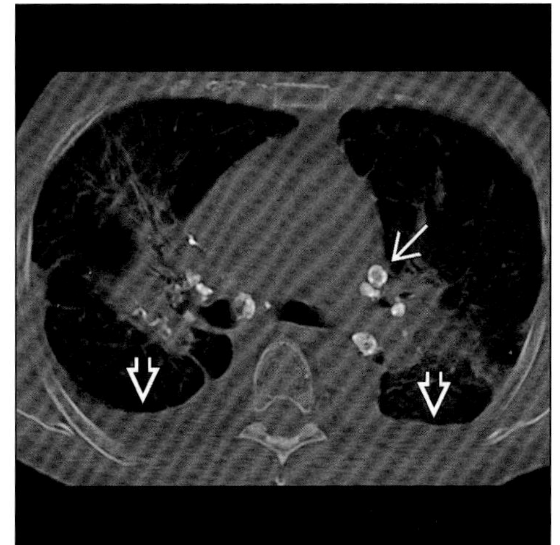

Treated Lymphoma

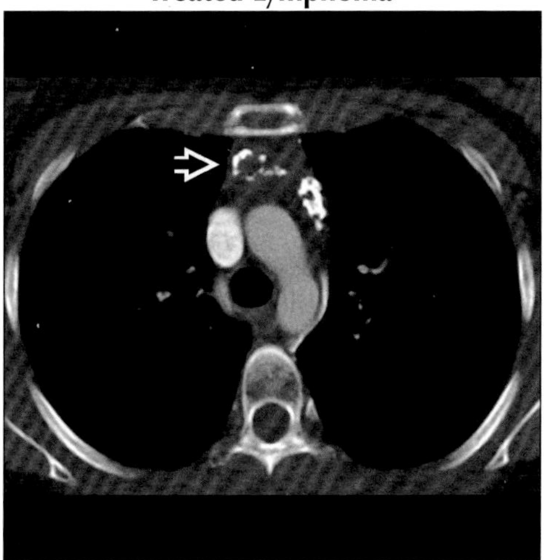

(Left) *Axial NECT shows bilateral hilar lymph nodes with an eggshell pattern of calcification ➔. There are associated perihilar lung opacities and bilateral pleural effusions ➔ in this patient with sarcoidosis.* ***(Right)*** *Axial CECT shows a partially calcified mass in the anterior mediastinum. Some of the calcifications are eggshell in distribution ➔. This can be seen in treated lymphoma, especially Hodgkin disease.*

Treated Lymphoma

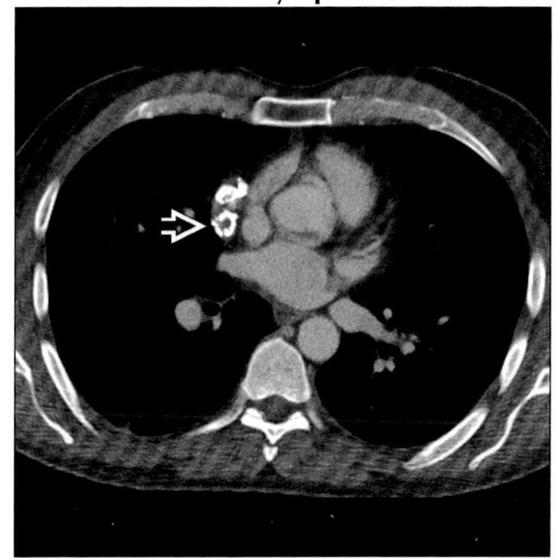

Fungal Infection

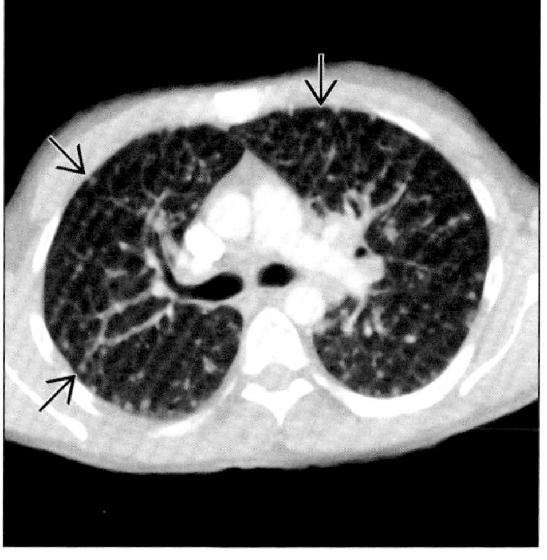

(Left) *Axial CECT shows a mass adjacent to the heart with internal eggshell calcifications ➔. This is another example of treated Hodgkin disease.* ***(Right)*** *Axial CECT shows nodules in all lobes ➔ in this patient with massive inhalation histoplasmosis. Fungal infection is often associated with lymphadenopathy, and an eggshell distribution of calcification has been described.*

Scleroderma

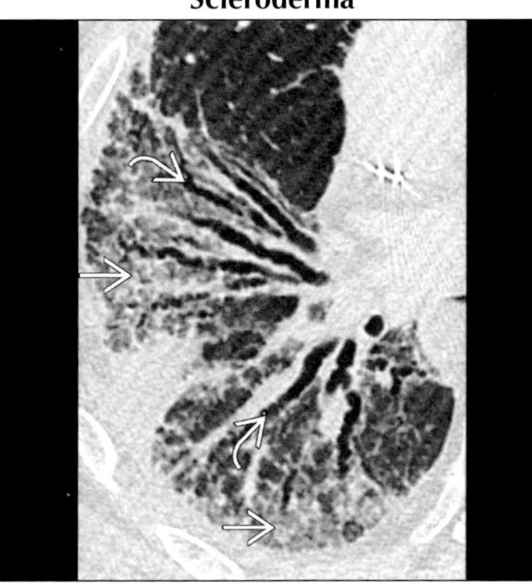

Amyloidosis

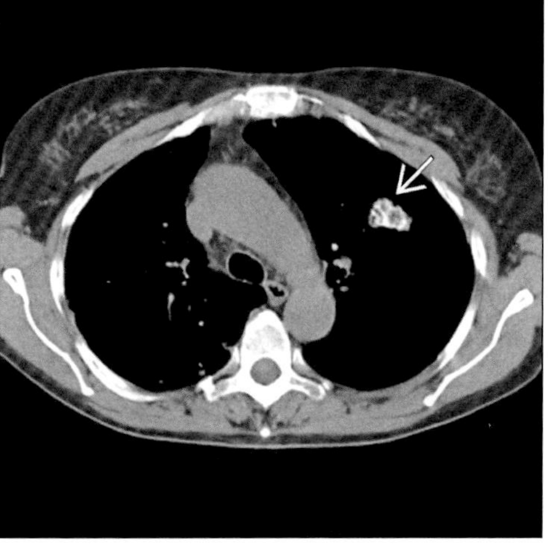

(Left) *Axial HRCT shows severe interstitial fibrotic changes ➔ and traction bronchiectases ➔ at the right lung base in bronchovascular distribution (NSIP pattern). This is a typical appearance of scleroderma, which has been reported to cause eggshell calcifications.* ***(Right)*** *Axial HRCT shows a left upper lobe mass with eggshell calcification ➔. There was also hilar and mediastinal lymphadenopathy. Lung biopsy revealed pulmonary amyloidosis.*

LYMPHADENOPATHY, HILUM

DIFFERENTIAL DIAGNOSIS

Common
- Bronchogenic Carcinoma
- Lymphoma
  - Non-Hodgkin Lymphoma
  - Hodgkin Lymphoma
- Metastasis
- Primary Tuberculosis
- Fungal Infection
- Sarcoidosis
- Chronic Heart Failure

Less Common
- Viral Infection
- Nontuberculous Mycobacteria
- Berylliosis
- Silicosis
- Amyloidosis
- Castleman Disease

Rare but Important
- Drug-Induced Lymphadenopathy

ESSENTIAL INFORMATION

Key Differential Diagnosis Issues
- Increased hilar density: Most common radiographic manifestation of hilar mass
- Lymphadenopathy: Common cause of unilateral or bilateral hilar enlargement
  - Considerable overlap in differential diagnosis
  - Unilateral hilar enlargement: Bronchogenic carcinoma, metastases, lymphoma, and infections
  - Bilateral hilar enlargement: Sarcoidosis (symmetric), metastases, lymphoma
- Enlarged pulmonary artery may mimic hilar mass
- CECT is recommended to evaluate hilar enlargement
  - Low-attenuation/minimal enhancement lymphadenopathy: Tuberculosis, nontuberculous mycobacteria, metastases (testicular tumors), and Hodgkin lymphoma

Helpful Clues for Common Diagnoses
- **Bronchogenic Carcinoma**
  - Invasive, spiculated, large, aggressive appearance
  - Associated pulmonary emphysema common
  - Associated mediastinal or contralateral lymphadenopathy
  - Usually solid, noncavitating, no avid contrast enhancement
  - Calcification rare
- **Lymphoma**
  - **Non-Hodgkin Lymphoma**
    - Bulky, bilaterally asymmetrical, mediastinal-hilar adenopathy
    - Slight to moderate uniform enhancement
  - **Hodgkin Lymphoma**
    - Homogeneous rounded or bulky soft tissue masses
    - May present with asymmetric hilar adenopathy and minimal mediastinal involvement
    - Nodes calcifying following radiation therapy (20%)
- **Metastasis**
  - Bronchogenic cancer: Hilar involvement (30%)
  - Distal primary tumors: Hilar metastases without mediastinal involvement are exceptional
    - Head & neck tumors, genitourinary track, breast, and malignant melanoma
- **Primary Tuberculosis**
  - Unilateral hilar or mediastinal adenopathy (unilateral in 80-90% of cases)
  - CECT: Lymph nodes show low-attenuation center and peripheral rim enhancement
- **Fungal Infection**
  - Histoplasmosis
    - Right middle lobe syndrome (encased bronchus)
    - Postobstructive pneumonia: Encased bronchus or broncholith
    - CECT: Enlarged lymph nodes show central low attenuation from caseous necrosis
  - Coccidioidomycosis
    - Bronchopneumonic infiltrates with hilar node enlargement (20%)
    - Rarely, bilateral hilar adenopathy occurs without parenchymal involvement
  - Paracoccidioidomycosis (*P. brasiliensis*)
    - More common in Latin American countries

  - Frequent enlargement of hilar and mediastinal lymph nodes
  - Complications: Suppuration and fistula formation, scarring and pulmonary fibrosis
- **Sarcoidosis**
  - Most common cause of bilateral symmetric hilar adenopathy
  - Radiograph shows 1, 2, 3, nodes (right paratracheal, right and left hilar), also called Garland triad
  - Must exclude lymphoma
  - Can rarely develop eggshell pattern of calcification
- **Chronic Heart Failure**
  - Mediastinal lymphadenopathy does not necessarily indicate malignancy or infectious process
  - Usually mild symmetric enlargement only

Helpful Clues for Less Common Diagnoses

- **Viral Infection**
  - Epstein-Barr virus
    - Splenomegaly in 50% of cases
    - Generalized lymphadenopathy (hilar and mediastinal involvement included)
  - Rubeola (measles)
    - Pulmonary infiltrates (55%) and hilar lymphadenopathy (74%) early in course
- **Nontuberculous Mycobacteria**
  - Extensive hilar (unilateral or bilateral) and paratracheal lymphadenopathy
  - ± parenchymal disease
  - Nodes undergo extensive necrosis
- **Berylliosis**
  - Sarcoid pattern in patient with exposure to beryllium
  - Hilar or mediastinal adenopathy (40%), always associated with lung disease
  - Nodes: Diffuse or eggshell calcification
- **Silicosis**
  - Silicosis and coal worker's pneumoconiosis (CWP) similar, lung disease usually less severe in CWP
  - Hilar and mediastinal lymphadenopathy common
  - Eggshell calcification (5%)
- **Amyloidosis**
  - Isolated finding or associated with interstitial involvement
  - May be massive
  - Adenopathy: Stippled, diffuse, or eggshell calcifications
- **Castleman Disease**
  - Hyaline-vascular type (> 90%): Children & young adults; focal mass; asymptomatic
  - Plasma cell type: 40-50 years old; adenopathy; systemic illness
  - CECT: Avid contrast enhancement (both forms)

Helpful Clues for Rare Diagnoses

- **Drug-Induced Lymphadenopathy**
  - Causative drugs: Phenytoin, bleomycin, carbamazepine, indomethacin, minocycline, interferon beta, and penicillin
  - Rare complication

Bronchogenic Carcinoma

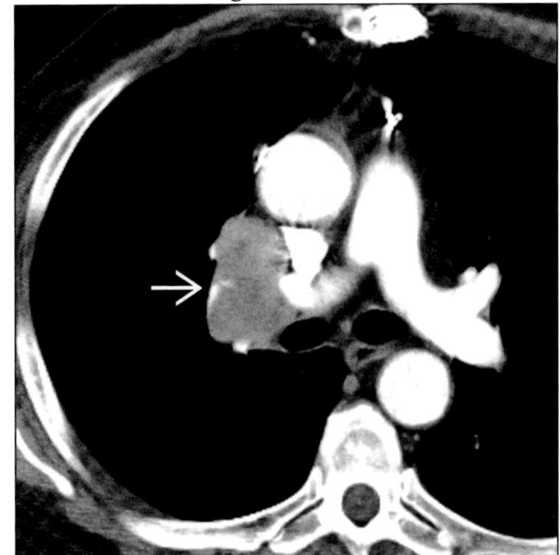

Axial CECT shows right hilar mass ➡ invading the mediastinum causing phrenic nerve paralysis and elevating the right hemidiaphragm (not shown).

Hodgkin Lymphoma

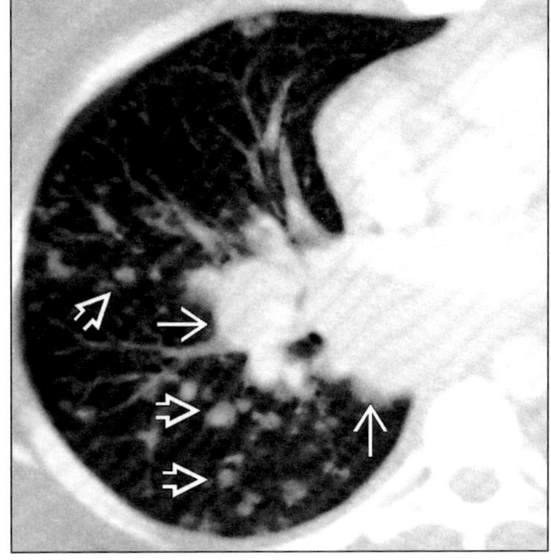

Axial CECT reveals large right hilar lymphadenopathy ➡, as well as multiple well-defined pulmonary nodules ⇨ in this patient with Hodgkin lymphoma.

LYMPHADENOPATHY, HILUM

Primary Tuberculosis

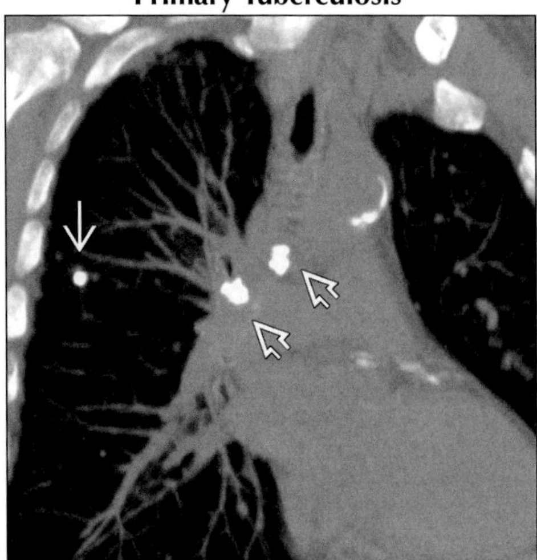

Primary Tuberculosis

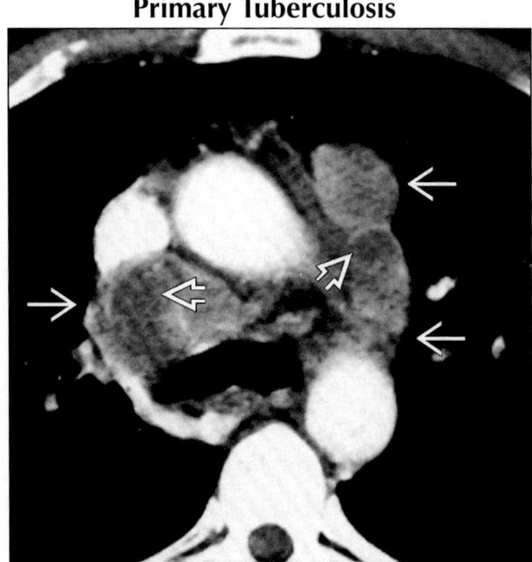

(Left) *Coronal NECT shows a calcified right upper lobe pulmonary nodule (Ghon focus) ➡ and calcified right hilar lymphadenopathy ➡. These findings represent the residua of a primary tuberculous infection. Such patients are typically not symptomatic or infectious.* ***(Right)*** *Axial CECT shows bilateral mediastinal lymphadenopathy in the right paratracheal and prevascular regions ➡. Note peripheral rim enhancement and hypodense necrotic center ➡.*

Fungal Infection

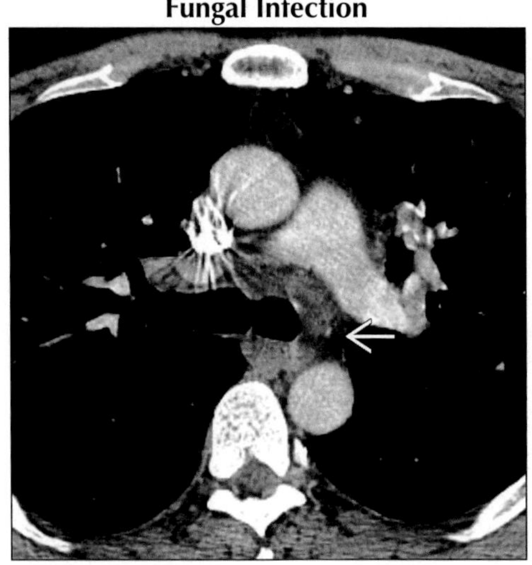

Fungal Infection

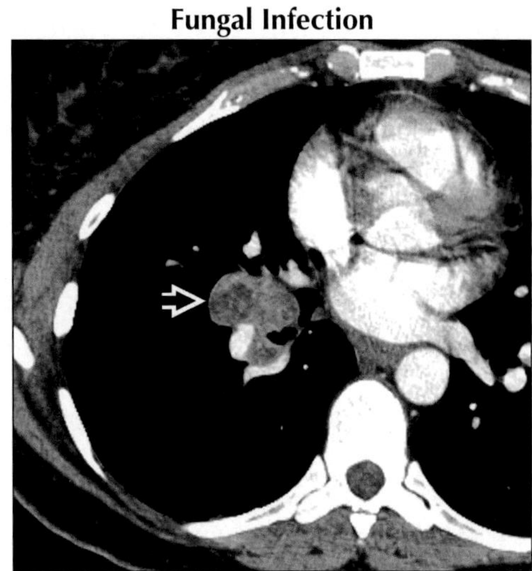

(Left) *Axial CECT shows mild generalized mediastinal and bilateral hilar lymphadenopathy ➡ in a young man with coccidioidomycosis.* ***(Right)*** *Axial CECT shows heterogeneous right hilar adenopathy ➡ in a young woman with histoplasmosis. A primary pulmonary site of infection is not always identified. These necrotic nodes often will heal with calcification.*

Sarcoidosis

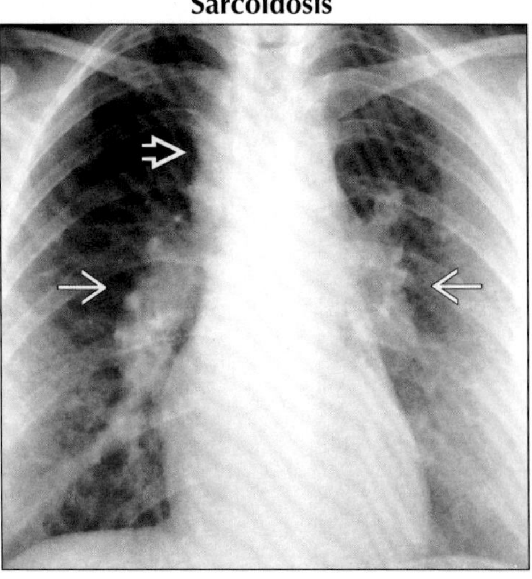

Chronic Heart Failure

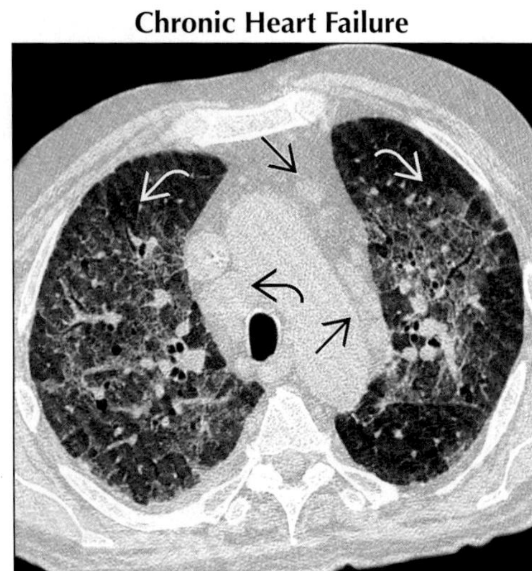

(Left) *Frontal radiograph shows enlarged bilateral hila with lobulated contours ➡ and right paratracheal lymphadenopathy ➡. This is the classic appearance of the Garland triad, which may be the only radiographic evidence of sarcoidosis.* ***(Right)*** *Axial HRCT shows bilateral diffuse ground-glass opacification in the nondependent upper lobes ➡. Note associated mild but diffuse right paratracheal ➡ and prevascular ➡ mediastinal lymphadenopathy.*

Berylliosis

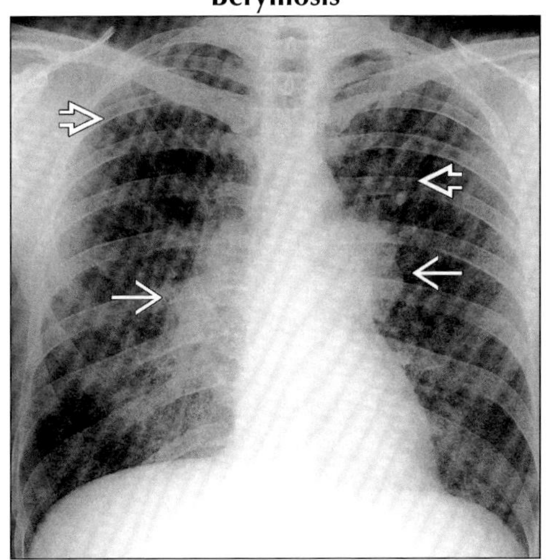

Silicosis

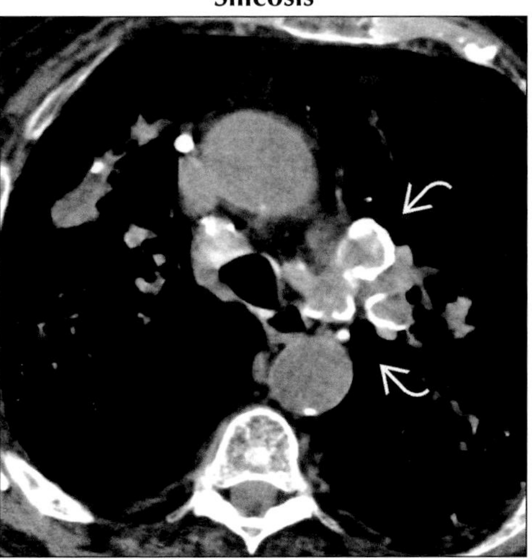

(Left) *Frontal radiograph shows typical radiographic features of diffuse interstitial lung disease due to berylliosis. Note bilateral hilar adenopathy* → *and diffuse nodular interstitial thickening* ⇨ *more profuse in the upper lung zones.* ***(Right)*** *Axial NECT shows multiple mediastinal lymph nodes with eggshell calcification* ↷ *in a patient with silicosis. Differential diagnosis includes sarcoidosis, berylliosis, or treated Hodgkin lymphoma.*

Amyloidosis

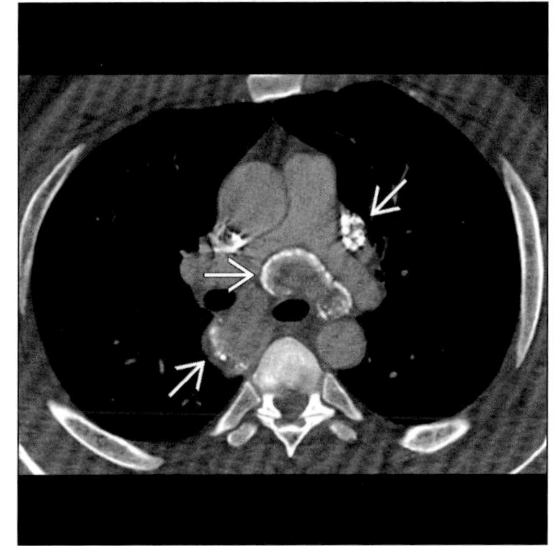

Amyloidosis

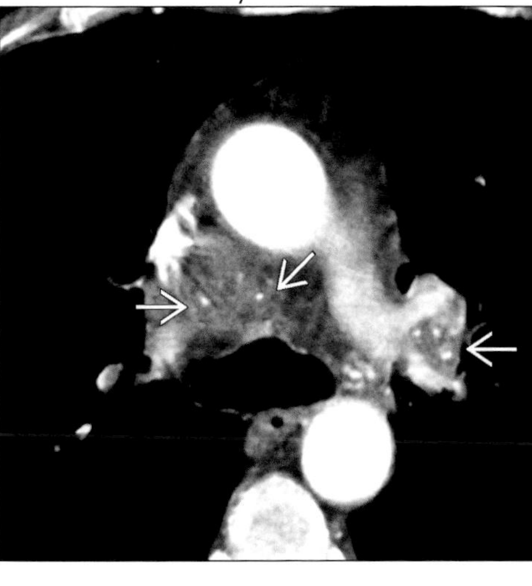

(Left) *Axial NECT shows multiple enlarged mediastinal lymph nodes that have rim calcification* →*. In this case, the lungs and airways were normal.* ***(Right)*** *Axial CECT shows bilateral hilar and mediastinal lymphadenopathy. Note associated multiple punctate calcifications* →*. In this case, the lungs and airways were also normal. Amyloidosis was confirmed by biopsy.*

Castleman Disease

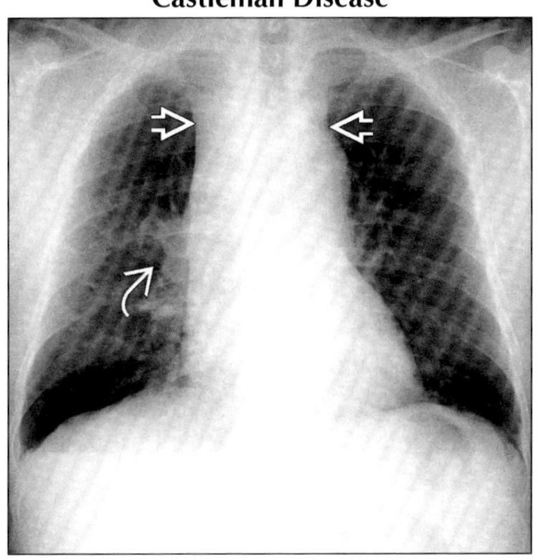

Castleman Disease

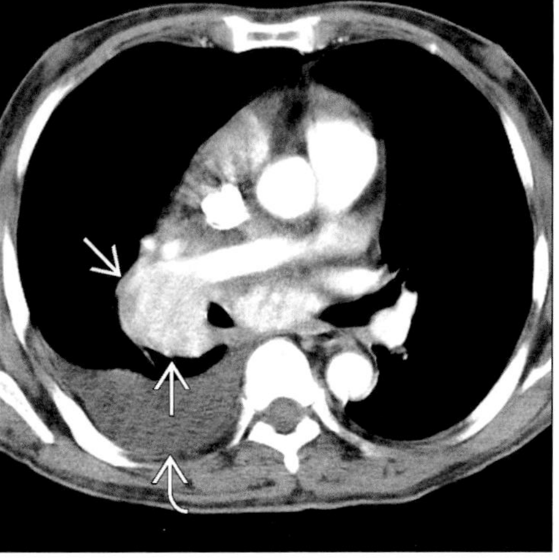

(Left) *Frontal radiograph shows diffuse mediastinal widening* ⇨ *and a right hilar enlargement* ↷*.* ***(Right)*** *Axial CECT of the same patient shows multiple avidly enhancing large right hilar and subcarinal lymph nodes* → *of Castleman disease, also called giant lymph node hyperplasia. Right pleural effusion* ↷ *is also present. The plasma cell variant of Castleman disease was demonstrated on biopsy.*

RETROTRACHEAL SPACE MASS

DIFFERENTIAL DIAGNOSIS

Common

- Vascular Anomalies
  - Aberrant Right Subclavian
  - Aberrant Left Subclavian
  - Double Aortic Arch
- Substernal Goiter
- Esophageal Disorders
  - Zenker Diverticulum
  - Achalasia
  - Foreign Body

Less Common

- Tracheal or Esophageal Masses
  - Esophageal Carcinoma
  - Esophageal Leiomyoma
  - Tracheal Neoplasms
- Nerve Sheath Tumors

Rare but Important

- Mediastinal Cysts

ESSENTIAL INFORMATION

Key Differential Diagnosis Issues

- Retrotracheal space
  - Lateral examination: Triangular area of lucency bounded
    - Posteriorly by spine (1st 4 thoracic vertebra)
    - Inferiorly by top of aortic arch
    - Anteriorly by posterior wall of trachea
    - Superiorly by thoracic inlet
  - Trachea is straight; convex bowing anteriorly is considered abnormal
  - Also known as Raider triangle after radiologist Louis Raider who originally described radiographic significance
  - Lesions in retrotracheal space may not be evident on frontal radiographs
    - Lesions may widen or disrupt posterior junction line
  - Lesions of retrotracheal space arise from normal contents
    - Esophagus, trachea, lymph nodes, lung, nerves (left recurrent laryngeal nerve, vagus nerve), thoracic duct
- Posterior tracheal band (or tracheoesophageal stripe)
  - Vertically oriented linear opacity < 4.5 mm in thickness (usually < 3 mm thickness)
  - Visible on lateral radiograph in 50%
  - Extends from thoracic inlet to carina
  - Components: Posterior tracheal wall, anterior esophageal wall, and mediastinal soft tissue
  - Tracheoesophageal stripe (TES) vs. posterior tracheal band (PTB); TES if
    - Stripe contains vertical fat radiolucency
    - Stripe passes below azygos arch

Helpful Clues for Common Diagnoses

- **Aberrant Right Subclavian**
  - Most common major aortic anomaly (0.5% of population)
  - Arises as last branch from left aortic arch
  - Origin often widened and known as diverticulum of Kommerell
    - Represents remnant of primitive distal right aortic arch
    - Seen in 60%
    - Aneurysmal when > 4 cm in diameter
  - Associated abnormalities
    - Congenital heart disease (CHD): Conotruncal anomalies, ventricular septal defects
    - Down syndrome with CHD; 37% have aberrant right subclavian
  - Surgical implications
    - Anomalous recurrent laryngeal nerve (nonrecurrent laryngeal nerve)
    - Thoracic duct may terminate on right
  - Most patients asymptomatic
  - Most common problem: Dysphagia (lusoria) from esophageal compression
- **Aberrant Left Subclavian**
  - Arises as last branch from right aortic arch
  - Most common type of right aortic arch (0.05% of population)
  - Associated abnormalities
    - Tetralogy of Fallot (70%)
    - Atrial septal defect or ventricular septal defect (20%)
    - Coarctation of aorta (7%)
- **Double Aortic Arch**
  - Most common vascular ring
  - Rarely associated with congenital heart disease
  - Results in tracheal &/or esophageal compression
  - Right arch is larger and positioned higher than left
- **Substernal Goiter**
  - Represents up to 7% of mediastinal tumors

- Usually has tracheal deviation on frontal radiograph
- Posterior to trachea (25%), predominant on right side
- Calcification in 25%
- High attenuation at CT due to natural iodine

- **Zenker Diverticulum**
  - Pulsion diverticulum at pharyngoesophageal junction
  - Descends into retrotracheal space posterior to trachea and esophagus
  - Size variable (0.5-8 cm)
  - May contain air or air-fluid level
  - May have findings of chronic aspiration
- **Achalasia**
  - Primary motility disorder of smooth muscle or secondary (e.g., Chagas disease)
  - Esophageal dilatation, usually marked, with air-fluid level in upper esophagus
  - CT: Smooth narrowing of distal esophagus
  - Smooth symmetric wall thickening (< 10 mm); any asymmetric thickening or frank mass consider carcinoma (pseudoachalasia)
- **Foreign Body**
  - Most common site of chronic esophageal foreign body is upper esophagus at level of thoracic inlet
  - Coins: Seen en face frontal and in profile on lateral views
  - CT useful for complications (perforation or abscess), may also be useful for nonradiopaque foreign body

Helpful Clues for Less Common Diagnoses

- **Esophageal Carcinoma and Leiomyoma**
  - Most common tumors of esophagus
  - Widening of tracheoesophageal stripe and presence of air-fluid level most common findings
- **Tracheal Neoplasms**
  - Rare, 2/3 either squamous cell carcinoma or adenoid cystic carcinoma
  - Adenoid cystic carcinoma more common in proximal 1/2 of trachea
  - May have either focal mass of tracheal wall or diffuse thickening of PTB
- **Nerve Sheath Tumors**
  - Neurofibroma or schwannoma
  - May occur along any peripheral nerve
  - In retrotracheal space: Recurrent laryngeal nerve, vagus nerve, phrenic nerve

Helpful Clues for Rare Diagnoses

- **Mediastinal Cysts**
  - Includes bronchogenic cysts, esophageal duplication cysts, thymic cysts, and thoracic duct cysts
  - None primarily located in region of retrotracheal space
  - Thoracic duct cyst
    - Rare, expands with fatty meals
    - Thin-walled, low-attenuation fluid characteristic

Aberrant Right Subclavian

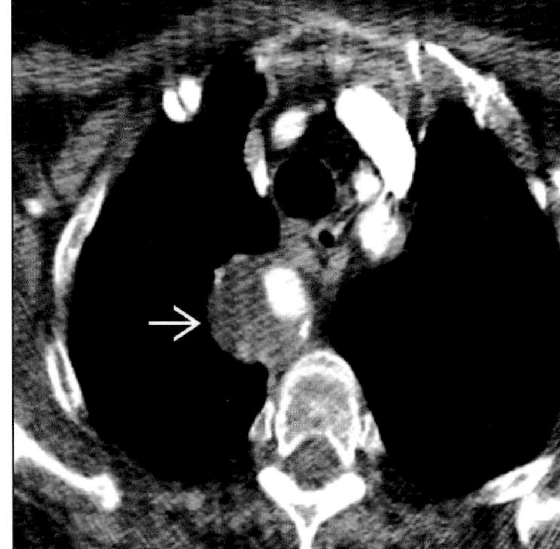

Axial CECT in the same patient shows partially thrombosed aneurysmal dilatation of diverticulum of Kommerell ➔.

Aberrant Right Subclavian

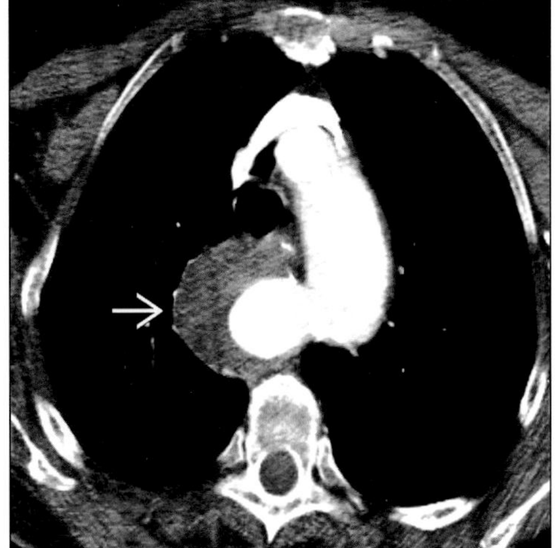

Axial CECT more inferiorly shows partially thrombosed aneurysmal diverticulum of Kommerell ➔. The diverticulum of Kommerell may become aneurysmal or may be site of dissection.

RETROTRACHEAL SPACE MASS

*(**Left**) Lateral radiograph shows a large mass in Raider triangle. Note that the trachea is bowed anteriorly. The most common cause of mass in retrotracheal triangle is aberrant right subclavian artery. (**Right**) Frontal radiograph shows a right paratracheal mass. There is no posterior junction line.*

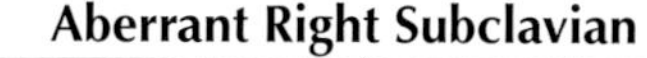

Aberrant Right Subclavian

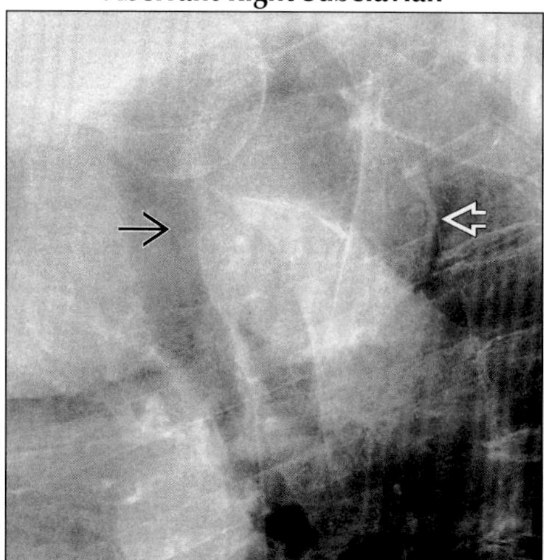

Aberrant Right Subclavian

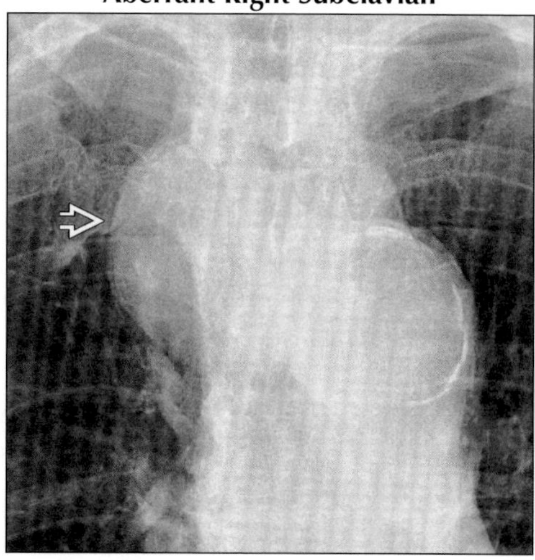

*(**Left**) Axial CECT shows left subclavian artery and dilated esophagus. (**Right**) Axial CECT more inferiorly shows right aortic arch and dilated aberrant left subclavian artery. Origin of aberrant artery is known as diverticulum of Kommerell. This patient suffered from dysphagia, known as dysphagia lusoria.*

Aberrant Left Subclavian

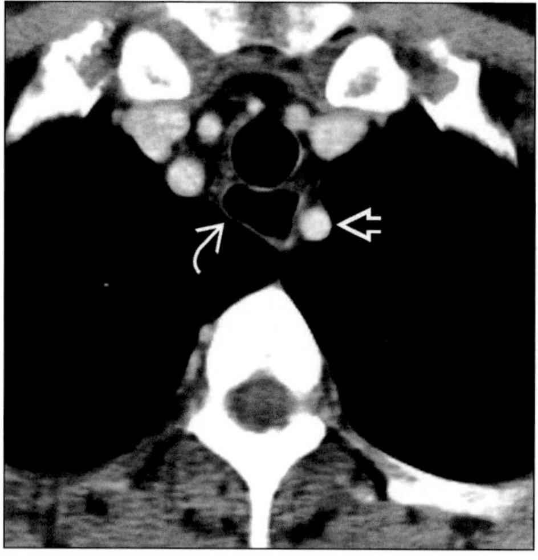

Aberrant Left Subclavian

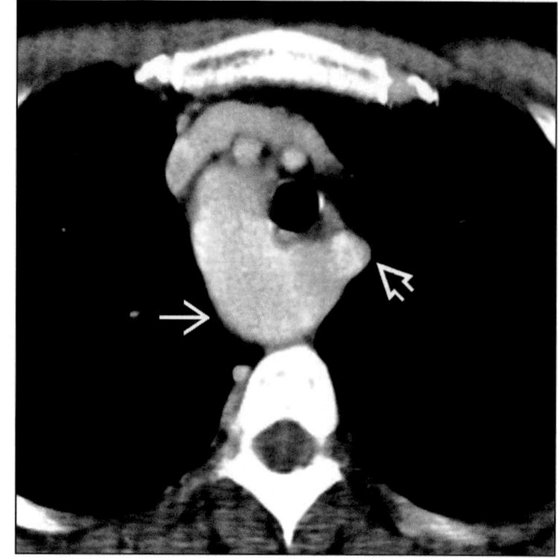

*(**Left**) Frontal radiograph shows a right paratracheal mass and what appears to be a small left aortic arch. (**Right**) Lateral radiograph shows a large mass in retrotracheal space. Trachea is slightly bowed anteriorly. Note that on both the frontal and lateral radiograph the tracheal caliber seems normal.*

Aberrant Left Subclavian

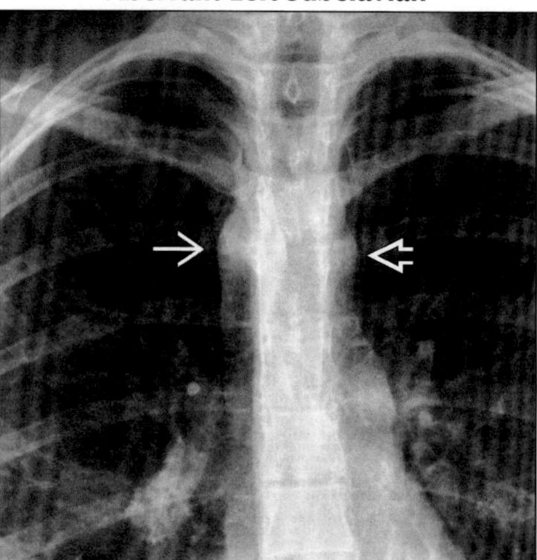

Aberrant Left Subclavian

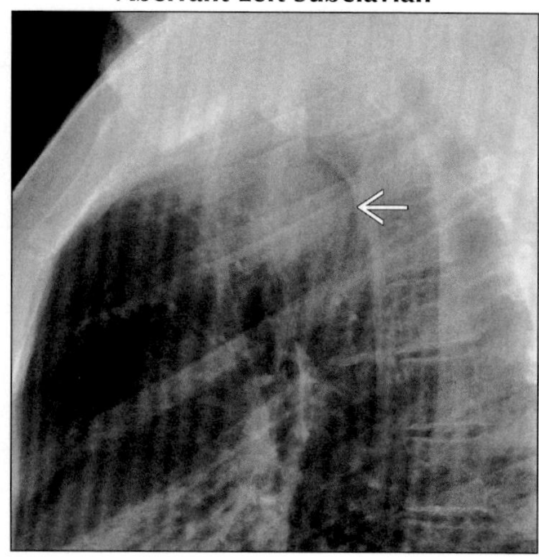

Aberrant Left Subclavian

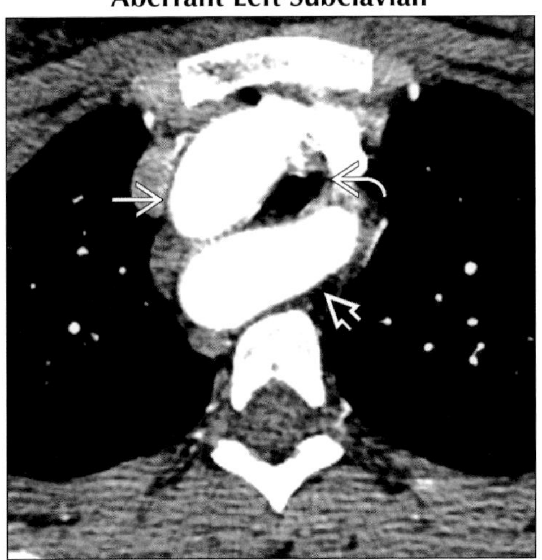

Aberrant Left Subclavian

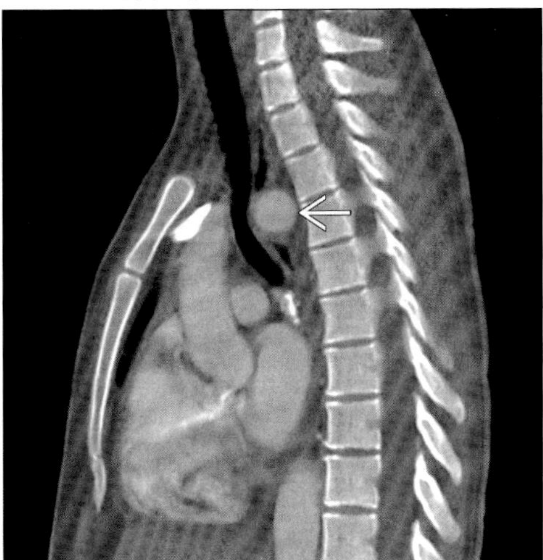

(Left) *Axial CECT in the same patient shows right aortic arch →, aberrant left subclavian artery →, and tracheal compression →. Symptoms of tracheal compression occur once the lumen is decreased 50%.* ***(Right)*** *Sagittal CECT reconstruction shows tracheal compression by aberrant left subclavian artery →. Long-term tracheal compression may lead to tracheomalacia of the compressed segment.*

Substernal Goiter

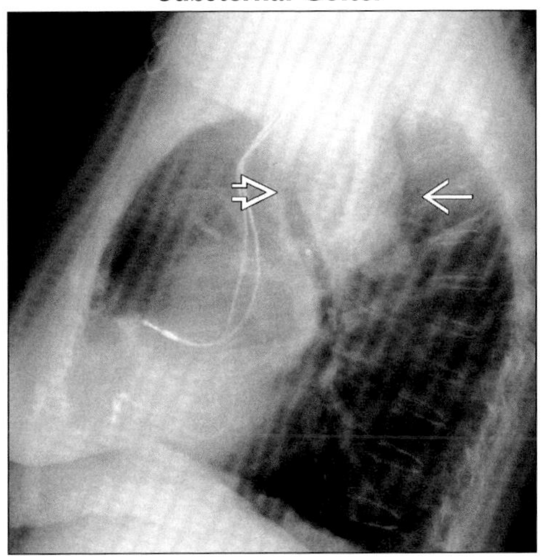

Substernal Goiter

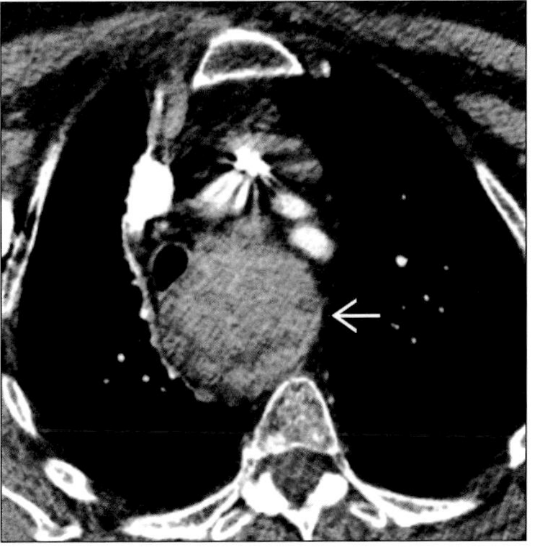

(Left) *Lateral radiograph shows a large mass → in the retrotracheal triangle. The trachea is bowed anteriorly →.* ***(Right)*** *Axial CECT shows a high-density heterogeneous mass arising from enlarged thyroid → and extending posteriorly into the retrotracheal space. Goiters can usually be visually traced to more cephalad thyroid tissue.*

Zenker Diverticulum

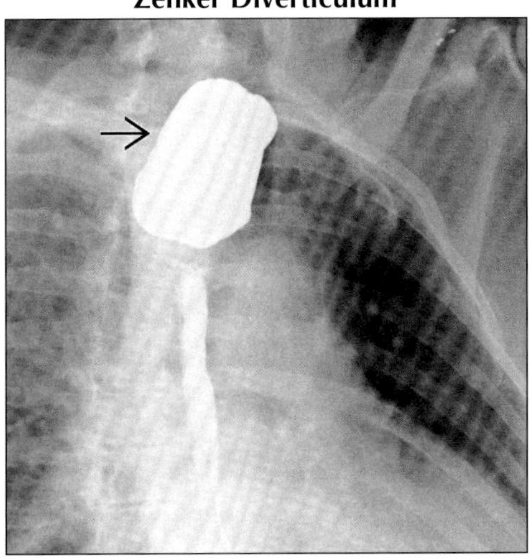

Zenker Diverticulum

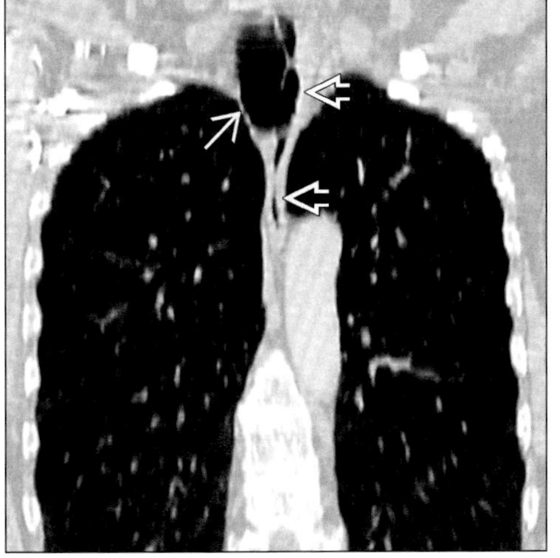

(Left) *Coronal oblique esophagram shows typical esophagram features of Zenker diverticulum. Note the barium-filled diverticulum → posterior to the trachea.* ***(Right)*** *Coronal NECT shows thin-walled, air-filled right paratracheal mass representing a Zenker diverticulum →, which communicates with the esophagus →.*

RETROTRACHEAL SPACE MASS

(Left) Lateral radiograph shows a large mass ➡ in the retrotracheal space. Trachea is bowed anteriorly ⇨. *(Right)* Frontal esophagram shows barium-filled Zenker diverticulum ➡ as the cause of the mass. Zenker may be fluid-filled, air-filled, or have an air-fluid level. Large Zenker diverticula often have signs of aspiration.

Zenker Diverticulum

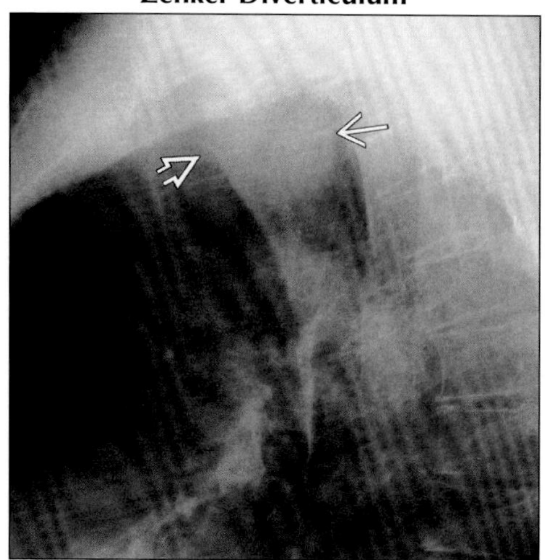

Zenker Diverticulum

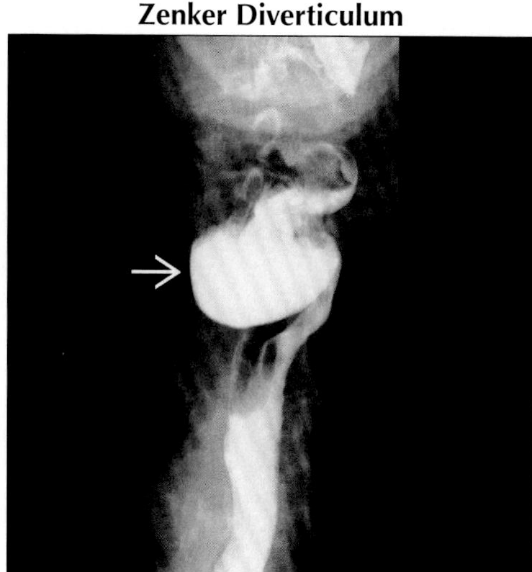

(Left) Lateral radiograph shows a mass in retrotracheal space. The mass contains some residual barium ➡. *(Right)* Axial CECT shows a contrast-filled mass ⇨ posterior to the trachea and esophagus ➡. Large Zenker diverticulum may lead to recurrent aspiration. Contrast-filled diverticulum has to be distinguished from large aortic aneurysm.

Zenker Diverticulum

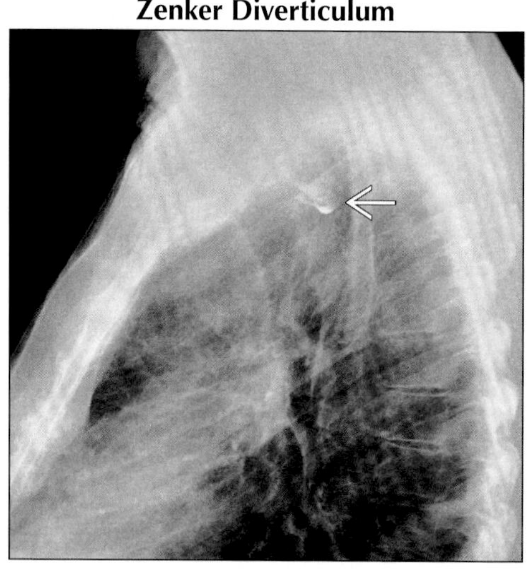

Zenker Diverticulum

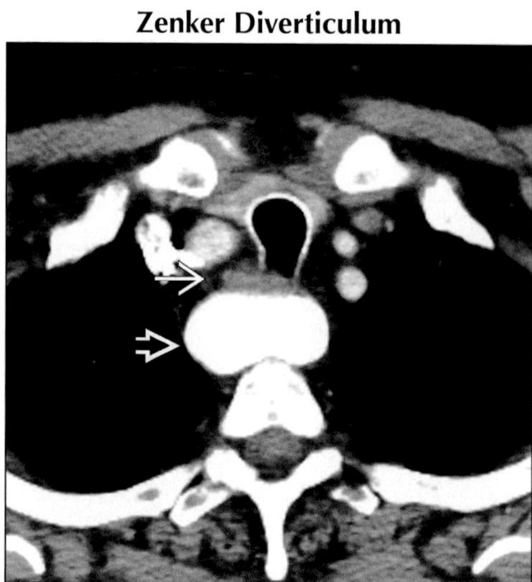

(Left) Lateral radiograph shows marked thickening of the tracheoesophageal stripe ⇨ that is 6 mm in width. Notice that the trachea is slightly bowed anteriorly. *(Right)* Frontal esophagram shows dilated esophagus from achalasia ➡. Air-fluid level is common with achalasia. Absence of gas in the stomach bubble also characteristic.

Achalasia

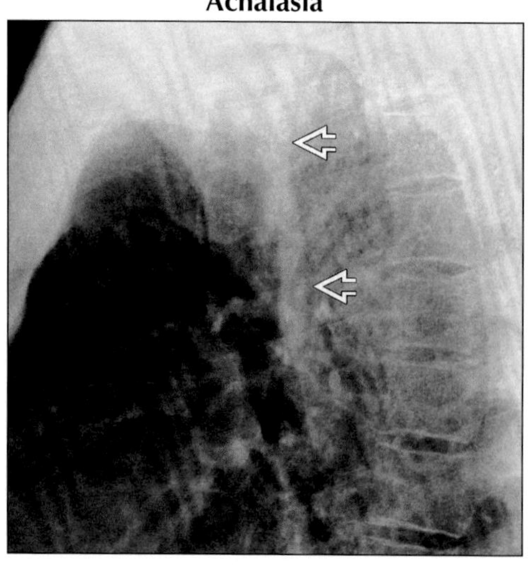

Achalasia

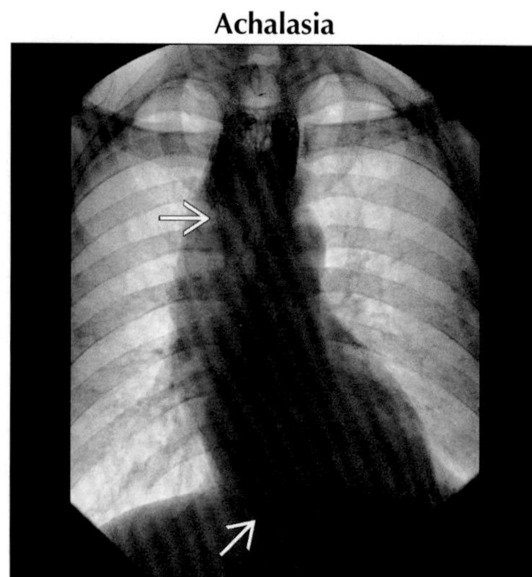

Foreign Body

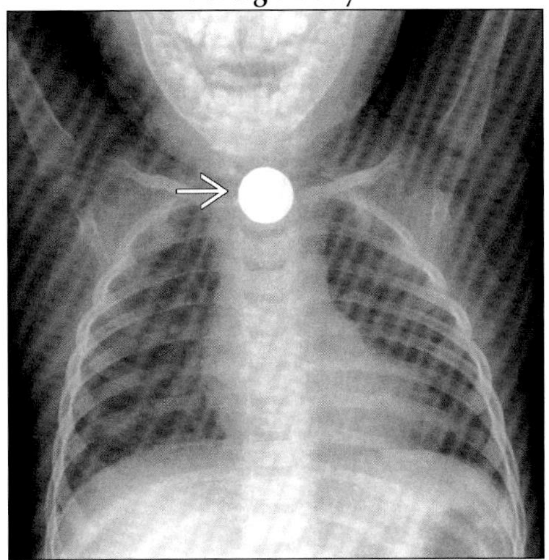

Foreign Body

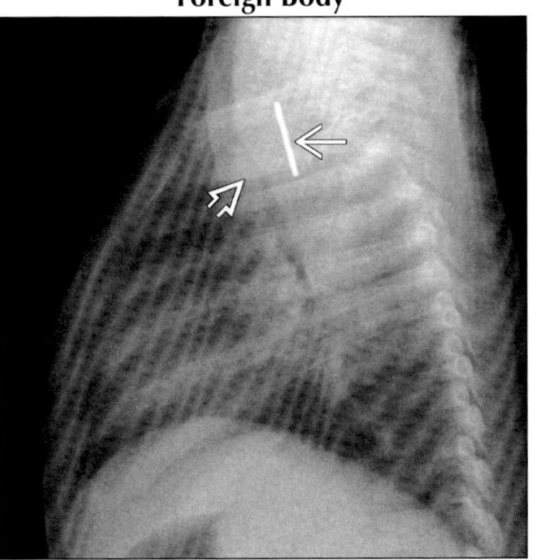

*(**Left**) Anteroposterior radiograph shows an en face coin ➡ lodged at the thoracic inlet. (**Right**) Lateral radiograph shows a coin ➡ in the retrotracheal space. Notice the marked airway narrowing ⇨ from the adjacent inflammatory reaction related to the chronic foreign body.*

Esophageal Carcinoma

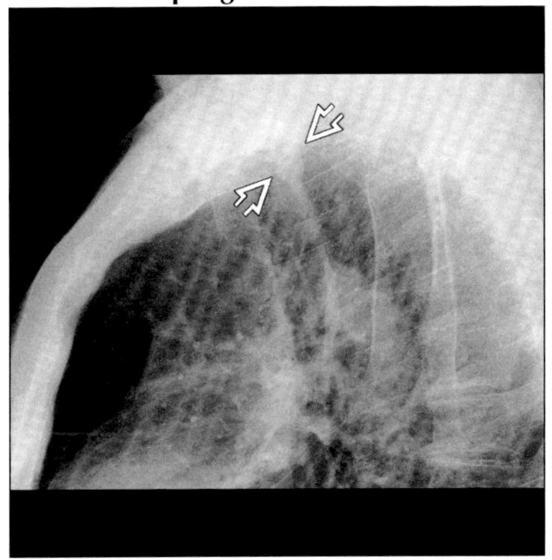

Esophageal Carcinoma

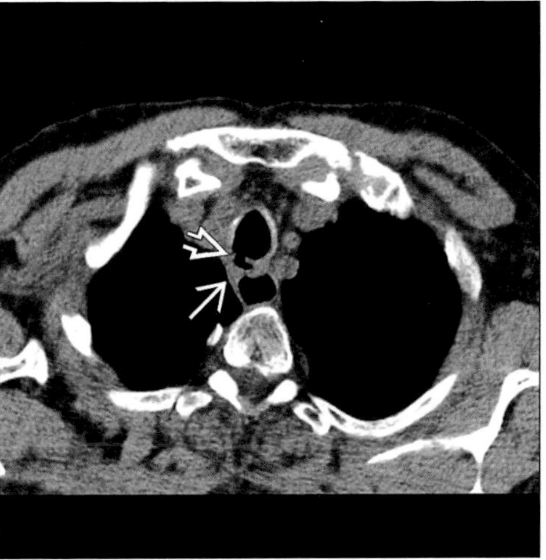

*(**Left**) Lateral radiograph shows a subtle mass ⇨ focally thickening the posterior wall of the trachea in the retrotracheal triangle. (**Right**) Axial NECT shows soft tissue thickening of the posterior wall of the trachea and anterior esophageal wall ➡. Note the fistulous tract ⇨. Diagnosis was an esophageal carcinoma. Esophageal tumors are more common than primary or secondary tracheal tumors.*

Nerve Sheath Tumors

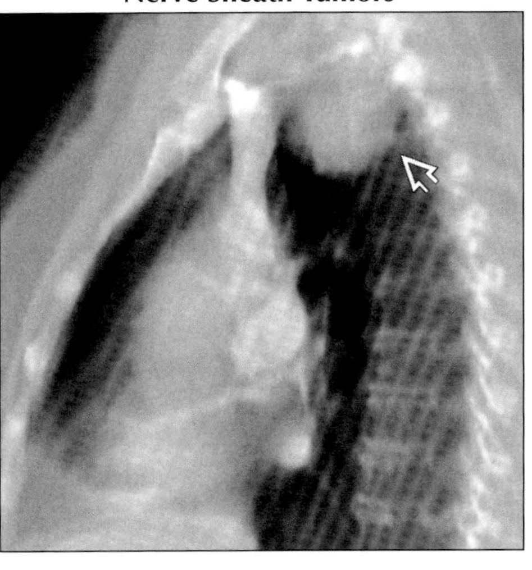

Nerve Sheath Tumors

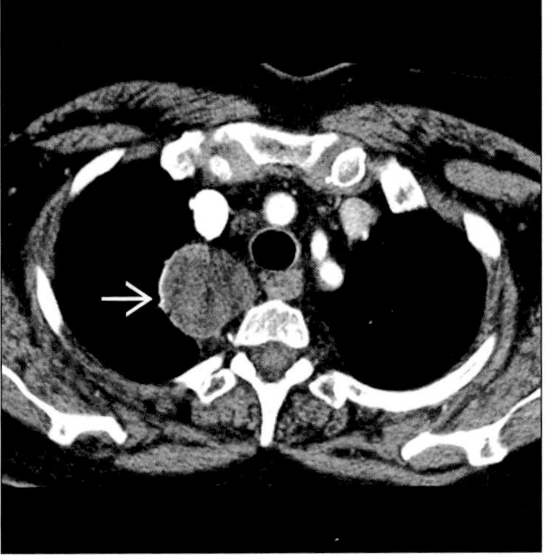

*(**Left**) Sagittal CECT reconstruction shows a large mass ⇨ in retrotracheal triangle. (**Right**) Axial CECT shows a low-density mass ➡ in the right superior mediastinum. Mass was a schwannoma. Nerve sheath tumors may have decreased attenuation due either to lipid or cystic degeneration. Calcification is seen in 10% of schwannomas. Nerve sheath tumors may have variable contrast enhancement.*

RETROCARDIAC MASS

DIFFERENTIAL DIAGNOSIS

Common

- Hiatal Hernia
- Descending Aortic Aneurysm
- Tortuosity (Aging) of Aorta
- Mediastinal Lymphadenopathy
- Postoperative State, Esophagus

Less Common

- Pulsion Esophageal Diverticulum
- Periesophageal Omental Hernia
- Achalasia
- Esophageal Perforation
- Paraesophageal Varices
- Benign Esophageal Tumors
- Esophageal Malignant Neoplasms
  - Carcinoma
  - Primary Esophageal Lymphoma
- Cystic Masses
  - Bronchogenic Cyst
  - Esophageal Duplication Cyst

Rare but Important

- Mediastinal Pancreatic Pseudocyst

ESSENTIAL INFORMATION

Key Differential Diagnosis Issues

- Retrocardiac mass with air-fluid level is characteristic of esophageal hiatal hernia
- Esophageal disorders may present radiographically as retrocardiac masses
- Should always consider vascular aneurysm
  - Aortic aneurysm may result in anterior, middle, or posterior mediastinum
  - Mediastinal mass with curvilinear calcification

Helpful Clues for Common Diagnoses

- **Hiatal Hernia**
  - Sliding hiatal hernia: Most common type
  - May be large containing stomach and portions of colon
  - Chest radiograph: Characteristic retrocardiac mass with or without air-fluid level
  - Widening of esophageal hiatus
- **Descending Aortic Aneurysm**
  - Focal or diffuse left paramediastinal or posterior mediastinal mass
  - Calcification in aneurysm wall (75%)
  - CECT: Allows accurate assessment of complications
  - MR: Similar to CT in diagnosis of aortic aneurysms
- **Tortuosity (Aging) of Aorta**
  - Increased prevalence in elderly population
- **Mediastinal Lymphadenopathy**
  - Common causes: Lymphoma, lymphocytic leukemia, metastases, and granulomatous infections
  - Giant lymph node hyperplasia (Castleman disease): Marked enhancement of single enlarged mediastinal lymph node group
- **Postoperative State, Esophagus**
  - Esophagectomy with gastric pull-up procedure
    - Gastric conduit is usually placed in paravertebral space of posterior mediastinum
  - Postsurgical complications
    - Postsurgical diaphragmatic hernia (omental fat ± colon)
    - Redundant conduit (excess length of gastric tube)
    - Mediastinitis due to anastomotic leak

Helpful Clues for Less Common Diagnoses

- **Pulsion Esophageal Diverticulum**
  - Large sac-like protrusion in epiphrenic region
  - Retrocardiac soft tissue mass often containing air-fluid level
- **Periesophageal Omental Hernia**
  - Omentum herniates through phrenicoesophageal ligament
  - Mimics lipomatous mediastinal tumor or esophageal lipoma
- **Achalasia**
  - Double contour of mediastinal borders: Outer borders of dilated esophagus project beyond shadows of aorta and heart
  - Dilatation of esophagus
  - Retained fluid, food debris, and air-fluid level
  - Aspiration pneumonia common
- **Esophageal Perforation**
  - Iatrogenic: Endoscopic procedures (80%-90%), trauma: Blunt trauma, foreign bodies: Impacted bones, spontaneous: Boerhaave syndrome, and neoplasms
    - Mediastinal fluid collections

- Extravasation of contrast medium into mediastinum
- Extraesophageal air (92%)

- **Paraesophageal Varices**
  - Right- or left-sided mediastinal soft tissue masses near diaphragm
  - Change in size and shape with peristalsis, respiration, and Valsalva maneuvers
  - CECT: Serpiginous contrast-enhanced structures
  - T1WI and T2WI MR: Multiple areas of flow void
- **Benign Esophageal Tumors**
  - Leiomyoma
    - Most frequent benign tumor of esophagus (distal esophagus)
    - Size: 2 cm to > 10 cm
    - Round/ovoid filling defect, outlined by barium
    - Amorphous or punctate calcifications
  - Esophageal GIST (GI stromal cell tumors)
    - Large mass
    - May ulcerate with gas and contrast medium entering cavity
- **Esophageal Malignant Neoplasms**
  - **Carcinoma**
    - Obscuration of periesophageal fat planes
    - Lobulated and irregular margins
    - Periesophageal and upper abdominal lymphadenopathy
  - **Primary Esophageal Lymphoma**
    - Less than 1% of all malignant esophageal neoplasms
    - Polypoid, ulcerated, and infiltrative
- **Cystic Masses**
  - **Bronchogenic Cyst**
    - Round, oval masses usually in right paratracheal or subcarinal region
    - CECT: Homogeneous water density mass with thin smooth wall (50%); indistinguishable from soft tissue lesions (50%)
    - MR: Homogeneous low signal intensity on T1WI and high signal intensity on T2WI
  - **Esophageal Duplication Cyst**
    - Majority occur in infants or children
    - Adjacent to or within esophageal wall
    - Ectopic gastric mucosa within cyst: May cause hemorrhage or perforation
    - CT or MR: Homogeneous water density mass in intimate contact with esophagus

Helpful Clues for Rare Diagnoses

- **Mediastinal Pancreatic Pseudocyst**
  - Location: 1/3 juxta- or intrasplenic, retroperitoneum, and mediastinum
  - Develops over a short time in patients with evidence of pancreatitis
  - NECT: Low-attenuation spherical or oblong mass in posterior mediastinum or adjacent thoracic cavity
  - CECT: Enhancement of thin fibrous capsule

Hiatal Hernia

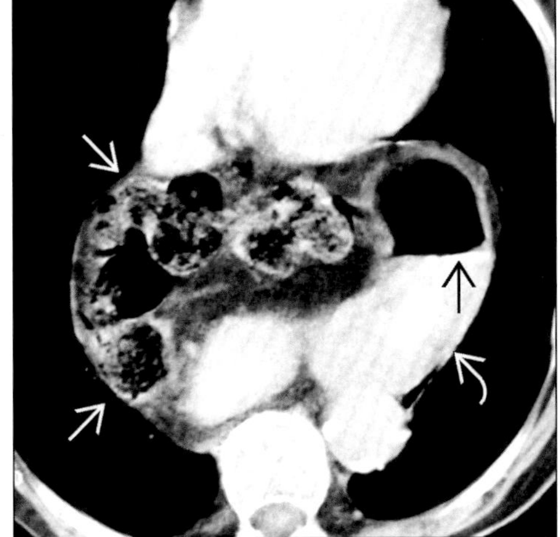

Axial CECT shows a large retrocardiac hiatal hernia containing the stomach ➔ and portions of the colon ➔. Note a visible air-fluid level within the stomach ➔.

Descending Aortic Aneurysm

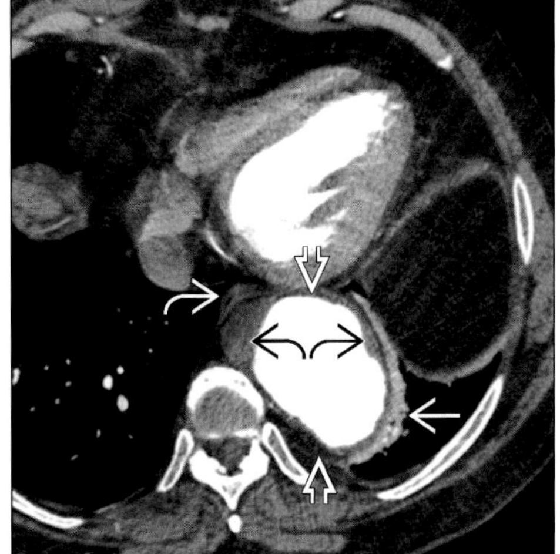

Axial CECT shows a large descending aortic aneurysm in a retrocardiac location ➔. Mural hematoma ➔ is seen. Note peripheral collapse of the LLL ➔. The esophagus is also anteriorly displaced ➔.

RETROCARDIAC MASS

(Left) Coronal CT reconstruction shows a markedly tortuous descending thoracic aorta ➔. When the distal part of the descending aorta elongates, it may manifest radiographically as a smooth, well-defined opacity in the retrocardiac area. *(Right)* Axial CECT shows retroesophageal enlarged lymph nodes ➔. The patient was a 65-year-old man with chronic lymphocytic leukemia.

Tortuosity (Aging) of Aorta

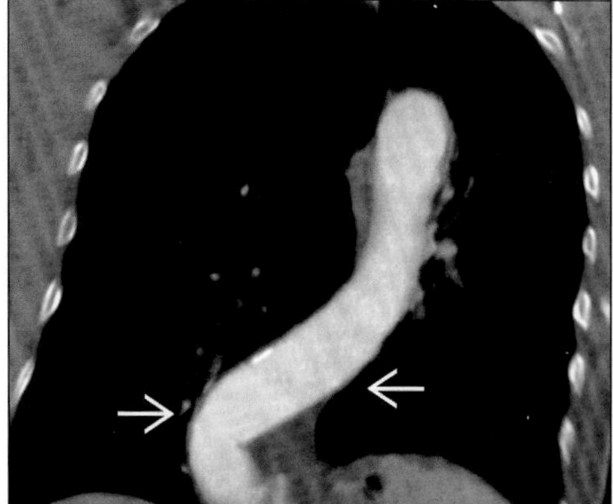

Mediastinal Lymphadenopathy

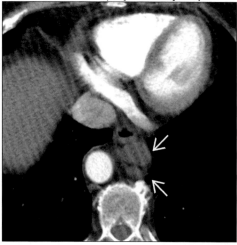

(Left) Sagittal CT reconstruction of CECT after esophagectomy shows a mildly dilated gastric conduit in the middle mediastinum ➔. Note the position of the gastric staple line ➔. Collapsed osteoporotic vertebral bodies are visible ➔. *(Right)* Sagittal CT reconstruction of NECT in an elderly patient with dysphagia and halitosis shows a large epiphrenic diverticulum ➔ containing contrast and retained food. Esophageal dysmotility is usually present.

Postoperative State, Esophagus

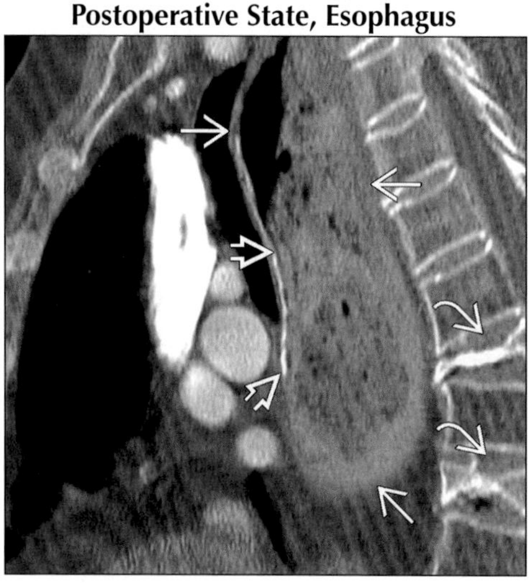

Pulsion Esophageal Diverticulum

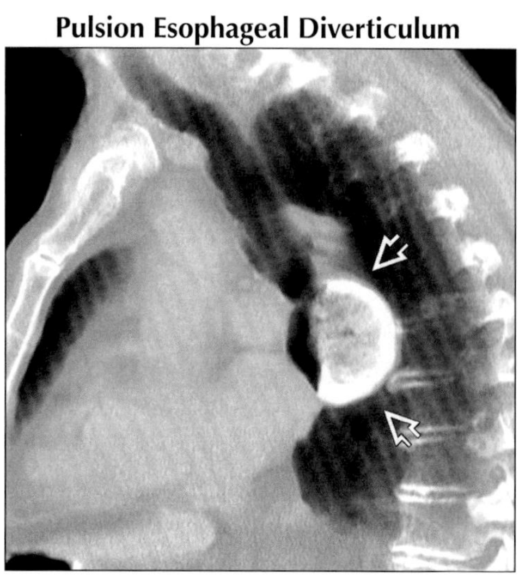

(Left) Axial CECT shows an omental hernia ➔ surrounding the distal esophagus ➔. Note small vessels within the omentum ➔. *(Right)* Axial NECT shows a large retrocardiac mass ➔ associated with luminal narrowing in the distal esophagus ➔. Findings are characteristic of infiltrating carcinoma. Focal extravasation of contrast ➔ indicates perforation/fistulization. A mediastinal paraesophageal inflammatory soft tissue mass is also visible ➔.

Periesophageal Omental Hernia

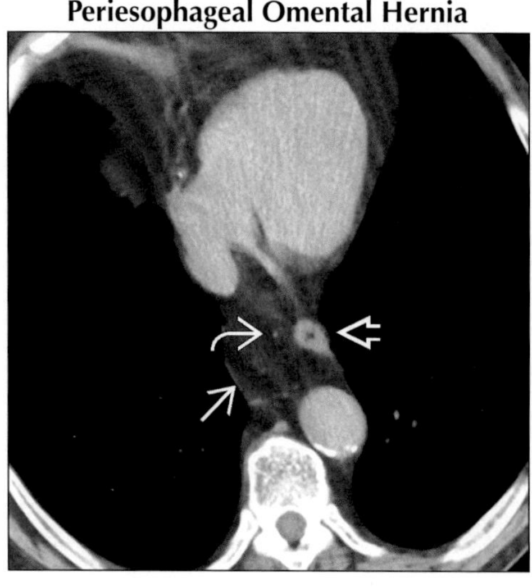

Esophageal Perforation

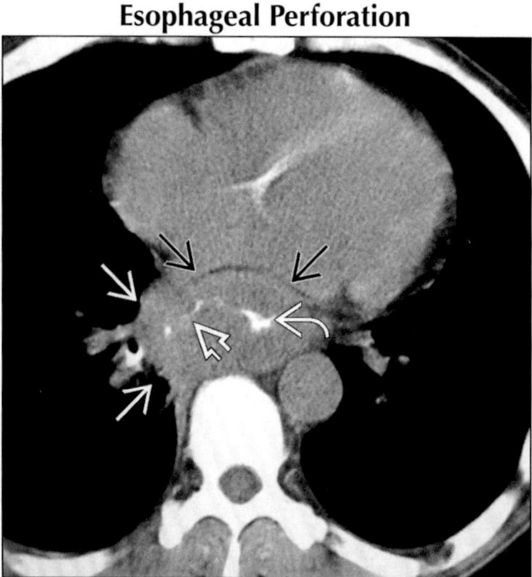

Paraesophageal Varices

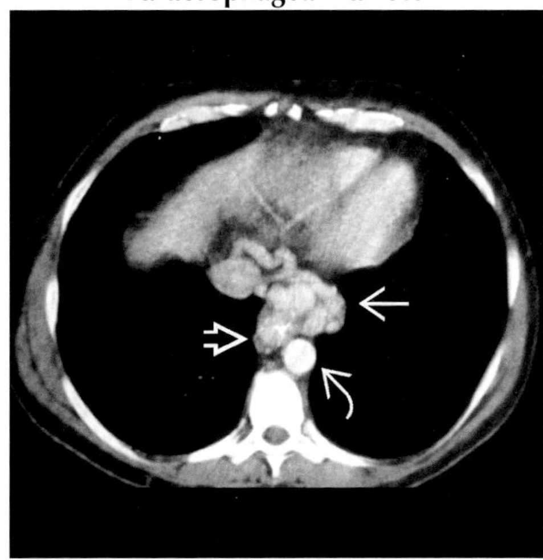

Benign Esophageal Tumors

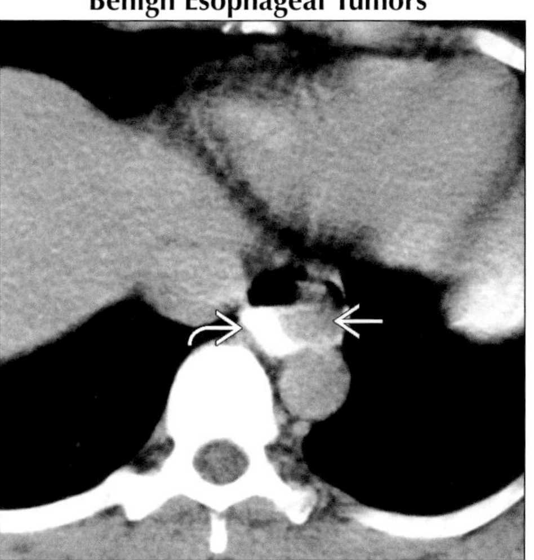

*(**Left**) Axial CECT in a 58-year-old man with upper GI bleeding shows multiple dilated, enhancing large paraesophageal varices ➡ to the left of the esophagus ➪ and anterior to the aorta ↷. (**Right**) Axial NECT in a middle-aged man with dyspepsia shows a round filling intraluminal soft tissue mass ➡ in the distal esophagus ↷. The mass was enucleated endoscopically and proved to be a benign leiomyoma.*

Primary Esophageal Lymphoma

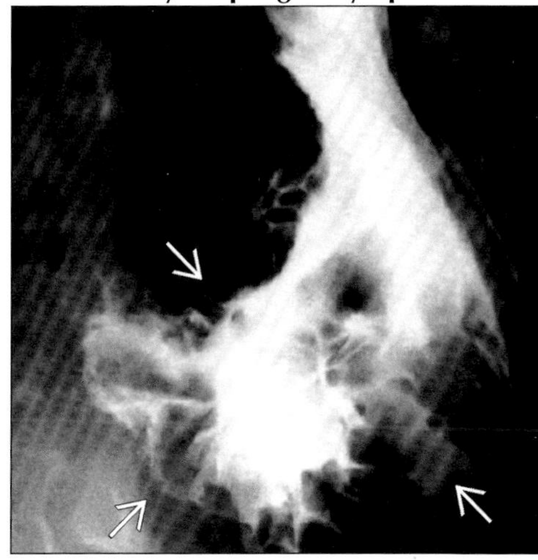

Primary Esophageal Lymphoma

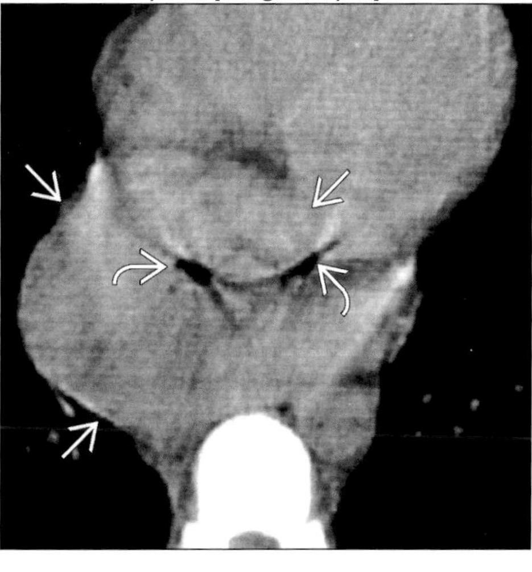

*(**Left**) Frontal esophagram in a 30-year-old man with AIDS shows a large ulcerated bulky mass in the lower 1/3 of the esophagus associated with a significant extramucosal component ➡. Patient complained of progressive retrosternal pain, dysphagia, vomiting, and mild hematemesis for 3 weeks. (**Right**) Axial NECT of the same patient shows a large bulky mass ➡ in the lower esophagus with central ulceration containing gas ↷.*

Esophageal Duplication Cyst

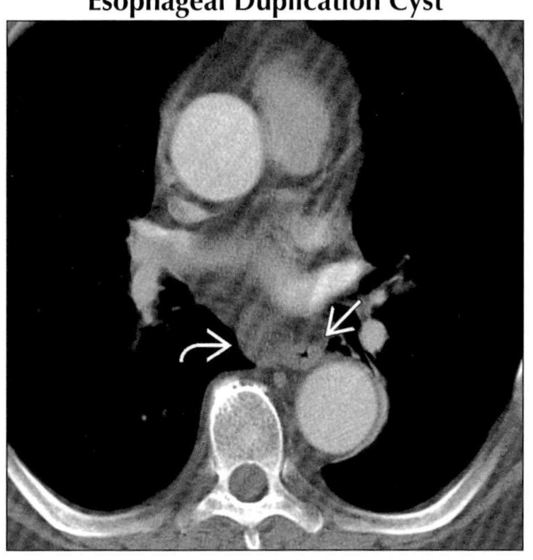

Mediastinal Pancreatic Pseudocyst

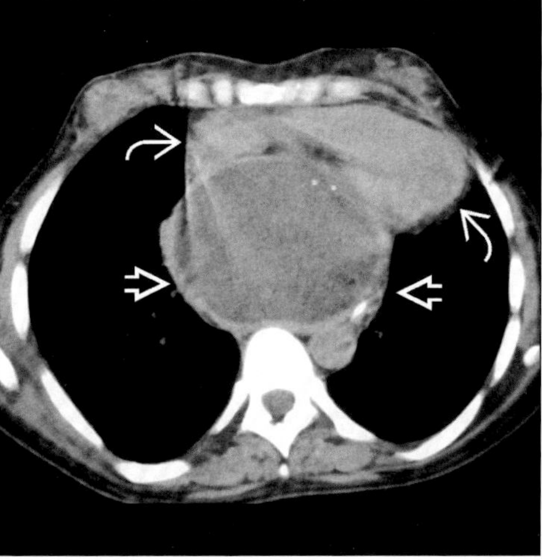

*(**Left**) Axial CECT shows the typical water attenuation of a smoothly marginated unilocular cyst ↷. Note the characteristic location adjacent to the esophagus ➡. (**Right**) Axial CECT in a 34-year-old woman with a previous history of pancreatitis shows a large cystic mass with smooth walls ➪ that displaces and compresses the heart ↷. (Courtesy N. Müller, MD.)*

LEFT COSTOVERTEBRAL ANGLE MASS

DIFFERENTIAL DIAGNOSIS

Common
- Bochdalek Hernia
- Aortic Aneurysm
- Lipoid Pneumonia
- Intralobar Sequestration
- Left Lower Lobe Collapse

Less Common
- Esophageal Varices
- Paraesophageal Hernia
- Nerve Sheath Tumors
- Sympathetic Ganglion Tumors
- Lateral Meningocele
- Esophageal Duplication Cyst

Rare but Important
- Extramedullary Hematopoiesis
- Esophageal Tear

ESSENTIAL INFORMATION

Key Differential Diagnosis Issues
- Mnemonic: **MASS IN LEFT CV**
  - **M**eningocele (lateral), **a**neurysm, **s**equestration, **s**ympathetic ganglion tumors
  - **I**ntraabdominal contents (hernias), **n**erve sheath tumors
  - **L**ipoid pneumonia, **e**xtramedullary hematopoiesis, **f**oregut malformations (esophageal duplication cyst), **t**rauma (esophageal tear)
  - **C**ollapse (left lower lobe), **v**arices

Helpful Clues for Common Diagnoses
- **Bochdalek Hernia**
  - Herniation through posteromedial pleuroperitoneal hiatus
  - Appearance depends on hernia contents and whether air is present within bowel
  - In adults: 66% left-sided, 33% right-sided; bilateral in 15%
- **Aortic Aneurysm**
  - Descending aortic aneurysm may be atherosclerotic, from dissection, mycotic, or traumatic from blunt chest trauma (pseudoaneurysm)
  - Curvilinear calcification should suggest aneurysm
  - If left pleural effusion, consider rupture
- **Lipoid Pneumonia**
  - Aspiration or inhalation of fatty or oily substances: Animal or vegetable oils, mineral oil laxatives, oil-based nose drops, and liquid paraffin
  - Chronic consolidation with low-attenuation areas (-30 to -150 HU)
  - Focal consolidation often mass-like
  - Favors dependent lung segments
- **Intralobar Sequestration**
  - Sequestration represents nonfunctioning lung tissue separated from normal lung
    - Receives its blood supply from a systemic artery, lacks normal communication with bronchi
  - Persistent left-sided (65%) paraspinal mass with history of recurrent pneumonia
  - Lung may contain solid, fluid, and cystic components (may have air-fluid level)
  - Systemic artery identification feeding lung is diagnostic
- **Left Lower Lobe Collapse**
  - Lobe collapses posteriorly, medially, and inferiorly; inferior displacement of hilum
  - Triangular paraspinal opacification silhouetting medial hemidiaphragm and descending aorta
  - In adults, must exclude endobronchial obstruction

Helpful Clues for Less Common Diagnoses
- **Esophageal Varices**
  - Secondary to portal hypertension, most commonly cirrhosis
  - Dilated, contrast-filled vessels adjacent to esophageal wall
  - May be unopacified on arterial phase imaging
  - Associated abnormalities: Cirrhotic liver, splenomegaly
- **Paraesophageal Hernia**
  - GE junction below diaphragm, gastric fundus intrathoracic
  - Protrusion usually anterior and lateral to esophagus
  - Smooth hemispherical retrocardiac mass, usually contains air or air-fluid level
  - May contain oral contrast
- **Nerve Sheath Tumors**
  - Neurofibromas or schwannomas
  - Round posterior mediastinal mass
  - Dumbbell extension into spinal canal (10%)

- Decreased attenuation due to lipid or cystic degeneration
- Calcification in 10% of schwannomas
- Variable contrast enhancement

- **Sympathetic Ganglion Tumors**
  - Age related: Neuroblastoma (< 3 years), ganglioneuroblastoma (3-10 years), ganglioneuroma (> 10 years)
  - Paragangliomas (extraadrenal pheochromocytomas) arise from sympathetic ganglia
  - Usually arise along sympathetic chain
  - Elongated vertical posterior mediastinal mass
  - Often intensely enhance with IV contrast
  - ~ 85% of neuroblastomas have calcification
- **Lateral Meningocele**
  - More common in neurofibromatosis type 1, 10% multiple
  - Right > left
  - Fluid attenuation; contiguous with thecal sac
  - Widens neural foramen, scoliosis common
  - Vertebral bodies often scalloped
  - Peripheral rim enhancement may occur
- **Esophageal Duplication Cyst**
  - Foregut malformation: Lung "bud" anomalies
  - Tubular, oriented vertically along esophagus
  - Cyst contents usually fluid: Increased attenuation may be due to mucoid, blood, or calcium oxalate contents
  - Often right-sided
  - Cyst wall may be thick and calcified
  - If ulcerated into esophagus or airway, will have air-fluid level
  - Cyst may contain gastric or pancreatic tissue that may cause hemorrhage, ulceration, or perforation

Helpful Clues for Rare Diagnoses

- **Extramedullary Hematopoiesis**
  - Associated with chronic anemias, especially sickle cell disease and thalassemia
  - Multiple lobulated posterior mediastinal masses, vertebral bodies often have prominent trabeculae (from marrow expansion)
  - Centered on vertebral bodies
  - Usually contain fat; calcification absent
  - Will enhance with contrast administration, often inhomogeneous
- **Esophageal Tear**
  - Etiology: Boerhaave syndrome, instrumentation, blunt chest trauma
  - Most common location: Left lateral wall of distal esophagus 2-3 cm above gastroesophageal junction
  - Air in left costovertebral angle (V-sign of Naclerio)
  - Associated findings: Periesophageal fluid collections, pleural effusion, consolidation or atelectasis of medial basilar segment left lower lobe
  - May have extravasation of oral contrast

Bochdalek Hernia

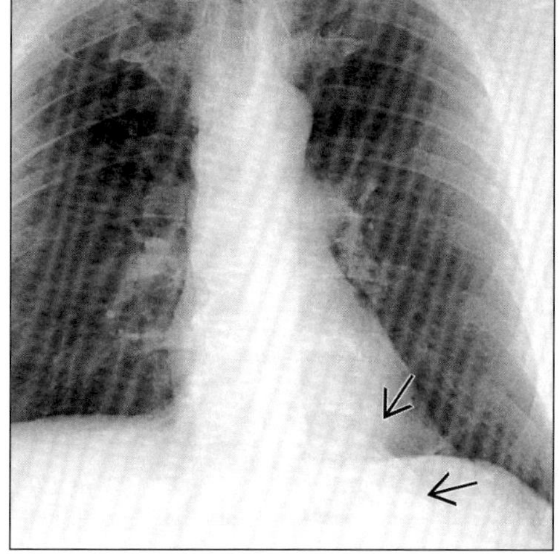

Frontal radiograph shows a well-defined left costovertebral mass ➔. Mass contains neither air nor calcification.

Bochdalek Hernia

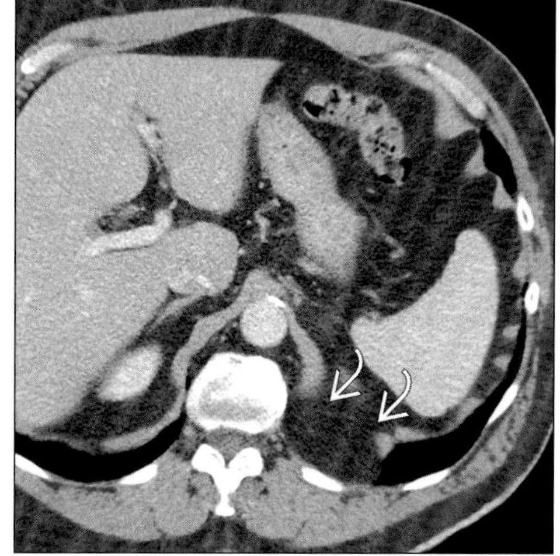

Axial CECT shows localized discontinuity of the hemidiaphragm ➔ with herniation of fat through diaphragmatic defect.

LEFT COSTOVERTEBRAL ANGLE MASS

*(**Left**) Axial CECT shows bowel and kidney ➔ in the left lower hemithorax. Diaphragmatic hernias can be very difficult to visualize on axial images only. (**Right**) Coronal CECT reconstruction shows herniation of bowel and kidney ➔ through posteromedial defect. Most Bochdalek hernias contain fat only but may contain kidney or bowel. Coronal and sagittal reconstructions are very useful for identifying diaphragmatic defects.*

Bochdalek Hernia

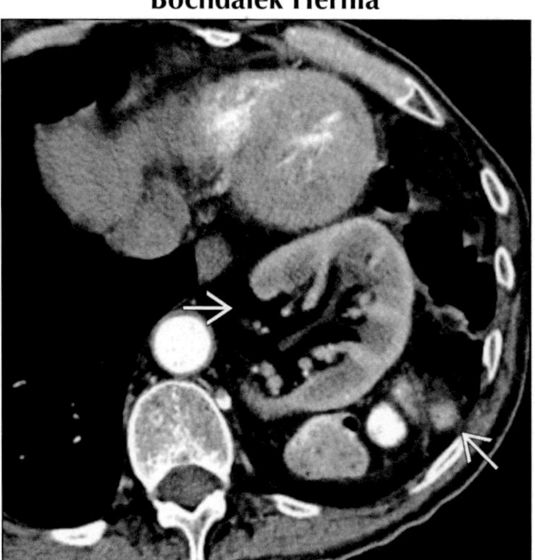

Bochdalek Hernia

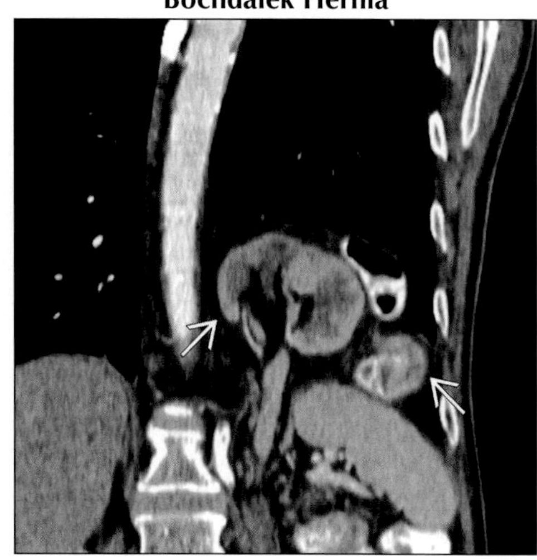

*(**Left**) Anteroposterior radiograph shows paraspinal widening ➔ in the left costovertebral angle. This patient was imaged supine on trauma board following a motor vehicle crash. (**Right**) Axial CECT shows paraspinal widening ➔ from hematoma and transection flap ➔. Traumatic aortic injury with pseudoaneurysm formation at the aortic hiatus is the 3rd most common location from blunt chest trauma, following aortic arch (isthmus) and ascending aorta.*

Aortic Aneurysm

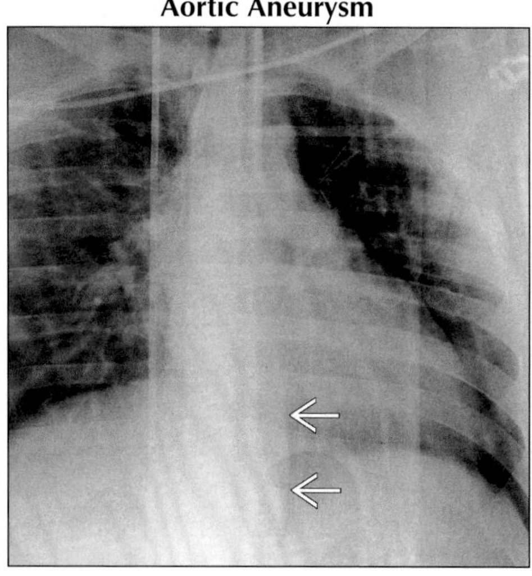

Aortic Aneurysm

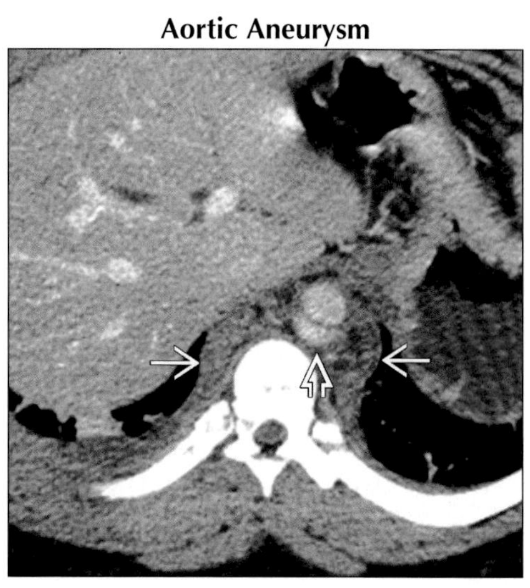

*(**Left**) Scout CECT shows focal chronic consolidation ➔ in the left lower lobe in an elderly woman. Patient took mineral oil daily for constipation. (**Right**) Axial CECT shows low-density, fat-containing consolidation ➔ in the left lower lobe from lipoid pneumonia. Lipoid pneumonia is often mass-like and may contain higher attenuation soft tissue. Patients are often asymptomatic.*

Lipoid Pneumonia

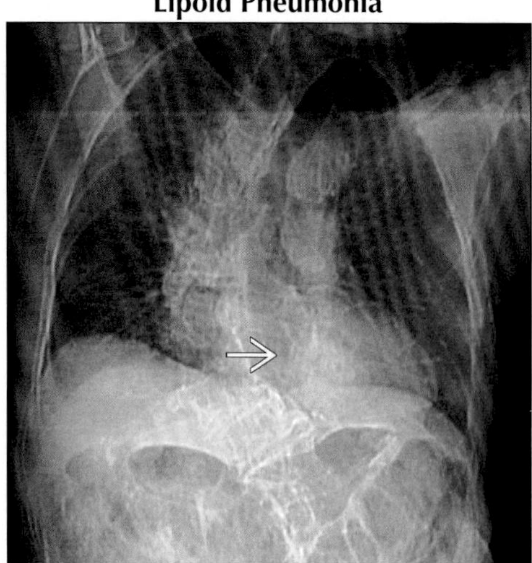

Lipoid Pneumonia

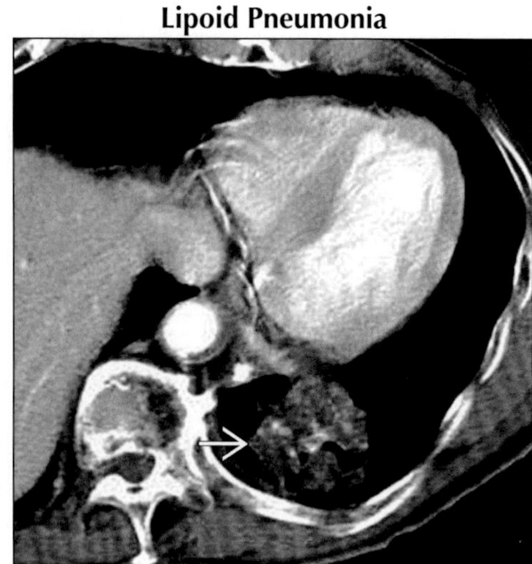

Intralobar Sequestration

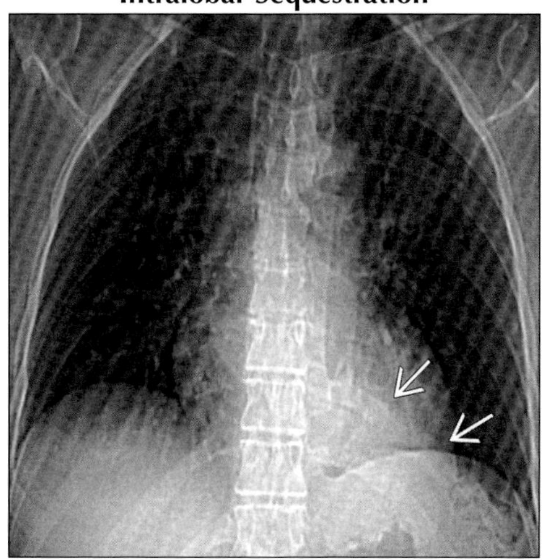

Intralobar Sequestration

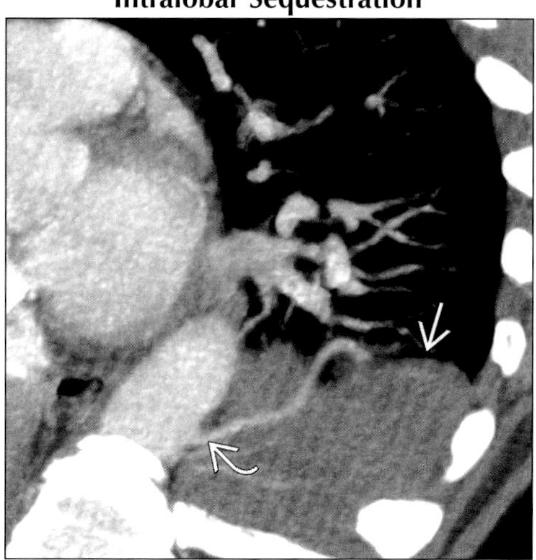

(Left) *Frontal radiograph shows a sharply marginated left costovertebral angle mass ➡, projecting behind the heart.* ***(Right)*** *Axial oblique CTA MIP reconstruction image shows a well-defined mass-like lesion ➡ in the lower left lobe together with the feeding vessels, which come directly from the aorta ➡. Systemic arterial supply is not always demonstrated if there are multiple small feeding arteries.*

Left Lower Lobe Collapse

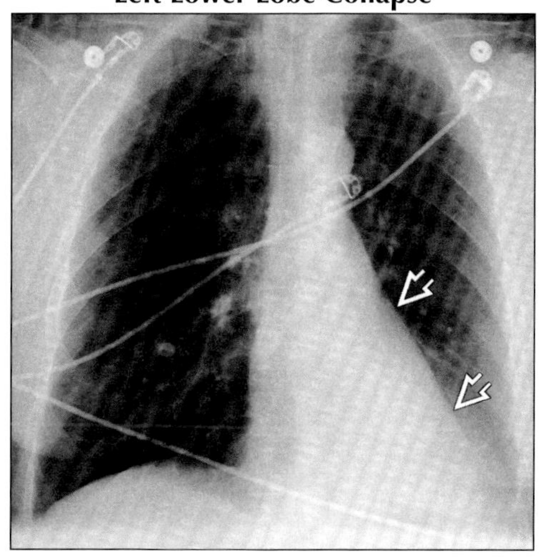

Left Lower Lobe Collapse

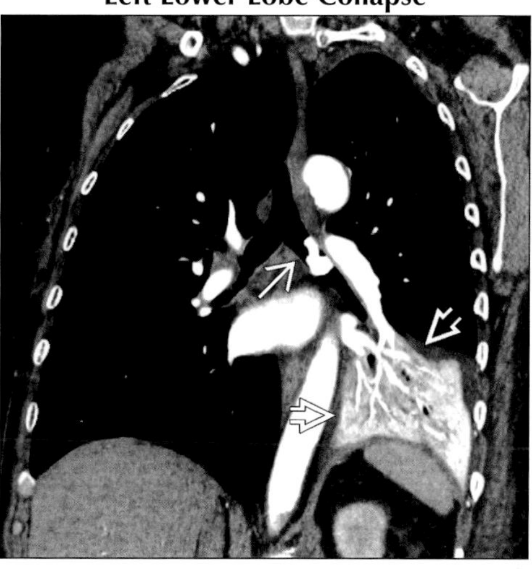

(Left) *Anteroposterior radiograph shows a triangular dense opacity in the left costovertebral angle ➡ that silhouettes left hemidiaphragm and descending aorta. Note that the left hemithorax is smaller than the right.* ***(Right)*** *Coronal CECT reconstruction shows the foreign body ➡ and collapsed left lower lobe ➡. Left hemidiaphragm is elevated. Aspirated bone was removed at bronchoscopy.*

Esophageal Varices

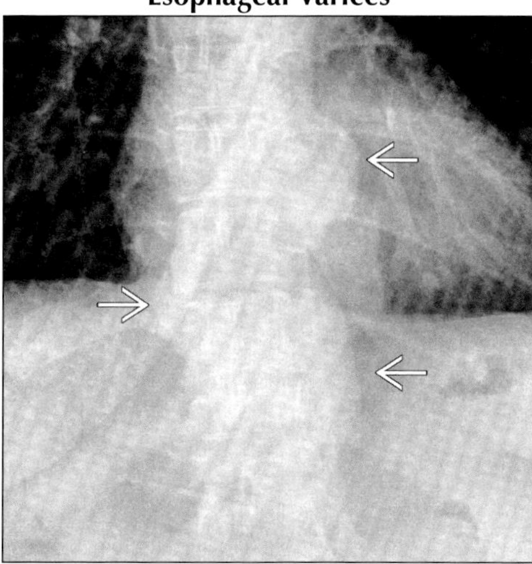

Esophageal Varices

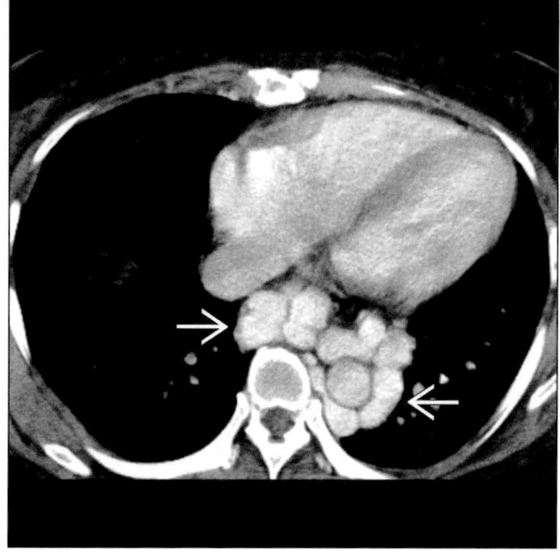

(Left) *Frontal radiograph shows lobulated, sharply defined posterior mediastinal masses ➡. Note that the masses have no consistent relationship to the adjacent vertebral bodies.* ***(Right)*** *Axial CECT shows multiple dilated varices ➡ from portal hypertension. Contrast-filled veins distinguish varices from nodes or other paramediastinal masses.*

LEFT COSTOVERTEBRAL ANGLE MASS

(Left) Frontal radiograph shows an abnormal thin-walled air-filled mass in the left costovertebral angle ➔. *(Right)* Axial CECT shows that the mass, representing the herniated stomach, fills with oral contrast ➔, alongside the esophagus ⇨. Small pleural effusion ↗ suggests strangulation. Paraesophageal hernias are more prone to strangulate than other hernias.

Paraesophageal Hernia

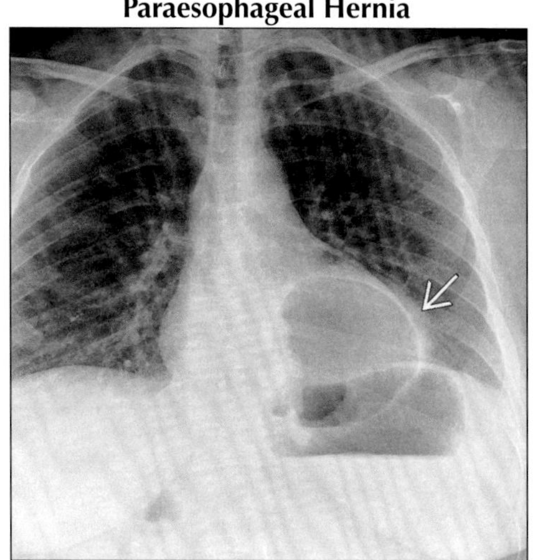

Paraesophageal Hernia

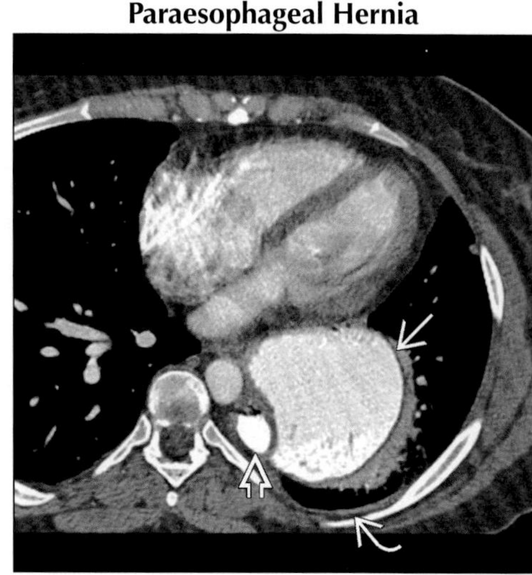

(Left) Frontal radiograph shows hyperinflation, scoliosis, and a focal posterior mediastinal mass ➔ in the left costovertebral angle. *(Right)* Axial CECT shows a well-defined low-attenuation mass ➔. The adjacent neural foramen is widened ↗. Mass is either a neurofibroma or schwannoma. Nerve sheath tumors are the most common cause of a posterior mediastinal mass.

Nerve Sheath Tumors

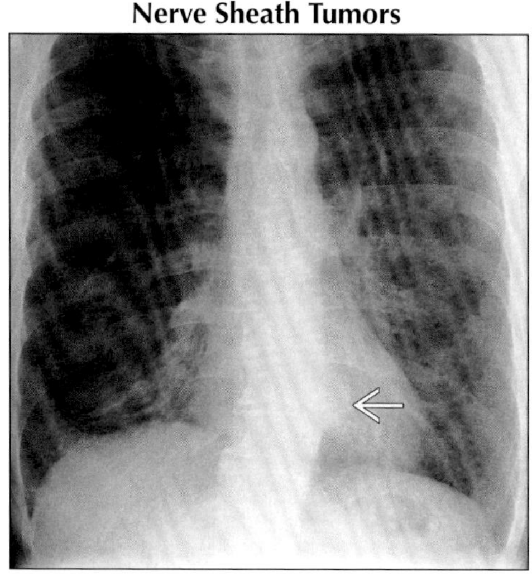

Nerve Sheath Tumors

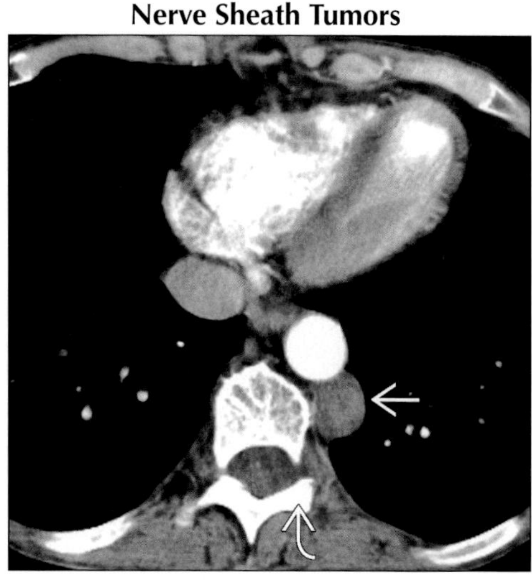

(Left) Frontal radiograph shows a paraspinal costovertebral mass ➔. The patient was hypertensive. *(Right)* Axial CECT shows an intensely contrast enhancing paraspinal mass ➔. Such an intensely enhancing mass must be differentiated from an aortic aneurysm. The diagnosis was paraganglioma.

Sympathetic Ganglion Tumors

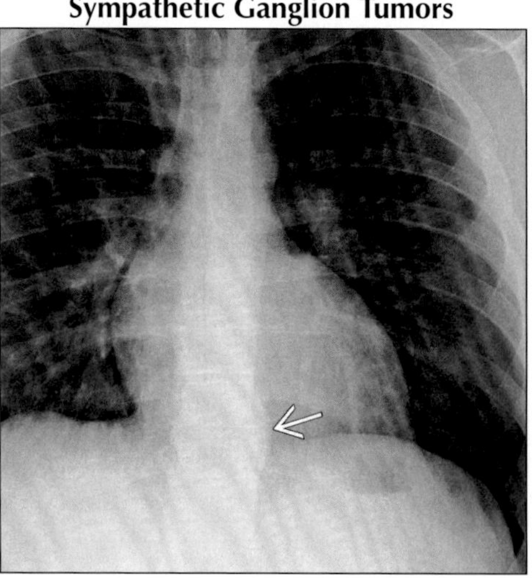

Sympathetic Ganglion Tumors

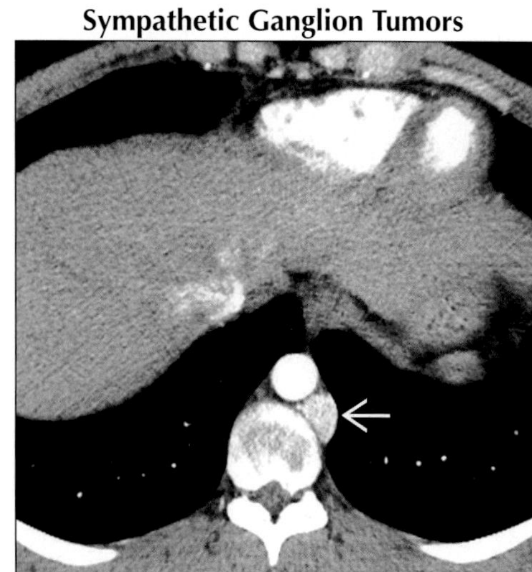

Esophageal Duplication Cyst

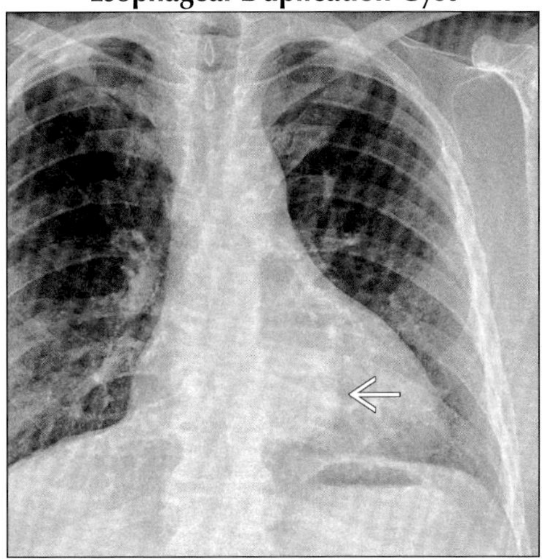

Esophageal Duplication Cyst

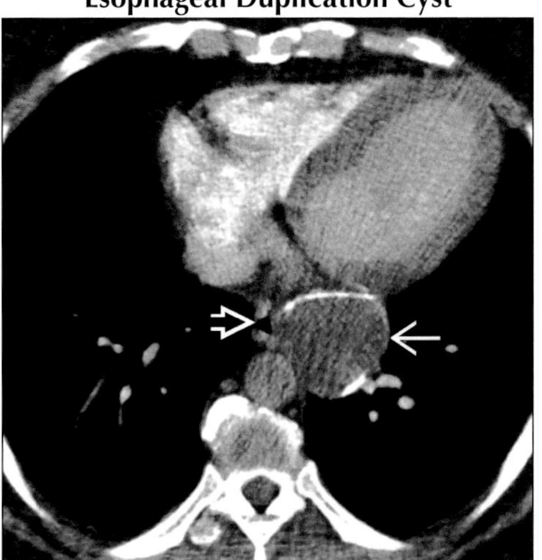

(Left) *Frontal radiograph shows a large, well-defined, left-sided costovertebral mass ➡.* ***(Right)*** *Axial CECT shows a periesophageal low-density mass with rim calcification ➡. The mass is adjacent to the esophagus ⇨ and aorta. Arterial phase imaging is necessary to ensure that the lesion is not an aortic aneurysm.*

Extramedullary Hematopoiesis

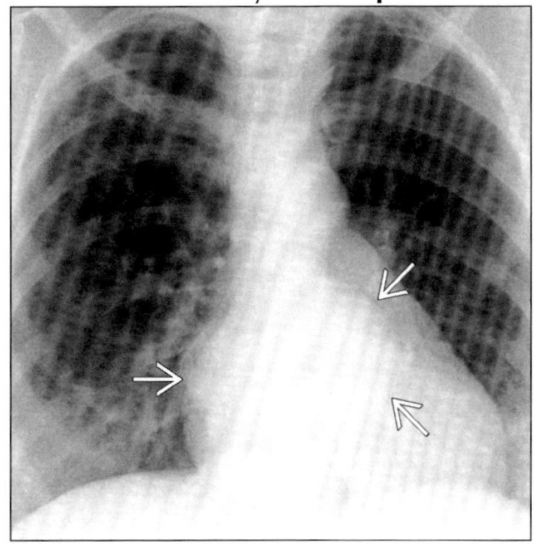

Extramedullary Hematopoiesis

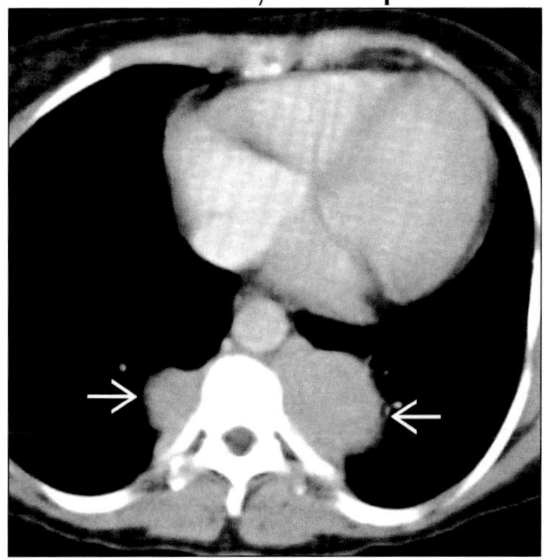

(Left) *Frontal radiograph shows paraspinal masses centered on the lower thoracic spine ➡. The heart is mildly enlarged.* ***(Right)*** *Axial CECT shows rounded and homogeneous soft tissue masses ➡ on both sides of the spine. Cardiac enlargement is from mild high output heart failure. Extramedullary tissue may enhance homogeneously or inhomogeneously. Often masses contain fat. Calcification is uncommon.*

Esophageal Tear

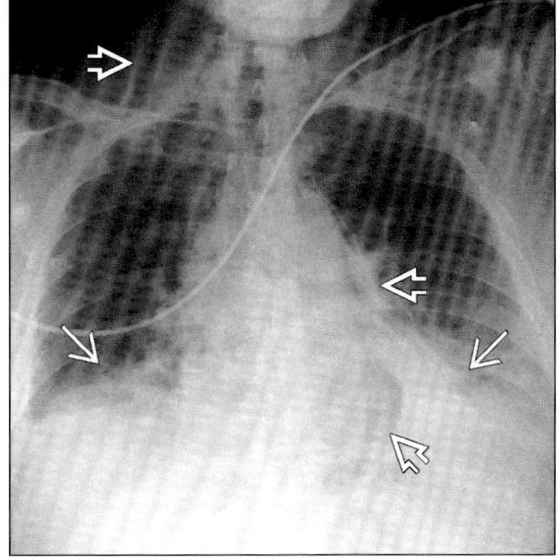

Esophageal Tear

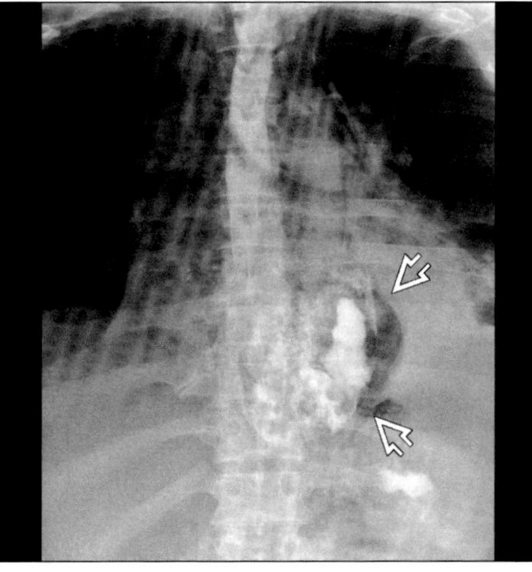

(Left) *Anteroposterior radiograph shows massive pneumomediastinum ⇨ and bibasilar atelectasis ➡. Note the largest collection of air is in the left costovertebral angle. This patient had blunt chest trauma.* ***(Right)*** *Frontal esophagram shows extravasation of air and contrast ⇨ into the left costovertebral angle. Esophageal tears are often missed with delayed diagnosis. One must maintain a high index of suspicion for this uncommon injury.*

CARDIOPHRENIC ANGLE MASS

DIFFERENTIAL DIAGNOSIS

Common
- Pericardial Cyst
- Pericardial Fat Pad
  - Lipomatosis
  - Pericardial Fat Necrosis
- Morgagni Hernia
- Adenopathy

Less Common
- Thymoma
- Right Middle Lobe Collapse
- Pectus Deformity

Rare but Important
- Fibrous Tumor of Pleura
- Impending Cardiac Volvulus

ESSENTIAL INFORMATION

Key Differential Diagnosis Issues
- Mnemonic: **FAT PAD**
  - **Fat**
  - **P**ericardial cyst, **A**denopathy, **D**iaphragmatic hernia

Helpful Clues for Common Diagnoses
- **Pericardial Cyst**
  - Benign disorder due to anomalous outpouching of parietal pericardium
  - 5-10% of all mediastinal masses
  - Location: Cardiophrenic angle
    - Right (70%), left (10-40%)
  - Size: 2-30 cm in diameter
  - Morphology: Round, sharp margins
  - Unilocular in 80%, 20% multiloculated
  - Wall imperceptible, noncalcified
    - No internal enhancement or enhancing rim
- **Pericardial Fat Pad**
  - Common normal finding can mimic pneumonia on radiographs
  - **Lipomatosis**
    - Exuberant deposition of unencapsulated adipose tissue in mediastinum
    - CT: Homogeneous fat attenuation, mass does not compress or invade adjacent structures
    - Does not enhance with contrast
    - May have enlarged pericardial fat pads
  - **Pericardial Fat Necrosis**
    - Rare benign condition of unknown etiology
    - Patients usually present with acute pleuritic chest pain
    - Imaging and pathologic features similar to those of fat necrosis in epiploic appendagitis
- **Morgagni Hernia**
  - Rare, 2% of all diaphragmatic hernias
  - Congenital defect through anterior parasternal hiatus between diaphragm muscle and ribs (space of Larrey)
  - Location: Primarily right-sided (heart limits herniation on left)
  - Smooth and sharply marginated
  - Commonly contains omental fat; may contain bowel, particularly transverse colon
    - Omentum contains vessels (compared to fat pads, which have sparse vessels)
    - Air in mass should suggest hernia
  - If there is pleural effusion, suspect strangulation of bowel in hernia sac
- **Adenopathy**
  - Lymphadenopathy from lymphoma most common cause in this location
    - Metastases from tumors of thorax or abdomen may also affect these nodes
  - Mantle radiation therapy: Cardiac blocker used to protect heart, area undertreated
    - "Recurrent fat pad" sign: Enlarging recurrent nodes from lymphoma in undertreated pericardial lymph nodes
    - Nodes may be irradiated since field was blocked initially
    - Appearance or enlargement of "fat pad" heralds development of adenopathy

Helpful Clues for Less Common Diagnoses
- **Thymoma**
  - Most common primary anterior mediastinal mass
  - Oval or lobulated mass
  - Homogeneous enhancement is common with small tumor, more heterogeneous enhancement for larger tumors
  - 1/3 have calcification present on CT, usually thin and linear within capsule
  - Cystic regions and necrosis are common (1/3), especially with larger tumors, and may be a dominant feature
  - Paraneoplastic syndromes in 40%

- Myasthenia gravis (35%), pure red cell aplasia (5%), hypogammaglobulinemia (10%)

- **Right Middle Lobe Collapse**
  - Right middle lobe smallest of all lobes
    - Indirect signs from collapse uncommon; hilar shift infrequent
    - Lobe collapses medially toward right heart border
  - Right middle lobe syndrome: Cicatrizing atelectasis of RML due to prior pneumonia and poor collateral drift
    - RML bronchus is small, susceptible to compression from adjacent lymphadenopathy
- **Pectus Deformity**
  - Pectus excavatum: 1 in 300-400 births, most common chest wall abnormality (90%)
  - Right heart border frequently obliterated because depressed sternum replaces aerated lung at right heart border
  - Heart displaced to left and rotated, may cause spurious cardiomegaly

Helpful Clues for Rare Diagnoses

- **Fibrous Tumor of Pleura**
  - Uncommon primary mesenchymal tumor of pleura
    - 80-85% benign, 15-20% malignant
    - Most common location: Inferior hemithorax
    - Often large (> 7 cm), grow very slowly over years
    - Lobulated, sharply marginated mass with longitudinal axis paralleling chest wall
    - Pedunculated lesions change location with position, a characteristic imaging feature
    - Rarely, pedicle may twist and detach tumor
    - Pleural effusion (20%), more common with malignant lesions
    - Calcification in 5%; calcification in malignant tumors more common (20%)
    - Tumors often enhance with contrast
    - Hypertrophic osteoarthropathy in 17-30%
    - Hypoglycemia rare (5%), known as Doege-Potter syndrome
    - Recurrence may occur even with benign tumors, requires long-term surveillance
- **Impending Cardiac Volvulus**
  - Herniation of heart into hemithorax
  - Generally takes 3 days for adhesions to form between cut edge of pericardium and heart
  - Usually occurs in immediate postoperative period
  - Most commonly presents with sudden shock
  - Prior to herniation, there may be a tight, spherical, cardiac bulge (like top of snow cone) as heart begins to herniate through pericardial defect

Pericardial Cyst

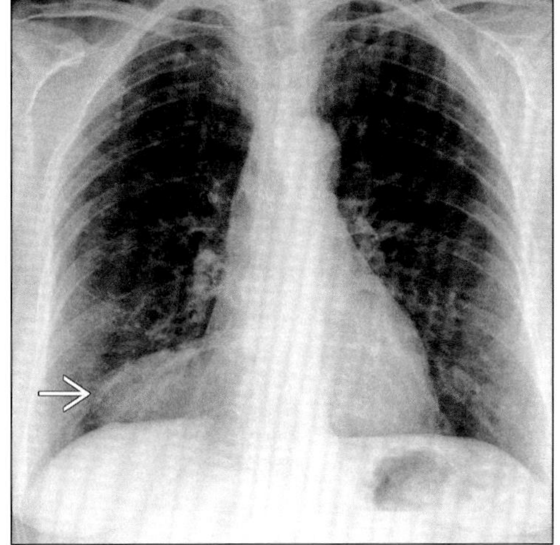

Frontal radiograph shows a mass ➔ in the right cardiophrenic angle. The right heart border is obscured.

Pericardial Cyst

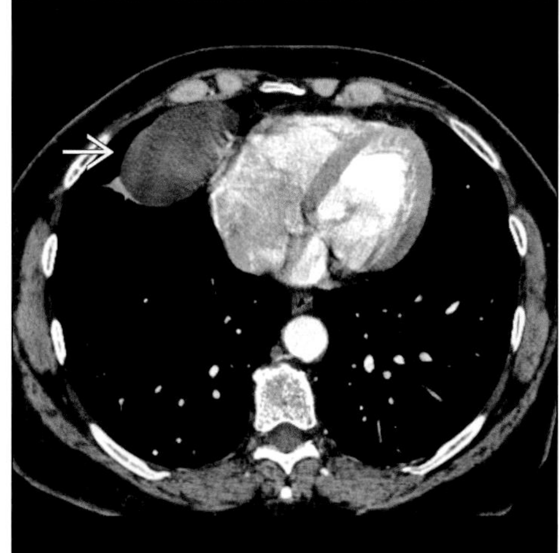

Axial CECT shows a sharply marginated, water density mass ➔ in cardiophrenic angle. The wall of the mass is imperceptible.

CARDIOPHRENIC ANGLE MASS

(Left) Frontal radiograph show a well-defined mass in the right cardiophrenic angle ➔. *(Right)* Axial CECT shows a fluid-filled thin-walled cystic lesion adjacent to the right ventricle ➔ with no mass effect on the heart. Cysts are typically nonseptated. Differential includes thymic cyst or bronchogenic cyst.

Pericardial Cyst

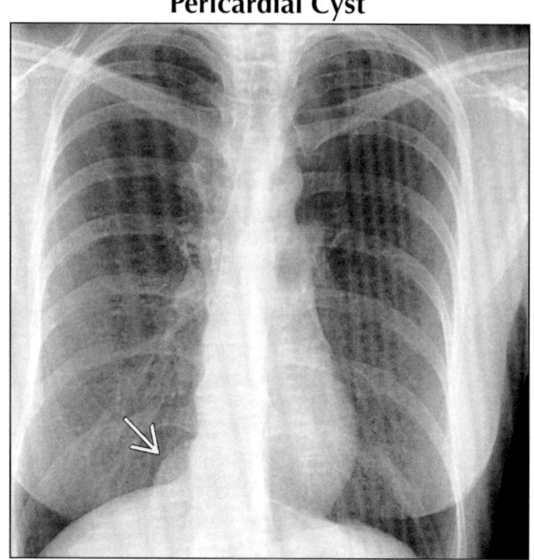

Pericardial Cyst

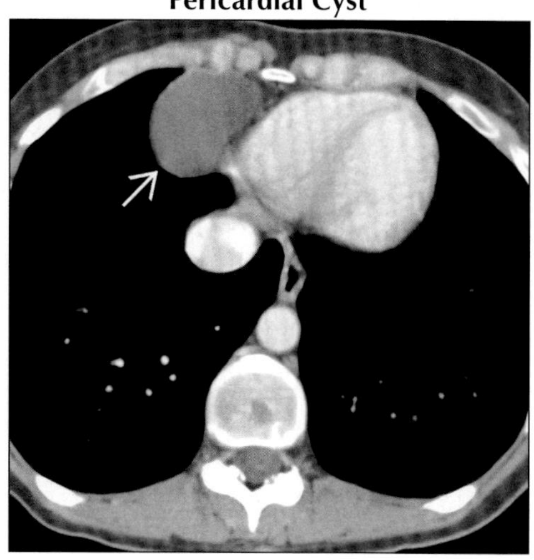

(Left) Anteroposterior radiograph shows diffuse mediastinal widening ➔. *(Right)* Coronal CECT reconstruction shows diffuse mediastinal widening from fat ➔ extending around both sides of the heart in the cardiophrenic angle. Lipomatosis is most commonly secondary to obesity.

Lipomatosis

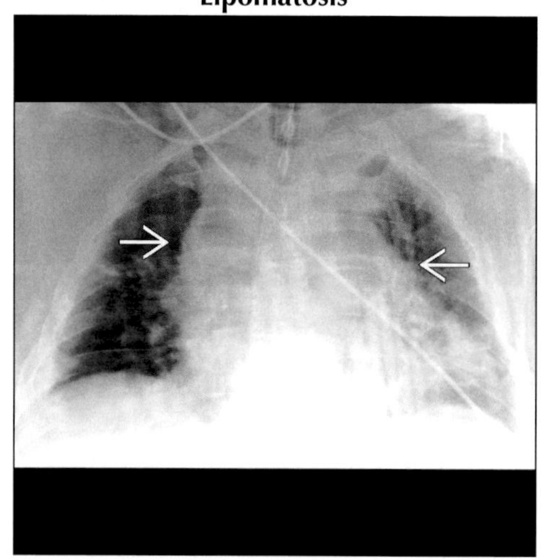

Lipomatosis

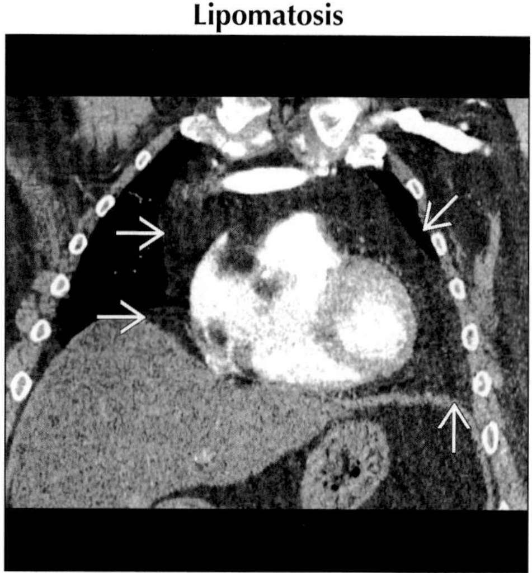

(Left) Axial NECT shows swirling high-density material in pericardial fat pad ➔ from pericardial fat necrosis. Note the small left pleural effusion ➔. *(Right)* Axial NECT more inferiorly shows swirling water density in pericardial fat pad ➔. This patient presented with acute chest pain, and follow-up showed resolution of these findings.

Pericardial Fat Necrosis

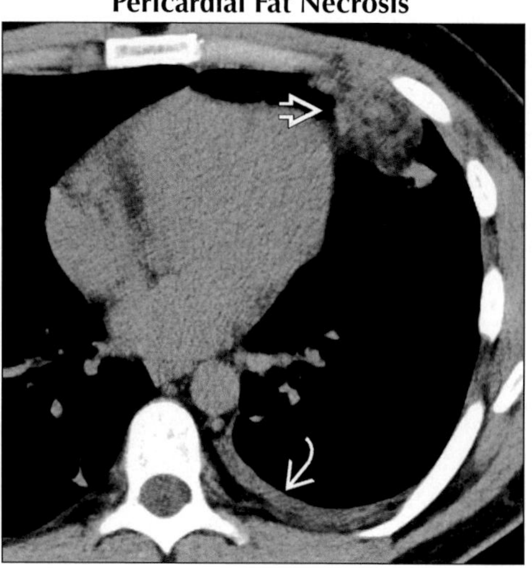

Pericardial Fat Necrosis

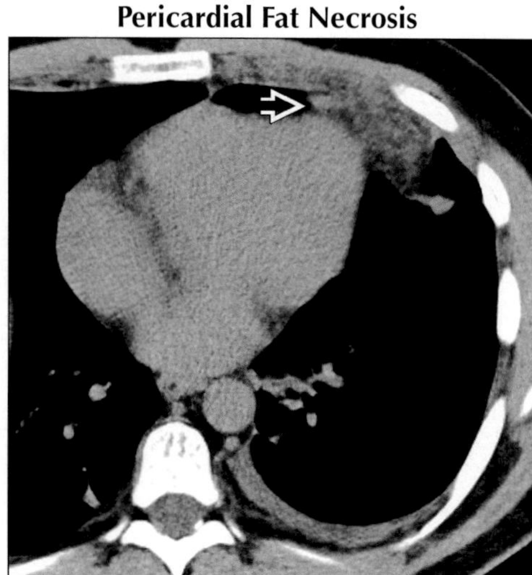

CARDIOPHRENIC ANGLE MASS

Morgagni Hernia

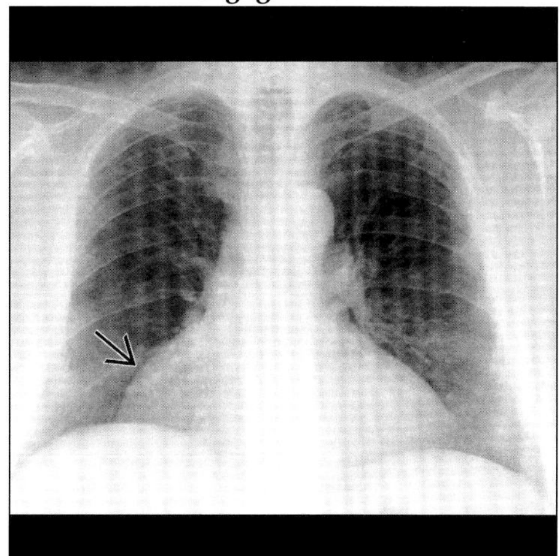

Morgagni Hernia

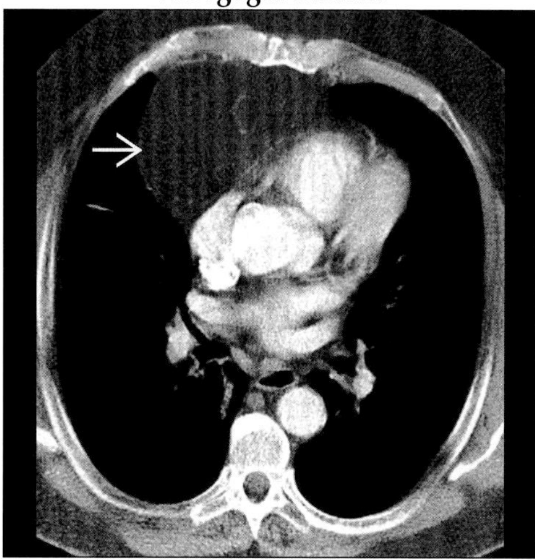

(Left) *Frontal radiograph shows abnormal opacity in the right costophrenic angle ⇨, which widens the right heart contour.* ***(Right)*** *Axial CECT shows herniation of peritoneal fat ➡ through Morgagni hiatus. Note that fat can be hard to visualize on mediastinal windows. Differential in this case includes an enlarged pericardial fat pad. Any soft tissue component raises the possibility of liposarcoma or thymolipoma.*

Morgagni Hernia

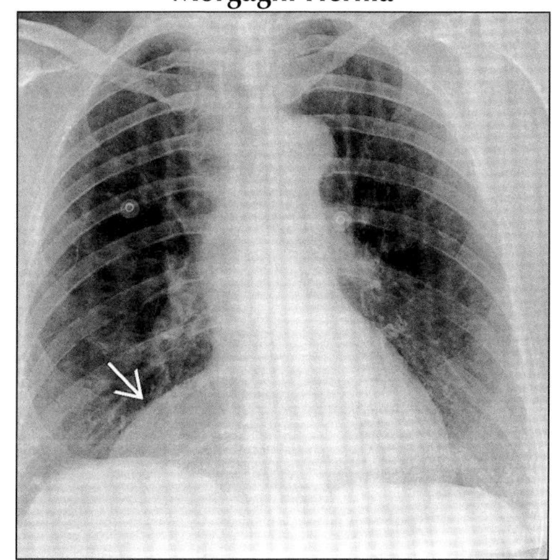

Morgagni Hernia

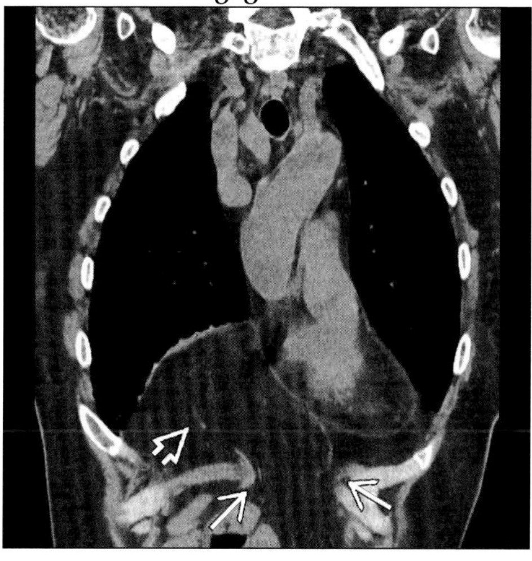

(Left) *Anteroposterior radiograph shows a sharply defined mass ➡ in the right costophrenic angle. The mass is somewhat lucent given its size.* ***(Right)*** *Coronal NECT reconstruction shows herniation of omental fat ⇨ through anterior Morgagni hiatus ➡. Coronal reconstructions are very advantageous in demonstrating diaphragmatic defects; the course of mesenteric vessels is also easier to visualize.*

Adenopathy

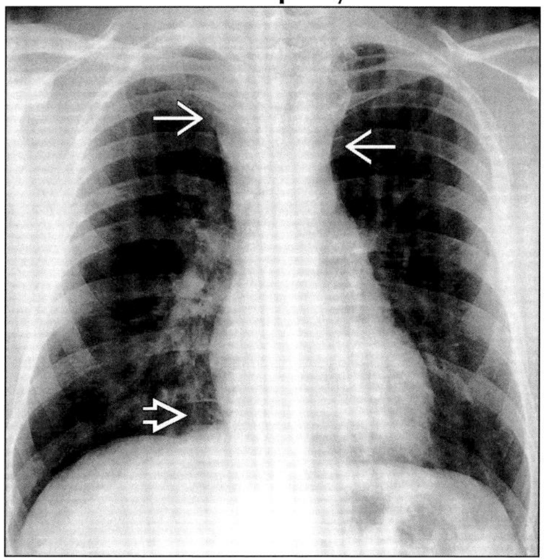

Adenopathy

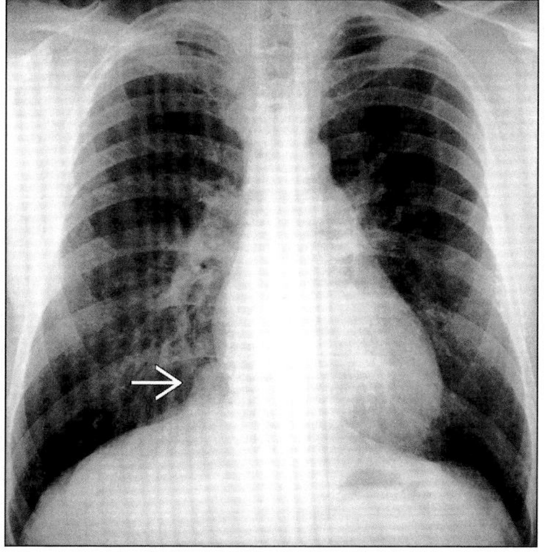

(Left) *Frontal radiograph shows superior mediastinal widening ➡ from Hodgkin disease. The right cardiophrenic angle is normal ⇨. This patient was treated with Mantle radiation therapy.* ***(Right)*** *Frontal radiograph months later shows resolution of mediastinal widening following radiation therapy. However, a new mass density ➡ has developed in the right cardiophrenic angle. The heart was blocked and received less radiation.*

CARDIOPHRENIC ANGLE MASS

Adenopathy

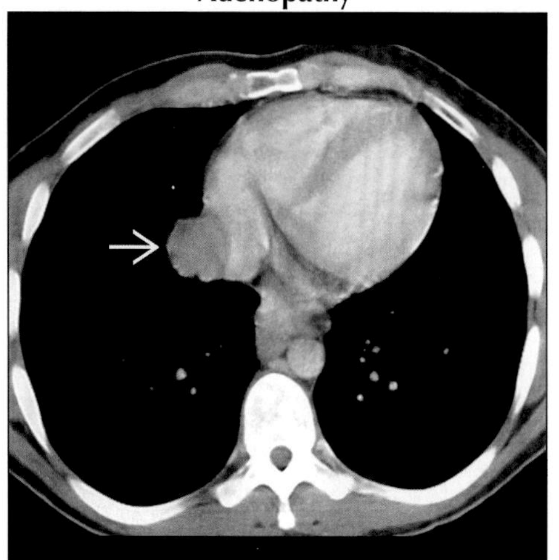

Adenopathy

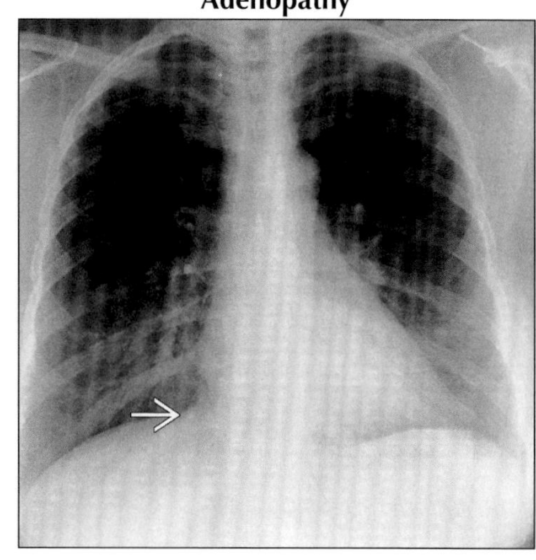

(Left) Axial CECT shows that the right cardiophrenic mass is solid ➔ impinging on the right atrium. This mass represented recurrent adenopathy. *(Right)* Frontal radiograph shows resolution of the mass in the right cardiophrenic angle ➔ following completion of additional radiation therapy.

Thymoma

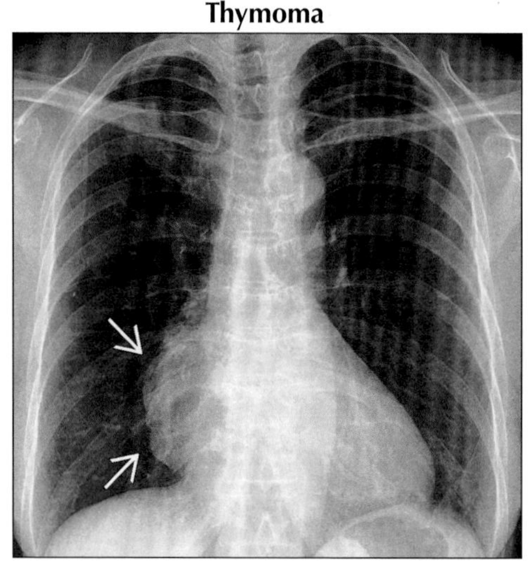

Thymoma

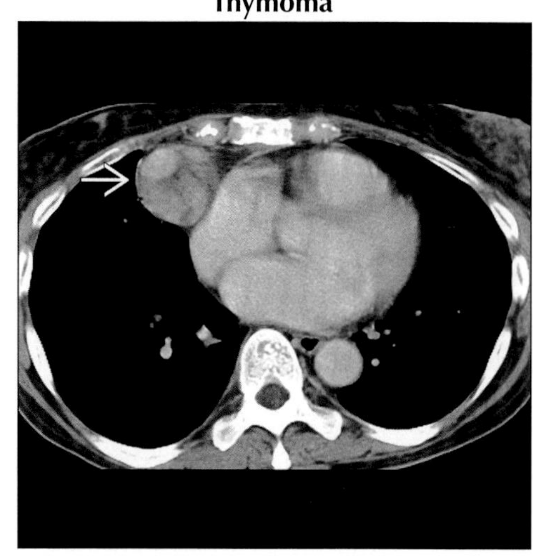

(Left) Frontal radiograph shows a large, sharply marginated mass ➔ overlying the right heart border and cardiophrenic angle. *(Right)* Axial CECT shows a contrast-enhancing, partially septated mass ➔ impinging on the right atrium. Thymomas can usually be connected to the more superiorly located thymic tissue.

Right Middle Lobe Collapse

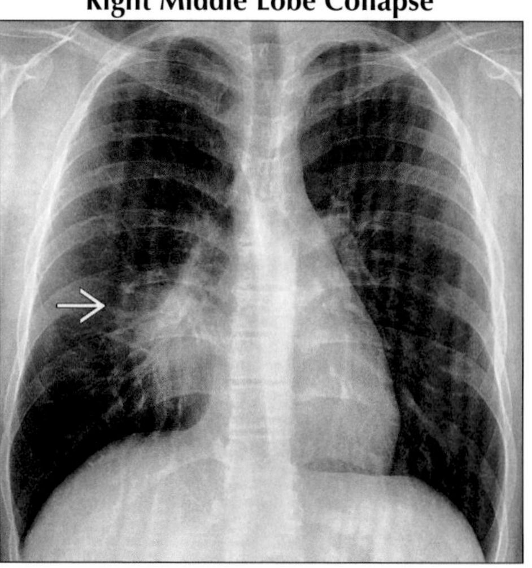

Right Middle Lobe Collapse

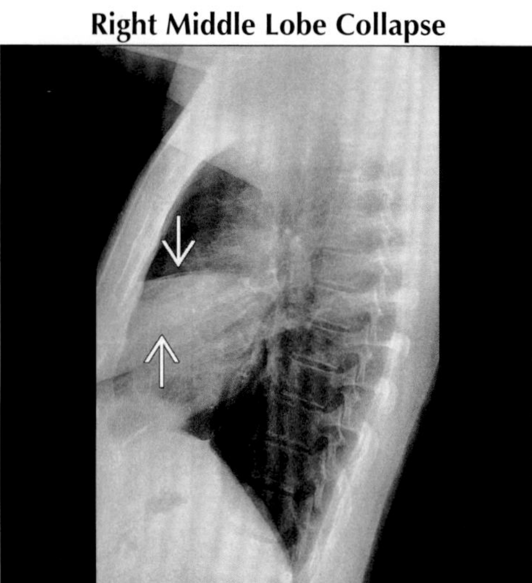

(Left) Frontal radiograph shows an ill-defined density ➔ overlying the right heart border. *(Right)* Lateral radiograph reveals that the density is the collapse of the right middle lobe sharply marginated by the major and minor fissures ➔. Lack of air-bronchograms suggests endobronchial obstruction. Carcinoid was diagnosed at bronchoscopy.

CARDIOPHRENIC ANGLE MASS

Pectus Deformity

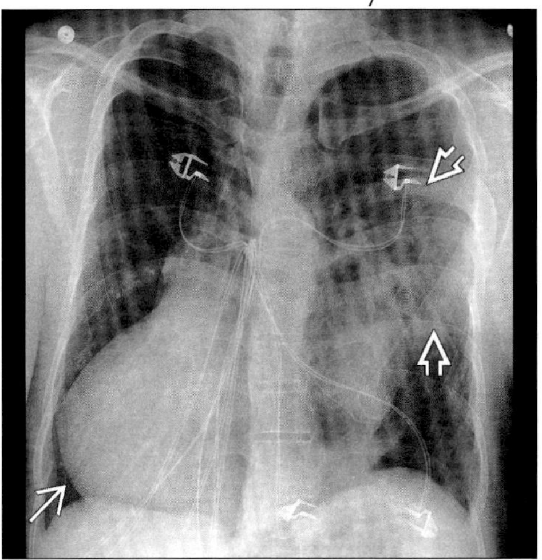

Pectus Deformity

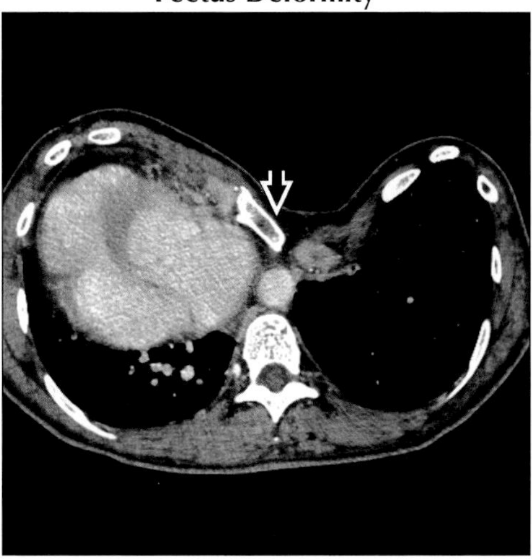

*(**Left**) Frontal radiograph shows the heart displaced into the right hemithorax ➡ and an ill-defined opacity ⇨ in the left hemithorax representing the normal added density of the oblique chest wall. (**Right**) Axial CECT shows severe pectus deformity ⇨ displacing the heart into the right hemithorax. This is a variant of typical pectus deformity, in which the heart is usually displaced to the left.*

Fibrous Tumor of Pleura

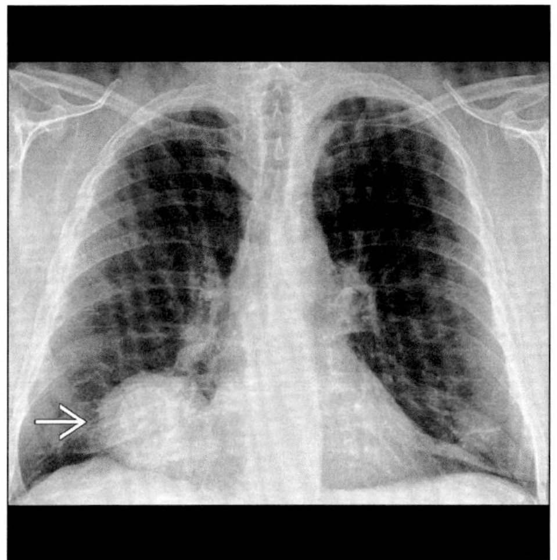

Fibrous Tumor of Pleura

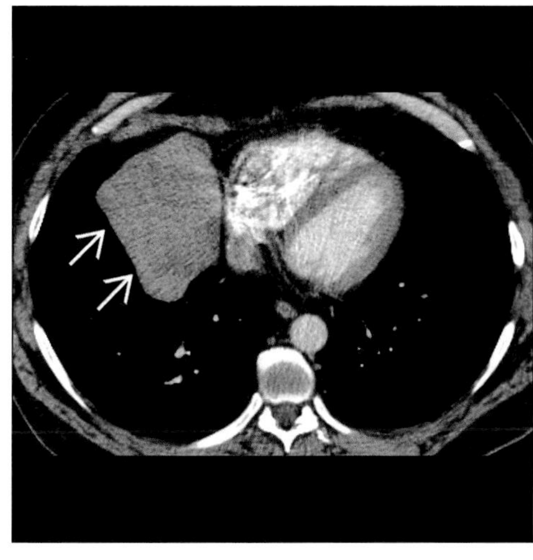

*(**Left**) Frontal radiograph shows a large, well-defined mass ➡ in the right cardiophrenic angle. (**Right**) Axial CECT shows a solid, somewhat lobulated mass ➡ in the right cardiophrenic angle. Fibrous tumors of the pleura are often attached to the pleura by a pedicle. The mass may shift with change in position. Like this tumor, most are large at the time of diagnosis.*

Impending Cardiac Volvulus

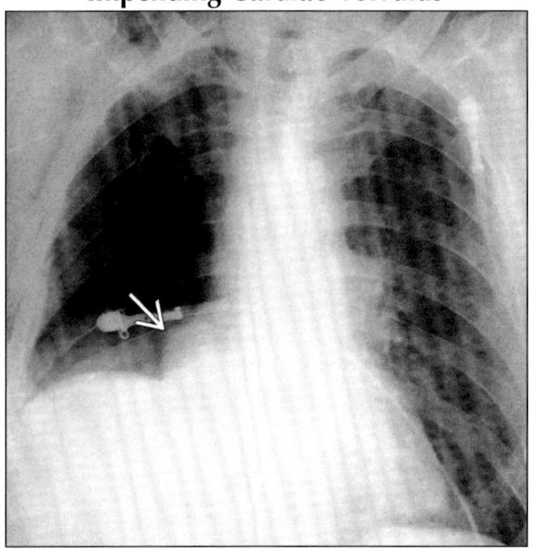

Impending Cardiac Volvulus

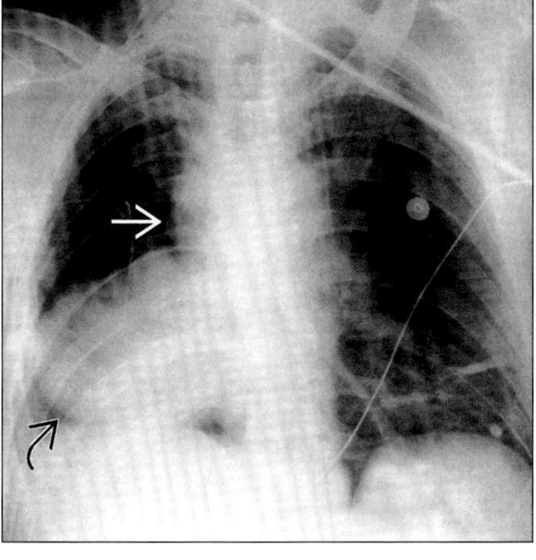

*(**Left**) Anteroposterior radiograph in the recovery room following right pneumonectomy demonstrates a focal contour abnormality ➡ in the right cardiophrenic angle. The mass is due to partial herniation of the heart through a pericardial defect. (**Right**) Anteroposterior radiograph hours later shows cardiac volvulus ↗. Widening of the superior mediastinum is due to superior vena cava obstruction ➡.*

SECTION 9
Pleura, Chest Wall, Diaphragm

ELEVATED HEMIDIAPHRAGM

DIFFERENTIAL DIAGNOSIS

Common
- Normal Variant
- Phrenic Nerve Paralysis or Injury
- Eventration of Diaphragm
- Diaphragmatic Weakness
- Lobectomy or Pneumonectomy
- Lobar Collapse

Less Common
- Subpulmonic Effusion
- Hepatomegaly
- Pleural, Diaphragmatic, or Abdominal Tumor
- Ascites
- Unilateral Lung Transplantation

Rare but Important
- Bochdalek Hernia
- Morgagni Hernia (Mimic)
- Diaphragmatic Tear (Mimic)

ESSENTIAL INFORMATION

Key Differential Diagnosis Issues
- Focal vs. uniform elevation
  - Causes of focal elevation
    - Eventration
    - Lobectomy
    - Diaphragmatic hernia
    - Diaphragmatic rupture
  - Causes of uniform elevation
    - Phrenic nerve paralysis
    - Diaphragmatic weakness
    - Unilateral lung transplantation
- Fluoroscopic evaluation of diaphragm helps distinguish phrenic nerve paralysis from other causes of weakness or eventration
  - Paradoxical motion is evident on forced inspiration (sniff maneuver) with phrenic nerve paralysis
  - Eventration shows no paradoxical motion

Helpful Clues for Common Diagnoses
- **Normal Variant**
  - Left hemidiaphragm is normally lower than right hemidiaphragm
  - Left hemidiaphragm can be slightly elevated or at same level as right hemidiaphragm in up to 10-15% of normal subjects
  - Dextrocardia or situs inversus: Left hemidiaphragm is at higher level
- **Phrenic Nerve Paralysis or Injury**
  - Uniform elevation
  - Paradoxical motion at fluoroscopy
  - Abnormal nerve conduction at electromyography studies
- **Eventration of Diaphragm**
  - Focal elevation
  - Focal muscle weakness or thinning
  - Typically right anterior diaphragm is affected
- **Diaphragmatic Weakness**
  - Indicates either neurogenic or muscular impairment
  - Can be reversible
  - Causes of diaphragmatic weakness
    - Recent surgery, typically cardiac surgery
    - Systemic lupus erythematosus (SLE): Vanishing lung syndrome from diaphragmatic myopathy
    - Guillain-Barré syndrome
    - Poliomyelitis
    - Polymyositis and dermatomyositis
- **Lobectomy or Pneumonectomy**
  - Will have definite clinical history
  - Mediastinal shift to side of surgery
  - Signs of prior thoracotomy or lung resection are usually evident
  - Pneumonectomy may show "whiteout" hemithorax and crowding of ribs
- **Lobar Collapse**
  - Direct or indirect signs of lobar collapse are visible

Helpful Clues for Less Common Diagnoses
- **Subpulmonic Effusion**
  - Lateral tenting (shouldering) on upright chest x-ray
  - Mobile or layering effusion on lateral decubitus radiographs
- **Hepatomegaly**
  - Differential considerations are same as uniform elevation of right hemidiaphragm
  - Most causes of hepatomegaly show abnormal liver function
- **Pleural, Diaphragmatic, or Abdominal Tumor**
  - Lobulated contour or focal apparent elevation
  - Associated pleural effusion in patients with pleural metastasis

- History of primary malignancy elsewhere
- Unusual cause of apparent elevation of hemidiaphragm

- **Ascites**
  - Ground-glass density with lack of gas-filled loops in upper abdomen
  - Clinical examination and US evaluation are often useful

Helpful Clues for Rare Diagnoses

- **Bochdalek Hernia**
  - Focal apparent elevation
  - Posterior in location; more common on left side
  - Can be small and incidental
- **Morgagni Hernia (Mimic)**
  - Focal apparent elevation of anterior right hemidiaphragm
  - Can appear as right cardiophrenic angle opacity or mass
  - Can mimic elevation of hemidiaphragm
  - CT is often confirmatory
    - Shows viscera or omentum traversing diaphragm
- **Diaphragmatic Tear (Mimic)**
  - Recent or remote history of trauma
  - Chest radiograph
    - Focal elevation of diaphragm
    - Air-filled bowel loops above expected level of diaphragm
    - NG tube above expected level of diaphragm
    - Contralateral shift of mediastinum
    - Collar sign: Focal constriction of bowel on barium examination as it traverses diaphragm
  - Chest CT
    - Viscera above diaphragm
    - Dependent viscera sign: Viscera no longer supported by posterior wall of diaphragm and lie in dependent position
    - Bowel, omentum, spleen, or liver in direct contact with underside of ribs
    - Can directly visualize diaphragmatic discontinuity
    - Collar sign: Focal constriction of bowel or liver as it traverses diaphragm
    - Coronal reformations very helpful
    - Often other compelling associated injuries

Alternative Differential Approaches

- Apparent focal elevation
  - Morgagni or Bochdalek hernia
  - Pericardial cyst
  - Lymphadenopathy
  - Lung mass
  - Pleural mass, especially those arising from visceral pleura, such as solitary fibrous tumor
  - Diaphragmatic tear
- Elevation associated with gas collection
  - Eventration
  - Phrenic nerve dysfunction
  - Empyema from gas-forming organisms
  - Paraesophageal hernia

Phrenic Nerve Paralysis or Injury

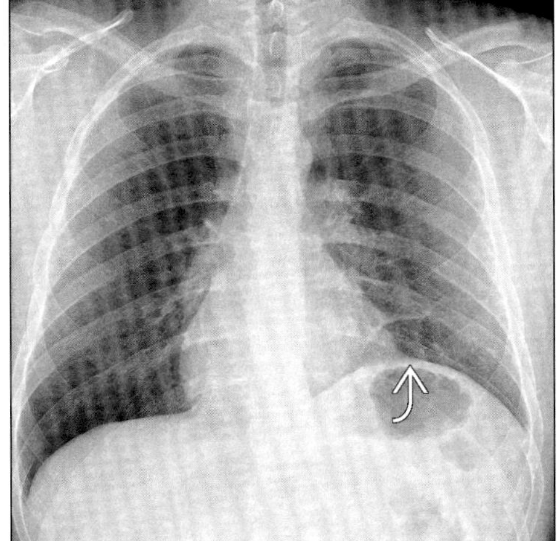

Frontal radiograph in a patient with Hodgkin disease shows uniform elevation of the left hemidiaphragm ➡ from phrenic nerve dysfunction. (Courtesy J.D. Godwin, MD.)

Phrenic Nerve Paralysis or Injury

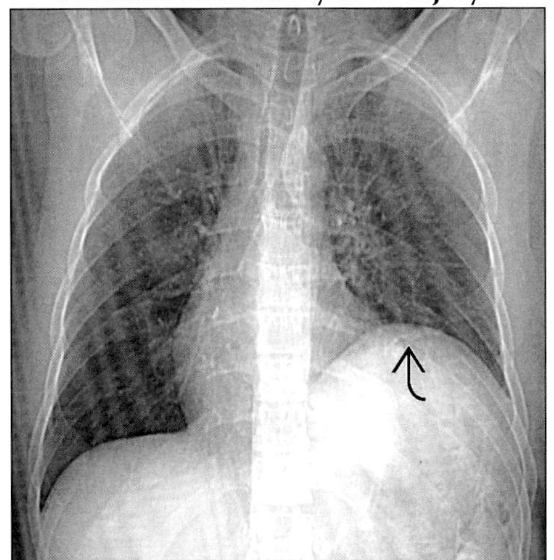

Anteroposterior NECT topogram from the same patient shows accentuation of uniform elevation ➡ of the left hemidiaphragm. Supine position acts as a stress on diaphragm.

ELEVATED HEMIDIAPHRAGM

Eventration of Diaphragm

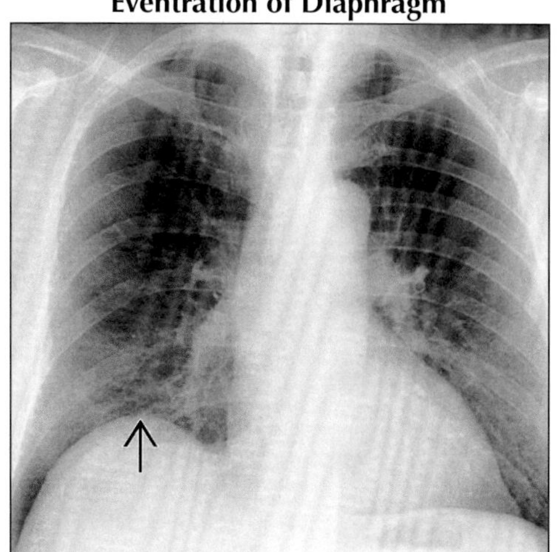

Eventration of Diaphragm

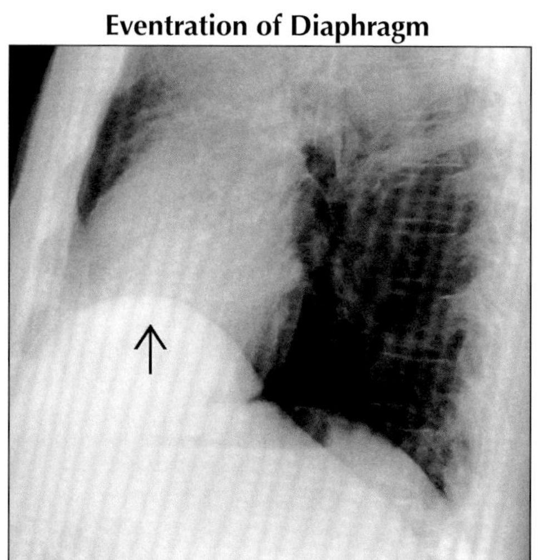

(Left) *Frontal radiograph shows focal elevation ⇨ of the right hemidiaphragm. The right and anterior location is typical of eventration.* ***(Right)*** *Lateral radiograph in the same patient demonstrates the anterior location ⇨ of eventration. Note that the posterior portion of each hemidiaphragm is normally positioned.*

Lobectomy or Pneumonectomy

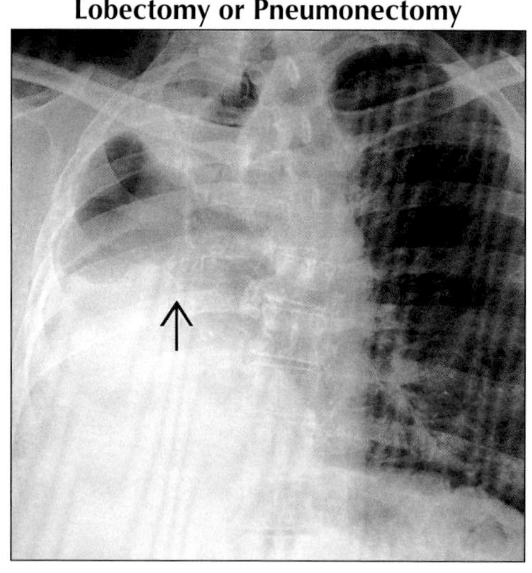

Lobectomy or Pneumonectomy

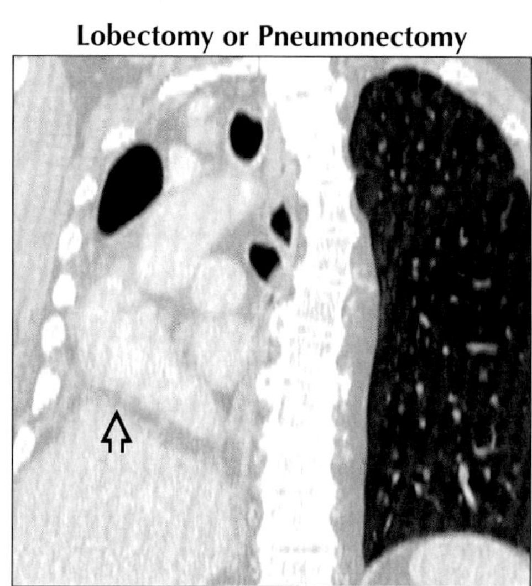

(Left) *Frontal radiograph shows features of a right pneumonectomy with elevation of the right hemidiaphragm ⇨ and shift of mediastinum to the ipsilateral side.* ***(Right)*** *Coronal CT reconstruction in the same patient confirms the findings seen on the chest radiograph with right pneumonectomy and displacement of mediastinal structures into the right hemithorax. Elevation of the right hemidiaphragm is clearly evident ⇨.*

Lobar Collapse

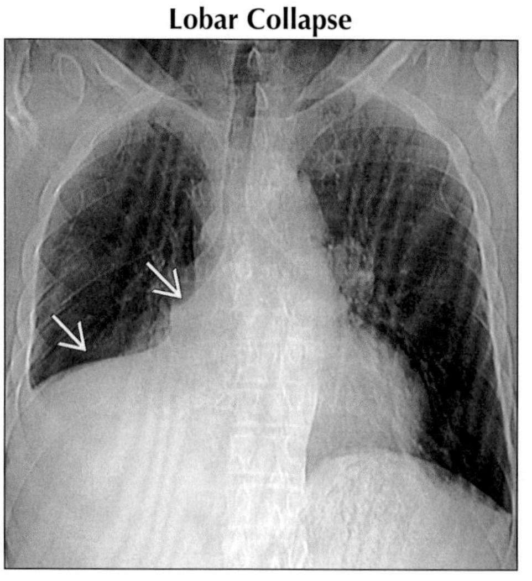

Lobar Collapse

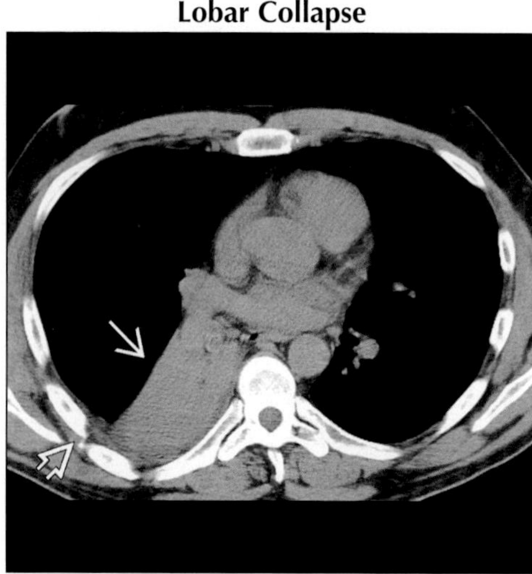

(Left) *Frontal radiograph shows apparent elevation of the right hemidiaphragm with a wedge-shaped opacity ➡ extending to the costophrenic angle, a typical appearance of combined right middle lobe and lower lobe atelectasis.* ***(Right)*** *Axial NECT shows collapse of the right middle lobe and right lower lobe ➡ from mucus plugs. Multiple acute right rib fractures ⇨ are also evident in this patient who had suffered blunt trauma.*

ELEVATED HEMIDIAPHRAGM

Pleural, Diaphragmatic, or Abdominal Tumor

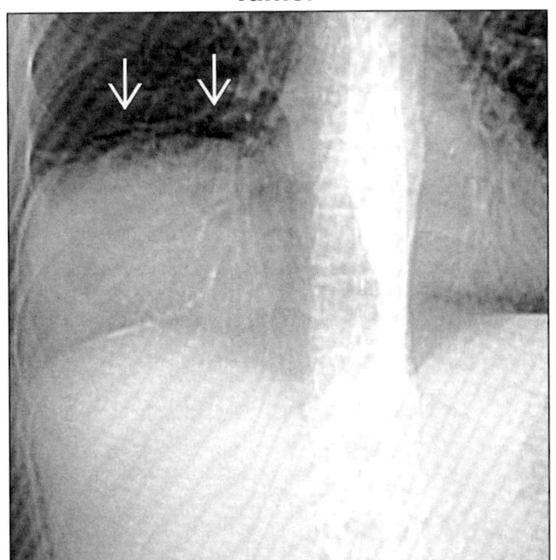

Pleural, Diaphragmatic, or Abdominal Tumor

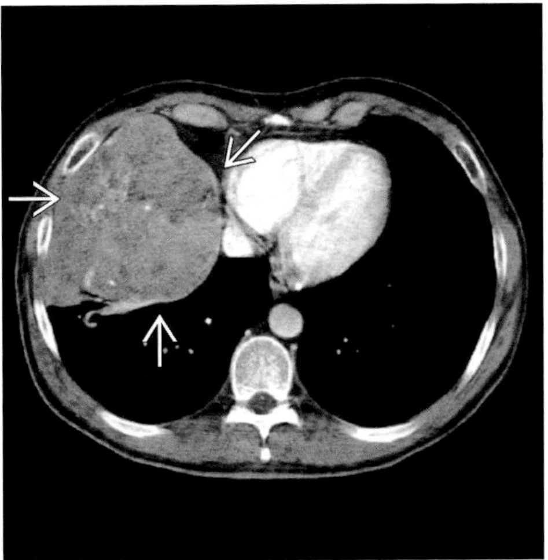

(Left) *Anteroposterior NECT topogram shows apparent elevation from a large pleural mass ➔. (Courtesy J.D. Godwin, MD.)* ***(Right)*** *Axial CECT in the same patient confirms the presence of a heterogeneously enhancing pleural tumor ➔, which proved to be a solitary fibrous tumor of the pleura. (Courtesy J.D. Godwin, MD.)*

Unilateral Lung Transplantation

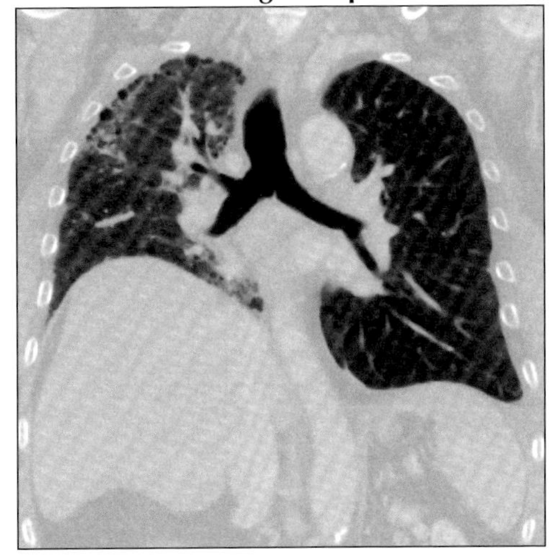

Bochdalek Hernia

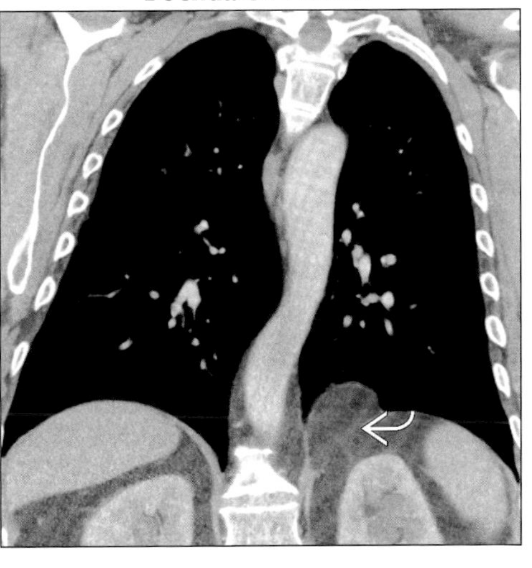

(Left) *Coronal CT reconstruction shows elevation of the right hemidiaphragm from right lung fibrosis and volume loss, a transplanted left lung with normal volume, and a hemidiaphragm at the expected level. (Courtesy J.D. Godwin, MD.)* ***(Right)*** *Coronal CT reconstruction shows herniation of abdominal fat through the Bochdalek foramen ➔. (Courtesy J.D. Godwin, MD.)*

Diaphragmatic Tear (Mimic)

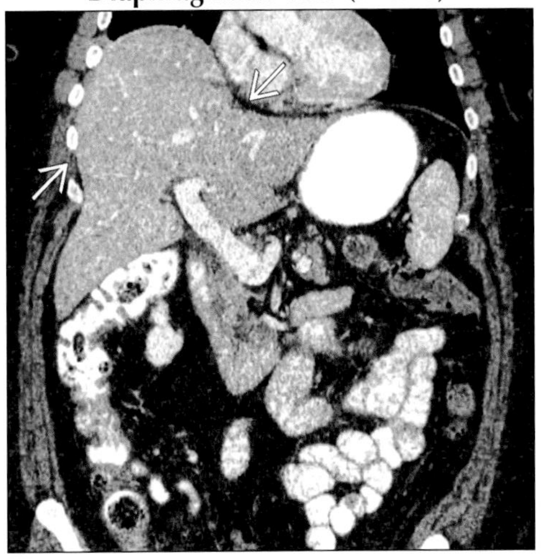

Diaphragmatic Tear (Mimic)

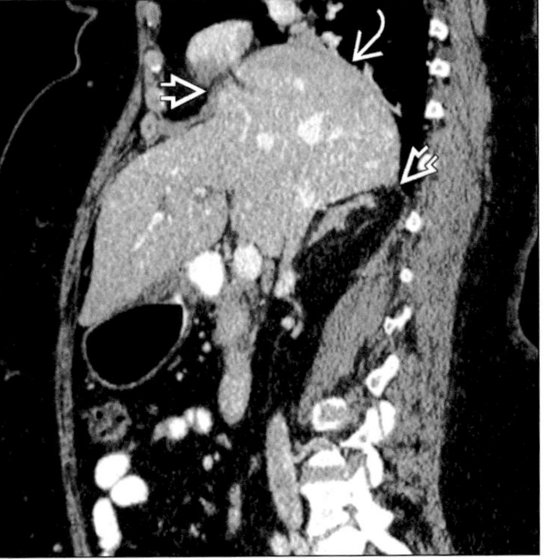

(Left) *Coronal CECT shows mushroom contour of herniated liver through a traumatic diaphragmatic tear ➔ with apparent elevation of the right hemidiaphragm.* ***(Right)*** *Sagittal CECT in the same patient shows thickened crura ➔ and liver herniation ➔ through the diaphragmatic defect.*

PNEUMOTHORAX

DIFFERENTIAL DIAGNOSIS

Common
- Spontaneous Pneumothorax
- Traumatic: Blunt or Penetrating Thoracic Injury
- Iatrogenic
- Obstructive Pulmonary Disease
- Interstitial Lung Diseases
- Connective Tissue Diseases
- Immunologic
- Infections
- Mimics of Pneumothorax

Less Common
- Metastases
- Pulmonary Infarction

Rare but Important
- Catamenial
- Birt-Hogg-Dubé Syndrome

ESSENTIAL INFORMATION

Key Differential Diagnosis Issues
- Most common symptoms: Sudden dyspnea and chest pain; may be asymptomatic
- Supine radiographic exams underestimate size and presence of air in pleural space
  - Radiographic findings
    - Deep sulcus sign
    - Hyperlucent anterior costophrenic sulcus over upper abdominal quadrant (subpulmonic)
    - Increased visualization of diaphragm and cardiac contour (anteromedial)
- Expiratory exam increases proportional size of pneumothorax to hemithorax volume: Aids detection of air in pleural space
- Spontaneous pneumothorax: Younger adults, tall individuals, and smokers
- Complications
  - Tension pneumothorax: Life-threatening complication
    - Radiographic findings (contralateral mediastinal shift) + hemodynamic compromise
    - Commonly seen in trauma or mechanical ventilation
  - Reexpansion pulmonary edema
    - Lung reexpansion can cause capillary leak
    - Common after large primary pneumothorax in younger patients
  - Pneumomediastinum
    - Most commonly in neonates
    - In adults being mechanically ventilated

Helpful Clues for Common Diagnoses
- **Spontaneous Pneumothorax**
  - Rupture of either small bullae or blebs
  - Familial pneumothorax: Occasionally reported
  - May be treated conservatively with chest tube drainage
- **Traumatic: Blunt or Penetrating Thoracic Injury**
  - Pneumothoraces result from alveolar compression, pulmonary laceration, tracheobronchial disruption, and barotrauma
    - Pulmonary lacerations in both blunt and penetrating trauma
    - Persistent pneumothorax due to air-leak or bronchopleural fistula
- **Iatrogenic**
  - Complication of biopsy procedures: Transthoracic needle aspiration (underlying emphysema), transbronchial biopsy, and colonoscopy
  - Complication of therapeutic procedures: Thoracentesis, central venous catheterization, mechanical ventilation, and tracheal intubation
  - Mechanical ventilation
- **Obstructive Pulmonary Disease**
  - Most common cause of secondary spontaneous pneumothorax
  - Complication of centrilobular or paraseptal pulmonary emphysema, asthma, and cystic fibrosis
- **Interstitial Lung Diseases**
  - Lymphangioleiomyomatosis (LAM): Pneumothorax develops in 80% of cases at some point
  - Langerhans cell histiocytosis: Pneumothorax develops in 25% of cases
  - Sarcoidosis
    - Associated with diffuse parenchymal disease
    - Necrosis of a subpleural granuloma
    - Bilateral, recurrent

- IPF: Pneumothorax or pneumomediastinum develops in 11% of cases
- **Connective Tissue Diseases**
  - Rheumatoid arthritis: Necrosis of subpleural necrobiotic nodules
  - Marfan syndrome: Pneumothoraces are commonly bilateral and recurrent; other respiratory abnormalities are bullae, cysts, and emphysema
  - Ehlers-Danlos syndromes: Pneumothorax is common in type IV Ehlers-Danlos syndrome; associated skeletal abnormalities are seen on chest radiograph
- **Immunologic**
  - Wegener granulomatosis
    - Usually associated with active vasculitis
    - Subpleural excavated nodules
  - Bronchocentric granulomatosis
    - Necrotizing granulomatous inflammation without associated vasculitis
    - Associated with allergic bronchopulmonary aspergillosis (50%)
- **Infections**
  - Bronchopleural fistula: May complicate necrotizing pneumonia (anaerobic, tuberculous, and pyogenic)
  - Postinfectious pneumatoceles resulting from *P. jiroveci* or *Staphylococcus*
  - Angioinvasive aspergillosis: Hematogenous dissemination with invasion of small arteries, vascular occlusion and often infarction
    - Particularly common in neutropenic stem cell transplant patients
  - Immunocompromised HIV(+) patients
    - *P. jiroveci*
- **Mimics of Pneumothorax**
  - Skin-folds, chest tube tracks, scapular edge, and rib companion shadow

Helpful Clues for Less Common Diagnoses

- **Metastases**
  - Metastatic sarcomas: Osteosarcoma, synovial cell sarcoma, angiosarcoma, and leiomyosarcoma
    - Frequently after induction of chemotherapy
- **Pulmonary Infarction**
  - Septic and aseptic emboli
    - Infective endocarditis in intravenous drug users

Helpful Clues for Rare Diagnoses

- **Catamenial**
  - Development of pneumothorax at time of menstruation from migrated endometrial tissue to pleura; 85-90% of cases occur on right
  - < 1/3 of cases associated with pelvic endometriosis
- **Birt-Hogg-Dubé Syndrome**
  - Dominantly inherited disease: Benign skin tumors, diverse types of renal cancer, pulmonary cysts (80%), and spontaneous pneumothorax

Spontaneous Pneumothorax

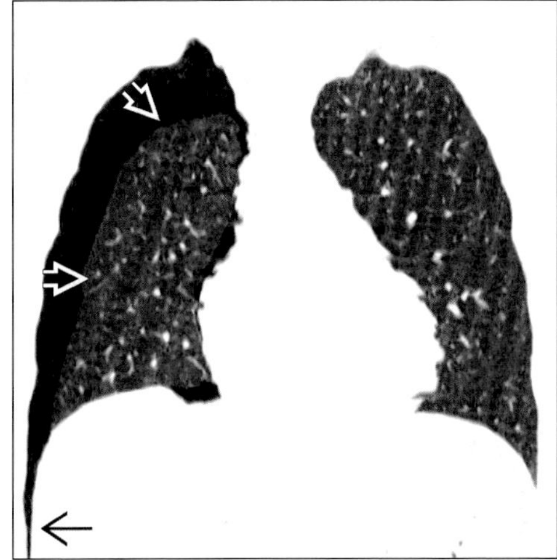

Coronal CT reconstruction shows a large anterior right pneumothorax ➔ causing the deep sulcus sign →.

Spontaneous Pneumothorax

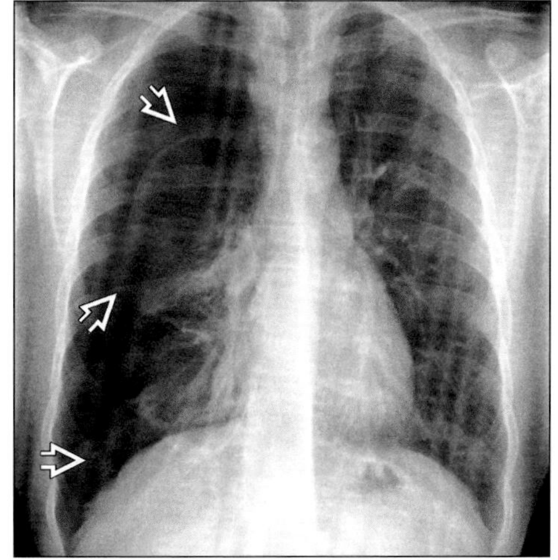

Frontal radiograph in full inspiration demonstrates a thin white line of the visceral pleura ➔ outlined by a large right pneumothorax. The patient was a 28-year-old male smoker.

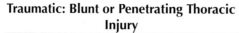

PNEUMOTHORAX

Traumatic: Blunt or Penetrating Thoracic Injury

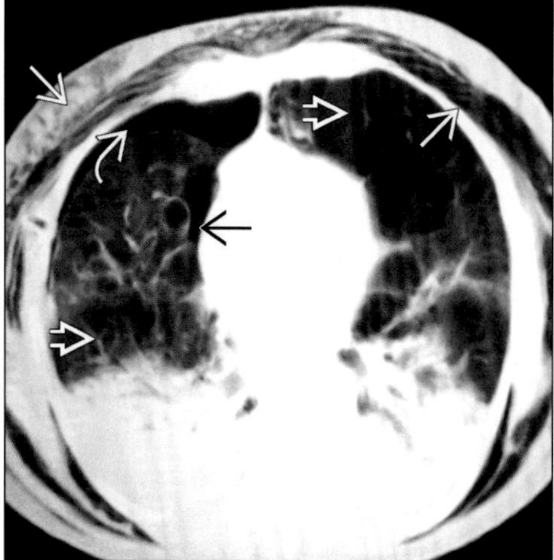

Traumatic: Blunt or Penetrating Thoracic Injury

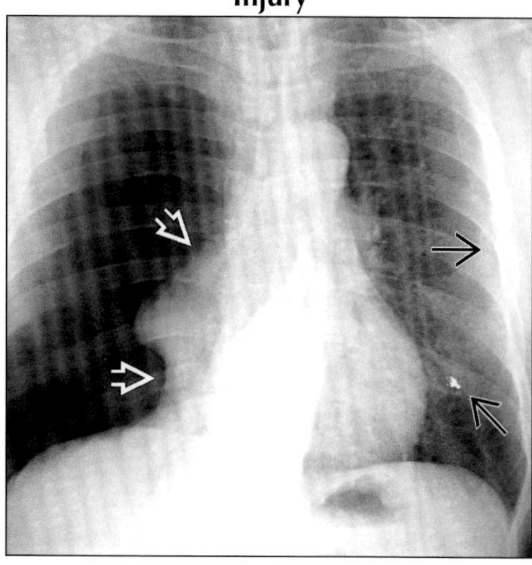

(Left) *Axial NECT shows a right pneumothorax and extensive subcutaneous emphysema. Note the subpleural small bullae in the right lung. Bilateral emphysematous changes are also demonstrated.* ***(Right)*** *Frontal radiograph shows a large right pneumothorax with mediastinal shift and collapse of the entire right lung. Note 2 small metallic bullet fragments in the left hemithorax.*

Interstitial Lung Diseases

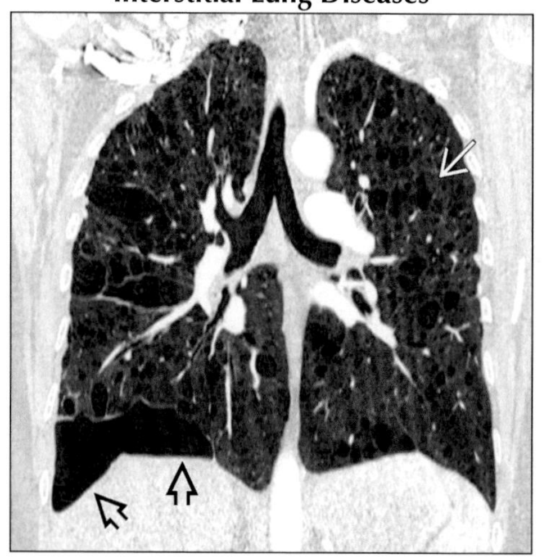

Interstitial Lung Diseases

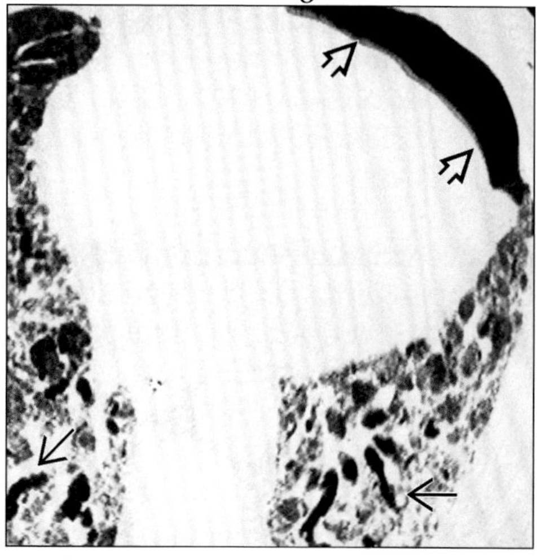

(Left) *Coronal NECT shows multiple thin-walled cysts scattered throughout both lungs. A loculated pneumothorax is seen in the right hemithorax. The findings are characteristic of lymphangioleiomyomatosis.* ***(Right)*** *Axial NECT shows a bilateral reticular pattern with traction bronchiectasis and a left pneumothorax. The patient had an accelerated UIP.*

Connective Tissue Diseases

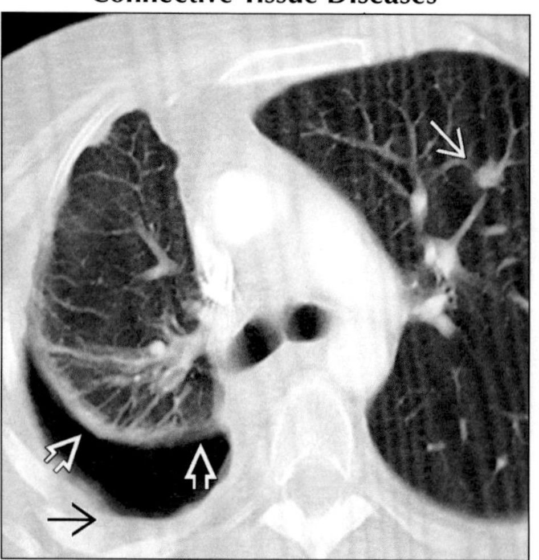

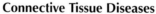

Immunologic

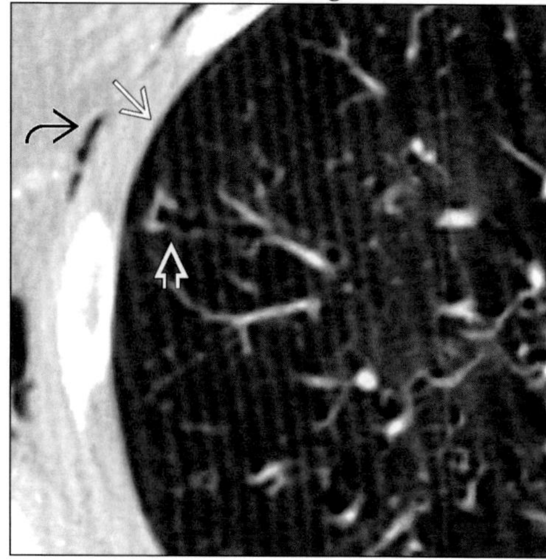

(Left) *Axial CECT (lung window) shows small hydropneumothorax in a 43-year-old woman with rheumatoid arthritis. The visceral pleura is markedly thickened. A small rheumatoid nodule is seen in the left lung.* ***(Right)*** *Axial NECT shows CT features of bronchocentric granulomatosis: Small right pneumothorax and subcutaneous emphysema. Note dilated airway puckered at the point of contact with the pleura.*

PNEUMOTHORAX

Infections

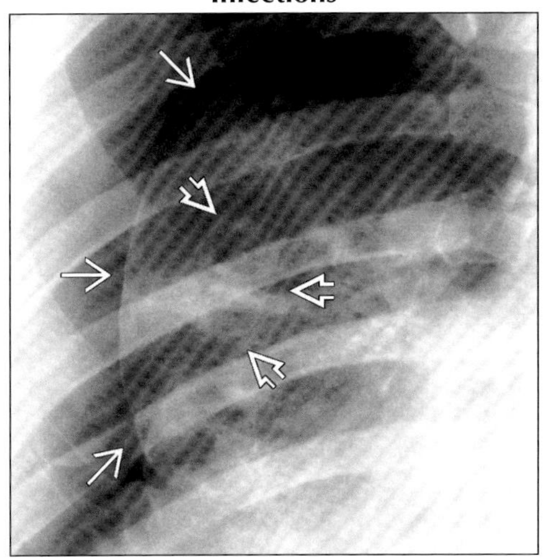

Infections

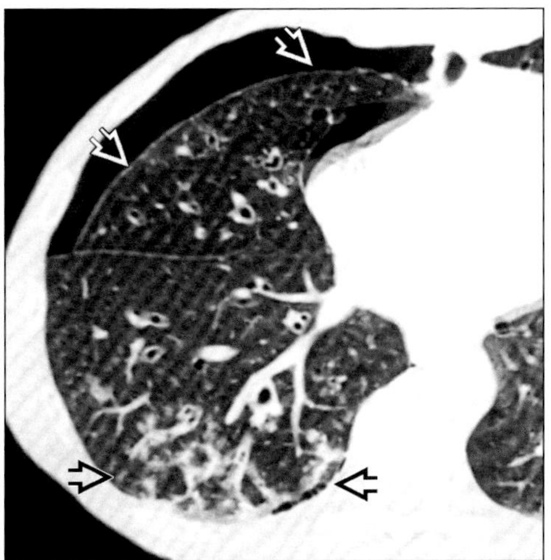

*(**Left**) Frontal radiograph shows a large right pneumothorax ➡ and multiple subpleural cysts ➡. This 45-year-old man was HIV(+) with prior history of P. jiroveci pneumonia. Pneumothorax was originated from rupture of one of the subpleural pneumatoceles. (**Right**) Axial NECT shows a right pneumothorax ➡. Multiple impacted bronchioles and "ill-defined" centrilobular nodules due to a bronchopneumonia were seen in the RLL ➡.*

Infections

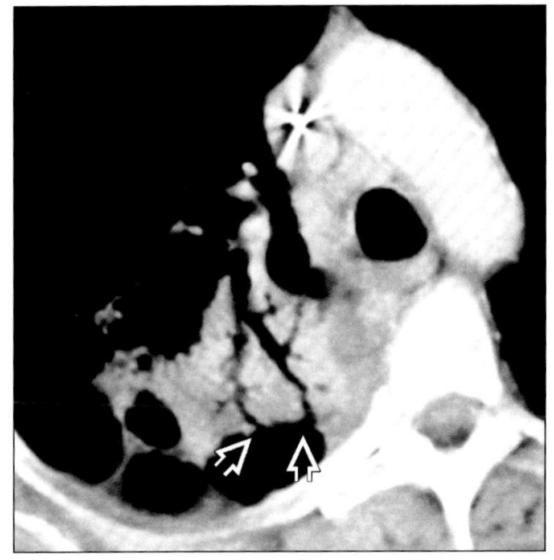

Mimics of Pneumothorax

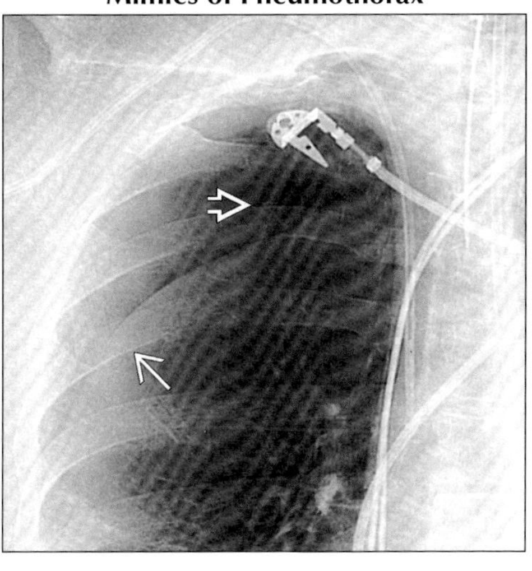

*(**Left**) Axial CECT shows a segmental consolidation in the posterior segment of the RUL. Direct communication between peripheral small bronchi and pleural cavity are nicely demonstrated ➡. (**Right**) Anteroposterior radiograph shows skinfold mimicking pneumothorax ➡. Note the skinfold is an edge rather than a line. Pulmonary vessels ➡ are seen coursing beyond the skinfold.*

Metastases

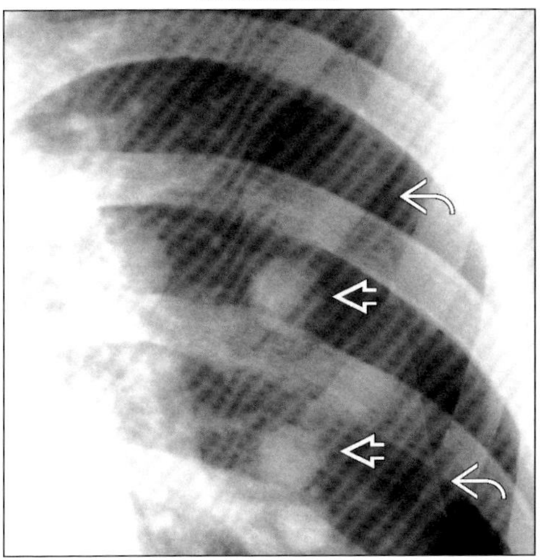

Catamenial

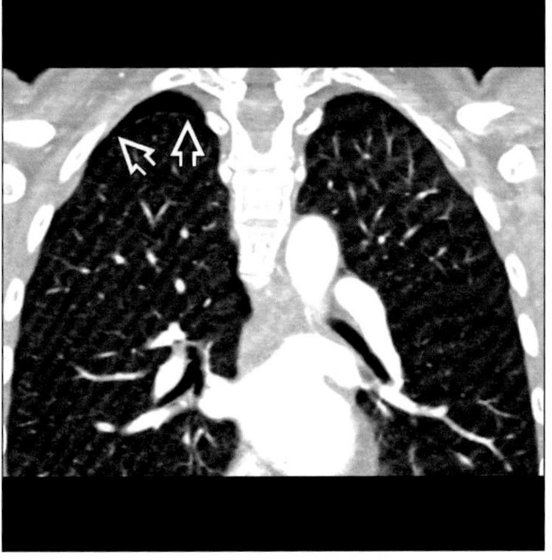

*(**Left**) Frontal radiograph shows a secondary left pneumothorax ➡. Several well-defined pulmonary nodules ➡ were also seen. This patient was a 27-year-old man who had an osteosarcoma. (**Right**) Coronal CECT shows subtle visceral pleural plaques ➡. While unproven, the plaques probably represent endometrial tissue.*

APICAL CAP

DIFFERENTIAL DIAGNOSIS

Common
- Normal Process of Aging
- Pancoast Tumor

Less Common
- Radiation Fibrosis
- Pleural Effusion (Supine Position)
- Lipoma or Extrapleural Fat

Rare but Important
- Aortic Transection
- Aspergilloma
- Pseudosequestration

ESSENTIAL INFORMATION

Helpful Clues for Common Diagnoses
- **Normal Process of Aging**
  - Sharp, smooth, or undulating margin, usually < 5 mm thick, often symmetric
  - Incidence increases with age
    - 40 years: 5%; 70 years: 50%
  - Incidence of right (22%) apical cap more common than left (17%) apical cap
  - Histology similar to pulmonary infarct
    - Age-related development probably due to chronic ischemia
  - Pathophysiology: Normal pulmonary artery pressure just sufficient to get blood to lung apex
- **Pancoast Tumor**
  - Asymmetric apical cap with convex margin > 5 mm thickness
  - Adjacent bone destruction of ribs (33%)

Helpful Clues for Less Common Diagnoses
- **Radiation Fibrosis**
  - For Hodgkin disease (mantle), breast cancer (supraclavicular nodes), head and neck cancers
- **Pleural Effusion (Supine Position)**
  - Apex in supine position most dependent portion of hemithorax
- **Lipoma or Extrapleural Fat**
  - Usually bilateral, enlarged body habitus, fat density at CT

Helpful Clues for Rare Diagnoses
- **Aortic Transection**
  - Left apical cap due to extravasation of blood in extrapleural space from related mediastinal bleeding or rib fractures
- **Aspergilloma**
  - Consider when new pleural thickening occurs adjacent to preexisting cavity, such as tuberculosis
  - Aspergilloma may not be radiographically evident
- **Pseudosequestration**
  - Refers to transpleural systemic-pulmonary artery anastomoses
  - Most commonly seen with severe pulmonary artery stenosis

Normal Process of Aging

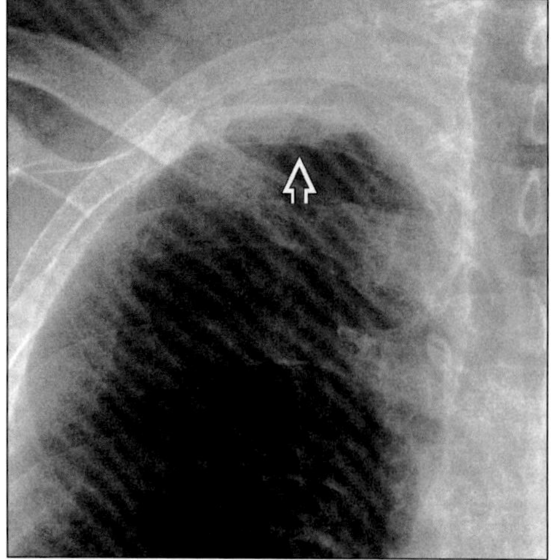

Frontal radiograph magnified view shows smooth right apical cap ⇨.

Normal Process of Aging

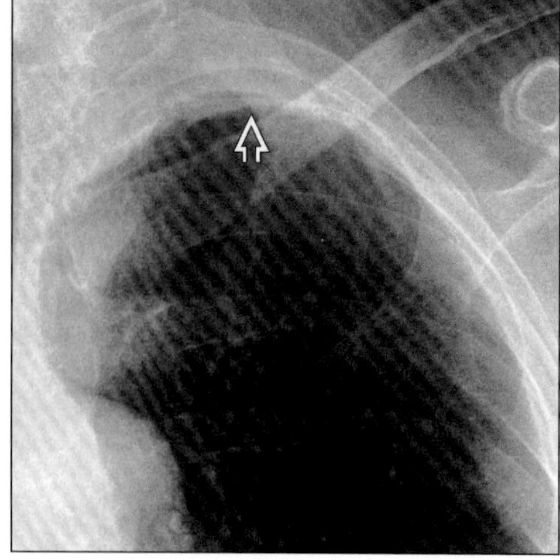

Frontal radiograph magnified view shows smooth left apical cap ⇨. Right apical cap is thicker than the left.

APICAL CAP

Pancoast Tumor

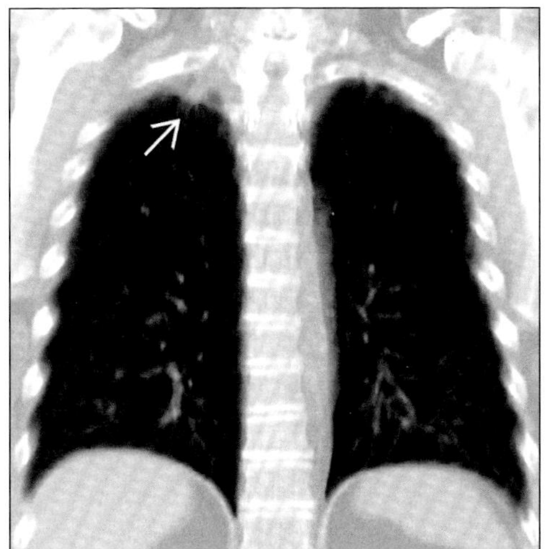

Radiation Fibrosis

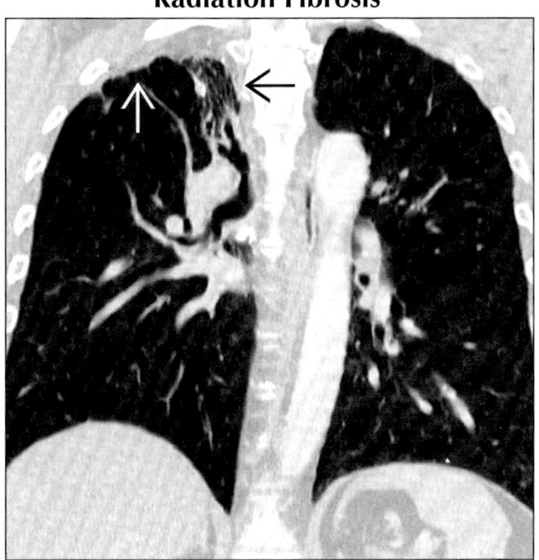

(Left) *Coronal NECT reconstruction shows focal apical thickening ➔. Edge is spiculated.* ***(Right)*** *Coronal CECT reconstruction shows right apical cap ➔ and volume loss of the right upper lobe ➔ from previous radiation therapy. Similar findings can be found with other causes of lung fibrosis, including tuberculosis or sarcoidosis.*

Pleural Effusion (Supine Position)

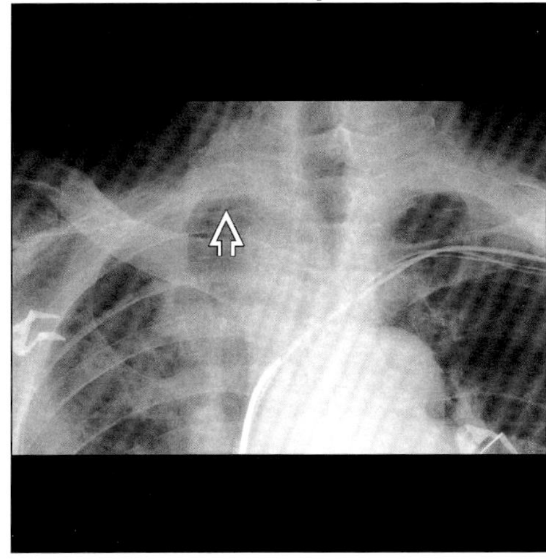

Aortic Transection

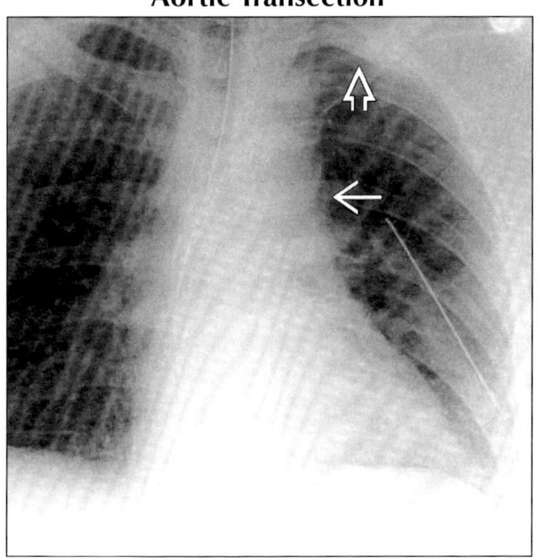

(Left) *Anteroposterior radiograph magnified view shows smooth right apical cap ➔. Right hemithorax is slightly more opaque than the left.* ***(Right)*** *Anteroposterior radiograph shows left apical cap ➔ and mediastinal widening and obscuration of aortic arch ➔ in a patient with blunt chest trauma.*

Aspergilloma

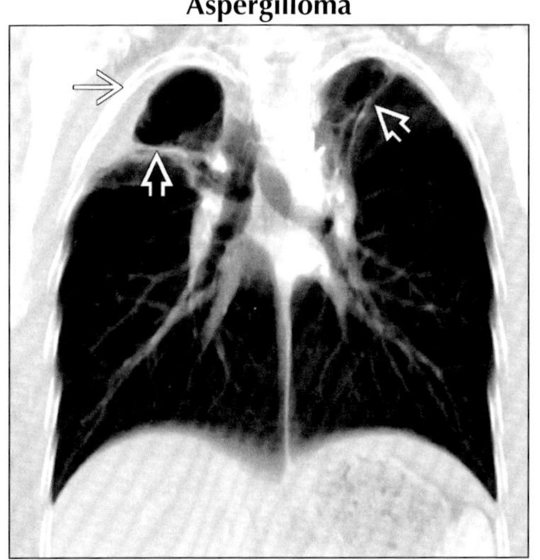

Pseudosequestration

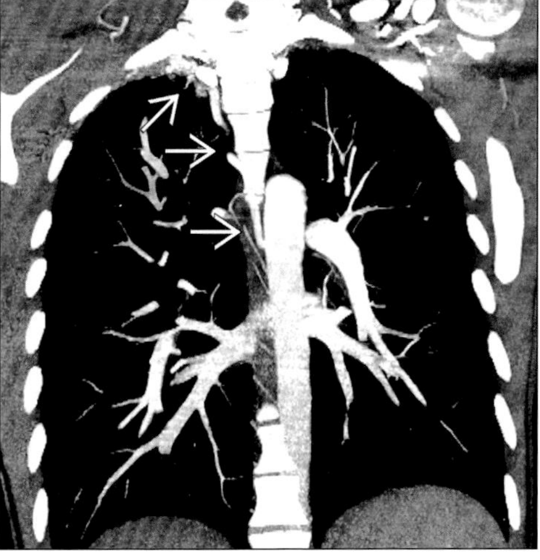

(Left) *Coronal CECT MIP reconstruction shows biapical cavities ➔ and right apical cap ➔. Even though there was no free fungus ball, pleural thickening adjacent to cavity suggests development of aspergilloma.* ***(Right)*** *Coronal CECT reconstruction shows enlarged collateral vessels ➔ resulting in a right apical cap. This patient had chronic obstruction of the right innominate artery.*

DIFFUSE PLEURAL THICKENING

DIFFERENTIAL DIAGNOSIS

Common
- Exudative Pleural Effusion
- Empyema
- Asbestos-related Pleural Disease
- Hemothorax
- Thoracotomy

Less Common
- Pleural Metastasis
- Radiation-induced Lung Disease
- Systemic Lupus Erythematosus
- Rheumatoid Arthritis
- Pleurodesis

Rare but Important
- Intrathoracic Drug Reaction
- Malignant Mesothelioma

ESSENTIAL INFORMATION

Key Differential Diagnosis Issues
- Definition of diffuse pleural thickening not standardized
- Commonly used definitions
  - Radiography
    - Extends more than 25% of chest wall
    - > 5 mm thickness at least at 1 site
    - Often involves costophrenic sulcus
  - CT
    - > 5 cm wide
    - > 8 cm craniocaudad extent
    - > 3 mm thick
- Less rigorous criteria may be appropriate
  - Lesser degree of pleural thickening may be functionally significant
- Extrapleural fat can mimic diffuse pleural thickening (fat attenuation)
  - Typically bilateral, symmetric, sparing costophrenic sulcus
- Often associated with parenchymal bands and rounded atelectasis

Helpful Clues for Common Diagnoses
- **Exudative Pleural Effusion**
  - Usually unilateral
  - Pleural thickening is late finding
    - Persists despite resolution of pleural effusion
  - Adjacent pneumonia or other pulmonary inflammation may present initially
    - Streptococcal and staphylococcal species most common
    - Nosocomial infection with gram-negative anaerobes and methicillin-resistant *Staphylococcus aureus* (MRSA)
  - Can calcify over time, though uncommon
- **Empyema**
  - Tuberculosis and streptococcal pneumonia most common causes
  - Usually unilateral
  - Pleural thickening is late finding
  - Adjacent pneumonia or other pulmonary inflammation may initially be present
  - Extensive calcification most commonly from tuberculosis
- **Asbestos-related Pleural Disease**
  - 10% of asbestos-exposed individuals affected
  - Distinct from pleural plaques
  - Affects primarily visceral pleura
  - Bilateral involvement more common than unilateral involvement
  - Often associated with significant restrictive respiratory impairment
  - Often associated with parenchymal bands and rounded atelectasis
- **Hemothorax**
  - Usually unilateral
  - Blunt or penetrating trauma
  - Iatrogenic
  - Parietal or visceral pleural thickening
    - Can develop rather quickly
    - Varying amount of residual pleural fluid
    - May calcify over time
  - Adjacent rib fractures suggestive
- **Thoracotomy**
  - Mild residual pleural thickening common
  - Usually smooth, mild thickening
  - Can result from postoperative hemothorax

Helpful Clues for Less Common Diagnoses
- **Pleural Metastasis**
  - ~ 90% of all pleural neoplasms
    - Lung carcinoma leading cause
    - Breast, ovary, and gastric carcinomas and lymphoma also common causes
  - Usually multiple
  - Can simulate benign pleural disease
  - Nodular, circumferential, and mediastinal pleural involvement suggestive of malignancy

- Associated pleural effusion common
- Can have lung or thoracic lymph node metastases

- **Radiation-induced Lung Disease**
  - Usually complication of radiation therapy for breast cancer, lung cancer, or lymphoma
  - Small residual pleural effusion may be present
  - Radiation-induced lung fibrosis often present in radiation field
- **Systemic Lupus Erythematosus**
  - Pleural thickening most common intrathoracic manifestation
    - Occurs in up to 30% in autopsy series
  - Unilateral more common than bilateral
  - Pleural effusion frequently present
- **Rheumatoid Arthritis**
  - Pleural diseases are most common intrathoracic manifestation
  - 40-70% pleural involvement in autopsy series
  - Pleural effusion may accompany pleural thickening
  - Unilateral more common than bilateral
- **Pleurodesis**
  - Variable degrees of pleural thickening and nodularity
    - Remain stable over time
    - May enhance with large amount of granulation tissue
  - Residual loculations of fluid common
  - High-attenuation deposits (from talc) mimic pleural calcification
    - Usually adjacent to dependent lung
    - May be lentiform

Helpful Clues for Rare Diagnoses

- **Intrathoracic Drug Reaction**
  - Numerous drugs linked to pleural effusions and thickening
  - Common agents include
    - Nitrofurantoin
    - Bromocriptine
    - Amiodarone
    - Procarbazine
    - Methotrexate
    - Bleomycin
    - Mitomycin
    - Dantrolene
  - Bilateral more common than unilateral
  - Generally resolve after cessation of therapy
- **Malignant Mesothelioma**
  - Most result from asbestos exposure
    - Latency of up to 40 years
  - Can simulate benign pleural disease
  - Nodular, circumferential, and mediastinal pleural involvement suggestive of malignancy
  - Mediastinum relatively "fixed" with little or no shift
  - Presence of pleural plaques biomarker of exposure
  - Associated pleural effusion may be present
  - Extrapleural spread
    - Chest wall, mediastinum, diaphragm

Exudative Pleural Effusion

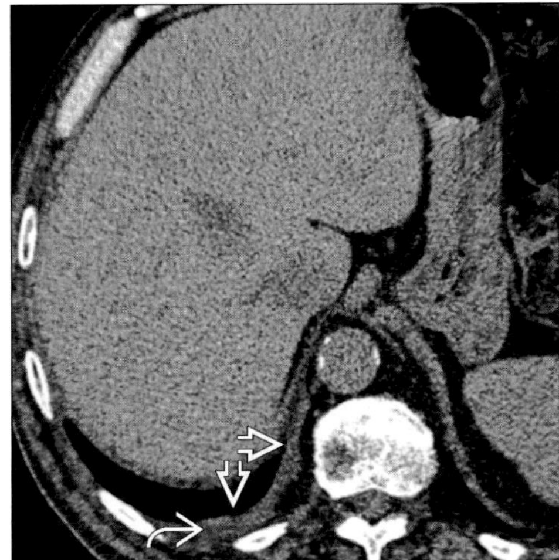

Axial NECT shows smooth right posterobasal pleural thickening ➡ with tiny residual effusion ➡ in this patient with recent pneumonia and parapneumonic effusion.

Asbestos-related Pleural Disease

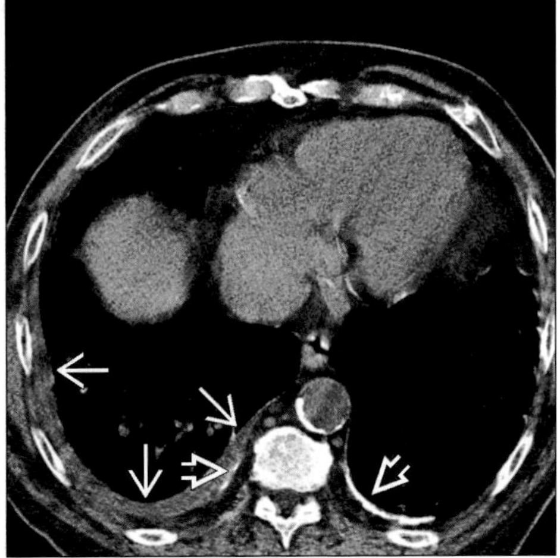

Axial NECT shows diffuse pleural thickening on the right ➡ in this patient with asbestos-related pleural disease. Note calcified plaques bilaterally ➡. Pleural thickening frequently leads to restrictive respiratory impairment.

DIFFUSE PLEURAL THICKENING

*(**Left**) Axial NECT shows bilateral pleural collections with associated pleural thickening in this patient with empyemas resulting from discitis. Loculations of gas are from thoracentesis. (**Right**) Coronal CT reconstruction shows pockets of pleural fluid in bilateral empyema from discitis of the thoracic spine. Gas is present in the right pleural space from thoracentesis.*

Empyema

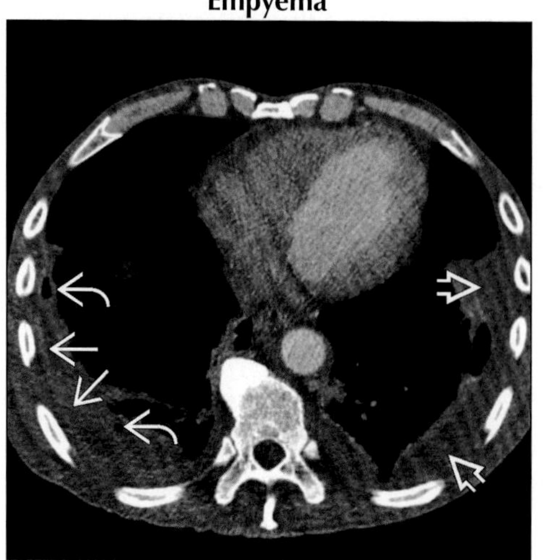

Empyema

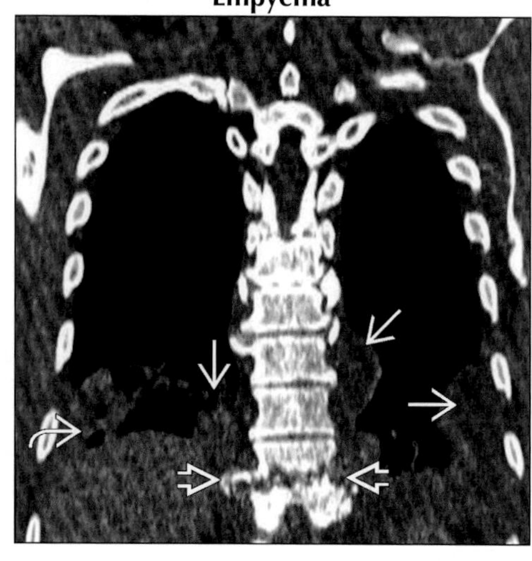

*(**Left**) Coronal CT reconstruction shows smooth right pleural thickening, which developed as a result of a large hemothorax. A portion of adjacent lung is compressed by the large hemothorax. (**Right**) Axial CECT shows thickening of the right paraspinal pleura in this patient who underwent right upper lobectomy for non-small cell lung carcinoma. Pleural metastases tend to be nodular and are often associated with a pleural effusion.*

Hemothorax

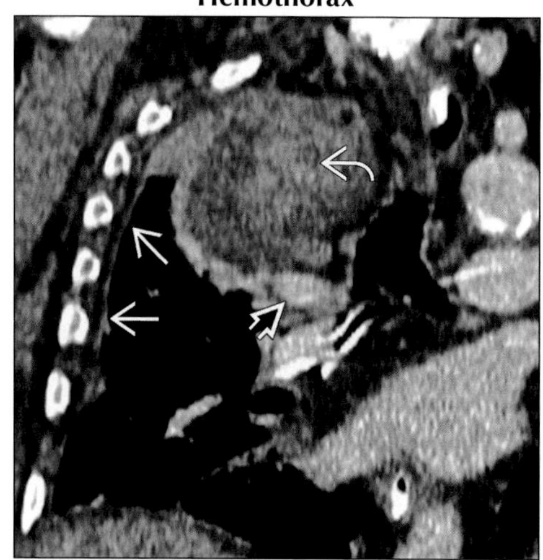

Thoracotomy

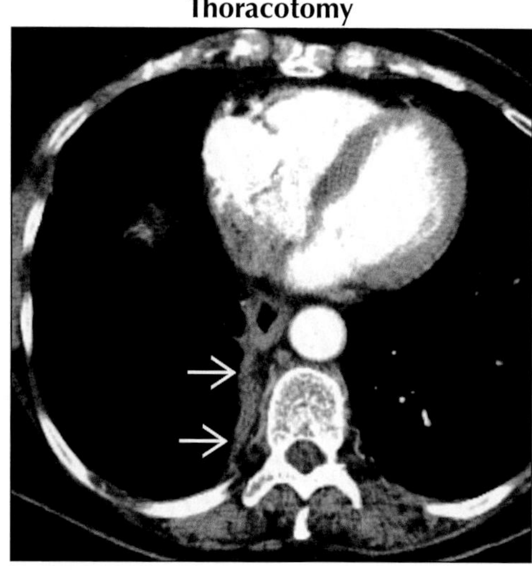

*(**Left**) Axial CECT shows extensive right pleural thickening in this patient with metastatic renal cell carcinoma. Note the circumferential, nodular distribution with involvement of the major fissure and mediastinal pleura. (**Right**) Coronal CT reconstruction shows extensive right pleural thickening and effusion in this patient with metastatic renal cell carcinoma. Note nodular mediastinal pleural thickening and a left lung metastasis.*

Pleural Metastasis

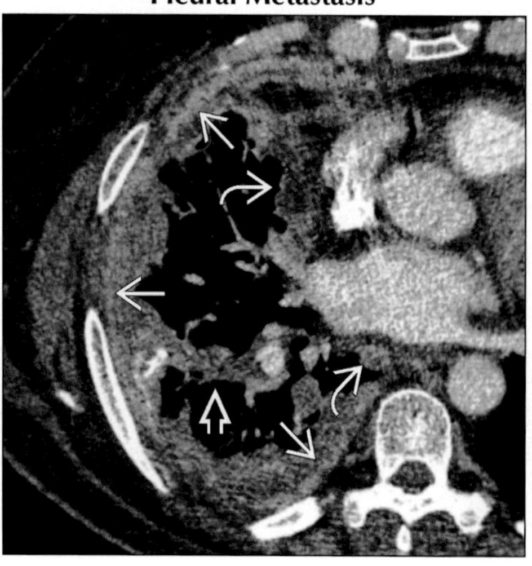

Pleural Metastasis

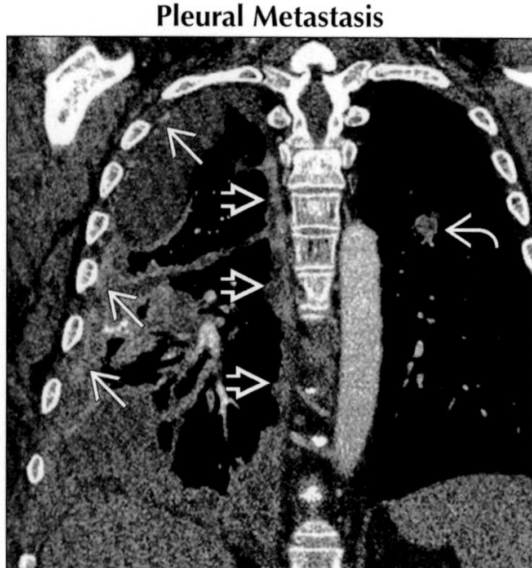

Radiation-induced Lung Disease

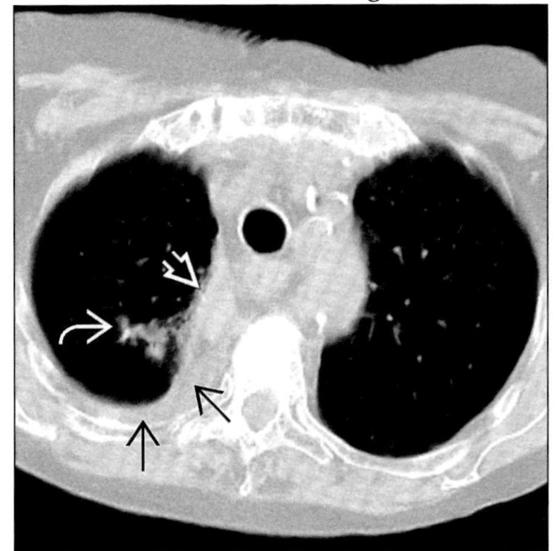

Systemic Lupus Erythematosus

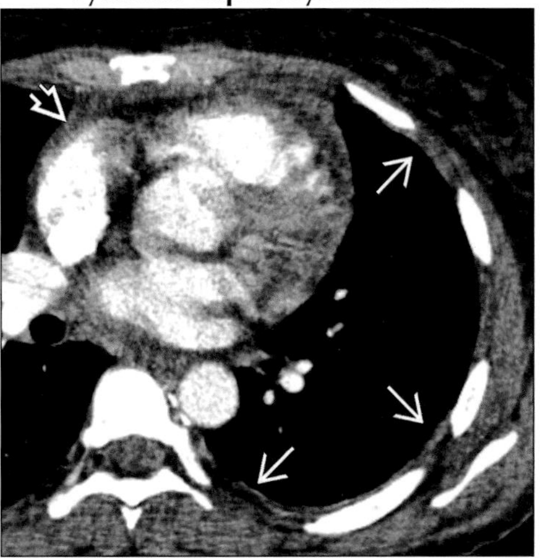

*(**Left**) Axial CECT shows smooth right pleural thickening ➝ adjacent to radiation fibrosis ➡ in this patient treated for lung cancer. Pleural thickening is typically limited to the radiation port but can be more extensive when more severe pleuritis develops. Note recurrent tumor ➡ just lateral to the radiated lung. (**Right**) Axial CECT shows smooth, mild left pleural thickening ➡ and a small pericardial effusion ➡. Serositis is common in lupus.*

Rheumatoid Arthritis

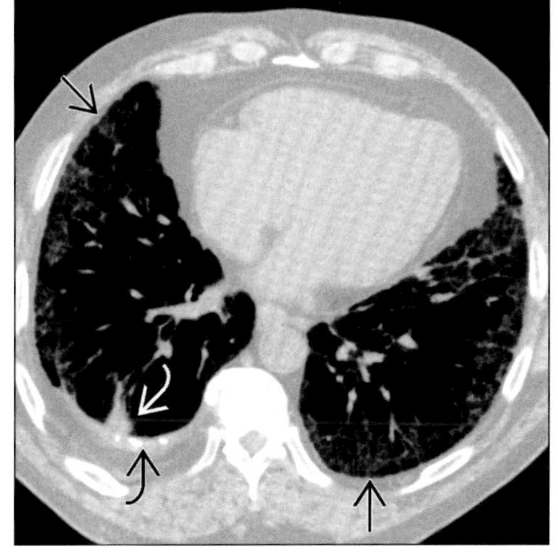

Pleurodesis

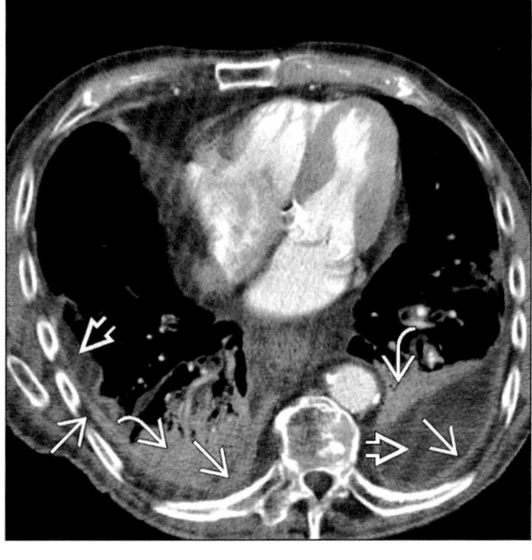

*(**Left**) Axial NECT shows right pleural thickening and calcification ➝ with adjacent rounded atelectasis ➡. Fairly extensive interstitial fibrosis is also present ➝. (**Right**) Axial CECT shows bilateral pleural thickening ➡ and small effusions ➡ in this patient who underwent talc pleurodesis for chronic pleural effusions resulting from yellow nail syndrome. Chronic lower lobe atelectasis ➡ is present bilaterally.*

Intrathoracic Drug Reaction

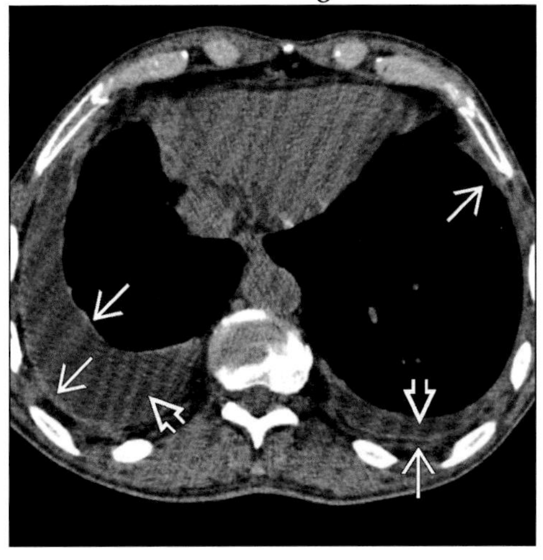

Malignant Mesothelioma

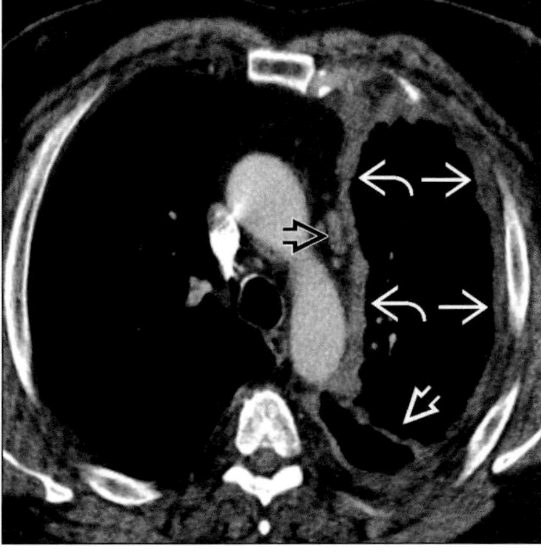

*(**Left**) Axial NECT shows bilateral pleural effusions ➡ with smooth visceral and parietal pleural thickening ➡ resulting from therapy with pergolide. The pleural effusions resolved upon cessation of the drug. (**Right**) Axial CECT shows circumferential left pleural thickening and nodularity ➡. Note involvement of the mediastinal pleura ➡ and major fissure ➡. Mediastinal lymphadenopathy is also present ➝.*

SPLIT PLEURA SIGN

DIFFERENTIAL DIAGNOSIS

Common
- Empyema
- Sterile Reactive Collection
- Malignant Effusion

Less Common
- Hemothorax
- Postsurgical
- Pleurodesis

Rare but Important
- Chronic Tuberculous Pleuritis

ESSENTIAL INFORMATION

Key Differential Diagnosis Issues
- Not specific for empyema
  - Can occur with other causes of loculated pleural fluid
- CECT
  - Enhancement of thickened inner visceral and outer parietal pleura
  - Thickened visceral and parietal pleural layers separated by fluid
  - Thickening of extrapleural fat

Helpful Clues for Common Diagnoses
- **Empyema**
  - Commonly associated with bacterial pneumonia
    - Gram positive bacteria (*Staphylococcus aureus* & *Streptococcus pneumoniae*): 50%
  - Transformation of parapneumonic effusion (not infected) into complicated effusion (infected but not purulent) and into empyema (frank pus)
  - CECT features
    - Pleural enhancement: Not seen in transudative effusions
    - High accuracy in differentiating empyema from lung abscess
- **Sterile Reactive Collection**
  - Smooth, thin pleural surfaces and homogeneous fluid density
- **Malignant Effusion**
  - Mesothelioma
    - Parietal and to lesser extent visceral pleura involvement
  - Metastases: Most common from breast, ovary, lung, and malignant thymoma
  - Pleural nodularity

Helpful Clues for Less Common Diagnoses
- **Hemothorax**
  - More uniform pleural thickening
- **Postsurgical**
  - Expected after lobectomy and pneumonectomy
- **Pleurodesis**
  - Often for malignant effusions
  - High attenuation areas in posterior basal regions of pleural space
  - Extension of talc deposits into fissures

Helpful Clues for Rare Diagnoses
- **Chronic Tuberculous Pleuritis**
  - Thick calcification

Empyema

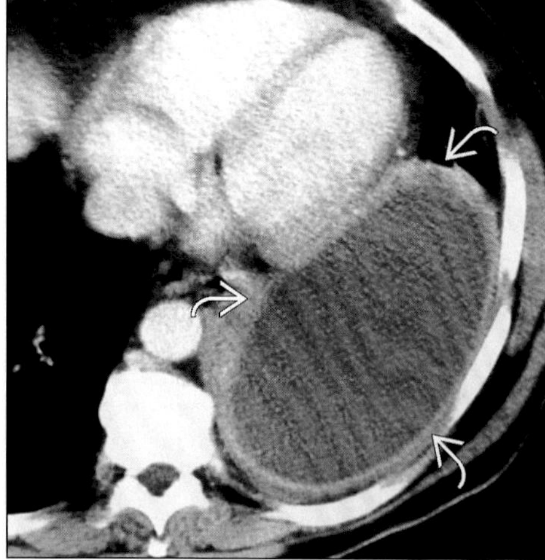

Axial CECT shows a large, loculated, left-sided pleural fluid with a typical split pleura sign ➔. Thoracocentesis showed empyema.

Sterile Reactive Collection

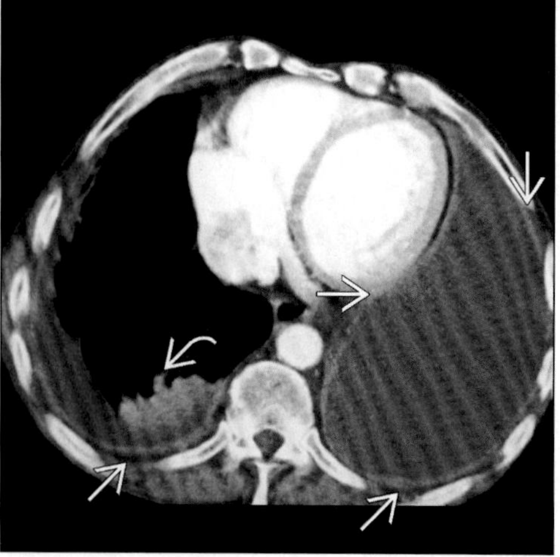

Axial CECT shows a smooth bilateral pleural thickening ➔ in a patient with asbestos exposure. Bilateral pleural effusion and a rounded atelectasis in the right lower lobe ➔ are also observed.

SPLIT PLEURA SIGN

Malignant Effusion

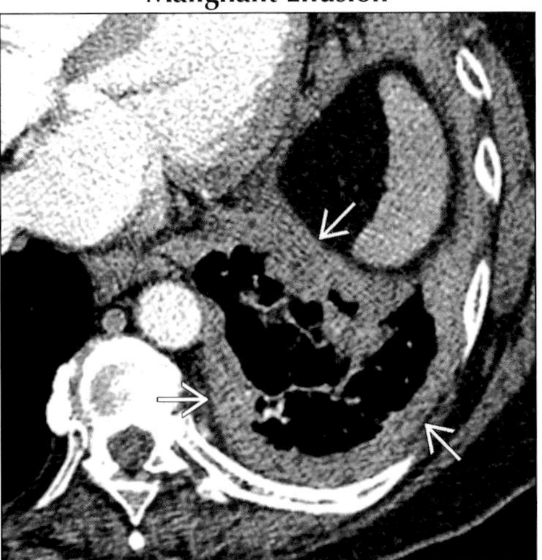

Hemothorax

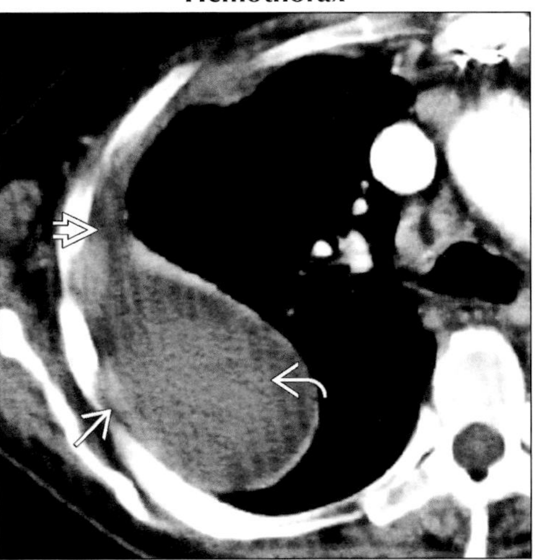

(Left) *Axial CECT shows diffuse pleural thickening affecting the left hemithorax* → *. Note the fluid collection appears somewhat nodular.* ***(Right)*** *Axial CECT in a patient on anticoagulant therapy shows heterogeneous attenuation of the right loculated pleural fluid collection* → *. The associated pleural thickening* → *is consistent with chronic loculated hemothorax. Note split pleura sign* → *.*

Postsurgical

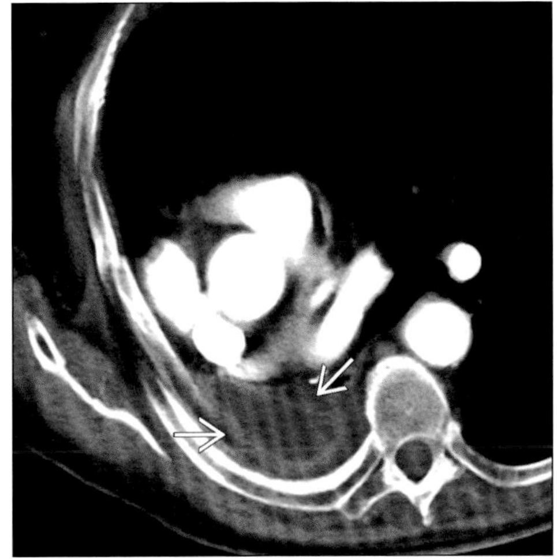

Pleurodesis

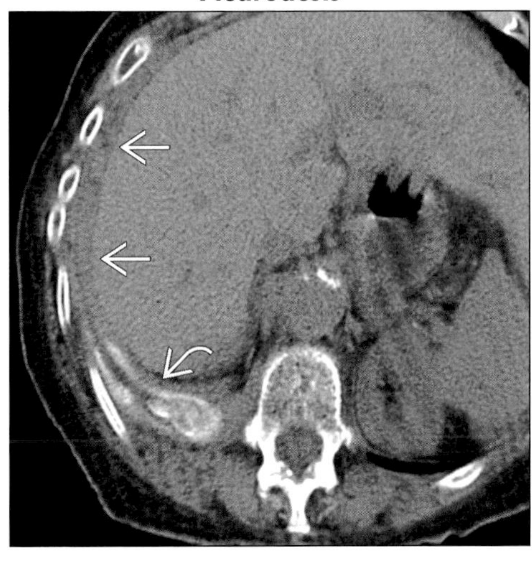

(Left) *Axial CECT shows typical findings of prior right pneumonectomy. There is a small, residual, lenticular, sterile fluid collection with associated parietal pleural thickening in the posterior right hemithorax* → *, showing the split pleura sign.* ***(Right)*** *Axial NECT shows talc deposition in both visceral and parietal pleura in the right posterior basal region* → *. Smooth thickening of the pleura is also visible* → *. This patient has a history of metastatic breast carcinoma.*

Chronic Tuberculous Pleuritis

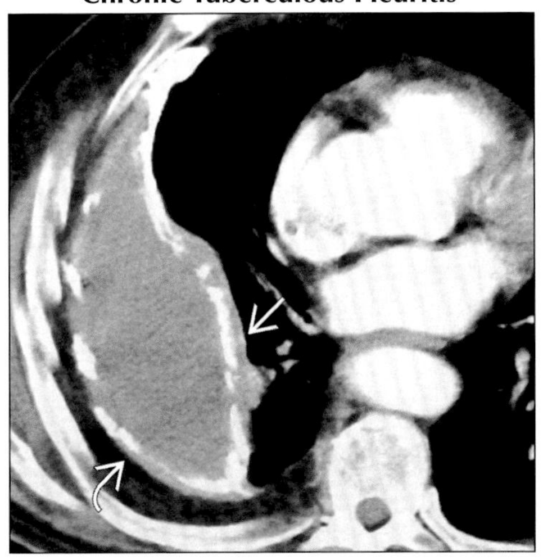

Chronic Tuberculous Pleuritis

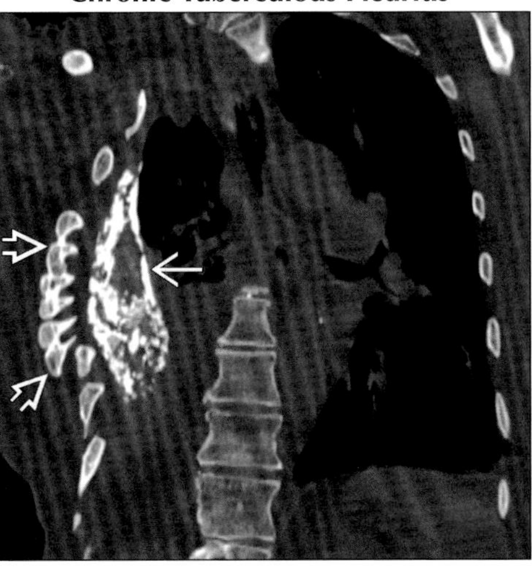

(Left) *Axial CECT shows a large loculated collection in the right hemithorax with extensive calcification of the visceral* → *and parietal* → *pleura (split pleura sign).* ***(Right)*** *Coronal NECT (bone window) shows marked reduction in volume of the right hemithorax, thick-walled calcified empyema (lenticular shape)* → *, fibrothorax, and periosteal thickening from chronic osteitis* → *.*

PLEURAL PLAQUES

DIFFERENTIAL DIAGNOSIS

Common
- Asbestos-related Pleural Disease
- Prior Empyema
- Prior Hemothorax or Other Injury to Pleura
- Pleural Effusion
- Extrapleural Fat

Less Common
- Pleural Metastases
- Primary Pleural Tumor
  - Malignant Mesothelioma
- Pleurodesis

Rare but Important
- Postcardiac Injury Syndromes

ESSENTIAL INFORMATION

Key Differential Diagnosis Issues
- Radiographs
  - Look for any associated abnormalities
    - Underlying lung disease: Lung cancer, metastases
    - Overlying chest wall disease or injury
    - Rib fractures
  - Detection of calcification is useful distinguishing feature
    - Asbestos-related plaque
    - Talc pleurodesis
    - Treated empyema or pleural tuberculosis
  - Distribution of "pleural thickening" helpful in determining etiology
    - Symmetric: Consider asbestos-related
    - Asymmetric: Less likely asbestos-related
  - In patients with asbestos exposure, must distinguish plaques from extrapleural fat
- CT
  - Most useful examination for distinguishing fat from fluid from solid thickening
  - Distinguishes true pleural disease from pleural-based lung abnormalities or chest wall disease
  - Look for any associated abnormalities
    - Underlying lung scarring, inflammation, or masses
    - Overlying rib fractures or callous around healed fractures, metastases, prior surgery

Helpful Clues for Common Diagnoses
- **Asbestos-related Pleural Disease**
  - Distribution
    - Hemidiaphragms
    - Paravertebral
    - Antero-/lateral
    - Bilateral and fairly symmetric
    - Parietal pleura, only rarely involves visceral pleura
    - Spares apices and costophrenic sulci
    - Well-demarcated elevations of pleura best seen in profile
  - Often calcified: Radiographic "holly leaf" sign
  - Large, thick plaques associated with round atelectasis
  - Biomarker of exposure to asbestos
  - Benign disease
  - Rarely extend more than 4 rib interspaces; 2-5 mm thick; relative symmetric involvement
  - Linear band of calcification when viewed in profile; irregular "holly leaf" configuration en face
- **Prior Empyema**
  - Adjacent lung abnormal, scarring from previous pneumonia
  - Usually unilateral
  - Focal or diffuse pleural scarring
  - Parietal and visceral involvement
  - Can be associated with prominent focal extrapleural fat, as a result of chronic pleural inflammation
- **Prior Hemothorax or Other Injury to Pleura**
  - Unilateral, multiple healed rib fractures
  - History or evidence of prior thoracotomy (resected rib)
  - History of prior thoracostomy tube
- **Pleural Effusion**
  - Small volume mimics thickened pleura
  - Free-flowing effusions will be mobile
    - Bilateral decubitus radiographs
    - Prone and supine CT
  - Loculated effusions should appear more lenticular
  - Involves fissures, apices, and costophrenic sulci, unlike asbestos-related pleural disease
  - Simple transudative effusions are near water attenuation
  - Exudative effusions have attenuation between water and soft tissue

- "Split pleura" sign
  - Enhanced or thickened pleura separated by lower attenuation fluid suggests empyema
- **Extrapleural Fat**
  - Fat attenuation on CT
  - Radiographs, most evident on lateral chest wall convexities
  - Symmetric, mid-lateral chest wall at level of 4th to 8th ribs; may extend into fissures
  - Associated with other fat deposition: Pericardial fat pads, widened mediastinum
  - No calcifications

Helpful Clues for Less Common Diagnoses

- **Pleural Metastases**
  - Usually known primary tumor, commonly adenocarcinoma
  - Typically nodular or "lumpy bumpy"
  - Extend into fissures
  - Effusions commonly associated
  - May be indistinguishable from mesothelioma
- **Malignant Mesothelioma**
  - Very similar or indistinguishable appearance to metastatic adenocarcinoma pleural metastases
    - Needs histologic differentiation
  - Almost all have history of asbestos exposure
  - Unilateral
  - Involves parietal and visceral pleura, pericardium
  - Circumferential, nodular thickening
    - Not usually focal like simple plaques
    - Markedly reduces volume of involved hemithorax
    - Often associated with asbestos-related plaques
    - Plaques can be engulfed by tumor
    - > 1 cm in thickness
  - Effusions common
    - May be very early presenting feature
- **Pleurodesis**
  - Mechanical or chemical irritation and inflammation of pleura to obliterate pleural space
    - Prevent fluid reaccumulation
    - Prevent spontaneous pneumothorax
    - Other agents include tetracycline or bleomycin
  - Usually unilateral
  - Can closely mimic appearance of asbestos-related pleural plaque

Helpful Clues for Rare Diagnoses

- **Postcardiac Injury Syndromes**
  - Dressler syndrome, post-myocardial infarction syndrome, post-cardiotomy pericarditis
    - Autoimmune phenomena occurring 1 month to 2 years after cardiac insult
  - Prior history of cardiac injury, myocardial infarction, or heart surgery
  - Usually pericarditis but can involve pleura resulting in pleurisy, pleural effusions

Asbestos-related Pleural Disease

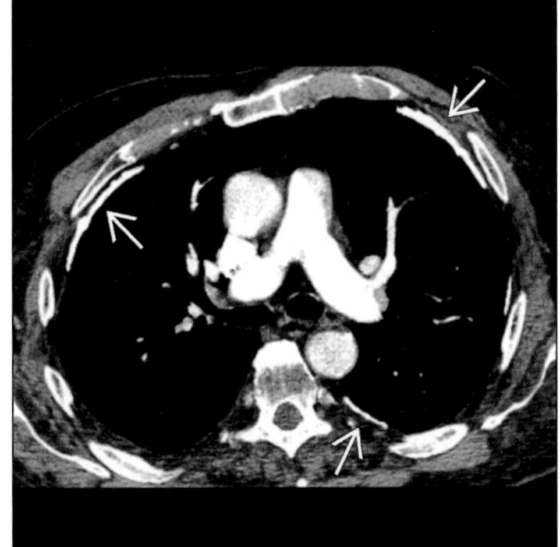

Axial CECT from a patient with long exposure to asbestos shows asbestos-related disease with focal calcified pleural plaques ➡ in a typical distribution pattern.

Asbestos-related Pleural Disease

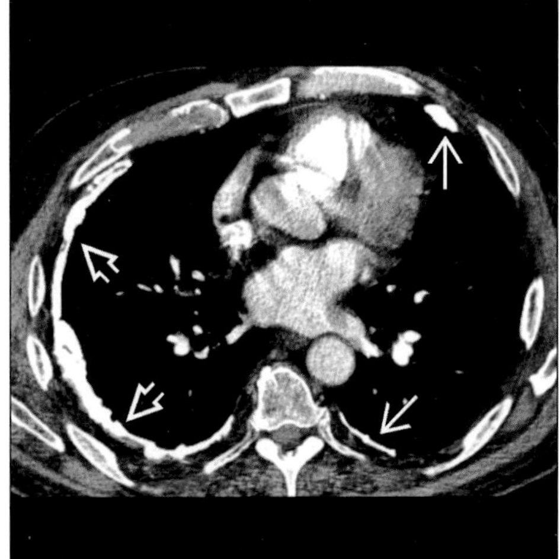

Axial CECT from a patient with a long exposure history to asbestos shows focal calcified pleural plaques ➡ and diffuse pleural thickening ➡ with volume loss of the right hemithorax.

PLEURAL PLAQUES

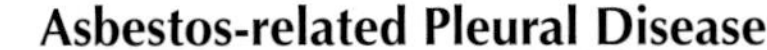

Asbestos-related Pleural Disease

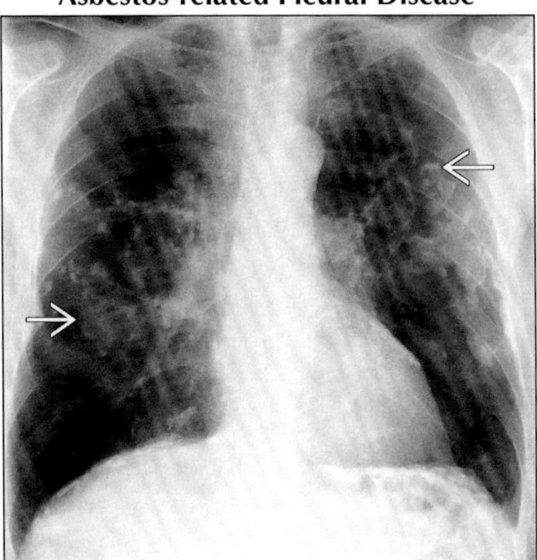

Asbestos-related Pleural Disease

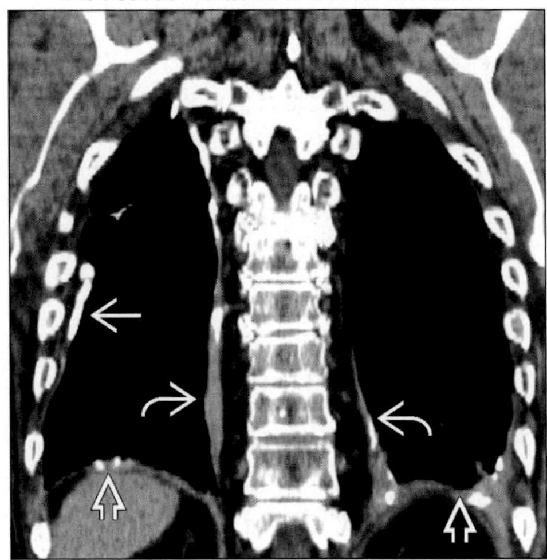

(Left) *Frontal radiograph shows typical calcified asbestos-related pleural plaques, in this case showing pleural plaque en face as the "holly leaf" sign* ➔. ***(Right)*** *Coronal NECT shows typical distribution for asbestos-related pleural plaques: Lateral chest wall* ➔*, hemidiaphragm* ➔*, and paravertebral* ➔.

Asbestos-related Pleural Disease

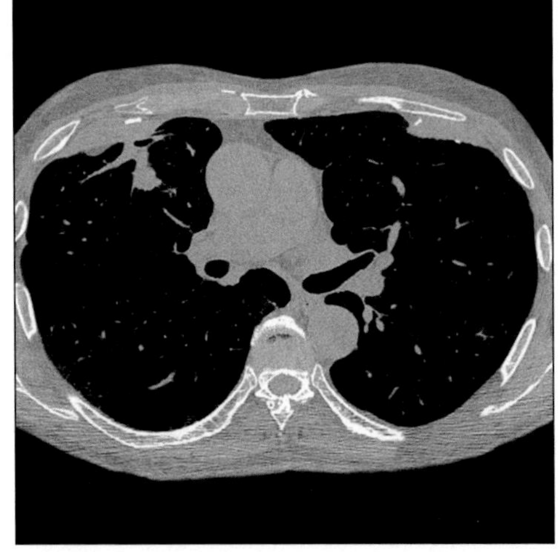

Asbestos-related Pleural Disease

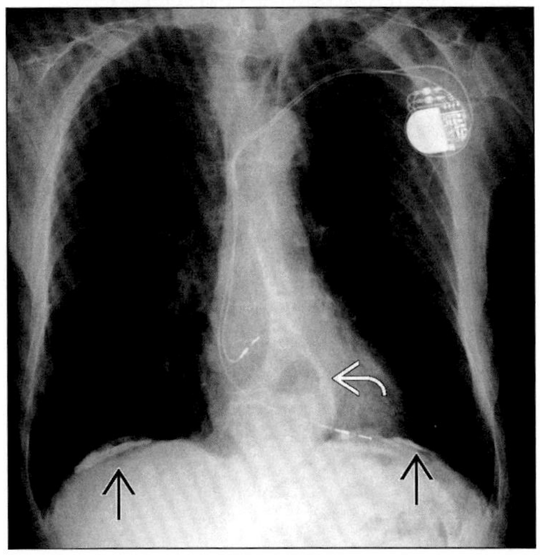

(Left) *Axial NECT shows typical bilateral, symmetric, thick, anterior pleural plaques with some calcification. In addition, note the associated rounded atelectasis in the right lung.* ***(Right)*** *Frontal radiograph shows typical bilateral, symmetric, calcified, asbestos-related pleural plaques, best seen over each hemidiaphragm* ➔*. Also note incidental hiatal hernia* ➔ *and bipolar pacemaker.*

Prior Empyema

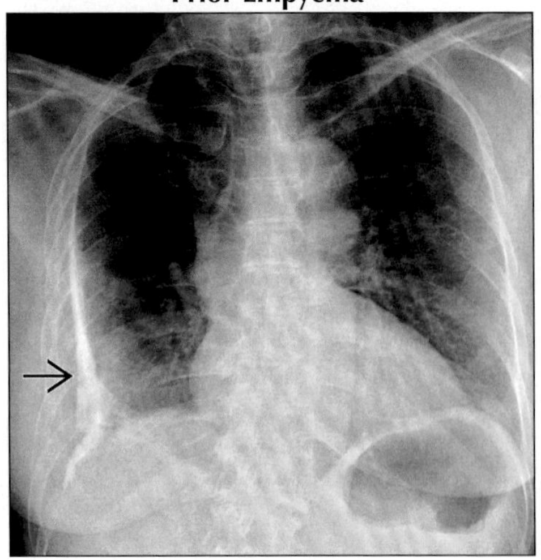

Prior Empyema

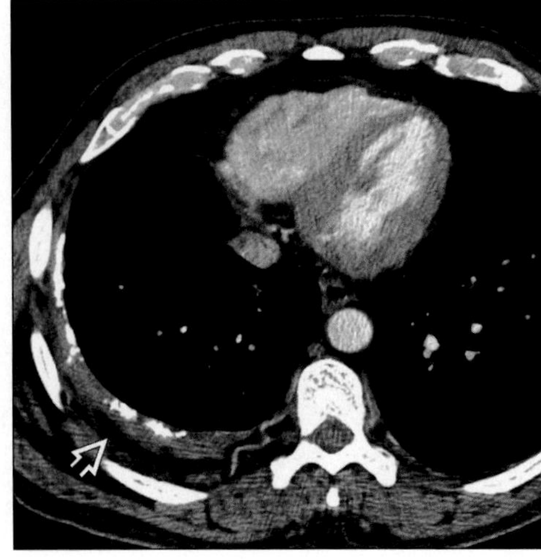

(Left) *Frontal radiograph shows extensive, dense, unilateral, right-sided calcification of pleura* ➔ *from this patient with prior treated pleural tuberculosis. Note there is no underlying lung abnormality in this case.* ***(Right)*** *Axial CECT shows extensive calcified pleural thickening in the right hemithorax from prior pleural tuberculosis. Note the underlying extrapleural fatty hyperplasia* ➔*, a common finding in patients with chronic pleural inflammation.*

Prior Hemothorax or Other Injury to Pleura

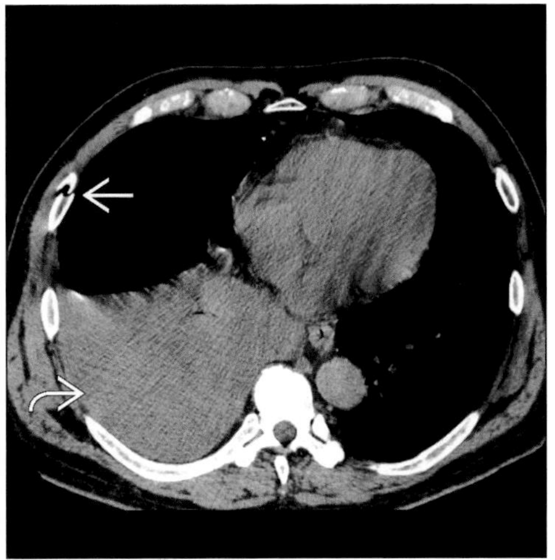

Pleural Effusion

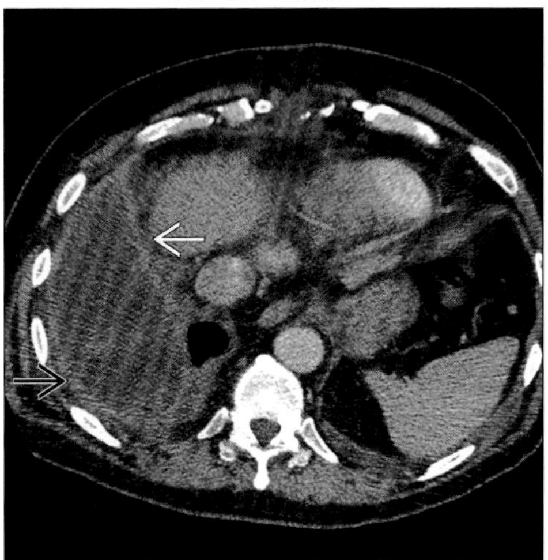

(Left) *Axial NECT shows typical CT features of hemothorax due to high-energy chest trauma, with moderate-sized hemothorax ➔ & rib fracture ➔. The right fluid collection is somewhat higher in attenuation (more like muscle) than simple water density.* ***(Right)*** *Axial NECT from a patient with empyema shows right-sided thickening of parietal ➔ & visceral pleura ➔ with lower attenuation fluid between the pleural layers, known as the "split pleura" sign.*

Pleural Metastases

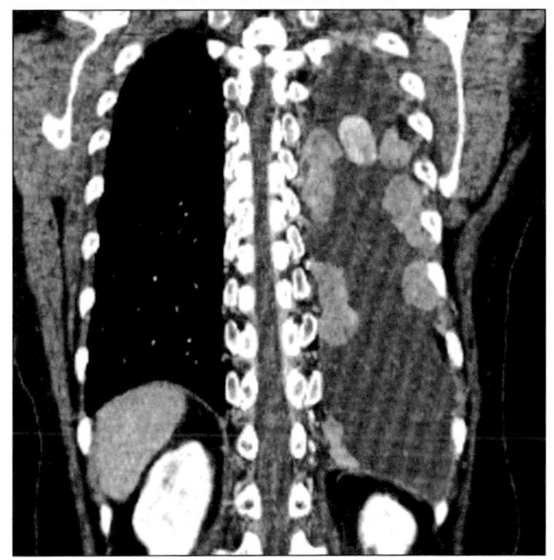

Pleural Metastases

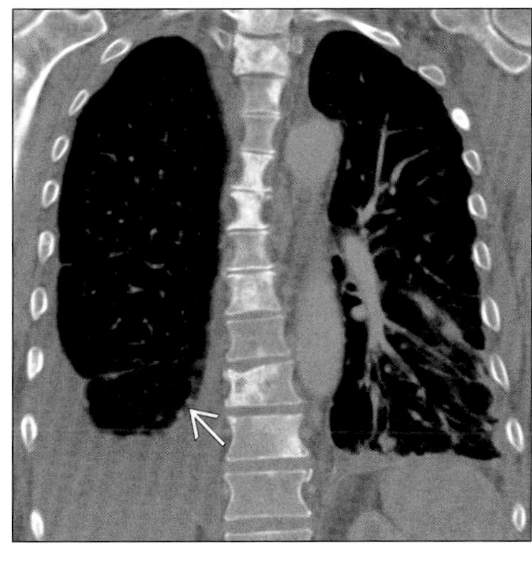

(Left) *Coronal CECT shows layering left pleural effusion and extensive nodular pleural metastases from a primary lung cancer.* ***(Right)*** *Coronal CT reconstruction from this patient with underlying primary lung cancer shows extensive bilateral pleural and lung metastases. Note the moderately large right pleural effusion and associated visceral pleural nodularity ➔.*

Pleurodesis

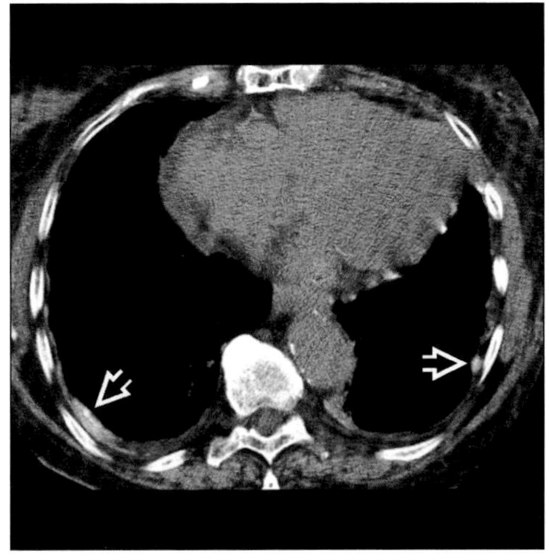

Postcardiac Injury Syndromes

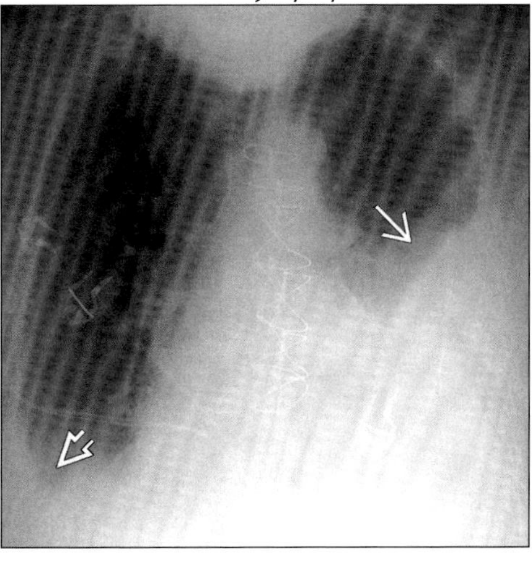

(Left) *Axial NECT shows typical CT features of bilateral, high-attenuation, focal pleural thickening from prior talc pleurodesis ➔. In this case, there is some focal pleural thickening along the right cardiac border as well.* ***(Right)*** *Anteroposterior radiograph shows typical radiographic features of pleural effusion due to postcardiac injury syndrome from median sternotomy 6 weeks earlier. Note the moderate to large left pleural effusion ➔ and small right pleural effusion ➔.*

PLEURAL MASS

DIFFERENTIAL DIAGNOSIS

Common
- Pleural Pseudotumor
- Pleural Plaque
- Pleural Thickening
- Empyema
- Rounded Atelectasis
- Subpleural Lung Cancer

Less Common
- Pleural Metastasis
- Pulmonary Infarctions (Subpleural)
- Extrapleural Abnormality
  - Benign or Malignant Chest Wall Mass
  - Extrapleural Hematoma
  - Fracture
- Pleurodesis

Rare but Important
- Lymphoma
- Malignant Mesothelioma
- Fibrous Tumor of Pleura

ESSENTIAL INFORMATION

Key Differential Diagnosis Issues
- Pleural vs. subpleural (pulmonary)
  - Pleural: Obtuse margins with chest wall, well-defined margins with lung, no air bronchograms
  - Subpleural (pulmonary): Acute margins with chest wall, ill-defined margins with lung, air bronchograms
- Differentiation of extrapleural vs. pleural abnormality can be difficult
  - Extrapleural component present if concomitant effect on extrapleural structures
    - Rib destruction in extrapleural tumor
    - Extension of mass into chest wall on CT
    - Internal displacement of extrapleural fat
- Incomplete border sign on radiograph highly suggestive of extrapulmonary (pleural or extrapleural) lesion
  - Margins partially sharp and partially unsharp

Helpful Clues for Common Diagnoses
- **Pleural Pseudotumor**
  - Loculated pleural fluid in interlobar fissure, usually minor fissure
  - History of congestive heart failure
  - Oval shape, peripheral tapering along margins of pseudotumor
- **Pleural Plaque**
  - Related to previous asbestos exposure
  - Bilateral focal regions of pleural thickening, ± calcification, often symmetric
  - Posterolateral, diaphragmatic, and pericardial preponderance; sparing of apices and costophrenic angles
- **Pleural Thickening**
  - Related to asbestos exposure, previous infection or inflammation, hemothorax
  - Usually smooth thickening of pleura, often diffuse, ± foci of calcification
  - May affect costophrenic angles; often broad extension as opposed to focality of pleural plaques
- **Empyema**
  - Pus in pleural space; most often from pneumonia/pulmonary abscess
  - Loculation, split pleura sign
    - Lenticular shape
    - Nondependent location
- **Rounded Atelectasis**
  - Definitive diagnosis on CT requires 4 findings
    - Pleural thickening, pleural effusion, or pleural plaque
    - Broad-based intimate attachment of mass-like consolidation to pleural abnormality
    - Volume loss
    - Comet tail (or hurricane) sign: Swirling of bronchovasculature into mass-like consolidation
- **Subpleural Lung Cancer**
  - Most common in upper lung zone (2/3 of primary lung cancers)
  - Spiculated margins, pleural tail, thick-walled cavitation
  - Hilar and mediastinal lymphadenopathy

Helpful Clues for Less Common Diagnoses
- **Pleural Metastasis**
  - Adenocarcinoma most common; drop metastases from invasive thymoma
  - Unexplained unilateral pleural effusion, irregular pleural thickening, and nodules ± enhancement
- **Pulmonary Infarctions (Subpleural)**

- Most often from pulmonary arterial embolism
- Usually in setting of superimposed cardiac dysfunction (cardiomyopathy, congestive heart failure)
  - Both pulmonary and bronchial arterial supply to lung reduced
- Lower lung predominant, peripheral/subpleural, wedge-shaped consolidation
- Resolves over months (retains its original shape) rather than patchy resolution as in pneumonia

- **Extrapleural Abnormality**
  - Mass effect on or destruction of extrapleural structures
  - Extrapleural hematoma
    - High association with rib fractures and elderly patients; sequela of blunt or penetrating trauma
    - Localized hyperdense fluid collection often internally displacing extrapleural fat stripe
    - Biconvex shape suggests arterial injury (usually intercostal)
- **Pleurodesis**
  - Iatrogenic fusion of visceral and parietal pleura; talc most often used
  - Treatment of recurrent pleural effusion (most often malignant etiology)
  - Unilateral high density foci, most often dependent
  - Associated pleural thickening (which can be nodular) or loculated pleural fluid

Helpful Clues for Rare Diagnoses

- **Lymphoma**
  - Concomitant mediastinal lymphadenopathy; ± pleural effusion
  - Can be difficult to differentiate pleural from extrapleural involvement
- **Malignant Mesothelioma**
  - Stigmata of previous asbestos exposure: Pleural plaques, pleural thickening, pleural effusion
  - Lobulated pleural thickening; small hemithorax
  - CT findings that suggest malignant pleural disease (mesothelioma or metastases)
    - Circumferential involvement of pleura, including visceral pleura
    - Involvement of mediastinal aspect of pleura
    - Nodularity
    - Thickness greater than 1 cm
- **Fibrous Tumor of Pleura**
  - Well-marginated, large pleural mass with avid enhancement (may be heterogeneous in larger tumors)
  - Margins with chest wall may be acute in large tumors
  - Majority arise from visceral pleura; up to half pedunculated; may be mobile

Pleural Pseudotumor

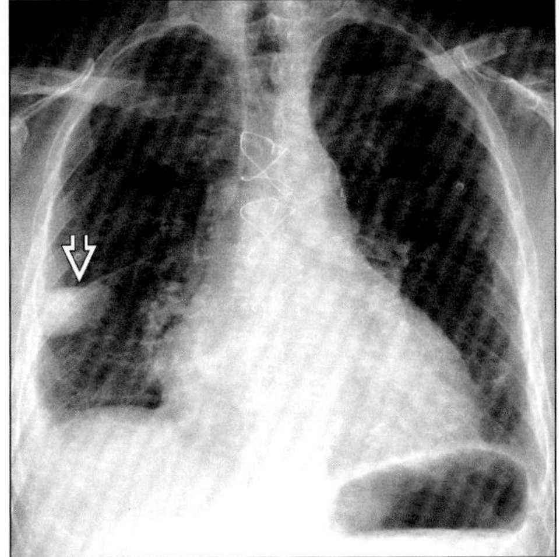

Frontal radiograph shows an oval mass ➡ in the peripheral mid right lung in this patient with cardiomegaly and history of heart failure.

Pleural Pseudotumor

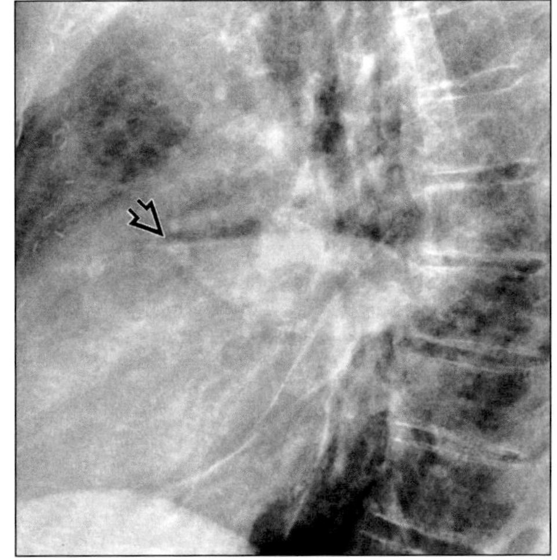

Lateral radiograph shows that the mass is located along the minor fissure and has tapered anterior and posterior margins (best seen anteriorly ➡). These findings are most consistent with a loculated pleural fluid collection.

PLEURAL MASS

*(**Left**) Lateral radiograph shows calcified pleural plaques ➔ along the anterior, posterior, and diaphragmatic aspects of the pleura. (**Right**) Frontal radiograph (magnified) shows the typical "holly leaf" appearance of an en face calcified pleural plaque on the anterior pleural surface.*

Pleural Plaque

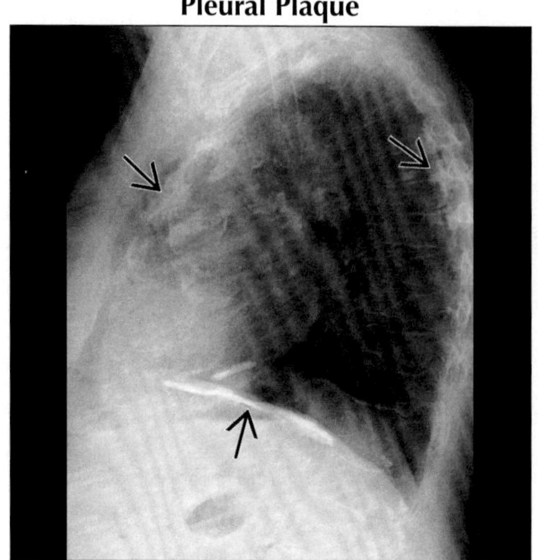

Pleural Plaque

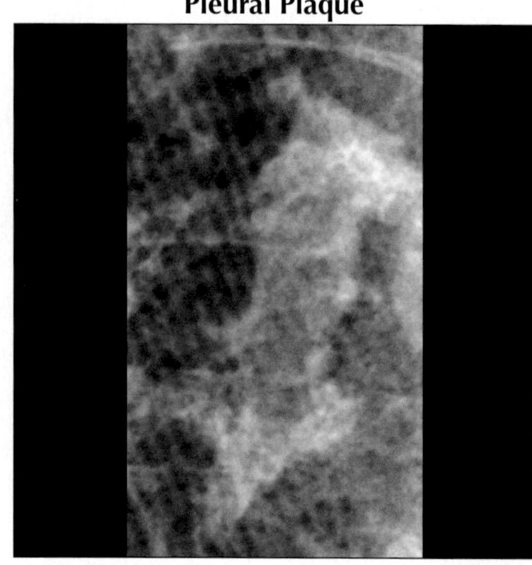

*(**Left**) Axial NECT shows partially calcified pleural thickening along majority of the right hemithorax ➔ resulting from previous inflammatory pleural effusion. Note associated hypertrophy of extrapleural fat ➔. (**Right**) Sagittal NECT shows partially calcified pleural thickening along the posterior aspect of the pleura ➔ and hypertrophy of extrapleural fat ➔. Parenchymal bands ➔ emanating from pleural thickening are precursors to round atelectasis.*

Pleural Thickening

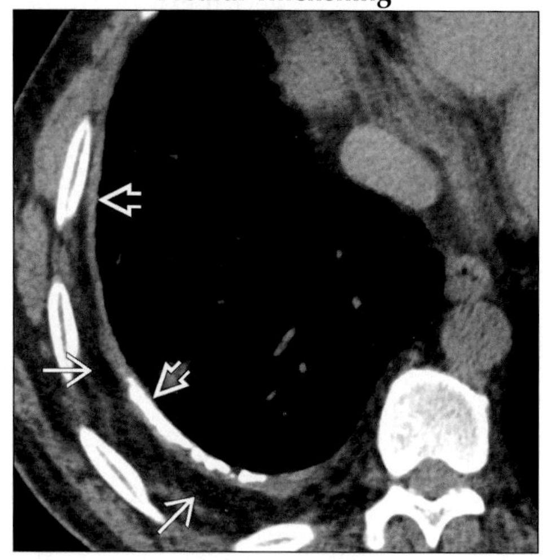

Pleural Thickening

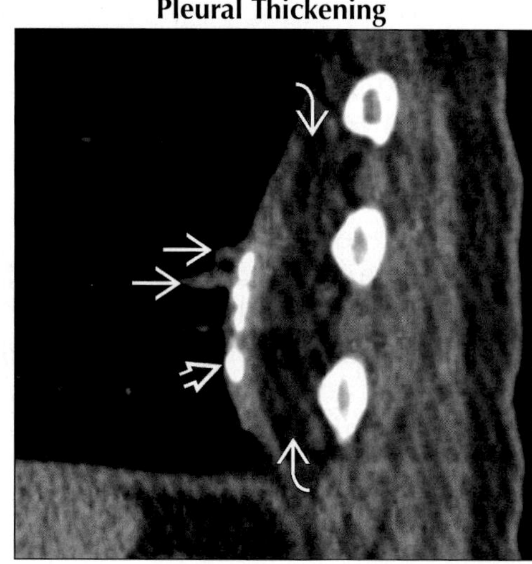

*(**Left**) Axial CECT shows loculated, low-density pleural fluid collections ➔ highly suggestive of empyema in this patient with pneumonia. Split pleura sign is not evident in this case. (**Right**) Axial CECT more inferiorly shows heterogeneous enhancement ➔ of the left lower lobe consistent with pneumonia (lower attenuation) and atelectasis (higher attenuation).*

Empyema

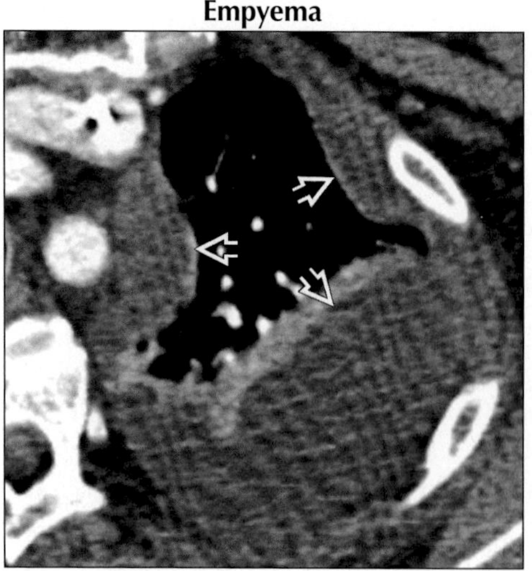

Empyema

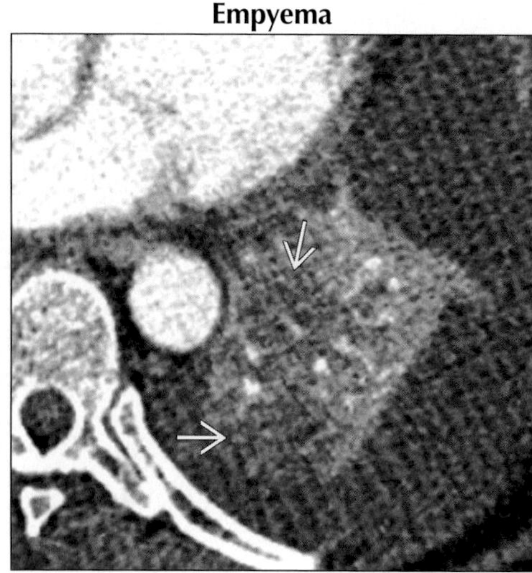

Rounded Atelectasis

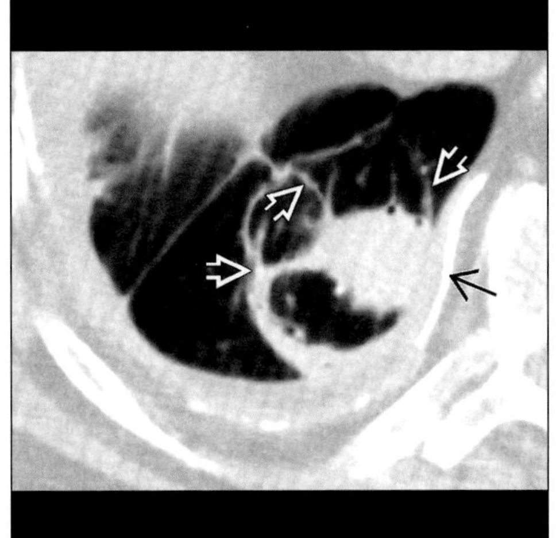

Rounded Atelectasis

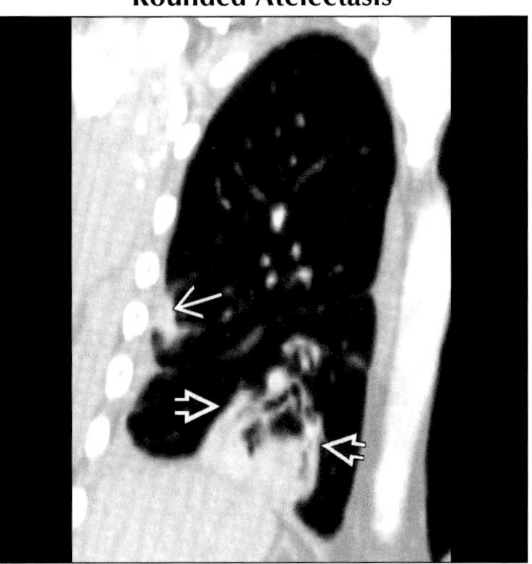

*(**Left**) Axial NECT shows a rounded mass in the right lower lobe with broad-based attachment to calcified pleural thickening →; there is characteristic swirling of the bronchovasculature into the mass-like consolidation ➔ (the comet tail sign). (**Right**) Coronal CECT shows a rounded mass in the right lower lobe with associated comet tail sign ➔. Early round atelectasis is also present more superiorly ➔. Rounded atelectasis is often multifocal.*

Subpleural Lung Cancer

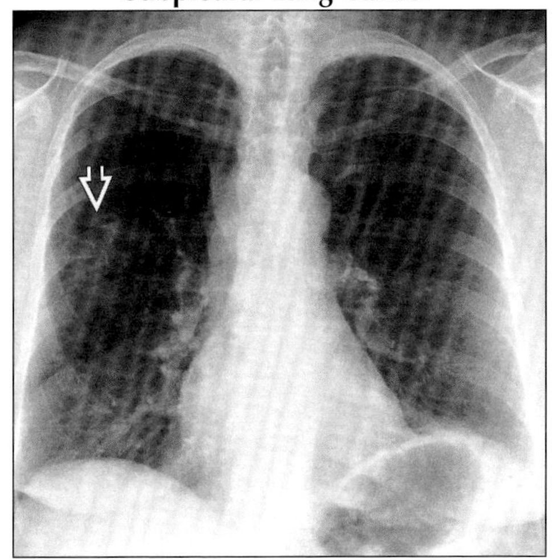

Subpleural Lung Cancer

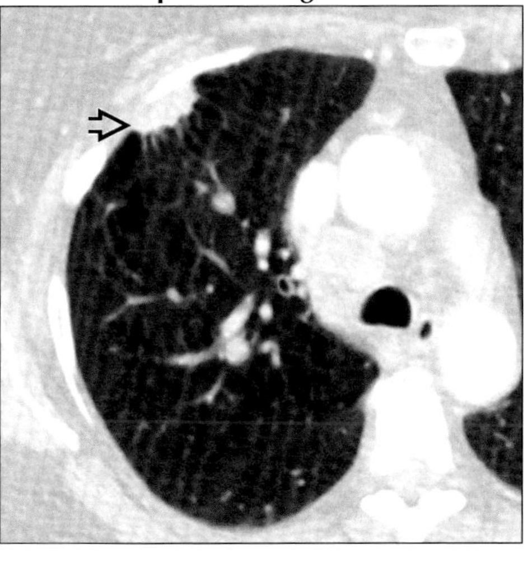

*(**Left**) Frontal radiograph shows an ill-defined opacity ➔ in the right mid lung, which persisted on follow-up. This subsequently proved to be lung cancer. (**Right**) Axial CECT shows a spiculated subpleural nodule ➔ in the right upper lobe, highly suggestive of bronchogenic carcinoma. Smoking-related centrilobular emphysema is also present.*

Subpleural Lung Cancer

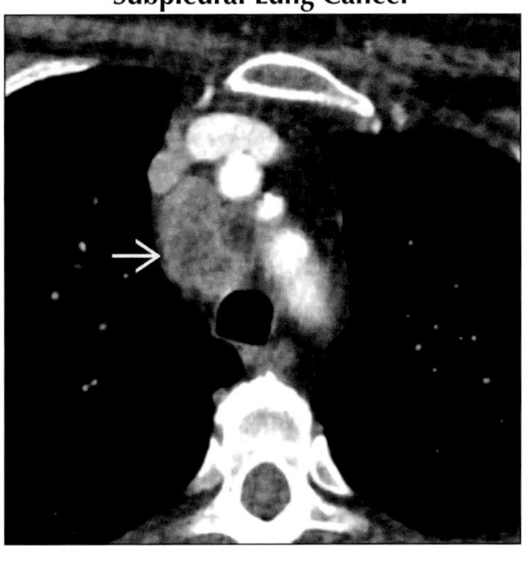

Pleural Metastasis

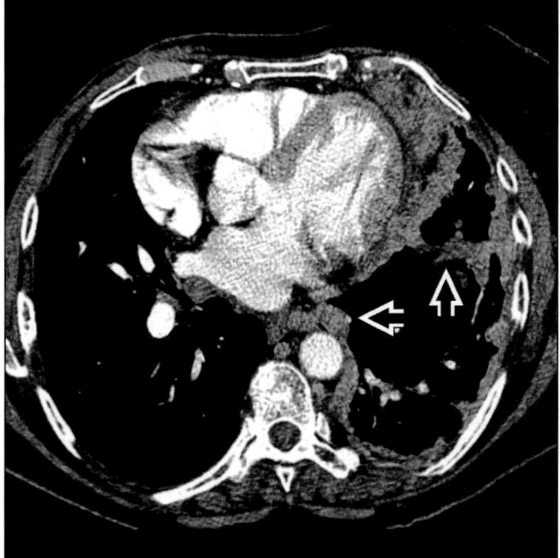

*(**Left**) Axial CECT from a patient with adenocarcinoma shows a markedly enlarged necrotic paratracheal (level IV) lymph node ➔. (**Right**) Axial CECT shows circumferential pleural nodularity ➔ extending into the left major fissure in this patient with metastatic breast adenocarcinoma.*

PLEURAL MASS

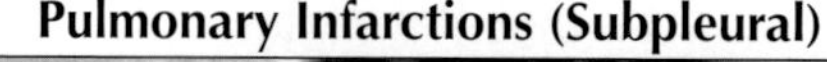

Pulmonary Infarctions (Subpleural)

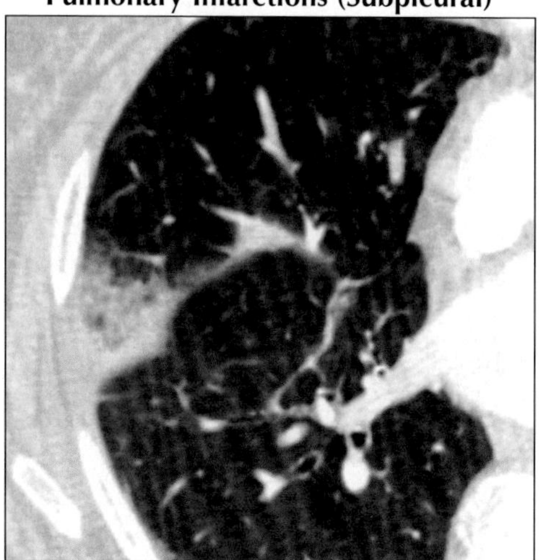

Pulmonary Infarctions (Subpleural)

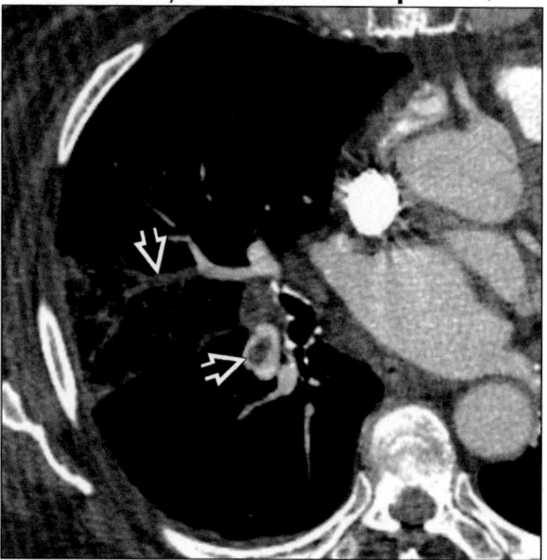

(Left) *Axial CECT shows subpleural focus of consolidation and ground-glass opacity in the right middle lobe, consistent with a pulmonary infarct.* ***(Right)*** *Axial CECT shows acute pulmonary arterial emboli ➔ in the right middle and lower lobes in this patient with a right middle lobe pulmonary infarct.*

Benign or Malignant Chest Wall Mass

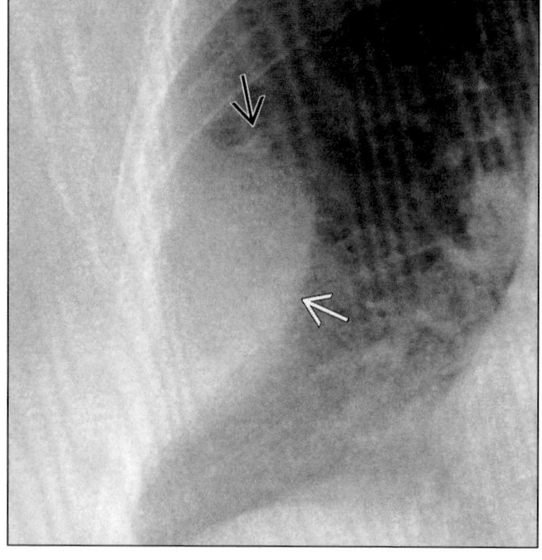

Benign or Malignant Chest Wall Mass

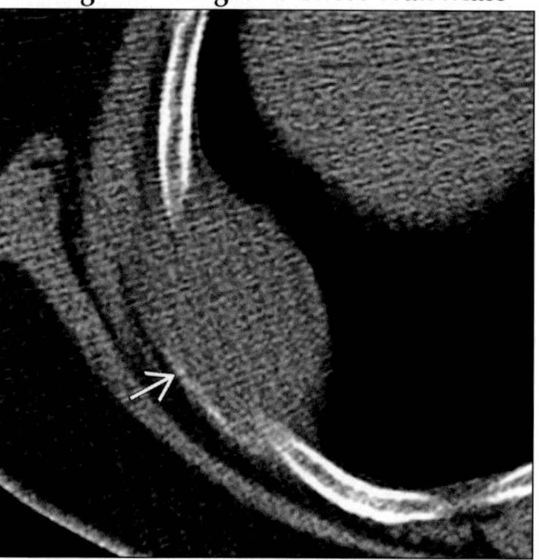

(Left) *Frontal radiograph shows an oval opacity in the right lateral chest. The opacity is poorly marginated superiorly ➔ but well marginated inferomedially ➔ (incomplete border sign), indicating that it is extrapulmonary.* ***(Right)*** *Axial NECT in the same patient shows that the extrapulmonary opacity is an extrapleural mass that has destroyed a posterolateral rib ➔. Pathologic findings were diagnostic of plasmacytoma.*

Extrapleural Hematoma

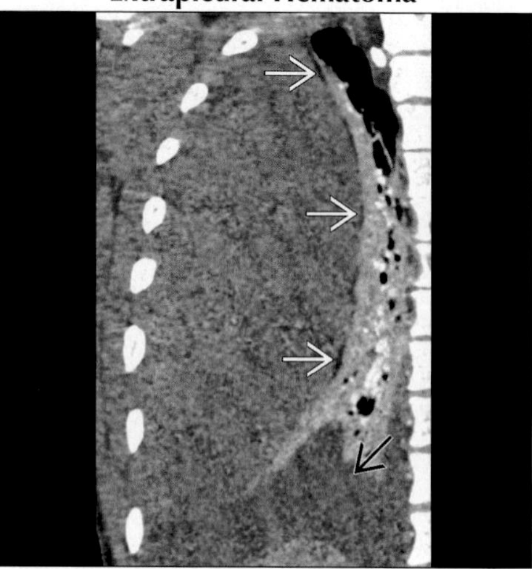

Fracture

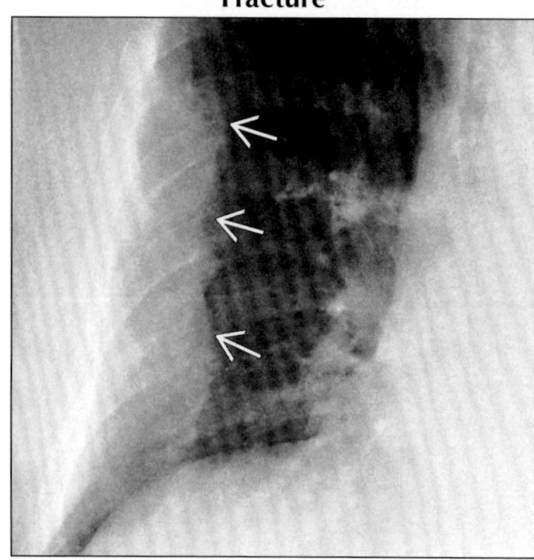

(Left) *Coronal CECT shows internal displacement of the extrapleural fat stripe ➔ by a large extrapleural hematoma. There is associated compressive atelectasis and a pleural effusion ➔.* ***(Right)*** *Frontal radiograph shows multiple displaced posterolateral rib fractures ➔. There is an oblong opacity along the right lateral hemithorax with poorly defined superior and inferior borders.*

Fracture

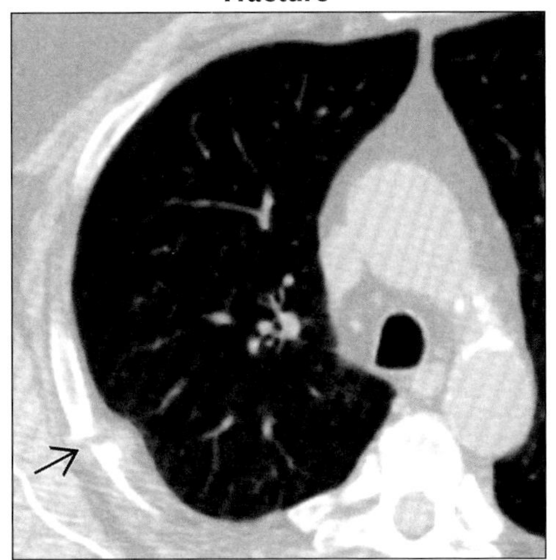

Pleurodesis

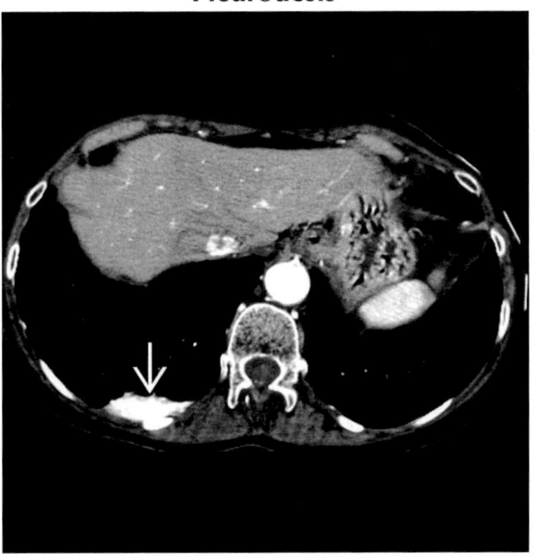

(Left) *Axial NECT in the same patient shows a displaced rib fracture ➔ with associated internal displacement of extrapleural structures, explaining the oblong opacity on chest radiograph.* ***(Right)*** *Axial CECT shows focal dependent high-density focus in the right posterior pleural space ➔ from talc pleurodesis.*

Lymphoma

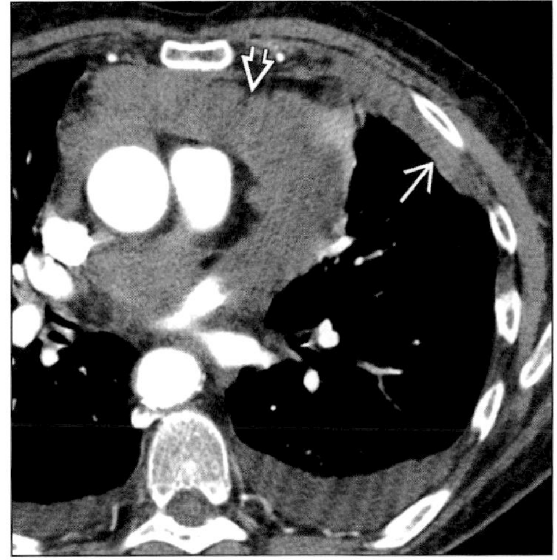

Malignant Mesothelioma

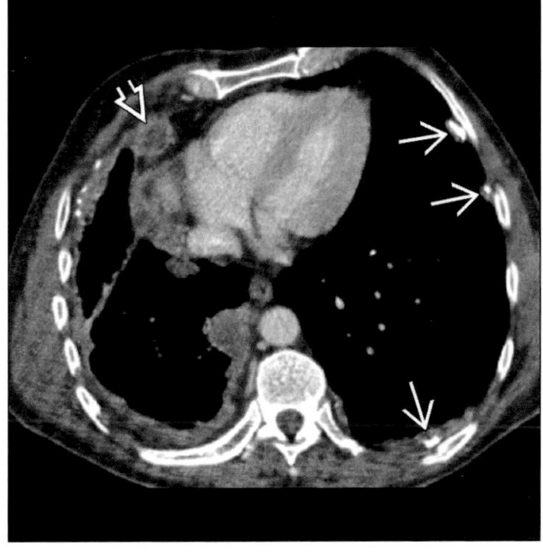

(Left) *Axial CECT shows a nodular, infiltrative mediastinal mass ➔ and a left anterior pleural or extrapleural mass ➔. Small pleural effusions are also present.* ***(Right)*** *Axial CECT shows calcified pleural plaques ➔ predominantly on the left. There is also a nodular, circumferential, right-sided pleural mass with extension into the right major fissure; the right hemithorax is small. An enlarged necrotic pericardial lymph node ➔ is also present.*

Malignant Mesothelioma

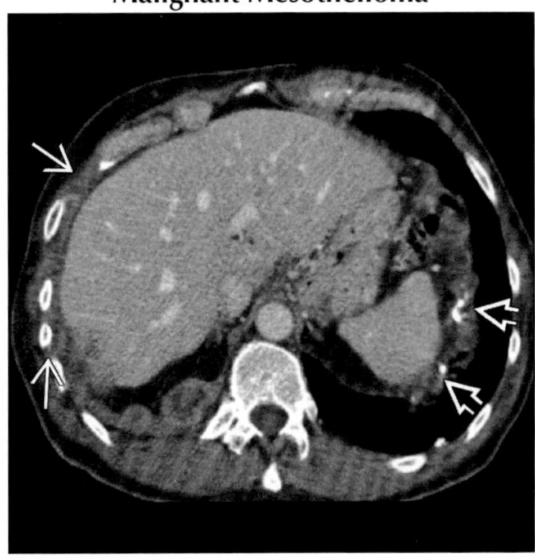

Fibrous Tumor of Pleura

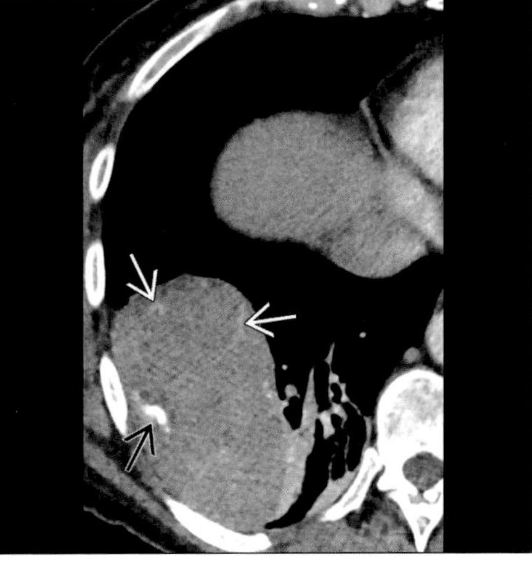

(Left) *Axial CECT shows extension of the nodular pleural thickening into the extrapleural chest wall ➔. Note calcified left-sided pleural plaques ➔.* ***(Right)*** *Axial CECT shows a large oval mass in the right lower lobe with a small focus of calcification ➔ and internal enhancing vessels ➔. Like many large fibrous tumors of the pleura, the margins of the mass with the chest wall are acute, which is more suggestive of a pulmonary mass. There is associated compressive atelectasis.*

PLEURAL CALCIFICATION

DIFFERENTIAL DIAGNOSIS

Common
- Asbestos-related Pleural Disease
- Empyema
- Exudative Pleural Effusion

Less Common
- Pleural Metastasis
- Hemothorax
- Pleurodesis
- Radiation-induced Lung Disease

Rare but Important
- Fibrous Tumor of Pleura

ESSENTIAL INFORMATION

Key Differential Diagnosis Issues
- Pleural plaques are usually the result of asbestos exposure
- Pleural thickening from any cause can calcify
  - Infection, hemorrhage, and asbestos account for most pleural calcification
  - Exuberant pleural calcification most commonly from tuberculosis
- Associated lung or chest wall findings may suggest underlying cause
- CT more sensitive than radiography

Helpful Clues for Common Diagnoses
- **Asbestos-related Pleural Disease**
  - Usually develops 20-30 years after exposure
  - Usually bilateral
  - Calcification occurs in ~ 15%
    - CT more sensitive than radiography for calcification
  - Characteristic locations
    - Posterolateral chest wall between 6th and 9th ribs
    - Dome of diaphragm
    - Mediastinal pleura, particularly over diaphragm
  - Diaphragmatic calcification highly suggestive of asbestos exposure
  - Unusual in apices or costophrenic sulci
  - Associated lung findings
    - Subpleural curvilinear opacities
    - Parenchymal bands
    - Rounded atelectasis adjacent to visceral pleural thickening
    - Interstitial fibrosis (asbestosis)
- **Empyema**
  - Usually unilateral
  - Tuberculosis most common cause worldwide
    - Pulmonary findings of TB present in about 85% with tuberculous empyema
    - Typically develops 3-6 months following primary infection
    - Caused by rupture of subpleural nidus of pulmonary infection into pleural space
  - Thickening of parietal and visceral pleura
    - May become sheet-like
    - Often most extensive posterolaterally
    - Residual effusion in ~ 15%
  - May lead to fibrothorax
    - Extensive calcification
    - Volume loss in affected lung (restrictive lung disease)
    - Compressive and rounded atelectasis
- **Exudative Pleural Effusion**
  - Usually unilateral
  - Calcification less common than with empyema
  - Associated pleural thickening
  - Adjacent pneumonia or other pulmonary inflammation may be present initially
  - Progression to empyema in 10% of patients hospitalized with pneumonia and parapneumonic effusion
    - *Streptococcus* and *Staphylococcus* species most common
    - Nosocomial infection with gram-negative anaerobes and methicillin-resistant *Staphylococcus aureus* (MRSA)
    - Up to 1/3 caused by anaerobic organisms

Helpful Clues for Less Common Diagnoses
- **Pleural Metastasis**
  - ~ 90% of all pleural neoplasms
  - Usually multiple
  - Calcified pleural metastases
    - Chondrosarcoma
    - Osteosarcoma
    - Sarcomatous mesothelioma
    - Adenocarcinomas (especially mucinous subtypes), including lung, breast, gastric, and ovarian
  - Associated pleural effusion in most
  - May have lung or thoracic lymph node metastases

- **Hemothorax**
  - Usually unilateral
  - Blunt or penetrating trauma
  - Iatrogenic
  - Parietal and visceral pleura calcification
    - Late finding
    - Can become sheet-like
    - Often most extensive posterolaterally
    - Varying amount of residual pleural fluid
  - Adjacent healed rib fractures suggestive
- **Pleurodesis**
  - High-attenuation deposits mimic pleural calcification
    - Usually adjacent to dependent lung
    - May be lentiform
  - Variable degrees of pleural thickening and nodularity
    - Remain stable over time
    - May enhance with large amount of granulation tissue
  - Residual loculations of fluid common
- **Radiation-induced Lung Disease**
  - Unusual complication of radiation therapy for breast cancer, lung cancer, or lymphoma
  - Associated with pleural thickening
  - Small residual pleural effusion may be present
  - Radiation-induced lung fibrosis often present in radiation field

Helpful Clues for Rare Diagnoses

- **Fibrous Tumor of Pleura**
  - Single well-defined soft tissue mass abutting pleura
    - 65-80% arise from visceral pleura
    - 20-35% arise from parietal pleural
    - Fissural origin not uncommon
    - ~ 50% arise from vascular pedicle (rarely evident on CT)
  - Variable size
    - Range from 1-36 cm, mean is 6 cm
  - Intermediate to high attenuation on unenhanced CT
    - Attributed to abundant capillary network and high density of collagen
  - Most exhibit intense contrast enhancement on CT and MR
    - Sparing in areas of necrosis or myxoid degeneration
  - Calcification in 7-25%
    - More common in larger tumors
    - Usually associated with necrosis
  - Pleural effusion in 25-37%
  - Paraneoplastic syndromes
    - Hypoglycemia in up to 7%
    - Clubbing of fingers in 4%
    - Resolve after tumor resection
  - ~ 12% malignant
    - Vascular pedicle less common with malignant tumors
    - Usually heterogeneous on unenhanced and contrast-enhanced CT and MR

Asbestos-related Pleural Disease

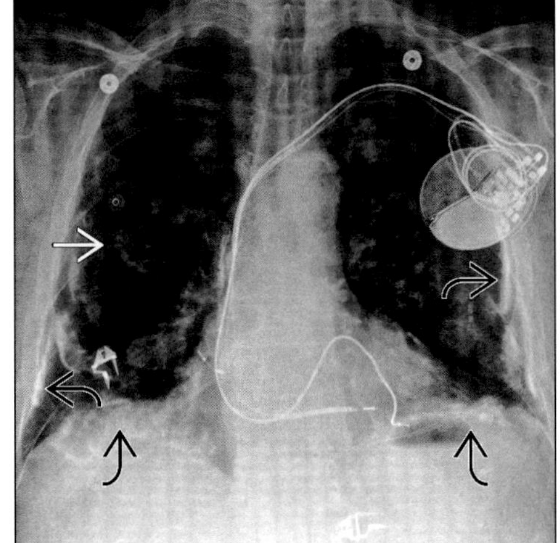

Frontal radiograph shows extensive calcified pleural plaques bilaterally both in tangent ⇾ and en face ➡. En face plaques often have a curled edge, similar to that of a holly leaf.

Asbestos-related Pleural Disease

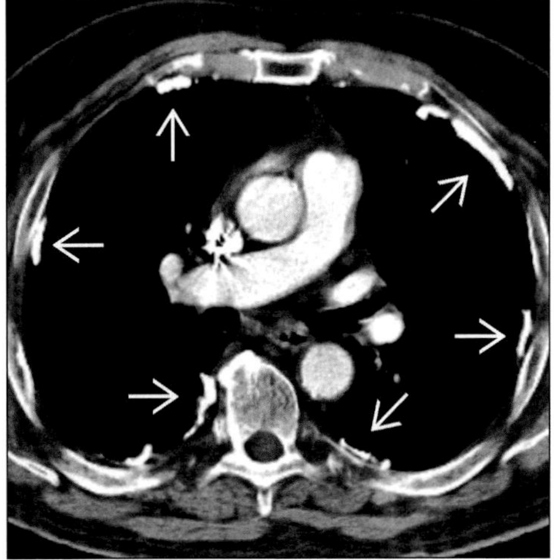

Axial CECT shows multiple calcified pleural plaques ➡. Note the characteristic locations along the anterolateral, posterior, and lateral chest wall pleura.

PLEURAL CALCIFICATION

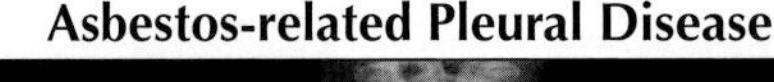

Asbestos-related Pleural Disease | **Asbestos-related Pleural Disease**

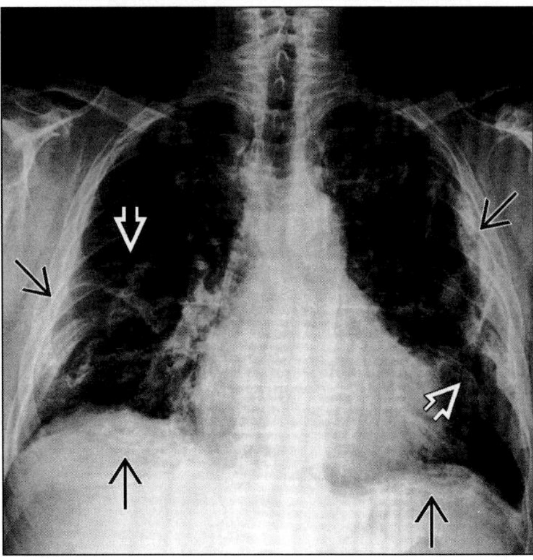

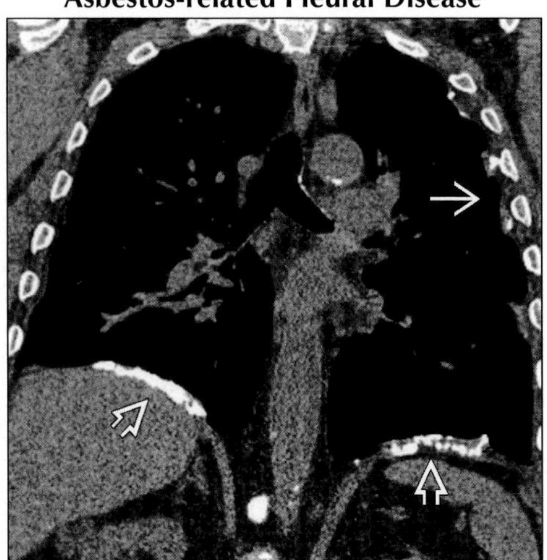

(Left) *Frontal radiograph shows extensive bilateral pleural plaques both in tangent and en face. Pleural plaques along the hemidiaphragms are almost always the result of asbestos exposure.* ***(Right)*** *Coronal CT reconstruction shows thick, partially calcified pleural plaques along the hemidiaphragms as well as along the left lateral chest wall. Bilateral pleural plaques are almost always the result of asbestos exposure.*

Empyema | **Empyema**

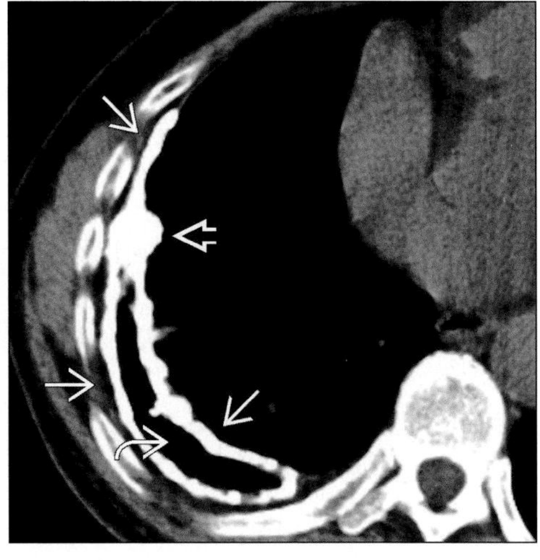

(Left) *Frontal radiograph shows extensive, coarse right pleural calcification in a patient with previous tuberculous empyema. Note mild right lung volume loss. Extensive pleural calcification is often the result of empyema, worldwide most commonly from tuberculosis.* ***(Right)*** *Axial NECT shows circumferential right pleural calcification in a patient with previous tuberculous empyema. The calcification can be smooth or nodular. Note chronic pneumothorax.*

Pleural Metastasis | **Pleural Metastasis**

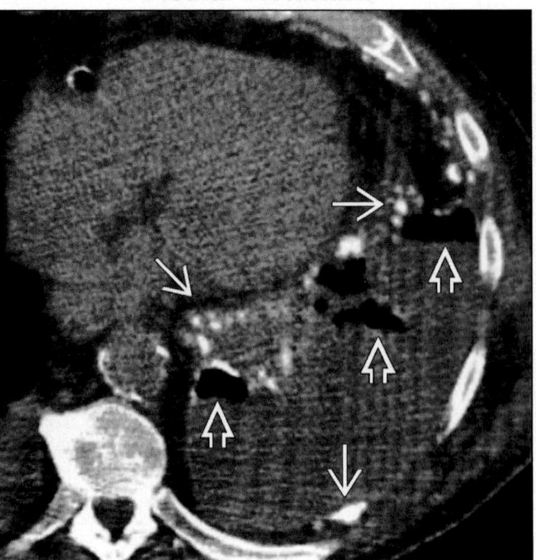

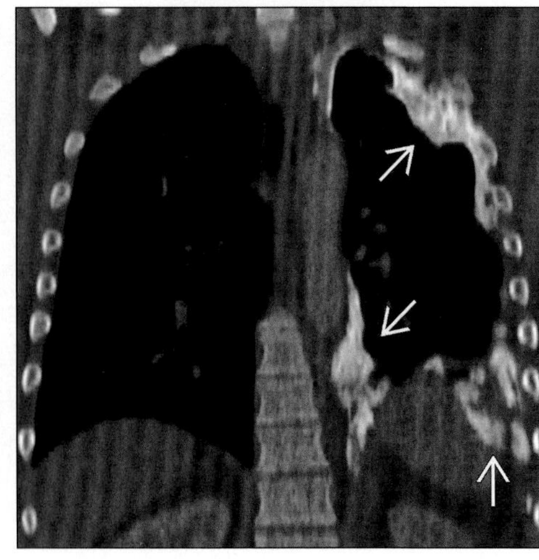

(Left) *Axial NECT shows extensive nodular pleural calcification and a larger pleural effusion from metastatic chondrosarcoma. Loculations of gas developed after diagnostic thoracentesis.* ***(Right)*** *Coronal CT reconstruction shows thick calcification of the left pleura resulting from metastatic osteosarcoma. Note the somewhat cloud-like calcific matrix produced by the tumor.*

PLEURAL CALCIFICATION

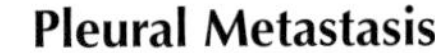

Pleural Metastasis

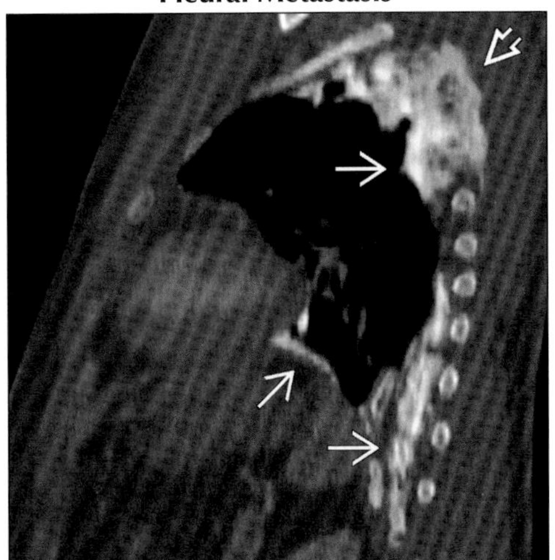

Hemothorax

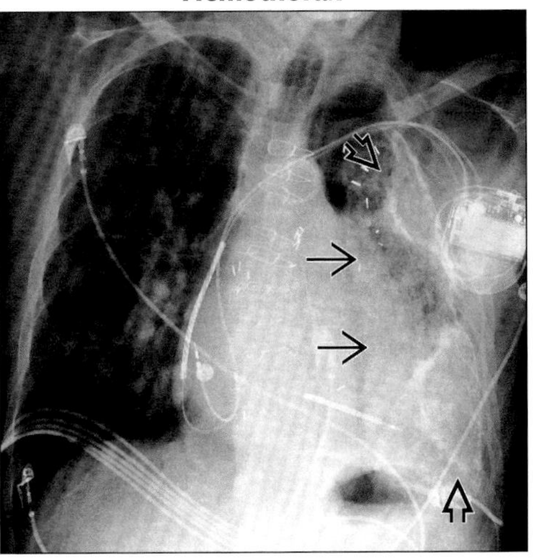

(Left) *Sagittal CT reconstruction shows extensive, thick left pleural calcification from metastatic osteosarcoma of the femur. Note extension into the chest wall apicoposteriorly.* ***(Right)*** *Frontal radiograph shows marked left pleural calcification, which is both sheet-like and nodular in this patient who suffered a postoperative hemothorax following cardiac surgery. Extensive pleural thickening or calcification can result in fibrothorax.*

Hemothorax

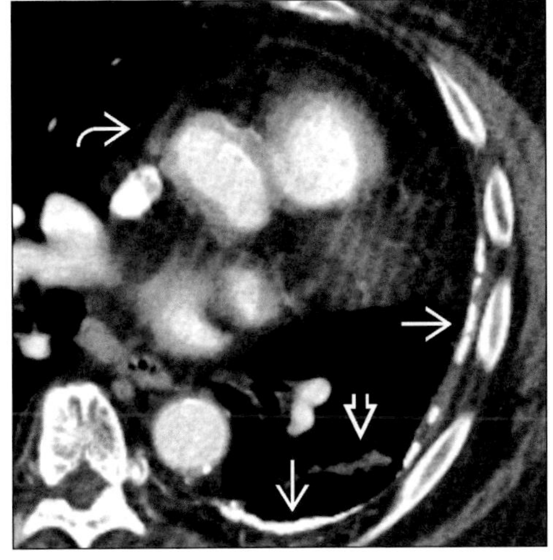

Pleurodesis

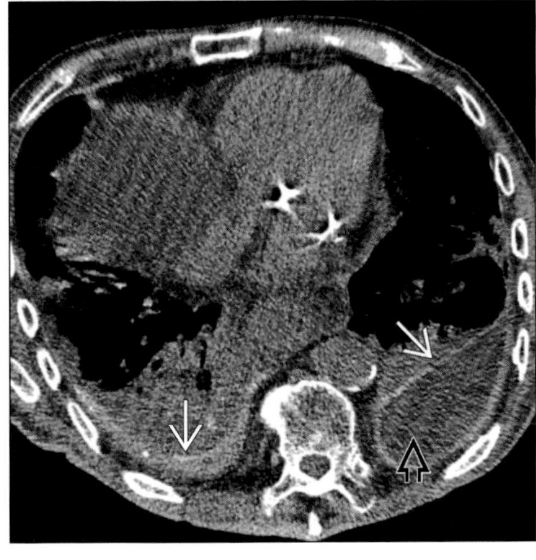

(Left) *Axial CECT shows left pleural thickening with calcification resulting from earlier traumatic hemothorax. A small band of linear atelectasis is in the left lower lobe. Note the leftward shift of the mediastinum.* ***(Right)*** *Axial NECT shows bilateral pleural thickening and calcification from talc pleurodesis in this patient with recurrent pleural effusions from yellow nail syndrome. Note the small residual pleural effusion on the left.*

Radiation-induced Lung Disease

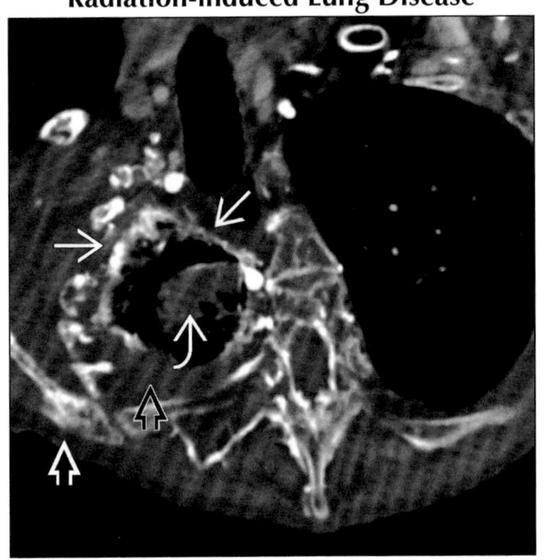

Fibrous Tumor of Pleura

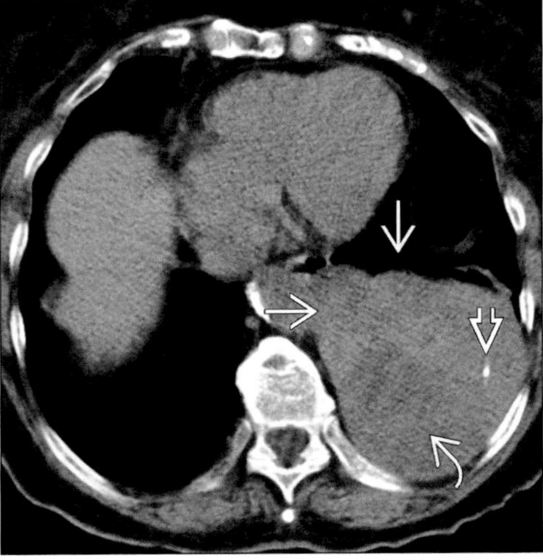

(Left) *Axial CECT shows nodular right apical pleural calcification and thickening resulting from external beam radiation therapy for breast carcinoma. Note the right apical radiation fibrosis, extrapleural tissue thickening, and osteitis of the scapula.* ***(Right)*** *Axial NECT shows a large soft tissue mass in the left pleural space containing both a small calcification and an area of lower attenuation, representing necrosis.*

UNILATERAL PLEURAL EFFUSION

DIFFERENTIAL DIAGNOSIS

Common
- Parapneumonic Effusion
- Neoplastic Diseases
  - Mesothelioma
  - Primary Lung Cancer
  - Breast Cancer
  - Pleural Metastases
  - Lymphoma
- Hepatic Cirrhosis
- Pancreatitis
- Trauma

Less Common
- Pulmonary Embolism
- Myxedema
- Rheumatoid Pleuritis
- Chylothorax
- Renal Disease
- HIV Infection

Rare but Important
- Catamenial Hemothorax
- Yellow Nail Syndrome

ESSENTIAL INFORMATION

Key Differential Diagnosis Issues
- Pleural effusions result from pleural, parenchymal, or extrapulmonary disease
  - Transudative effusions: Imbalance of hydrostatic and oncotic forces
  - Exudative effusions: From pleural diseases or decreased lymphatic drainage
- CT generally more sensitive than radiography for detection of relatively small volumes of pleural fluid
- Pleural pseudotumor: Accumulation of pleural fluid within interlobar fissure; vanishing tumors: Disappearance of effusions after treatment
  - Fluid in fissure has curvilinear edge concave to hilum
  - Minor fissure pseudotumor may be mistaken for pulmonary mass
- Large and massive pleural effusions are more likely to be malignant
  - Half of malignant effusions do not reveal any pleural finding apart from effusion
  - Pleural nodules and circumferential pleural thickening are highly specific for malignancy
- Ultrasonography: Useful to demonstrate pleural loculations
  - Fibrinous septations are better visualized on ultrasound than on CT scans

Helpful Clues for Common Diagnoses
- **Parapneumonic Effusion**
  - Bacteria
    - In CAP, most commonly associated organisms are gram-positive aerobic bacteria
    - In nosocomial infections, gram-negative aerobes (*H. influenzae, E. coli, P. aeruginosa*, and *Klebsiella*)
    - CECT: Pleural thickening and loculated fluid; split pleura sign of empyema: Fluid between enhancing thickened pleural layers
  - Tuberculosis
    - Thick pleural rind: Usually unilateral
  - Fungi
    - Rare causes of pleural effusion
- **Neoplastic Diseases**
  - **Mesothelioma**
    - Pleural thickening (89%)
    - Unilateral pleural effusion (87%)
    - Mediastinal pleural thickening (85%)
  - **Primary Lung Cancer**
    - Almost always ipsilateral pleural effusions
    - Infrequently bilateral
  - **Breast Cancer**
    - Ipsilateral pleural effusion in 83% of cases
  - **Pleural Metastases**
    - Adenocarcinoma most common tumor to metastasize to pleura
    - Thymomas may result in pleural dissemination: "Drop metastases"
    - CT: Irregular pleural thickening and small nodules at interlobar fissures
    - CECT: Variable enhancement
  - **Lymphoma**
    - Prevalence of pleural disease in both Hodgkin and non-Hodgkin lymphoma is similar (26-31%)
    - Usually occurs as part of disseminated disease
    - Contrast enhancement of parietal pleura
    - Coexistent involvement of parietal pleura, paraspinal region, and extrapleural space

UNILATERAL PLEURAL EFFUSION

- **Hepatic Cirrhosis**
  - Associated with transdiaphragmatic movement of ascites
  - Right-sided, unilateral 70%; left sided 15%; bilateral 15%
  - Small to massive
- **Pancreatitis**
  - Usually left-sided (70%) or bilateral (15%)
  - > pleural fluid amylase level is not specific indicator of pancreatitis
  - Pleural amylase values may be elevated in
    - Acute pancreatitis, pancreatic pseudocyst, rupture of esophagus, and ruptured ectopic pregnancy
    - Approximately 10% of malignant effusions have raised pleural amylase levels (especially adenocarcinoma)
- **Trauma**
  - CT of acute hemothorax: Fluid-fluid level or increased density of pleural fluid

Helpful Clues for Less Common Diagnoses

- **Pulmonary Embolism**
  - Pleural effusions in 30-50% of patients
    - Unilateral and small (85%)
    - Pleuritic pain: 75% of patients with pleural effusion
  - No specific pleural fluid characteristics
    - Pleural fluid red blood cell count > 100,000/mm^3 suggests malignancy, pulmonary infarction, or trauma
- **Myxedema**
  - Massive cardiomegaly (pericardial effusion) and thoracic inlet mass (goiter)
  - Unilateral or bilateral pleural effusions; small to moderate in size
- **Rheumatoid Pleuritis**
  - Middle-aged men with positive rheumatoid factor
- **Chylothorax**
  - Presence of chyle in pleural space: Malignancy (lymphoma and metastases), trauma, post-surgery, tuberculosis, LAM, sarcoidosis, and amyloidosis
- **Renal Disease**
  - Peritoneal or hemodialysis
    - Like ascites-related pleural effusions, usually on right
- **HIV Infection**
  - Causes of effusions: Kaposi sarcoma (30%), parapneumonic effusion (28%), tuberculosis (14%), *Pneumocystis jiroveci* pneumonia, and lymphoma

Helpful Clues for Rare Diagnoses

- **Catamenial Hemothorax**
  - Occurs in 14% of patients with pleural endometriosis
    - 85-90% occur on right (only 5% occur bilaterally)
- **Yellow Nail Syndrome**
  - Rhinosinusitis, pleural effusions, bronchiectasis, lymphedema, and yellow nails

Mesothelioma

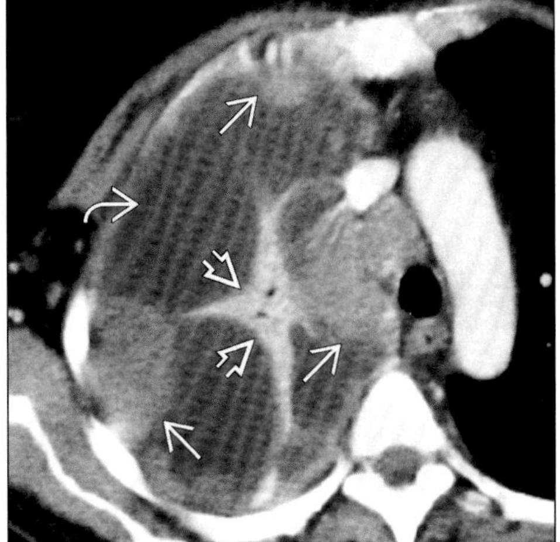

Axial CECT shows lobulated pleural thickening ➔, loculated pleural effusion ➔, and compressed right upper lobe collapse ➔ from malignant mesothelioma in the right hemithorax.

Primary Lung Cancer

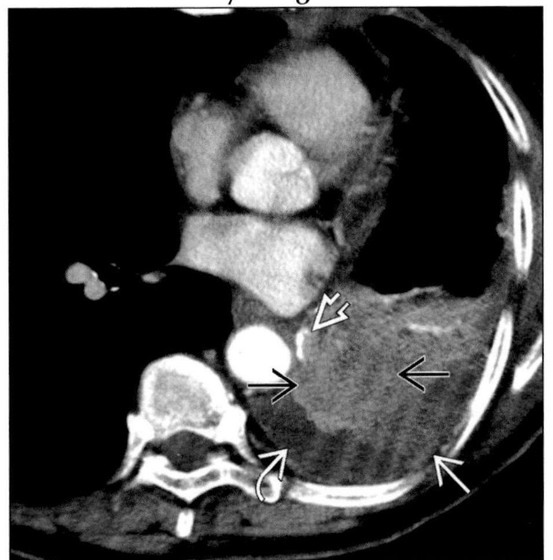

Axial CECT shows metallic clips ➔ from a previous LLL lobectomy for lung cancer. Years later, a left pleural effusion ➔ and pleural thickening ➔ were observed and a 2nd primary lung cancer was diagnosed ➔.

UNILATERAL PLEURAL EFFUSION

*(**Left**) Axial CECT shows a moderate right pleural effusion ➡ and diffuse nodular pleural thickening ➡. The patient has a right breast carcinoma also visible ➡. (**Right**) Axial CECT shows a moderately sized right pleural effusion ➡ and multiple enhancing metastatic tumor implants on the parietal pleura ➡.*

Pleural Metastases

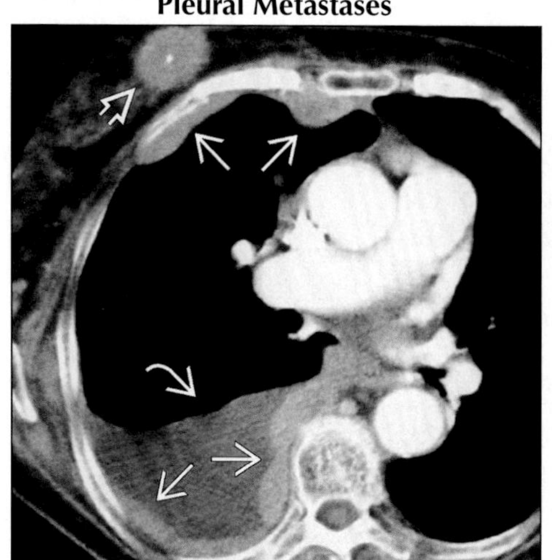

Pleural Metastases

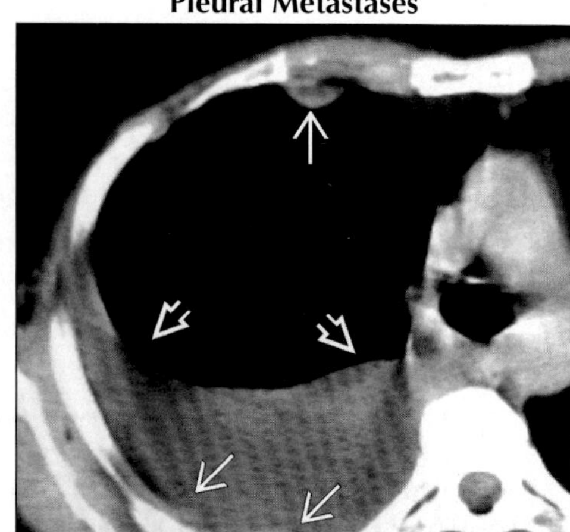

*(**Left**) Axial NECT shows a large anterior mediastinal thymoma ➡. Findings of nodular pleural implants ➡ and pleural effusion ➡ are consistent with invasive thymoma and "drop metastases." (**Right**) Axial CECT in a patient with diffuse B-cell lymphoma shows an enhancing periaortic mass ➡ contiguous with parietal pleural thickening ➡ and moderate left pleural effusion ➡. The patient did not present with adenopathy elsewhere in the body.*

Pleural Metastases

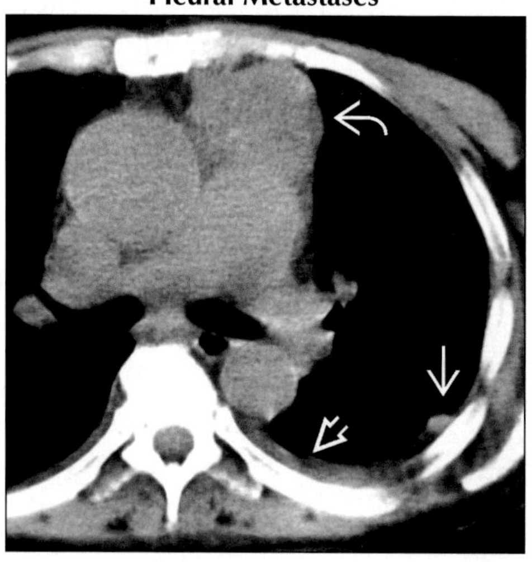

Lymphoma

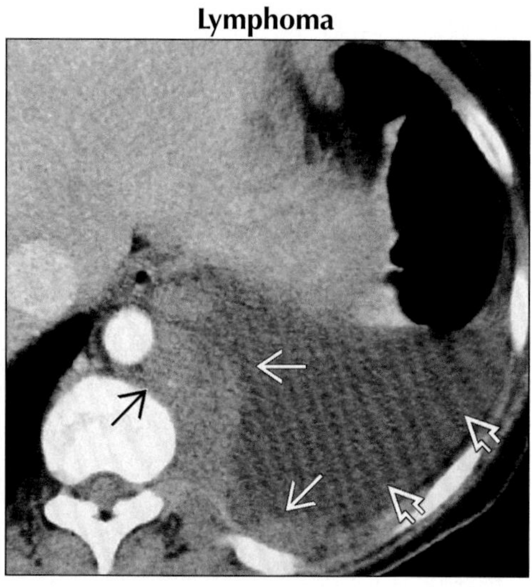

*(**Left**) Frontal radiograph shows loculated fluid in the minor ➡ and major ➡ fissures simulating a mass. Fluid is also seen in the right costophrenic sulcus ➡. The patient also had ischemic heart disease. (**Right**) Axial CECT corresponding image shows a large loculated fluid collection within a distended major fissure ➡. Moderate right pleural effusion is confirmed ➡.*

Hepatic Cirrhosis

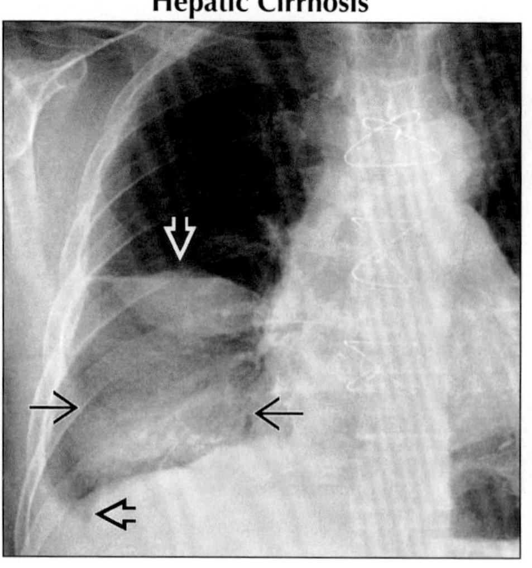

Hepatic Cirrhosis

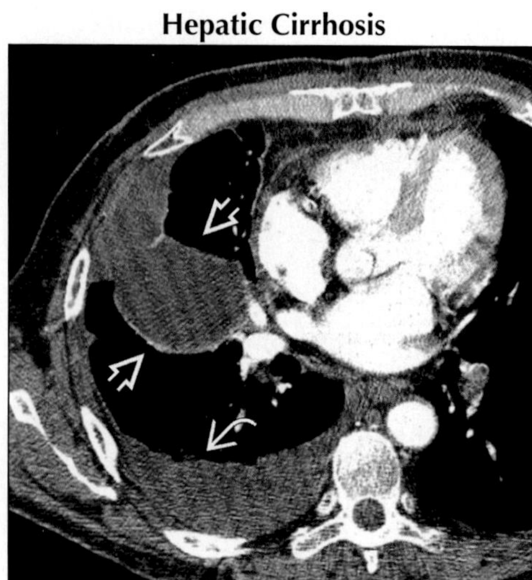

UNILATERAL PLEURAL EFFUSION

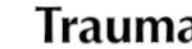

Trauma

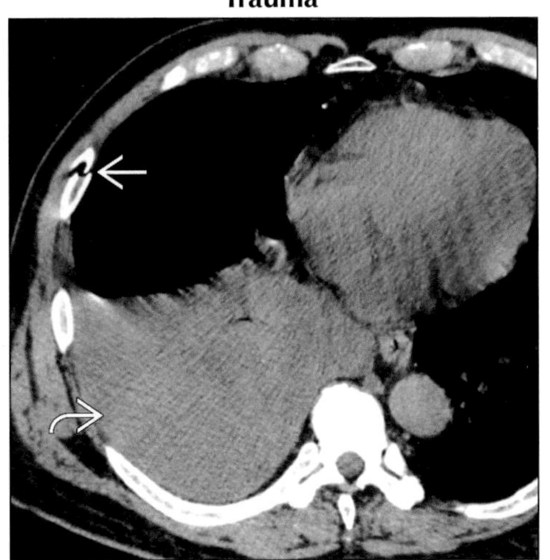

Pulmonary Embolism

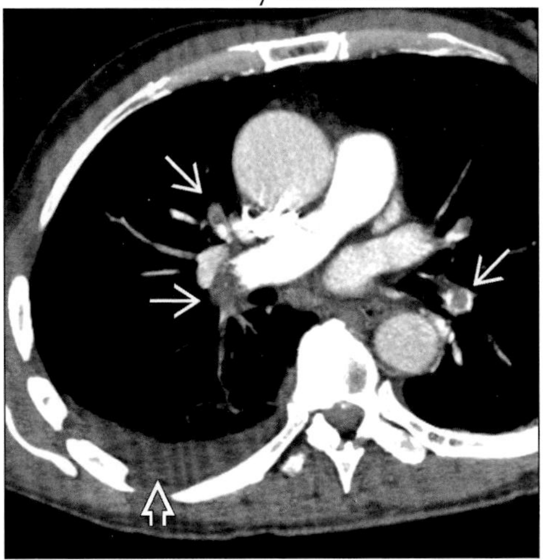

(Left) *Axial NECT shows a rib fracture ➔ and a moderately sized right pleural fluid collection. The pleural fluid shows relatively high attenuation ➔, suggestive of hemothorax.* ***(Right)*** *Axial CECT shows bilateral multiple pulmonary emboli ➔. A right small pleural effusion is also visible ➔.*

Myxedema

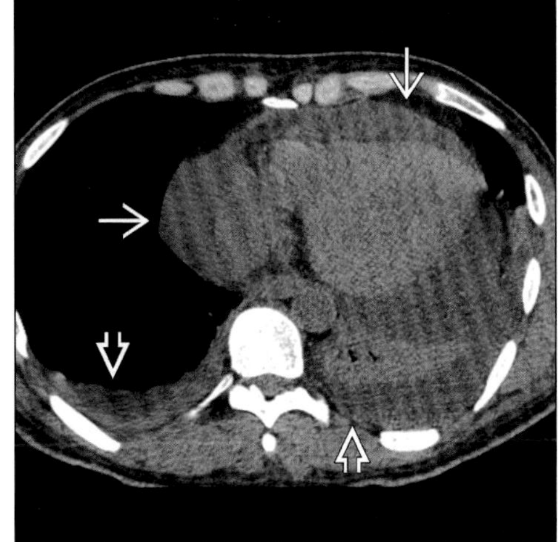

Rheumatoid Pleuritis

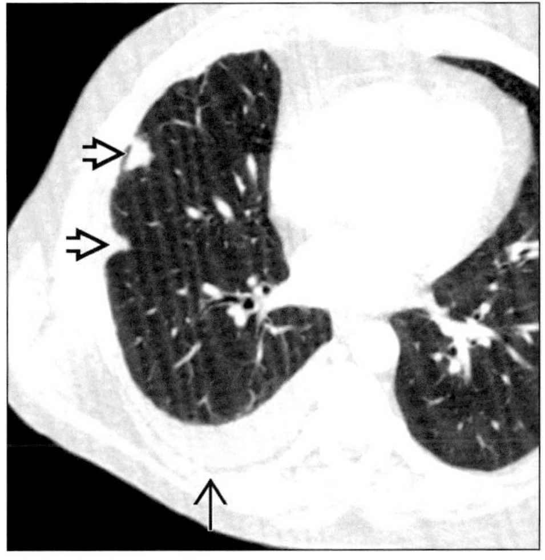

(Left) *Axial NECT shows large pericardial effusion ➔ and bilateral pleural effusion ➔, left greater than right, as well as associated left lower lobe collapse.* ***(Right)*** *Axial CECT (lung window) shows a chronic exudative right effusion ➔ and peripheral right middle lobe rheumatoid nodules ➔. (Courtesy H.T. Winer-Muram, MD.)*

Chylothorax

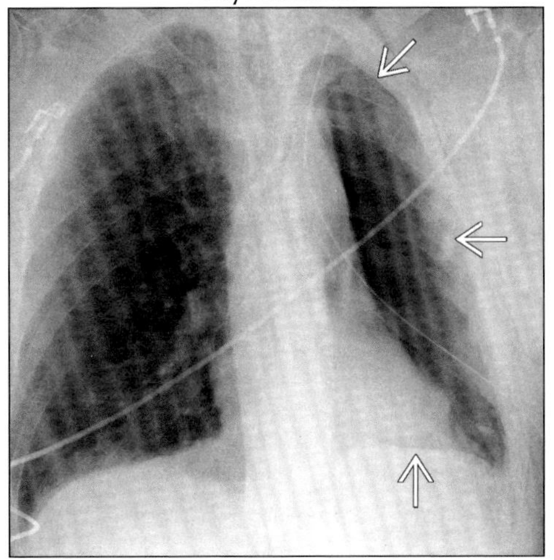

Chylothorax

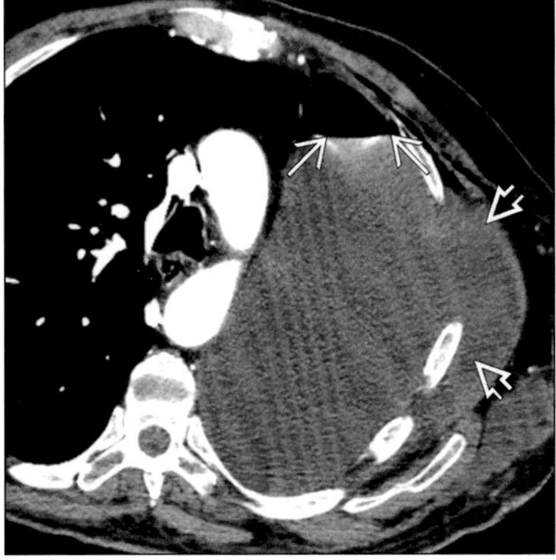

(Left) *Frontal radiograph shows immediate normal postoperative left pneumonectomy appearance. Space completely air-filled ➔.* ***(Right)*** *Axial CECT 9 days following pneumonectomy. Space is almost completely fluid-filled; a small air-fluid level is visible ➔. Note decompression of fluid in the pneumonectomy space through the thoracotomy defect into the chest wall ➔.*

BILATERAL PLEURAL EFFUSION

DIFFERENTIAL DIAGNOSIS

Common
- Congestive Heart Failure
- Postcardiac Injury Syndrome
- Infection
- Renal Disease
- Metastatic Malignant Pleural Disease
- Lymphoma
- Trauma/Iatrogenic
- Lupus Pleuritis
- Abdominal Surgery

Less Common
- Asbestos-related Pleural Disease
- Pregnancy-related

Rare but Important
- Diffuse Pulmonary Lymphangiomatosis
- Venoocclusive Disease
- Drug-induced Pleuritis

ESSENTIAL INFORMATION

Key Differential Diagnosis Issues
- Congestive heart failure (CHF) leading cause of bilateral pleural effusion
- Small pleural effusions are not readily identified on conventional chest radiographs
  - Meniscus sign on PA radiograph (> 200 mL)
  - Pleural effusions can be entirely overlooked on supine radiographs
  - Lateral decubitus chest radiograph: Useful for detecting small pleural effusions if clinically indicated
- CT scans
  - Should be performed with contrast enhancement
  - No reliable distinction between exudates and transudates
  - Can usually differentiate between benign and malignant pleural thickening
- CT criteria for differentiating pleural fluid from ascites
  - Interface sign: Fluid outside diaphragm is pleural; inside diaphragm, ascites
  - Diaphragm sign: Indistinct interface between pleural effusion and liver owing to diaphragm
  - Displaced-crus sign: Crus is anteriorly and laterally displaced from spine by pleural effusion
  - Bare-area sign: Pleural fluid may extend behind liver at level of bare area

Helpful Clues for Common Diagnoses
- **Congestive Heart Failure**
  - Pulmonary venous hypertension essential for pleural fluid development
  - Cardiomegaly, pulmonary vascular congestion, interstitial and alveolar edema
  - Pleural effusion mainly derives from excess interstitial pulmonary fluid
  - Bilateral effusions, relatively equal size
- **Postcardiac Injury Syndrome**
  - Combination of pericarditis, pleuritis, and pneumonitis after variety of myocardium and pericardium injuries
    - Post-myocardial infarction syndrome (Dressler syndrome)
    - Post-pericardiotomy syndrome: Pleuropulmonary reaction following extensive pericardiotomy
  - Pleural effusion (80%): Bilateral or unilateral with nearly equal frequency
- **Infection**
  - Loculation suggests empyema
  - Large effusions suggest anaerobic, gram-negative organisms, or *S. aureus*
- **Renal Disease**
  - Nephrotic syndrome
    - Due to hypoalbuminemia, hypervolemia, and increased hydrostatic pressures
    - Commonly subpulmonary and recurrent
- **Metastatic Malignant Pleural Disease**
  - Lung, breast, ovary, and stomach
  - Unexplained pleural effusion in patient with malignancy
  - CT: Irregular pleural thickening and small nodules (implants)
    - Metastases may have variable enhancement
- **Lymphoma**
  - Bilateral pleural effusion in 50%
  - Chylothorax occasionally encountered
- **Trauma/Iatrogenic**
  - Hemothorax
    - Blunt or penetrating chest trauma
  - Esophageal perforation
    - Causes: Idiopathic, iatrogenic, traumatic, and neoplastic

- Clinically may simulate myocardial infarction or acute aortic dissection
- Extraluminal air and bilateral pleural effusions

- **Lupus Pleuritis**
  - > 50% of patients with SLE will have pleural disease at some time in course of their disease
  - Pleural disease usually painful
  - Exudative pleural effusion usually small, either bilateral or unilateral
- **Abdominal Surgery**
  - Small early effusions common within 3 days after surgery (70%); bilateral (63%)
  - Clinically not significant
  - Predisposing factors: Upper abdominal surgery and postoperative atelectasis

Helpful Clues for Less Common Diagnoses

- **Asbestos-related Pleural Disease**
  - In approximately 3% of asbestos-exposed individuals
  - Unilateral or bilateral and generally of small volume (< 500 mL)
  - Over 50% asymptomatic
  - As early as 1 year after exposure (mean latency = 30 years)
  - May predispose to rounded atelectasis
- **Pregnancy-related**
  - Antenatally and in immediate postnatal period
  - Normal finding on chest radiograph within 24-48 hours of delivery
    - Small and bilateral
    - Due to hypervolemia and high intrathoracic pressures from Valsalva maneuvers

Helpful Clues for Rare Diagnoses

- **Diffuse Pulmonary Lymphangiomatosis**
  - Rare disease of lymphatic system affecting individuals under 20 years; progressive disease with poor prognosis
  - Term used when abnormalities are restricted to chest
    - CT: Thickening of interlobular septa, infiltration of mediastinal fat, areas of ground-glass opacity, and uni- or bilateral chylous effusions
- **Venoocclusive Disease**
  - Rare cause of pulmonary hypertension affecting postcapillary (venous) pulmonary circulation
  - CT features: Smooth interlobular septal thickening, ground-glass opacity, and enlarged central pulmonary arteries with normal-caliber veins
  - Moderate to small bilateral pleural effusions
- **Drug-induced Pleuritis**
  - Number of medications may cause exudative pleural effusions: Amiodarone, nitrofurantoin, phenytoin, methotrexate, cyclophosphamide, and carbamazepine
  - Full list at http://www.pneumotox.com

Congestive Heart Failure

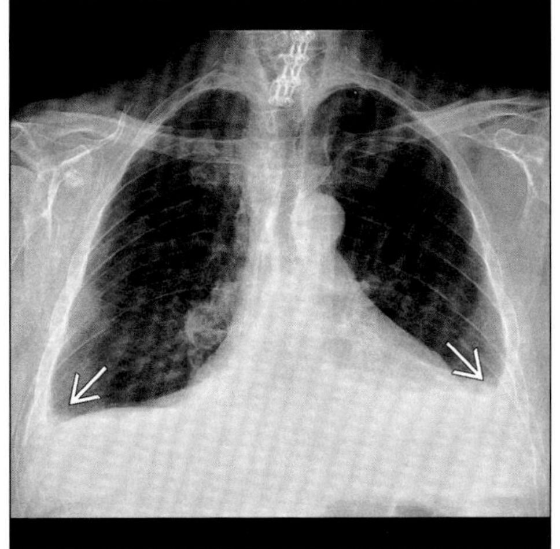

Frontal radiograph in a patient with prior myocardial infarctions and chronic CHF shows blunting of both costophrenic angles ➔, representing bilateral pleural effusions.

Congestive Heart Failure

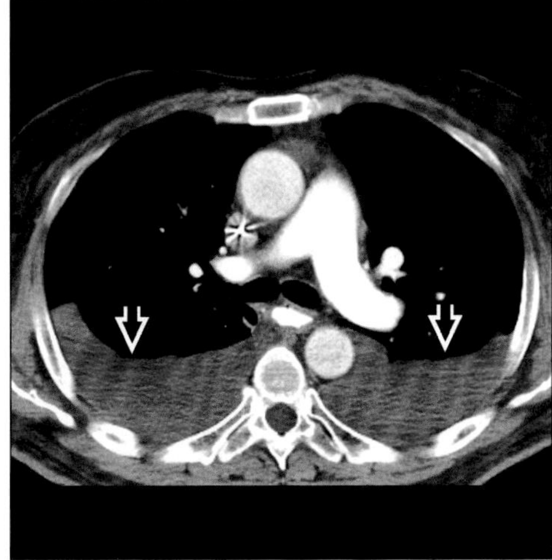

Axial CECT of the same patient shows bilateral large pleural effusions layering out posteriorly in both hemithoraces ➔. The pleural surfaces are smooth, thin, and partially imperceptible.

BILATERAL PLEURAL EFFUSION

Postcardiac Injury Syndrome

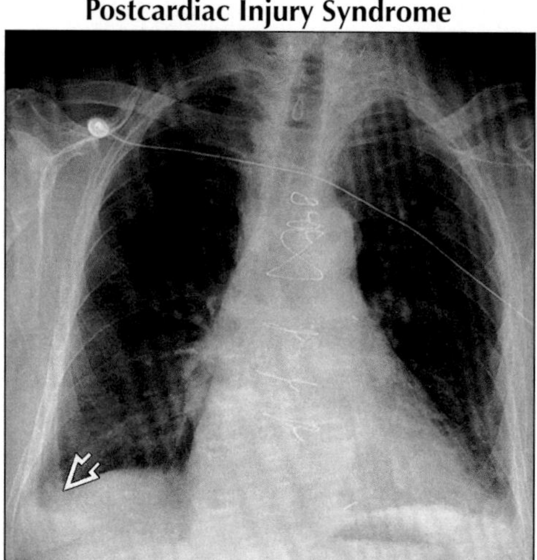

Postcardiac Injury Syndrome

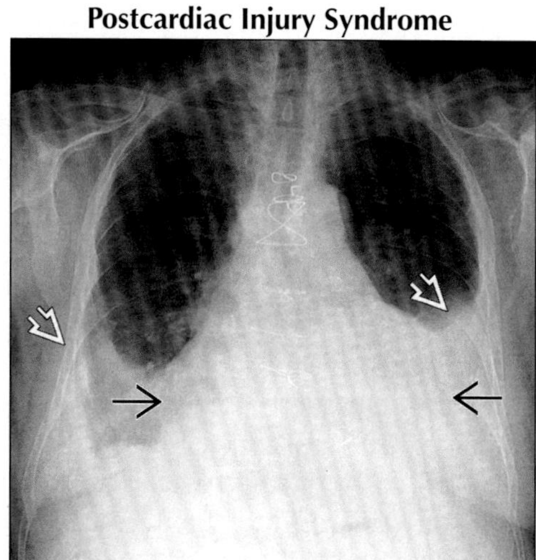

(Left) *Frontal radiograph immediately following median sternotomy and coronary artery bypass surgery shows a small right pleural effusion ➪, a normal postoperative appearance.* ***(Right)*** *Frontal radiograph of the same patient obtained 2 weeks later shows a significant enlargement of the heart silhouette →. Bilateral pleural effusion is also clearly visible ➪. The patient was diagnosed with Dressler syndrome.*

Infection

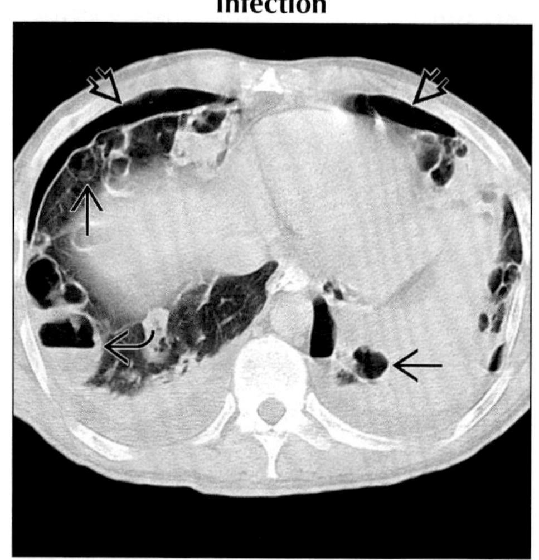

Metastatic Malignant Pleural Disease

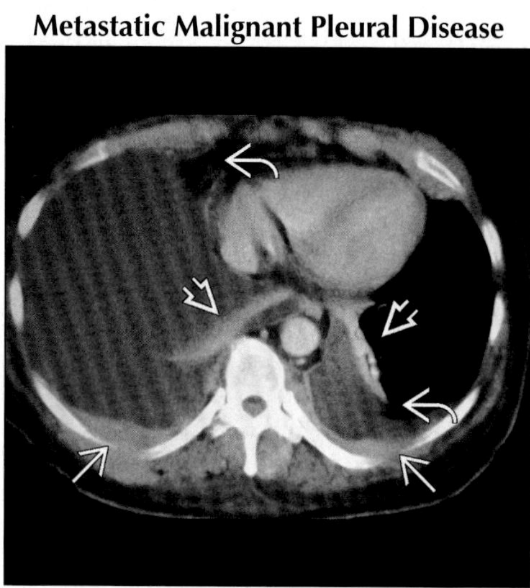

(Left) *Axial NECT shows multiple bilateral cavitating lung nodules → from staphylococcal pneumonia. Some nodules contain fluid levels ↪. Bilateral hydropneumothoraces are demonstrated ➪.* ***(Right)*** *Axial CECT shows bilateral pleural effusion ➔ and small areas of smooth pleural thickening ➔ in a patient with colonic adenocarcinoma. Compressive bilateral subsegmental atelectasis is also seen in both lower lobes ➪.*

Lymphoma

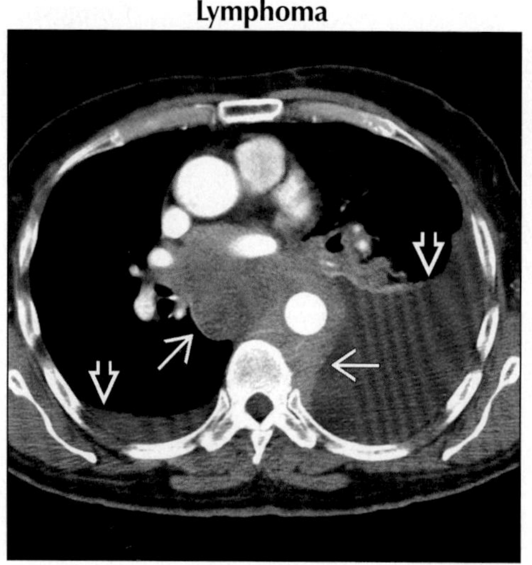

Trauma/Iatrogenic

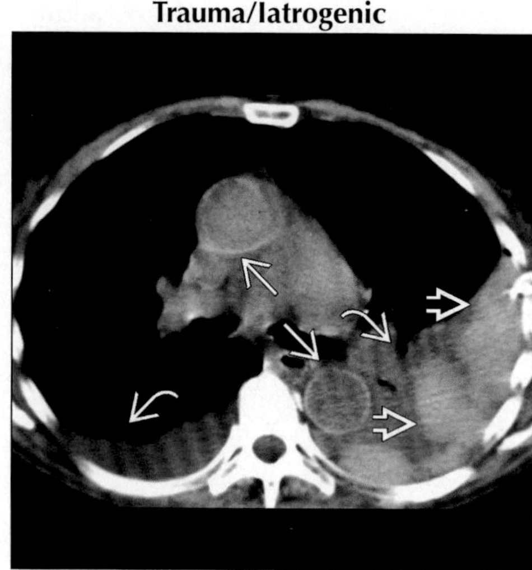

(Left) *Axial CECT shows a soft tissue middle mediastinal and left paravertebral mass, representing non-Hodgkin lymphoma and surrounding the aorta ➔ without associated displacement. Bilateral pleural effusion is also seen ➪.* ***(Right)*** *Axial NECT shows bilateral moderate pleural effusion ➔ with dependent high attenuation material ➪ indicating hemothorax. The thin hyperdense aortic wall ➔ is due to acute anemia.*

BILATERAL PLEURAL EFFUSION

Lupus Pleuritis

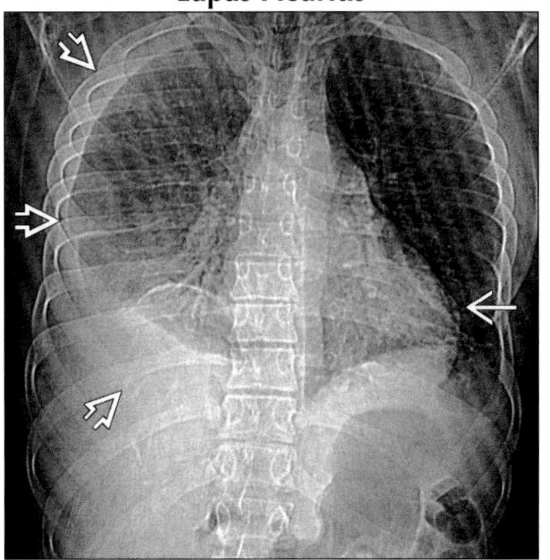

Lupus Pleuritis

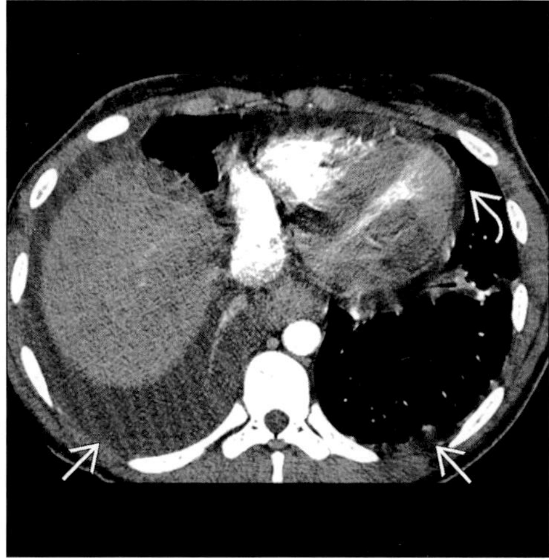

(Left) *Anteroposterior scanogram shows large right pleural effusion ➡ and cardiomegaly ➡.* ***(Right)*** *Corresponding CECT shows bilateral pleural effusions ➡, especially large on the right, and a small pericardial effusion ➡, all related to multi-organ serositis.*

Diffuse Pulmonary Lymphangiomatosis

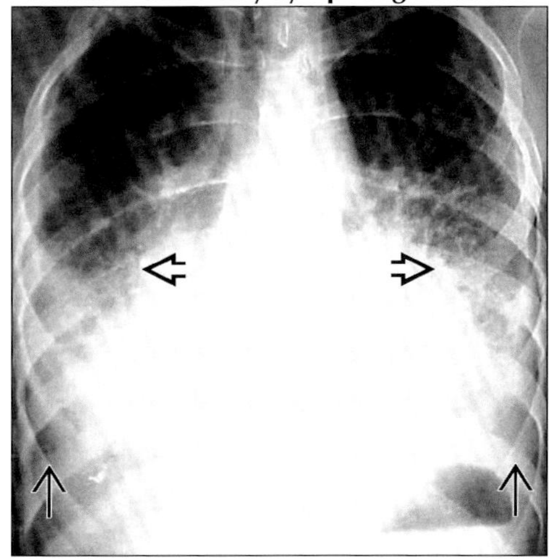

Diffuse Pulmonary Lymphangiomatosis

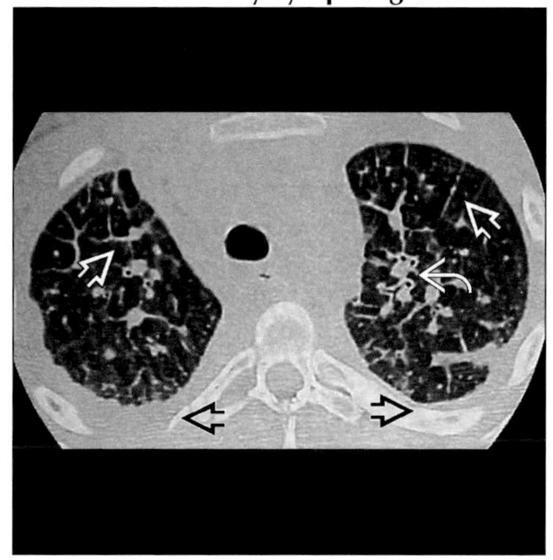

(Left) *Anteroposterior radiograph shows enlarged and hazy perihilar structures ➡ with moderate-sized bilateral pleural effusions ➡.* ***(Right)*** *Axial NECT shows marked thickening of the bronchovascular bundles ➡ in a patient with diffuse pulmonary lymphangiomatosis. Smooth septal thickening ➡ and bilateral pleural effusion ➡ are also visible. (Courtesy D. Escuissato, MD.)*

Drug-induced Pleuritis

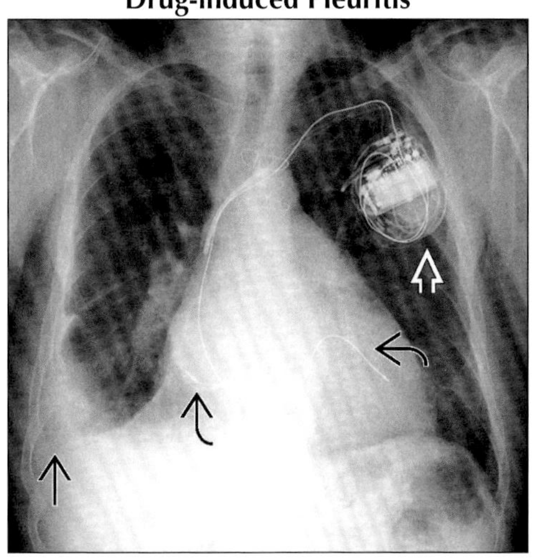

Drug-induced Pleuritis

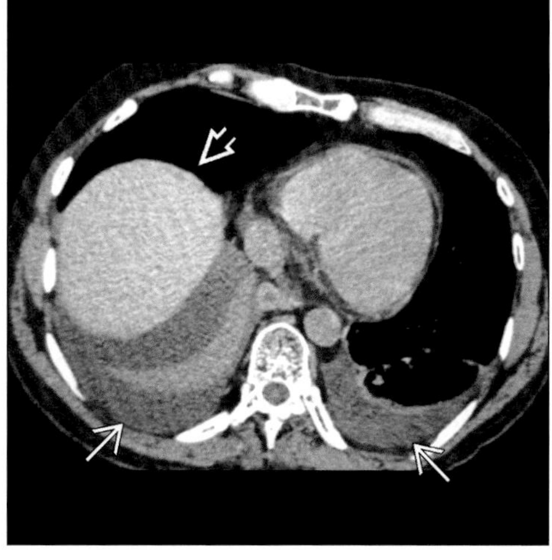

(Left) *Frontal radiograph shows cardiomegaly, pacemaker ➡ with intracardiac wires ➡, and a right pleural effusion ➡ that was longstanding.* ***(Right)*** *Axial NECT of the same patient shows bilateral pleural effusion ➡ that persisted despite treatment for congestive heart failure. Thoracentesis showed an exudative effusion. The hepatic high attenuation ➡ is the result of amiodarone treatment. Diagnosis: Amiodarone-induced pleuritis.*

THORACIC ABNORMALITIES ASSOCIATED WITH ACUTE/CHRONIC LIVER DISEASE

DIFFERENTIAL DIAGNOSIS

Common
- Varices
- Alpha-1 Antiprotease Deficiency
- Hepatic Hydrothorax
- Noncardiac Pulmonary Edema

Less Common
- Hepatopulmonary Syndrome
- Portopulmonary Hypertension
- Cystic Fibrosis
- Hepatocellular Carcinoma Metastases
- Sarcoidosis

Rare but Important
- Lymphocytic Interstitial Pneumonia
- Amiodarone Pulmonary Toxicity
- Heterotaxy Syndrome

ESSENTIAL INFORMATION

Key Differential Diagnosis Issues
- Elevated right hemidiaphragm may be secondary to underlying liver disease

Helpful Clues for Common Diagnoses
- **Varices**
  - Most common complication of portal hypertension
  - Radiographic clues: Small liver, splenomegaly, lower paraspinal widening
  - CT: Serpiginous vessels surrounding thickened distal esophageal wall
    - Vessels may be unopacified on arterial phase imaging
  - Rarely, portal veins may decompress into pulmonary veins across pleural adhesions or inferior pulmonary ligament leading to right-to-left shunt
    - Splenopneumopexy: Obsolete surgical procedure of left hemidiaphragm with abrasion of spleen and left lower lobe allowing collaterals to develop
- **Alpha-1 Antiprotease Deficiency**
  - Inherited (autosomal dominant) deficiency of alpha-1 antitrypsin (A1AT)
    - Hepatic A1AT expressed in liver, released into circulation
    - In deficiency, A1AT accumulates in liver leading to cirrhosis
    - 5-10% of patients > 50 years old with A1AT have cirrhosis
  - CT: Panlobular emphysema, primarily in lower lung zones
    - Mild cylindrical bronchiectasis also common (40%)
  - Pulmonary function preserved until 5-6th decade in nonsmokers (3rd decade in smokers)
  - Emphysema major cause of death in smokers
  - Liver disease major cause of death in nonsmokers
- **Hepatic Hydrothorax**
  - Definition: Pleural effusion in cirrhosis in absence of cardiopulmonary disease
  - Prevalence in cirrhotic patients (5-10%)
  - Right pleural effusion (85%), left (13%), bilateral (2%)
  - May occur in absence of ascites
- **Noncardiac Pulmonary Edema**
  - Seen in up to 40% with fulminant hepatic failure
  - High mortality rate

Helpful Clues for Less Common Diagnoses
- **Hepatopulmonary Syndrome**
  - Triad of chronic liver disease (usually cirrhosis), increased alveolar-arterial oxygen gradient on room air, intrapulmonary vascular dilatation
  - May be related to liver's inability to break down circulating vasodilators (thought to be nitric oxide)
  - Prevalence 20% in those awaiting orthotopic liver transplantation
  - CT: Dilated peripheral arteries (2x larger than adjacent bronchi), primarily in lower lobes
  - V/Q scan: Macroaggregated albumin bypasses lungs and results in systemic activity in brain and kidneys
  - Reversible after orthotopic liver transplantation
- **Portopulmonary Hypertension**
  - May be related to liver's inability to break down circulating vasoconstrictive agents
  - Not related to severity of liver disease
  - Prevalence: 2-5% in patients with cirrhosis
  - CT findings identical to other causes of pulmonary hypertension: Enlarged central pulmonary arteries, attenuation of peripheral pulmonary arteries, mosaic attenuation

- Mean survival 15 months
- Relative contraindication to orthotopic liver transplantation

- **Cystic Fibrosis**
  - Hereditary disorder (autosomal recessive) that affects chloride transport
  - Airways primarily affected
    - Bronchiectasis usually predominant in upper lobes
  - Up to 40% have focal biliary cirrhosis, 10% go on to develop biliary cirrhosis
- **Hepatocellular Carcinoma Metastases**
  - Typical manifestation is multiple variable-sized pulmonary nodules
  - Proclivity of hepatocellular carcinoma to invade veins may give rise to intravascular metastases
- **Sarcoidosis**
  - Drug complication of interferon therapy in patients with hepatitis C infection
  - Sarcoid primarily affects chest (75%) or skin
  - Radiographic findings identical to typical sarcoidosis, ranging from symmetric hilar adenopathy to perilymphatic nodularity

Helpful Clues for Rare Diagnoses

- **Lymphocytic Interstitial Pneumonia**
  - Part of a spectrum of lymphoproliferative disorders
  - Association between primary biliary cirrhosis and Sjögren syndrome
  - CT: Ground-glass opacities (100%), poorly defined centrilobular nodules
    - Thin-walled cysts most distinctive finding (80%), involve < 10% of total lung, may be only finding
- **Amiodarone Pulmonary Toxicity**
  - Antiarrhythmic agent with 3 iodine molecules
  - Toxicity is dose related and accumulates in liver and lung
    - Acute presentation: High-opacity areas of lung consolidation
    - Chronic presentation: Diffuse interstitial thickening
- **Heterotaxy Syndrome**
  - Situs describes position of cardiac atria and viscera
  - Atrial situs best determined by location of liver
  - Situs ambiguous or heterotaxy syndrome
    - Asplenia: Right-sided symmetry
    - Polysplenia: Left-sided symmetry
  - If discordant location of stomach bubble and cardiac apex, then consider asplenia or polysplenia

Varices

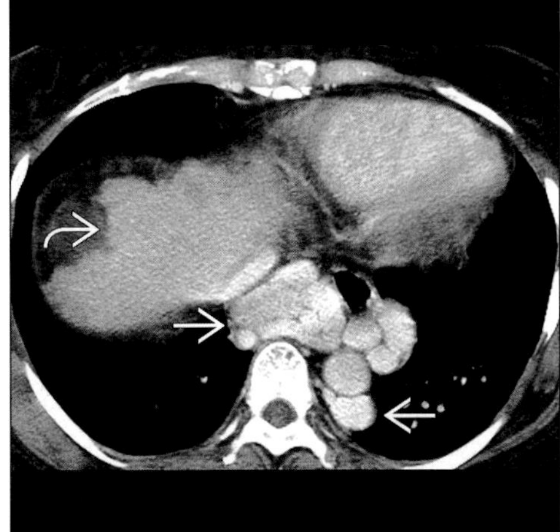

Axial CECT shows enlarged, contrast-enhancing paraesophageal varices ➡. The liver is small and cirrhotic ➡. Note that the varices are as large as the descending aorta.

Varices

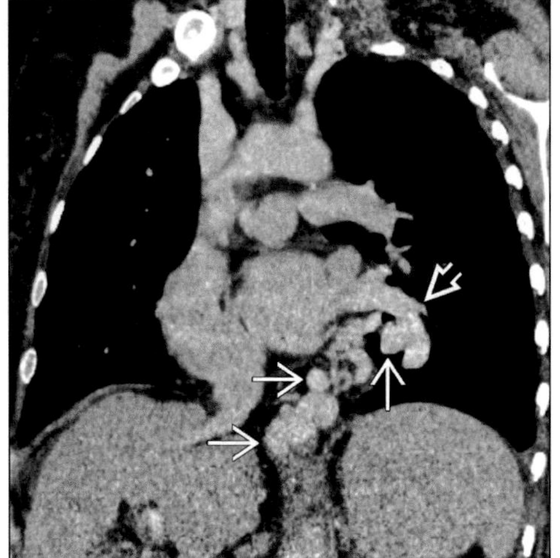

Coronal oblique CECT reconstruction shows varices ➡ draining into left pulmonary vein ➡ and causing a right-to-left shunt. Varices entered lung through inferior pulmonary ligament.

THORACIC ABNORMALITIES ASSOCIATED WITH ACUTE/CHRONIC LIVER DISEASE

*(**Left**) Axial HRCT shows basilar distribution of panlobular emphysema ➡. Peripheral pulmonary vessels are attenuated and sparse. (**Right**) Axial NECT shows cirrhotic liver ➡ and tube ➡ from percutaneous portovenous shunt. Small bilateral pleural effusions ➡ are also seen. There was no ascites. Patient had no cardiac or respiratory disease.*

Alpha-1 Antiprotease Deficiency

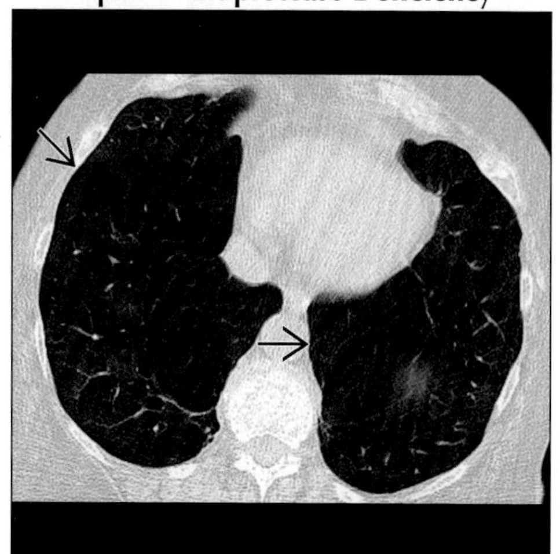

Hepatic Hydrothorax

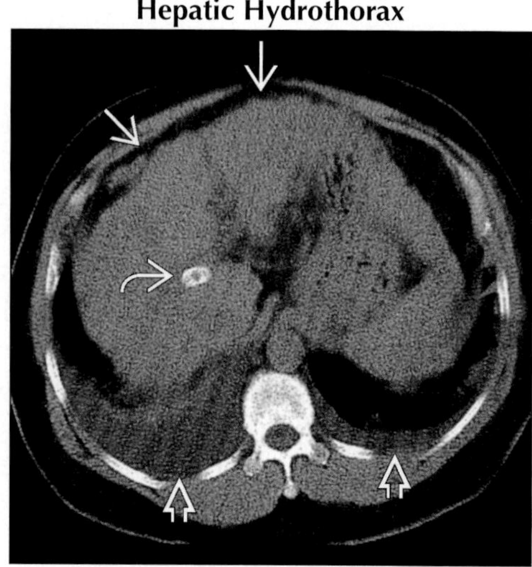

*(**Left**) Anteroposterior radiograph shows peripheral consolidation from noncardiac pulmonary edema in this patient with fulminant hepatic failure. (**Right**) Axial CECT shows enlarged tortuous pulmonary vessels ➡. Tortuous peripheral vessels come almost to the edge of the lung and are larger in diameter than adjacent airways ➡. Patient had platypnea (dyspnea in upright position relieved in supine position).*

Noncardiac Pulmonary Edema

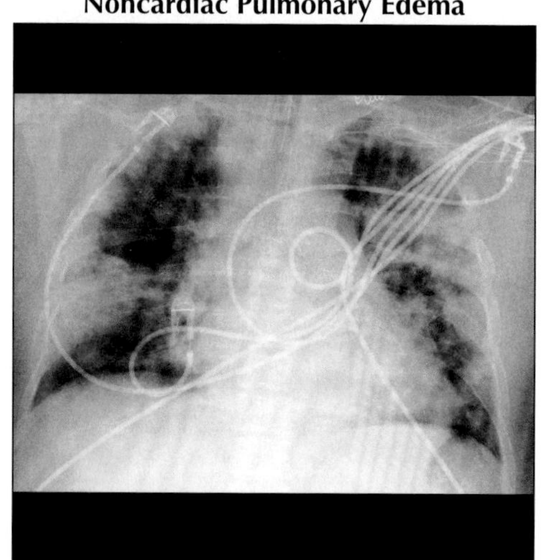

Hepatopulmonary Syndrome

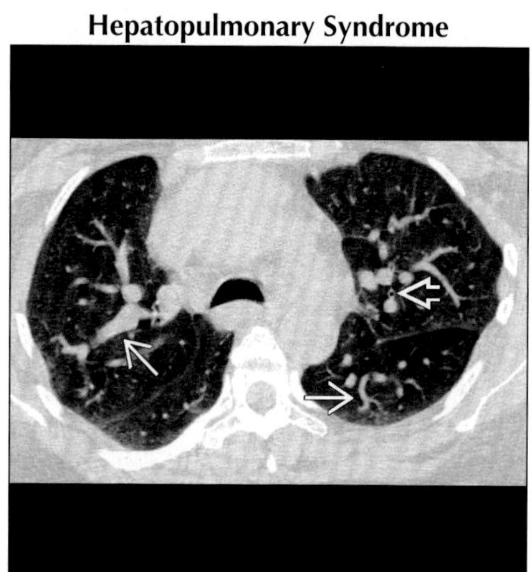

*(**Left**) Frontal radiograph shows enlarged main pulmonary artery ➡. Liver is small ➡ from cirrhosis. Enlarged spleen distorts the stomach bubble ➡. (**Right**) Coronal NECT reconstruction shows diffuse bronchiectasis ➡ and small cirrhotic liver ➡. Secondary biliary cirrhosis develops because of long-term partial or total obstruction of the larger bile ducts.*

Portopulmonary Hypertension

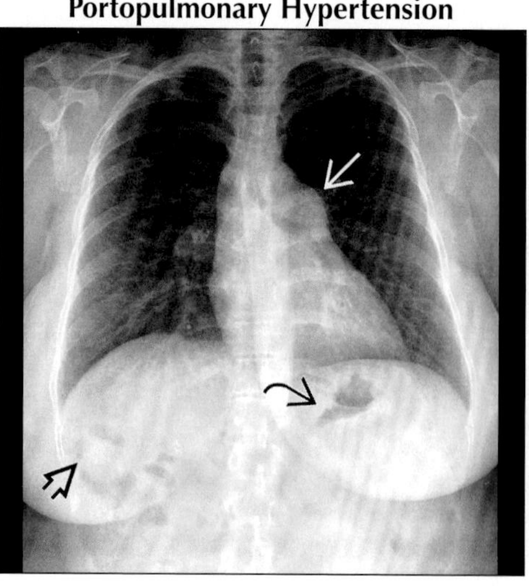

Cystic Fibrosis

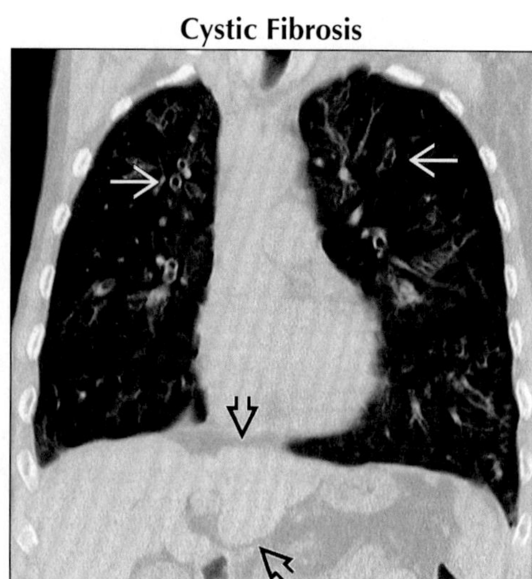

Hepatocellular Carcinoma Metastases

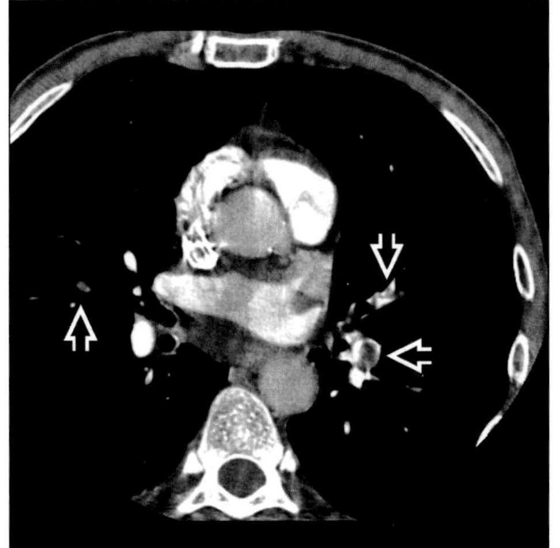

Hepatocellular Carcinoma Metastases

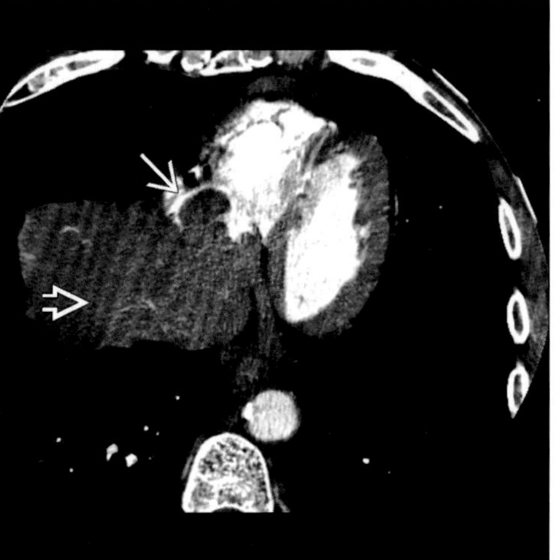

*(**Left**) Axial CECT shows multiple pulmonary emboli ➡ from tumor emboli. Patient had cirrhosis. Venous pulmonary emboli are uncommon in patients with cirrhosis because of the liver's inability to produce clotting factors. (**Right**) Axial CECT more inferiorly shows mass in the right atrium ➡ arising from direct extension of hepatoma ➡ through hepatic veins.*

Sarcoidosis

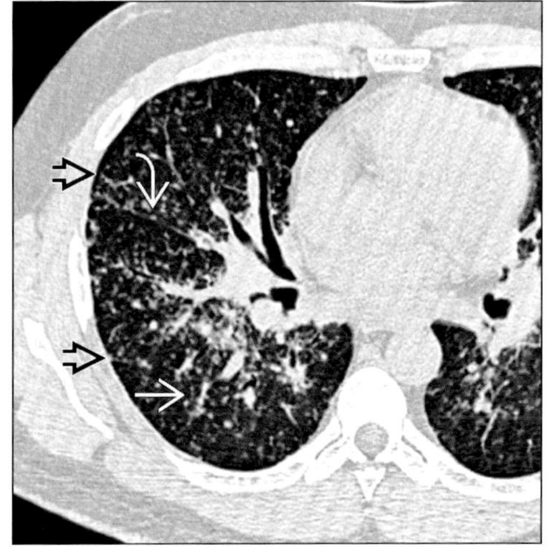

Lymphocytic Interstitial Pneumonia

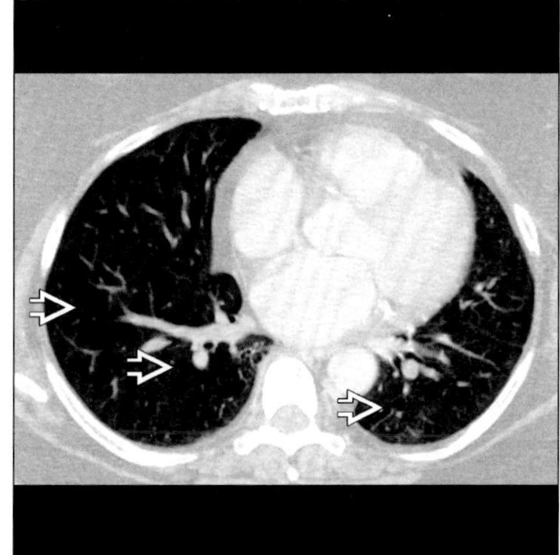

*(**Left**) Axial HRCT shows perilymphatic distribution of nodules on interlobular septa ➡ and the major fissure ➡. Note the beaded vessel ➡ that represents peribronchovascular disease. (**Right**) Axial CECT shows a few small scattered cysts ➡ in a patient with Sjögren syndrome. 75% of patients with primary biliary cirrhosis have signs of the sicca complex. 5% of patients with Sjögren syndrome have mitochondrial antibodies.*

Amiodarone Pulmonary Toxicity

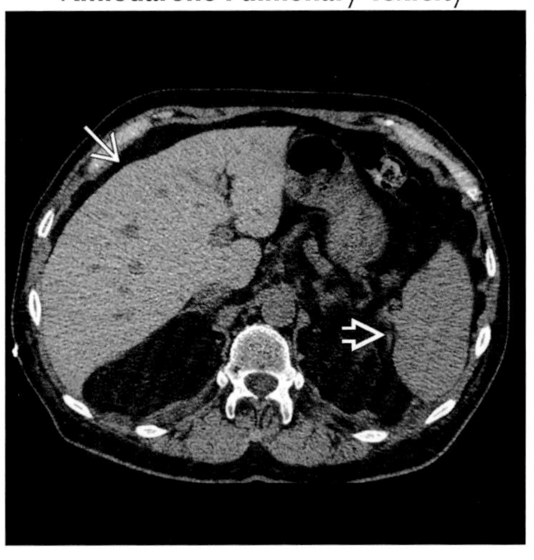

Heterotaxy Syndrome

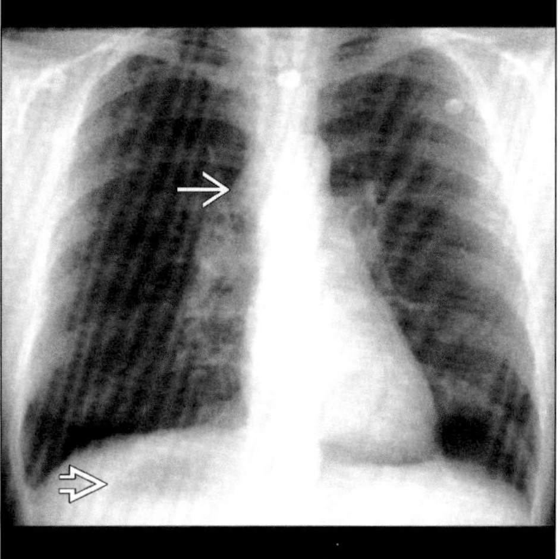

*(**Left**) Axial NECT shows high liver density ➡ compared to spleen ➡. Amiodarone contains 3 iodine molecules and accumulates in the liver and lung. (**Right**) Frontal radiograph shows enlargement of the azygous arch ➡. Note the stomach bubble ➡ under the right hemidiaphragm. Discordance between the site of the stomach bubble and cardiac apex suggests a heterotaxy syndrome, which in this patient proved to be polysplenia.*

RENOPULMONARY SYNDROMES

DIFFERENTIAL DIAGNOSIS

Common

- Uremic Pulmonary Edema
- Uremic Pericarditis
- Diffuse Alveolar Hemorrhage (DAH)
  - Wegener Granulomatosis
  - Goodpasture Syndrome
  - Systemic Lupus Erythematosus
  - Microscopic Polyangiitis
- Renal Cell Carcinoma

Less Common

- Lymphangiomyomatosis
- Metastatic Pulmonary Calcification
- Sarcoidosis

Rare but Important

- Sickle Cell Disease
- Birt-Hogg-Dubé Syndrome
- Erdheim Chester Disease

ESSENTIAL INFORMATION

Key Differential Diagnosis Issues

- Recognition of renal osteodystrophy in chronic renal failure (CRF)
  - Bone resorption
    - Erosion of distal clavicles
  - Osteopenia (50%)
    - Compression fractures (5-25%)
    - Rib fractures (5-25%)
  - Osteosclerosis of axial skeleton (10-30%)
    - Vertebral bodies: Band-like areas of sclerosis of superior and inferior endplates ("rugger jersey" spine)
  - Brown tumors (1%): Lytic expansile lesions, cortical, usually solitary
  - Soft tissue calcification
    - Periarticular and symmetric
- Pleural effusions common in CRF
  - From overhydration, left ventricular (LV) failure, nephrotic syndrome, autoimmune disease, peritoneal dialysis
- Cardiomegaly common in CRF
  - From overhydration, LV failure, high output failure, pericardial disease, underlying disease causing renal failure

Helpful Clues for Common Diagnoses

- **Uremic Pulmonary Edema**
  - Batwing central pulmonary opacities classic but not specific
  - From LV failure, overhydration, anemia, hypoproteinemia, high output AV fistula, diffuse alveolar damage (uremic lung)
- **Uremic Pericarditis**
  - Includes acute pericarditis, pericardial effusions, cardiac tamponade, constrictive pericarditis
  - Injury from toxic metabolites from renal failure, underlying disease, drug toxicity
  - Cardiomegaly in 95%
- **Diffuse Alveolar Hemorrhage (DAH)**
  - From small-vessel vasculitis affecting lung and kidney
  - Acute onset batwing consolidation in anemic patient
  - Hemoptysis (66%), may be mild
  - Radiology-pathology correlation
    - Hemorrhage into alveolar spaces (ground-glass opacities to consolidation)
    - Blood removed from alveoli by macrophages (2-3 days)
    - Macrophages migrate into interstitium (septal thickening)
    - Macrophages removed by lymphatics (7-14 days) (lungs return to normal)
  - **Wegener Granulomatosis**
    - Hemorrhagic presentation in 8%
    - May occur in absence of cavitary nodules
  - **Goodpasture Syndrome**
    - May follow influenza-type illness
    - Males (M:F = 9:1), often smokers
  - **Systemic Lupus Erythematosus**
    - Autoimmune disorder characterized by antinuclear antibodies, females (M:F = 1:10)
    - Hemorrhage in 2%, may be fatal
    - Renal involvement in 60-90%
    - Unexplained small bilateral pleural effusions and cardiomegaly
  - **Microscopic Polyangiitis**
    - Variant of polyarteritis nodosa
    - Pulmonary hemorrhage (10-30%)
    - Glomerulonephritis (80-100%)
- **Renal Cell Carcinoma**
  - Propensity for metastasizing to uncommon locations (e.g., mediastinal nodes, endobronchial, intravascular) in addition to typical locations (lung, pleura, bone)

Helpful Clues for Less Common Diagnoses

- **Lymphangiomyomatosis**

- Nonneoplastic hamartomatous proliferation of atypical muscle cells
- Women of child-bearing age
- Radiographic manifestations
  - Thin-walled cysts: Diffuse, bilateral, and uniform in size; cysts increase in number and size as disease progresses, results in hyperinflation
  - Spontaneous pneumothorax (40%)
  - Small chylous pleural effusions
- Renal angiomyolipomas (20-50%): Small (< 1 cm), multiple, bilateral

- **Metastatic Pulmonary Calcification**
  - Calcium deposition in normal tissue
  - Tropism for tissues with relative alkaline pH: Upper lung zones, gastric wall, kidney medulla
  - Due to hypercalcemic condition, most commonly chronic renal failure
  - HRCT: Mulberry-shaped nodules of amorphous calcification 3-10 mm in diameter in centrilobular location
- **Sarcoidosis**
  - 3.5% develop nephrolithiasis, may be presenting feature
  - Hypercalciuria (50%), hypercalcemia (20%)
  - Pulmonary macrophages produce calcitriol
  - Stones more common in sunny months

Helpful Clues for Rare Diagnoses

- **Sickle Cell Disease**
  - Due to abnormal hemoglobin, which deforms when deoxygenated
  - Nephropathies: Papillary necrosis, renal infarcts, pyelonephritis, renal medullary carcinoma
  - Radiographic manifestations
    - Lungs: Variable-sized opacities due to pneumonia, atelectasis, or infarcts; interstitial thickening from edema
    - Cardiac: Cardiomegaly
    - Skeletal: Osteonecrosis of humeral heads, H-shaped vertebra (10%), enlarged ribs (marrow expansion), bone sclerosis (bone infarcts)
    - Abdomen: Small or absent spleen
- **Birt-Hogg-Dubé Syndrome**
  - Facial papules (fibrofolliculomas)
  - Renal tumors: Range from oncocytomas to renal cell carcinoma
    - May be bilateral and multifocal
  - Lungs: Thin-walled cysts, predominantly lower lobes, few in number
    - Lung cysts closely associated with interlobular septa or visceral pleura
- **Erdheim Chester Disease**
  - Non-Langerhans cell histiocytosis
  - Skeletal: Bilateral symmetric osteosclerosis of metaphyses and diaphyses, especially long leg bones (sparing epiphyses)
  - Renal: Perirenal fat effaced by soft tissue, bilateral and symmetric
  - Lungs and pleura: Smooth thickening of visceral pleura and fissures, usually bilateral and symmetric
  - Cardiac: Cardiac enlargement from pericardial or cardiac involvement

Uremic Pulmonary Edema

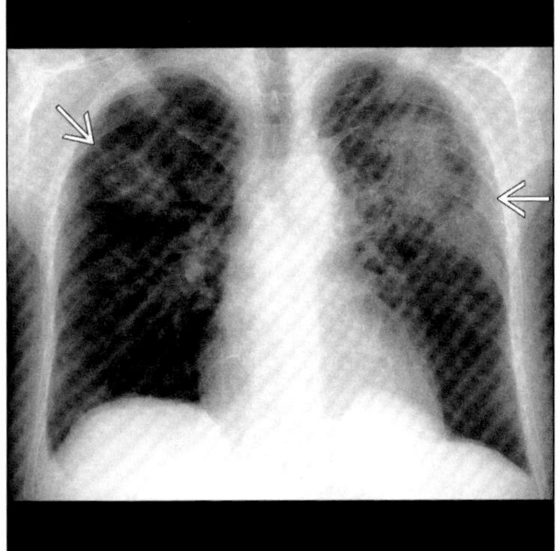

Frontal radiograph shows central batwing consolidation ➔. Edema is most common, but differential includes hemorrhage and infection. Other patterns of edema are common.

Uremic Pericarditis

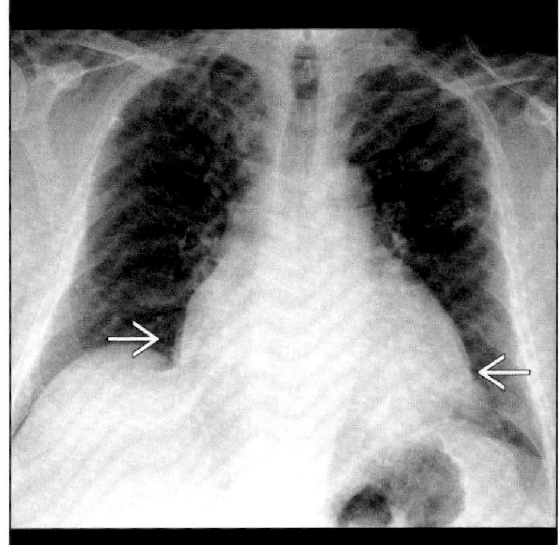

Frontal radiograph shows mild cardiomegaly ➔. Cardiomegaly is common with renal disease and may be due to left ventricular failure, pericarditis, or secondary to underlying disease.

RENOPULMONARY SYNDROMES

*(**Left**) Axial CECT shows moderate pericardial effusion ➡. Tubular shape of the right ventricle ➡ suggests mild constriction or tamponade. Pericardial disease may be secondary to uremic toxins, underlying disease (like SLE), or drugs used to treat underlying disease. (**Right**) Axial CECT shows multiple foci of pericardial calcification ➡. Right atrium is enlarged ➡. The patient had symptoms of constrictive pericardial disease.*

Uremic Pericarditis

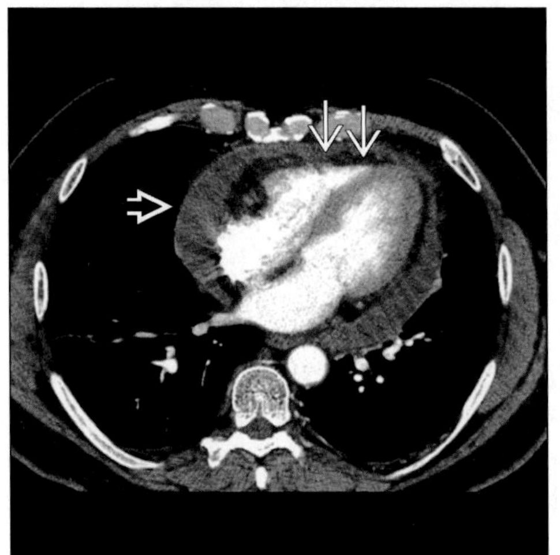

Uremic Pericarditis

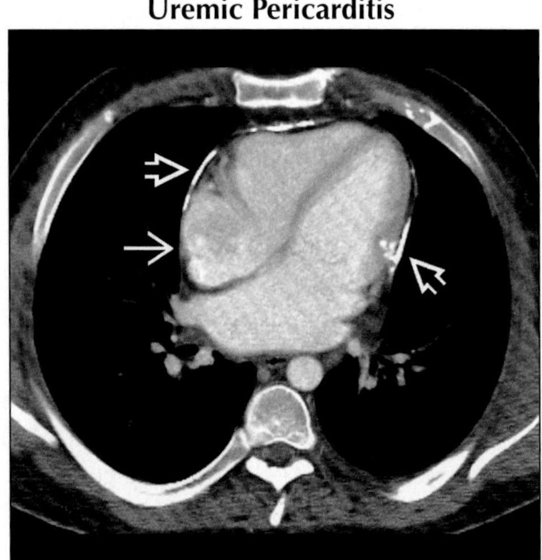

*(**Left**) Anteroposterior radiograph shows diffuse pulmonary consolidation ➡ in a batwing pattern. Most common vasculitis that results in hemorrhage is Wegener. Other Wegener manifestations: Cavitary nodules or airway thickening may be absent. (**Right**) Axial NECT shows central pulmonary consolidation with peripheral sparing ➡ from acute pulmonary hemorrhage. Peripheral sparing is common with diffuse alveolar hemorrhage*

Wegener Granulomatosis

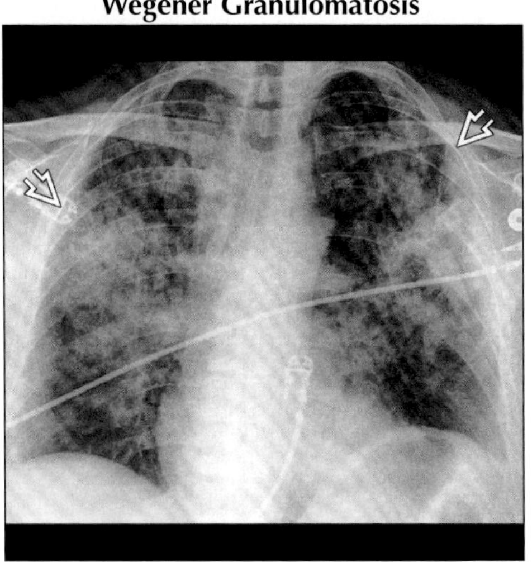

Wegener Granulomatosis

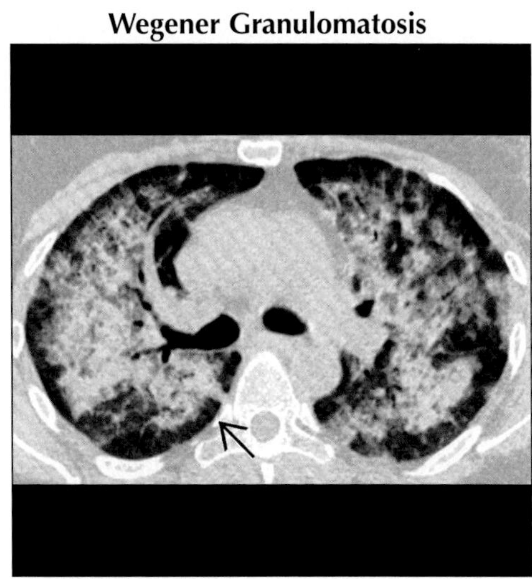

*(**Left**) Frontal radiograph shows central perihilar basilar opacities ➡ and a dialysis catheter ➡. (**Right**) Axial HRCT shows diffuse ground-glass opacities ➡ involving all lobes. Lucencies ➡ represent underlying emphysematous spaces in this patient with glomerulonephritis. Percutaneous renal biopsy showed Goodpasture. CT of pulmonary hemorrhage will range from mild ground-glass opacities to dense consolidation, depending on severity of bleeding.*

Goodpasture Syndrome

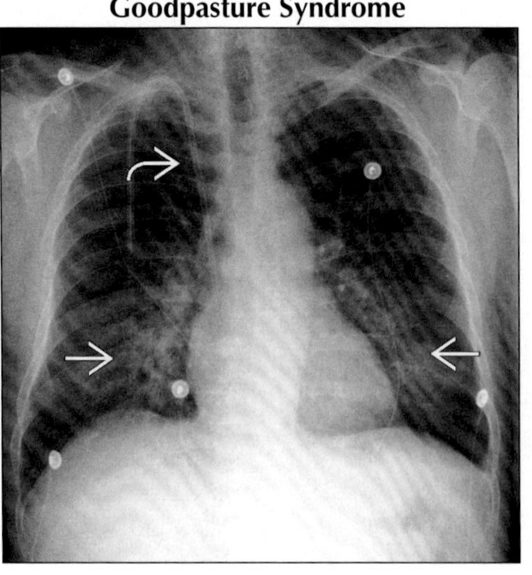

Goodpasture Syndrome

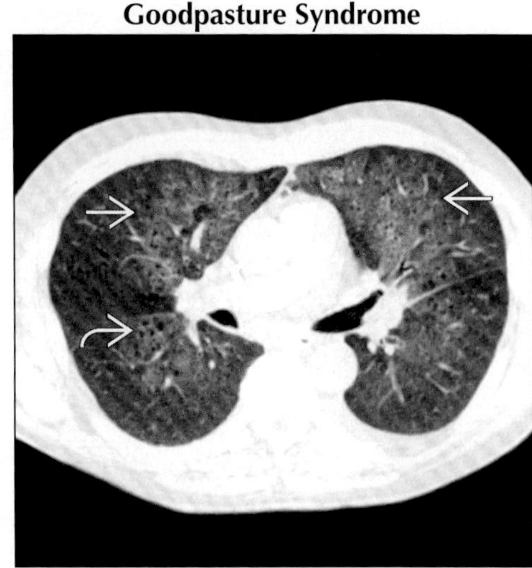

Systemic Lupus Erythematosus

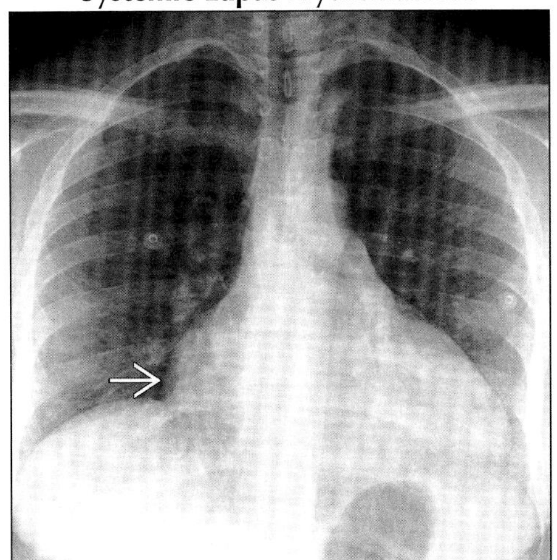

Systemic Lupus Erythematosus

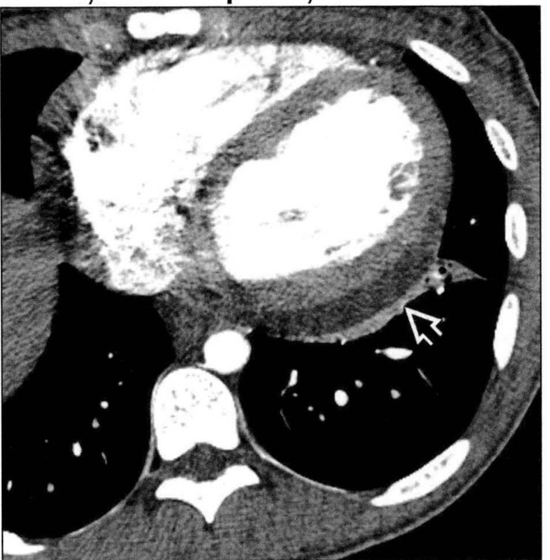

(Left) *Frontal radiograph shows cardiomegaly ➡. Most common manifestation of lupus is pleural thickening or effusions. Pulmonary disease is uncommon, and etiology is usually secondary to pneumonia, hemorrhage, and lupus pneumonitis.* ***(Right)*** *Axial CECT shows moderate-sized pericardial effusion ⇨ and mild dilatation of left ventricle. Left ventricular enlargement may be secondary to renal failure.*

Renal Cell Carcinoma

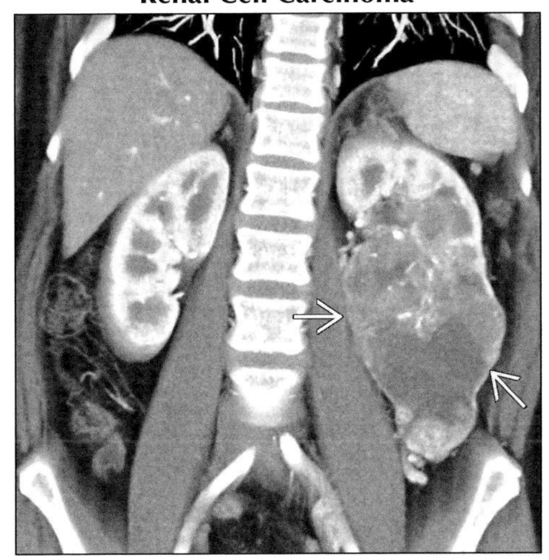

Renal Cell Carcinoma

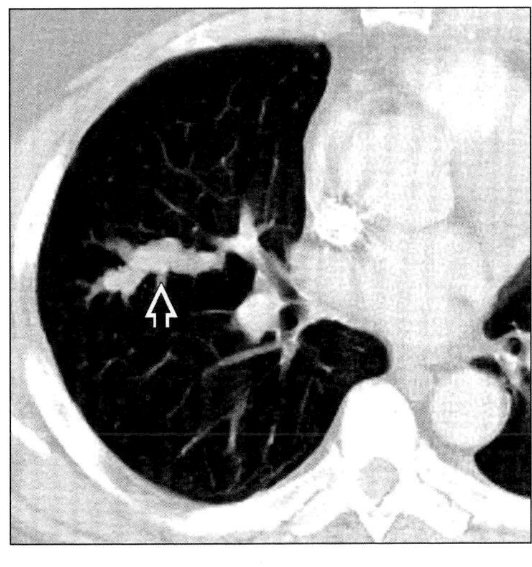

(Left) *Coronal CECT shows a large mass ➡ replacing all but the upper pole of the left kidney. Renal cell carcinoma has a propensity to invade renal veins and IVC. Most common metastases are lung (multiple pulmonary nodules), lymphangitic tumor, pleura, and bone.* ***(Right)*** *Axial CECT shows enlarged lobulated pulmonary arteries ⇨ from intravascular renal cell metastases. Metastasis conforms to the shape of the pulmonary artery.*

Lymphangiomyomatosis

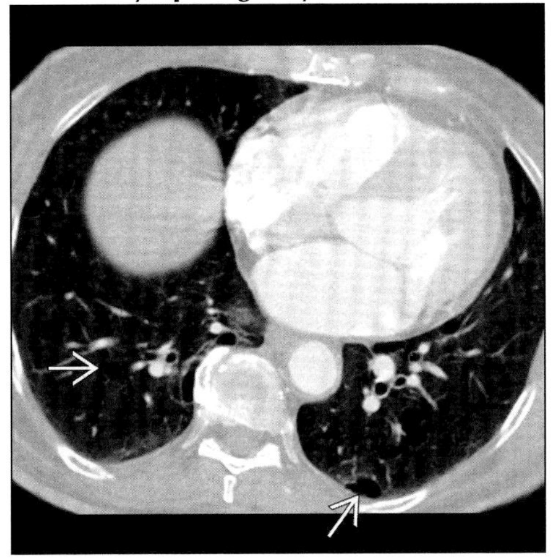

Lymphangiomyomatosis

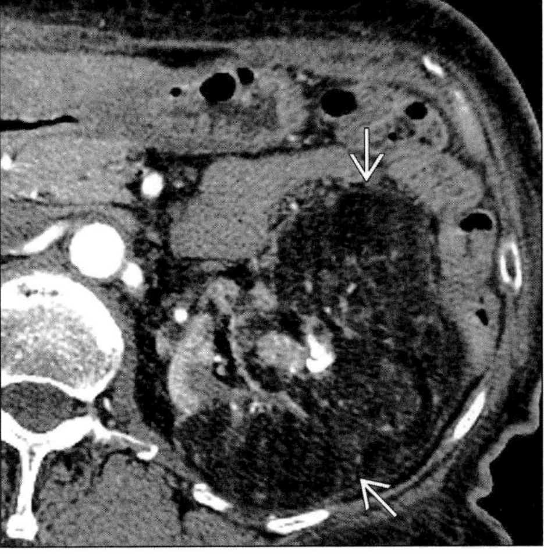

(Left) *Axial CECT shows small scattered cysts ➡ throughout the lower lobes. Cysts were distributed uniformly throughout the lung. Cysts are all similar in size. Subpleural cysts may cause spontaneous pneumothorax.* ***(Right)*** *Axial CECT shows an inhomogeneous fatty mass in the left kidney ➡ from an angiomyolipoma. Fat in the mass is diagnostic of angiomyolipoma. Tumors may be bilateral.*

RENOPULMONARY SYNDROMES

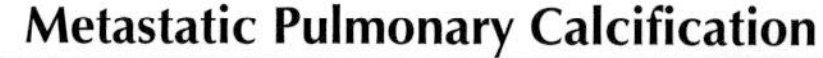

Metastatic Pulmonary Calcification

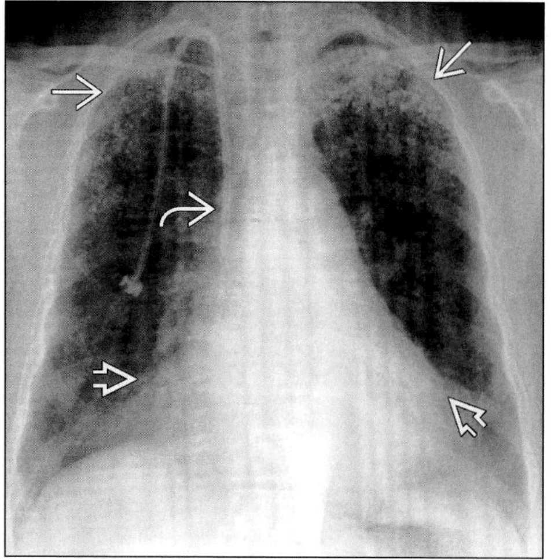

Metastatic Pulmonary Calcification

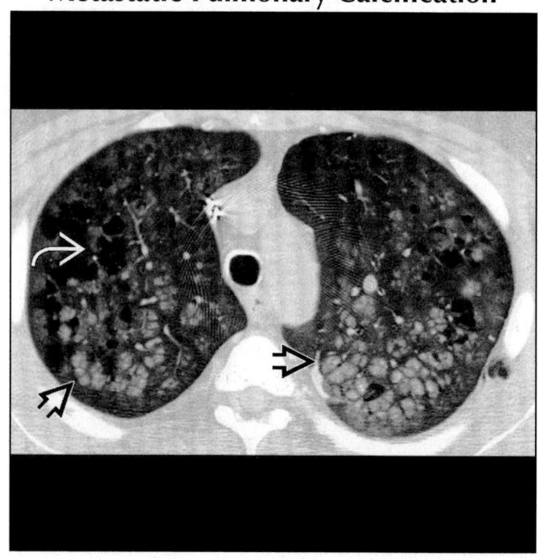

(Left) *Frontal radiograph shows multiple nodules in the upper lobes →, mild cardiomegaly ⇨, and dialysis catheter ↪. Differential would include infection (especially tuberculosis) and sarcoidosis.* ***(Right)*** *Axial NECT shows emphysema ↪ and clustered rosettes of high-density calcification ⇨. Metastatic pulmonary calcification can be seen with any cause of hypercalcemia. Onset may be chronic or develop over days.*

Sarcoidosis

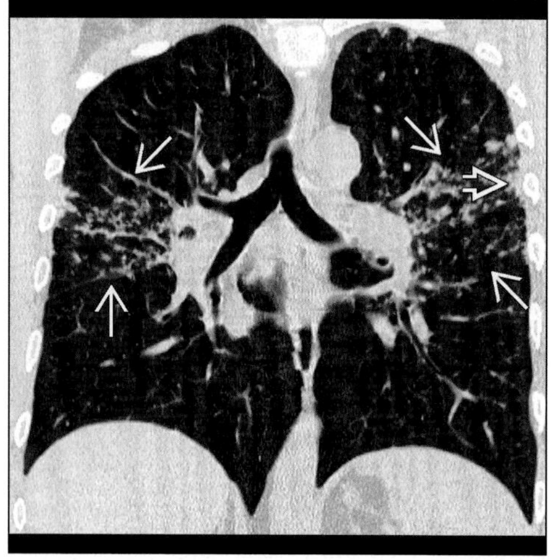

Sarcoidosis

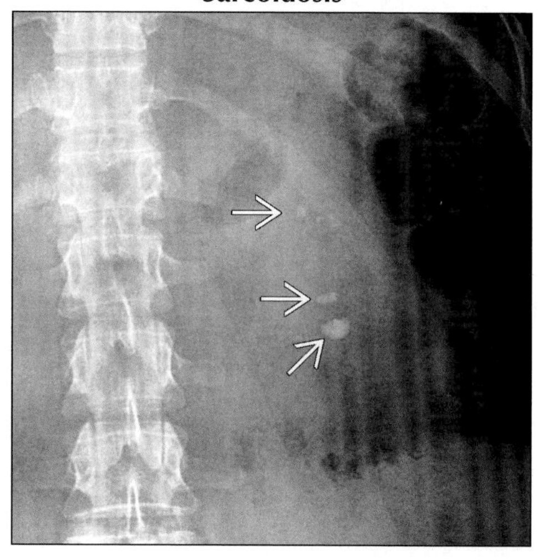

(Left) *Coronal HRCT shows peribronchial nodules → and subpleural nodules forming pseudoplaques ⇨. Bronchovascular distribution is characteristic of sarcoidosis. Chronic disease has a proclivity for the upper lung zones.* ***(Right)*** *Radiograph shows shows multiple opaque renal stones →. Renal stones are not uncommon in sarcoidosis. Indeed, stones are more common in the spring and summer when the patient is exposed to sunlight.*

Sickle Cell Disease

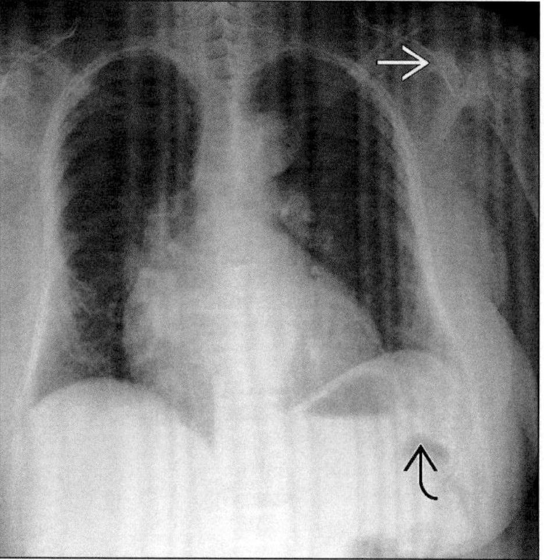

Sickle Cell Disease

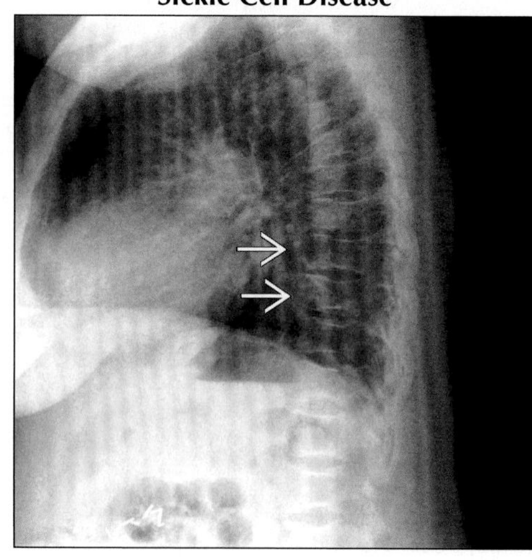

(Left) *Frontal radiograph shows an enlarged heart with evidence of right ventricular hypertrophy and pulmonary arterial hypertension, absence of spleen ↪, and avascular necrosis of left humeral head →.* ***(Right)*** *Lateral radiograph shows H-shaped vertebral bodies →. Vertebral body changes are different from that seen in renal osteodystrophy. Cardiomegaly (from chronic anemia and high output failure) is the most common thoracic manifestation of sickle cell disease.*

Sickle Cell Disease

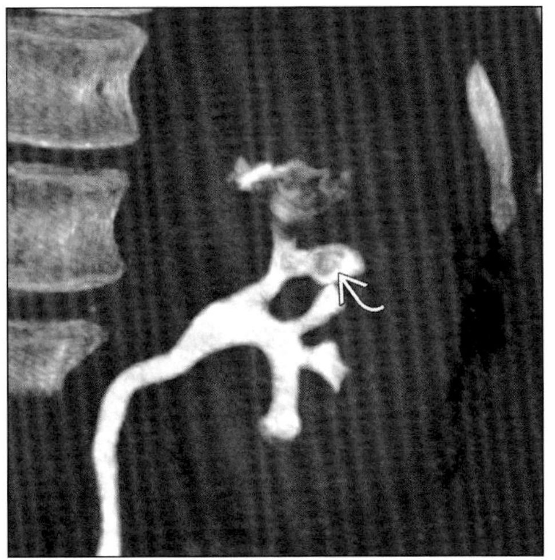

Sickle Cell Disease

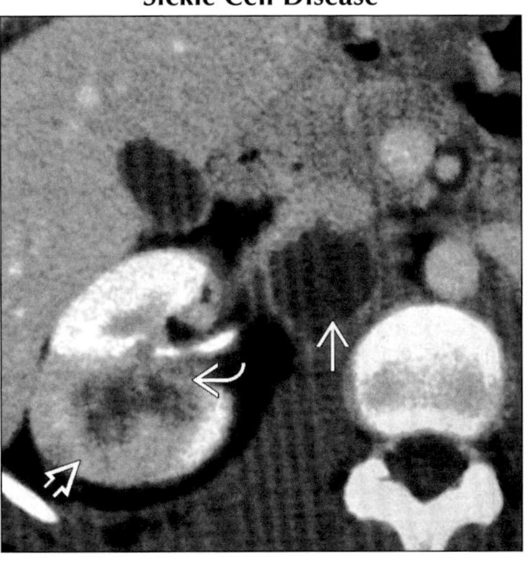

(Left) *Coronal CECT shows clubbing of the calyces, sloughed papillae within the collecting system, and amorphous debris within the upper pole calyces of the left kidney. These are classic findings indicating papillary necrosis in these patients.* ***(Right)*** *Axial CECT shows infiltrating renal medullary carcinoma, with central extension into the renal hilum. Note IVC thrombus. Tumor is almost exclusively seen in patients with sickle cell disease.*

Birt-Hogg-Dubé Syndrome

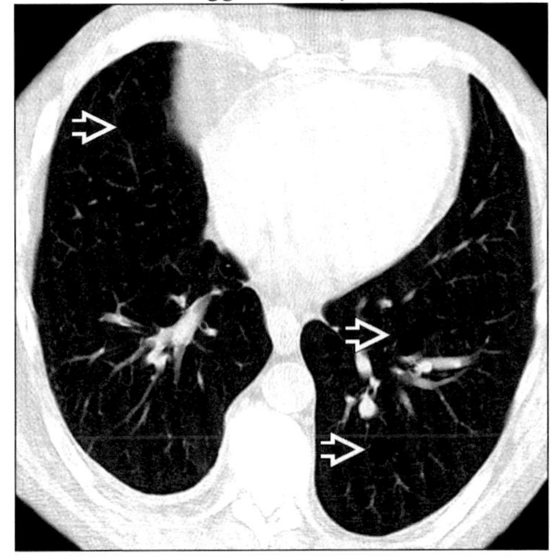

Birt-Hogg-Dubé Syndrome

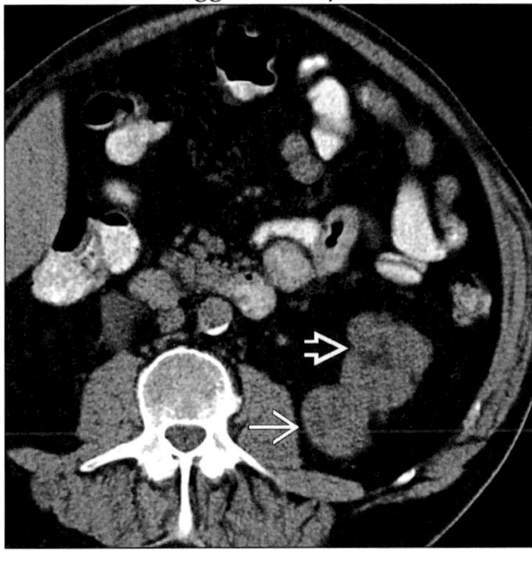

(Left) *Axial CECT shows few variable-sized thin-walled cysts. Cysts are often adjacent to fissures or pleura and may lead to spontaneous pneumothorax. Cysts are more common in lower lung zones.* ***(Right)*** *Axial NECT shows normal kidney and exophytic renal cell carcinoma. Birt-Hogg-Dubé is autosomal dominant. Family members should be screened for renal tumors.*

Erdheim Chester Disease

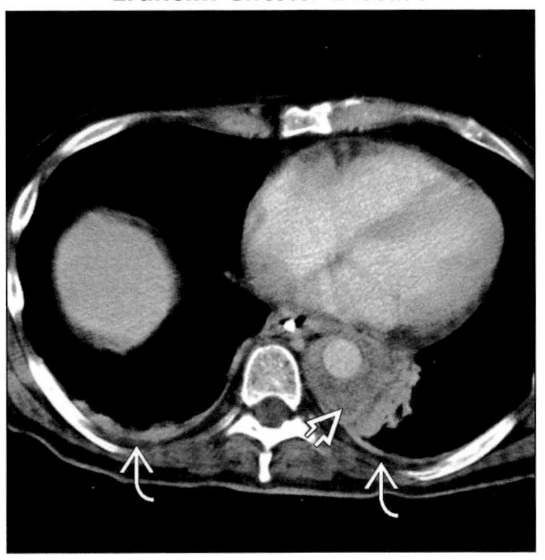

Erdheim Chester Disease

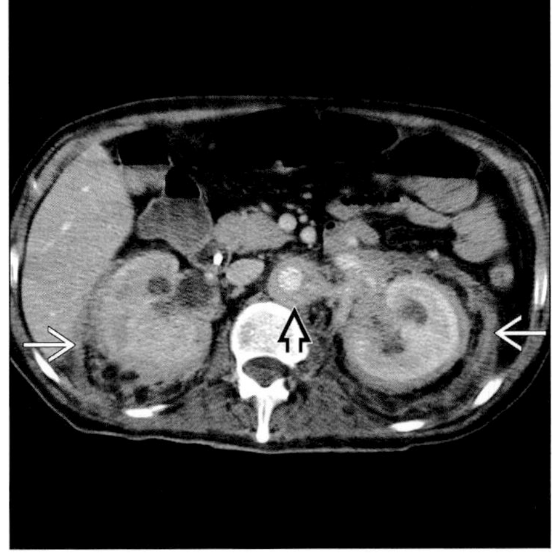

(Left) *Axial NECT shows marked coating of the aorta and bilateral pleural thickening. Aortic coating involved the long segment of the aorta.* ***(Right)*** *Axial NECT shows perirenal and periaortic infiltration typical of Erdheim Chester disease. Perirenal disease may lead to renal failure. Most common manifestation of Erdheim Chester disease is symmetric osteosclerotic bone disease. Systemic disease is seen in 50%.*

PULMONARY CUTANEOUS SYNDROMES

DIFFERENTIAL DIAGNOSIS

Common

- Infections
  - Tuberculosis, Coccidioidomycosis, Histoplasmosis, Aspergillosis, Zygomycoses, Herpes Zoster
- Superior Vena Cava Syndrome

Less Common

- Wegener Granulomatosis
- Hypertrophic Osteoarthropathy
- Fat Embolism Syndrome
- Hereditary Hemorrhagic Telangiectasia

Rare but Important

- Neurofibromatosis Type 1

ESSENTIAL INFORMATION

Key Differential Diagnosis Issues

- Imaging depends upon associated condition
- With pulmonary cutaneous infections, usually disseminated disease

Helpful Clues for Common Diagnoses

- **Infections**
  - Patients typically immunocompromised
  - **Tuberculosis**: Primary cutaneous tuberculosis, lupus vulgaris, scrofuloderma
    - Primary tuberculosis may show unilateral hilar lymphadenopathy, unilateral pulmonary consolidation, pleural effusion
    - Reactivation tuberculosis shows fibrocavitary disease in upper lobes
    - Miliary disease uncommon but indicates hematogenous dissemination
  - **Coccidioidomycosis**: Nonspecific erythema nodosum
    - Nonspecific patchy segmental consolidation, hilar or paratracheal lymphadenopathy
    - 5% have persistent consolidation or fibrocavitary changes
    - Remote disease shows single thin-walled cavity or nodule in periphery of upper lobe
    - Miliary pattern suggests disseminated disease
  - **Histoplasmosis**: Cutaneous findings variable and include erythema multiforme and erythema nodosum
    - Imaging findings of acute histoplasma pneumonia nonspecific; solitary or multifocal airspace opacity, ipsilateral hilar and mediastinal lymphadenopathy
    - Subcentimeter calcified or noncalcified pulmonary granulomas often persist after resolution of pneumonia
    - Chronic cavitary disease indistinguishable from reactivation tuberculosis
  - **Aspergillosis**: Only angioinvasive disease can manifest cutaneously
    - Classic presentation as nodule surrounded by "ground-glass" opacity; halo sign
    - Consolidation and cavitation often progressive with prolonged infection
  - **Zygomycoses**: Particularly *Mucor* species
    - Commonly involves paranasal sinuses and orbit but can include any tissue
    - Can spread hematogenously or directly from lung or sinus
    - Most commonly seen in patients with diabetes mellitus
- **Superior Vena Cava Syndrome**
  - Impaired venous drainage of head, neck, and upper extremities due to obstruction to flow in superior vena cava
    - Facial plethora, arm swelling, dyspnea, cough, dilated chest veins
  - External compression more common than in situ thrombosis
  - Classically small cell lung cancer
    - 2-4% incidence of SVC syndrome with any lung cancer or non-Hodgkin lymphoma, 10% incidence with small cell lung cancer
  - Chest radiograph shows mediastinal widening
  - Chest CT confirms obstruction of major veins and associated dilation of collateral vessels

Helpful Clues for Less Common Diagnoses

- **Wegener Granulomatosis**
  - Small to medium vessel autoimmune vasculitis
  - Nearly all patients have upper airway or lung involvement

- Skin involvement includes palpable purpura, subcutaneous nodules, ulcers, digital infarcts and gangrene, pyoderma, rheumatoid papules, urticaria, gingival hyperplasia
- Multiple pulmonary nodules without zonal predominance, 50% with cavitation
- Diffuse or focal tracheal thickening or narrowing

- **Hypertrophic Osteoarthropathy**
  - Clubbing, periostitis of distal phalanges, pachydermia
  - Primary disease also called pachydermoperiostosis
    - Rare, hereditary
  - Secondary disease most commonly seen with lung cancer
  - Associated pulmonary diseases include
    - Primary lung malignancy, most commonly non-small cell lung cancer
    - Cystic fibrosis
    - Idiopathic pulmonary fibrosis
    - Uncommon with asthma or COPD
  - Small minority with cyanotic heart disease, infective endocarditis, inflammatory bowel syndrome, thyroid disease, HIV
- **Fat Embolism Syndrome**
  - Gradual onset petechial rash, respiratory distress, altered mental status, 24-48 hours after long bone fracture
  - Other findings include tachycardia, renal failure, anemia, thrombocytopenia
  - Can also complicate pancreatitis and administration of total parenteral nutrition
  - Imaging features are nonspecific, ranging from normal to diffuse parenchymal consolidation
- **Hereditary Hemorrhagic Telangiectasia**
  - Telangiectasis tends to be located in head, neck, and distal upper extremities
  - History/symptoms include epistaxis, hemoptysis, subarachnoid hemorrhage or seizure, gastrointestinal bleeding
  - Most common findings in lung are arteriovenous malformations

Helpful Clues for Rare Diagnoses

- **Neurofibromatosis Type 1**
  - Multiple discrete cutaneous and subcutaneous neurofibromas, café au lait spots
  - Skeletal abnormalities: Kyphoscoliosis, bowed legs, skull defects and anomalies of skull shape, pulsating or nonpulsating exophthalmos, orbital displacement, macrodactyly
  - Thoracic cage deformities, such as pectus excavatum and pseudoarthrosis, coarctation of aorta
  - Associated with multiple endocrine neoplasia type 2B and a variety of other neoplasms

Infections

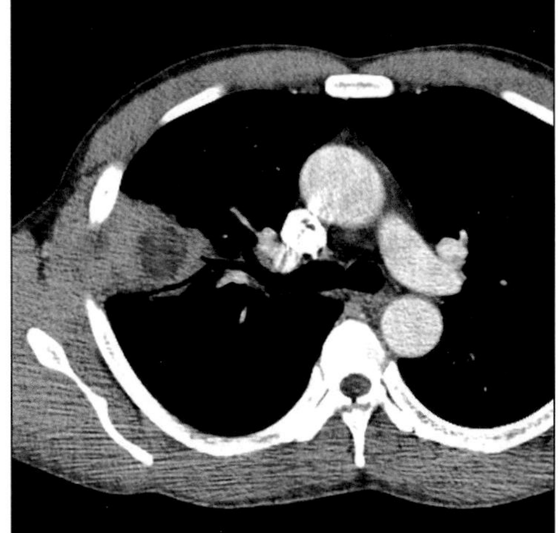

Frontal radiograph shows a focal necrotizing pneumonia in the right upper lobe, invading the chest wall, in this patient with histoplasmosis infection.

Infections

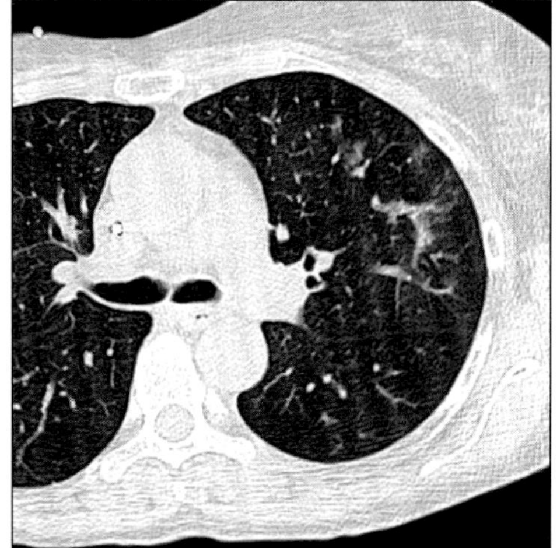

Axial CECT in an immunocompromised patient shows left upper lobe patchy consolidation with surrounding ground-glass opacity, subsequently proven to be invasive aspergillosis.

PULMONARY CUTANEOUS SYNDROMES

Infections

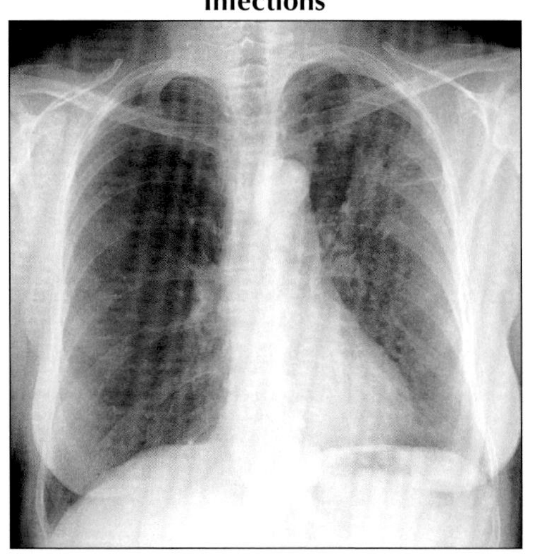

Infections

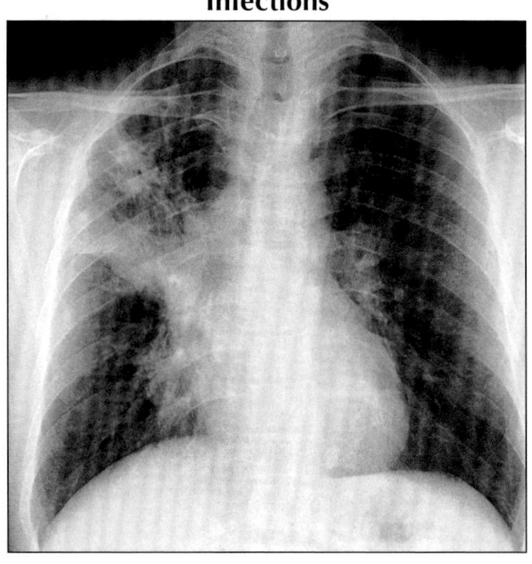

(Left) *Frontal radiograph shows nonspecific focal consolidation in the left upper lobe, subsequently shown to be coccidioidomycosis infection in this patient with recent travel to the United States desert southwest.* ***(Right)*** *Frontal radiograph shows typical features of reactivation tuberculosis with extensive right upper lobe fibronodular disease with volume loss. It is crucial to assess for endobronchial spread of disease in these patients.*

Infections

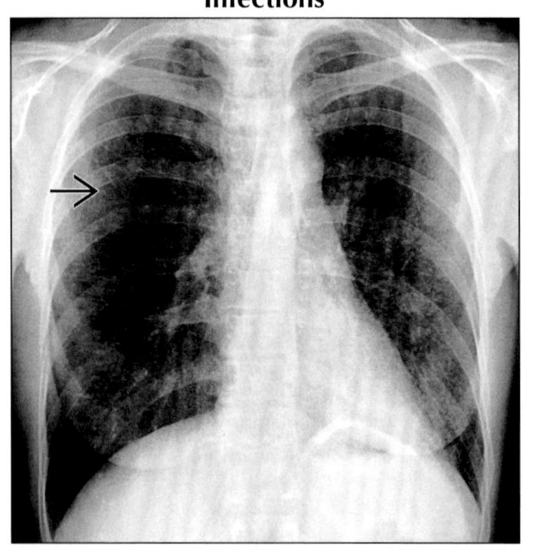

Infections

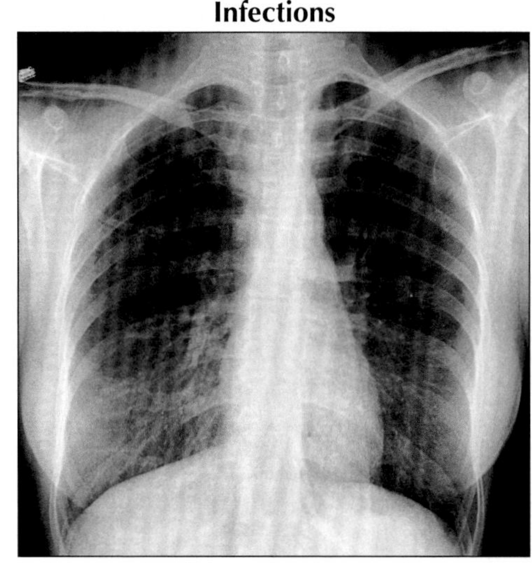

(Left) *Frontal radiograph shows innumerable randomly distributed small millet-seed-sized nodules ➔ throughout both lungs in this patient with miliary tuberculosis.* ***(Right)*** *Frontal radiograph shows soft tissue swelling and several air-fluid levels in the base of the right neck resulting from tuberculous lymphadenitis, so-called scrofula. This can be an isolated finding with normal lungs or associated with mediastinal lymphadenopathy.*

Infections

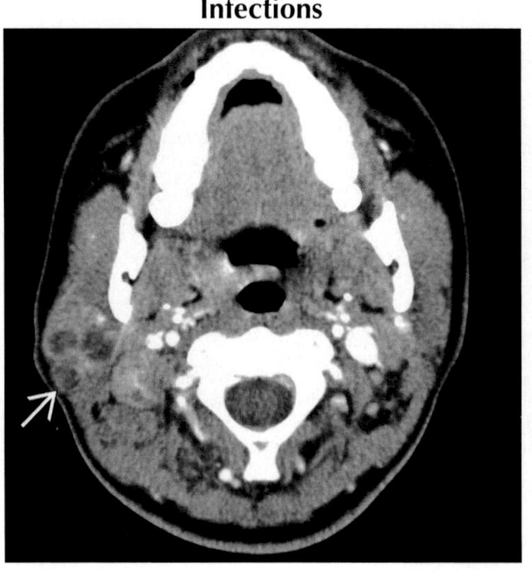

Infections

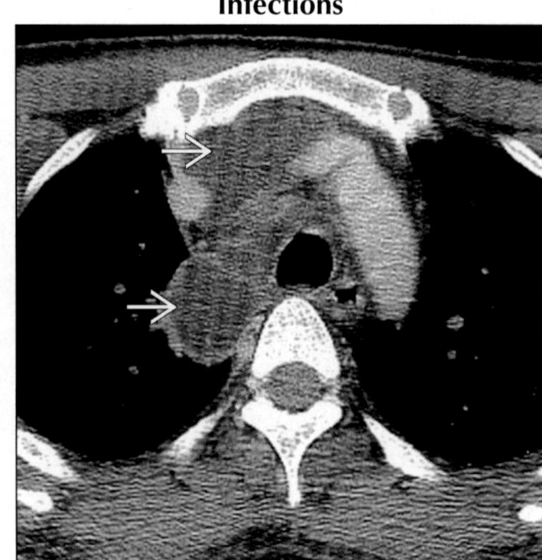

(Left) *Axial CECT through the lower neck shows multiple necrotic right-sided lymph nodes ➔ due to mycobacterial, usually tuberculous, lymphadenopathy, so-called scrofula. These can form a "cold abscess" with chronic draining fistulas to the skin.* ***(Right)*** *Axial NECT from this patient with primary tuberculosis shows several large areas of low-attenuation fluid with lymphadenitis in the neck and mediastinum ➔.*

Superior Vena Cava Syndrome

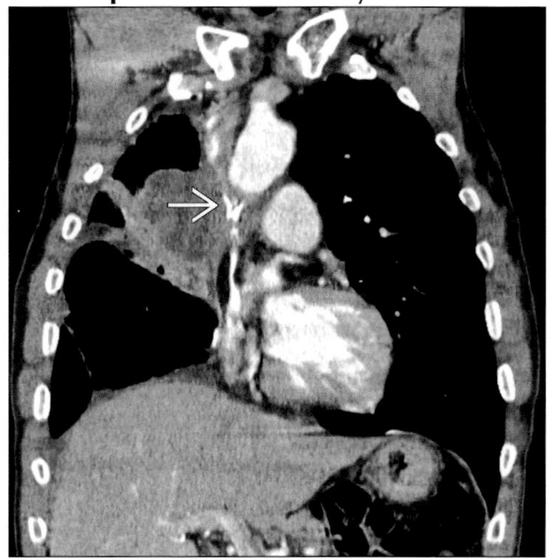

Wegener Granulomatosis

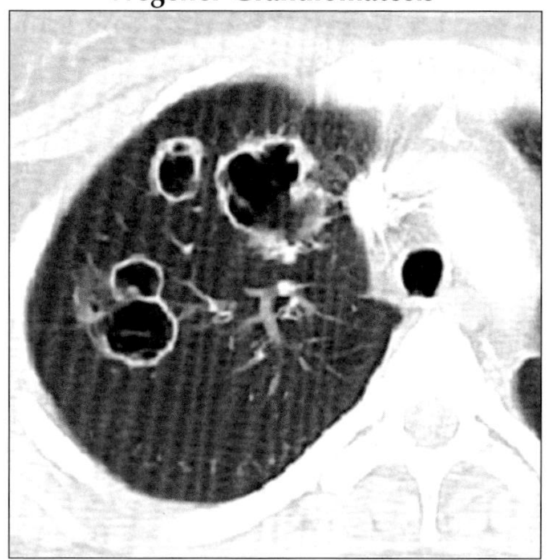

(Left) *Coronal CECT shows a large right hilar mass with some right upper lobe volume loss due to small cell lung cancer. Note the compression and distortion of the superior vena cava ➡. The patient presented with upper extremity and facial plethora.* ***(Right)*** *Axial CECT shows multiple cavitating masses in the right upper lobe from this patient with Wegener granulomatosis. This patient also showed other noncavitating masses in other portions of the lungs.*

Hereditary Hemorrhagic Telangiectasia

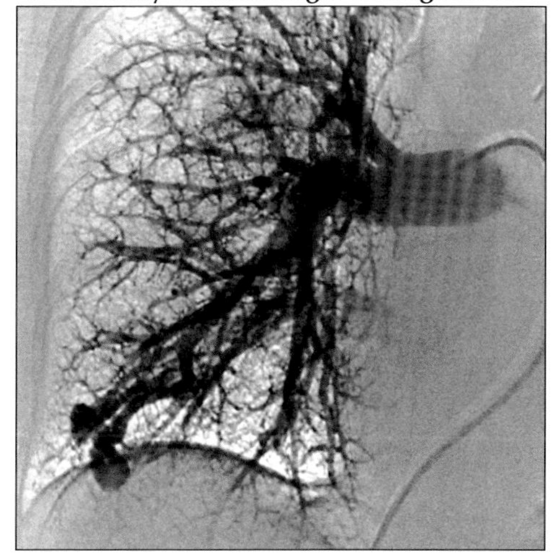

Hereditary Hemorrhagic Telangiectasia

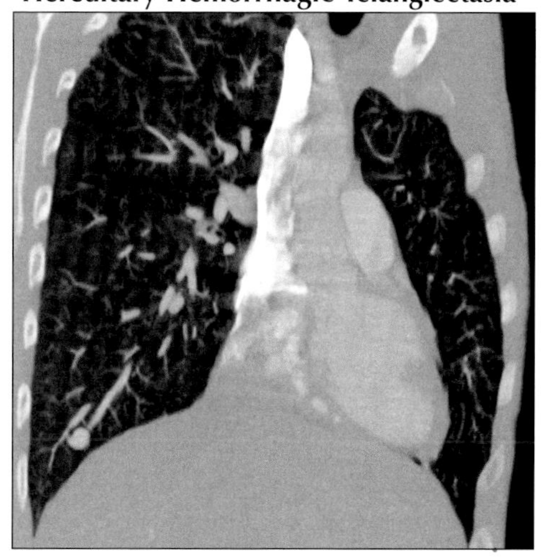

(Left) *Angiography shows large right lower lobe arteriovenous malformation, subsequently shown to be shunting 8% of the cardiac output. This was a solitary malformation in this case but are often multiple.* ***(Right)*** *Coronal oblique CECT from the same patient shows the pulmonary arteriovenous malformation in the right lower lobe as a solitary finding.*

Neurofibromatosis Type 1

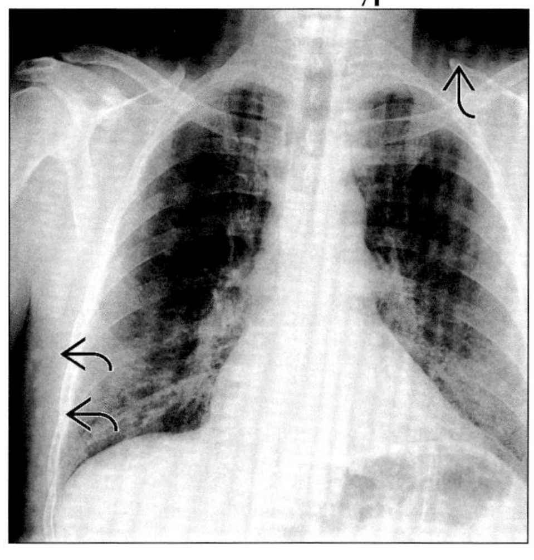

Neurofibromatosis Type 1

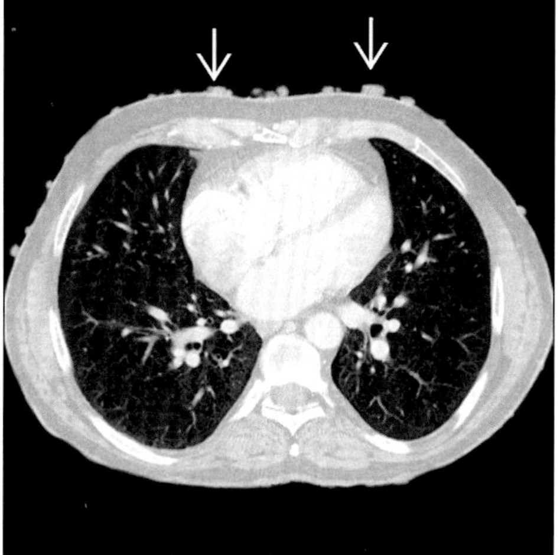

(Left) *Frontal radiograph shows multiple neurofibromas on the skin ↗. The remainder of the thoracic cage was normal, but these patients can show so-called ribbon ribs resulting from multiple plexiform neurofibromas.* ***(Right)*** *Axial CECT shows multiple cutaneous neurofibromas ➡ in this patient with neurofibromatosis 1. There is underlying centrilobular pulmonary emphysema.*

RIB DESTRUCTION

DIFFERENTIAL DIAGNOSIS

Common
- Metastases
- Multiple Myeloma
- Bronchogenic Carcinoma

Less Common
- Osteomyelitis
- Ewing Sarcoma

Rare but Important
- Chondrosarcoma
- Osteosarcoma
- Askin Tumor
- Empyema Necessitatis
- Langerhans Cell Histiocytosis
- Lymphoma
- Other Sarcomas

ESSENTIAL INFORMATION

Key Differential Diagnosis Issues
- Age of patient
  - ≤ 30 years old
    - Ewing sarcoma
    - Askin tumor
    - Langerhans cell histiocytosis
    - Osteosarcoma
  - ≥ 40 years old
    - Metastatic disease
    - Multiple myeloma
    - Bronchogenic carcinoma
- Differentiate from benign causes that may expand ribs but do not destroy cortex
  - Fibrous dysplasia, enchondroma, brown tumor

Helpful Clues for Common Diagnoses
- **Metastases**
  - Most common cause of rib destruction in adults
  - Ribs contain red marrow so highly vascular
  - Polyostotic (multiple lesions)
  - History of primary tumor
  - Most common tumors to metastasize to rib are breast, lung, kidney, or thyroid carcinoma
  - Most common solitary rib metastasis secondary to thyroid or renal cell carcinoma
- **Multiple Myeloma**
  - 2nd most common cause of rib destruction in adults
  - Most common bone manifestation is generalized osteopenia
  - Solitary expansile lytic lesion may indicate solitary plasmacytoma
  - Biopsy required for definitive diagnosis
- **Bronchogenic Carcinoma**
  - Rib destruction secondary to Pancoast tumor or hematogenous metastases
  - Pancoast tumor
    - Syndrome of ipsilateral arm pain, Horner syndrome, and ipsilateral hand muscle wasting
    - Superior sulcus tumor invades apical fat to involve brachial plexus and sympathetic ganglia
    - Rib destruction is best sign to definitively diagnose chest wall invasion
    - MR occasionally used to assess for neurovascular invasion

Helpful Clues for Less Common Diagnoses
- **Osteomyelitis**
  - May be difficult to distinguish from Ewing sarcoma or Askin tumor
  - Aggressive lytic lesion with wide zone of transition
  - ± soft tissue mass
  - Usually occurs in association with empyema, pneumonia, or chest wall infection
  - Chronic osteomyelitis
    - ± periosteal reaction
    - ± sclerosis of involved ribs
- **Ewing Sarcoma**
  - 5-15% arise in ribs
  - Adolescents and young adults usually present with painful chest wall mass
  - Small round blue cell tumor
  - Radiographic patterns
    - 80% are lytic with bone destruction
    - 10% are mixed lytic/blastic lesions
    - 10% are sclerotic
    - 40% have expanded rib
    - Most have disproportionately large soft tissue mass compared to osseous involvement
    - Intrathoracic component ≥ extrathoracic component
    - Metastasizes most commonly to bone
  - Epicenter on rib

- Heterogeneity of mass reflects tumor necrosis
- Bone scintigraphy demonstrates increased activity in affected rib and helps diagnose metastatic disease

Helpful Clues for Rare Diagnoses

- **Chondrosarcoma**
  - Patient 30-60 years old ± chest wall pain
  - Occurs anteriorly or near costochondral junction
  - Radiographs and CECT show
    - Large mass with bone destruction
    - ± soft tissue involvement
    - Chondroid matrix (rings and arcs calcification)
- **Osteosarcoma**
  - Patient 10-30 years old with painful mass
  - Bone destruction secondary to heterogeneous soft tissue mass
  - ± cloud-like osteoid matrix
  - Lung is most common site of metastatic disease
    - Metastases may calcify
- **Askin Tumor**
  - Form of primitive neuroectodermal tumor (PNET)
  - Arises in soft tissues of thorax
  - Children and young adults present with chest wall pain
  - Radiographs show
    - Heterogeneous mass ± rib destruction
    - Rib destruction less common than Ewing sarcoma
    - ± pleural effusion
    - Metastasizes to lung and bone
- **Empyema Necessitatis**
  - Empyema that subsequently invades through chest wall
  - Most common related bony abnormality
    - Rib sclerosis or periosteal reaction secondary to chronic osteomyelitis
  - Organisms can be remembered by BATMAN pneumonic as BATMAN breaks through barriers
    - *Blastomyces*
    - *Actinomyces*
    - *Tuberculosis* (75% of cases)
    - *Mucor*
    - *Aspergillus*
    - *Nocardia*
- **Langerhans Cell Histiocytosis**
  - Expansile lytic lesion
  - No sclerotic rim
  - Polyostotic
  - ± soft tissue mass
- **Lymphoma**
  - Heterogeneous or homogeneous soft tissue mass
  - ± mediastinal lymphadenopathy
  - Extrathoracic disease is common
  - 30% have lung involvement
  - Peaks in 5th-8th decades of life
- **Other Sarcomas**
  - Rib destruction seen with
    - Rhabdomyosarcoma, malignant fibrous histiocytoma, and synovial sarcoma

Metastases

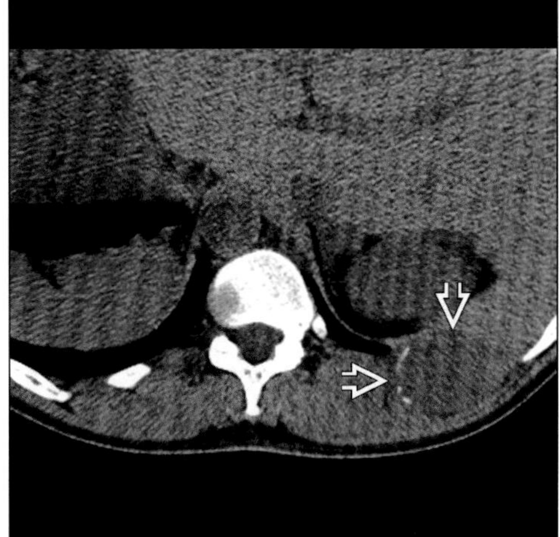

Axial NECT shows an expansile lytic rib lesion with large soft tissue component ⇨. Lower sections (not shown) revealed a heterogeneous mass in the kidney in this patient with proven renal cell carcinoma.

Metastases

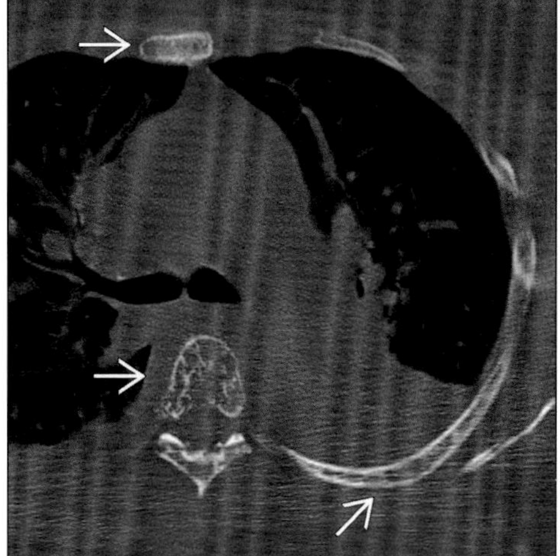

Axial NECT shows multiple lytic bone lesions within the ribs, vertebral body, and sternum →. This patient had a history of breast cancer and was experiencing bone pain.

RIB DESTRUCTION

(Left) Axial CECT shows a large enhancing soft tissue mass destroying a left posterior rib ➔. Note ring-enhancing hypervascular liver metastasis ➔ with central low density. There are also lung metastases ➔ in this patient with metastatic renal cell carcinoma. (Right) Axial CECT shows an expansile soft tissue mass involving a posterior rib ➔. This proved to be a solitary plasmacytoma on biopsy.

Metastases

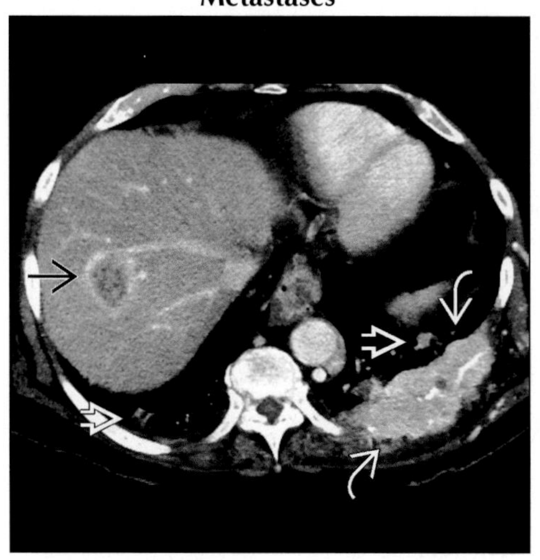

Multiple Myeloma

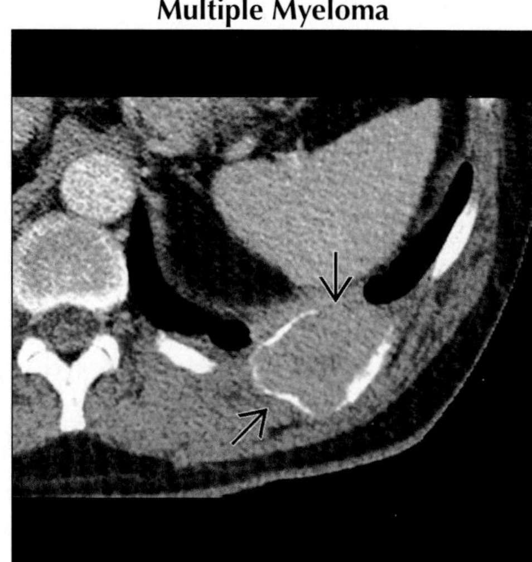

(Left) Frontal radiograph shows a left hilar mass ➔ with infiltrative lateral margins. Note associated left lung volume loss, indicated by elevation of the hemidiaphragm. There is a destructive and expansile right rib lesion ➔ indicating stage IV disease. Seeing this rib lesion illustrates the importance of not succumbing to satisfaction of search. (Right) Axial CECT shows a destructive rib metastasis ➔ in this patient with non-small-cell carcinoma.

Bronchogenic Carcinoma

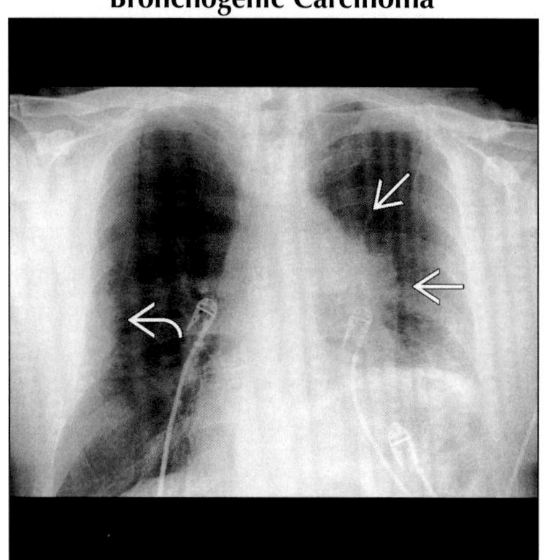

Bronchogenic Carcinoma

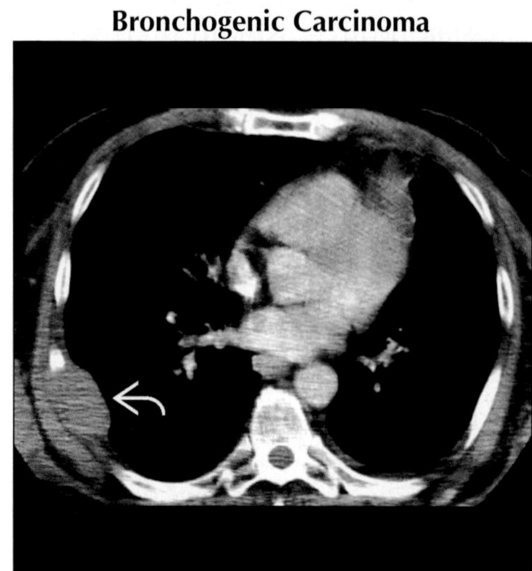

(Left) Frontal radiograph shows a right apical mass ➔ with relative preservation of right lung volume. Right 1st rib destruction ➔ is seen on closer inspection, thus decreasing the likelihood that the mass represents a pneumonia. This patient was subsequently diagnosed with a Pancoast tumor. (Right) Coronal CECT shows extensive destruction of ribs with sclerosis ➔. Note the soft tissue tract extending from the ribs to the overlying skin ➔.

Bronchogenic Carcinoma

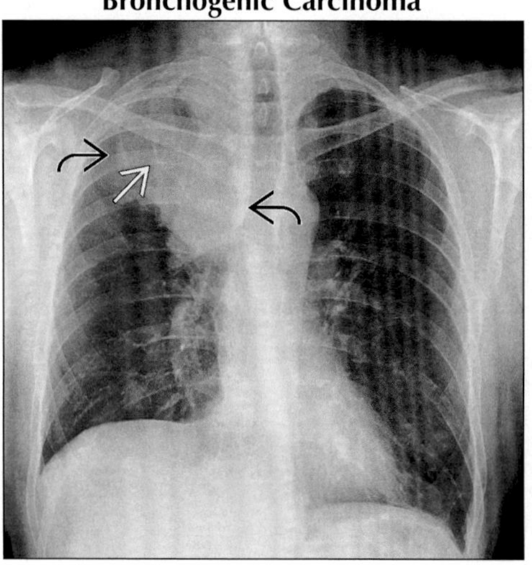

Osteomyelitis

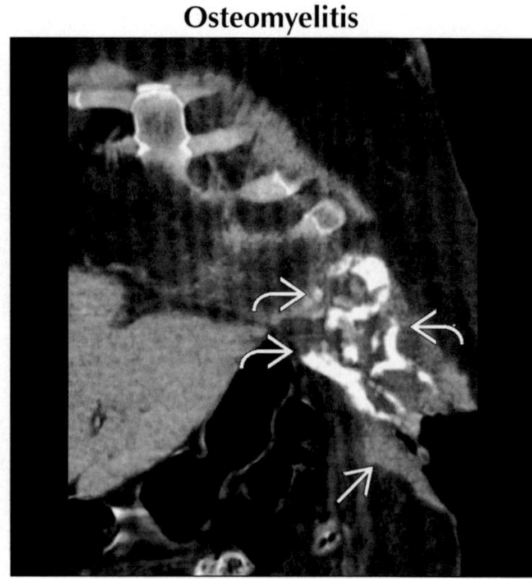

RIB DESTRUCTION

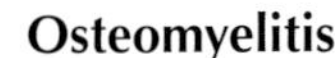

Osteomyelitis

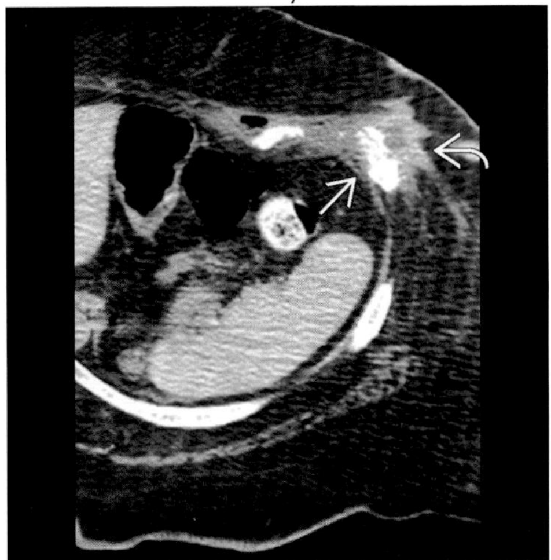

Osteomyelitis

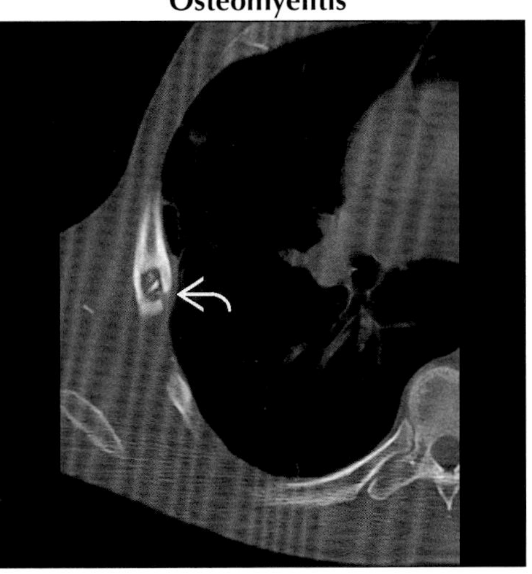

(Left) *Axial CECT shows a soft tissue lesion with central low density* ➡ *that communicated with a tract to the left chest wall. Note underlying rib distortion and sclerosis* ➡*, which indicates the presence of rib osteomyelitis.* ***(Right)*** *Axial NECT shows a lytic and expansile rib lesion. Note loss of cortex medially* ➡*. This was associated with a skin infection and phlegmon (not shown), thus helping to confirm that the lesion was secondary to infection.*

Ewing Sarcoma

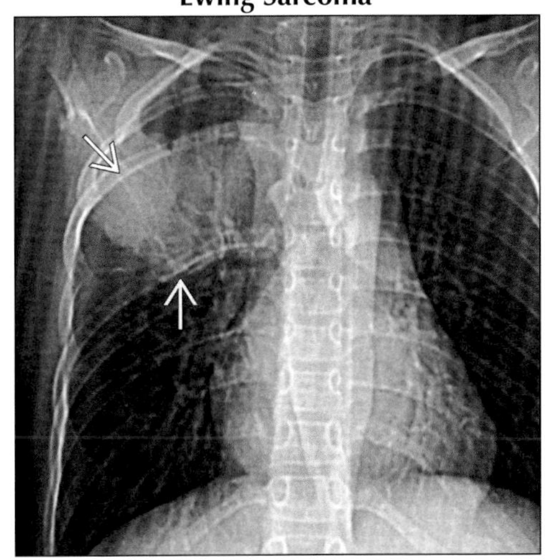

Ewing Sarcoma

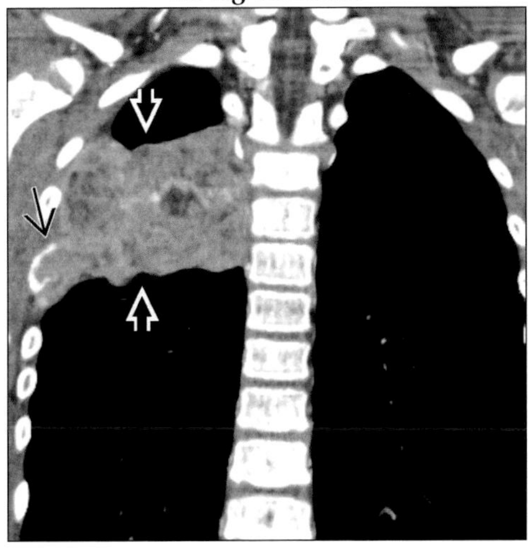

(Left) *Frontal scout image shows a large right chest wall mass with associated posterior 5th rib destruction* ➡ *in this teenage patient.* ***(Right)*** *Coronal CECT from the adjacent scout image demonstrates the large heterogeneous soft tissue mass* ➡ *causing underlying rib destruction* →*. Askin tumor could have a similar presentation, but it is less commonly associated with rib destruction.*

Ewing Sarcoma

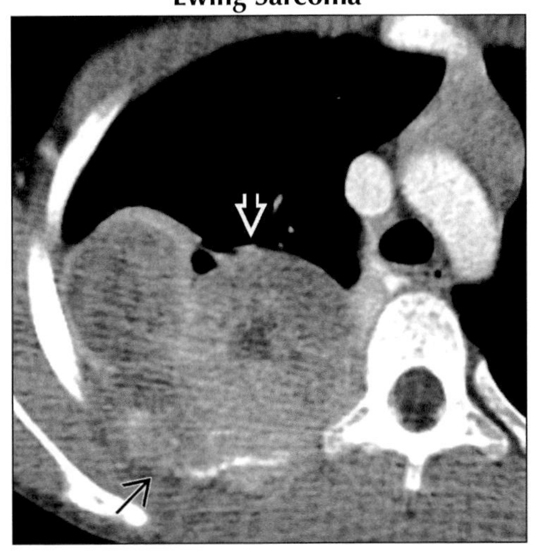

Ewing Sarcoma

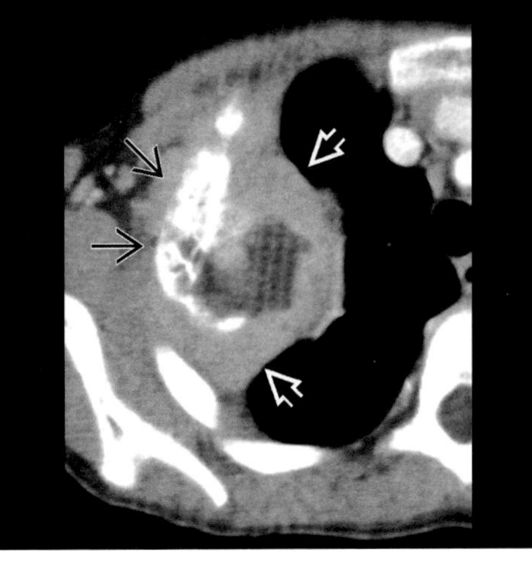

(Left) *Axial CECT shows a large mass* ➡ *with associated rib destruction* →*. The mass projects into the thoracic cavity. The key differential point is the age of the patient (15 years).* ***(Right)*** *Axial CECT shows a large mass with associated central low density* ➡ *that likely indicates necrosis. Note sclerotic and expanded rib* → *as the site of origin of the mass. Infection with osteomyelitis could be eliminated from the differential based on history.*

RIB DESTRUCTION

*(**Left**) Lateral radiograph shows an anteriorly located nodular opacity ➩. No definite chondroid matrix is seen, and differential would include a mediastinal or lung nodule. (Courtesy D. Godwin, MD.) (**Right**) Axial NECT in the same patient shows a soft tissue nodule occurring at the costochondral junction causing rib destruction ➩. There is associated calcification within the lesion ↶. (Courtesy D. Godwin, MD.)*

Chondrosarcoma

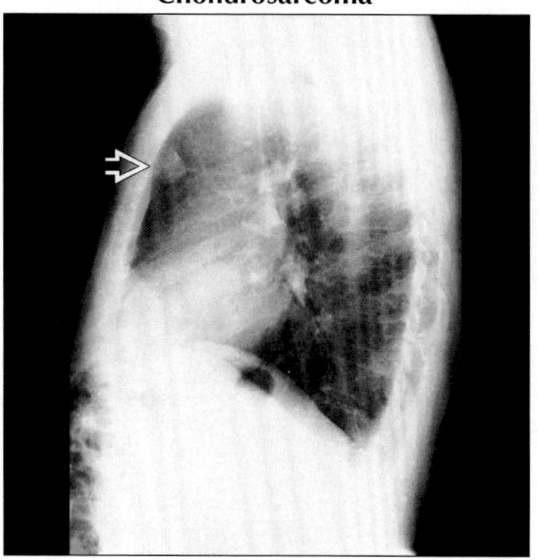

Chondrosarcoma

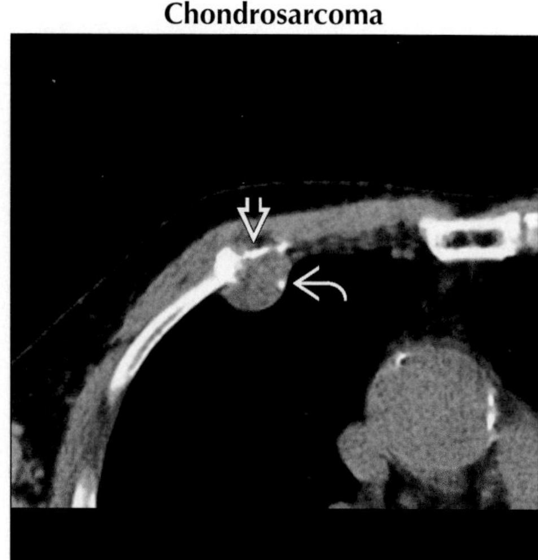

*(**Left**) Coronal NECT shows a large mass with osteoid matrix ➩. Note that the epicenter of the lesion is within the chest wall, which causes mild underlying rib destruction. (**Right**) Axial NECT shows cloud-like osteoid matrix → extending anteriorly from the costochondral junction. Given the location, chondrosarcoma would be difficult to exclude as a diagnosis. (Courtesy D. Godwin, MD.)*

Osteosarcoma

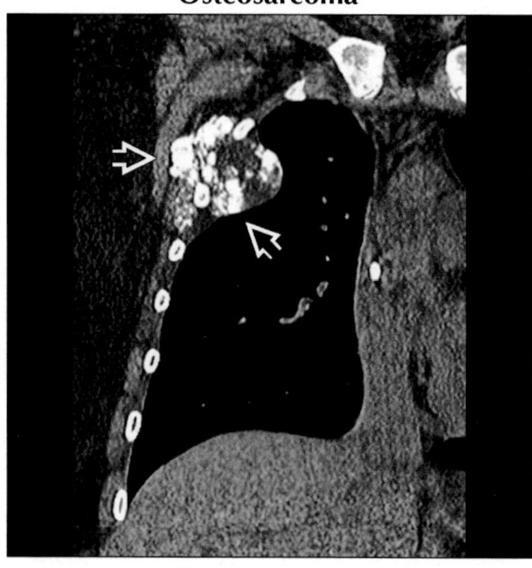

Osteosarcoma

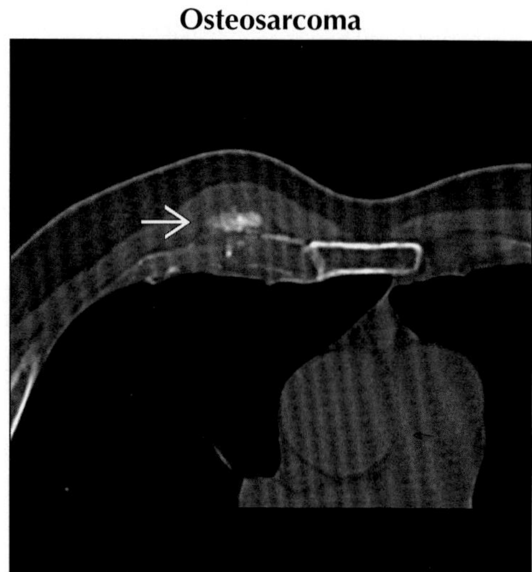

*(**Left**) Frontal radiograph shows a large chest wall mass → with destruction of the left 7th rib. Patient age and symptoms are the main distinguishing characteristics. Ewing sarcoma could have an identical appearance and requires tissue for final diagnosis. (**Right**) Axial CECT shows a homogeneous mass → with epicenter within the left chest wall. Note underlying rib sclerosis and cortical breakthrough.*

Askin Tumor

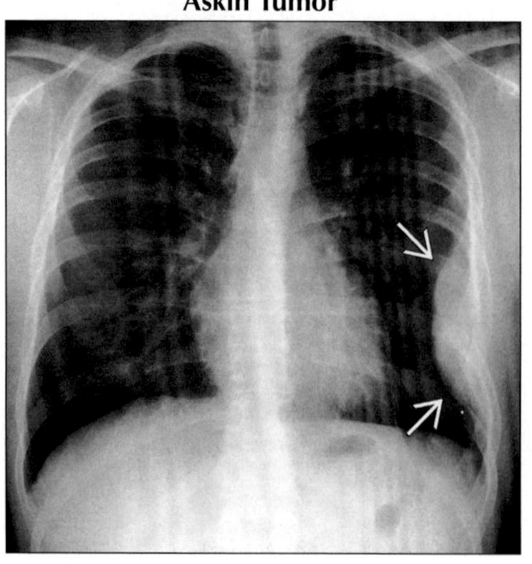

Askin Tumor

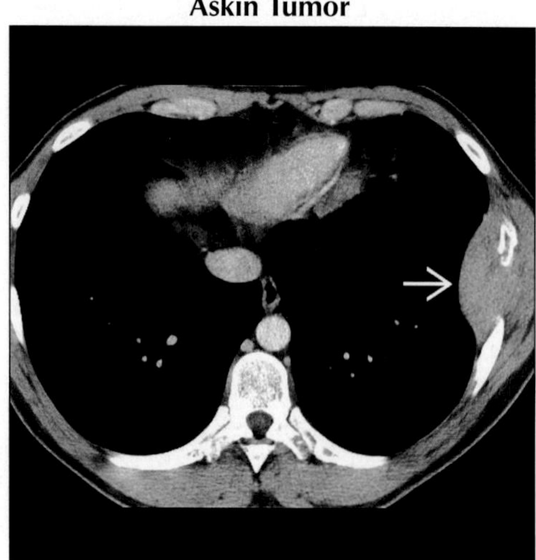

RIB DESTRUCTION

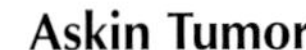

Askin Tumor

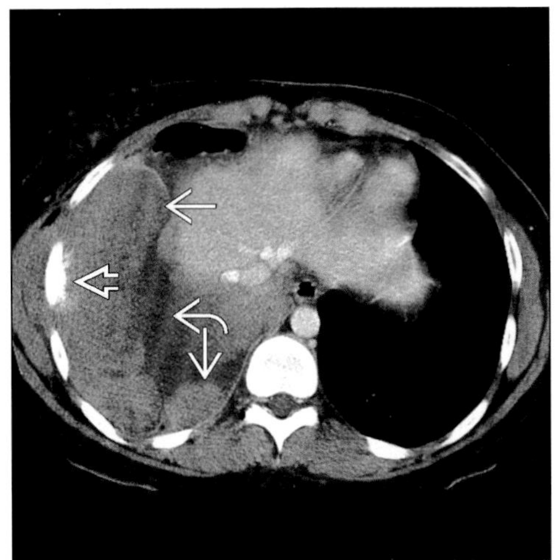

Empyema Necessitatis

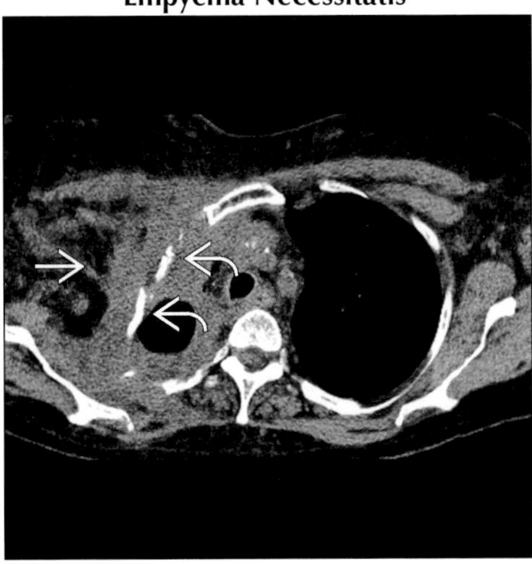

(Left) *Axial CECT shows a large lobulated mass → in the right hemithorax with extension into the chest wall surrounding a rib →. Key component in this case is the patient's age (13 years). Note associated right pleural effusion →.* ***(Right)*** *Axial NECT shows extension of soft tissue stranding → into the chest wall. There are deformities of the right anterior and lateral ribs → from chronic osteomyelitis in this patient with nocardial infection.*

Empyema Necessitatis

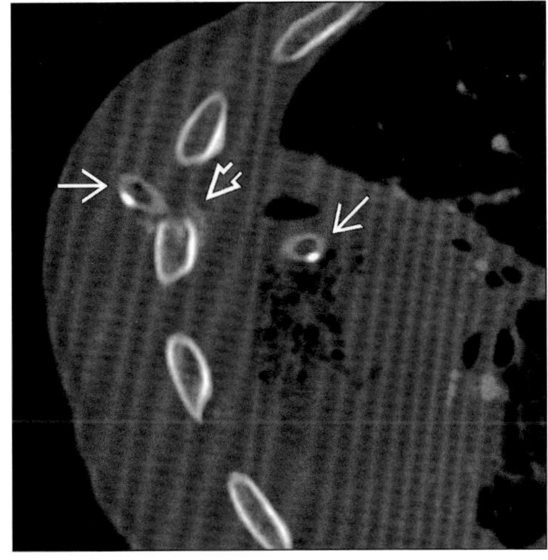

Empyema Necessitatis

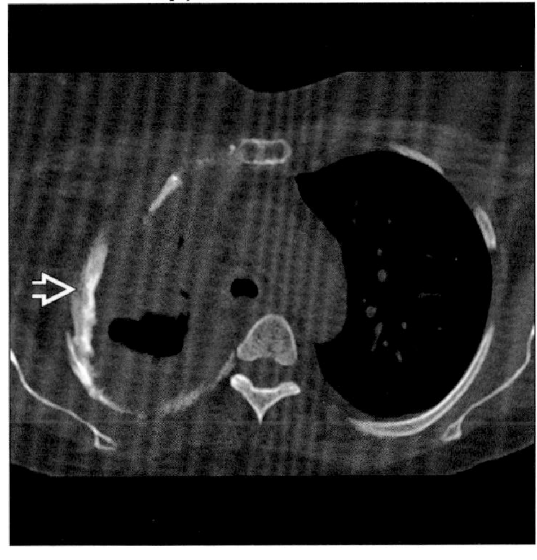

(Left) *Axial CECT shows a right-sided chest tube → and periosteal reaction → indicating associated osteomyelitis from chest wall extension of right empyema. Note right-sided hydropneumothorax with loculated air. Empyema necessitatis is most commonly due to M. tuberculosis infection.* ***(Right)*** *Axial NECT shows typical CT features of empyema necessitatis from nocardiosis. Bone windows show chronic periostitis → indicating osteomyelitis.*

Langerhans Cell Histiocytosis

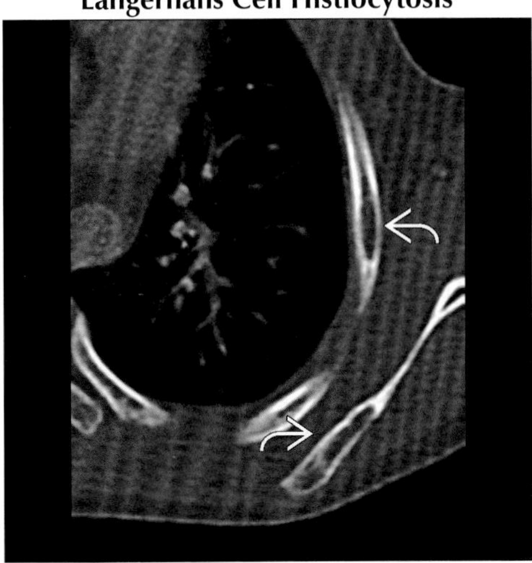

Lymphoma

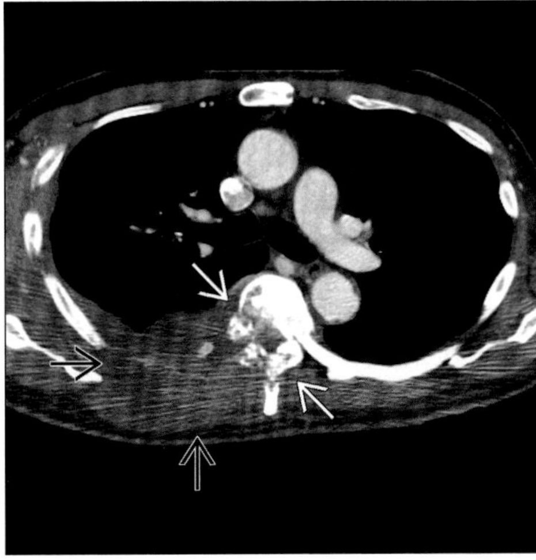

(Left) *Axial NECT shows lytic lesions in the rib and scapula →. There is no associated soft tissue mass. Skeletal survey revealed additional lesions in the skull and long bones. Age of patient and polyostotic bone lesions narrows the differential diagnosis.* ***(Right)*** *Axial CECT shows an inhomogeneous soft tissue mass → destroying a right posterior rib and half of a vertebral body →. This proved to be an unusual case of diffuse large B-cell lymphoma.*

BELL-SHAPED CHEST

DIFFERENTIAL DIAGNOSIS

Common
- Neonatal or Early Childhood Insult

Less Common
- Down Syndrome
- Muscular Disorders

Rare but Important
- Rickets
- Intrauterine Oligohydramnios
- Skeletal Dysplasia
- Giant Omphalocele

ESSENTIAL INFORMATION

Key Differential Diagnosis Issues
- Definition
  - Narrow upper chest with outward bowing of lower chest
  - Obliquely directed posterior ribs
- Caused by disorders resulting in cerebral or muscular dysfunction
- Clinical history key in diagnosis

Helpful Clues for Common Diagnoses
- **Neonatal or Early Childhood Insult**
  - Conditions leading to hypotonia
    - Sepsis, dehydration, infantile respiratory distress syndrome, spinal cord injury, and intracranial hemorrhage
  - Transient occurrence secondary to traversing birth canal
  - Paralytics for mechanical ventilation

Helpful Clues for Less Common Diagnoses
- **Down Syndrome**
  - Hypotonia and bell-shaped thorax ↓ in severity with age
  - Thoracic skeletal manifestations
    - Bell-shaped chest in 80%
    - Multiple manubrial ossification centers in 80%
    - 11 rib pairs in 30%
    - 58% chance of Down syndrome with above 3 findings
  - Gastrointestinal malformations
    - Duodenal atresia/web, tracheoesophageal fistula, omphalocele, Hirschsprung disease, and imperforate anus
  - Cardiac malformations
    - Endocardial cushion defect, ventricular septal defect, atrial septal defect, tetralogy of Fallot, and patent ductus arteriosus
  - Atlantoaxial instability in 14% of patients secondary to laxity of transverse ligaments
    - Diagnose with flexion/extension radiography
- **Muscular Disorders**
  - Spinal muscular atrophy
    - Progressive lower motor neuron degeneration
    - Multiple subtypes with varying ages of presentation
    - Autosomal recessive
    - Recurrent respiratory infections
    - Chest shape progressively ↑ in severity with most extreme example of bell-shaped thorax
  - Muscular dystrophy
    - Primary muscle breakdown
    - Varying age of presentation and disease severity depending on type of muscular dystrophy
    - ± rapidly progressive scoliosis
  - C-shaped scoliosis leads to respiratory insufficiency
    - Treat with long-segment fusion

Helpful Clues for Rare Diagnoses
- **Rickets**
  - Widened growth plates
  - Osteomalacia
  - Metaphyseal cupping and fraying
  - Deformed costochondral junctions (rachitic rosary)
- **Intrauterine Oligohydramnios**
  - Long-term oligohydramnios leads to pulmonary hypoplasia with muscular hypotonia
  - Causes
    - Renal abnormalities, urinary bladder obstruction, posterior urethral valves, or asymmetric growth retardation
  - Fetal ultrasound
    - Amniotic fluid index (AFI) is defined by 4 largest AP fluid pockets in each quadrant
    - AFI ≤ 6 cm is diagnostic of oligohydramnios
- **Skeletal Dysplasia**

BELL-SHAPED CHEST

- Abnormal skeletal development with muscular hypotonia
- Diagnosis important for prognosis and genetic counseling
- Skeletal survey useful in diagnosing and classifying skeletal dysplasias
- Important definitions
  - Rhizomelia implies proximal limb shortening (humerus and femur)
  - Mesomelia implies middle limb shortening (radius/ulna and tibia/fibula)
  - Acromelia implies distal limb shortening (hands and feet)
- Achondroplasia
  - Most common short-limbed dwarfism and nonlethal skeletal dysplasia
  - Autosomal dominant
  - Prenatal ultrasound demonstrates rhizomelic shortening
  - ↓ AP vertebral body diameter
  - ↓ interpediculate distance in lower lumbar spine
  - Tombstone-shaped iliac bones
  - Frontal bossing
  - Small foramen magnum
- Camptomelic dysplasia
  - Enlarged skull
  - ± 11 rib pairs
  - Late ossification of mid-thoracic pedicles
  - Hypoplastic scapulae
  - Bowed long bones
  - Tall and narrow iliac wings
- Jeune syndrome
  - Acromelic shortening
  - Short ribs with high clavicular position
  - Cone-shaped epiphyses of middle and distal phalanges
  - "Trident" acetabulum with 3 downward projecting spurs
  - Normal spine
  - ± ossified capital femoral epiphyses in infancy
- Cleidocranial dysplasia
  - Abnormal membrane bone development
  - Autosomal dominant
  - Absent or dysplastic clavicles
  - Widened pubic symphysis
  - Squared iliac wings
  - Wormian bones
  - Persistent metopic suture
- Thanatophoric dysplasia
  - In utero or early neonatal death
  - Sporadic disorder
  - Rhizomelic shortening
  - ± prenatal ultrasound demonstrates cloverleaf-shaped skull
  - Polyhydramnios
  - "Trident" acetabulum
  - Platyspondyly (a.k.a. flat vertebral bodies)
  - Short ribs
  - Telephone-receiver-shaped femurs
  - Metaphyseal flaring

- **Giant Omphalocele**
  - Herniated bowel and liver covered by peritoneal lining
  - High association with cardiovascular abnormalities

Neonatal or Early Childhood Insult

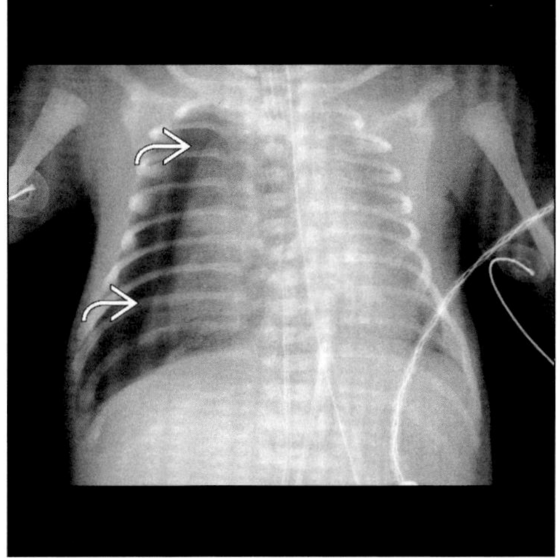

Frontal radiograph shows a bell shaped chest with right-sided pneumothorax ➔ in a 2-day-old premature triplet with infantile respiratory distress syndrome (IRDS).

Neonatal or Early Childhood Insult

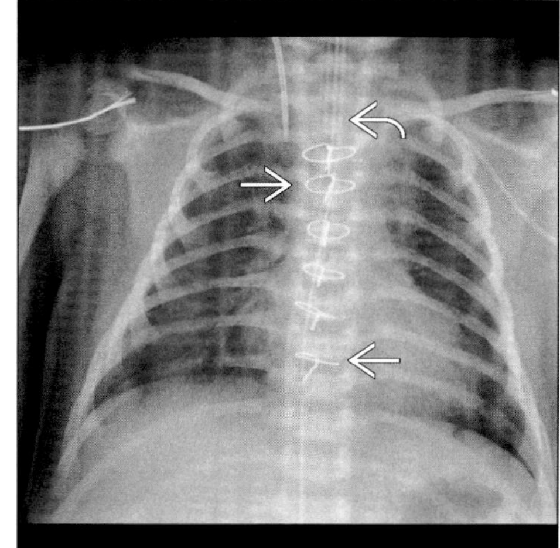

Frontal radiograph shows median sternotomy wires ➔ in this 14-day-old patient status post coarctation repair. Bell-shaped thorax is presumed secondary to paralytics from intubation ➔.

BELL-SHAPED CHEST

Neonatal or Early Childhood Insult

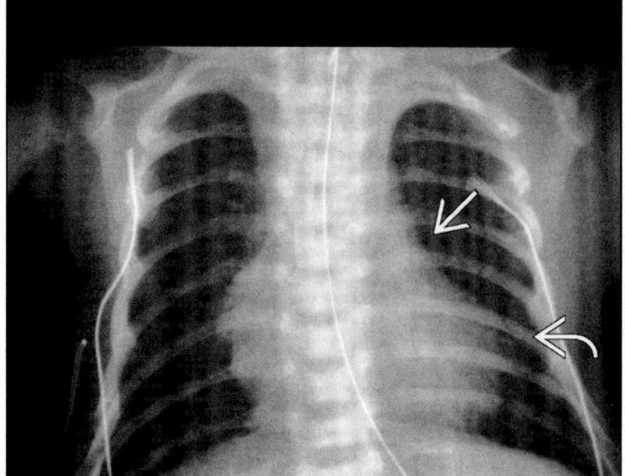

Down Syndrome

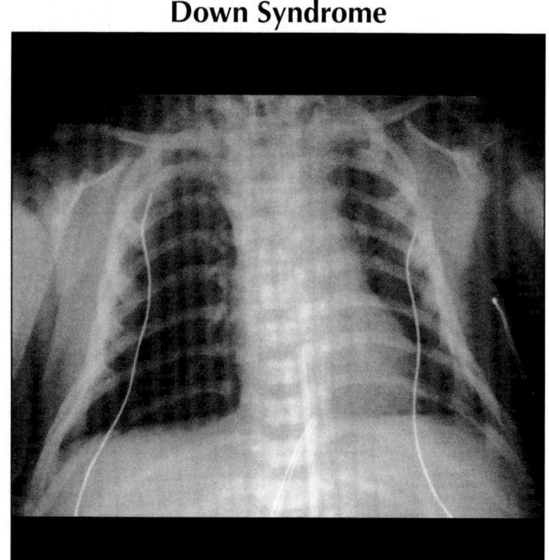

(Left) *Frontal radiograph shows a boot-shaped heart with upturned cardiac apex ➔ secondary to right ventricular hypertrophy. Note decreased pulmonary vasculature and a small main pulmonary artery ➔, which is characteristically seen in tetralogy of Fallot. The small pulmonary artery is secondary to pulmonary stenosis or atresia.* ***(Right)*** *Frontal radiograph shows a narrow upper and wider lower thorax. This patient was hypotonic at birth.*

Down Syndrome

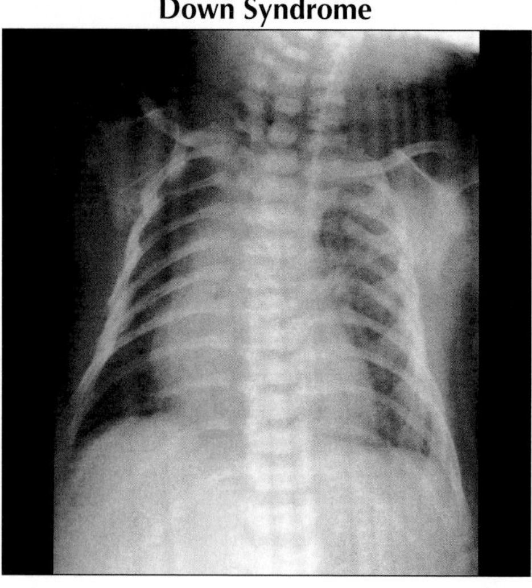

Down Syndrome

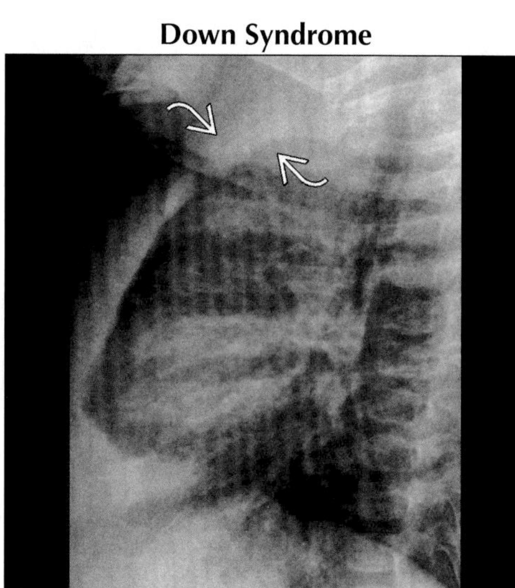

(Left) *Frontal radiograph shows a bell-shaped chest in Down syndrome. Features that allow diagnosis are clinical history and 11 rib pairs.* ***(Right)*** *Lateral radiograph in the same patient shows a double manubrial ossification center ➔. Symptomatic or asymptomatic atlantoaxial instability is an important radiographic finding seen on cervical spine imaging in 13% of cases (not shown).*

Down Syndrome

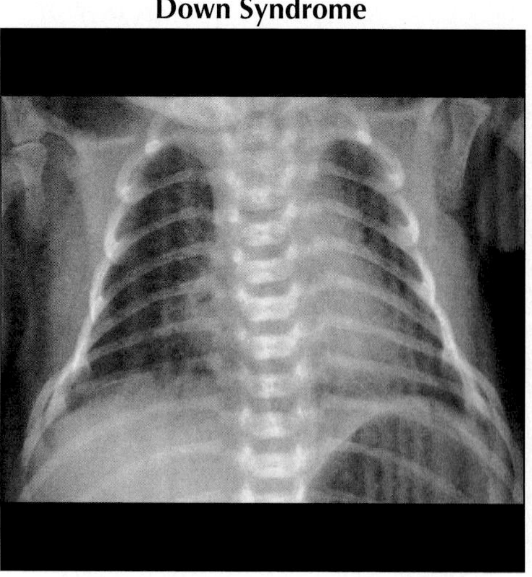

Muscular Disorders

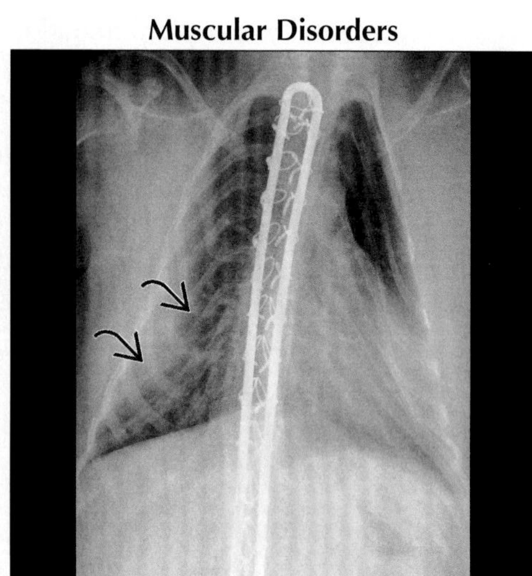

(Left) *Frontal radiograph shows characteristic bell-shaped thorax, which is present in 80% of Down syndrome patients. Patients outgrow the chest appearance as their hypotonia decreases with age. Other clues to diagnosis include 11 rib pairs, also seen in this case.* ***(Right)*** *Frontal radiograph shows characteristic obliquely directed posterior ribs ➔ and narrow upper thorax. The most severe cases of bell-shaped thorax occur in spinal muscular atrophy.*

BELL-SHAPED CHEST

Muscular Disorders

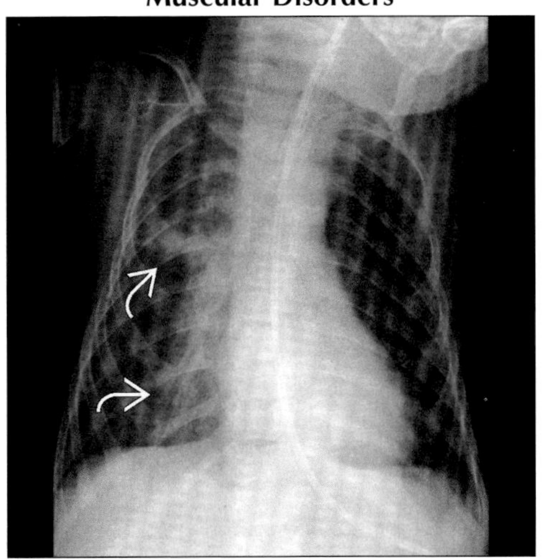

Muscular Disorders

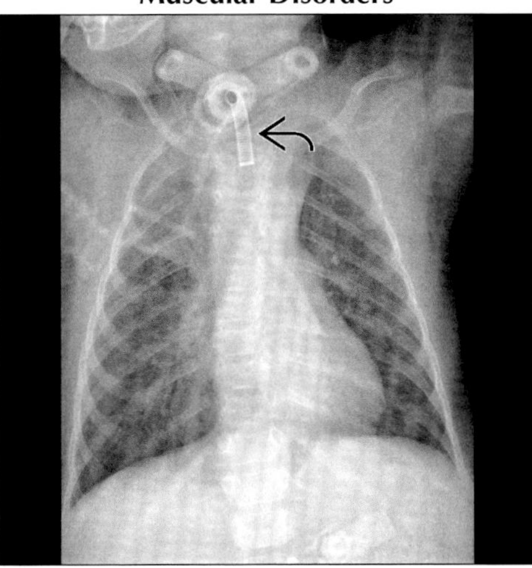

*(**Left**) Frontal radiograph shows a child with spinal muscular atrophy and early appearance of a bell-shaped thorax. Right upper and middle lung opacities are secondary to atelectasis &/or pneumonia ➔, findings associated with weakened cough and hypotonia. (**Right**) Frontal radiograph in the same child years later shows progressive narrowing of the upper thorax. Note tracheostomy tube secondary to respiratory distress ➔.*

Muscular Disorders

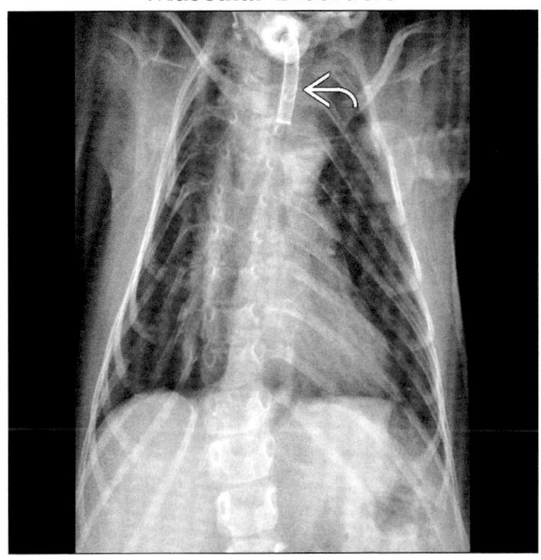

Muscular Disorders

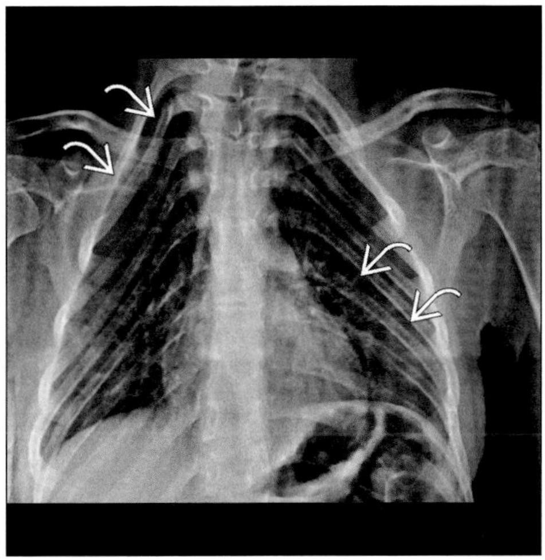

*(**Left**) Frontal radiograph shows further progression of bell-shaped thorax in the same patient. Note tracheostomy tube ➔. There is worsening convex right C-shaped scoliosis and osteoporosis, findings seen in neuromuscular disorders. (**Right**) Frontal radiograph shows obliquely directed posterior ribs ➔ and a narrow upper thorax in this patient with cerebral palsy. Chest shape is secondary to hypotonia.*

Muscular Disorders

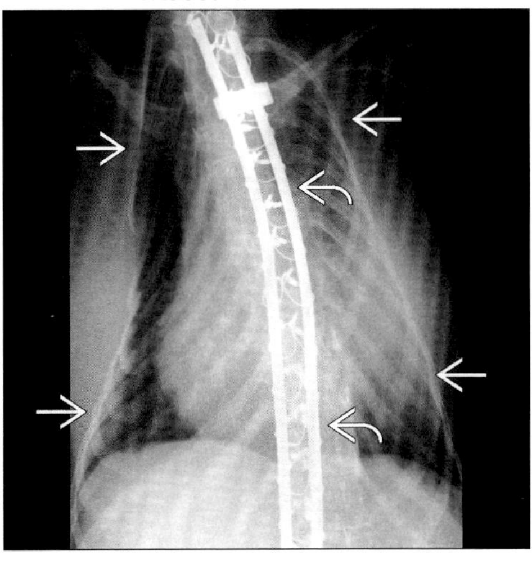

Rickets

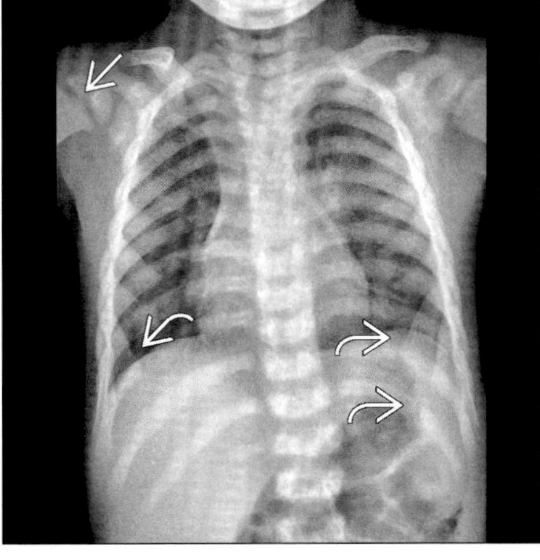

*(**Left**) Frontal radiograph shows elongated thorax with bell-shaped appearance ➔. Note spinal fusion ➔, which is commonly used to treat C-shaped scoliosis in order to improve respiratory capacity. (**Right**) Frontal radiograph shows metaphyseal fraying and growth plate widening best seen in the right humerus ➔. Note osteomalacia indicated by bowing of the anterior ribs at their insertion sites on the diaphragm ➔, the so-called Harrison groove.*

BELL-SHAPED CHEST

(Left) Anteroposterior radiograph shows metaphyseal fraying and irregularity of the distal radius and ulna ➔. Note abnormal bone mineral density with coarsened appearance representing osteomalacia. *(Right)* Frontal radiograph shows small lungs secondary to prolonged intrauterine oligohydramnios diagnosed by fetal ultrasound. Causes of oligohydramnios include renal anomalies, posterior urethral valves, and bladder obstruction.

Rickets

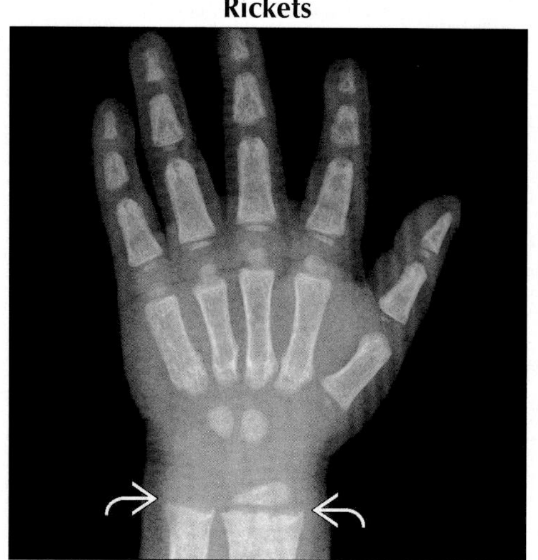

Intrauterine Oligohydramnios

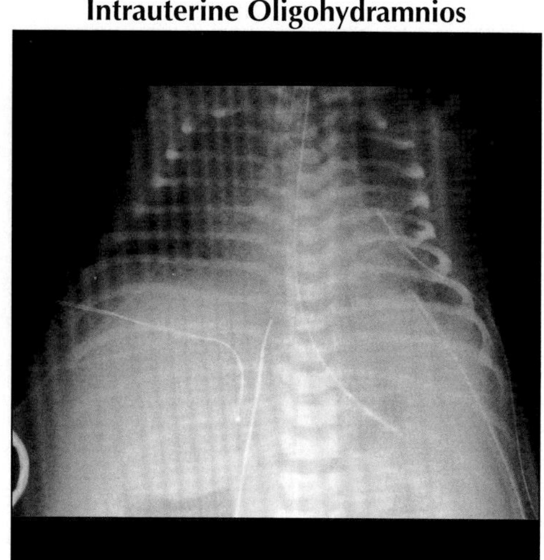

(Left) Frontal radiograph shows a small thorax ➔, rhizomelic limb shortening (short humeri and femurs), telephone-receiver-shaped femurs ➔, and platyspondyly ➔. These are all characteristic findings of thanatophoric dysplasia. *(Right)* Frontal radiograph shows short ribs with long high-riding clavicles and bell-shaped chest. Note normal vertebral bodies ➔ and normal-appearing humeri. A trident acetabulum confirmed Jeune syndrome.

Skeletal Dysplasia

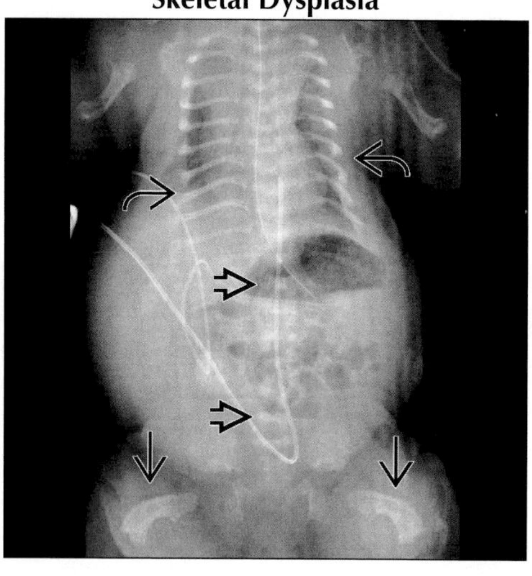

Skeletal Dysplasia

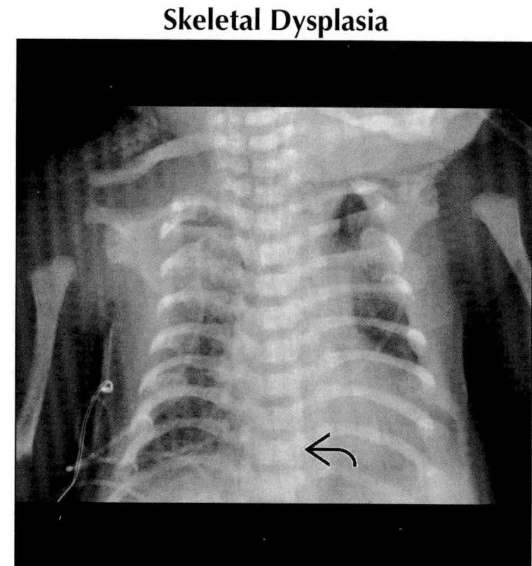

(Left) Frontal radiograph shows characteristic "trident" acetabulum with 3 downward pointing spurs ➔ in this case of Jeune syndrome. Note normal appearance to the spine. "Trident" acetabulum can also be seen in thanatophoric dysplasia and chondroectodermal dysplasia. *(Right)* Frontal radiograph shows short ribs ➔ and metaphyseal flaring ➔. Thanatophoric dysplasia is the most common lethal neonatal skeletal dysplasia.

Skeletal Dysplasia

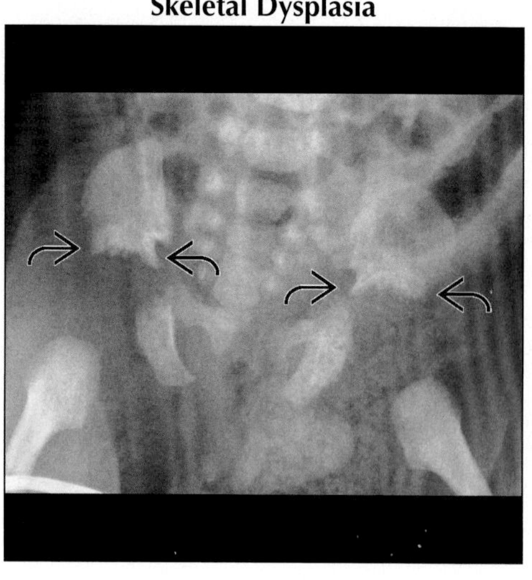

Skeletal Dysplasia

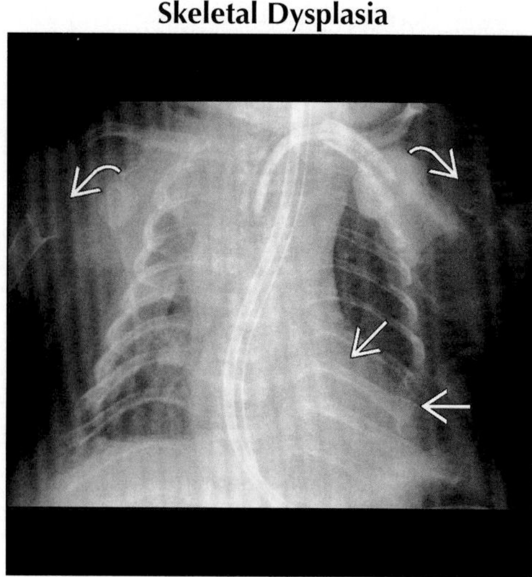

Skeletal Dysplasia

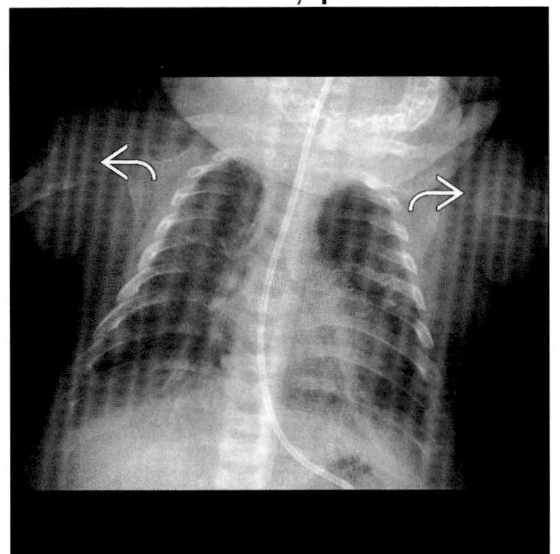

Skeletal Dysplasia

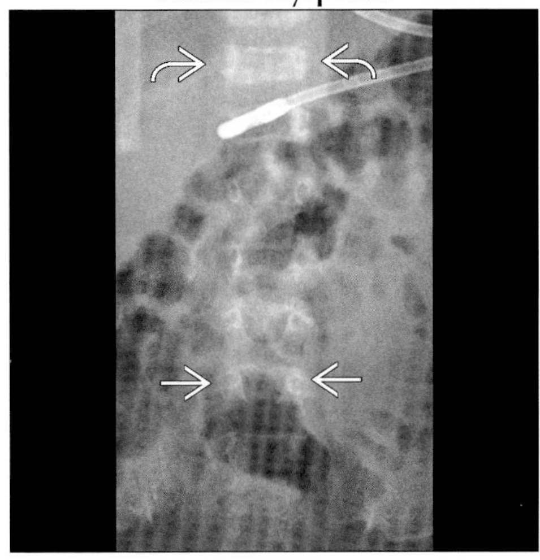

(Left) *Frontal radiograph shows short ribs and bell-shaped thorax. Note metaphyseal cupping of the humeri ➔ in this patient with achondroplasia.* ***(Right)*** *Anteroposterior radiograph of the spine shows decreasing interpediculate distance in the lower lumbar spine ➔ compared to the lower thoracic spine ➔, which is characteristic of achondroplasia. This predisposes the patient to symptomatic spinal stenosis.*

Skeletal Dysplasia

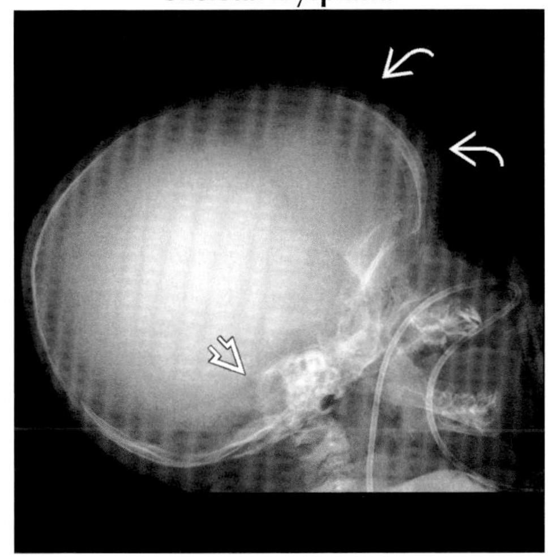

Skeletal Dysplasia

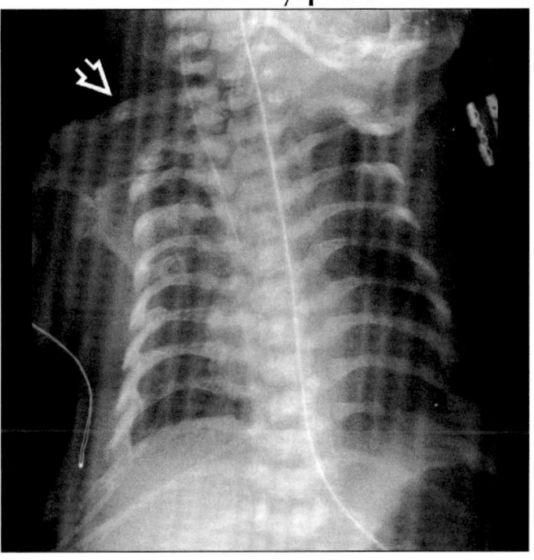

(Left) *Lateral radiograph shows an enlarged skull with frontal bossing ➔ in this case of achondroplasia. There is a small skull base ➔.* ***(Right)*** *Frontal radiograph shows bell-shaped chest with short ribs, normal spine, and high clavicular position ➔. Other important findings seen on the skeletal survey (not shown) are cone-shaped epiphyses of the middle and distal phalanges and early ossified capital femoral epiphyses in this case of Jeune syndrome.*

Giant Omphalocele

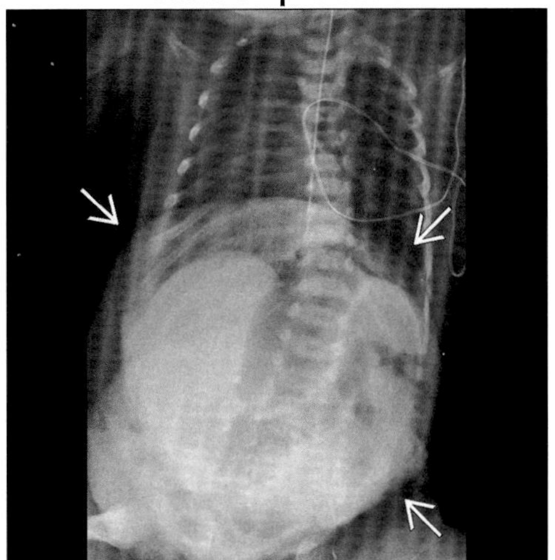

Giant Omphalocele

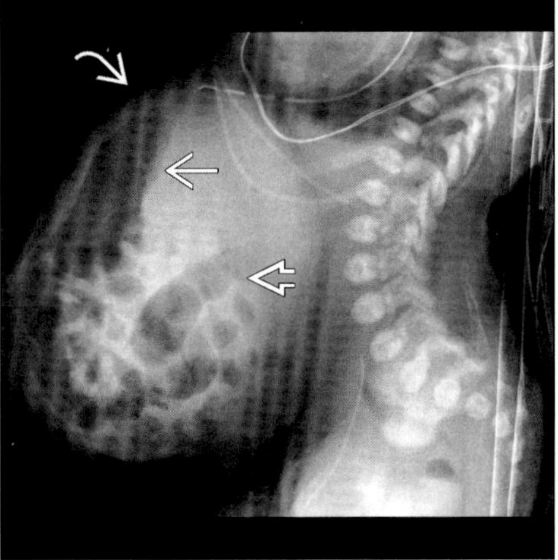

(Left) *Frontal radiograph shows an abnormal chest shape caused by a large omphalocele ➔. Omphalocele has a high association with chromosomal and cardiovascular abnormalities.* ***(Right)*** *Lateral radiograph shows a large omphalocele ➔ containing multiple gas-filled bowel loops ➔ and stomach ➔. This results in an abnormal chest configuration, as seen on the previous image.*

SOFT TISSUE CALCIFICATIONS

DIFFERENTIAL DIAGNOSIS

Common
- Dystrophic Calcification

Less Common
- Metastatic Calcification
- Chondrocalcinosis

Rare but Important
- Tumoral Calcinosis
- Neoplasm

ESSENTIAL INFORMATION

Key Differential Diagnosis Issues
- Includes skin, subcutaneous fat, muscle, and connective tissues; not mediastinum
- Calcification refers to calcium deposition without specific structural organization
- Ossification refers to calcium deposition with formation of medullary space and cortex
- It is not always possible to distinguish between calcification and ossification
- Clinical history usually important in establishing diagnosis

Helpful Clues for Common Diagnoses
- **Dystrophic Calcification**
  - Accounts for approximately 95% of soft tissue calcification
  - Underlying inflammatory disorder, not metabolic disease
  - Commonly from trauma or infection; may progress to heterotopic ossification
    - Also connective tissue disorders, such as scleroderma, SLE, dermatomyositis
  - Usually amorphous in appearance; can be focal or quite extensive

Helpful Clues for Less Common Diagnoses
- **Metastatic Calcification**
  - Associated with systemic metabolic disease, chronic renal failure, hypercalcemia
  - Can appear speckled or large and globular
  - Associated with calcification of other structures, including vessels and heart valves
- **Chondrocalcinosis**
  - Dystrophic calcification of cartilage, often due to calcium pyrophosphate dihydrate deposition disease (CPPD)
  - Seen in shoulder joint and intervertebral discs

Helpful Clues for Rare Diagnoses
- **Tumoral Calcinosis**
  - Rare familial condition
  - Large, round or amorphous, periarticular calcifications; dependent sedimentation levels may be present
  - Shoulder joint is commonly affected
- **Neoplasm**
  - Primary bone neoplasm may invade soft tissues
  - Consider osteosarcoma, chondrosarcoma, hemangiomas
  - Distant metastases to soft tissues are very rare

Dystrophic Calcification

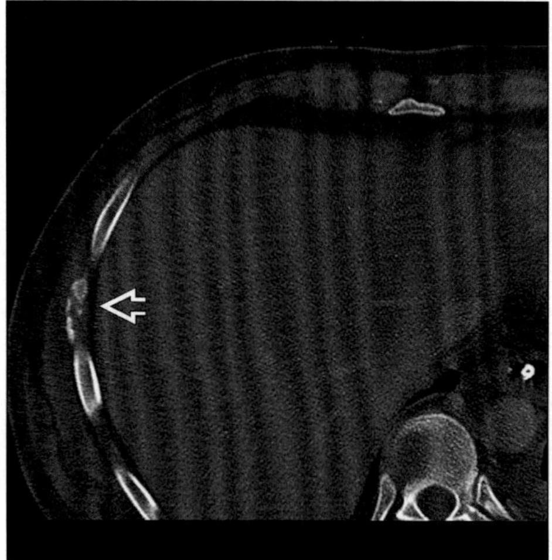

Axial CECT shows amorphous dystrophic calcification in the right intercostal space ⇨ which is traumatic in origin, caused by placement of an intercostal tube.

Dystrophic Calcification

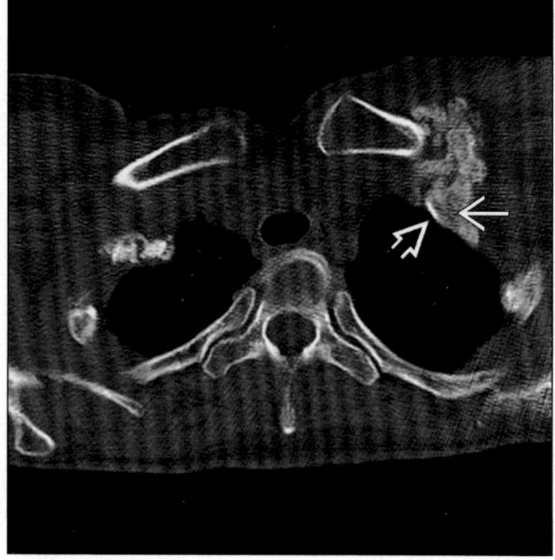

Axial NECT shows dystrophic calcification due to prior trauma. Notice the formation of cortex ⇨ and a medulla →, indicating progression to heterotopic ossification.

SOFT TISSUE CALCIFICATIONS

Metastatic Calcification

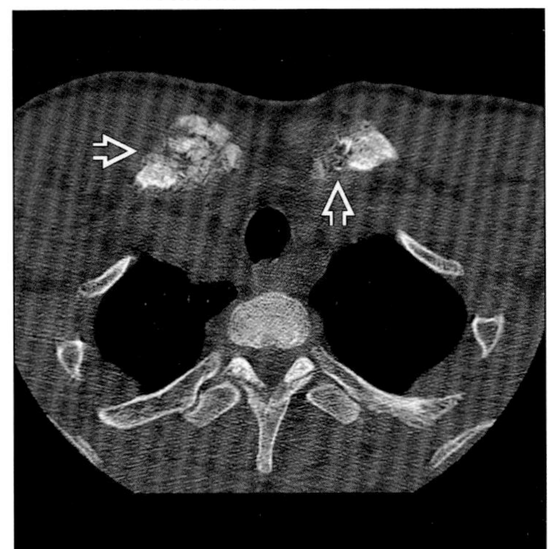

Chondrocalcinosis

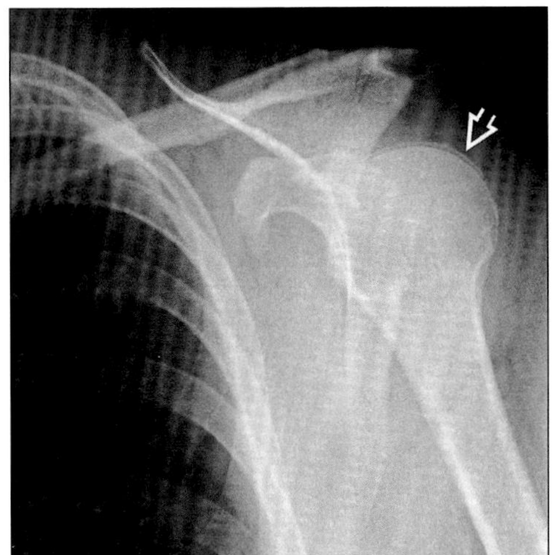

*(**Left**) Axial NECT shows amorphous metastatic calcifications near the sternal heads of the clavicles ➡, which were caused by end-stage renal disease. Clinical history is important to the diagnosis. (**Right**) Frontal radiograph shows chondrocalcinosis superior to the left humeral head ➡ in a patient with calcium pyrophosphate dihydrate deposition disease (CPPD). This may be a subtle finding.*

Tumoral Calcinosis

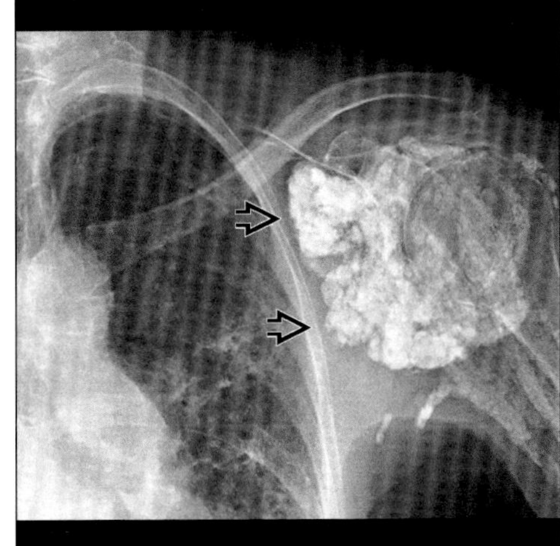

Neoplasm

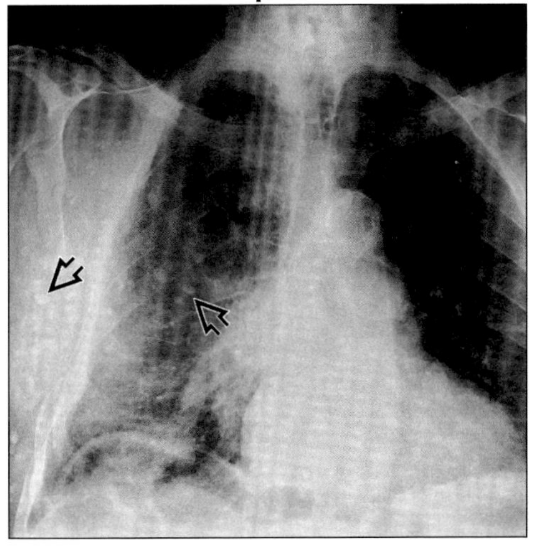

*(**Left**) Frontal radiograph shows extensive round and amorphous calcifications centered around the left shoulder joint ➡. This is a typical appearance of tumoral calcinosis. (**Right**) Frontal radiograph shows numerous round calcifications projecting over the right hemithorax ➡. Also notice the increased density and thickness of the right-sided soft tissues compared with the left.*

Neoplasm

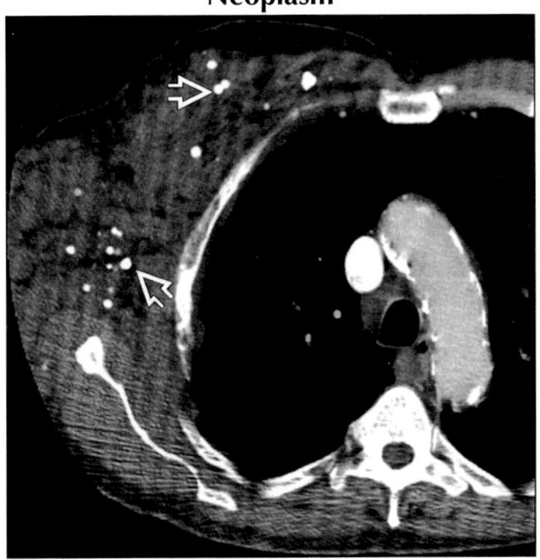

Neoplasm

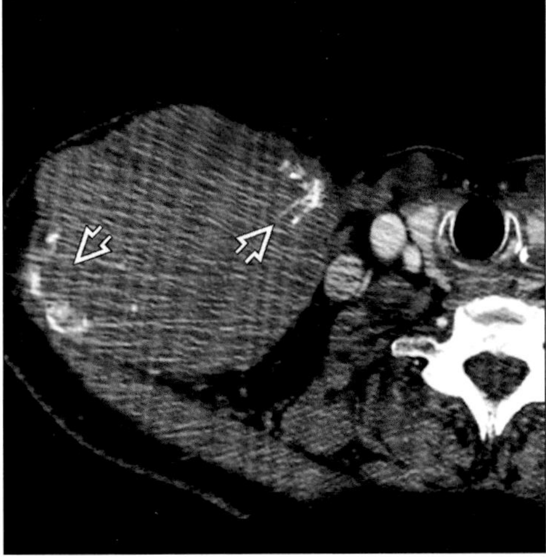

*(**Left**) Axial CECT in the same patient shows a large soft tissue mass with numerous internal round calcifications ➡, consistent with phleboliths. This is a typical appearance of a soft tissue hemangioma. (**Right**) Axial CECT shows a large soft tissue mass with internal calcification ➡. The calcifications within this mass actually represent the destroyed right clavicle from a primary bone lymphoma.*

CHEST WALL INVASIVE DISEASES

DIFFERENTIAL DIAGNOSIS

Common

- Primary Tumors
  - Lung Cancer
  - Mesothelioma
- Metastases

Less Common

- Actinomycosis
- Empyema Necessitatis
  - Tuberculosis
- Primary Rib Tumors
  - Chondrosarcoma
  - Osteosarcoma
- Lymphoma
- Soft Tissue Sarcomas
  - Fibrosarcoma and Malignant Fibrohistiocytoma

Rare but Important

- Primary Chest Wall Infection: Necrotizing Fasciitis
- Primitive Neuroectodermal Tumor (Askin Tumor)
- Deep Fibromatoses
  - Aggressive Fibromatosis
  - Musculoaponeurotic Fibromatoses
  - Desmoid Tumors
- Sternal Osteomyelitis

ESSENTIAL INFORMATION

Key Differential Diagnosis Issues

- Consider clinical presentation, natural history, and patient age at presentation
- Empyema necessitatis: Fluid collections in pleura and chest wall
- Necrotizing fasciitis
  - Signs of inflammation may not be apparent (early stage) if bacteria are deep within soft tissues
  - Subcutaneous air (gas-forming organisms) commonly present
- Chondrosarcoma is most common malignant primary bone tumor of chest wall in adults
- Soft tissue sarcomas are indeterminate by imaging features
- Fibromatosis may be component of Gardner syndrome (familial adenomatous polyposis)

Helpful Clues for Common Diagnoses

- **Lung Cancer**
  - Pancoast tumor: Traverses lung apex and may involve lower trunks of brachial plexus
  - May involve pleura, intercostal nerves, adjacent ribs, and vertebrae
    - Findings of invasion: Rib destruction, encasement of nerves or blood vessels
- **Mesothelioma**
  - Circumferential pleural involvement (including mediastinal pleura)
  - Pleural fluid 95%
  - CT findings of chest wall invasion: Obscuration of fat planes, infiltration of intercostal muscles, periosteal reaction, and bone destruction
  - May also invade mediastinum and diaphragm
- **Metastases**
  - Frequent history of primary tumor
  - Common primaries: Lung, kidney, breast, and prostate

Helpful Clues for Less Common Diagnoses

- **Actinomycosis**
  - Rod-shaped bacterium, anaerobe, sulfur granules
  - Traverses fascial planes from lung to pleura to chest wall
  - May create fistulas
- **Empyema Necessitatis**
  - Mycobacterium tuberculosis
    - Contiguous spread from underlying pleural or pulmonary lesions
    - May create fistulas
- **Primary Rib Tumors**
  - Chondrosarcoma, osteosarcoma
    - Lesions can be osteolytic, osteoblastic, or both
    - Scattered flocculent calcifications
    - Large lobulated excrescent mass arising from rib
    - Chest wall extension: Soft tissue mass
- **Lymphoma**
  - Direct extension into anterior chest wall from anterior mediastinal lymph nodes
  - Isolated chest wall lesions without direct extension can occur
  - Chest wall mass with rib destruction: Lytic or sclerotic

- May grow around sternum or ribs without destroying them
- **Soft Tissue Sarcomas**
  - Fibrosarcoma and malignant fibrohistiocytoma
    - Malignant fibrous histiocytoma: Most common malignant soft tissue sarcoma in adults
    - Similar CT and MR appearances

Helpful Clues for Rare Diagnoses

- **Primary Chest Wall Infection: Necrotizing Fasciitis**
  - Rapidly spreading infection of subcutaneous tissue
  - Uncommon but potentially fatal condition
  - Tissue necrosis and gas formation
  - Spontaneous or in patients with diabetes, immunosuppression, post trauma, or surgery
  - *Staphylococcus aureus*, *Pseudomonas aeruginosa*
- **Primitive Neuroectodermal Tumor (Askin Tumor)**
  - Large chest wall mass in adolescent or young adult
  - Rib destruction, pleural thickening or pleural effusion and focal invasion of lung
  - MR should be performed to delineate soft tissue involvement
- **Deep Fibromatoses**
  - Aggressive fibromatoses
    - Can be very large with high tendency to recur after treatment
    - Rarely intrathoracic
    - CT features: Enhancing soft tissue mass that may be iso- or slightly hypodense to surrounding muscle
    - MR features: Isointense on T1-weighted images and heterogeneously hyperintense on T2-weighted images; shows bands of low signal on all sequences
  - Musculoaponeurotic fibromatoses
    - Chest wall involvement (10-28%)
    - Solitary or multicentric
  - Desmoid tumors
    - Soft tissue masses with poorly defined margins
    - Most frequently located in abdomen (50%)
    - Chest wall (8-10%)
    - Very rarely intrathoracic
- **Sternal Osteomyelitis**
  - Primary
    - Intravenous illicit drug users
  - Secondary
    - After median sternotomy for cardiac surgery (0.5-5%)
    - CT is imaging method of choice
    - CT features: Irregularity of bony sternotomy margins, bony sclerosis, and peristernal soft tissue masses with abscess formation

Lung Cancer

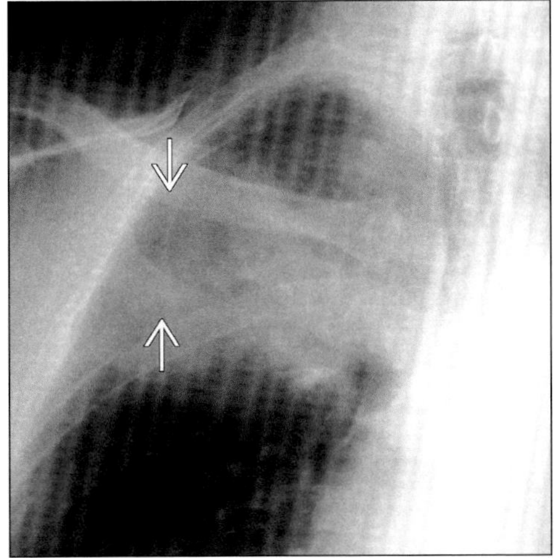

Anteroposterior radiograph shows a large opacity in the upper part of the right hemithorax. Osteolysis of the 3rd and 4th ribs ➡ is also seen in this patient with Pancoast tumor.

Mesothelioma

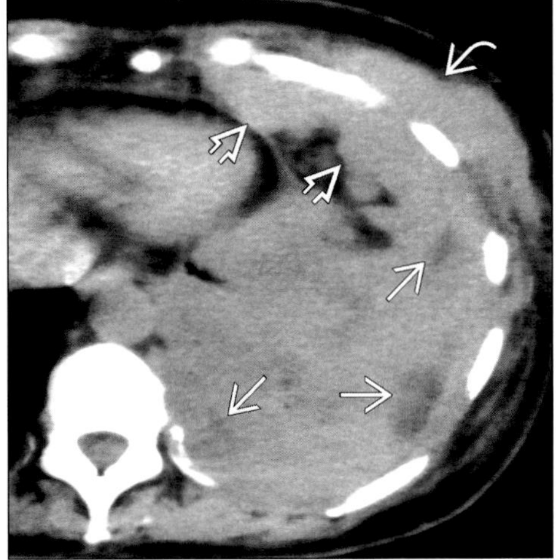

Axial NECT shows a large heterogeneous mass with areas of necrosis ➡ in the left hemithorax. Diffuse nodular pleural thickening ➡ and chest wall infiltration ➡ is seen.

CHEST WALL INVASIVE DISEASES

*(**Left**) Anteroposterior radiograph shows a large mass ➡ with associated osteolysis of the posterior arch of the 3rd rib ➡. The patient was a 4-year-old boy with an adrenal neuroblastoma. (**Right**) Axial CECT shows bilateral areas of consolidation in the anterior portions of the upper lobes ➡. Significant anterior chest wall involvement is observed ➡. Note a moderate left pleural effusion with associated thickening of the parietal pleura ➡.*

Metastases

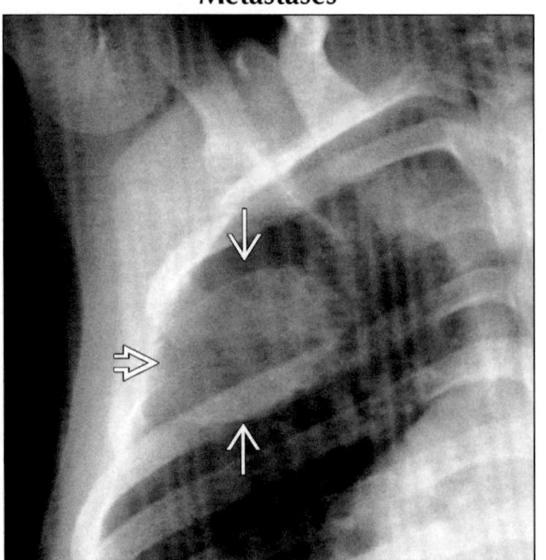

Actinomycosis

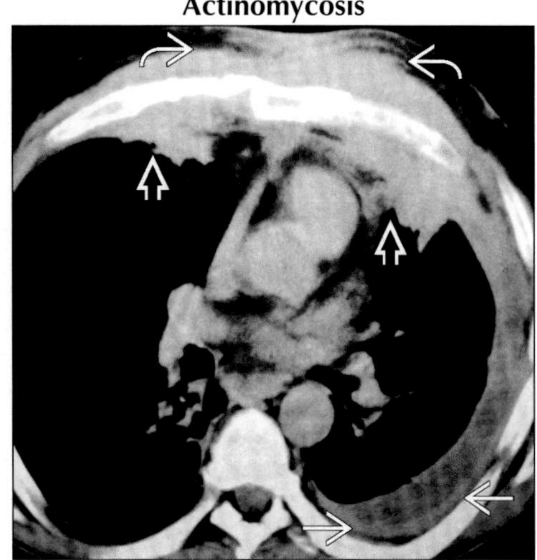

*(**Left**) Axial T1WI C+ FS MR shows a large fluid collection in the apex of the right hemithorax ➡. A "tubular" shadow is seen crossing the soft tissues of the posterior chest wall ➡. This was a 54-year-old man who presented with tuberculous pleurocutaneous fistula in his back ➡. (**Right**) Axial T2WI FS MR in the same patient shows a hyperintense fistula ➡ connecting the pleural collection ➡ with subcutaneous tissue in the left paravertebral area ➡.*

Empyema Necessitatis

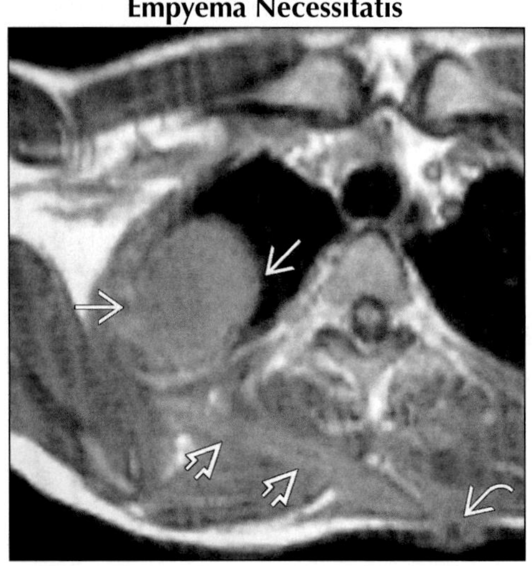

Empyema Necessitatis

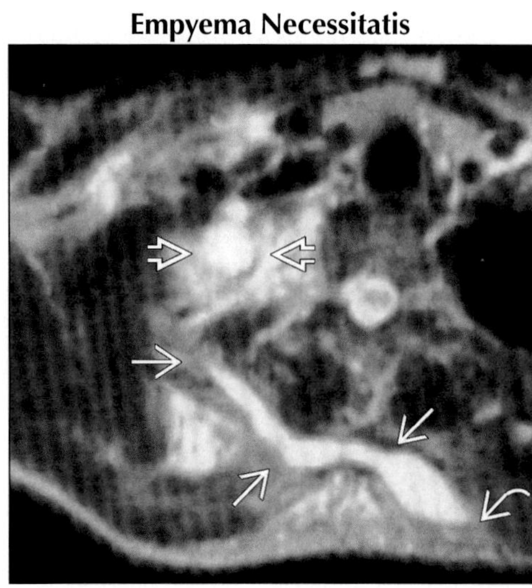

*(**Left**) Axial NECT shows a low-density mass with coarse calcification ➡ arising from the right 7th rib and protruding and infiltrating the anterior chest wall ➡. (**Right**) Axial NECT shows a focal extrapulmonary mass with associated rib destruction ➡ and soft-tissue infiltration ➡. The mass is densely mineralized showing osseous component ➡, a finding characteristic of osteosarcoma.*

Chondrosarcoma

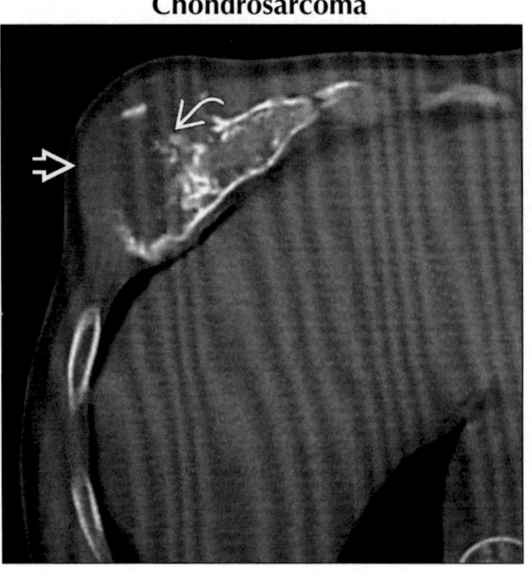

Osteosarcoma

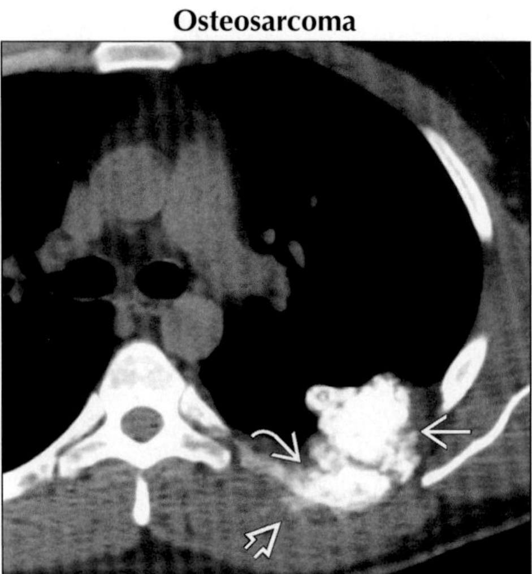

Lymphoma

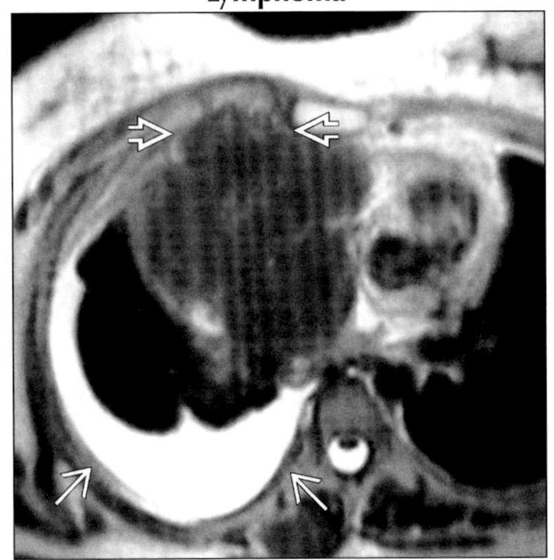

Primary Chest Wall Infection: Necrotizing Fasciitis

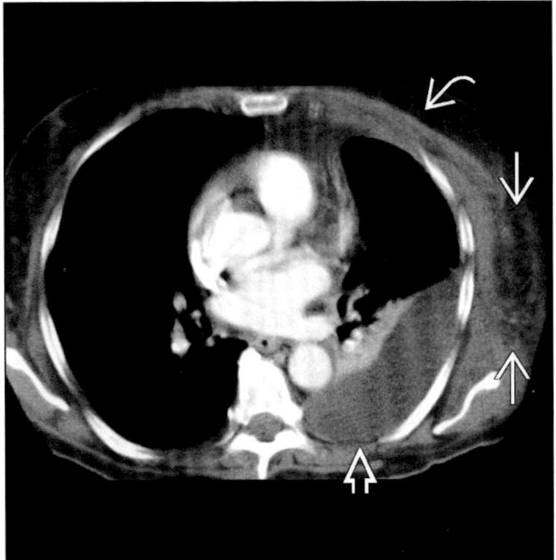

(Left) *Axial T2WI FS MR shows a large heterogeneous anterior mediastinal mass invading the chest wall ➡. Subsequently this patient was diagnosed with invasive lymphoma. A moderate pleural effusion is also visible ➡.* ***(Right)*** *Axial CECT shows an ill-defined soft tissue infiltration in the left chest wall ➡, with loss of normal soft tissue planes. Thickening at anterior chest wall musculature ➡ and left pleural effusion are also seen ➡.*

Primitive Neuroectodermal Tumor (Askin Tumor)

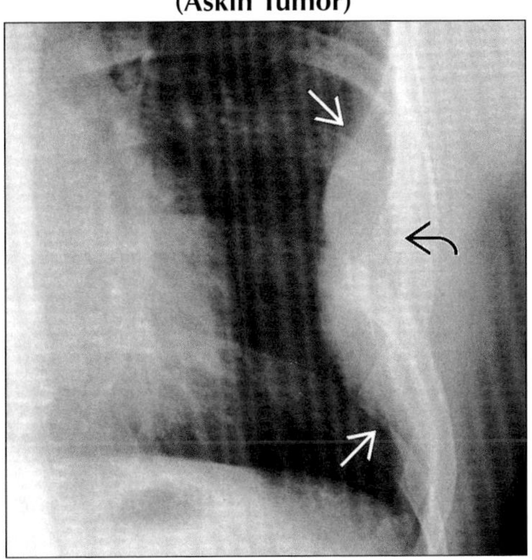

Primitive Neuroectodermal Tumor (Askin Tumor)

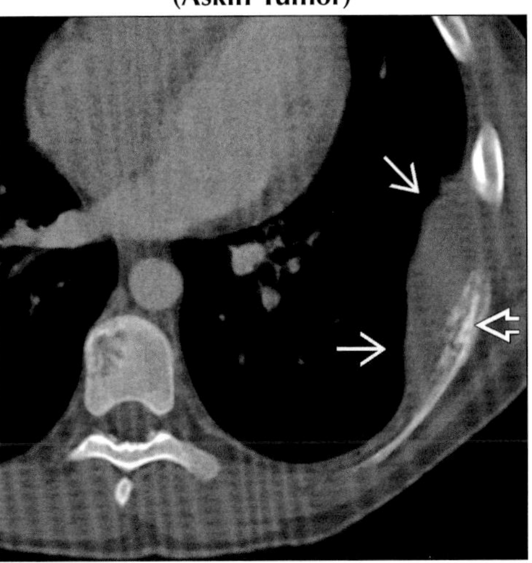

(Left) *Frontal radiograph shows a large chest wall mass ➡ with lytic destruction of the left 7th rib ➡. Note the obtuse angles of the mass, with the lung indicating its extrapulmonary location.* ***(Right)*** *Axial CECT shows a homogeneous mass ➡ centered on the rib destruction. Bone window better shows lytic rib destruction ➡. There is obliteration of the endothoracic fat stripe as well.*

Aggressive Fibromatosis

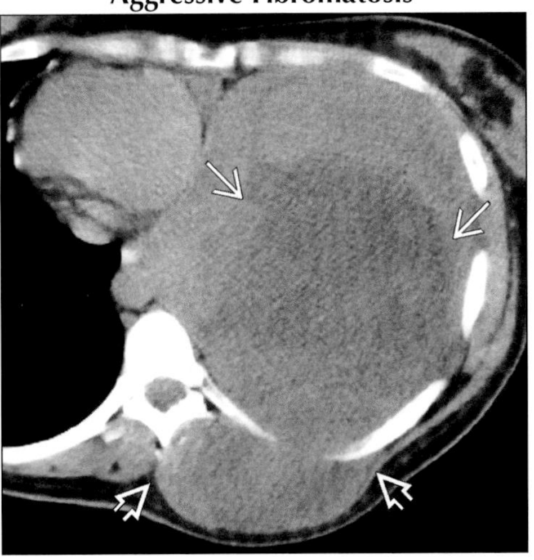

Sternal Osteomyelitis

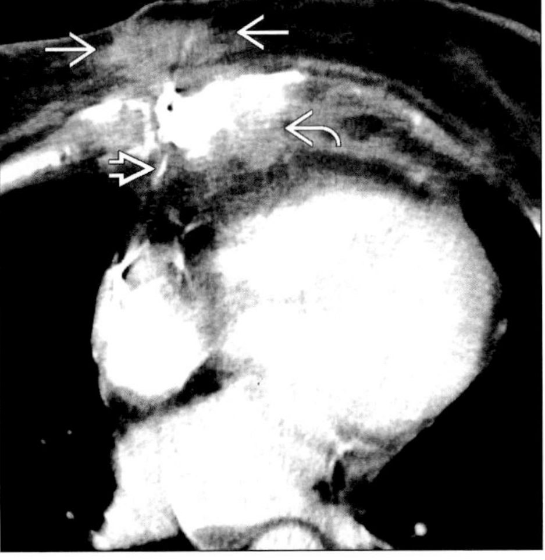

(Left) *Axial NECT shows a large, heterogeneous mass with low attenuation from necrosis ➡. This is aggressive fibromatosis in a 48-year-old woman. Note the intra- and extrathoracic component ➡.* ***(Right)*** *Axial CECT shows bone destruction of the sternum ➡ and presternal swelling with soft tissue infiltration ➡ in a patient who underwent previous sternotomy for cardiac surgery. Note adjacent sternal wires ➡. Diagnosis was β-hemolytic Streptococcus organisms.*

SECTION 10
Heart

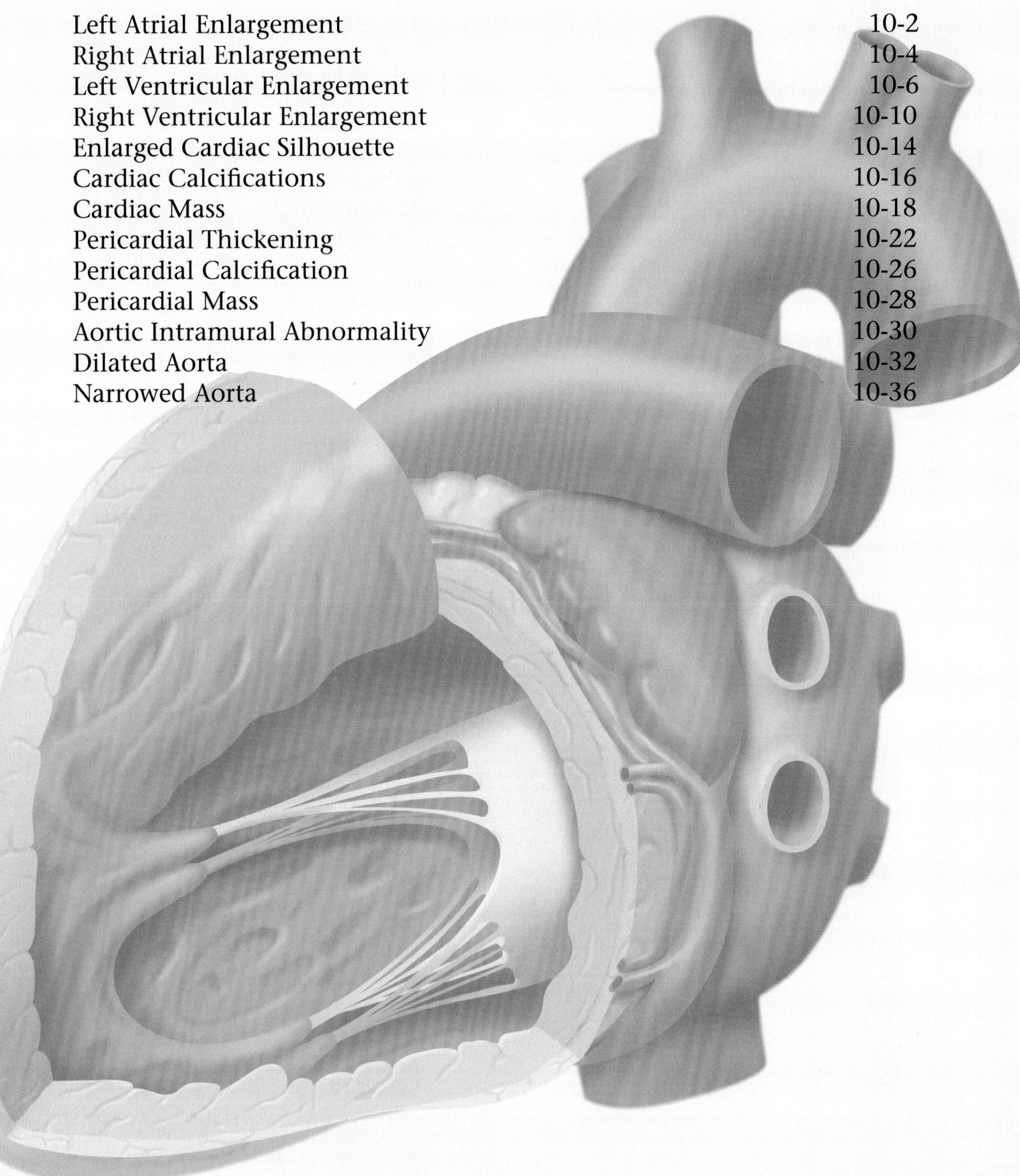

LEFT ATRIAL ENLARGEMENT

DIFFERENTIAL DIAGNOSIS

Common
- Left Heart Failure
- Mitral Valve Disease
- Chronic Atrial Fibrillation

Less Common
- Left to Right Shunts

Rare but Important
- Constrictive Pericarditis/Restrictive Cardiomyopathy

ESSENTIAL INFORMATION

Key Differential Diagnosis Issues
- Radiograph: Double density sign, splaying of carina, superior displacement of left main bronchus, posterior esophageal displacement, enlarged LA appendage
- Aortic root diameter: LA short axis ratio should be near 1:1
- Rightward displacement of interatrial septum suggests LA enlargement
- Normal volume = 22 ± 5 mL/m^2

Helpful Clues for Common Diagnoses
- **Left Heart Failure**
  - Chronic ischemia, diabetes, and chronic hypertension most common etiologies
  - Diastolic heart failure can exist with normal LV end diastolic volume and ejection fraction
- **Mitral Valve Disease**
  - Stenosis
    - Coexistent edema suggests valve area is less than 1 cm^2 (normal 4-6 cm^2)
    - Calcified leaflets not to be confused with mitral annular calcification
  - Regurgitation
    - Often coexists with stenosis and calcified valve
    - Absence of calcifications suggests prolapse or ruptured papillary muscle
- **Chronic Atrial Fibrillation**
  - Exclude LA appendage thrombus on contrast exams
  - Senescent dilation may lead to A-fib

Helpful Clues for Less Common Diagnoses
- **Left to Right Shunts**
  - Qp:Qs ratio does not equal 1
  - VSD does not cause LA dilation unless large
  - ASD only with Eisenmenger physiology in advanced age
  - PDA will also have LV enlargement

Helpful Clues for Rare Diagnoses
- **Constrictive Pericarditis/Restrictive Cardiomyopathy**
  - Tubular-shaped ventricles are disproportionally smaller than atria
  - Constrictive pericarditis suggested by focal or diffuse pericardial thickening > 4 mm or calcification in presence of heart failure
  - Restrictive cardiomyopathy suspected in absence of pericardial thickening

Left Heart Failure

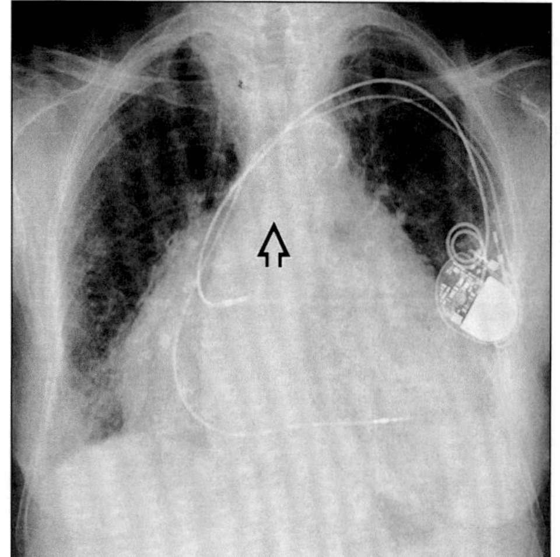

Frontal radiograph shows cardiomegaly with left atrial and ventricular enlargement in a patient with heart failure. Note splaying of the carinal angle (normal < 90°) ⇨.

Left Heart Failure

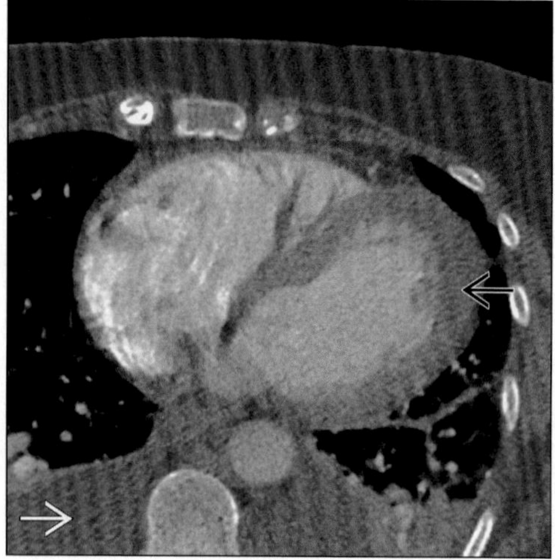

Axial CECT in a patient with diastolic heart failure and left atrial enlargement from uncontrolled hypertension shows pleural effusion ➡ and concentric LV thickening ⇨.

LEFT ATRIAL ENLARGEMENT

Mitral Valve Disease

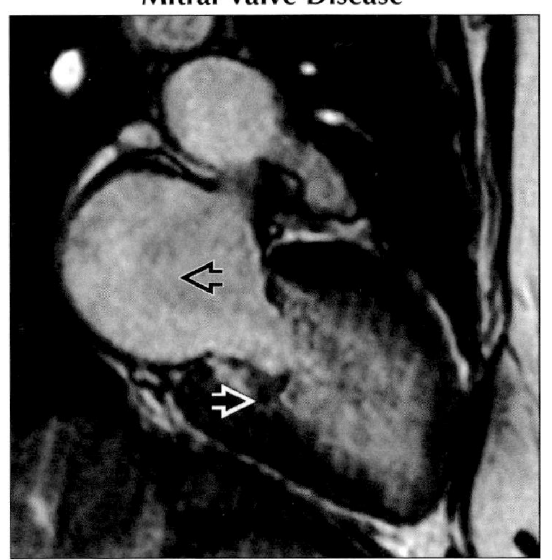

Mitral Valve Disease

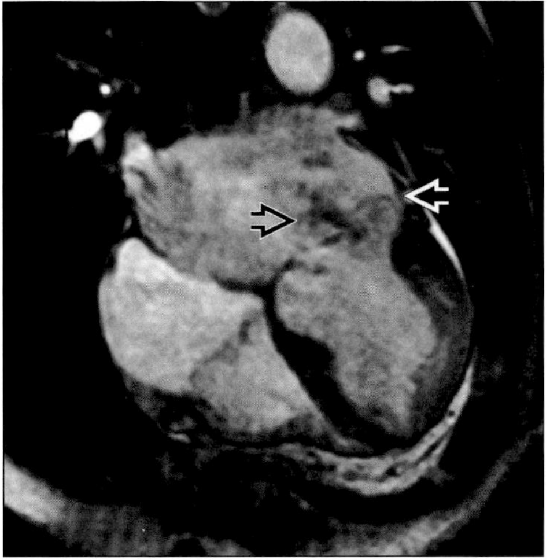

(Left) *Vertical long axis bright-blood cine shows calcified mitral valve with both mitral stenosis and regurgitation in a patient with rheumatic heart disease. Left atrial enlargement is present.* ***(Right)*** *Four chamber bright-blood cine shows prolapse of the mitral valve with a regurgitant jet.*

Chronic Atrial Fibrillation

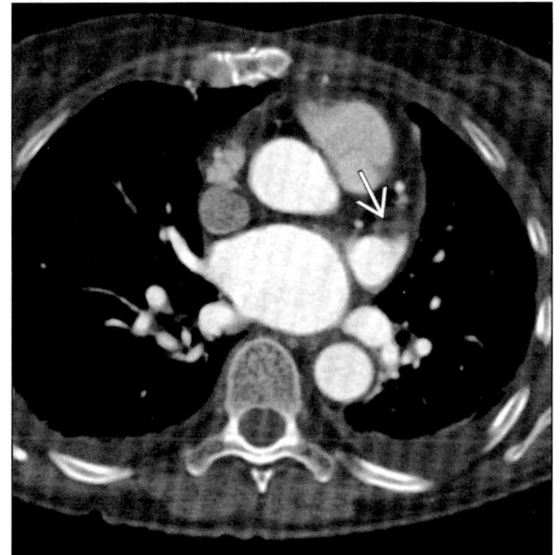

Left to Right Shunts

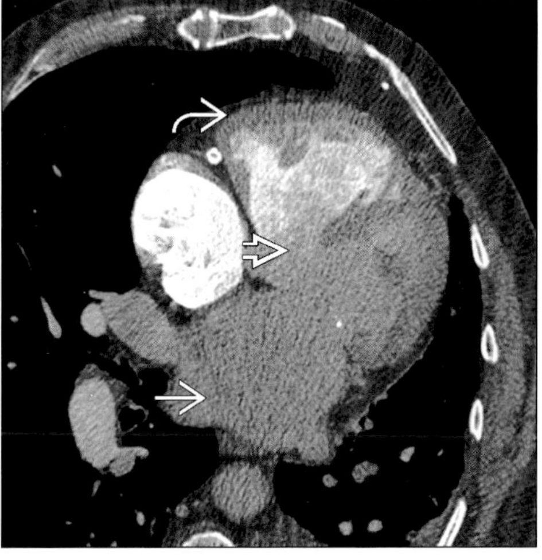

(Left) *Axial cardiac CT shows a filling defect (thrombus) in the left atrial appendage of a patient with enlarged left atrium. Appendages of a patient with chronic atrial fibrillation should be inspected for thrombus.* ***(Right)*** *Four chamber CT shows large membranous VSD with left atrial enlargement. RV hypertrophy reflects longstanding elevated right-sided pressure.*

Constrictive Pericarditis/Restrictive Cardiomyopathy

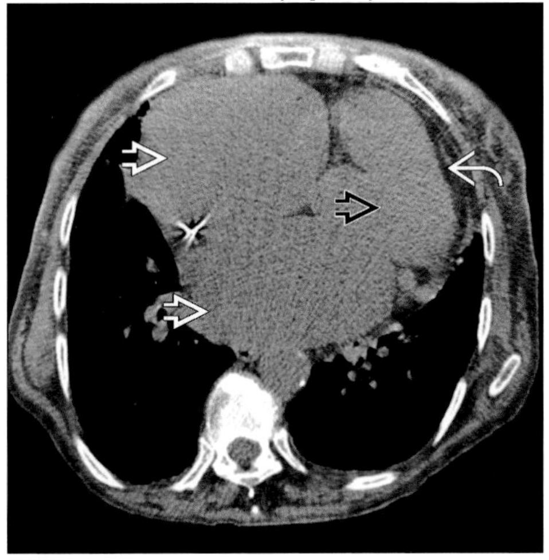

Constrictive Pericarditis/Restrictive Cardiomyopathy

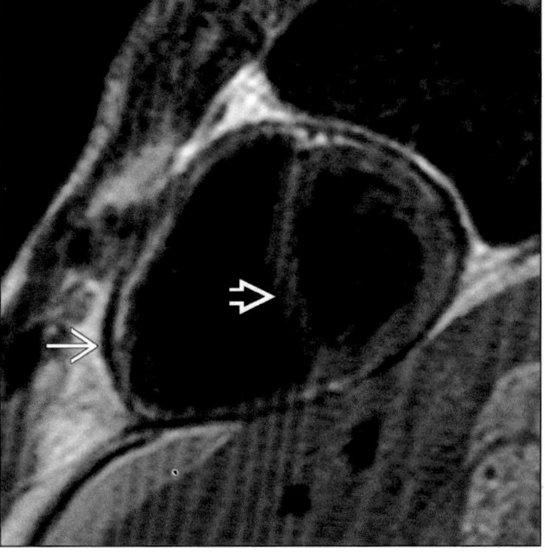

(Left) *Axial unenhanced CT shows biatrial enlargement with small ventricles and a normal pericardium in a patient with restrictive cardiomyopathy from sarcoidosis.* ***(Right)*** *Short-axis black blood mid-chamber image shows pericardial thickening and flattening of the interventricular septum in a patient with constrictive pericarditis. Left and right atrial enlargement were also present.*

RIGHT ATRIAL ENLARGEMENT

DIFFERENTIAL DIAGNOSIS

Common

- Secondary Causes of Right Ventricle Enlargement
- Tricuspid Valve Disease
- Chronic Atrial Fibrillation

Less Common

- Left to Right Shunt

Rare but Important

- Right Atrial Mass
- Ebstein Anomaly

ESSENTIAL INFORMATION

Key Differential Diagnosis Issues

- Radiograph shows rightward displacement of right-lower heart contour
- End diastolic volume (maximum volume) > 90 mL/m^2 highly specific for enlargement

Helpful Clues for Common Diagnoses

- **Secondary Causes of Right Ventricle Enlargement**
  - Pulmonary hypertension suggested by aorta:PA ratio < 1:1 or main PA > 2.9 cm
  - Failure suggested by coexistent coronary artery disease
- **Tricuspid Valve Disease**
  - Regurgitation commonly due to myxomatous degeneration, rheumatic heart disease in older population
  - Increased serotonin levels in carcinoid syndrome can generate fibrous tricuspid leaflet plaques that cause regurgitation
- **Chronic Atrial Fibrillation**
  - Diagnosis suggested by ECG abnormality
  - Right atrial appendage should be examined for thrombus

Helpful Clues for Less Common Diagnoses

- **Left to Right Shunt**
  - MR PA:aorta flow ratio > 1
  - Atrial septal defect (ASD)
    - MR bright-blood cine likely to show flow jet except in large ASD
  - Ventricular septal defect (VSD)
    - Most common left to right shunt but often not hemodynamically significant or spontaneously closes by adulthood
  - Partial anomalous pulmonary venous return
    - Most commonly from right upper lobe to SVC seen best on CT or MRA

Helpful Clues for Rare Diagnoses

- **Right Atrial Mass**
  - Myxoma: Soft, pliable mass, connected to interatrial septum by thin stalk
  - Most often intermediate low T1-weighted signal, high T2-weighted signal
- **Ebstein Anomaly**
  - Apical displacement of septal and posterior tricuspid leaflets with atrialization of proximal right ventricle
  - Coexistent tricuspid regurgitation and stenosis common

Secondary Causes of Right Ventricle Enlargement

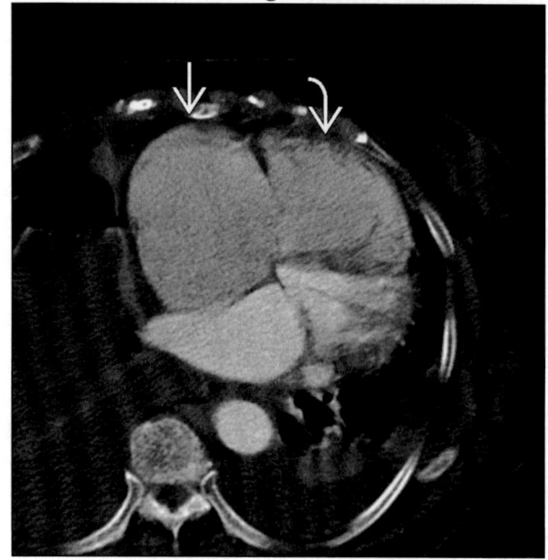

Axial enhanced CT shows RA ➔ and RV ➔ enlargement due to primary pulmonary hypertension and right heart failure. Left heart function is normal. On this admission, patient presented with atrial fibrillation.

Tricuspid Valve Disease

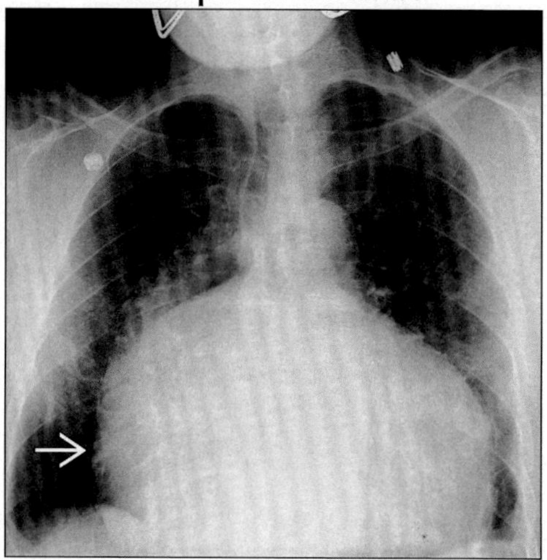

Frontal radiograph shows enlarged cardiac silhouette in a patient with RA and RV enlargement. Note marked lateral displacement of the right heart border ➔.

RIGHT ATRIAL ENLARGEMENT

Tricuspid Valve Disease

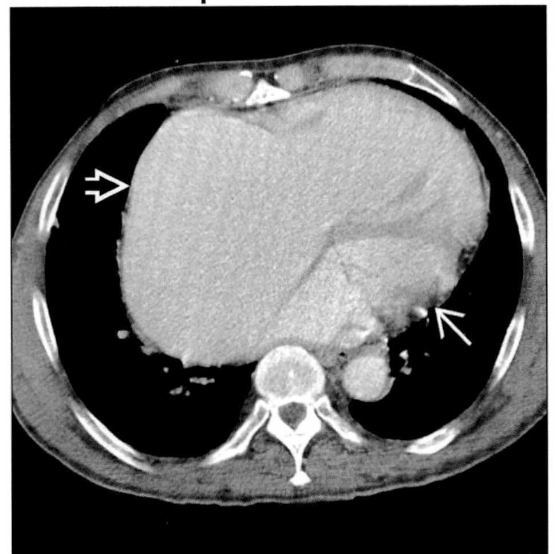

Tricuspid Valve Disease

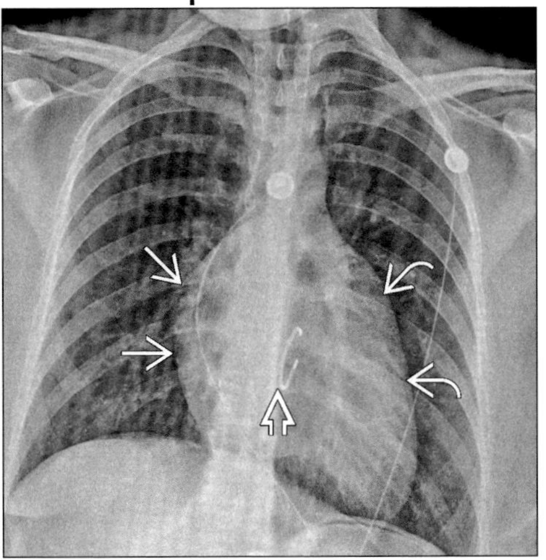

(Left) Axial enhanced CT shows marked RA enlargement in a patient with severe tricuspid regurgitation. Note the massive right heart enlargement ➡ and normal LV ➡. *(Right)* Frontal radiograph shows displaced cardiac contours of both RA ➡ and RV ➡ enlargement in a patient with repaired pulmonary atresia and tricuspid regurgitation ➡.

Left to Right Shunt

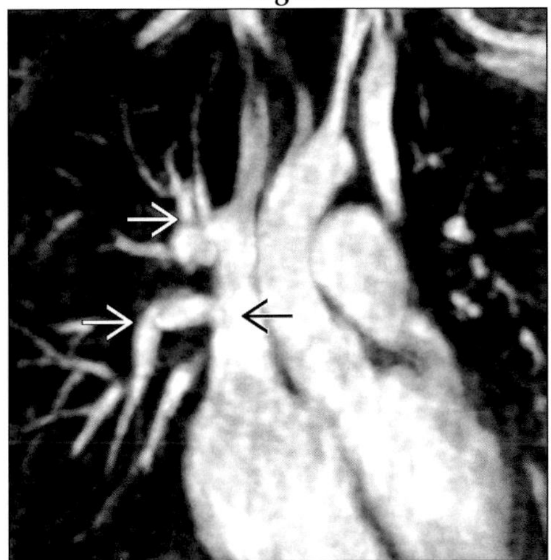

Left to Right Shunt

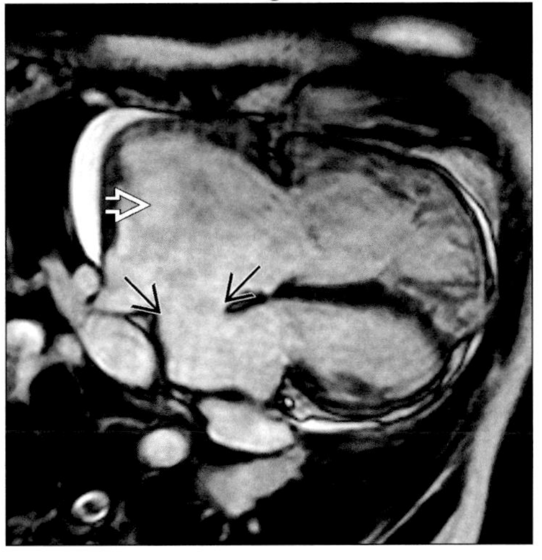

(Left) 3D MRA shows right upper lobe venous return ➡ entering the SVC ➡. Right atrial enlargement was present. This patient did not have a sinus venosus defect. *(Right)* Four chamber MR cine shows large ASD ➡ with RA enlargement ➡. Note that no flow jet is present in this large atrial septal defect. Qp:Qs was 2.2.

Right Atrial Mass

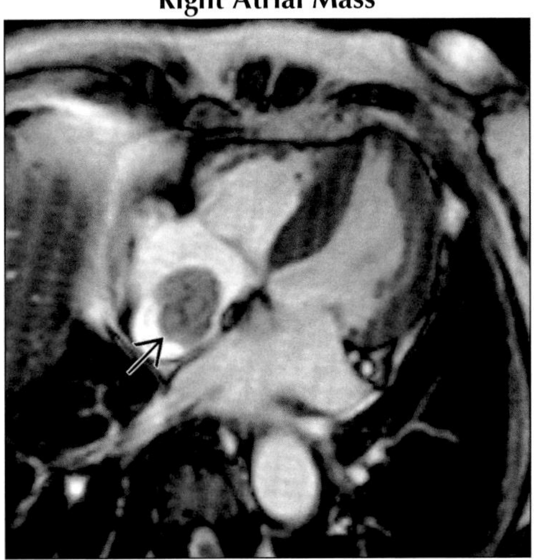

Ebstein Anomaly

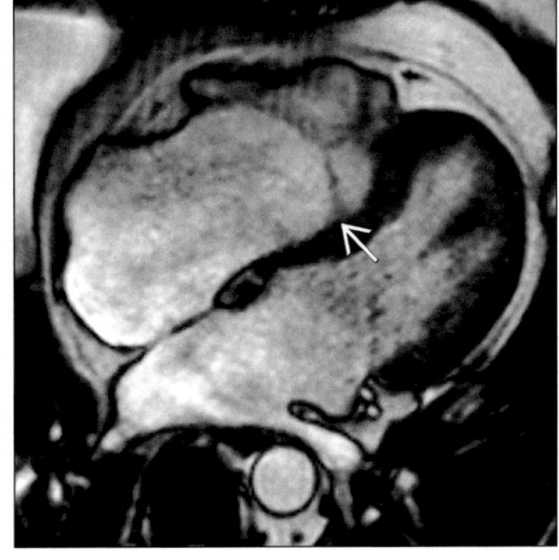

(Left) Four chamber cine MR shows a right atrial mass that attaches to the intraatrial septum ➡, a path-proven right atrial myxoma. Although not in this case, these masses can obstruct the AV valve and cause chamber enlargement. *(Right)* Four chamber cine MR shows downward displacement of the tricuspid leaflet ➡, giving the appearance of an enlarged RA. This adult was an undiagnosed case of Ebstein anomaly with tricuspid regurgitation and an ASD.

LEFT VENTRICULAR ENLARGEMENT

DIFFERENTIAL DIAGNOSIS

Common
- Heart Failure
- Aortic Regurgitation
- Mitral Regurgitation
- Acute Myocardial Infarction

Less Common
- Patent Ductus Arteriosus
- Coarctation of Aorta
- Idiopathic Dilated Cardiomyopathy
- Hypertrophic Cardiomyopathy
- Amyloidosis

Rare but Important
- Athlete's Heart
- Pregnancy-induced Dilated Cardiomyopathy
- Alcohol-induced Dilated Cardiomyopathy

ESSENTIAL INFORMATION

Key Differential Diagnosis Issues
- Determination of LV chamber enlargement
  - Radiographic
    - Normal cardiothoracic ratio ≤ 0.5 on PA and ≤ 0.6 on AP at deep inspiration
    - Leftward and downward displacement of left heart border
    - LV extending 2 cm posterior to IVC border (Hoffman-Rigler sign) on lateral view
  - Cross sectional
    - LV volume is best measured qualitatively, not quantitatively, when only axial planes are available
    - Reliable measurements require double oblique planes, usually short axis
    - Normal internal LV diameter at base is 3.9-5.3 cm for females and 4.2-5.9 cm for males
    - 2-dimensional Simpson rule of discs in short axis or 3D auto-segmented are most reproducible
    - Less reliable: Biplane method of Simpson rule and area length rule
    - Volume > 130 mL in females and > 200 mL in males is highly specific for pathologic enlargement
- Determination of LV wall thickness
  - End-diastolic wall thickness > 1.2 cm is pathologic
  - LV mass > 104 gm/m^2 in females or 119 gm/m^2 in males is specific for pathology
- Pitfalls
  - Radiographic LV enlargement may be mimicked by pericardial effusion, poor lateral positioning, or pericardial fat pad
  - Misidentification of end diastole most frequent cause of erroneous left ventricular size measurement
  - Cardiac volume may be affected by pre-imaging administration of β blockers or nitroglycerin

Helpful Clues for Common Diagnoses
- **Heart Failure**
  - Ischemic cardiomyopathy most common etiology, followed by diabetes and hypertension
  - EF < 40%
  - Multivessel coronary artery calcifications or stenosis
  - Evidence of prior infarct, subendocardial fat
  - If retrospective gated CT or MR performed, myocardium can be evaluated for evidence of hibernation
  - Subendocardial or transmural delayed enhancement present in coronary artery distribution indicates ischemia
  - If delayed enhancement excludes subendocardial layer, nonischemic etiologies should be considered
- **Aortic Regurgitation**
  - Bicuspid valve or calcified aortic valve
  - Incomplete coaptation of cusps during diastole
  - Regurgitant jet present on bright-blood MR
- **Mitral Regurgitation**
  - Mitral valve calcifications
  - Dilated left atrium
  - Isolated right upper lobe edema is rare manifestation resulting from regurgitant jet
- **Acute Myocardial Infarction**
  - Enlarged cardiac silhouette compared to recent prior
  - Supporting clinical information, troponin leak, ECG changes, or typical chest pain

Helpful Clues for Less Common Diagnoses
- **Patent Ductus Arteriosus**

- Initially, enlarged main pulmonary arteries; later, LV, LA, and ascending aortic enlargement
- LV enlargement with dilated ascending aorta in absence of valvular disease
- Best seen in gated CT or 3D MRA
- MR Qp:Qs ratio < 1:1

- **Coarctation of Aorta**
  - Associated with bicuspid valve
  - Hemodynamic narrowing represented by dilated intercostal collaterals
  - Not to be confused with pseudocoarctation, a tortuous arch without hemodynamic narrowing
  - Undiagnosed cases in adults often occur when narrowing distal to left subclavian take-off
- **Idiopathic Dilated Cardiomyopathy**
  - Age often < 60 years
  - Diagnosis of exclusion
    - Significant coronary artery occlusion or myocarditis to be excluded
  - MR delayed enhancement present in approximately 40% of cases, most commonly mid-myocardial
  - EF < 40% &/or fractional shortening < 25%
- **Hypertrophic Cardiomyopathy**
  - LVOT view shows MR with systolic anterior motion of mitral valve leaflet
  - Asymmetric septal, apical, and concentric variants exist
  - In concentric variant, differential includes hypertensive heart disease/aortic stenosis, amyloidosis, and sarcoidosis
  - Patchy mid myocardial enhancement in areas of LV thickening and RV insertion into LV
- **Amyloidosis**
  - Patients typically > 65 years
  - Increased LV wall thickness with poor or normal contractility
  - Diffuse subendocardial perfusion defect
  - Delayed enhancement inversion recovery sequences show equal relaxation times between blood pool and myocardium

Helpful Clues for Rare Diagnoses

- **Athlete's Heart**
  - Occurs in athletes who engage in prolonged aerobic activity
  - End-diastolic wall thickness: End-diastolic volume > 0.15 in young patient with dilated heart suggests athlete's heart
  - LV volume will decrease following 3 months of deconditioning
- **Pregnancy-induced Dilated Cardiomyopathy**
  - Postpartum LV enlargement and hypokinesis
  - Follow-up imaging in 3 months may show resolution
- **Alcohol-induced Dilated Cardiomyopathy**
  - Accompanying clinical history
  - Follow-up imaging will show resolution if acute

Heart Failure

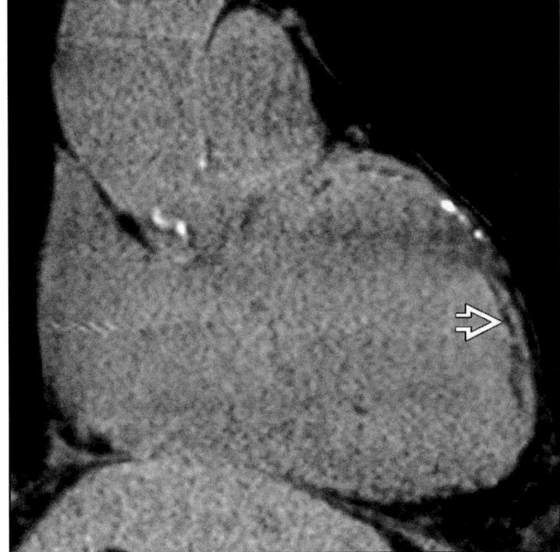

Coronal oblique NECT of ischemic heart failure shows LV enlargement with subepicardial fat ⇨, predominantly in an LAD distribution, representing prior infract.

Heart Failure

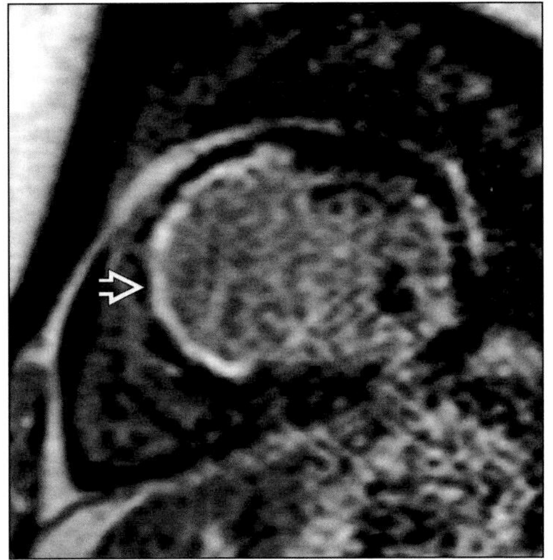

Short axis inversion recovery MR through the LV mid-chamber shows dilated LV with late Gd enhancement in a LAD distribution ⇨, compatible with ischemic cardiomyopathy.

LEFT VENTRICULAR ENLARGEMENT

*(**Left**) Four chamber bright-blood MR in a patient with history of long uncontrolled standing hypertension shows a mildly dilated LV with diffuse wall thickening. This will eventually progress to an appearance indistinguishable from other dilated CM. (**Right**) Diastolic phase LVOT contrast-enhanced CT shows markedly dilated LV without aortic valve disease. This patient had depressed EF and densely calcified coronary arteries, indicating ischemic cardiomyopathy.*

Heart Failure

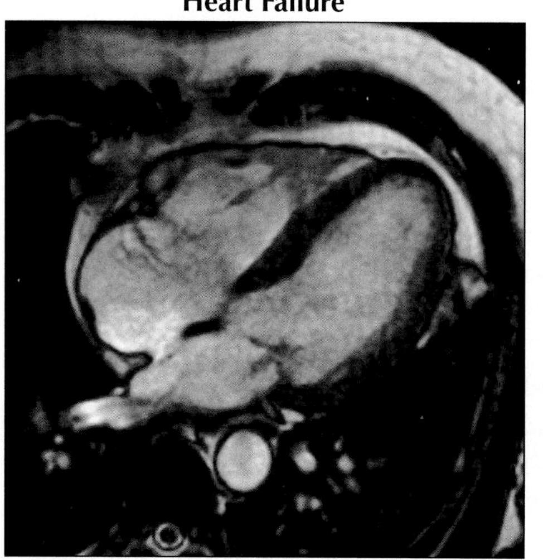

Heart Failure

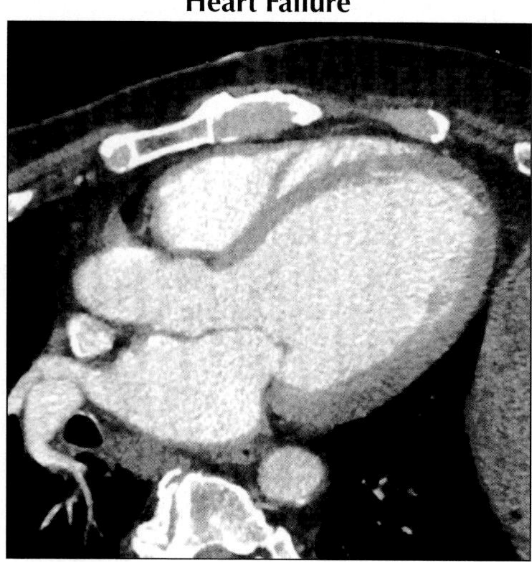

*(**Left**) Coronal cine MR shows a turbulent jet originating at the aortic valve, directed toward the LV chamber ➨. (**Right**) Systolic phase LVOT cine MR image of mitral regurgitation shows low signal corresponding to regurgitation ➡ due to mitral valve prolapse. The prolapsing leaflet is seen ➨ with a regurgitant jet directed at the septum.*

Aortic Regurgitation

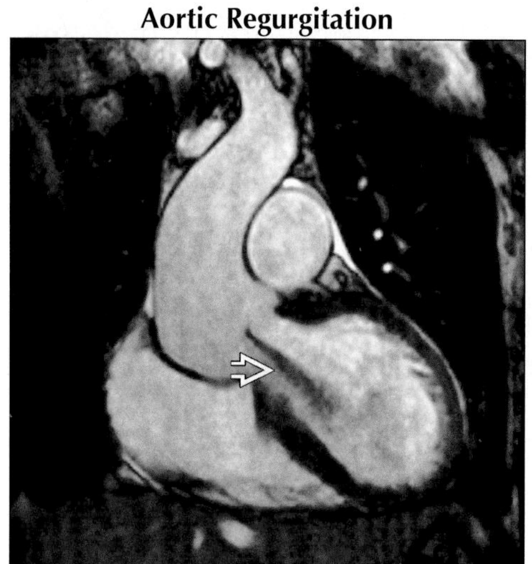

Mitral Regurgitation

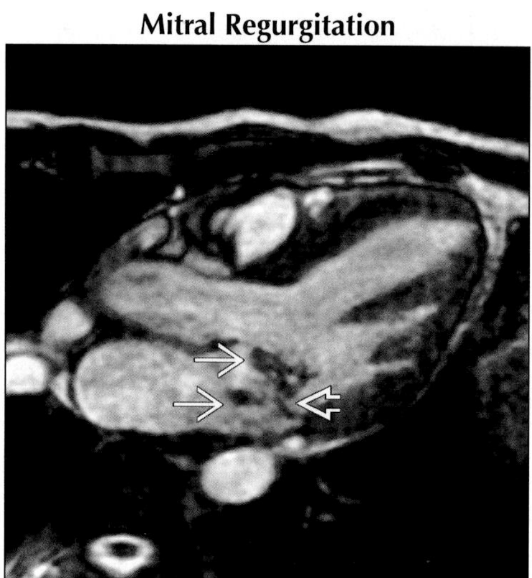

*(**Left**) Inversion recovery FSE MR short axis image through the LV mid-chamber shows mid-myocardial LAD distribution late gadolinium enhancement ➨. Hypointense subendocardium indicates acute MI associated microvascular obstruction ➡. (**Right**) Four chamber view CTA shows dilation of the left atrium and left ventricle from chronic volume overload (due to left to right shunting across the patent ductus arteriosus, not shown).*

Acute Myocardial Infarction

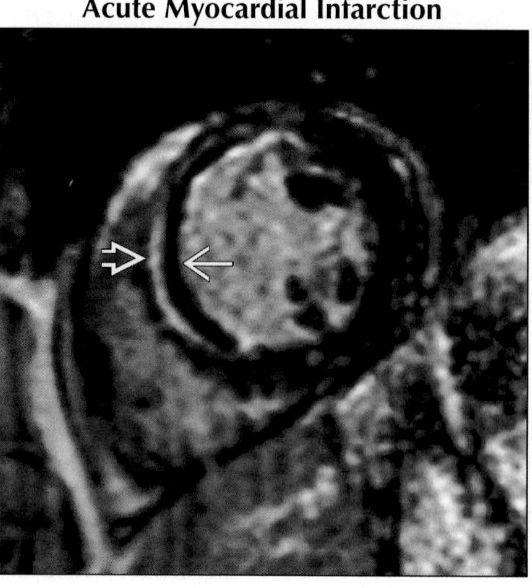

Patent Ductus Arteriosus

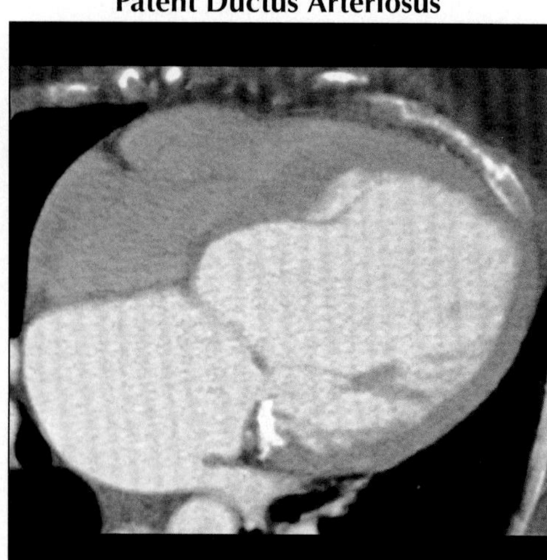

Patent Ductus Arteriosus

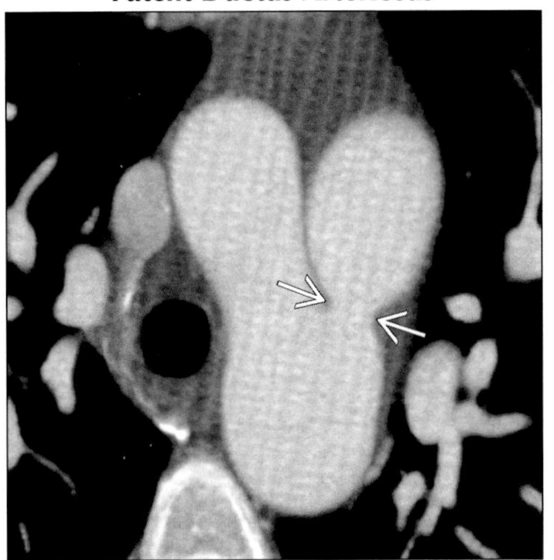

Coarctation of Aorta

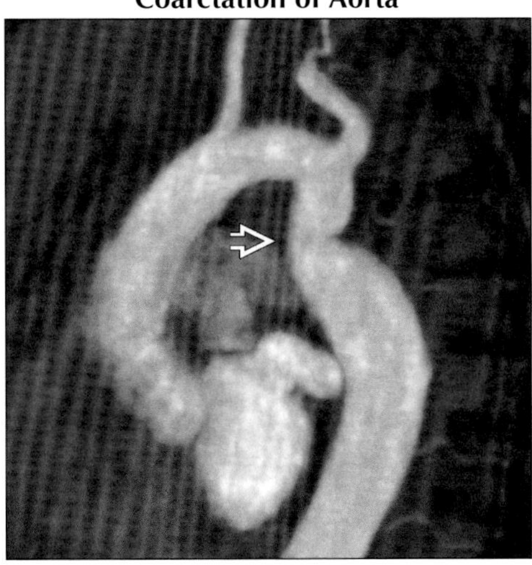

(Left) *Axial oblique CTA shows a connection ➡ between the proximal descending aorta and the pulmonary artery, diagnostic of a patent ductus arteriosus. Left to right shunt resulted in LV enlargement.* ***(Right)*** *Sagittal T1WI C+ FS MR shows focal narrowing distal to the left subclavian take-off ⇨. Presence of intercostal collaterals and LV enlargement indicated a hemodynamically significant stenosis, differentiating it from pseudocoarctation.*

Idiopathic Dilated Cardiomyopathy

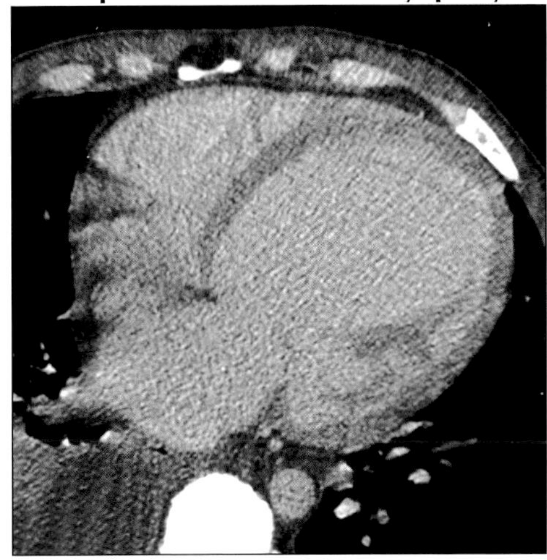

Idiopathic Dilated Cardiomyopathy

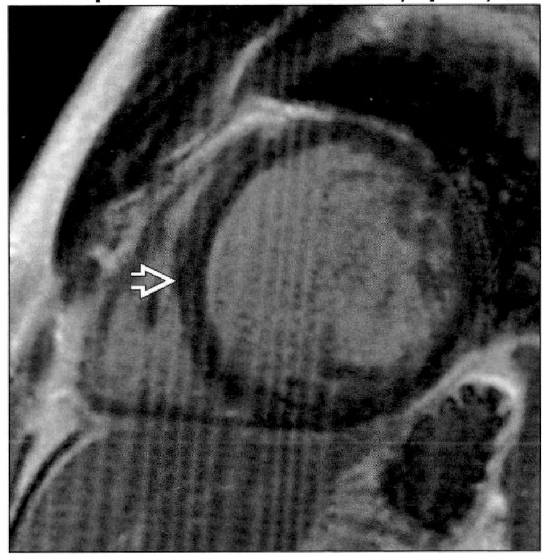

(Left) *Axial NECT from a 41-year-old man with symptoms of heart failure shows LV dilation without CAD. Cardiomyopathy etiology was not found and a diagnosis of idiopathic dilated cardiomyopathy was made.* ***(Right)*** *Inversion recovery FSE MR short axis view shows septal mid-myocardial enhancement in a patient with dilated cardiomyopathy ⇨.*

Hypertrophic Cardiomyopathy

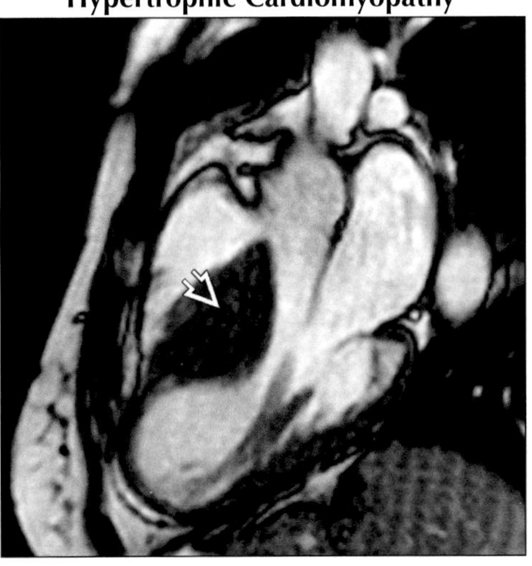

Amyloidosis

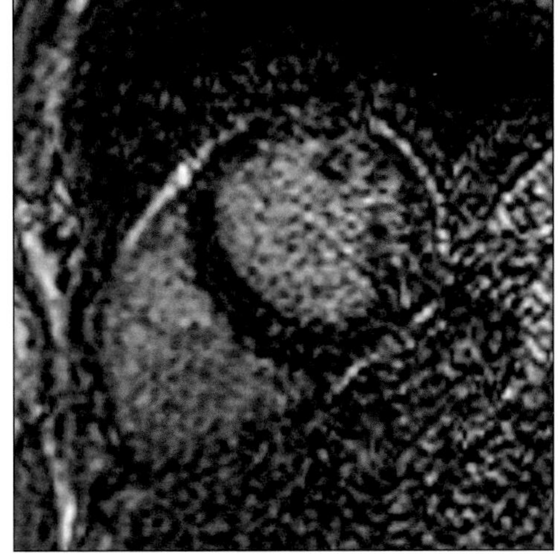

(Left) *MR cine diastolic phase LVOT bright-blood image of asymmetric variant hypertrophic cardiomyopathy shows asymmetric thickening of interventricular septum at base ⇨. Study should be interrogated for fibrosis & SAM.* ***(Right)*** *Inversion recovery FSE MR short axis through LV mid-chamber 10 min after Gd shows near equal relaxation of blood pool & myocardium. Finding is caused by altered Gd concentration kinetics due to presence of amyloid protein.*

RIGHT VENTRICULAR ENLARGEMENT

DIFFERENTIAL DIAGNOSIS

Common
- Left Heart Failure
- Secondary Pulmonary Hypertension
- Right Heart Failure

Less Common
- Left to Right Shunt
- Right Heart Valvular Disease
- Primary Pulmonary Arterial Hypertension

Rare but Important
- Arrhythmogenic Right Ventricular Dysplasia
- Congenital Heart Disease
  - D-transposition of Great Vessels with Atrial Switch
  - Tetralogy of Fallot (TOF) with Pulmonic Regurgitation or Stenosis

ESSENTIAL INFORMATION

Key Differential Diagnosis Issues
- Quantitative determination of right ventricle dilation
  - Normal end diastolic volume = 75 ± 13 mL/m^2 for adolescent to adult
  - Volumes best measured with bright-blood cine MR in axial or short axis plane or retrospectively gated CT
- Radiographic signs of RV dilation
  - Leftward displacement and flattening of left heart contour on frontal view
  - Filling of retrosternal clear space and posterior displacement of left ventricle on lateral view
  - Flattening of interventricular septum only during diastole suggests volume overload
  - Flattening of interventricular septum during systole and diastole suggests pressure overload with or without volume overload
- Quantitative determination of right ventricular hypertrophy
  - Wall thickness > 5 mm suggests hypertrophy
  - Normal right ventricular free wall mass = 26 ± 5 g/m^2

Helpful Clues for Common Diagnoses
- **Left Heart Failure**
  - Ischemic cardiomyopathy and diabetes mellitus most common
  - Multi-vessel coronary artery calcifications/disease
  - LV and LA enlargement
  - Pulmonary edema
  - Prior myocardial infarction, LV delayed enhancement, or LV endomyocardial fat
  - Diastolic heart failure more commonly associated with elevated LA pressure
- **Secondary Pulmonary Hypertension**
  - Main pulmonary artery > 2.8 cm if < 50 years, main pulmonary artery:ascending aorta ratio > 1 if > 50 years
  - RV mass/(LV + septum mass) > 0.6 suggests pulmonary hypertension
  - MR delayed contrast enhancement at RV wall insertion into interventricular septum
  - Suspect if interstitial lung disease, chronic obstructive pulmonary disease, or chronic pulmonary embolism
  - Suspect if mitral valve stenosis present
    - Calcified mitral valve leaflets
    - High flow jet on MR vertical long axis cine
    - Left atrial dilation
    - MR short axis mitral valve area < 2.5 cm on cine and elevated peak velocity on through plane phase contrast
    - Cardiac masses, such as atrial myxoma, can cause valve occlusion
- **Right Heart Failure**
  - Markedly enlarged RV with relatively normal LV
  - Right atrial enlargement
  - Enlarged IVC/SVC and ascites
  - Ischemic cardiomyopathy suggested by proximal right coronary artery occlusive disease or left circumflex disease when left-dominant coronary anatomy present

Helpful Clues for Less Common Diagnoses
- **Left to Right Shunt**
  - Atrial septal defect (ASD)
    - 2nd most common left to right shunt but most likely to cause dilated RV
    - Coexistent RA enlargement
    - MR bright-blood cine short axis or 4-chamber stack without skip throughout interatrial septum may show flow jet
    - Large ASD may not show flow jet on bright-blood cine

- MR phase contrast determines main pulmonary artery:aorta flow > 1
- In cases of sinus venous ASD, look for partial anomalous pulmonary venous return

○ Ventricular septal defect (VSD)
- Most common left to right shunt but often not hemodynamically significant or spontaneously closes by adulthood
- Best investigated with methods similar to ASD

• **Right Heart Valvular Disease**

○ Valvular calcifications indicate stenosis or regurgitation

○ Phase contrast MR to determine pressure gradients and regurgitant fractions most helpful

○ Isolated enlargement of left pulmonary artery suggests pulmonary stenosis

• **Primary Pulmonary Arterial Hypertension**

○ Pulmonary artery > 25 mmHg, pulmonary capillary wedge pressure < 15 mmHg, pulmonary vascular resistance > 2.4 mN x s/cm^5

○ Absence of secondary cause of pulmonary hypertension

○ Distinction between primary and secondary causes is critical because therapeutic pulmonary vasodilators are deleterious in secondary causes

○ Imaging findings suggesting primary pulmonary hypertension
- Normal lung volumes and parenchyma
- Normal left heart size and absence of valvular calcifications

Helpful Clues for Rare Diagnoses

• **Arrhythmogenic Right Ventricular Dysplasia**

○ Diagnosis requires presence of sufficient major and minor criteria, many of which are not related to imaging

○ Major imaging criteria: Severe RV dilation, localized RV aneurysms, fibrofatty replacement of myocardium

○ Minor imaging criteria: Mild RV dilation, regional RV hypokinesis, RV microaneurysms

• **Congenital Heart Disease**

○ **D-transposition of Great Vessels with Atrial Switch Repair**
- RV hypertrophy and enlargement as a result of acting as systemic ventricle
- Prognosis and further therapy determined by changes in RV function and size

○ **Tetralogy of Fallot (TOF) with Pulmonic Regurgitation or Stenosis**
- Pulmonary regurgitation &/or stenosis and in post-repair TOF patients
- RV dilation severe in cases of pulmonary atresia
- Regurgitant fraction best appreciated quantitatively with through-plane MR phase contrast of main PA

Left Heart Failure

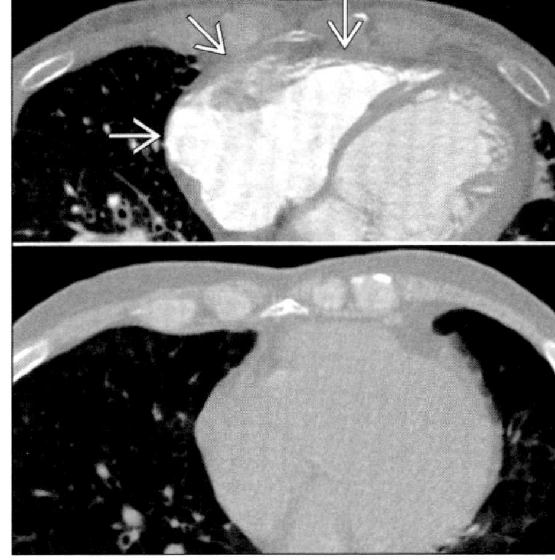

Axial CT unenhanced baseline (bottom) and enhanced CT during an episode of heart failure exacerbation (top) shows RA and RV enlargement ➡. Note edema-related peribronchial thickening.

Secondary Pulmonary Hypertension

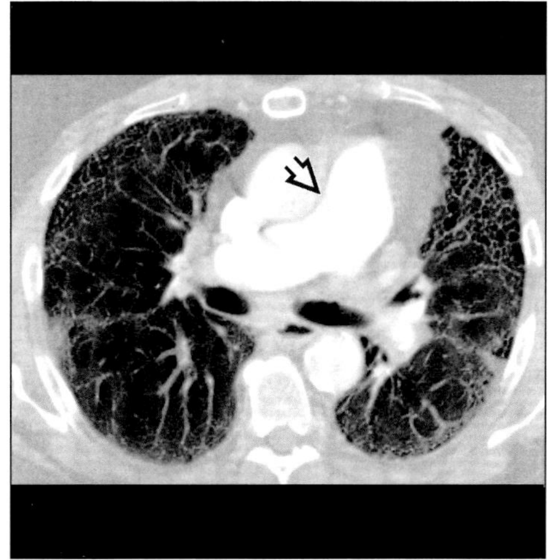

Axial HRCT shows honeycombing in idiopathic pulmonary fibrosis with an enlarged pulmonary artery ➪ reflecting secondary pulmonary hypertension, which can lead to RV dilation.

RIGHT VENTRICULAR ENLARGEMENT

*(**Left**) Coronal enhanced CT shows enlarged pulmonary artery → and mosaic perfusion → in a patient with documented chronic pulmonary embolism. (**Right**) Frontal radiograph shows right ventricle enlargement → with enlarged pulmonary artery →.*

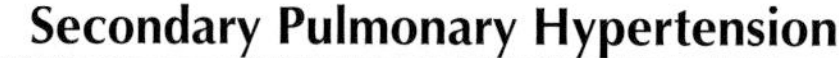

Secondary Pulmonary Hypertension

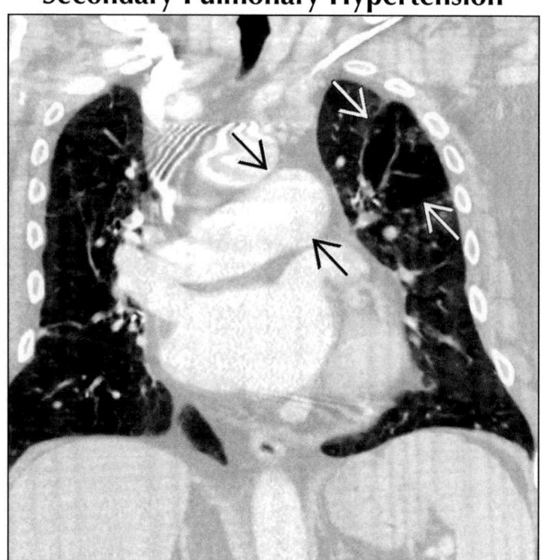

Secondary Pulmonary Hypertension

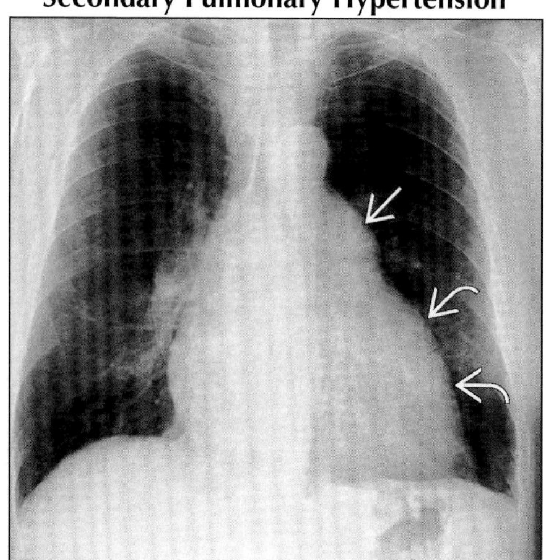

*(**Left**) Axial HRCT shows typical CT features of progressive massive fibrosis from talcosis. Note focal high-density opacities → of progressive massive fibrosis, as well as dilated pulmonary artery → from pulmonary hypertension, which can lead to RV enlargement. (**Right**) Four chamber cine MR shows turbulent mitral jet during diastole →. Left atrial enlargement is present. This patient had secondary pulmonary hypertension and RV enlargement.*

Secondary Pulmonary Hypertension

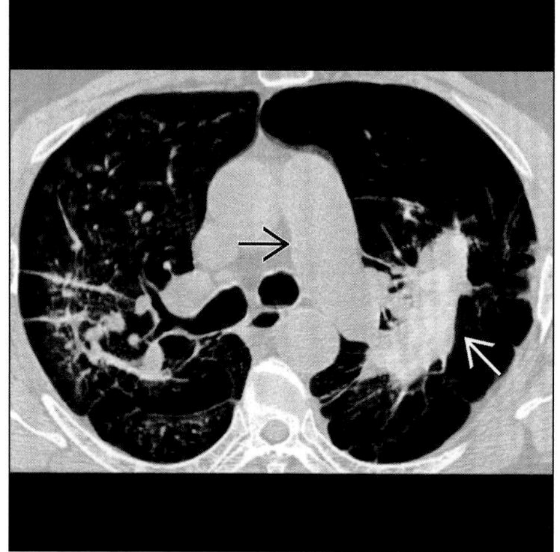

Secondary Pulmonary Hypertension

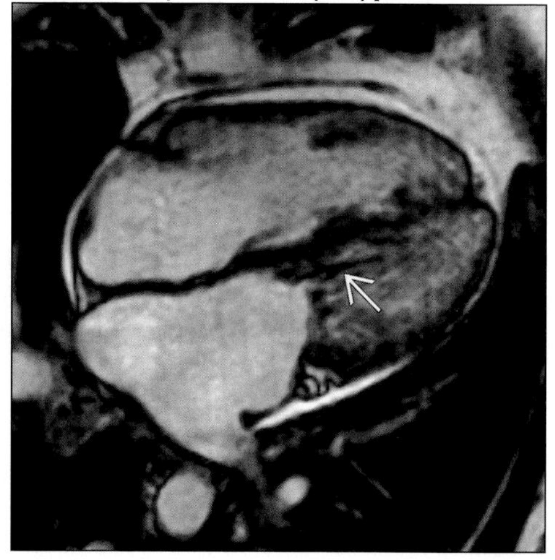

*(**Left**) Axial unenhanced CT shows dilation of the IVC →, greater than twice the diameter of the aorta →. The patient also had dilated SVC and right atrium. This indicated elevated right atrial pressure. (**Right**) Four chamber cine MR shows a large ASD with right atrial and ventricular enlargement. Note that no turbulent jet was present because the ASD was so large. Qp:Qs ratio was 2.2.*

Right Heart Failure

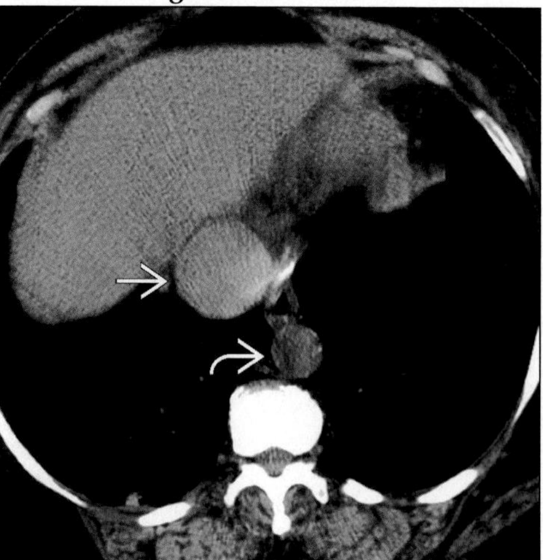

Left to Right Shunt

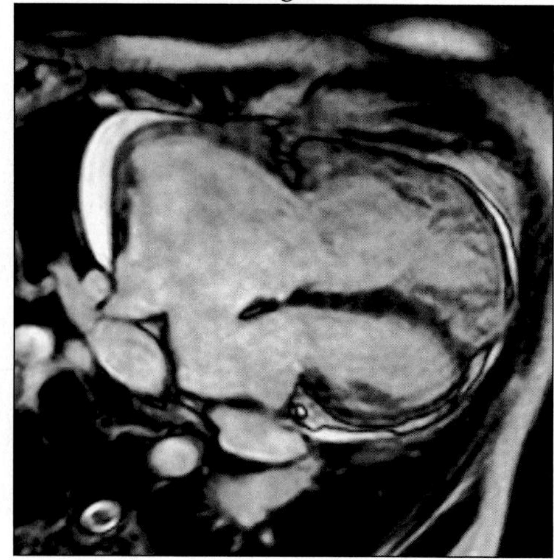

RIGHT VENTRICULAR ENLARGEMENT

Right Heart Valvular Disease

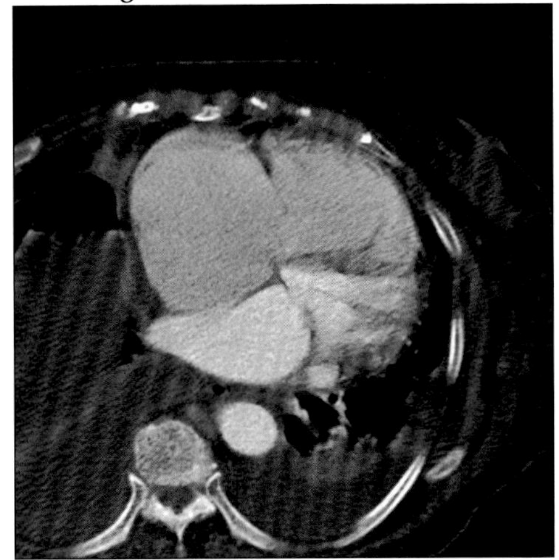

Right Heart Valvular Disease

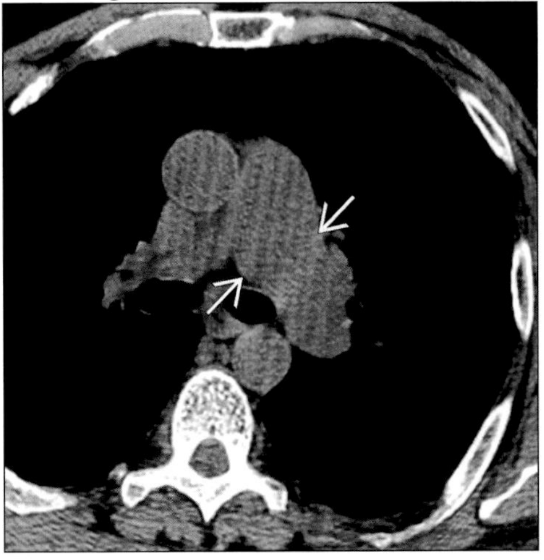

(Left) Axial enhanced CT shows RA and RV enlargement in a patient with tricuspid regurgitation. A regurgitant flow jet was also seen on MR. MR derived stroke volume and pulmonary artery forward flow was used to calculate the regurgitant fraction. *(Right)* Axial unenhanced CT shows isolated enlargement of the left main pulmonary artery ➡. This patient had pulmonary artery stenosis and RV enlargement.

Primary Pulmonary Arterial Hypertension

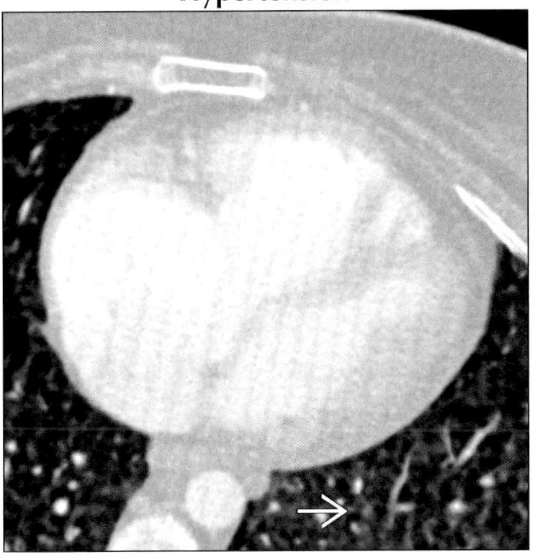

Arrhythmogenic Right Ventricular Dysplasia

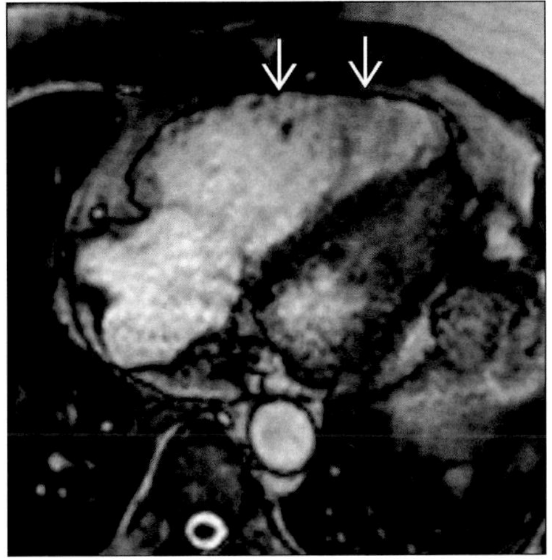

(Left) Axial enhanced CT shows RV enlargement in a patient with pulmonary capillary hemangiomatosis. Note the poorly defined centrilobular ground-glass opacity nodules ➡. *(Right)* Horizontal long axis cine MR shows severe right ventricle enlargement ➡ in a patient with ARVD. This patient also had global hypokinesis. These findings represent major imaging criteria.

D-transposition of Great Vessels with Atrial Switch

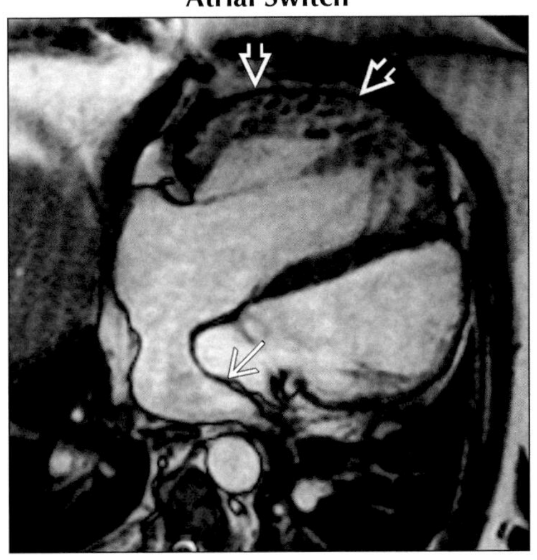

Tetralogy of Fallot (TOF) with Pulmonic Regurgitation or Stenosis

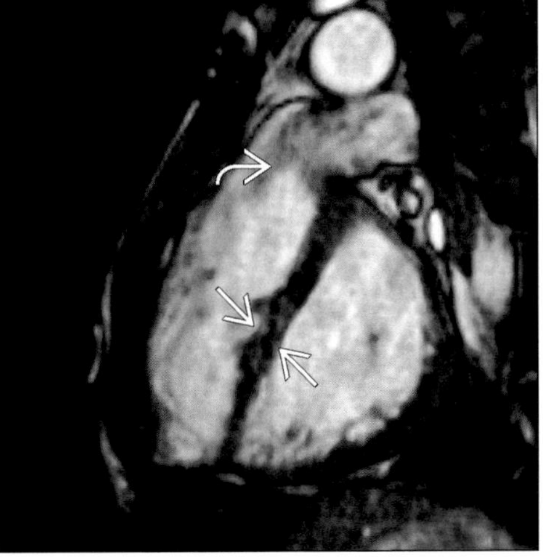

(Left) Four chamber cine MR in a patient with D-TGA with atrial switch shows an atrial baffle ➡. The RV supplies the systemic circulation, leading to dilation and hypertrophy ➡. *(Right)* RVOT cine MR in a patient with corrected tetralogy of Fallot shows flattening of the interventricular septum ➡ and pulmonic regurgitation ➡. Flattening indicates increased right-sided pressure compared to the LV.

ENLARGED CARDIAC SILHOUETTE

DIFFERENTIAL DIAGNOSIS

Common
- Ischemic Cardiomyopathy
- Valvular Disease
- Heart Failure Exacerbation
- Pericardial Effusion

Less Common
- Nonischemic Dilated Cardiomyopathy
- Pericardial Mass

Rare but Important
- Left Ventricle Aneurysm

ESSENTIAL INFORMATION

Key Differential Diagnosis Issues
- Pericardial space fluid: Globular enlargement
- Cardiac chamber enlargement: Characteristic contour abnormality such as filling of retrosternal clear space in right ventricle enlargement
- Pericardial mass: Focal contour irregularity

Helpful Clues for Common Diagnoses
- **Ischemic Cardiomyopathy**
  - Sub-endocardial fat or calcium, left ventricle (LV) wall thinning in coronary distribution, dense coronary calcifications
  - MR shows subendocardial or transmural delayed enhancement in coronary artery distribution
- **Valvular Disease**
  - Valvular calcifications most common
  - MR cine or phase contrast shows flow jets
- **Heart Failure Exacerbation**
  - Coexistent signs of pulmonary edema
- **Pericardial Effusion**
  - New globular heart enlargement on radiograph, fluid-density pericardial fluid on CT
  - Hemopericardium suggested by high-density pericardial fluid or neoplasm history (lung, breast, melanoma)

Helpful Clues for Less Common Diagnoses
- **Nonischemic Dilated Cardiomyopathy**
  - Dilated LV, thin wall, EF < 40%
  - Either no delayed enhancement present or enhancement is not subendocardial
- **Pericardial Mass**
  - Pericardial cyst: Circumscribed fluid density at right more than left cardiophrenic angle
  - Pericardial fat pad: Fat density most commonly at right cardiophrenic angle

Helpful Clues for Rare Diagnoses
- **Left Ventricle Aneurysm**
  - True aneurysm
    - Post infarct wall thinning, dilatation, and associated thrombus
    - Most often present along apical anterior or lateral wall
  - False aneurysm
    - Ruptured myocardium contained by pericardial adhesions at inferior-basal wall
    - Neck narrower than internal diameter

Ischemic Cardiomyopathy

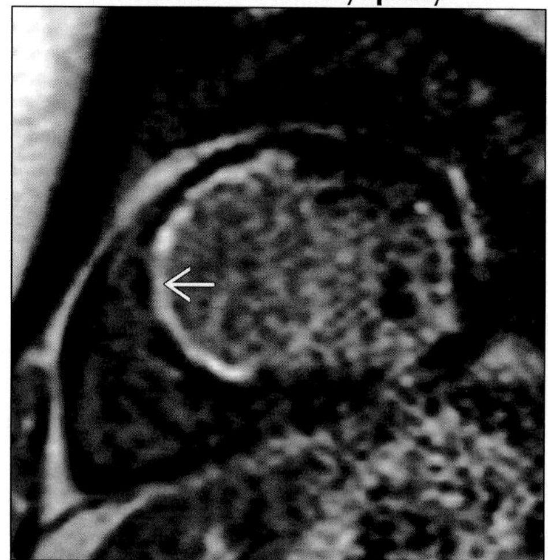

Short axis delayed gadolinium-enhanced image shows subendocardial enhancement ➔ in the septal and anterior wall at the base. The patient had hypokinesis and wall thinning at this location.

Valvular Disease

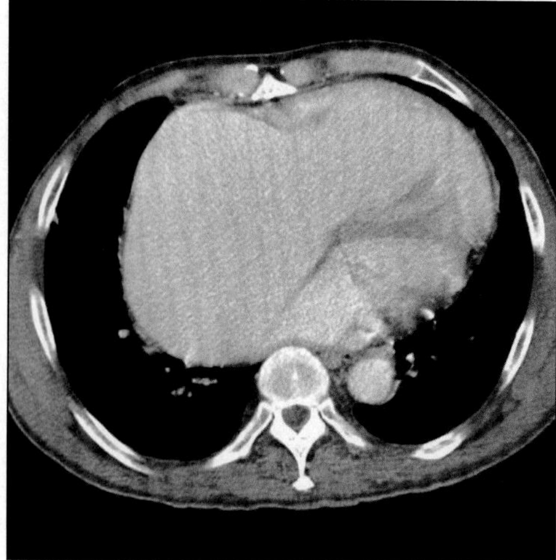

Axial enhanced CT shows an enlarged right atrium in a patient with severe tricuspid regurgitation. Radiograph showed rightward deviation of the right heart border. Regurgitant jet was seen on MR.

Heart Failure Exacerbation

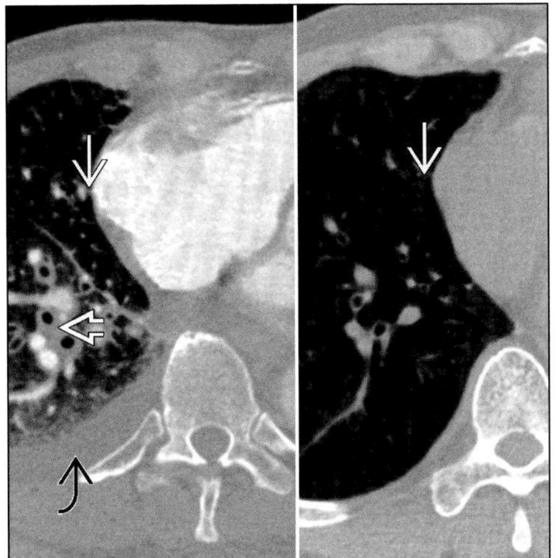

Pericardial Effusion

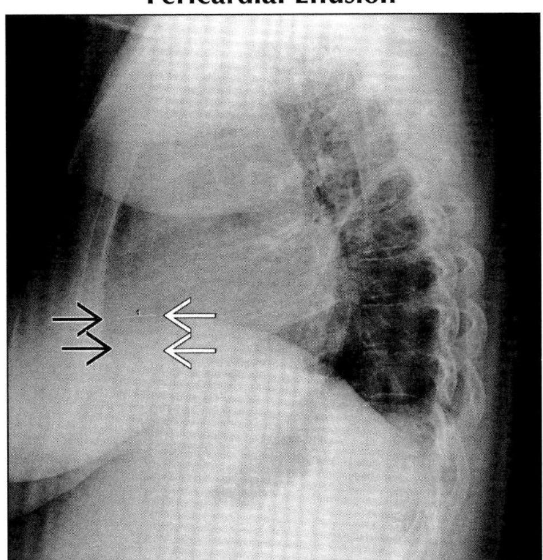

(Left) *Baseline axial unenhanced CT (right) and contrast-enhanced CT during an episode of heart failure exacerbation (left) shows enlargement of the cardiac silhouette ➡, peribronchial thickening ⇨, and right pleural effusion ⤴. Cardiac silhouette was enlarged on radiography.* ***(Right)*** *Lateral radiograph shows filling of the retrosternal clear space. Epicardial ➡ and pericardial → fat are separated by fluid (line), which appears radiopaque.*

Nonischemic Dilated Cardiomyopathy

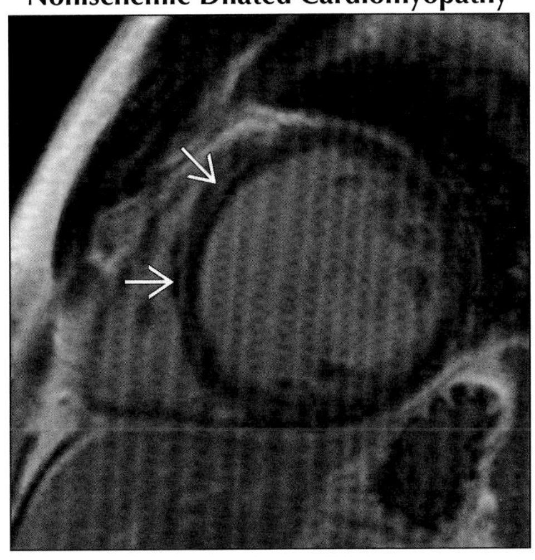

Pericardial Mass

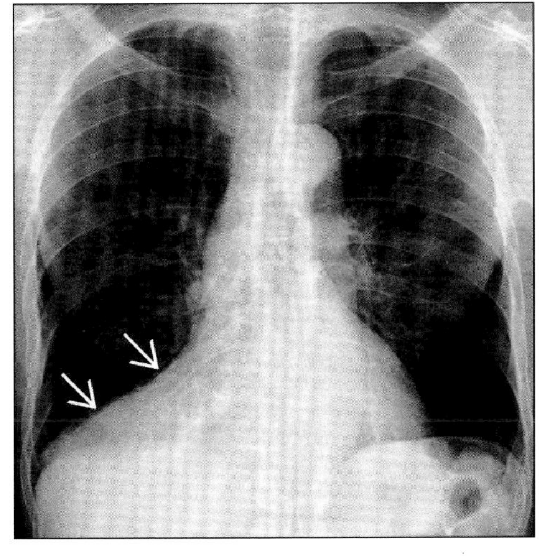

(Left) *Short delayed Gd-enhanced image shows mid myocardial enhancement ➡ in a noncoronary artery distribution. Patient had a depressed ejection fraction but no evidence of coronary artery disease.* ***(Right)*** *Frontal radiograph shows a right cardiophrenic angle opacity ➡ with well-defined margins. CT exam showed fat attenuation tissue representing a unilateral large pericardial fat pad.*

Pericardial Mass

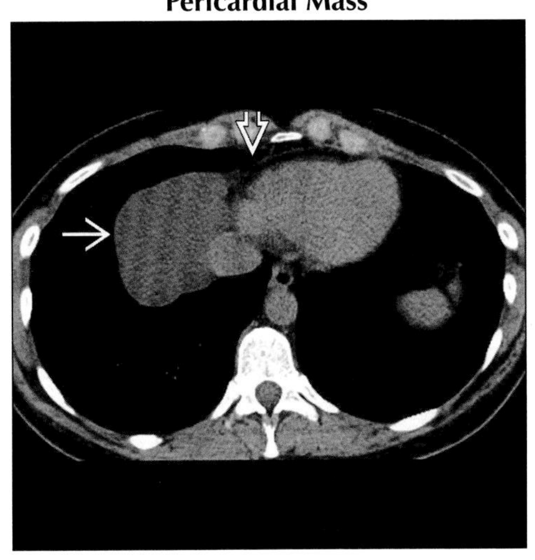

Left Ventricle Aneurysm

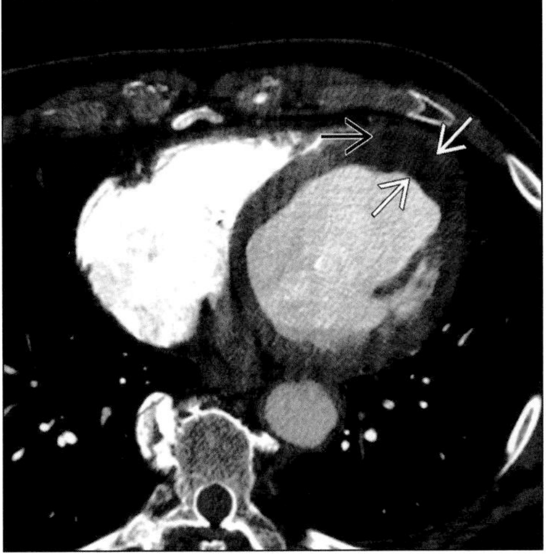

(Left) *Axial NECT shows typical CT features of cystic cardiophrenic mass from a pericardial cyst. Low-density, well-marginated fluid is seen in the right cardiophrenic angle ➡. Pericardial fat plane ⇨ is undisturbed.* ***(Right)*** *Axial enhanced CT shows dilation of the LV with a rim of low density. Patient had a true aneurysm of the LV with adjacent thrombus ➡. Note the true endocardial contour →.*

CARDIAC CALCIFICATIONS

DIFFERENTIAL DIAGNOSIS

Common
- Coronary Artery
- Mitral Valve
- Aortic Valve

Less Common
- Pericardial
- Myocardial
- Other Cardiac Valves and Chambers

Rare but Important
- Mass

ESSENTIAL INFORMATION

Key Differential Diagnosis Issues
- Most common pitfall is misidentifying which anatomic structure is calcified
- Cardiac calcifications more common in dialysis patients

Helpful Clues for Common Diagnoses
- **Coronary Artery**
  - Curvilinear, parallel lines most commonly in proximal coronary arteries and at vessel branch points
  - Amount of calcium correlates with amount of coronary plaque but not degree of stenosis
  - Presence correlates with risk of future cardiac events
- **Mitral Valve**
  - Annular calcifications: Associated with mitral valve insufficiency
  - Valvular calcifications: Suggests stenosis, most often due to rheumatic heart disease
- **Aortic Valve**
  - Calcification burden correlates with stenosis severity
  - Bicuspid valve: Young patient, coexistent coarctation
  - Degenerative: > 60 years old, risk factor for coronary atherosclerosis
  - Rheumatic heart disease: Coexistent mitral valve stenosis, > 35 years old

Helpful Clues for Less Common Diagnoses
- **Pericardial**
  - Associated with constrictive pericarditis
- **Myocardial**
  - Indicates prior infarction; myocardial fat will likely be present
- **Other Cardiac Valves and Chambers**
  - Tricuspid valve: Most commonly due to rheumatic heart disease, mitral and aortic valve will likely be calcified
  - Pulmonary valve: Most commonly due to congenital pulmonary stenosis
  - Atrial calcifications: Associated with severe atrial dilation

Helpful Clues for Rare Diagnoses
- **Mass**
  - Chronic thrombus: Atrial appendage or adjacent to infarcted myocardium
  - Metastasis: History of primary tumor
  - Atrial myxoma: Look for characteristic location and attachment

Coronary Artery

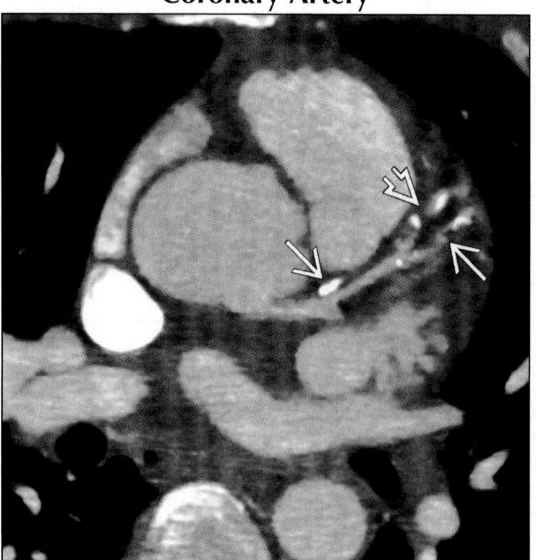

Axial oblique enhanced CT MIP shows discrete calcifications in a linear arrangement ➔ in a patient with LAD atherosclerosis. Note the presence of noncalcified plaque ➔.

Mitral Valve

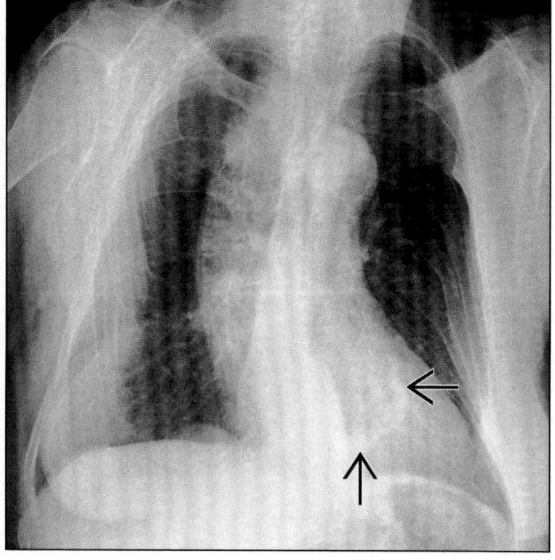

Frontal radiograph shows characteristic C-shaped calcification ➔ indicating mitral valve annular calcification. This calcification pattern is not associated with stenosis.

CARDIAC CALCIFICATIONS

Mitral Valve

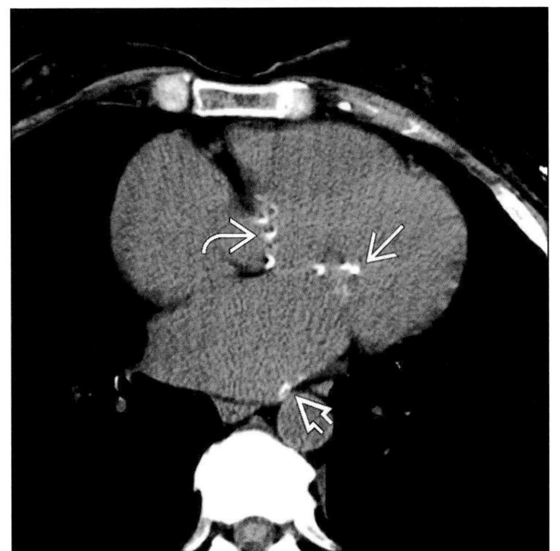

Aortic Valve

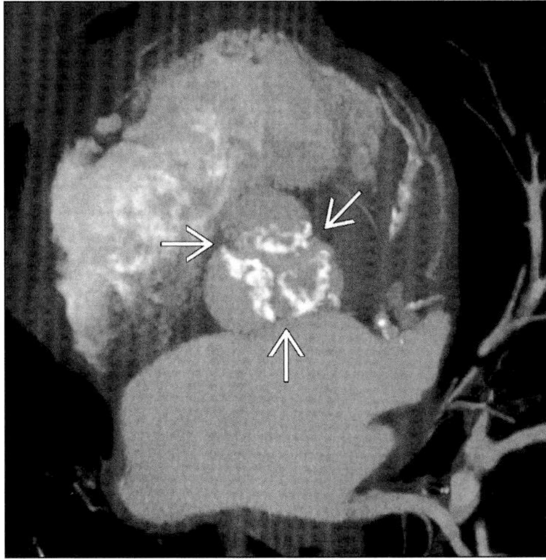

(Left) *Axial unenhanced CT shows mitral valve leaflet calcifications in a patient with mitral stenosis ➡ presumed to be due to rheumatic heart disease. Note the enlarged left atrium and left atrial calcifications ⇨. Patient also has aortic stenosis ↪.* ***(Right)*** *Double oblique enhanced CT MIP shows dense calcifications of the aortic valve cusps ➡ in a patient with severe aortic stenosis. Calcium burden correlates with severity of stenosis.*

Pericardial

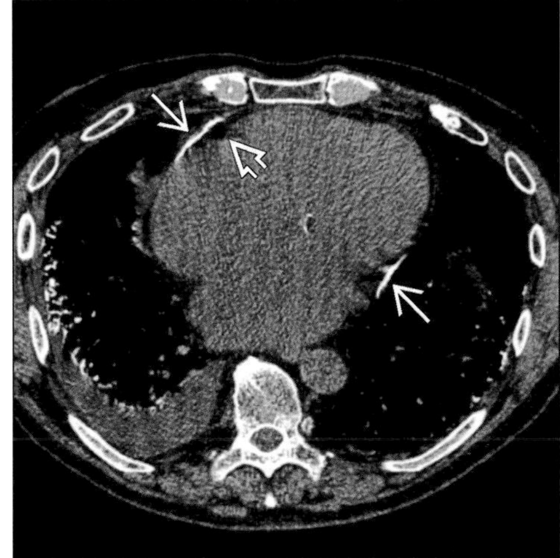

Myocardial

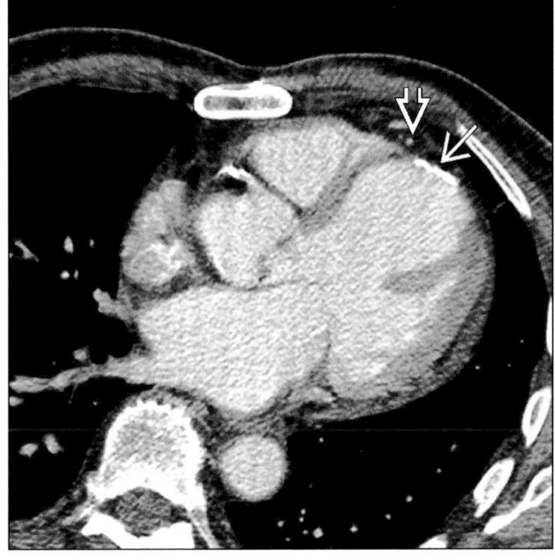

(Left) *Axial unenhanced CT shows pericardial calcification ➡ at the atrioventricular groves, the most characteristic location. Note epicardial fat ⇨ to differentiate from coronary calcium.* ***(Right)*** *Left ventricular outflow view shows apical calcification ➡ and wall thinning in a patient with prior myocardial infarction. Note epicardial fat to differentiate from pericardium ⇨. Wall motion abnormality was present (not shown).*

Mass

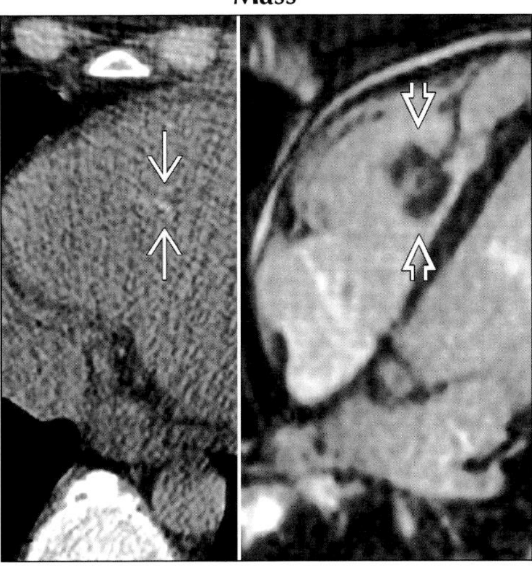

Mass

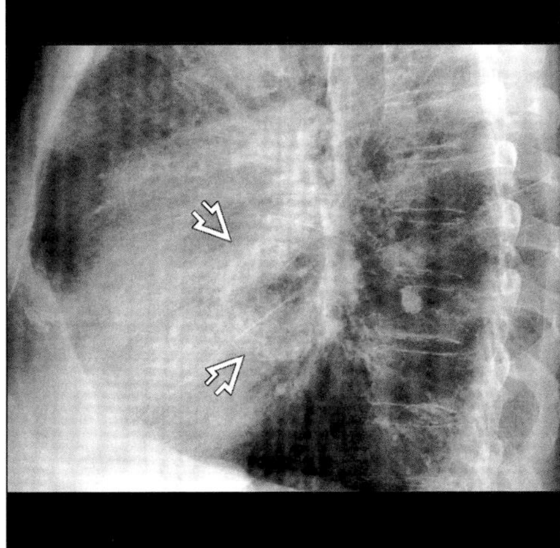

(Left) *Axial unenhanced CT (left) and bright blood MR (right) shows a new calcification ➡ in the RV of a 40-year-old patient with remote history of pulmonary embolus. This calcification corresponded to the presence of a chronic thrombus ⇨.* ***(Right)*** *Lateral radiograph shows curvilinear calcification ⇨ in the left atrium in a patient with left atrial myxoma.*

CARDIAC MASS

DIFFERENTIAL DIAGNOSIS

Common
- Thrombus
- Cardiac Metastases

Less Common
- Myxoma

Rare but Important
- Sarcoma
- Rhabdomyoma
- Fibroma
- Hemangioma

ESSENTIAL INFORMATION

Key Differential Diagnosis Issues
- Clinical impact is most affected by determination of possible malignancy
  - Etiology of cardiac masses often cannot be distinguished with imaging
  - Mass prevalence, coupled with ancillary findings and clinical history, is best tool in generating focused differential
  - Thrombus is most common cardiac mass
  - Malignant:benign ratio ~ 60:1
  - Metastasis:primary cardiac tumor ratio = 40:1
  - Primary benign:primary malignant ratio = 3:1
  - Primary cardiac neoplasm prevalence reported at 1 per 3,000 to 100,000 in autopsy series
- Malignant vs. benign
  - Heterogeneous MR signal is nonspecific and can be seen in benign or malignant neoplasms
  - Most lesions are T2 hyperintense and T1 isointense to myocardium
  - Malignant tumors more often have moderate to strong enhancement than benign masses
  - Multi-chamber involvement or extension into adjacent structures suggest malignant mass
  - Myxomas (benign) are usually heterogeneous
  - Pleural or pericardial effusion suggests primary cardiac malignancy or metastasis
  - In absence of effusion, primary malignancy is less common and metastasis is very uncommon
  - Right heart mass suggests metastasis

Helpful Clues for Common Diagnoses
- **Thrombus**
  - MR signal characteristics vary based on age of thrombus
  - Chronic thrombus T1 and T2 hypointense
  - Acute thrombus T1 and T2 hyperintense
  - Thrombus will not enhance on post-Gd images; best determined on subtraction post-Gd images
  - Enhancement with vessel expansion suggests tumor thrombus
  - Thrombus will remain dark on delayed enhancement images using long inversion time (500 ms) due to T2* shortening
  - Signal intensity will decrease when employing gradient echo sequences vs. spin echo due to T2* shortening
  - Commonly occur adjacent to area of heart wall hypokinesis or wall thinning
  - Commonly occur in atrial appendages
  - Associated with history of myocardial infarction or atrial fibrillation
  - Polypoid thrombi more likely to embolize than smooth peripheral thrombi
- **Cardiac Metastases**
  - In adults, most commonly lung, breast, lymphoma, esophagus, and melanoma primary
  - In children, most commonly leukemia, lymphoma, neuroblastoma, Wilms, hepatoblastoma, and sarcoma
  - Approximately 90% are clinically silent
  - Autopsy series of cancer patients show prevalence of approximately 7%
  - Imaging features are variable; diagnosis suggested by history of above malignancies

Helpful Clues for Less Common Diagnoses
- **Myxoma**
  - LA:RA ratio about 4:1; bilateral (4%), RV (8%)
  - 10% of cases due to autosomal dominant inheritance
  - Many cases cause pseudo-mitral valve disease
  - Approximately 50% will prolapse across AV valve
  - ~ 15% with calcification
  - Lobulated:smooth contour ratio approximately 3:1

Helpful Clues for Rare Diagnoses

- **Sarcoma**
  - Most patients are symptomatic, complaining of dyspnea
  - Most patients present with metastasis
  - Angiosarcoma most common pathology at 33%
  - Angiosarcoma most commonly in right atrium
  - Other sarcoma histologies preferentially intracavitary in left atrium
  - Commonly occur between 3rd and 5th decades
  - Lesion morphology is variable ranging from infiltrative to endocardial
  - Intense heterogeneous contrast enhancement
  - Heterogeneous, mostly intermediate T1W signal and heterogeneous, mostly high T2W signal
- **Rhabdomyoma**
  - Most common benign tumor in pediatric population
  - High T2W signal and intermediate T1W signal
  - Multiple lesions are often present
  - Myocardial/intramural location
  - 50% of patients have coexistent tuberous sclerosis
- **Fibroma**
  - 2nd most common benign tumor in pediatric population
  - Focal bulge, most commonly in ventricular wall, extending toward cardiac lumen
  - Involved myocardium is hypokinetic
  - Myocardial/intramural location
  - Solitary
  - Calcification common
  - T1 iso- or hyperintense compared to myocardium
  - T2 hypointense compared to myocardium
  - MR and CT contrast enhancement similar to myocardium or nodular peripheral enhancement
  - Present in 10-15% of patients with Gorlin syndrome
    - Autosomal dominant disease with propensity to develop multiple neoplasms, such as basal cell cancers and medulloblastomas
- **Hemangioma**
  - Patients usually asymptomatic
  - Heterogeneous attenuation on unenhanced CT
  - Hyperenhancement on enhanced CT
  - T1 isointense compared to myocardium
  - T2 hyperintense compared to myocardium
  - Isointense to blood pool on balanced steady-state free precession

Thrombus

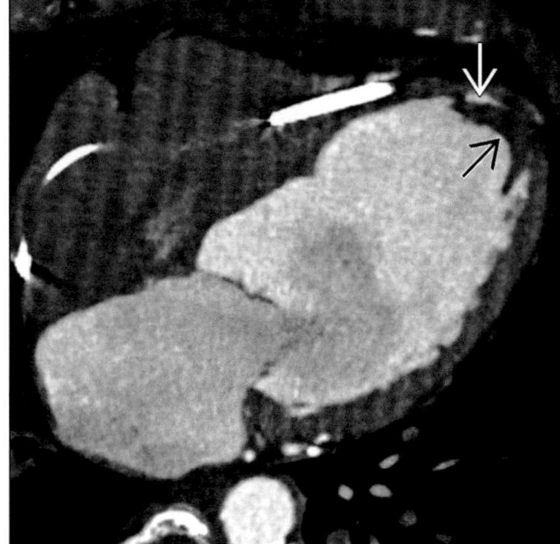

Axial contrast-enhanced CT shows a filling defect in the left ventricular apex ⇨ with adjacent calcifications ➡ and wall thinning. This patient had a prior myocardial infarct and apical hypokinesis.

Thrombus

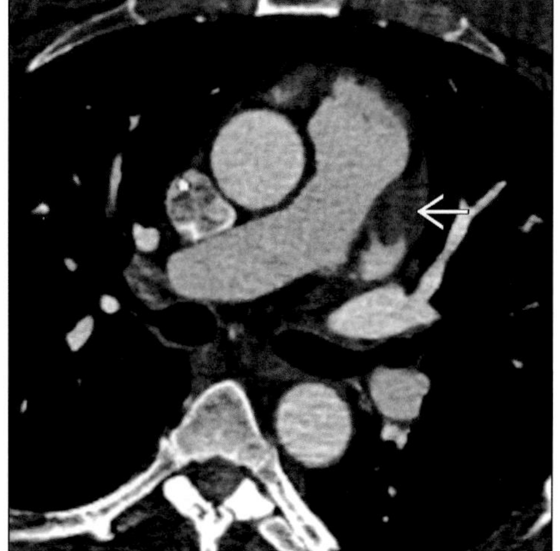

Axial enhanced CT shows a well-marginated filling defect in the left atrial appendage ➡ in a patient with atrial fibrillation. Atrial appendages are common locations for thrombi.

CARDIAC MASS

*(**Left**) Filling defect ➔ is seen in the inferior right atrium in a young patient with testicular cancer. Although any malignancy can metastasize to the heart, this is not commonly reported for this histology. This intracardiac mass resolved after anticoagulation. (**Right**) Four chamber plane at the level of the coronary sinus, delayed Gd-enhanced image using an inversion time of 500 ms, in the same patient shows a low signal intensity of the filling defect ➔.*

Thrombus

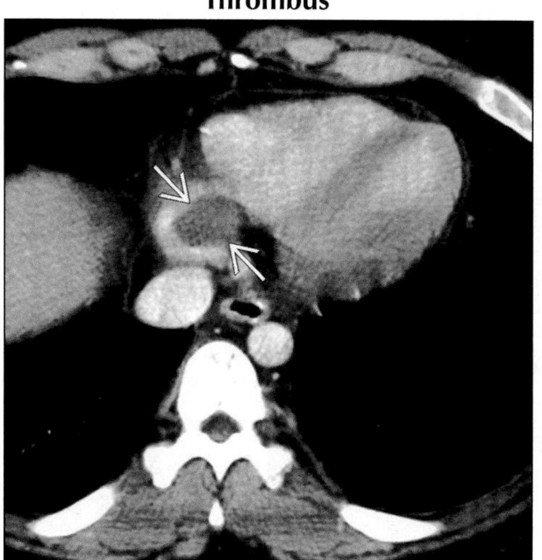

Thrombus

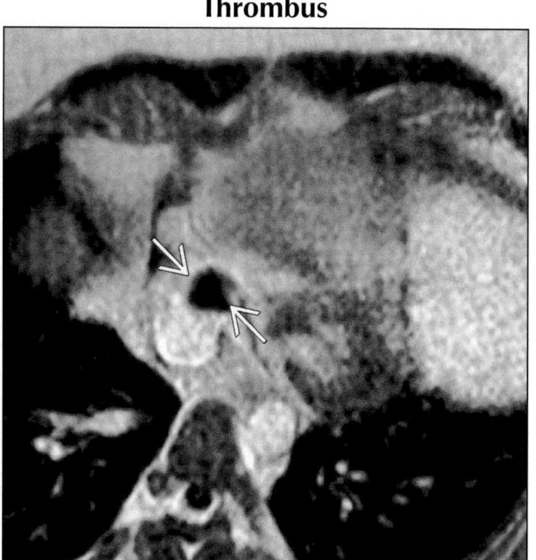

*(**Left**) Frontal radiograph in a patient with known metastatic melanoma shows deviation of the left heart border ➔ (new compared to 1 month prior). Further imaging showed cardiac metastasis. (**Right**) Axial enhanced CT in the same patient with metastatic melanoma shows diffuse hepatic metastasis and expansion of the anterior wall of the left ventricle ➔. Note heterogeneous contrast attenuation.*

Cardiac Metastases

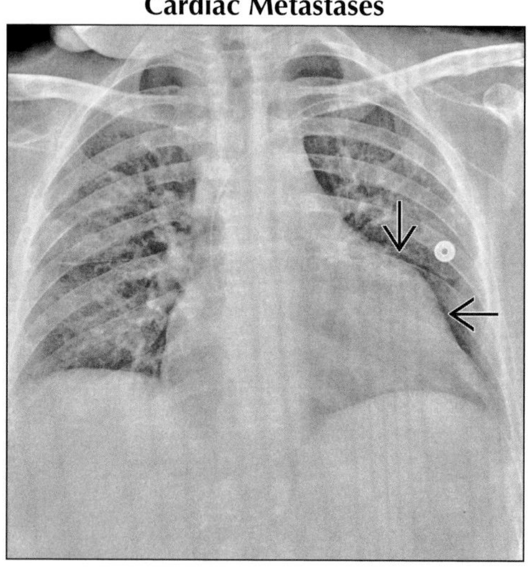

Cardiac Metastases

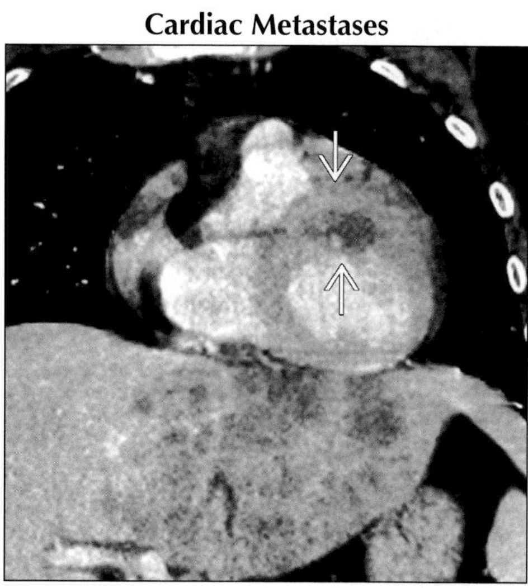

*(**Left**) Axial enhanced CT shows a heterogeneous mass in right and left atrium ➔. Although sparing of the fossa ovalis ➔ suggests lipomatous hypertrophy of intraatrial septum, heterogeneous enhancement, soft tissue attenuation, and involvement of both atria indicate malignancy. (**Right**) Short axis post-Gd enhanced T1-weighted image shows an enhancing mass ➔ in the left atrium, which represented metastatic B-cell lymphoma.*

Cardiac Metastases

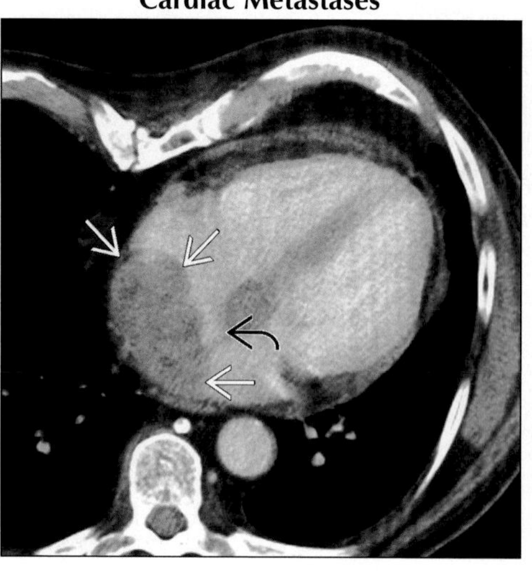

Cardiac Metastases

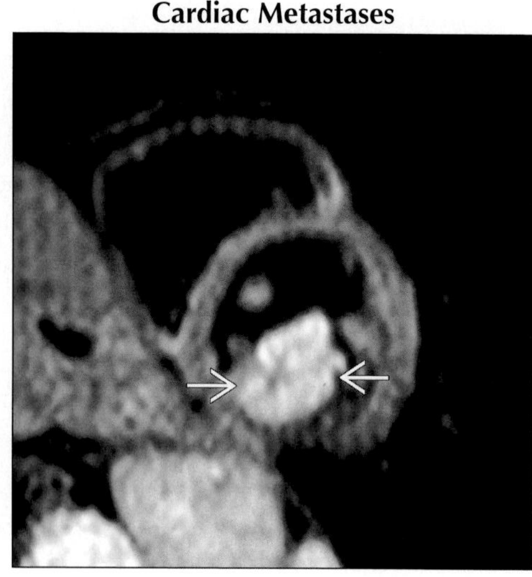

CARDIAC MASS

Myxoma

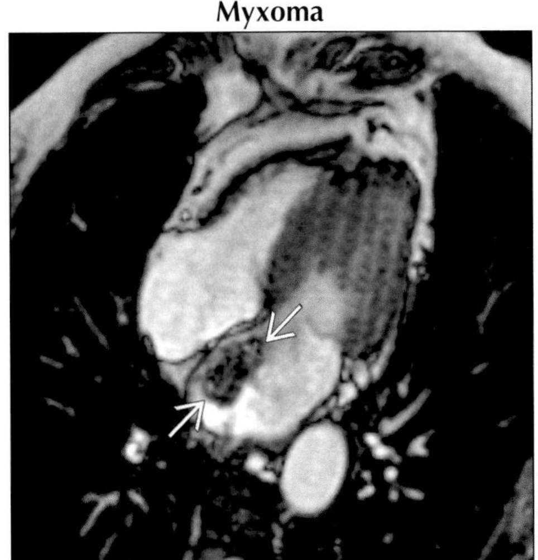

Sarcoma

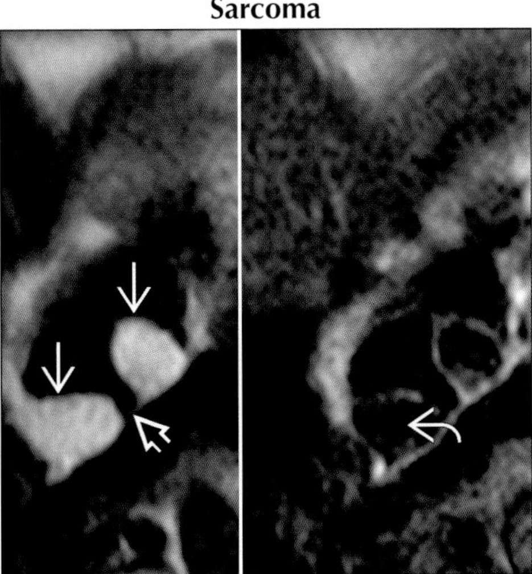

(Left) *Four chamber bright-blood image shows filling defect in LA ➡. Mass was mobile and appeared tethered to intraatrial septum, presumably by a thin stalk.* ***(Right)*** *Four chamber black-blood MR without (left) and with (right) fat suppression shows lipomatous hypertrophy of intraatrial septum ➡. Note sparing of fossa ovalis ➡ and near complete loss of signal with fat suppression ➡. This is benign but may be confused with a cardiac mass.*

Sarcoma

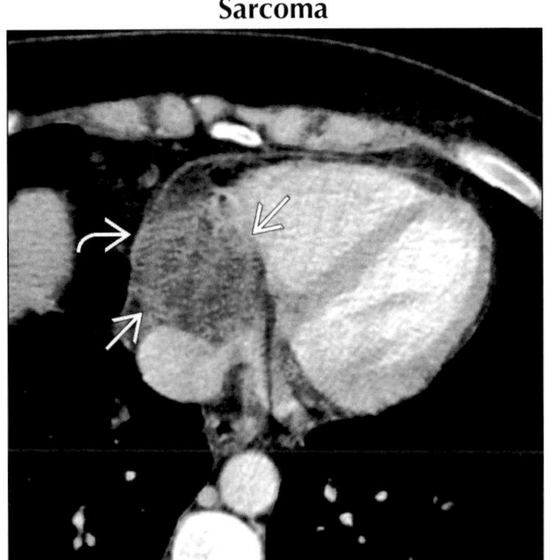

Sarcoma

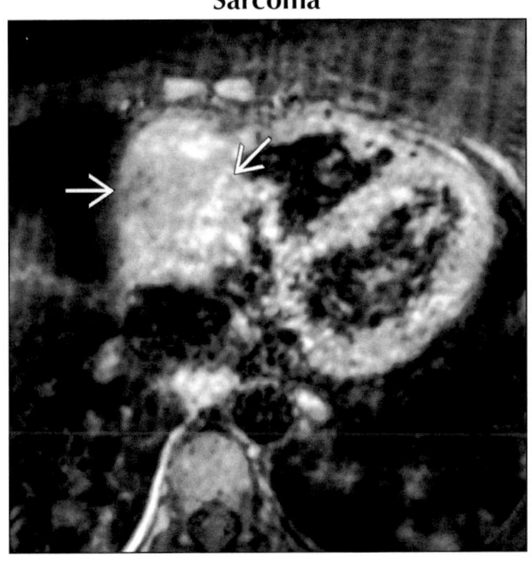

(Left) *Axial enhanced CT shows a heterogeneous enhancing mass filling the right atrium ➡ with extension into the pericardium and obliteration of the epicardial fat ➡. There was no pericardial effusion. Pathology revealed an angiosarcoma.* ***(Right)*** *Axial post-Gd enhanced MR in the same patient shows heterogeneous contrast enhancement ➡. The right atrium is the most common location for cardiac angiosarcoma.*

Sarcoma

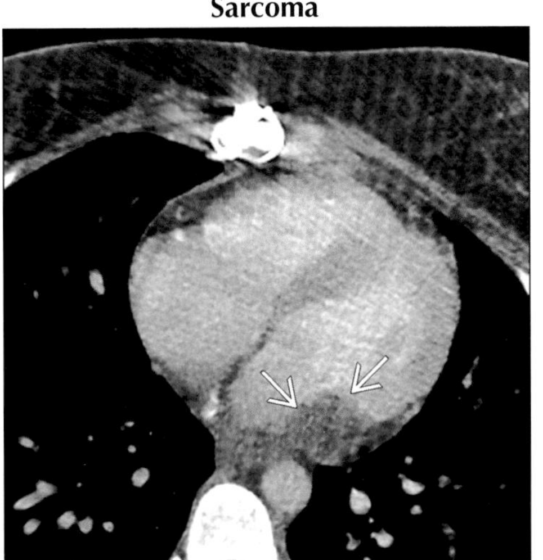

Hemangioma

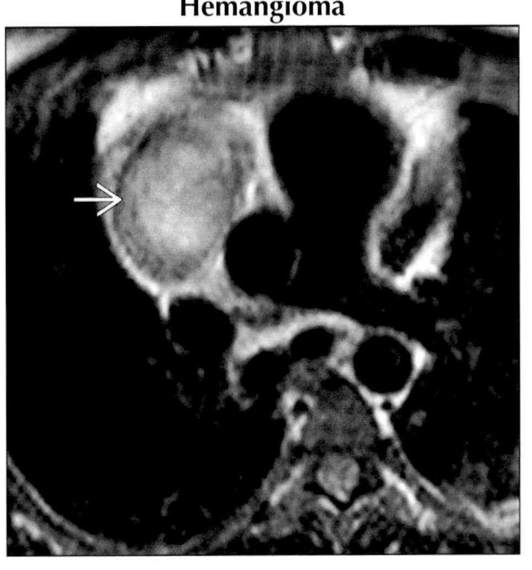

(Left) *Axial enhanced CT shows left posterior atrial wall thickening with a lobulated contour ➡. The mass has a broad attachment base. Resection demonstrated a leiomyosarcoma.* ***(Right)*** *Axial T2-weighted black-blood MR shows a high signal right atrial mass ➡. Note the heterogeneous enhancement following IV contrast administration. Surgical removal revealed hemangioma.*

PERICARDIAL THICKENING

DIFFERENTIAL DIAGNOSIS

Common
- Small Pericardial Effusion (Mimic)
- Malignancy
- Infectious-Idiopathic Pericarditis

Less Common
- Cardiac Surgery
- Uremic Pericarditis
- Radiation-induced Pericarditis

Rare but Important
- Connective Tissue Disease
- Post Myocardial Infarction

ESSENTIAL INFORMATION

Key Differential Diagnosis Issues
- Pericarditis often accompanied by effusion, which significantly aids in diagnosis
  - Hemorrhagic effusion: Malignancy, post myocardial infarction most common
  - Large simple effusion: Infection, idiopathic, and malignancy most common
  - Symptomatic effusion: Malignancy and acute pericarditis most common
- Large effusion without significant thickening makes infectious cause unlikely
- Determination of pericardial thickening
  - Abnormally thickened pericardium ≥ 4 mm with ≥ 6 mm highly specific
  - LV pericardium thinner than RV, > 2 mm may represent abnormal thickening
  - Thickening may be focal, commonly adjacent to atrioventricular groove
- MR imaging features
  - Normal pericardium, low T1W, low T2W, no enhancement
  - Abnormal pericardium, low T1W, high T2W, post-contrast enhancement
- Pericardial thickening in presence of heart failure symptoms is very suggestive of constrictive pericarditis
  - Coexistence of pericardial calcifications further increases suspicion for constrictive pericarditis
  - Imaging features suggesting constriction
    - IVC: Descending aorta ratio ≥ 2; SVC: Descending aorta ratio ≥ 1, coronary sinus dilation, and ascites
    - Biatrial enlargement with normal-sized, tubular-shaped ventricles
    - Septal bounce with respiratory variation in septal wall motion

Helpful Clues for Common Diagnoses
- **Small Pericardial Effusion (Mimic)**
  - Small pericardial effusion on CT can mimic thickening
  - Presence of pulmonary edema, pleural effusions suggest small pericardial effusion is present
  - Observe fluid in pericardial recess or pooling in dependent pericardium
  - High T2W, low T1W signal on MR if simple effusion
  - Pericardial fluid differentiated from soft tissue on inversion recovery sequences
    - Fluid is dark on phase preserved images, bright on magnitude images, indicating long T1
  - Hemorrhagic effusions demonstrate high T1W and absence of enhancement
- **Malignancy**
  - Most commonly from lung cancer, breast cancer, and lymphoma
  - In patients with history of malignancy, ~ 50% of pericardial thickening is due to other causes (most commonly idiopathic)
  - ~ 5% of presenting pericarditis is due to undiagnosed malignancy
  - Nodular pericardium, often enhancing
  - MR shows high T2W signal
- **Infectious-Idiopathic Pericarditis**
  - Pericardial friction rub, fever, and response to NSAIDs
  - Pericardial thickening with enhancement and possible effusion
  - May result in rapid accumulation of serous or serosanguineous pericardial fluid, increasing risk of tamponade
  - Idiopathic pericarditis
    - Diagnosis of exclusion, thought to be most often due to undiagnosed viral infection
  - Infectious pericarditis
    - In developed world, viral and bacterial etiologies are most common
    - Although rare in developed world, tuberculosis remains major cause for pericarditis in developing countries
    - Tuberculous disease of pericardium also presents with mediastinal lymphadenopathy

Helpful Clues for Less Common Diagnoses

- **Cardiac Surgery**
  - Post pericardiotomy syndrome
    - Febrile illness secondary to inflammatory reaction involving pleura and pericardium
  - Patients have history of surgery opening pericardium
  - Aseptic loculated, simple and hemorrhagic effusions all occur
- **Uremic Pericarditis**
  - Occur in patients with chronic renal dysfunction on dialysis or patients with acute renal failure
  - Fibrinous pericarditis caused by accumulated toxins, resolves after dialysis
  - Associated with hemorrhagic effusions
- **Radiation-induced Pericarditis**
  - Radiation pericarditis only seen with > 40 Gy of mediastinal radiation, most commonly delivered in lymphoma and lung cancer treatment
  - Current radiotherapy protocols for breast cancer does not cause pericarditis, unlike older treatment protocols
  - Radiation pericarditis can occur within weeks to decades after exposure
  - Subset may present decades later with recurrent effusions and progressive fibrosis and thickening
  - Associated with rapid accumulation of pericardial fluid and collagen deposition causing pericardial fibrosis, mostly in parietal pericardium
  - Fibrosis will often be present in adjacent tissue
  - Pleural thickening and calcifications will be sharply demarcated, contained within radiation field
- **Connective Tissue Disease**
  - Most commonly rheumatoid arthritis and systemic lupus
  - Most common cardiac manifestation of systemic lupus erythematosus, with 50% developing pericardial effusion at some point
  - Pericarditis can occur with almost any connective tissue disease

Helpful Clues for Rare Diagnoses

- **Post Myocardial Infarction**
  - Larger MI and lack of reperfusion therapy increases risk
  - Immediate form: Within 1 week
    - 5% of patients who receive thrombolytics, 15% of patients who do not
  - Late form: > 1 week post infarct
    - Associated with recurrent bouts of pericarditis, fever (Dressler syndrome)
    - Affects approximately 0.5% of post MI patients who receive thrombolytics, 4% of patients who do not receive thrombolytic therapy

Small Pericardial Effusion (Mimic)

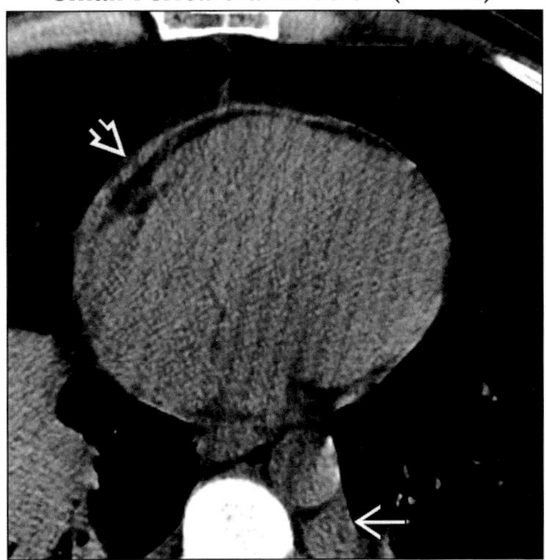

Axial unenhanced CT shows what appears to be smooth pericardial thickening ⇨. This is small pericardial effusion that later resolved. Note pleural effusion ➡.

Small Pericardial Effusion (Mimic)

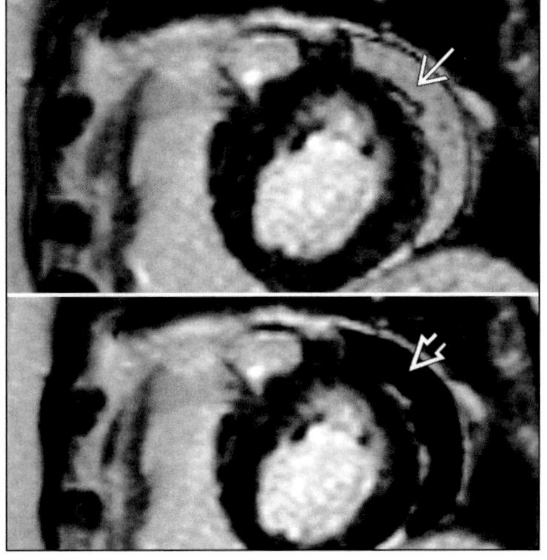

Short axis magnitude (top) and phase preserved (bottom) inversion recovery images show fluid can be identified as high signal on magnitude images ➡ and low signal on phase preserved images ⇨.

PERICARDIAL THICKENING

Malignancy

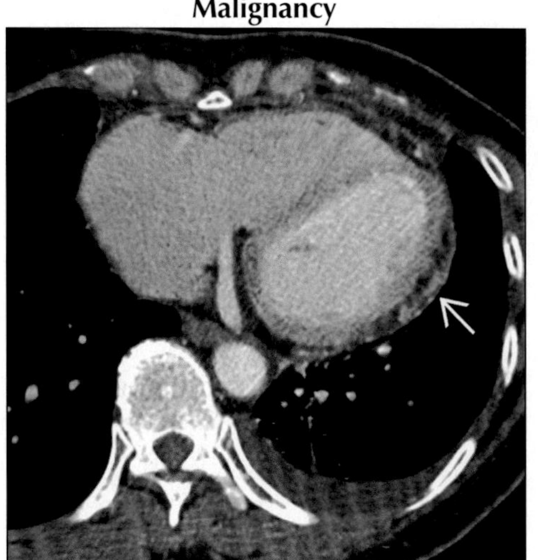

Malignancy

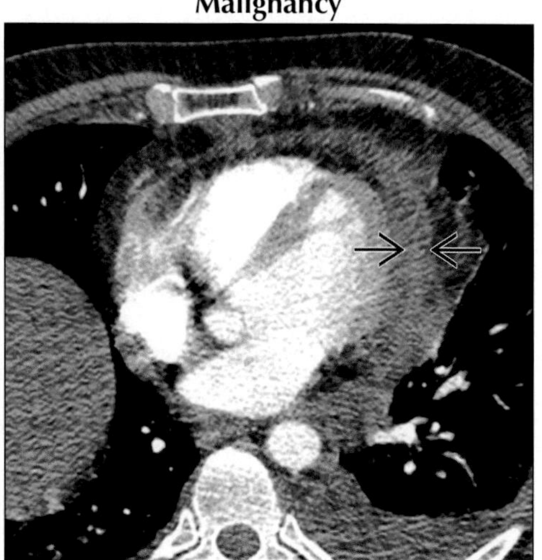

(Left) *Axial enhanced CT shows a nodular pericardium in a patient with biopsy-proven metastasis to the pericardium ➡. Nonmalignant pericardial thickening is smooth.* ***(Right)*** *Axial enhanced CT shows diffuse pericardial thickening ➡ in a patient with lymphomatous involvement of the pericardium.*

Malignancy

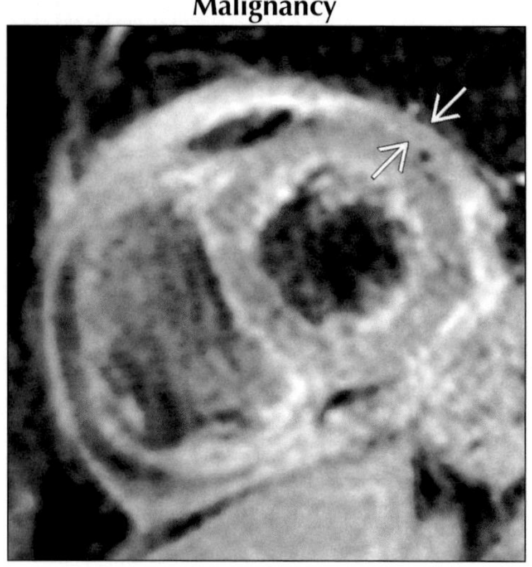

Infectious-Idiopathic Pericarditis

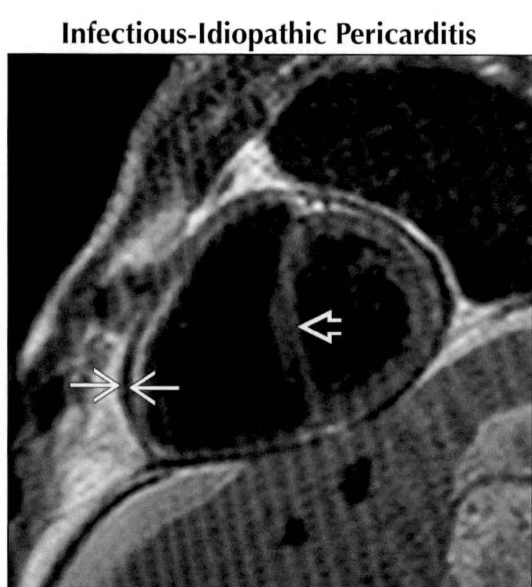

(Left) *Short axis T1W fat-saturated post-Gd MR in a patient with metastatic ovarian cancer and pericardial thickening shows diffuse enhancement of the pericardium ➡. Patient was found to have malignant effusion.* ***(Right)*** *Short axis MR black-blood image shows pericardial thickening ➡ in a patient with remote pericarditis now presenting with pericardial constriction. Note flattening of the interventricular septum ➡.*

Infectious-Idiopathic Pericarditis

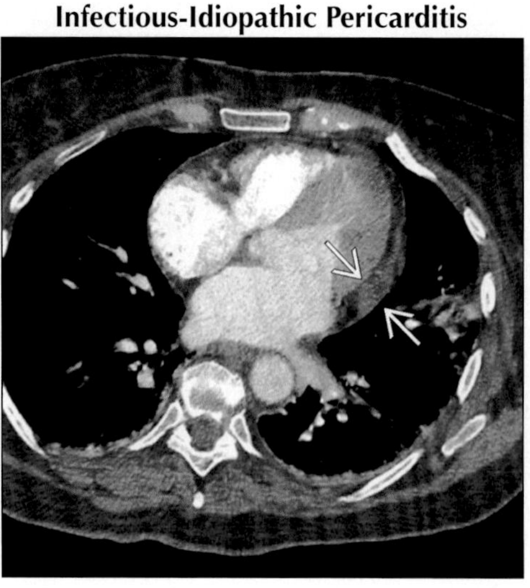

Infectious-Idiopathic Pericarditis

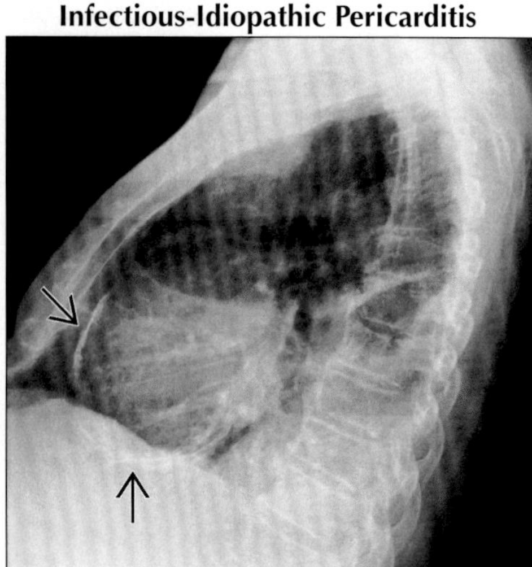

(Left) *Axial CT shows pericardial thickening, particularly in the left atrioventricular grove ➡ in a patient with idiopathic pericarditis. The atrioventricular is the most common location for pericardial thickening.* ***(Right)*** *Lateral chest radiograph shows pericardial calcifications ➡. Although pericardial thickening cannot be seen on radiographs, the presence of pericardial calcifications implies prior pericarditis.*

PERICARDIAL THICKENING

Cardiac Surgery

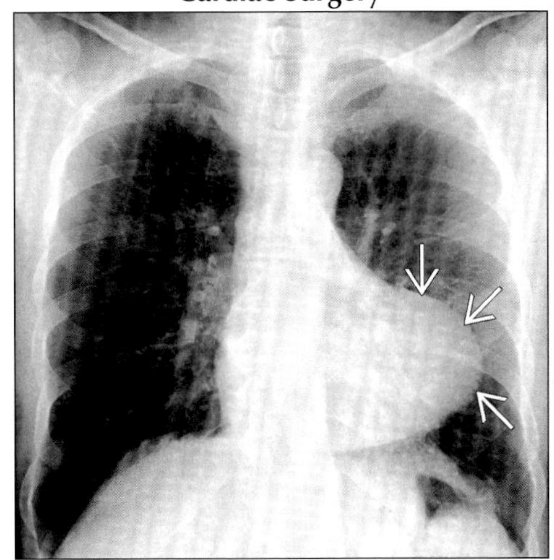

Cardiac Surgery

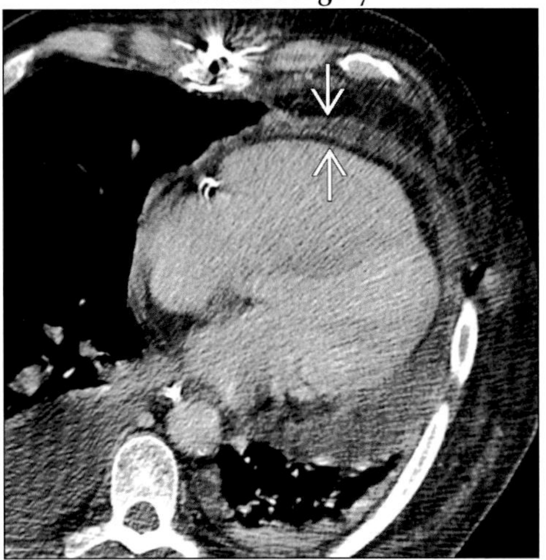

(Left) *Frontal radiograph shows abnormal left cardiac contour ➔. Patient was 1 year post cardiac surgery. Although differential includes herniation via pericardial defect or LV aneurysm, pericardial adhesions and thickening were present.* ***(Right)*** *Axial enhanced CT from a different patient shows pericardial thickening and small effusion ➔ in a patient status post cardiac surgery for repair of a right atrial defect.*

Cardiac Surgery

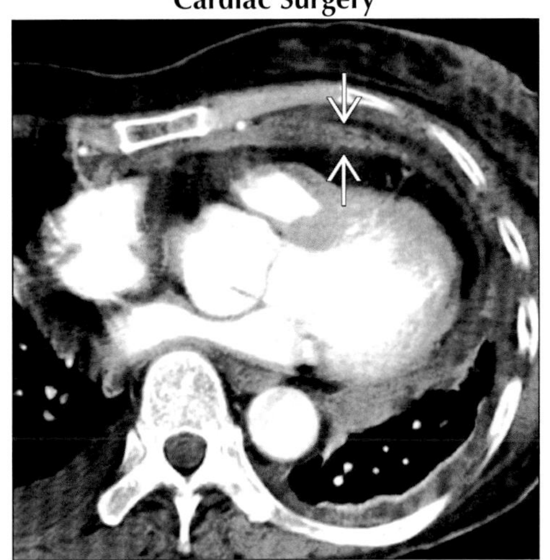

Radiation-induced Pericarditis

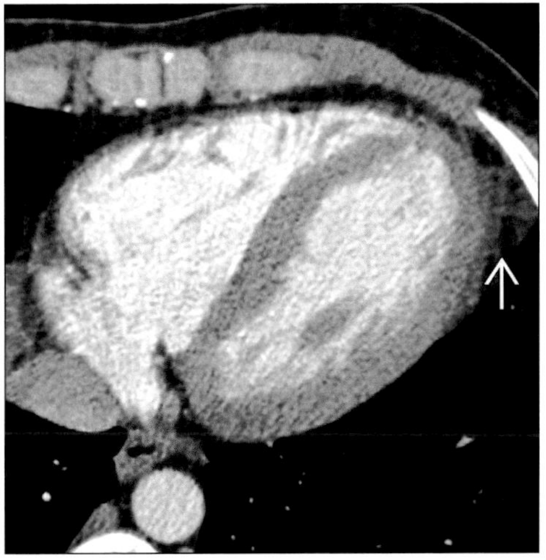

(Left) *Axial enhanced CT shows pericardial thickening and effusion ➔ in a patient status post cardiothoracic surgery. Final diagnosis was post pericardiotomy syndrome.* ***(Right)*** *Axial enhanced CT shows focal pericardial thickening at the cardiac apex with inflammatory stranding of the adjacent pericardial fat ➔. Patient had received > 40 Gy of radiation to the abdomen, which included only the cardiac apex.*

Radiation-induced Pericarditis

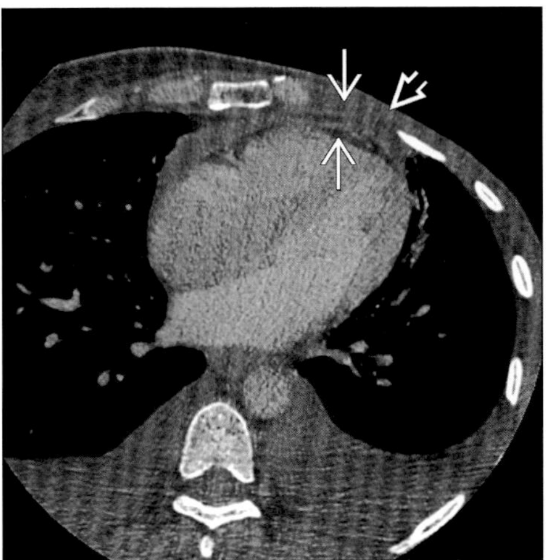

Connective Tissue Disease

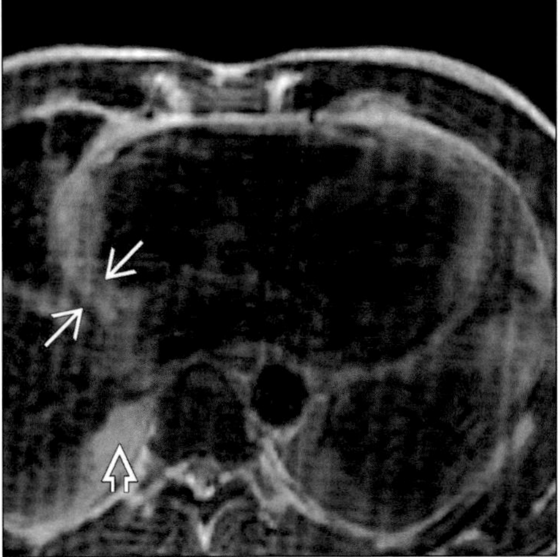

(Left) *Axial enhanced CT shows pericardial thickening in the anterior pericardium ➔ in a patient who received radiation for breast cancer. Note fibrosis of the adjacent soft tissues ⇨.* ***(Right)*** *Axial T2W black-blood image shows pericardial fluid and thickening ➔ in a patient with Still disease and symptoms of pericarditis. Note pleural effusions ⇨.*

PERICARDIAL CALCIFICATION

DIFFERENTIAL DIAGNOSIS

Common
- Prior Pericarditis

Less Common
- Prior Hemopericardium

Rare but Important
- Prior Radiation

ESSENTIAL INFORMATION

Key Differential Diagnosis Issues
- Any cause of chronic or prior pericarditis may cause pericardial calcification
- Calcification features or distribution limited in identifying etiology, history most helpful
- Calcifications adjacent to pericardium are often mistaken for pericardial calcifications, particularly when overlying left ventricle
- Constrictive pericarditis: Pericardial calcification with dilated IVC, SVC, atria, tubular ventricles, and hepatic vein contrast reflux
- Reporting spatial location of calcifications assist in planning surgical therapy

Helpful Clues for Common Diagnoses
- **Prior Pericarditis**
  - Although TB is uncommon in developed world, it is a common cause of calcified pericardium in developing world
    - Characteristically thick, irregular, amorphous calcifications predominantly over anterior and inferior RV
  - Uremic pericarditis: Eggshell calcification pattern
  - Idiopathic: Diagnosis of exclusion; often result of undiagnosed viral infection

Helpful Clues for Less Common Diagnoses
- **Prior Hemopericardium**
  - Most commonly from trauma, malignancy, or surgery
  - Metastasis
    - Far more common than primary tumors
    - Nodular pericardium with coexistent hemopericardium
    - Lung cancer, breast cancer, and lymphoma account for 75% of cases

Helpful Clues for Rare Diagnoses
- **Prior Radiation**
  - Acute and chronic forms of radiation pericarditis can lead to calcification
  - Radiotherapy must exceed 40 Gy, a dose most commonly delivered for Hodgkin disease or lung cancer
  - Acute pericarditis can occur weeks to months after radiation
  - Acute pericarditis is generally symptomatic
  - Chronic pericarditis does not occur before 6 months
    - More often leads to constrictive physiology but can be asymptomatic
  - Fibrosis of adjacent mediastinal adipose tissue

Prior Pericarditis

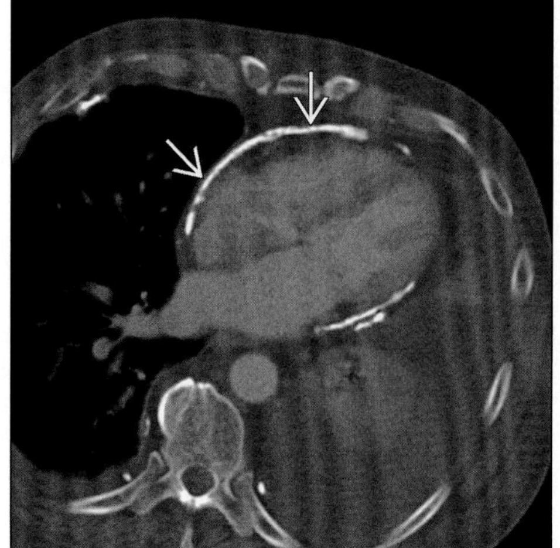

Axial enhanced CT shows dense pericardial calcifications of the pericardium ➔. Cardiac chambers appear normal in size. Compare with postsurgical appearance in figure to the right.

Prior Pericarditis

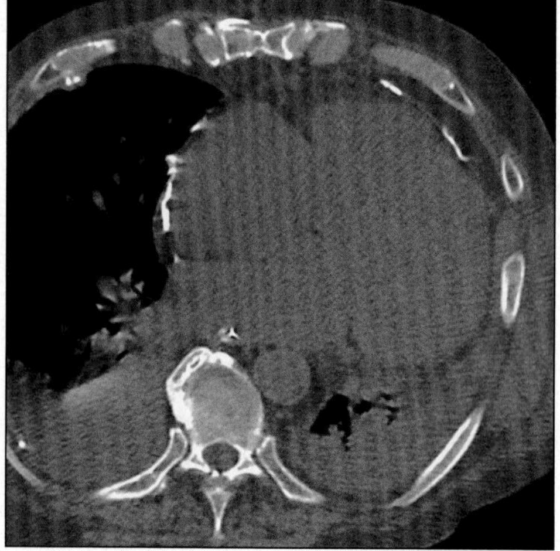

Axial enhanced CT shows the same patient shown on the left but after pericardial stripping. Cardiac enlargement illustrates the degree of anatomic distortion caused by pericardial constriction.

PERICARDIAL CALCIFICATION

Prior Pericarditis

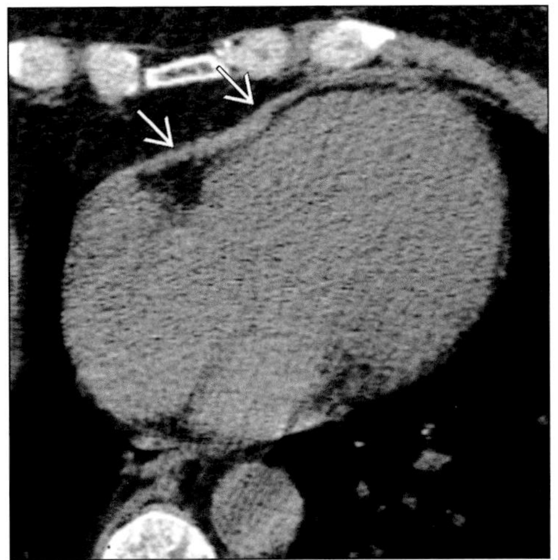

Prior Pericarditis

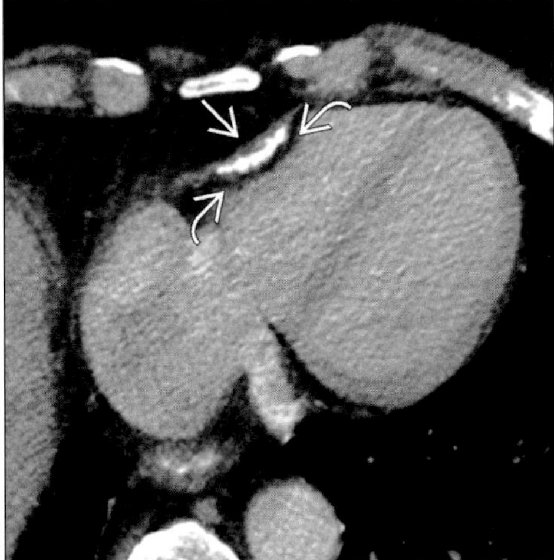

*(**Left**) Axial unenhanced CT shows pericardial thickening ➡ in a patient with chronic pericarditis due to rheumatoid arthritis. Chronic pericarditis can lead to calcifications. (**Right**) Axial enhanced CT in the same patient 10 years later shows development of pericardial calcifications ➡ in region of longstanding pericardial thickening. Note focal constriction on right ventricle ➡.*

Prior Pericarditis

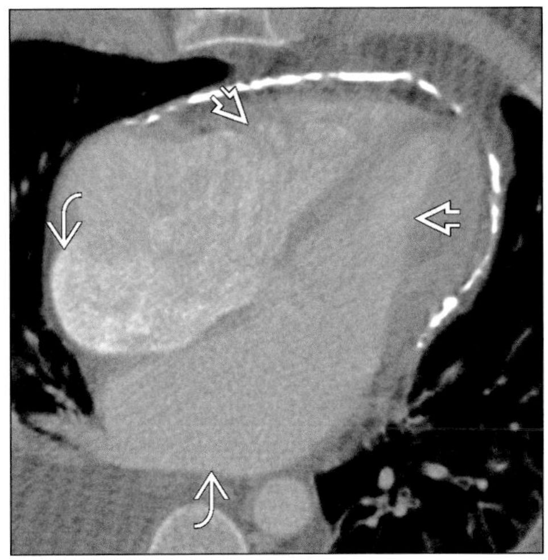

Prior Pericarditis

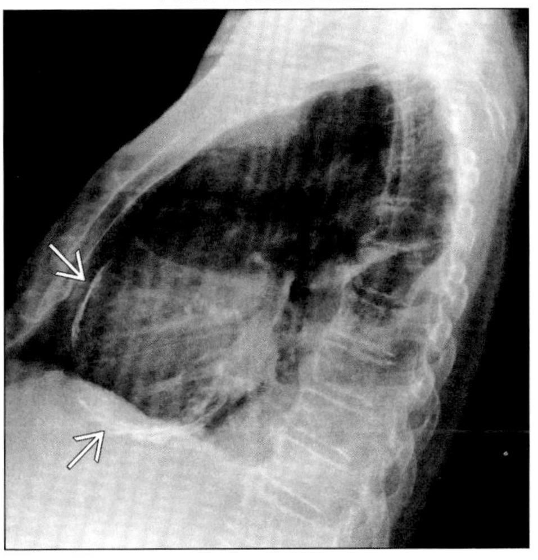

*(**Left**) Axial enhanced CT shows apical predominant pericardial calcifications in a 45-year-old patient with history of tuberculosis. Note tubular ventricles ➡ and dilated atria ➡. (**Right**) Lateral radiograph shows pericardial calcifications of the anterior and inferior wall ➡ in a patient with suspected remote pericarditis.*

Prior Hemopericardium

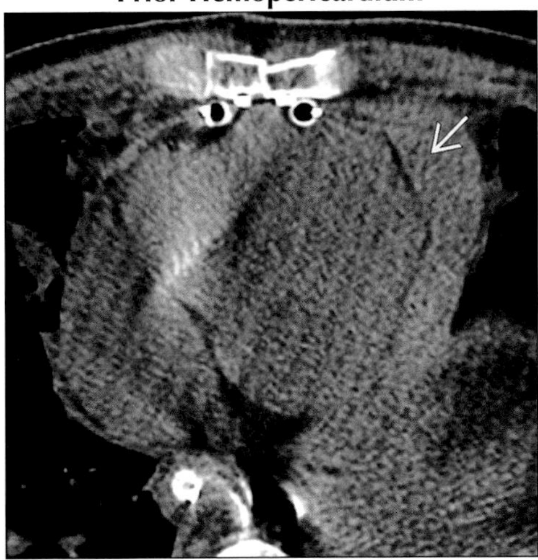

Prior Radiation

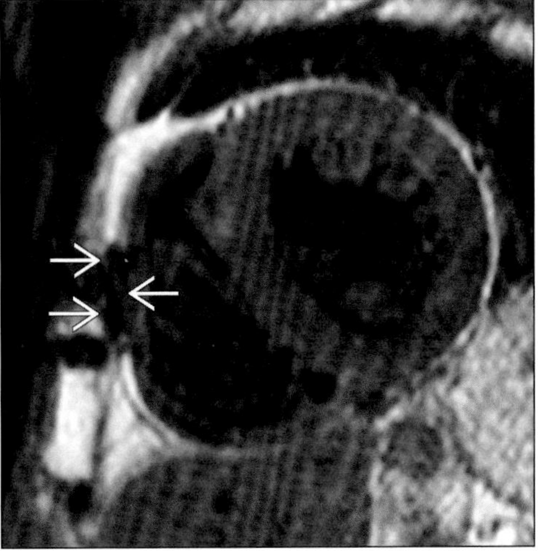

*(**Left**) Axial unenhanced CT shows high-density pericardial fluid ➡ in patient with hemopericardium. Although this represents the acute presentation, these patients may develop pericardial calcifications. (**Right**) Short axis black blood MR shows signal loss at the anterior pericardium ➡ in a patient with focal pericardial calcification from prior mediastinal radiation. Signal loss is greater with gradient echo sequences as apposed to the spin echo sequence shown here.*

PERICARDIAL MASS

DIFFERENTIAL DIAGNOSIS

Common
- Metastatic Disease
- Loculated Fluid or Focal Thickening

Less Common
- Benign Primary Pericardial Tumors

Rare but Important
- Primary Pericardial Mesothelioma
- Other Malignant Primary Pericardial Tumors

ESSENTIAL INFORMATION

Key Differential Diagnosis Issues
- Diagnostic evaluation should focus on distinction between neoplastic and nonneoplastic etiology
- Loculated fluid or thickening can easily be confused with neoplastic pericardial mass
- If patient has history of breast cancer, lung cancer, or lymphoma cancer, focal thickening is equally likely to be metastatic tumor versus other cause
- Without history of cancer, undiagnosed malignancy should be considered less likely
- Absence of enhancement or low-density fluid suggest nonneoplastic etiology

Helpful Clues for Common Diagnoses
- **Metastatic Disease**
  - Far more common than primary tumors
  - Nodular, enhancing pericardium; mediastinal adenopathy
  - Lung, breast, and lymphoma account for 75% of cases
- **Loculated Fluid or Focal Thickening**
  - Low-density, well-circumscribed fluid suggests pericardial cyst
  - Thick, enhancing wall surrounding fluid suggests abscess

Helpful Clues for Less Common Diagnoses
- **Benign Primary Pericardial Tumors**
  - Teratoma: Most common benign tumor, heterogeneous CT attenuation
    - Most often in children
  - Lipoma: Encapsulated fat, high T1W signal decreased with fat suppression
  - Hemangioma: Strong contrast enhancement
  - Fibroma: Low T1W and T2W signal; no contrast enhancement

Helpful Clues for Rare Diagnoses
- **Primary Pericardial Mesothelioma**
  - Most common primary neoplasm of pericardium
  - Represents 50% of all primary pericardial tumors, 1% of all malignant mesothelioma
  - Diffuse nodular pericardial thickening with calcification and associated effusion
- **Malignant Primary Pericardial Tumors**
  - Lymphoma, sarcoma, and liposarcoma most common histologies
  - Large, enhancing mass associated with hemopericardium

Metastatic Disease

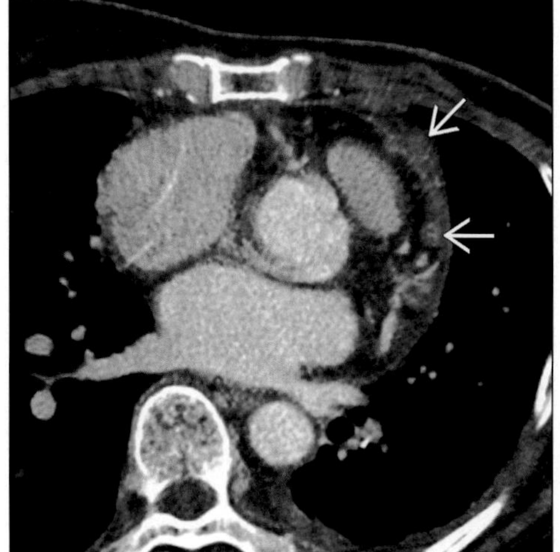

Axial enhanced CT shows nodular enhancing pericardial masses ➔ in a patient with known metastatic lung cancer. These patients can present with hemopericardium.

Loculated Fluid or Focal Thickening

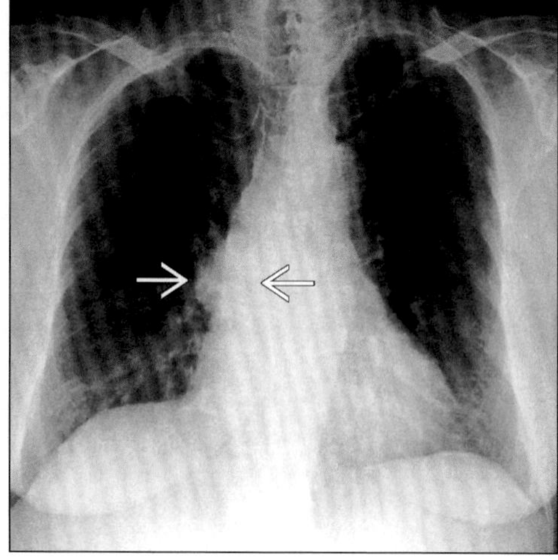

Frontal radiograph shows a rounded opacity superimposed upon the right heart border ➔. On CT this was found to represent a pericardial cyst.

Loculated Fluid or Focal Thickening

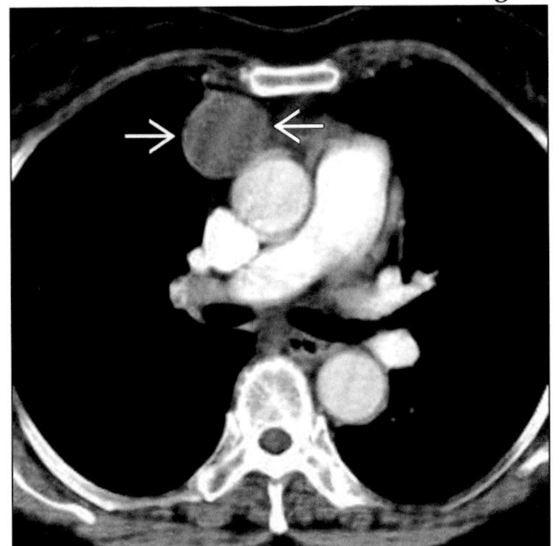

Loculated Fluid or Focal Thickening

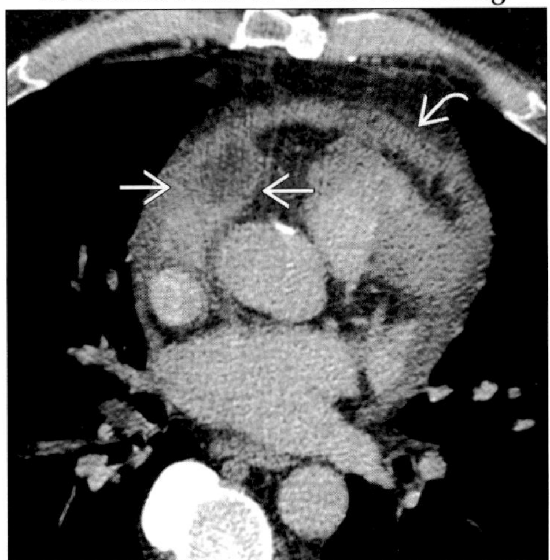

(Left) *Axial enhanced CT of the chest shows a pericardial cyst as a well-circumscribed, thin-walled fluid collection ➔ adjacent to the right atrium without adjacent inflammatory stranding.* ***(Right)*** *Axial enhanced CT from a patient with a pericardial abscess shows a fluid collection adjacent to the right atrial appendage ➔. The collection has thick, enhancing walls and there is associated pericardial thickening ➔ and inflammatory stranding.*

Benign Primary Pericardial Tumors

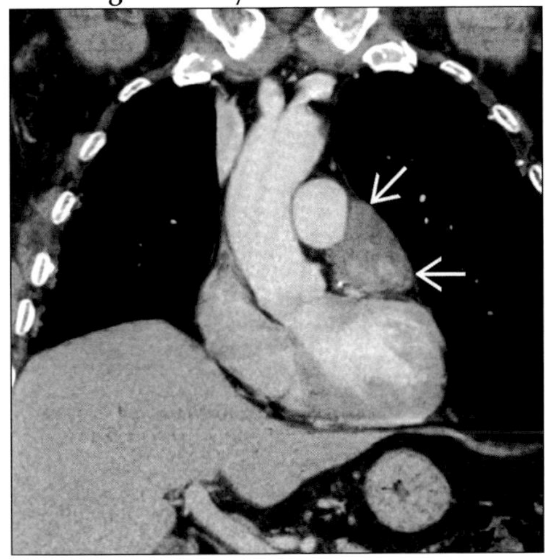

Benign Primary Pericardial Tumors

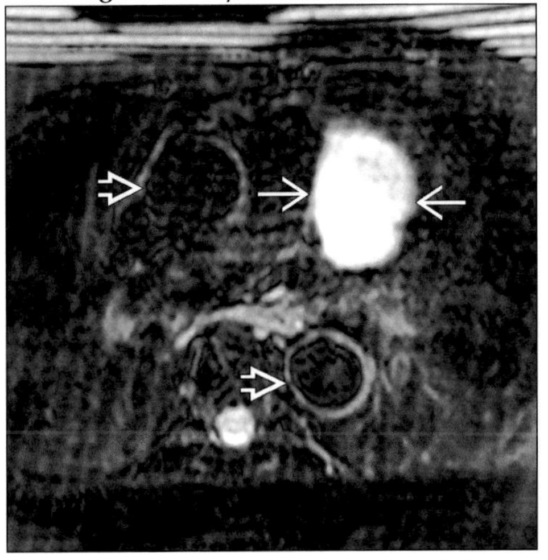

(Left) *Coronal enhanced CT from a patient with a pericardial hemangioma shows heterogeneous contrast enhancement of a pericardial mass adjacent to the left atrial appendage ➔. Fat planes adjacent to the pericardium are preserved, a benign feature.* ***(Right)*** *Axial T2WI fat-saturated MR shows high signal adjacent to the left atrial appendage ➔ in a patient with a hemangioma. Note the aorta as an anatomic landmark ➔.*

Other Malignant Primary Pericardial Tumors

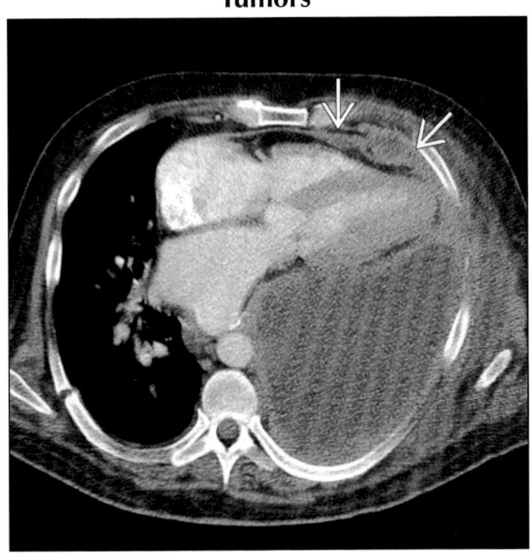

Other Malignant Primary Pericardial Tumors

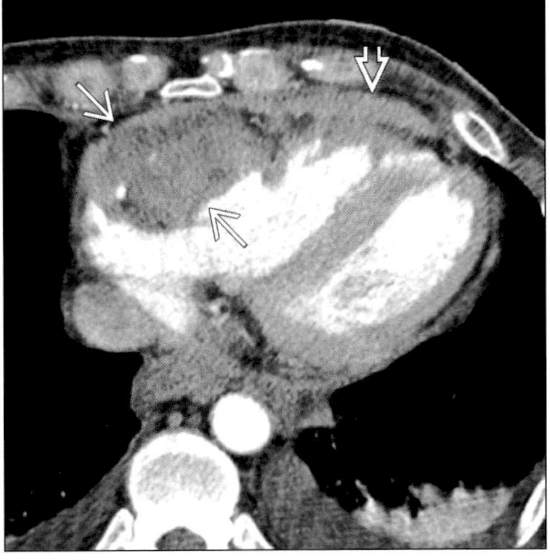

(Left) *Axial enhanced CT shows extension of a pleural mesothelioma along the anterior pericardium ➔. Pericardial extension of a primary pleural mesothelioma is far more common than a primary pericardial tumor.* ***(Right)*** *Axial enhanced CT from a patient with lymphoma shows a right-sided heart mass that extends from the pericardium to the right ventricle lumen ➔. Note the hemopericardium ➔.*

AORTIC INTRAMURAL ABNORMALITY

DIFFERENTIAL DIAGNOSIS

Common
- Atherosclerosis/Adherent Thrombus
- Aortic Dissection

Less Common
- Aortic Intramural Hematoma
- Penetrating Atherosclerotic Ulcer

Rare but Important
- Takayasu/Giant Cell Arteritis
- Radiation

ESSENTIAL INFORMATION

Key Differential Diagnosis Issues
- Aortic wall should measure < 4 mm
- Aortic wall should be isointense to lumen

Helpful Clues for Common Diagnoses
- **Atherosclerosis/Adherent Thrombus**
  - Concentric diffuse involvement vs. spiral involvement of intramural hematoma
  - Aorta often tortuous with atherosclerotic disease in branch vessels
- **Aortic Dissection**
  - Intimal flap readily seen on contrast CT as unenhanced line through lumen
  - Intraluminal calcifications on noncontrast CT suggest diagnosis and represent displaced intimal calcifications
  - "Beak" sign: False lumen side of dissection flap meets outer wall with acute angle
  - "Cobweb" sign: False lumen traversed by media fibers
  - Confusion with pulsation artifact at aortic root avoided by inspecting coronal images

Helpful Clues for Less Common Diagnoses
- **Aortic Intramural Hematoma**
  - Hyperdense aortic wall compared to lumen when acute, isodense when old
  - Check LV chamber for hypodense blood to avoid pitfall of confusion anemia
  - Patient more likely to progress to dissection with coexistence of ulcer-like projections
  - Most commonly in descending aorta
- **Penetrating Atherosclerotic Ulcer**
  - Luminal irregularity
  - Must extend beyond expected contour of intima
  - Outer aortic wall thickening indicates acuity

Helpful Clues for Rare Diagnoses
- **Takayasu/Giant Cell Arteritis**
  - Radiographically indistinguishable, differentiated based on age (Takayasu < 50 years, giant cell > 50 years)
  - FDG PET can determine active disease
  - Aortic caliber will be reduced
  - Subclavian stenosis is hallmark finding
  - Pulmonary artery strictures and mesenteric vessel stenosis are common
- **Radiation**
  - Vascular calcifications confined to radiation field
  - Radiation history will be present

Atherosclerosis/Adherent Thrombus

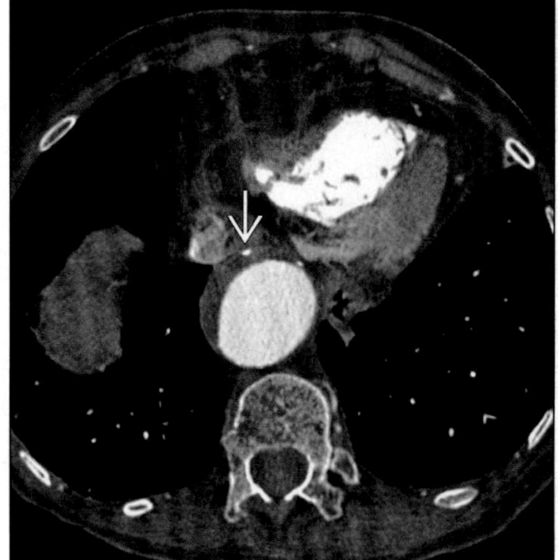

Axial enhanced CT shows mural thrombus in an otherwise dilated aorta. Note that intimal calcifications are on the outer edge of the thrombus ➡.

Aortic Dissection

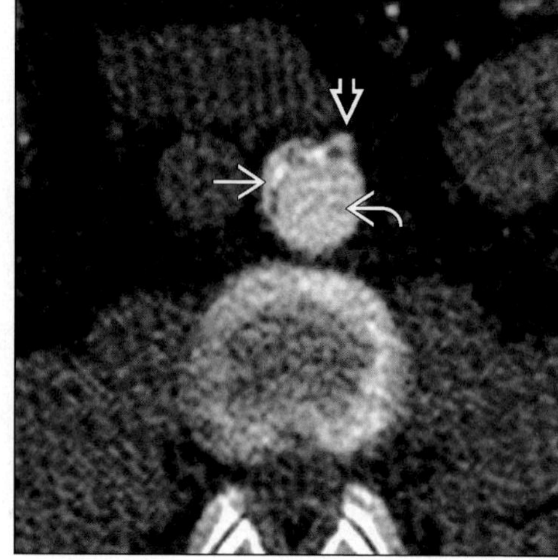

Axial enhanced CT shows a severely displaced dissection flap, compressing the true lumen and occluding the SMA ⇨. Note true lumen ➡ and false lumen ↪. This was treated with fenestration.

AORTIC INTRAMURAL ABNORMALITY

Aortic Dissection

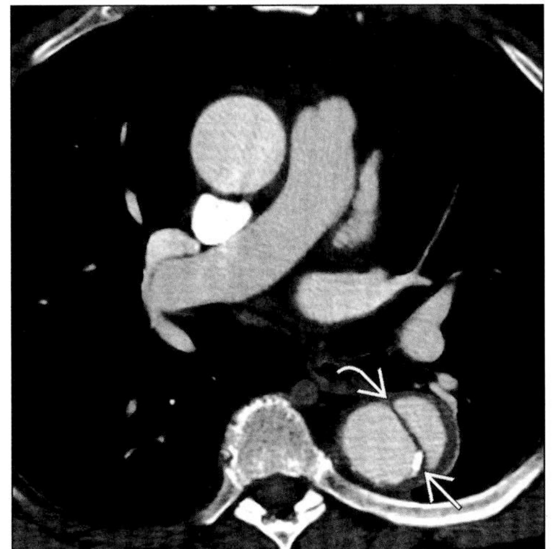

Aortic Intramural Hematoma

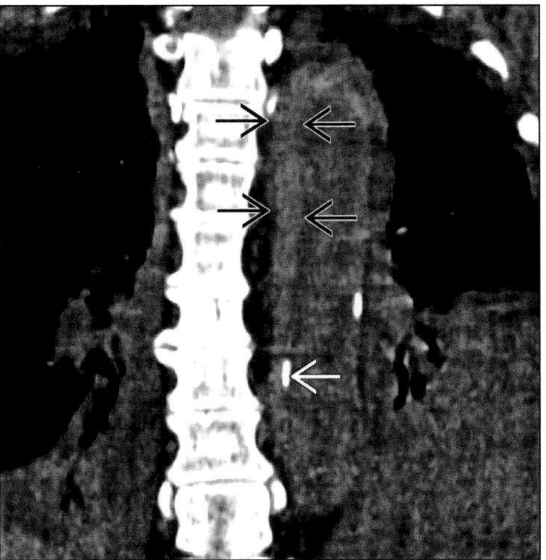

(Left) *Axial enhanced CT shows a dissection flap ➦ in the descending aorta with a displaced intimal calcification ➡. The dissection did not involve the arch and was managed medically.* ***(Right)*** *Coronal unenhanced CT shows asymmetric thickening and hyperdense ➡ aortic wall, representing the hematoma. Note the displaced intimal calcification ➡.*

Aortic Intramural Hematoma

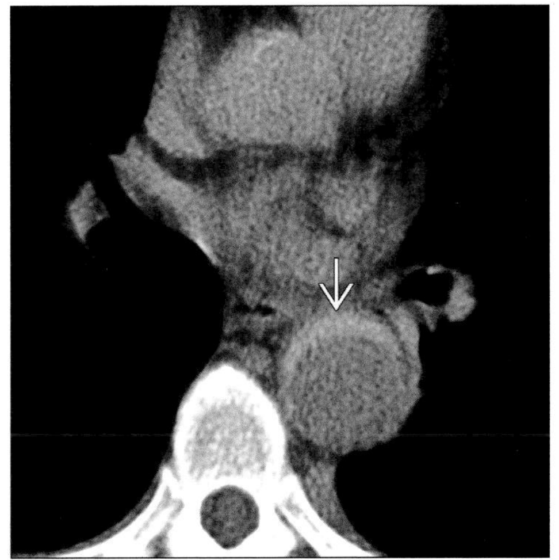

Penetrating Atherosclerotic Ulcer

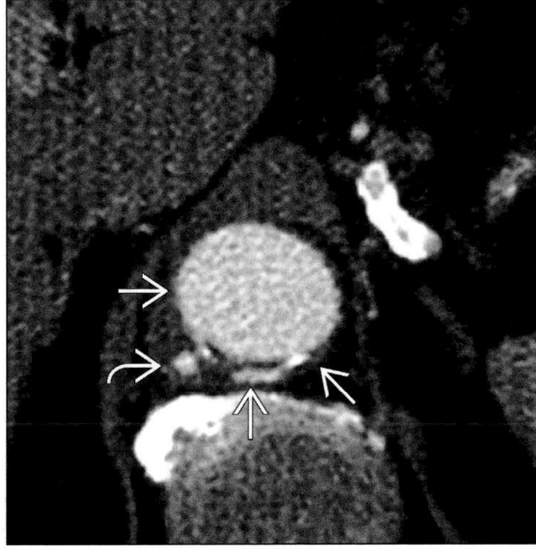

(Left) *Axial enhanced CT shows hyperdense, thickened aortic wall ➡ in a hypertensive patient who presented to the ER with back pain. This finding can be missed on an enhanced exam.* ***(Right)*** *Axial enhanced CT shows a small focus of contrast ➦ extending beyond the expected aortic wall ➡. Adjacent wall thickening suggested it is likely acute and explains the patient's back pain.*

Takayasu/Giant Cell Arteritis

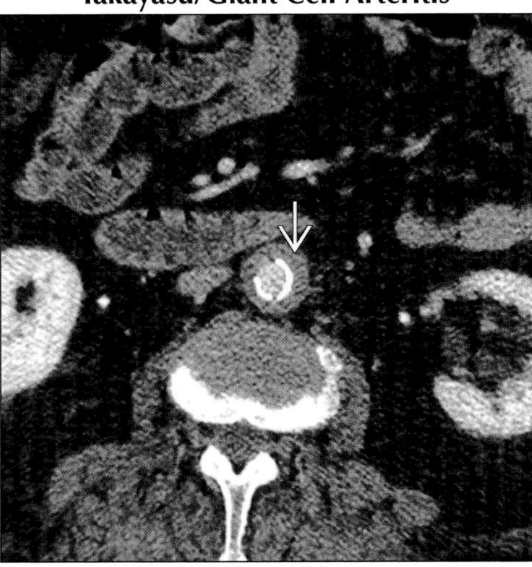

Radiation

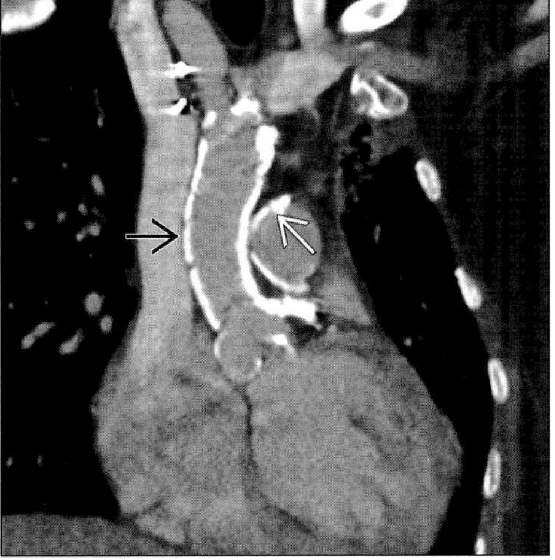

(Left) *Axial enhanced CT shows thickened aortic wall ➡ with inner intimal calcifications. Although causing aortic narrowing, this may progress to aneurysmal dilation.* ***(Right)*** *Double oblique enhanced CT shows dense aortic ➡ and pulmonary artery ➡ calcifications in a patient who received prior mediastinal radiation. Vascular calcifications were not present elsewhere. Note that calcifications are spatially confined to the radiation field.*

DILATED AORTA

DIFFERENTIAL DIAGNOSIS

Common
- Atherosclerotic
- Degenerative
- Aortic Stenosis

Less Common
- Aortic Dissection
- Pseudoaneurysm
  - Mycotic Aneurysm
  - Penetrating Atherosclerotic Ulcer
  - Post-Traumatic Pseudoaneurysm

Rare but Important
- Collagen Vascular Diseases
- Connective Tissue Disease
- Syphilis

ESSENTIAL INFORMATION

Key Differential Diagnosis Issues
- Pathology indicated by outer diameter measurements
  - Measurements providing high specificity for pathology
    - Ascending > 4.5 cm
    - Proximal descending > 3.2 cm
    - Ascending:descending ratio > 1.5:1
    - Isthmus:hiatus ratio > 1.4:1
    - Aorta should taper throughout course; focal distal diameter increase of > 50% is abnormal
- Morphology
  - Saccular (false aneurysm): Dissection, mycotic, post-traumatic, penetrating atherosclerotic ulcer (PAU)
  - Fusiform (true aneurysm): Atherosclerosis, valvular disease
- Location
  - Ascending aorta: Valvular pathology, dissection, connective tissue disease, syphilis
  - Descending aorta: Dissection, PAU, atherosclerotic, mycotic, post-traumatic
- Distance of aneurysm from major branch vessels determines feasibility of stent placement
- Tortuosity, calcification, and minimum luminal diameter of iliac arteries determine vascular access strategy
- Diameter of proximal and distal aneurysm determines selection of stent size
- Etiology of aneurysm (mycotic, inflammatory, or atherosclerotic) influences decision to treat surgically or endovascular

Helpful Clues for Common Diagnoses
- **Atherosclerotic**
  - Descending aorta: Tortuous, diffuse intimal calcifications, mural thrombus, focal dilation
  - Caused by intimal disease with fibrous replacement of underlying media
  - Coexistent small and medium vessel atherosclerosis
- **Degenerative**
  - Systemic hypertension: Leads to accelerated elastic fiber fragmentation and smooth muscle degeneration
  - Ascending aortic dilation with relative preservation of root diameter
  - Older patients
- **Aortic Stenosis**
  - Dense calcifications of aortic valve
  - Grade of stenosis related to valve area
    - > 2.0 cm^2: No hemodynamically significant stenosis
    - 2–1.5 cm^2: Mild stenosis
    - 1.5–1 cm^2: Moderate stenosis
    - < 1 cm^2: Severe stenosis
  - Aortic bicuspid-related stenosis
    - Young patient with calcified valve despite paucity of vascular calcifications elsewhere
    - Prevalence of 1:1,000: Men more commonly affected
    - Associated with aortic coarctation and patent ductus arteriosus
    - Prone to dissection

Helpful Clues for Less Common Diagnoses
- **Aortic Dissection**
  - Intimal calcifications displaced toward aortic lumen: Can be appreciated on unenhanced study
  - False lumen expands, leading to aortic dilation
  - Majority of patients present with systemic hypertension
  - Intimal flap seen on enhanced CT, 3D MRA, or MR black-blood sequence
  - May occur in areas of prior intramural hematoma or penetrating atherosclerotic ulcer
- **Pseudoaneurysm**

- **Mycotic Aneurysm**
  - Saccular configuration, irregular lumen, larger than PAU
  - Adjacent abscess or inflammation
  - More common etiology in young patients with thoracic aortic aneurysms
  - Most commonly caused by bacterial infection (*Staphylococcus* and *Salmonella*) at site of prior aortic defect
  - Patients will have prior history of sepsis, IV drug use, endocarditis
- **Penetrating Atherosclerotic Ulcer**
  - Diffuse atherosclerotic disease present
  - Penetration of contrast beyond expected outer aortic wall contour
  - Adjacent inflammatory stranding and wall thickening present
  - On MR, slow-flowing blood may make PAU appear thrombosed; phase contrast or MRA will more accurately characterize
  - New PAU found with adjacent inflammation may indicate cause of symptoms in patients presenting with chest pain
- **Post-Traumatic Pseudoaneurysm**
  - History of high-energy blunt trauma
  - Aortic contour abnormality at ligamentum arteriosum
  - Can less commonly occur at aortic root or hiatus
  - Calcifications indicate remote trauma

Helpful Clues for Rare Diagnoses

- **Collagen Vascular Diseases**
  - Takayasu/giant cell arteritis
    - Radiographically indistinguishable; Takayasu suspected in age < 40 years, giant cell suspected in age > 40 years
    - Wall thickening and enhancement present
    - Branch vessel involvement present, classically subclavian stenosis
    - Although most commonly causes stenosis, aneurysms can develop
    - May also present with pulmonary artery stenoses
- **Connective Tissue Disease**
  - Marfan syndrome, Ehlers-Danlos syndrome
  - Connective tissue defect of aortic wall
  - Annuloaortic ectasia present with ascending aorta dilation creates "tulip bulb" appearance
  - Aortic root dilation often results in aortic regurgitation at presentation
- **Syphilis**
  - Occurs in tertiary syphilis
  - Frequency in develop world has markedly decreased
  - Often manifest as descending aortic aneurysm although abdominal aortic aneurysm and sinus of Valsalva aneurysms occur
  - Chronic inflammation leads to obliterative endarteritis causing ischemia of media and adventitia

Atherosclerotic

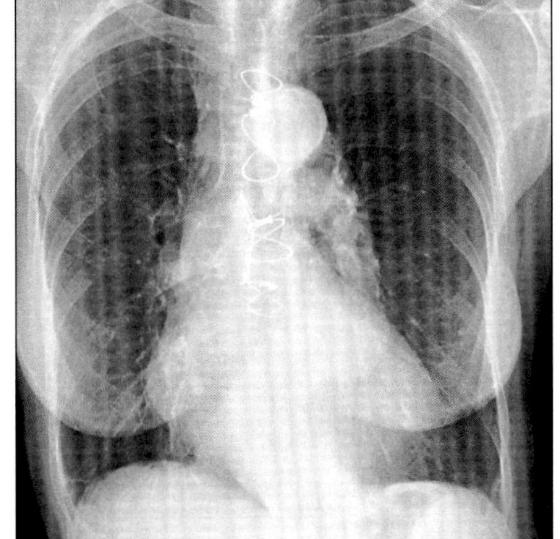

Frontal radiograph shows a dilated tortuous aorta with diffuse calcifications. Intimal disease further exacerbates medial degeneration by increasing wall stress and restricting blood flow.

Atherosclerotic

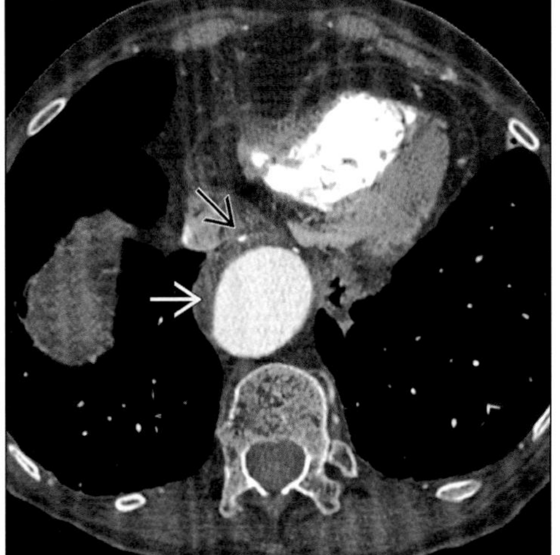

Axial enhanced CT shows intimal disease with mural thrombus ➡ and intimal calcifications ⇨. This patient had a diffusely dilated and tortuous aorta.

DILATED AORTA

(**Left**) Coronal enhanced CT shows extravasation of contrast ➡ from a dilated abdominal aorta. Note extravasated blood ➡, which can easily be detected with unenhanced CT. (**Right**) Axial enhanced CT shows dilated abdominal aorta with extensive mural thrombus ➡. Calcifications ➡ occur when the thrombus is chronic and does not represent displaced intimal calcifications.

Atherosclerotic

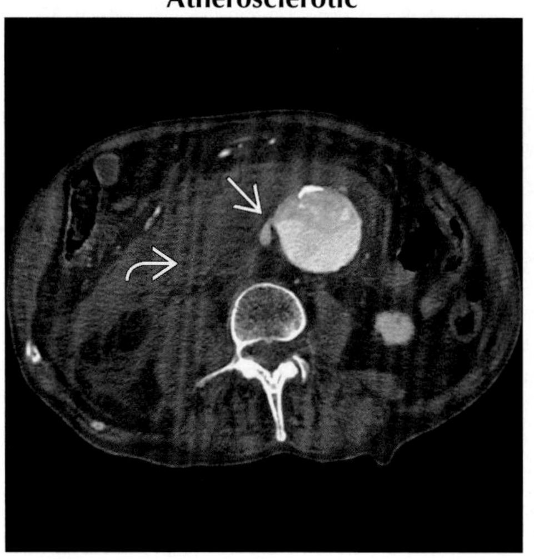

Atherosclerotic

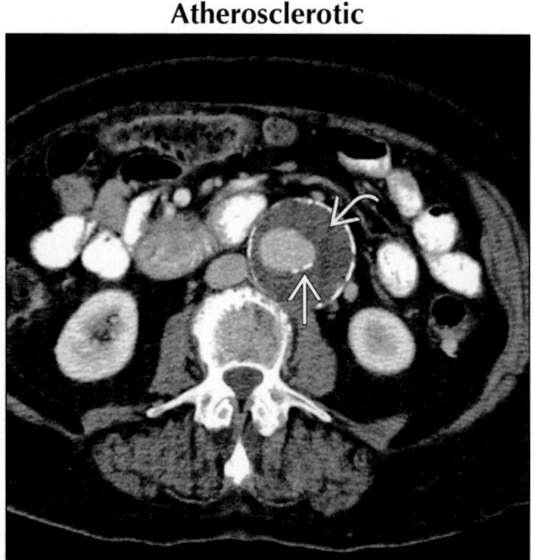

(**Left**) Lateral radiograph shows diffuse aortic calcifications ➡ in a patient with longstanding hypertension and a dilated ascending aorta. (**Right**) Double oblique cine MR image shows a bicuspid aortic valve ➡ in a young patient with a dilated ascending aorta. This image can be used to calculate valve area to quantify stenosis.

Degenerative

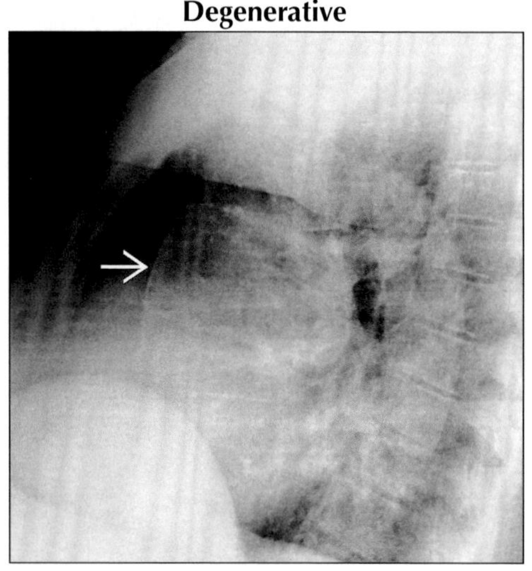

Aortic Stenosis

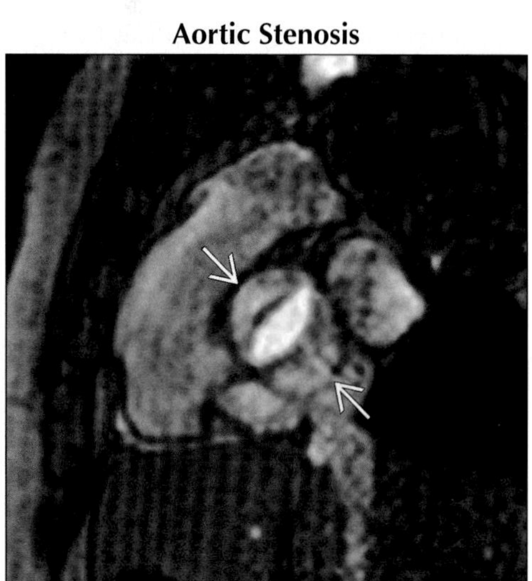

(**Left**) Left ventricular outflow view enhanced CT shows calcifications on the aortic cusps ➡ in an older patient with an ascending aortic aneurysm. (**Right**) Axial enhanced CT shows ascending aortic false lumen dilation ➡ in acute dissection. Note "bird beak" sign ➡ and "cob web" sign ➡, which help identify the false lumen ➡. Patient had a bicuspid valve and was treated with a modified Bentall procedure.

Aortic Stenosis

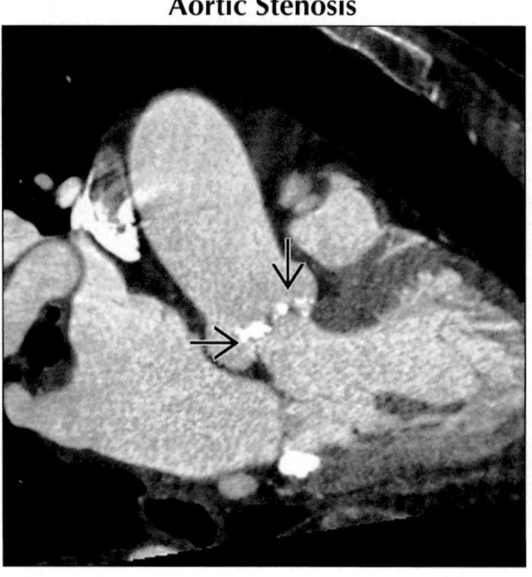

Aortic Dissection

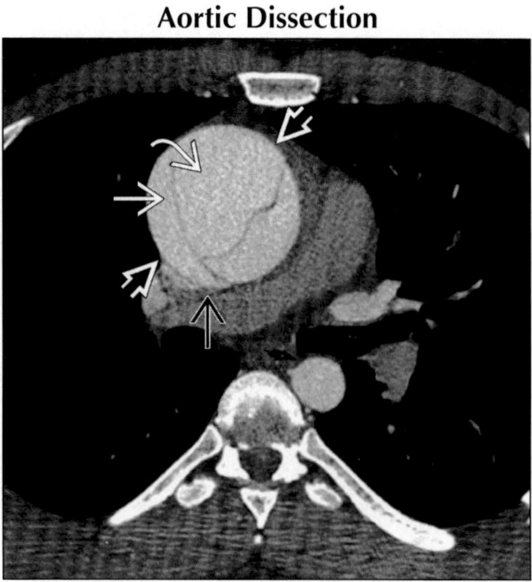

Aortic Dissection

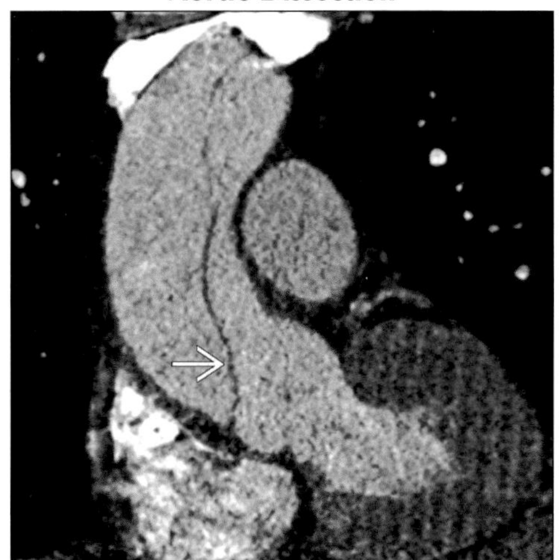

Mycotic Aneurysm

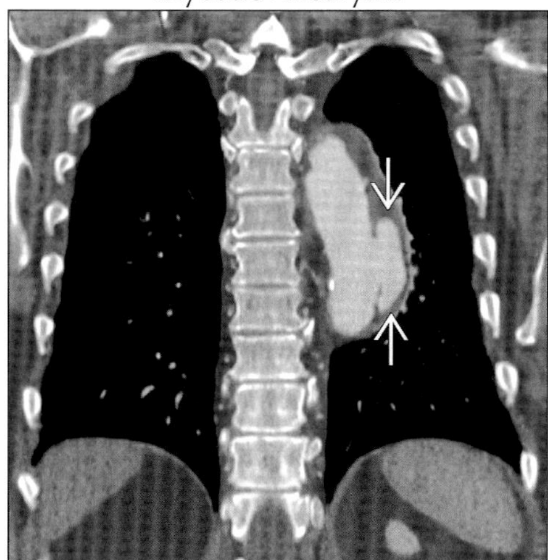

*(**Left**) Double oblique enhanced CT shows dilation of the ascending aorta in a hypertensive patient presenting with anterior chest pain. Note intimal flap ➔. This patient was treated with emergent surgery. (**Right**) Coronal enhanced CT shows pseudoaneurysm in the mid descending aorta ➔ thought to be a mycotic aneurysm. Aside from this aneurysm, there was a paucity of disease throughout the remaining aorta.*

Penetrating Atherosclerotic Ulcer

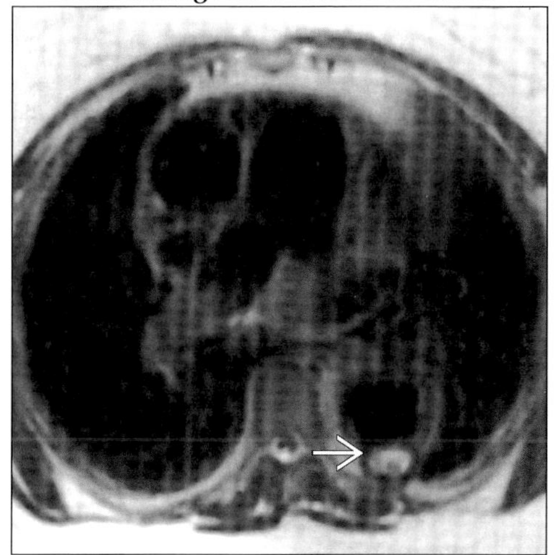

Penetrating Atherosclerotic Ulcer

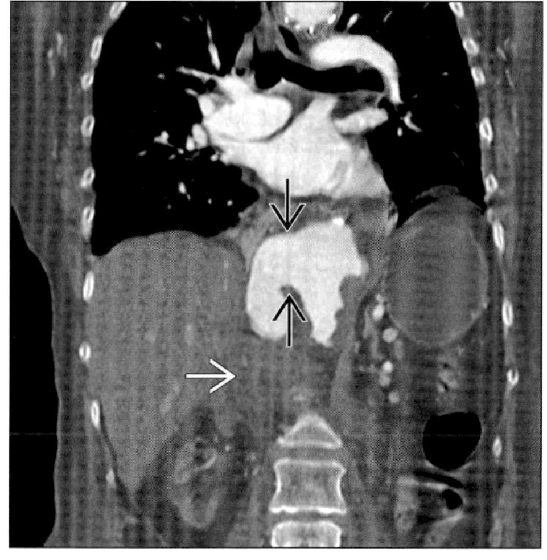

*(**Left**) Axial black-blood MR shows an aortic wall defect ➔ that extends beyond the expected contour of the aortic lumen. High signal in this penetrating aortic ulcer is due to slow-flowing blood and not thrombosis. (**Right**) Coronal enhanced CT shows a previously diagnosed penetrating atherosclerotic ulcer ➔ that progressed to frank rupture. Note extravasated blood ➔.*

Post-Traumatic Pseudoaneurysm

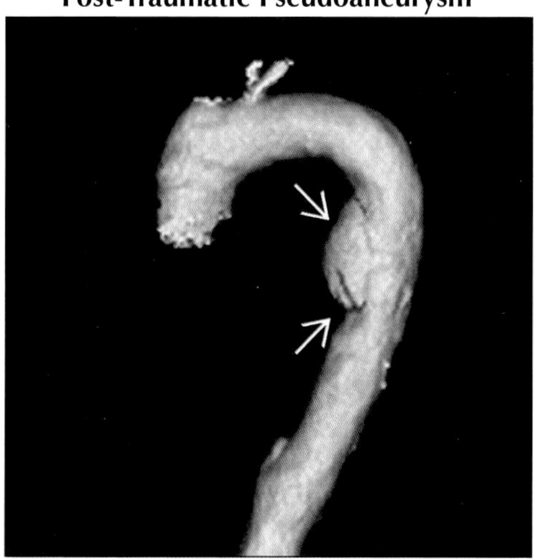

Connective Tissue Disease

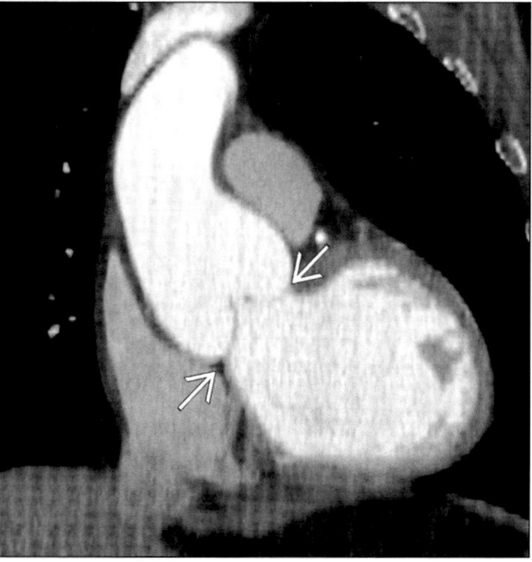

*(**Left**) Volume rendered image shows focal dilation ➔ of the aortic lumen at the level of the ligamentum arteriosum. This patient suffered a high-speed deceleration injury and presented with a traumatic pseudoaneurysm. The patient was treated with endovascular repair. (**Right**) Double oblique coronal left ventricular outflow view shows aortic root dilation ➔ and loss of sinotubular junction morphology in a patient with Marfan disease.*

DIFFERENTIAL DIAGNOSIS

Common
- Coarctation of Aorta
- Pseudo-coarctation

Less Common
- Large Vessel Vasculitis

Rare but Important
- Extrinsic Aortic Compression

ESSENTIAL INFORMATION

Key Differential Diagnosis Issues
- Focal outer diameter narrowed in coarctation or vasculitis
- Diffuse outer diameter narrowing can occur in vasculitis
- Normative data should be consulted to exclude common pitfall of misinterpreting normal aortic dimension for small body as abnormal
- For > 45 years, aorta considered abnormally small if diameter at level of main pulmonary artery < 24 mm for ascending and < 18 mm for descending aorta
  - Larger diameters may still be abnormal if older age, larger body surface area (BSA), or male

Helpful Clues for Common Diagnoses
- **Coarctation of Aorta**
  - Focal narrowing occurs below ductus arterious in adults, at ductus arterious with arch hypoplasia in neonates
  - Dilated collaterals (intercostal, internal thoracic) indicate hemodynamically significant coarctation
  - Treated coarctation patients can have restenosis
  - Associated with bicuspid aortic valve, Turner syndrome, Marfan syndrome
- **Pseudo-coarctation**
  - Redundant aorta with narrowing distal to left subclavian origin without hemodynamic effect
  - No rib notching, cardiomegaly, or collateral vessels
  - Dilated brachiocephalic artery and high arch often present

Helpful Clues for Less Common Diagnoses
- **Large Vessel Vasculitis**
  - Variable segment length narrowing
  - Branch vessel narrowing is common
  - Periaortic thickening and enhancement
  - Periaortic FDG uptake implies active disease
  - < 40 years implies Takayasu, > 40 years implies giant cell arteritis

Helpful Clues for Rare Diagnoses
- **Extrinsic Aortic Compression**
  - Retroperitoneal fibrosis, neurofibromatosis, sarcomas, other neoplasms

Coarctation of Aorta

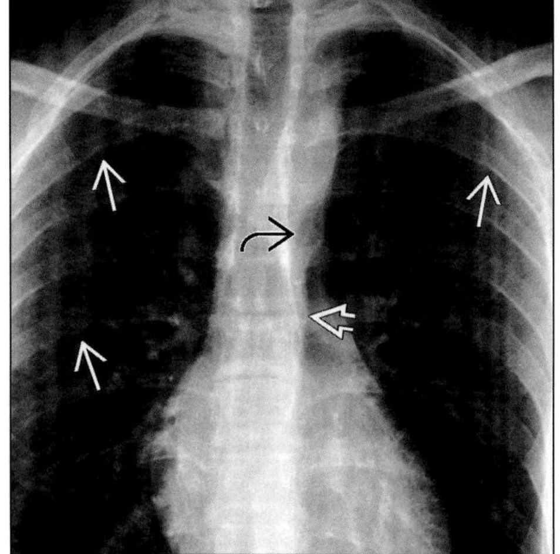

PA radiograph shows subtle areas of rib notching ➡. Note the rapid narrowing of the proximal descending thoracic aorta ↪, which then returns to normal size more distally ➡.

Coarctation of Aorta

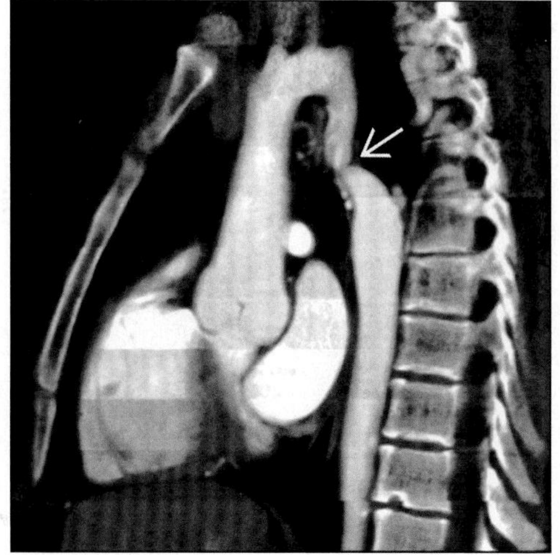

Sagittal multiplanar CT reformat from the same patient shows focal narrowing of the aorta distal to the ductus arteriosus ➡. Prominent collaterals were present (not shown).

Pseudo-coarctation

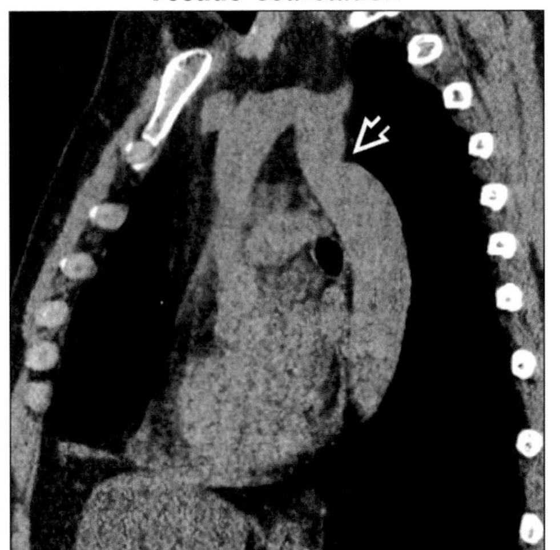

Extrinsic Aortic Compression

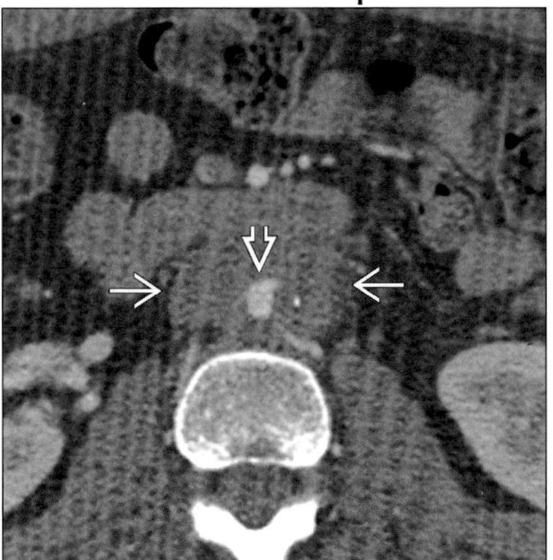

*(**Left**) Sagittal oblique unenhanced CT shows focal mild narrowing of the aorta ➡ in a patient with pseudo-coarctation. The aorta appears redundant. No collateral vessels were present. (**Right**) Axial enhanced CT shows extrinsic compression of the aorta ➡ by retroperitoneal soft tissue ➡ in a patient with retroperitoneal fibrosis.*

Large Vessel Vasculitis

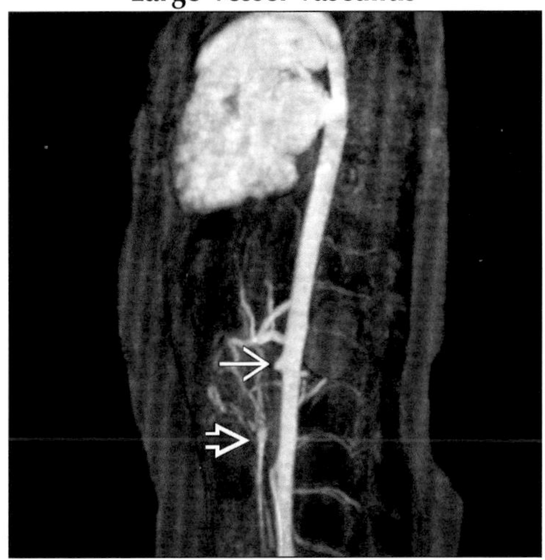

Large Vessel Vasculitis

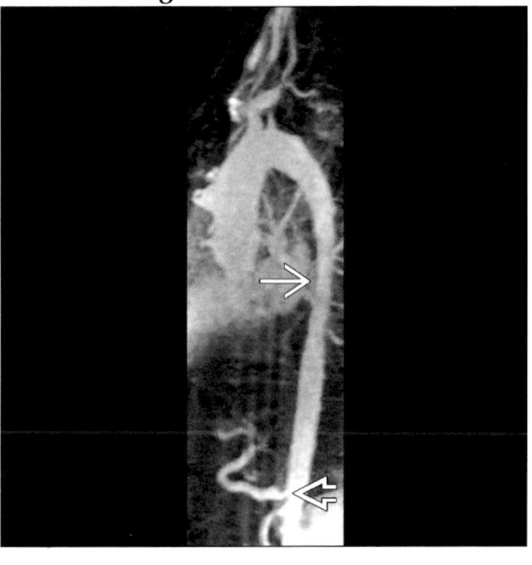

*(**Left**) Coronal oblique contrast-enhanced MRA shows a diffusely narrowed aorta occlusion of the superior mesenteric artery ➡. Note reconstituted SMA ➡. (**Right**) Sagittal oblique MIP MRA from a patient with Takayasu arteritis shows tapered narrowing of the mid-descending thoracic aorta ➡. Celiac artery origin stenosis is also present ➡.*

Large Vessel Vasculitis

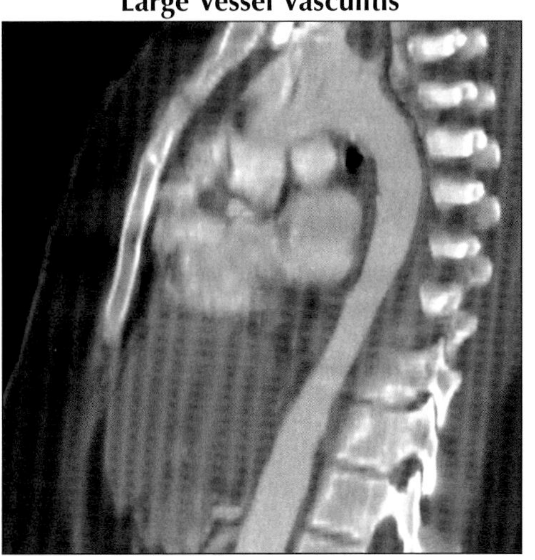

Large Vessel Vasculitis

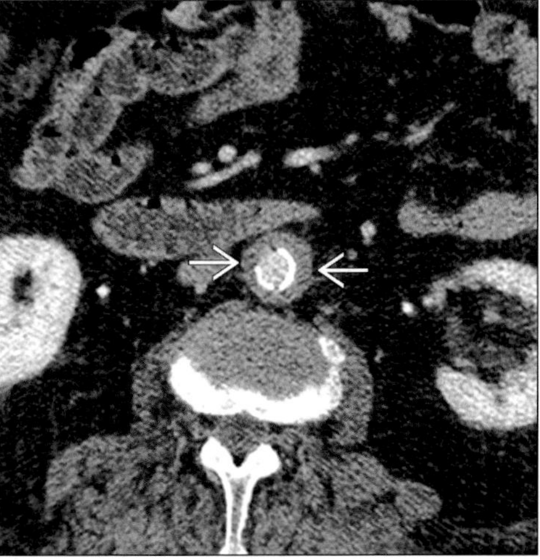

*(**Left**) Sagittal oblique MIP enhanced CT shows tapered narrowing of the mid-descending aorta with wall thickening in a patient with Takayasu arteritis. Note the absence of atherosclerotic disease. (**Right**) Axial enhanced CT shows a narrowed aorta with circumferential wall thickening ➡. Branch vessel stenoses were also present. This patient was older than 40 years and was diagnosed with giant cell arteritis.*

INDEX

A

INDEX

INDEX

B

INDEX

C

INDEX

D

INDEX

E

INDEX

INDEX

INDEX

I

INDEX

K

L

INDEX

INDEX

INDEX

INDEX

N

O

INDEX

INDEX

INDEX

INDEX

R

S

INDEX

INDEX

INDEX

Y

Z